Nursing Care
of Children

Nursing Care of Children

EIGHTH EDITION

Florence G. Blake, R.N., M.A.

Professor of Pediatric Nursing, Graduate Program,
University of Wisconsin, Madison

F. Howell Wright, M.D.

Professor of Pediatrics, University of Chicago

Eugenia H. Waechter, R.N., Ph.D.

Assistant Professor of Maternal-Child Nursing,
School of Nursing,
University of California at San Francisco

J. B. LIPPINCOTT COMPANY

PHILADELPHIA / TORONTO

To the memory of

Dorothy Gaehr Wright

who contributed much to this and preceding editions through

her perceptive criticism, wise counsel and patient encouragement

Preface

In response to evolutionary changes throughout the field of nursing, the title of this 8th edition shifts from *Essentials of Pediatric Nursing* to *Nursing Care of Children*. Today a true science of nursing is being delineated founded upon scientific principles and a growing body of nursing research. Such professional intervention is truly "nursing care." The future of this discipline lies in the identification of new roles for nurses as integral members of, and with greater responsibilities to, teams delivering health care of increasing excellence. Also reflected in the title change is the focus of the book upon the child within his family and community, whether in health or during illness.

The introductory material on the fundamental principles of the nursing care of children has been extensively revised and expanded to include discussion of some of the special problems of hospitalized children who come from various cultural backgrounds and minority groups. To work effectively with children and their families who have cultural orientations different from her own, the nurse must understand how the child's early experiences modify his response to illness and hospitalization. The delivery of health services to children and families must also take into account the rapid changes occurring in our society.

Until recently the emotional problems related to death and dying have been avoided in nursing curricula. An awakening of interest and concern about this difficult area of nursing has stimulated the inclusion of a section designed to help the nurse meet the needs of children who are approaching the end of life.

The chapters devoted to normal growth and development which introduce each of the units draw theory from several schools of thought. Intellectual development and functioning are emphasized because they determine to a considerable extent the individual child's understanding of illness and hospitalization and dictate the nursing intervention which will be most helpful to him. Many new illustrations portray stages in normal development. Bibliographies in these and other chapters are not limited to literature within the health professions but are drawn from other sources having direct application to the nursing care of children.

To provide easy reference and maintain an unbroken flow of the text, some of the tables of values and the longer descriptions of nursing procedures have been placed in the Appendix. A dosage table of commonly used drugs has been added.

Childhood illness encroaches upon many disciplines —embryology, biochemistry, obstetrics, neonatology, immunology and infectious disease, hematology, cardiology, surgery, neurology, dermatology, psychiatry and adolescent medicine. Without running to excessive length, an introductory text must of necessity be selective in its approach and depend heavily upon brief explanations and adequate references to more intensive reading. We hope that we have maintained a proper balance in the extent of treatment of the more commonly encountered disorders and the synoptic dismissal of those which are less common. To this end we have, for instance, expanded the treatment of surgical and orthopedic disorders while reducing the space devoted to conditions such as poliomyelitis that are fading from the medical scene. Pathophysiologic content has been expanded throughout.

We wish to acknowledge with sincere gratitude assistance obtained from many sources. Mr. David Miller and others of the J. B. Lippincott Co. have been most skillful and helpful in directing our efforts. Innumerable colleagues in the fields of nursing, pediatrics and other disciplines both at the University of California, the University of Chicago and elsewhere have been most gracious in lending illustrations and critical appraisal of our material. Particular thanks are due to Dr. Harry Shirkey for permission to use some of the material so laboriously collected for the table on drug dosages and to Beryl M. Peters for her assistance in numerous ways throughout the preparation of the book. Mrs. Gertrude Inouye has been a continual aid in correspondence and the preparation of manuscripts and tables. Many superb photographs were supplied by Carol Baldwin. And finally, we express our indebtedness to the many parents and children who permitted us to use them or their pictures in the preparation of appropriate illustrative material.

Florence G. Blake
F. Howell Wright
Eugenia H. Waechter

Contents

Nursing Care
of Children

UNIT 1

Introduction to Nursing Care of the Child

1

Growth and Development of Maternal and Child Health Services

There was a time not so long ago when the specialties of pediatrics and pediatric nursing did not exist, for the special services for the protection of children which we now take for granted have evolved largely during the past hundred years. Previously, hospitals for children or separate departments for their care in general hospitals were rare. Old records disclose that as many as six or eight children were sometimes confined in one bed and that children might be placed in the same bed with critically ill adults.*

The trend toward eradicating such gross neglect of children began in 1802 when the first children's hospital was erected in Paris. The Hospital for Sick Children built in Great Ormond Street in London was the first of its kind in an English-speaking country. Three years later the first hospital for children in America opened in Philadelphia. Today we have many children's hospitals in the United States, and most large general hospitals provide a special unit for the care of young patients. Even in small suburban hospitals the trend is away from the practice of confining children with adults. This chapter will describe briefly some of the movements and developments out of which have grown the present complex of special health and social services designed to aid children and their families.

THE RISE OF PEDIATRICS AS A SPECIALTY

Throughout the history of medicine many famous physicians have shown in their writings an interest in the maladies of children. But only in the 19th century, first on the continent of Europe and later in the United States, did physicians appear who devoted the major portion of their professional interest to children. Prior to that time the emphasis was on the

disease, not the patient. The fact that illness occurred in a child rather than an adult was of comparatively little significance to the physician or the nurse. It should not be inferred that medical personnel of that era had no understanding of their child patients as persons. Many of them were intuitive psychologists with deep insight into the relationship between personality and disease. However, such knowledge came out of their living experiences rather than from the medical and nursing texts and curricula. No scientific facts about the special emotional needs of sick children had yet been accumulated, nor had a science of pediatrics been delineated.

Toward the middle of the 19th century Dr. Abraham Jacobi came to this country from Germany where a trend toward specialization in children's disease had already begun. Dr. Jacobi was convinced that disease in children was sufficiently different from that in adults to warrant special study. It was largely through his efforts that the clinical investigation which led ultimately to the specialty of pediatrics was initiated. He opened a clinic for children and began to lecture on the diseases to which they are prone. In 1870 he received from the College of Physicians and Surgeons the first appointment in America as Professor of Diseases of Children, and in 1888 he played a leading role in the founding of the American Pediatric Society.

Also prominent in the small group of able physicians who helped to establish the fledgling specialty was Dr. L. Emmett Holt. His writings, both lay and professional, rapidly became international reference standards. The textbook of pediatrics which he wrote in 1896 is still used today after a series of modernizing revisions.

Another landmark in the history of pediatrics was the establishment, also in 1888, of the first department of pediatrics at Harvard University, headed by Dr.

* Stokes, Joseph: Pediatrics. *In* The Choice of a Medical Career, p. 22. Philadelphia, Lippincott, 1961.

Thomas Morgan Rotch. Other medical schools gradually followed this lead, but the Golden Age of pediatrics did not begin until the first full-time chair was established at Johns Hopkins University for Dr. John Howland in 1913. Dr. Stokes says, "The joining of laboratory and clinical investigation was the key to this development, and its leavening influence was spread through the other academic centers by a corps of such able investigators and teachers as Park, Gamble, Powers, Blackfan, Marriott, Kramer, Davidson and others."* Eventually, departments of pediatrics appeared in all of the medical schools in the country. At first many were mere adjuncts of a department of medicine, but, with the introduction of full-time clinical chairs, they began to gain autonomy and to initiate intensive research programs of their own.

Recognition of the need for special instruction of nurses in the care of children roughly parallels the development of separate units for the care of children which appeared first in foundling homes, then in children's hospitals and finally in the pediatric units within general hospitals. Associated with some of the earliest children's hospitals—those in Philadelphia, Denver, Boston and New York for instance—schools were established which were devoted to the training of nurses in the care of sick children. But it was not until departments of pediatrics were firmly established in medical schools that pediatrics became a compulsory part of the undergraduate nursing school curriculum. Although supplementary courses for registered nurses were given in many children's hospitals, university graduate study of pediatric nursing did not appear until the fourth decade of this century.

The rapidly expanding volume of knowledge that accompanied the growth of pediatric departments and the increasing complexity of technics of diagnosis and treatment soon led to the appearance of subspecialties within the broad field of pediatrics. These centered about the diseases of particular organ systems, e.g., pediatric neurology, pediatric cardiology, pediatric hematology and pediatric endocrinology. The attack on children's problems has been bolstered further by the incorporation into pediatric departments of specialists whose basic training is in other fields such as surgery, psychiatry, psychology, nutrition, physiotherapy, occupational therapy, social work, biochemistry, microbiology, pathology and genetics. Thus the modern children's hospital or pediatric department has become a complex aggregation of teams of specialists working to improve the health services available to children through the discovery of new knowledge and the training of capable personnel. An important component of these teams is the nurse who not only renders direct bedside care to the children concerned but also func-

tions as a liaison between children, physicians, parents and other professional and ancillary workers who are involved in the provision of care.

CHANGING ATTITUDES TOWARD HOSPITAL CARE

At the turn of the century the causes of many diseases which are now controlled were unknown and, consequently, prevention was ineffectual. The resulting loss of life was shocking, particularly among women who contracted childbed fever and infants suffering from diarrhea and infectious diseases. The rate of sickness was correspondingly high and posed both a threat to society and a challenge to the medical profession.

Understandably, childbirth in hospitals was greatly feared. Ignorance of the cause of disease and the phenomenon of birth gave rise to a multitude of superstitions and misconceptions, generated in an effort to explain the unknown. Everyone finds it difficult to accept mystery and uncertainty, particularly in relation to such important events as pregnancy, birth and death. When cause and effect are not clear, gaps in understanding are likely to be filled in by the fantasies of well-meaning but uninformed people. Medical misfortune was once regarded as a punishment for one's sins or as a visitation from evil spirits. Even today, in spite of better dissemination of medical knowledge, the nurse meets these attitudes, often fortified by old wives' tales about charms and rituals designed to protect the mother and the child from mishap during pregnancy and delivery. Most of these superstitions, though harmless and frequently amusing, too often are believed and serve as a basis for the anxieties of expectant parents or for the self-recrimination of those who have produced an abnormal child. Similarly, superstitious notions may account for some of the irrational responses to hospitalization and treatment which are encountered by medical personnel.

Quite apart from the misconceptions that surrounded disease, the care of hospitalized children 40 years ago was set in a framework of rigid policies in regard to nursing procedures, isolation, bed rest and visiting regulations. These policies were dictated in part by the nature of the diseases prevalent and by firm convictions about what was necessary for the sick child. Infection ran rampant, unimpeded by antibiotics which had yet to be discovered. Illnesses were not only of greater severity, but the patients also remained infectious for long periods of time, and the danger of cross-infection within the hospital was ever present. Only by isolation technics could the spread of infection be controlled, and rigid rules were enforced to prevent the intermingling of illnesses. Visitors, regarded as a hazard to the proper maintenance of isolation technic, were discouraged. The general prevalence of nutritional disturbances and the pro-

---

* *Ibid.*, p. 31.

longed periods of illness and convalescence fostered a concentration on arbitrary orders for feeding and the administration of fluids in an attempt to prevent dehydration and wasting. The nursing routines and relatively simple treatments of those days were conducted with ritualistic attention to detail. Not only fear of cross-infection but a firm belief in the virtue of prolonged "absolute bed rest" kept children isolated from each other and confined—often by restraining jackets—to the area of their own beds.

The volume of severe illness constantly kept the staff so engaged in the care of desperately ill children that there was little time to consider the individual child's needs for play, companionship and emotional support from his parents. Almost of necessity, nurses and physicians acquired a veneer of casual unconcern, under which they suppressed the worry and the frustration of their responsibilities. Parents were avoided, because they threatened this defense and because the staff felt poorly prepared to deal with the anxieties which were revealed during visiting hours.

Advances in medical knowledge and diffusion of health education to the public during the past quarter century have wrought drastic changes in the use of hospitals and the manner in which patients are handled. The discovery of antibiotics has made hospital delivery so safe that a high proportion of women now avail themselves of the technical safeguards offered. Instruction about the basic facts of pregnancy and delivery has done much to dispel the superstitious notions once held, although these have not been eradicated completely. Antibiotics, public health measures and public education have resulted in a tremendous reduction in the amount and the severity of infectious disease so that fewer children require hospital treatment for these illnesses, and the period of isolation and convalescence can be shortened. Their places in hospitals are being taken by children for whom newer technics offer relief from previously uncorrectable malformations, by those who require complicated diagnostic measures, and by those whose chronic diseases can be ameliorated by newer drugs. Isolation is still required, but it tends to be briefer and less restrictive. New knowledge of nutrition has provided the means through which deficiency disease can be abolished, has reduced the incidence of gastrointestinal disorders in small infants and given greater facility to the maintenance of fluid and caloric balance during the course of a disease. A drastic revision of attitudes toward bed rest now encourages early ambulation after many operations and some forms of medical illness, eliminating some of the physical and emotional depression which used to follow restraint during prolonged convalescence.

In addition to these improvements in medical knowledge which have permitted changes in the methods of dealing with the hospitalized child, great advances have taken place in the understanding of children and their parents. The rising interest in the psychology of Freud, Jung and Adler eventually spread into the fields of pediatrics and public health and stimulated intensive study of human development from conception through the child-rearing age. The stages of personality development were described from infancy to adulthood, and there followed a better appreciation of the child's psychological needs at the various stages of growth. At the same time, a deeper understanding was gained of the emotional and psychosomatic disorders of childhood and of their methods of treatment. The psychology of women during the reproductive cycle also became the subject of intensive study, resulting in a better understanding of the personality changes and emotional needs of women during the child-bearing period. In many medical centers interest is now focused on the needs, frustrations and relative ignorance of expectant couples, women in labor and parents seeking help in rearing their young children. Today the mother is considered to be a unique person; she is the central figure in the family and, as such, has a profound influence on the mental health of each of its members.

Research in the field of child psychiatry also has drawn attention to the special emotional needs of parents and children at times when the latter are sick or handicapped. Hospital personnel have come to regard the child and his family as mutually dependent on each other. Because of the family's deep involvement with the child and his health problems, their anxieties require as much attention as do those of the child himself. It has been found that the anxiety of many parents can be allayed by enlisting them as active members of the health team.

Increased concentration on the emotional needs of the child in the hospital has sharpened the insight of staff members and has stimulated them to devise methods of care that make possible a constructive adjustment to illness and hospitalization rather than one that results in psychic trauma.*

Current practice in the care of hospitalized children recognizes the importance of adequate preparation for admission and such upsetting experiences as venepuncture, anesthesia and injection. The therapeutic value of play is acknowledged, and toys from home are welcomed as an important link with the child's family. New and interesting toys are also available from the hospital collection. When isolation precautions are not in force, group play and occupational therapy under

---

* The terms "constructive adjustment," "mastery" and "coping" indicate modes of adaptation which conserve energy and ensure to the child a continuation of warm relationships with others, respect for himself and maximal opportunities for further personality development. Experiences that cannot be handled without residual feelings of fear, anger, distrust, helplessness or revenge are commonly defined as psychic traumas or traumatic experiences. The words "unhealthy adjustment" designate a mode of adjustment that results in nonconstructive expenditure of energy and interference with the maintenance of self-esteem and healthy relationships with other people.

the supervision of trained workers is available. The supportive effect of school work for the older child with a prolonged illness has led many hospitals to provide bedside or classroom instruction by qualified teachers. The sanitary bleakness that used to mark the hospital environment is relieved by attractive and colorful decoration of patient rooms and by informal clothing worn by some members of the staff.

Freud's followers have emphasized the need of the infant and the young child for an intimate, warm sustained relationship with his mother or a permanent mother substitute. Recognizing this, hospitals are liberalizing their visiting hours and, in many instances, are providing facilities for mothers to room-in with their young children. Where rooming-in facilities are not provided, some services are attempting to limit the number of personnel to whom the child must relate by a case method of assignment. In this way a greater effort is being made to help the child to master his fears and uncertainties so that he may emerge from the period of hospitalization with increased inner strength to cope with stress.

Growing recognition of the potential unfortunate effects of hospitalization on both the child and his family has stimulated a trend toward a minimal hospital stay and, whenever possible, the substitution of outpatient treatment and home care which avoids separating the child from his family and local community. As a result, public health nursing services and instruction of mothers in home care are growing in importance. Public health nursing in particular has taken on new dimensions in providing follow-up care and support of the family.

EXPANSION OF COMMUNITY HEALTH AND PROTECTIVE PROGRAMS

During the past century there has been a drastic change in the attitudes of society toward children. At the start of the Industrial Revolution the child enjoyed no more legal status than that of a chattel which his parents could use as they saw fit. He could be put to work for long hours and under frightful conditions on farms or in mines, canneries and factories. Neither national nor local government had the right or the conscience to interfere as long as parents permitted such abuses. Children bereft of families were sheltered in orphanages and institutions, many of which became notorious for harsh treatment and penurious management. The foundling homes of the day were poorly protected against epidemics of disease, and, even during the 19th century, some of them lost more than 50 per cent of the infants consigned to their care. The lack of public conscience concerning the exploitation of children and the cruel and unsympathetic treatment to which they were often subjected has been well depicted in the writings of Charles Dickens. These novels aroused public concern not only in England, the scene of the conditions described,

but also in America where child labor laws were soon enacted to thwart the most serious forms of exploitation.

One of the first public efforts in behalf of children was the White House Conference of 1909 convened by President Theodore Roosevelt. At this and the subsequent conferences, which have met every 10 years, representatives from Federal agencies, national, state and local voluntary organizations and citizens' groups (including youth as well as adults) assemble in Washington to study the needs of children and to make recommendations for the creation of new services or the extension of existing ones. The agenda includes plans not only for children who are ill, handicapped, delinquent or deprived of parental care, but also methods of protecting the growth potential of those who are our healthiest young citizens. Thus, the delegates to the White House Conference of 1960 discussed ways to help children and youth to "realize their full potential for a creative life in freedom and dignity." Great stress was placed on the importance of assisting the youth of the nation to acquire values, ideals and integrity which would not only elevate their own feelings of personal dignity but also prepare them for successful careers as parents.

The last two White House Conferences emphasized the responsibility of society to help the family to maintain its integrity. During the past 10 years much interest and research have been directed toward uncovering the problems which beset the American family of every class and ethnic origin and of perfecting methods of alleviating the stress to which they are subjected.

Families in all strata of our society have been affected by the many social and economic forces which gradually have transformed this country into an industrial nation during the past 200 years. The migration of millions of families from farms and small towns, first to the large cities, then to suburbia and exurbia and now to the newly developing "megalopolis" has contributed to family disorganization. Whereas in 1800, two thirds of American families lived in rural areas, today it is estimated that less than 10 per cent of our population lives on or from the land.

Isolation of the nuclear family from the former extended family and the current mobility of nuclear family units have worked sweeping changes in social structure, values and mores which have far-reaching implications for the family. The rural family was an economically productive entity where home and place of work were physically united. Because of its isolation from larger communities, the family group of that time was also a biosocial and extended group with greater emphasis on family tradition and continuity. Task orientations and gender identifications of family members were well defined with a minimum of ambiguity between masculine and feminine roles. Along with its productive function, the family unit also accepted responsibility for large aspects of education, for occupational training of its youth and for the care of its aged members. Interdependence and geographical stability deeply affected the influence of transmission of family values and mores upon the younger generation.

The family of today is in transition, both geographically and socially. Because of horizontal mobility and decreasing size of the nuclear family, there is an intensification of relationships with exclusive dependence on the immediate family. At the same time, vertical mobility often results in avoidance of extended family members. Absence of the father for long periods of the day has resulted in a less clear-cut role model for his sons. No longer are the roles within families as clear-cut as the traditional ones of 100 years ago. Mothers in increasing numbers are pursuing careers and children are exposed to many influences outside the home at a much younger age. Mobility also provides for diversity of contacts for parents, for the development of different interests and for spatial separation. The former functions of the family as an economic and educational unit have been curtailed, whereas the importance of the child to provide emotional satisfactions and family perpetuity and to insure meaning to life has increased.

Despite such influences on the family in an increasingly complex society, the basic unit continues to have vitality. The new space age demands stronger and more resolute individuals, better equipped educationally and socially. American families are responding to the challenges and demands of our expanding world and are finding new resources in selected friendship groupings, in educational and social endeavors that are community provided and in supportive services. The family of today, however, is still vulnerable. It is a vital responsibility of professional personnel committed to the optimum development of children to support endeavors which have as their goal the integrity of the family unit.

The challenge of replacing some of the support which vanished with the extended family is being met in part by governmental and voluntary agencies. The Children's Bureau of the Department of Health, Education and Welfare has taken a prominent role in the development of many programs designed to improve the welfare of children.

The Children's Bureau was established in 1912 as a direct result of the first White House Conference. It was charged by Congress to investigate and report on "all matters pertaining to the welfare of children and child life among all classes of our people." Its early studies emphasized the hazards of childbirth and early infancy and led to improvements in prenatal supervision, obstetric care, infant feeding and general sanitation.

In the early 1930s the Bureau investigated the effects of the economic depression on children and sponsored a national conference to stimulate interest in child health and nutrition, from which arose the school lunch program implemented by the Federal Emergency Relief Administration. The Bureau made proposals for legislation to expand existing programs for children, and in 1935 these proposals served as a basis for the children's provisions under the Social Security Act. The legislation authorizes financial aid to the states to support the development of maternal and child health programs, services for crippled children and child welfare programs (Aid to Families with Dependent Children). The Children's Bureau accepted the responsibility for administering the grants and for supplying information and technical assistance in implementing the programs.

As larger yearly appropriations from the government have become available it has been possible for the objectives of programs to be broadened. In many states the crippled children's services, originally restricted to children with orthopedic handicaps, have progressively included rheumatic fever, congenital heart disease, cleft palate, speech and hearing disorders, epilepsy and such chronic diseases as nephrosis, cystic fibrosis of the pancreas and diabetes.

Similarly, the maternal and child health programs have increased the number of prenatal and well-child services and have provided centers for the care of prematurely born infants.

Successive amendments to the Social Security Act have allowed expansion of the Children's Bureau programs. In 1960, grants for research projects in child welfare were authorized, and in 1963 similar provisions were made to support projects relating to maternal and child health and crippled children's services.

Amendments of 1963 authorized special project grants for maternity and infant care. These programs provide prenatal care for women who have or are likely to have physical problems during pregnancy and childbirth, or who are in circumstances which are likely to increase the health hazards for them or for their infants. Delivery and postnatal care for the mother and health care for the infant are provided, as well as family planning services. These programs are available only to those unlikely to receive care because of economic or other reasons beyond their control.

In 1965, amendments to the Social Security Act authorized funds to support special projects for comprehensive health care for children and youth who would not otherwise receive it. These programs include preventive medical, dental and emotional health care, diagnosis, treatment and follow-up care.

In addition to providing leadership and guidance for these state-administered programs, the Children's Bureau over the years has assisted mothers and children in the United States and throughout the world by collecting facts about children in order to identify the urgent problems and by working with public and voluntary agencies to solve them. It promulgates standards for maternal and child care, initiates supporting legislation, provides consultation services and disseminates literature to parents explaining normal growth and development and the special needs of children with handicaps.

Recognition of the changing needs of children has by no means been limited to the Children's Bureau. Public sensitivity to the problems in this field is reflected in the burgeoning of programs of assistance supported by state and local governments and by private agencies.

School health programs now include more than the provision of a hot lunch for students. Parents are urged to obtain for their children periodic medical examinations and immunization against the preventable diseases. Many schools maintain a nurse and/or a physician to implement this program and to conduct screening examinations for tuberculosis and defects of sight and hearing. Psychologists are present in the larger school systems not only to study problems of learning but to consider the emotional adjustment of students as well. The attitude toward children with handicaps is being modified by the realization that many of them can profit more by attending regular school than by segregation into special classes or separate schools.

Growing recognition of the interdependence of social, economic and physical factors upon the educational achievement of the child has led to the creation of Head Start programs which attempt to prepare socially and economically deprived preschool children for successful entry into the school system. Head Start projects are aimed at increasing emotional and social development through varied experiences which broaden the horizons of the child and increase his understanding of the world in which he lives. The programs are planned to include parent participation, provision of one or more hot meals each day and comprehensive health services for the children.

The growing rate of poisonings among small children exposed to dangerous drugs and chemicals in their homes has stimulated the establishment of Poison Control Centers in many of the large cities where, usually under the aegis of a medical school, statistics are compiled and methods of treatment are evaluated. These centers supply immediate advice to physicians or other individuals caring for children who have ingested poisons.

The special requirements of premature infants have led to the establishment of centers where they may receive expert care from personnel versed in the particular needs of these most vulnerable infants. Specially designed incubators or ambulances permit the safe transport of prematures from the place of birth to centers many miles away.

In many states regional heart centers have been established at which are concentrated pediatricians and surgeons capable of dealing with congenital malformations. Here children can receive the benefit of new and complicated technics for the diagnosis and correction of any defects which were inoperable only a decade ago. Similar facilities are available for children with congenital or traumatic orthopedic disorders that require difficult surgical operations or complicated mechanical prostheses. In the rehabilitation of such children a new philosophy is emerging which attempts to consider the individual child, his concept of himself and his place in the community and the family. Successful rehabilitation thus seeks not only to correct the physical disability itself but to prepare the child for a role of maximal satisfaction in society.

The problems of mentally retarded children are receiving increased recognition from government and private sources. Research into the causes of retardation and its diagnosis has been stimulated by monetary grants from a variety of sources. Improved facilities for the physical care of such children in institutions have been supplemented with newer technics of teaching which attempt to bring out the maximal potential within each child. Supportive services for the parents of retarded children living in the home have also been established with a view to helping both the child and the family in which he lives.

The important contribution of the many social agencies that offer support to families and children cannot be overlooked. Some provide general service to families, while others have more restricted goals such as the placement of children for adoption or the provision of day care for children of working mothers. Many are engaged in attempts to combat the rise of juvenile delinquency by providing recreational outlets in underprivileged neighborhoods through camps, settlement houses and neighborhood clubs. Others are striving for new solutions to the problem by working directly with the youth involved in delinquency.

Health services directed toward children are offered in a wide variety of settings which is constantly expanding as new methods of reaching those children not yet under care are constantly sought. The opportunities for the nurse engaged in the care of children are endless, challenging and rewarding.

BIBLIOGRAPHY

Ackerman, N.: Treating the Troubled Family, New York, Basic Books, Inc., 1966.

American Academy of Pediatrics: Care of Children in Hospitals, Evanston, Ill., 1960.

Brittian, C. V.: Preschool programs for culturally deprived children, Children 13:130, 1966.

Christensen, H. T., (Ed.): Handbook of Marriage and the Family, Chicago, Rand McNally and Co., 1964.

Egan, M. C.: Combating malnutrition through maternal and child health programs, Children 16:67, 1969.

Erickson, F.: The need for a specialist in modern pediatric nursing, Nurs. Forum 4:24, 1965.

Glickman, E.: Professional social work with headstart mothers, Children *15*:59, 1968.

Hales-Tooke, A.: Improving hospital care for children, Children *15*:116, 1968.

Handel, G. (Ed.): The Psychosocial Interior of the Family, Chicago, Aldine Pub. Co., 1967.

Keliher, A. V.: Parent and child centers—what they are, where they are going, Children *16*:63, 1969.

Murphy, L. B.: The consultant in a day-care center for deprived children, Children *15*:97, 1968.

Rainwater, L.: Family Design, Chicago, Aldine Pub. Co., 1965.

Swallow, K. A., and Davis, G. H.: 645 days of maternity and infant care, Children *14*:141, 1967.

U. S. Dept. Health, Education and Welfare: Five Decades of Action for Children, Washington, D. C., U. S. Gov't Printing Office, 1967.

————: Your Children's Bureau: The Bureau's Current Programs (pamphlet), Washington, D. C., U. S. Gov't Printing Office, 1964.

2

Fundamental Principles of the Nursing Care of Children

THE ROLE OF THE NURSE IN SUPPORTING THE HEALTH OF CHILDREN

Social Background

Rapid social changes occurring both within the United States and around the world during the past decade have significant implications for the nursing profession. As an important member of the health team, the pediatric nurse is being asked to assume increasing responsibilities in an expanding role which includes guidance and counseling of mothers and supervision of the health of their children. Some of the factors which affect the profession of nursing, and of pediatric nursing in particular, are described below.

All who deal with human problems are concerned about the phenomenal growth in population. In the United States the 200 million mark has been passed and, although the rate of increase is slowing, the youthfulness of our population will result in further expansion. The larger number of women of childbearing age will soon increase the proportion of children in the total population. To provide for their adequate care a disproportionate increase in the number of nurses (and paramedical personnel) will be needed, for the production of physicians is a slower process by virtue of the number of years of training required. Inevitably, nurses will assume an increasing part of the services to ill children and will play more significant roles in the promotion of physical and mental health among the relatively well.

The previous chapter has indicated some of the stresses imposed upon family life as our society becomes increasingly mobile, as it moves from an agricultural environment into the complexities of urban and suburban living, and as it loses the built-in support and guidance of the old-fashioned family which included more than the nucleus of parents and children. The nurse counseling such modern families will have to adapt to a wide range of attitudes which depend upon racial, cultural, religious and economic differences among her clientele. She will also have to evaluate the impact of protracted absence of traveling fathers, the problems of mothers who work and commit their children to the care of sitters or day nurseries, the lack of adequate play space and recreational facilities often in the face of an increase in leisure time, and many other difficulties which arise out of the modern environment.

Within the hospital setting the nurse has a particularly important opportunity to influence the physical, emotional and intellectual outcome of the child under stress because she is the closest to him both spatially and emotionally during this critical period.

Through exposure to television programs, paperback books and articles in newspapers and magazines, parents today are becoming more sophisticated in their medical knowledge. To meet their expectations of a high level of professional competence, nurses will have to draw upon a better knowledge of pediatrics and improve their facility in discussing such issues as family planning, genetic counseling, child rearing and appropriate methods of referral to social and medical agencies.

With the phenomenal growth of scientific knowledge and improvements in methods of communication, the modern nurse will have a tremendous opportunity to contribute meaningfully to the problems of children not only in her own country, but all over the world. This book is directed toward furthering the understanding of the nature and nurture of children and of the environmental influences which affect their development.

Philosophical Orientation to the Nursing Care of Children

The philosophy underlying the nursing care of children must be related to, and based upon, an orientation to the nursing profession in general. Nursing as a science and practice is now at a crossroads. Some believe that its future development should concentrate upon the administrative functions of the nurse in the delivery of health care. Others believe that the theory and science of nursing must be developed in relation to direct service to patients. There is also difference of opinion as to the emphasis that should be given to new functions which will of necessity be delegated to nurses by physicians. Undoubtedly, both aspects of the profession will need to be developed. However, nursing research must be largely concerned with the problems of direct patient care, which is the heart and core of nursing and a basic prerequisite to the assumption of administrative responsibilities. It is to this aspect of pediatric nursing that the contents of this book are devoted.

The nursing care of children entails an understanding of the child as a developing person with unique ways of feeling and thinking, and with his own individual methods of coping with his environment. Empathy for her patients will be fostered in the degree to which the pediatric nurse learns to understand and accept her own attitudes and feelings and to appreciate the way in which she handles *her* problems. With such self-understanding she will be able to recognize and make explicit the origin and meaning of the behavior she observes in her hospitalized patients. Backed by theoretical knowledge and skill in its application, she will then be able to intervene in a constructive manner.

Disciplines allied to nursing have made great strides toward the understanding of human growth and development. Nursing must push even further to build a scientific and theoretical basis for its unique discipline. By the synthesis and extension of those concepts dealing with the interpersonal relationships of people under stress and by the study of nursing practices, the body of nursing theory will be advanced and the nurse will acquire enthusiasm for further study and research contributions.

UNDERSTANDING OF GROWTH AND THE DEVELOPMENTAL PROCESS

In contrast to the nursing of adults, pediatric nursing deals with individuals who are going through a period of rapid change. Whereas the adult's body will alter relatively little during the remainder of his life, the child must accommodate to more than a 3-fold increase in length and an approximate 20-fold increase in weight between birth and adolescence. Simultaneously, his muscular and intellectual skills and his emotional controls progress from the rudimentary state

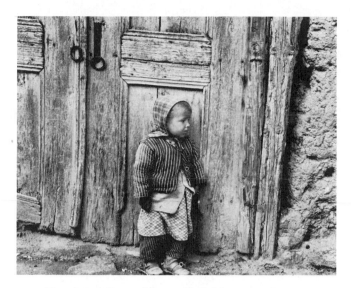

FIG. 2-1. The problems of children in other parts of the world have a new and significant importance to the modern pediatric nurse. This child of an Aegean village must combat problems of poverty, lack of adequate nutrition and other obstacles to optimum physical and mental development. (Carol Baldwin)

of the newborn to the complex, highly integrated level of the adult.

The term "growth and development" is used to encompass the changes that take place during the dramatic transition from the helpless state of earliest infancy to physical and emotional maturity. Strictly speaking, *growth* implies an increase in size, while *development* denotes an improvement in skill and functional capacity. For example, the child's brain increases very little in size (growth) after the age of 6, but the operations that it can perform (development) continue to advance throughout the person's lifetime. Since it is often difficult to make a clear distinction between growth and development, it has become common practice to use the terms jointly or even interchangeably.

The rapid changes which a child undergoes in response to the growth impulse complicate the task of evaluating his physical health and progress. Any standard against which he is measured must take due account of his age. Some allowance also must be made for individual variations in rate of growth and development. Thus, in assessing the growth of a 1-year-old boy, it is not expected that his weight will exactly match the 22 pounds which is average for his age. But if his weight falls outside the range of 19½ to 25½ pounds, the figure begins to assume significance when it is understood that four-fifths of all 1-year-old males fall within these boundaries. In the same way the evaluation of developmental progress must be made in terms of a normal *range* rather than a precise average. An infant who fails to sit without assistance at 8 months should not be considered abnormally slow merely because the average age for this achievement is 7 months. However, if the child still is not sitting by 12 months of age, the delay exceeds the normal range, and a reason must be sought. Ranges are more cumbersome than averages, but without them individuality may be maligned unjustly.

The growth and development of a child is a complex but orderly process. For purposes of description, it usually is divided into physical, physiologic, motor, intellectual, emotional and social aspects. These last three components may be combined into what is often referred to as *psychosocial development*. The separation of these facets of growth is admittedly artificial, for they are closely interrelated and interdependent. For instance, psychosocial development does not occur independently of physical and motor development but is greatly influenced by it just as growth of the body is affected by the quality of the child's interpersonal relationships. Motor development (walking, for example) depends on normal growth of bone and muscle (physical), supplied by adequate food and energy (physiologic) and guided by the developing nervous system (intellectual). In extreme instances it may be impeded by maternal neglect (emotional) or by the cultural norms of a society which overprotects its infants (social). If maternal neglect occurs, not only is motor development slowed but there is also retardation in psychosocial development.

For a given child these several aspects of growth do not necessarily proceed at the same rate. A child who is growing slowly in the physical aspects of height and weight often outstrips his peers in motor achievement and social adaptation. Or an intellectually precocious schoolboy may lag behind in athletic skills and social adjustment. Thus, proper understanding of the child depends on an evaluation of the several phases of his growth and the manner in which they interrelate.

To fulfill her role as a part of the health team, the nurse must have knowledge of physical development and of the intrafamily and community relationships which contribute to the development of a healthy personality. Information on this subject introduces each of the following units of the text:

Unit II. The Newborn (Conception to 1 Month)
Unit III. The Infant (1 Month to 1 Year)
Unit IV. The Toddler (1 to 3 Years) and the Preschool Child (3 to 6 Years)
Unit V. The School Age Child (6 to 13 Years)
Unit VI. The Adolescent (13 to 18 Years)

In the first section of each unit the authors deal with the physical and physiologic changes that can be anticipated during the period of the child's life under discussion. In general these aspects of growth are readily measured and can be referred to as standards of healthy growth with some degree of exactitude. In the second section are discussed the food requirements necessary to provide building materials for the growing body and to supply energy for its operations. In the final sections are treated those phenomena which depend on the development of the central nervous system—the motor skills, the intellectual powers and the emotional sensitivity to the environment which constitute the unique biologic heritage setting the human child apart from all other animals.

The final section of each unit introductory chapter is based on Erikson's ground plan in the human life cycle.* Listed in Table 1 are the steps identified in man's psychosocial development and the *core problems* or *crises* with which he struggles at the various stages in his life. In addition to these major problems the child has a multitude of other tasks to accomplish. Although distinct in themselves, when accomplished they contribute immeasurably to the successful resolution of core problems. These tasks, such as learning to climb, for instance, are those which are commonly referred to as *developmental tasks*.

As will be noticed in Table 1, each core problem has a negative as well as a positive counterpart. In the initial stage of psychosocial development the negative counterpart of the core problem (mistrust) is conquered through a mutually satisfying mother-child relationship. As the child progresses through subsequent stages of development, his relationships expand first to others within the family and then later to persons in the world beyond his home. In the initial stages of development only family members influence the solution the child makes to his problems. Later other persons who become emotionally significant to him will influence the outcome of his efforts to reach a higher level of maturity.

Support of the Child's Growth Potentials

Successful conquering of the negative counterparts of each core problem or crisis prepares the child to undertake the next step in development. However, Erikson points out that the negative counterparts of

Table 1. The Eight Stages in the Life Cycle of Man*

Period of Life	The Core Problem or Crisis (The positive counterpart appears first followed by the negative one)
1. Infancy: (birth to 1 year)	Trust vs. mistrust
2. Early childhood: (the toddler age 1-3 years)	Autonomy vs. shame and doubt
3. Play age: (the preschool years 3-6 years)	Initiative vs. guilt
4. School age: (6-13 years)	Industry vs. inferiority
5. Adolescence: (13-18 years)	Identity vs. identity diffusion
6. Young adulthood	Intimacy vs. isolation
7. Adulthood	Intimacy vs. self-absorption
8. Senescence	Integrity vs. disgust

* Adapted from Erikson, Erik: Youth and the life cycle, Children 7:43-50, March-April, 1960.
For a discussion of the last three stages the reader is referred to the references on pages 48-9, of the bibliography at the end of chapter 6 and to Duvall, Evelyn M.: Family Development, ed. 3, Philadelphia, Lippincott, 1967.

* Erikson, Erik: Childhood and Society, ed. 2, New York, Norton, Inc., 1963.

the core problems are never *completely* or *permanently* conquered. Instead they must be reconquered continuously throughout life "in the same way that the body's metabolism resists decay."* He continues by saying:

All that we learn [in the process of growing-up†] are certain fundamental means and mechanisms for retaining and regaining mastery. Life is a sequence not only of developmental but also of accidental crises. It is hardest to take when both types of crisis coincide.

In each crisis, under favorable conditions, the positive is likely to outbalance the negative, and each reintegration builds strength for the next crisis. But the negative is always with us to some degree in the form of a measure of infantile anxiety, fear of abandonment—a residue of immaturity carried throughout life, which is perhaps the price man has to pay for a childhood long enough to permit him to be the learning and the teaching animal, and thus to achieve his particular mastery of reality.‡

The accidental crises to which Erikson refers include, of course, the crisis of illness. The effects of illness on the growing child who is simultaneously at the height of his struggle with a core problem in his development is a subject with which the pediatric nurse must be deeply concerned. Awareness of the particular developmental problem with which the child is faced is important for the nurse because she will become a part of his environment during such a crisis. If she has a broad base for the understanding of human development and needs, she will be in a position to affect the child's solution of his problems.

Erikson makes another point which has a bearing on the nursing care of children. He says that the adult who undergoes serious surgery has to repeat the battle with the negative counterparts of each stage of psychosocial development in the process of recovery. This is also true for the child, not only when he has undergone a major surgical operation but also when he has suffered from a severe illness. Massive regression—often to the earliest level of psychosocial development —is not uncommon during the acute phase of an illness. During this stage of illness, a large proportion of the child's energy is concentrated on his fight against disease and on adaptation to treatment. *An important major principle of nursing care is to respect the child's need to regress and to help him to accept dependence on others if he resists this.*

Another important major principle of nursing care is *awareness of the child's need for help in reconquering the negative counterpart of the core problem in the stage of development to which he has regressed.* Then, as he moves ahead into each of the stages through which he passed prior to the time he became ill, his previously formed means of retaining and regaining mastery must be *recognized* and *supported in accordance with his particular needs.* When these principles are applied in the care of the sick child, the experience of illness can serve to strengthen his adaptive capacities rather than retard his progress toward maturity.

The nurse must also be deeply concerned with the level of cognitive functioning at which the child is operating when he is under the stress of illness and hospitalization. The meanings which new experiences hold for a child are deeply affected by the concepts which he has attained, by the level of his understanding of causality and by his thinking processes. His reactions to procedures and his methods of dealing with stress are similarly affected. The nurse who is assisting the child in gaining mastery of unfamiliar experiences and who is concerned in communicating with children and in supporting their growth in intellectual capacity must, therefore, also be knowledgeable regarding the principles of intellectual development. These are included in the discussion of each developmental level throughout the book.

The introductory sections of each unit suggest some of the ways in which knowledge of growth and development can be used in the guidance of children who are in the particular stage of development under discussion. There are no prescriptions which meet the needs of *all* children at a particular level of development. Principles of guidance must be adapted to the particular requirements of the individual child because each has his own characteristic way of dealing with problems as a result of his unique constitutional heritage and past experiences.

At the beginning of this chapter it was pointed out that individual differences in rate of growth as well as the interrelationships between the different aspects of development have to be taken into account when appraising a child's physical health status. More than age must also be taken into account in assessing the child's level of psychosocial adjustment.

The foregoing points, are especially true when care is being planned for the sick, the convalescent or the handicapped child, for he has a health problem to which he must adjust.

However, understanding the sequence of physical development and the intellectual and emotional aspects of behavior which tend to occur in response to the problems of each age period will serve to guide the nurse in appraising the level at which the child is functioning during the various stages of his illness and adjustment to the hospital. It also provides a guide to the detection of physical, intellectual and psychological signs indicative of the child's readiness to advance toward the level of development at which he happened to be before he became ill. Furthermore, it will familiarize the nurse with the gratifications and learning experiences which *all* children, including those who are afflicted with a physical handicap, need for healthy personality development.

---

* Erikson, Erik: *Ibid.*, p. 44.
† The words within the brackets are the authors'.
‡ Erikson, Erik: *Ibid.*, p. 44.

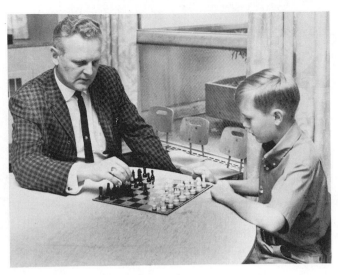

Fig. 2-2. Visits from his father are important to the school aged boy. Competitive games requiring concentration and the use of strategy become popular in this age group. (Bill Bargagliotti)

The nurse will find many additional uses for her knowledge of growth and development in the care of children if she studies each of her patients with the following questions in mind: (1) In what respects does the child's illness or handicap interfere with the reception of gratifications which are necessary for optimal growth at his particular age level? (2) In what specific ways does his health problem interfere with the learning which normally takes place at his particular age level? (3) What substitute experiences might be provided to protect the child's growth potentials?

The introductory section of each unit also emphasizes the vital functions of the parents in the protection of their children's physical growth potentials, in the shaping of their personalities and thinking abilities, and in the provision of support during periods when the children require care and education outside the home. This discussion has been included not only because it is essential for the understanding of the process of psychosocial development but also because it provides insight into the emotional investment that parents make in their children. With sensitivity to the meaning which children have to parents, the nurse can better appreciate the emotional impact of illness and abnormality.

A third major principle of pediatric nursing is the protection of family interpersonal relationships. To protect the child's growth potentials to the fullest, the nurse must take into account the situation of the parents, not only because they make up the most important part of their child's environment but also because they are important people in their own right. Parents, too, are in the process of development. They require help (1) in working out constructive relationships with each other and with their children, (2) in acquiring satisfaction and competence in child-rearing, and (3) in learning to cope with their feelings and responsibilities when their children are ill or handicapped. It is the child's intra-family relationships which to a great extent make him what he is. They will also influence to a considerable degree the kind of adjustment that he will make to his health problems and to the necessary treatment.

PROVISION OF PHYSICAL SUPPORT

The process of pediatric nursing is a series of activities specifically planned to influence the child's environment in ways which support him in moving in the direction of physical health and constructive adjustment to his problems. Physical care includes the following considerations: (1) understanding of the health problems that tend to occur during the various stages of the child's development, of the treatment disease requires, and of the way in which disease can be prevented; (2) skill in observing the patient's physical and psychological responses to his disease and to the various kinds of treatment measures which are instituted; (3) skill in interpreting the significance of the symptoms of disease which are observed; (4) judgment in executing responsibilities to the patients and their parents and to the other members of the health team; (5) understanding of the principles underlying physically supportive and comforting care which children require; and (6) ability to evaluate the effectiveness of the physical care provided.

The nurse's curative and comforting skills are as important today as they were a century ago. Meticulous, comforting bodily care not only supports the child in his fight against disease and alleviates the distressing symptoms which it produces but also strengthens him emotionally. It reassures him that he will be protected, cared for and cherished as a person. It prevents the needless expenditure of energy which occurs when his bodily needs are frustrated.

The pediatric nurse must acquire special skills because she works with patients who are developing in all spheres. Particular gentleness in the care of the body is imperative, not only because of the delicacy of the tissues but also because of the message which gentleness always transmits. The provision of physical care is an important mode of communication with the child because he is perceptive to the feeling the nurse conveys by her manner of touching and moving him and by her handling of painful parts of his body. Because of the child's extreme perceptiveness to physical cues, he responds more intensively to rough or careless handling. This is particularly true when he is overwrought, frightened or angry and is facing a painful treatment or is being restrained from aggressive physical expression of his feelings.

The purpose of setting up procedures and working out routines for care of children is to ensure safety

FIG. 2-3. This boy has special needs arising from his inability to use either of his arms. Mutual understanding between nurse and patient is not achieved from one contact; it grows from a succession of experiences which make it possible for the two persons to become attuned to each other.

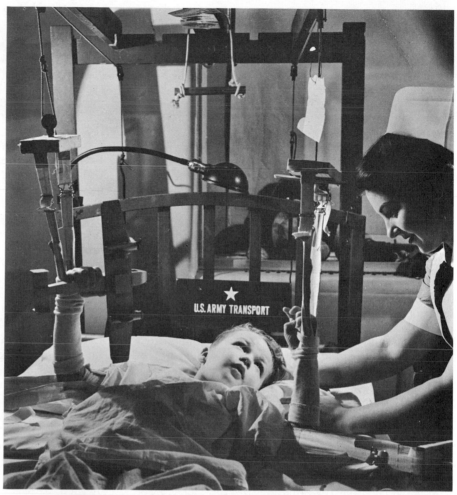

and maximum comfort. Ensuring safety requires adherence to the principles underlying the procedure and implies manual skills, initiative and imagination in finding ways to help children cope constructively with their feelings. Many general procedures designed to protect children in pediatric units are presented in the Appendix or mentioned as they relate to treatment of specific conditions.

As the nurse works with children, she will need and want to develop her powers of observation and that undefined discerning quality which signals changes in her patient's condition. The latter quality is derived from experience. Though originally intuitive, it should become conscious in order to provide concrete data to support the conclusions the nurse draws concerning the condition of her patients and their particular needs. It also provides the rationale for her future actions and for formulation of goals of care and evaluation of nursing intervention. True evaluation of the nurse's work can only be made in relation to conscious and specific goals to be accomplished.

The young child, unlike the adult, is unable to detect or to describe changes within his body or to report chilliness, nausea or a feeling of impending danger. He can *feel* changes within himself and reacts more intensely to them than does the adult, but his only means of signalling his distress is through crying, restlessness, irritability or withdrawal from his environment. The nurse must be alert to these nonverbal cues. On the other hand, some acutely ill children give few behavioral cues to changes within their bodies. In such cases, the nurse must be particularly alert in detecting changes in temperature, blood pressure, intracranial pressure, etc. She must be forever watchful to detect alterations in her patient's physical state, for *they take place quickly in children* —often without warning.

PROVISION OF EMOTIONAL SUPPORT

To provide emotional support to the child, the nurse must understand the emotional impact of illness and hospitalization on children of different age levels and on their parents. She must have knowledge of the child's background of family experiences, the course of his development and the manner in which previous experience affects his reaction to illness, treatment and hospitalization. A pediatric nurse should: (1) have self-awareness and constructive attitudes toward herself and toward those with whom she works; (2) help the child and his parents at the time of admission to the hospital; (3) observe the child's responses to disease and to the hospital milieu; (4) study his parents' reactions in order to give assistance where it is most needed; (5) help the child to maintain his trust in the provision of emotional support; and (6) help to coordinate the joint efforts of the health team and the child's family toward achievement of their common purpose.

Emotional support becomes paramount when illness strikes or when a child or an adult is facing a major change in himself or in his life situation. *Such situations create stress or a change in the body which activates psychic activity aimed toward restoration of the person's homeostatic balance.* Illness and all its discomforts create problems of adjustment (stress) for the child and his parents. Stress is also encountered during normal development throughout life. Some of such problems are simply solved; others are complex and often require the assistance of others in the helping professions.

Emotional support, the heart of nursing, can only be given within the context of a constructive relationship. Strength comes only from people who are of emotional importance and who have knowledge of the child's problems, strengths and needs. All children who are hospitalized, particularly those under 6 years of age, must have a nurse on whom they can rely in the absence of their parents. Children confer trust only upon nurses who have earned confidence by conscious effort in a continuing relationship (Fig. 2-3).

Nursing care of children calls for constant exercise of intelligence and imagination by the nurse. She must cope with the changes of normal development and also with the behavioral changes and the needs precipitated by illness and by handicapping conditions. She must also deal with parents whose need for support varies as their child's situation changes.

Providing continuity of nursing care for the patient also makes possible greater professional development of the student. It provides opportunities for her (1) to see for herself the physical and behavioral changes that occur during the various stages of a person's illness, (2) to evaluate the effects of her care on her patient's physical progress and behavior, (3) to learn to manage wisely the emotional interaction occurring between herself and her patient, and (4) to become more competent in carrying out the steps entailed in the nursing process.

"Emotional support" refers to those components of nursing care which aid in ego development and in effective ego functioning. The ego is that portion of an individual's personality which is involved in testing reality and in directing needed adjustments in behavior. At birth, a child is endowed with inherent energy often called "instinctual drives." This term designates biologic urges or needs characteristically directed toward one of two major goals: (1) obtaining pleasure and (2) striking out against frustration. A healthy infant instinctively protests when his need for food is frustrated. Urges toward pleasure (love) and toward aggressiveness when thwarted are biologically determined. When a baby's basic biologic needs are satisfied by a giving mother, his tension diminishes. This state of fulfillment later expands into the wish to be loved and eventually to give love in return. However, when his needs are unfulfilled, he expresses his frustration primitively in an undifferentiated aggressive response. When the urge toward pleasure (love) and aggression are opposed, or in conflict, anxiety results which is expressed in behavioral change.

These built-in universal drives, largely genetically determined, are components of the *nature* of the infant or the part of the personality technically called the *id*. The instinctual drives vary in quality and intensity so that even at birth each child has his own peculiar individuality. He also has his own unique response to stimulation and an individual activity pattern. Immediately after birth the infant begins to interact with his surroundings, though at first he is unable to distinguish himself from his environment. The efforts made by persons around the child (chiefly the mother at first or any person who is providing care) in appeasing, assuaging, encouraging and helping him to redirect, modify or control his innate impulses constitute *socialization* and assist in active personality formation implied by the term *nurture*.

While opinions differ concerning the exact extent to which the ultimate personality depends on its inherited nature, there is little doubt that the quality of the nurture it receives has a considerable influence on the final outcome. Thus, the optimal guidance of the child during the formative years requires an appreciation of his basic nature and a long-range view of efforts to modify it.

The mother is the child's primary source of nurture, particularly during the early years. The act of mothering in all its main aspects is highlighted throughout this text to show the important role that the mother plays in the protection of her child's unique endowment and in helping him to modify his inborn impulses toward complete and immediate gratification and uncontrolled aggressive responses to frustration. Special attention to mothering is also given in order to increase the nurse's insight into the needs of the child when he is separated from his mother. Stress on mothering also serves to point up the importance of the nurse's role in supporting the mother-child relationship both in health and during periods of illness.

The development of the child's ego is guided by the socialization he receives, by his experiences within the home and larger society, by the development of his intellectual capacities and by the growth of his nervous system. As he reacts to the optimum in levels and quality of environmental stimulation, his responses become modified or altered into directions approved by the society within which he exists. Personality development is influenced beneficially by mutually satisfying experiences with his mother and others of significant importance to him. The ego matures in a healthy manner when the important persons in the child's life: (1) understand growth and the developmental process, (2) perceive his physical and psychological readiness to adapt to new learning experiences which strengthen his adaptive capacities, (3) introduce new learning experiences at this time, (4) understand his point of view, and (5) supply the physical and emotional support which makes it possible for him to conquer the negative counterpart of each core problem.

The ego has many functions. As previously stated, it tests reality; that is, it preserves the individual's orientation to the world as it actually is. It is considered to mediate between the demands of the original inborn impulses and realistic societal demands in order to assure maximum gratification with minimum censure from the conscience.

The *conscience* (or technically the *super-ego*) is considered to develop from the ego after several years of experience with the demands of society. During the earliest years of the child's life, his parents represent this society which imposes certain requirements on him. Later, parental standards and expectations, bolstered by experiences with others outside the home, become internalized into the personality of the child. He then begins to take over the task of modification and control of impulses in order to exist in harmony with the culture in which he lives.

When the ego is functioning effectively, it determines the manner in which the person will respond to basic impulses, to conflicts within his personality and to conflicts between his desires and the demands of his environment. The ego has been referred to as "the executive of the personality."* It is that part of the psychic structure which collects all the data it can from observing the demands of the id, the conscience and the outer world and then works out a realistic plan of action. The most important task of the ego is to preserve harmony between all parts of the personality and between the person and his environment. When it has strengths† to fulfill its functions efficiently and smoothly, the individual is said to be well adjusted and in emotional equilibrium. His basic needs and desires are satisfied; he has energy to work, to play and to love; and he has the emotional equilibrium that he requires to solve his daily problems. If he happens to become ill, he will have strength to fight disease and will be able to turn to others for help if he needs it.

However, if the person's original nature and impulses, reality demands and conscience (id, ego and super-ego) are in conflict, the person is said to have a problem in adjustment, or to be "maladjusted." He will have little energy for work, play and love, and, if he is ill, recuperation may be slowed considerably. He also will be chronically discontented with himself and with his world. Such internal conflicts impede growth and development of both the body and the mind.

A manifestation of such clashes within the personality is anxiety. Anxiety is very similar to fear, but there is a difference. Fear stems from some objective danger which can be readily perceived: for instance, fear of a painful procedure. On the other hand, the causes of anxiety are much more obscure; the threat originates within the person, and it may be very difficult to determine its underlying basis.

Up to a point, anxiety, like fear, can be beneficial in that it warns the individual of some impending danger and stimulates him to take positive steps to overcome it. However, if anxiety is unduly intense or prolonged, it can have a destructive effect on the personality.

Freud originally postulated that the arousal of anxiety triggers the ego into erecting mechanisms of defense to preserve the individual's emotional equilibrium. Although Freud was mainly concerned with *repression*, his daughter, Anna, later extended this theoretical formulation to describe numerous mechanisms by which the ego defends the person against acute anxiety. She described those defenses which safeguard the person's relationship with himself and others, conserve energy, provide gratification and contribute toward further self-realization and productivity as *constructive defenses*. Those mechanisms, however, which threaten the person's relationship to himself and others, consume large quantities of energy, restrict the reception of pleasure and lessen potentials for full growth of adaptive capacities were designated as *unhealthy defenses*. Some of these defenses are described later in the text as they relate to methods used by children in dealing with problems associated with illness and physical handicaps.

In the last several years, some psychoanalysts have been distinguishing between defense mechanisms, utilized by the ego to maintain equilibrium, and *coping mechanisms,* which are ego directed efforts toward active mastery of the anxiety producing situation. It is not the behavior seen *per se* that differentiates defensive activity from coping activity, but rather the underlying mechanisms which delineate the type of ego functioning. Coping behavior is described as flexible, purposive and implying underlying choice, whereas defense mechanisms are considered as almost automatic, rigid, and triggered by the present as a result of past experience. Although present behavior is largely determined by the past, coping implies adap-

---

* Hall, Calvin S.: A Primer of Freudian Psychology, New York, New American Library of World Literature, Inc., 1954.

† Throughout this text ego strengths will also be referred to as "inner resources" or "adaptive capacities."

tive behavior, an evaluation of the present, reality orientation, awareness and control by the individual. In the ego's use of defensive maneuvers, however, it is considered that there is usually some distortion of the present in terms of the past with accompanying lesser degrees of awareness. Throughout the text, differentiation of coping and defensive activity will be made whenever it seems appropriate.

The ego may lack strength because of immaturity, as in the case of the young child or the older child or adult who has been deprived of growth-producing interpersonal relationships. The ego may also be weakened when its normal executive powers are being diverted to deal with illness and the frightening unknowns of a new environment. Under such circumstances the anxious person is hard pressed in dealing with anxiety. He must draw heavily on the assistance of those who care for him to solve his problems and to regain his emotional equilibrium. Such assistance is in effect emotional support. The particular form which such support must take varies from person to person depending on the severity of the individual's problems, the stage of development he is in, and his capacity for dealing with his problems and the anxiety that they provoke.

The newborn has no ego resources to use in coping with anxiety; his only psychological defense is his cry. His psychic structure is unformed. For him emotional support must contain elements which are different from those required by the well-adjusted school-age child. If the anxious person is wisely supported, the danger serves to strengthen his power to cope with stress, not only for the present but also in the future. Anxiety is not pathologic; it is essential for growth in adaptive powers. It is only when the tasks of the ego exceed its strength and the individual is given no support in coping with his problem that anxiety becomes a deterrent to progress in the direction of health. (The word *mastery* refers to problem solving which results in healthy growth and development rather than in maladjustment.)

SUPPORT FOR THE CHILD'S INTELLECTUAL GROWTH POTENTIAL

Just as the child goes through different phases in emotional development, so also does he advance in intellectual development through various levels of concept formation and thinking styles. In the fairly recent past, it was held that intelligence was firmly fixed by genetic inheritance and could not be altered substantially by experiences after birth. The term "intelligence" still defies precise definition since it comprises a multitude of different skills, abilities and types of behavior. The measurement of intelligence is also inexact in the early years of life and bears little correlation with later measurements of mental abilities.

The assumptions of fixed intelligence and constant I.Q. were based on Charles Darwin's theory of natural selection. This idea was bolstered by the intelligence testing movement, which selected tests on the premise that the characteristics measured were stable and therefore that the testing would be highly predictive of later intellectual performance.

Later evidence however, based on the measurement of the I.Q. of identical twins raised apart, showed substantial differences in performance. This finding, plus evidence from longitudinal studies of the past 20 years which indicate variations in the performance of intellectual tasks at different testing periods, highlight the effect of environmental factors on intellectual growth and current functioning. The studies done with children subjected to an unstimulating environment in orphanages and foundling homes also added impetus to the growing conviction that subsequent intelligence and problem-solving abilities are significantly affected by early environmental factors and by cumulative experience.

The theory of predetermined development was an outgrowth of the concept of recapitulation—that in individual development, all the earlier stages of evolution of the species are re-traversed. This notion received support from the finding of cephalocaudal and proximodistal anatomical and behavioral development of lower forms of life, suggesting that certain behavioral skills in children, such as walking or stair climbing could not be altered by experience or practice. The normative approach to child development, in which there is concern with describing characteristics of children at a particular age based on the premise of genetically predetermined development, logically then advocated child rearing practices geared toward non-interference with the child's inherent developmental capacities.

Recent observations however, have indicated that children raised in orphanages rarely creep and are delayed in walking. It was also found that although improvement in motor skills did occur with maturation of the nervous system, they were also accelerated by practice. This observation with children was paralleled by the finding that animals require practice or learning, along with maturation, to develop normal sequences of behavior.

This evidence has resulted in the emphasis in the last few years on the importance of preverbal experience, or *primary learning*, in the development of intelligence, as distinguished from later learning and problem solving ability. It emphasizes that although inheritance plays an important part in intellectual behavior, the level of ultimate functioning is a result of a continuous interaction between the organism and its environment.

Earlier theories of motivation for behavior have also been affected by these findings and by recent developments in neuropsychology. Although in the past it has been accepted that the brain is inactive unless stimulated, it has recently been demonstrated that portions of brain tissue which have no direct connection to incoming nerve fibers are continuously active. Although an individual *is* often motivated by a need to return to former equilibrium, particularly when he is under severe stress or coping with debilitating illness or pain, the realization is growing that not all observed behavior is so motivated. In the absence of acute stress, children and adults are observed to seek out new opportunities to learn, to explore novel situations and to acquire new experiences. Thus they have an inner motivation toward healthy growth in addition to the need for return to homeostasis when inner or environmental forces disrupt emotional balance. It is also implied that this need to search out and master new experience is an inherent part of the nature of the child. Exploration of the novel or unusual is stimulated by an *incongruity* between the current stimulus and past experience. Thus the child is motivated to explore situations which do not match his memory of the familiar. Repeated encounters, however, transform the new experience into the expected, and attention thereafter diminishes. This phenomenon has been termed *habituation* to a stimulus.

Just as the first years of life have been emphasized in discussing the child's emotional development, so his preverbal experiences are stressed here while considering his intellectual growth. In both areas, subsequent progress is affected by early events. Great efforts have been made in recent years to counteract cultural deprivation and to enrich the learning opportunities of all children through preschool education and in nurseries and Head Start programs.

Also underlying this concern with learning opportunities for young children are the many reports in the past several years of the effects of sensory deprivation on the immature and mature organism. The finding that newborn animals need experience or learning along with maturation to perform normally expected behavior (such as pecking sequences in young chicks) has been previously mentioned. It has also been demonstrated that even such basic behavior as reaction to painful stimulation in animals can be altered by sensory restrictions of the early environment. The cumulative results of such studies strongly suggest that sensory organs and nerve fibers need early sensory stimulation in order to develop normally both structurally and functionally.

Further evidence which supports the conviction of the organism's dependence on his environment for normal intellectual functioning as well as for emotional responses comes from the numerous studies of adults subjected to periods of severe sensory deprivation. Several general conclusions can be drawn from these isolation studies, although individual interpretation is made difficult by differences in methodology. Disturbances in thought processes, problem solving, perception and psychological processes were regularly reported throughout these experiments in isolating individuals from normal sensory experiences. Clearly, even the mature adult is dependent on his environment to a degree hitherto unrecognized. The child is even more dependent on his environment, for he is much more vulnerable, particularly when ill, and his ego capacities are much lower.

The hypothesis of *critical periods* drawn from these findings also has implications for nursing care. In the studies with controlled environmental stimulation in young animals, an optimum time period for sensory stimulation or experience to be of maximum benefit was observed. The hypothesis implies that the quantity or quality of desired learning will be diminished after that time period is passed during which environmental stimulation has the most profound effects. These studies are continuing at present and have the potential for increasing our understanding of child development. The concept is not unfamiliar, for it has been suggested also by investigators of emotional development in children. It may well be that the critical period for any sort of learning or development is that time when maximum capacities—sensory, motor and motivational as well as psychological—are first present.

SEQUENCES IN INTELLECTUAL DEVELOPMENT

Jean Piaget, one of the foremost investigators of intellectual development in children, in describing the various stages in development of intellectual processes from birth through adolescence, has advanced immeasurably our understanding of children and of their behavior. Throughout his voluminous writings he emphasizes: (1) the sequential nature of changes in intellectual behavior and (2) the continuous interaction between the child and his environment.

His discussion of changes in intellectual behavior emphasizes learning opportunities through which new experience is *assimilated,* along with the necessary *accommodation,* or modification of previous mental structures resulting from that experience. He also stresses continuity and gradualness of change, the hierarchal nature of development (the building of higher mental capacities upon former structures) and the importance of novelty (curiosity) and active experimentation in learning.

The sequences in intellectual development described by Piaget correspond rather roughly in time span to those described for emotional development. However, it must again be emphasized that age or maturation alone, divorced from learning experiences, is not sufficient in this sphere. Each of the following periods is subdivided into stages of more specific changes in the child's reasoning. These will be elaborated throughout the text as indicated to enhance understanding of the child's behavior as it affects nursing care.

The *sensorimotor period* lasts from birth until the child is roughly between 18 months and two years of age. Beginning with reflexive behavior, the child

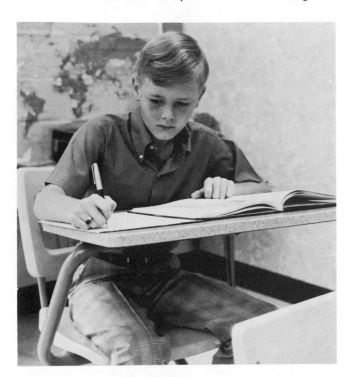

Fig. 2-4. Some hospitals have school rooms as well as teachers for the convalescent child, thus enabling him to keep up with his class and also providing a change of routine along with the peer support of a classroom situation. (Bill Bargagliotti)

gradually develops intentionality of behavior and interest in novelty. During this stage, the young child is unable to form concepts *per se,* but utilizes symbols and symbolic play and imitation. This phase is of great importance, however, for the child is learning to differentiate himself from the environment, the "me" from the "not me." Discovery of the universe outside himself leads to interest in objects, learning that objects exist when he cannot see them, and beginning experimentation.

The second stage, roughly from 18 months to about 4 years of age, is termed the *symbolic* or *preconceptual* phase. In this period and during the earlier phase, the child is extremely *egocentric;* i.e., he has difficulty in appreciating the point of view of others although he is now developing beginning ability in this direction. During this stage the child develops language, imagination or *symbolic function,* and is concerned with imitation and learning through play.

In the *intuitive phase,* beginning at approximately 4 years of age and lasting until roughly 7 years of age, the child is engrossed in forming concepts. Through finding contradictions between new situations and his past experience, and coping with them, he enlarges former concepts and forms new ones. He can now fill gaps in his knowledge through active ques-

tioning and experimentation. From interaction with his environment, he is no longer as completely dependent on visual perception in making judgments. When he becomes proficient in this, he enters the stage of *concrete operations.*

This stage of development, beginning at approximately the age of 7 or 8 years, continues until adolescence. Now children cease to be as totally egocentric; i.e., they have the ability to communicate in language with shared topics and mutual give and take and are able to see the viewpoint and perspective of others. The child's judgment of time becomes less confused and his conception of space is more like that of the adult. In many ways, however, the thinking of the child at this stage still differs substantially from that of the adult. He is very much concerned with the present, or *concrete,* and must have objects to manipulate to make logical relationships. He is still unable to project into the future—that is, to hypothesize—and operates on "trial and error."

The stage of *formal operations* comes into being when the child is about 11 or 12 years of age. Now the child has the ability to consider possibilities even if he has not experienced them in a real situation. The adolescent is no longer bound to what he can see and handle; he can consider hypotheses, or what may or may not be true, and what would follow if they were true. He can argue and follow an argument and see many varieties and alternative ways of running the world or of achieving his immediate intentions. He is also better able to use logic in deductive and inductive reasoning without resorting to observation.

Implications for the Nurse

Supporting the child in intellectual growth and mastery implies the provision and modification of current experience to enhance the child's understanding and to assist in his coping strategies. It also implies safeguarding and enhancing the child's potential for future growth and intellectual functioning and accomplishments. The observations of Piaget and others interested in this area of the child's development have many implications for the nurse working with children. In order to understand the communications of children and the meaning of their behavior, she must have knowledge regarding their general thinking processes. Conceptions of space, time and causality and early egocentrism have great import for children's responses to illness and hospitalization. They also give direction for nursing intervention and suggest ways of dealing with children to enhance real communication with them. Motivation for the child's behavior may be inherent in the way in which he processes the information he receives. The methods he uses for coping with unfamiliar experiences are affected by his understanding and perception of them. However, the nurse also must realize that the child with whom she is dealing is an individual, and she should not apply generalizations without careful observation to determine *his* perception and understanding and *his* particular patterns of growth.

One of the most important of implications to be drawn is the previously mentioned need of children for stimulation and interactional experiences with their environment in order to function effectively and to develop adequately. As each developmental level is discussed in the remainder of this book, further attention is given to support for the child's intellectual growth potentials. Specific nursing actions are suggested as they apply to particular circumstances of the ill or handicapped child.

The Student in Relation to the Learning Process. The student also is learning and experiencing new situations. Although she is applying realized intellectual capacities in assimilating new knowledge and experience, she also needs support in stressful situations and the understanding of others in order to achieve her full potential of helpfulness to children and their parents. The capacity to give fully of herself will not be possible during this beginning period. It takes time to learn to deal with the tensions aroused when working with anxious children and their parents. Children who are ill and separated from their parents need constant attention and their reactions can be unnerving. It is frustrating to see a deformed child or one in acute distress without knowledge of how to lessen his despair. It also requires fortitude, especially when giving care which unavoidably inflicts pain.

Working with frightened, angry, dependent and grief-stricken children and parents takes great energy and patience. The nurse is bombarded by powerful emotions and cannot always be cool, poised and objective. It is understandable for her to be anxious and hurt when the child directs anger or aggression toward her or to feel inadequate in the face of grief.

Sometimes the nurse shields herself from pain by physically withdrawing from the situation, or she may develop a blind spot in her own perception. At the beginning of her pediatric experience, resorting to these escape devices can be expected at times but habitual flight would cripple the nurse as an effective helper. It would limit her opportunities to develop her potentialities for motherliness, to detect symptoms of stress and to give appropriate support. It would also leave the child and his parents to bear their problems alone.

Acquiring awareness and tolerance of one's own feelings and those of parents and children requires motivation and time. Knowledge must first be assimilated before it can be used and although the nurse may react intensely at first, she will gradually acquire insight into the frustrations of hospitalized children and of their need to express their fury periodically.

She will also learn that by accepting their aggression as well as their affection, she can become more helpful to them.

The nurse who can be charitable toward her early reactions, feelings of helplessness and frustration and accept them as a natural part of learning will find that she is beginning to enjoy her work, she has fewer conflicts and more capacity for giving. The practice of introspection can improve her performance through understanding and tolerance of her feelings as the natural consequences of past experiences. With the insight that *everyone* behaves on this basis, she will be less inclined to pass judgments on herself and others and more able to use her energy to change attitudes that interfere with her work.

RESPONSES TO STRESSFUL SITUATIONS

The term *stress* is now widely used to denote any of a variety of physical and psychological subjective responses of an individual implying intense reaction to an experience and changes in usual behavior. Stress is a normal phenomenon and occurs throughout life as a result of the strains of living itself, from expected crises in development or from other occurrences containing a threat to the individual's physical or psychological integrity. It involves two major factors: (1) the quality and quantity of the force or *stressor* exerted upon the individual, and (2) the capacity of the individual to cope with it.

The threat to the individual may originate within himself through disease or malfunctioning of a part of the body or from conflicts within his psychological structure. It may also be imposed from without through his social, cultural or physical environment. For stress to be experienced, the individual must become aware of the threat or make an appraisal of the situation. In addition, stress can be experienced if the situation is appraised as capable of harm, although in reality it may be benign. If the threat seems to be overwhelming or coping capacities are weak, the usual defensive maneuvers may occur to protect the individual against experiencing anxiety.

Psychological stress involving threat may not be directly observable but must often be inferred from antecedent conditions. The threat must be relevant to the individual's goals and values. Its main characteristics are two-fold: (1) It is *anticipatory* and future oriented and (2) it is brought about by *cognitive processes* involving perception, learning, memory, judgment and thought. One of the distinctions between physiologic and psychological stressful situations is that in the latter there is anticipation of harm not yet present. It is not the present which constitutes the threat, but cues in the environment which herald future damage. Threat can also vary in degree in a continuum which is a function of many factors: age of the individual, amount, imminence and likelihood of anticipated harm, cultural expectations of behavior, etc. The personality of the individual, his beliefs, past experiences and goals contribute to the great individual differences in the appraisal of a threatening situation. The threat usually involves frustration of a motive; and the more severe and basic the threat or motive, the more universal is the stress reaction and therefore the more predictable.

The physiologic aspects of stress reactions have been carefully documented and include changes in the electroencephalographic pattern, changes in the autonomic system including alterations in breathing, heart rate and blood pressure, vascular changes (pallor, flushing) and changes in hormonal activity involving mainly the hypothalamus and adrenal cortex.

Parental Reaction to Stress

As previously mentioned, parental reactions to a child's illness or deformity and to his need for hospitalization will show wide variation. Such a situation touches basic emotions, goals and needs and therefore can be anticipated. The factors which will influence each parent's manner of coping involve: (1) the seriousness and immediacy of the threat to their child, (2) situational constraints (some action tendencies may be unacceptable to parents), (3) the ego resources of each parent, (4) former experiences with illness and hospitalization, (5) individual styles or tendencies toward a particular method of coping with threat and (6) individual beliefs and values.

In most instances, the nurse can expect negatively toned affect (expressions of anger or fear), motor-behavorial reactions (agitation, etc.) and alterations in usual adaptive functioning. Although affect may not be expressed verbally, it is usually possible to infer emotion through "body language" even though the person is not aware that he is communicating his distress. The nurse can anticipate that the mother's perception will be narrowed so that she can attend only to the situation at hand and may have difficulty in hearing or in interpreting what is said to her. Her usual performance will be impaired, more so in complex situations, so that she may sometimes appear confused or helpless or unable to do for her child what would be easily accomplished at home.

Parents as well as children need a nurse who understands the stress that they are undergoing. The nurse must never forget that parents (or any lay person) cannot regard illness, deformities or handicaps with her professional knowledge and objectivity. While the nurse may know that an illness is not really serious, or that a certain deformity can be corrected by surgery, she should not assume that parents know this. She may have knowledge that tells her the mother has no realistic cause to feel guilty, fearful or angry. The mother's feelings may be irrational from the nurse's point of view, but to the mother they are real or she would not be distressed.

One of the most universal reactions of parents is guilt. Some parents may resent the financial burden or feel self-pity. Many may see the child's illness or deformity as catastrophic for themselves and feel resentful. Others may feel ashamed of the child's deformity and anticipate being ostracized. Many will feel grief and dread seeing their child in pain.

Many mothers may fear that their relationship to their child is endangered and some will consider the nurse as a rival and fear that their child may transfer his affection to her. Some parents are anxious lest hospitalization arouse the child's hostility toward them for abandoning him and resent the fact that they are not permitted to stay and care for him. This is particularly true of mothers of infants and young children because at this stage the mother and child are mutually dependent. When the mother is not allowed to minister to her child, she becomes frustrated, for she feels both aggressive and needing of approval. She also feels dependence on the doctors and nurses and apprehensive lest something she did caused her child's illness. Such conflicting feelings inevitably create anxiety.

Although many mothers have superb ego resources, the nurse should expect all of them to suffer varying degrees of anxiety. Some may manifest this by discussing seemingly unrelated problems because even minor difficulties seem insurmountable at this time. They may then seek understanding and relief from tension as a support in coping with the present problem.

When the nurse is able to listen to expressions of anxiety or anger without making the mother feel guilty or becoming anxious herself, she will notice that the mother will become more relaxed. *It is therapeutic to accept passively the mother's anxiety, to the degree in which it is appropriate to the current situation.* When the child's illness abates, most mothers solve other problems easily because they have surplus energy to deal with them. However, if the anxiety continues unabated, the nurse could quite reasonably suspect that there is more to it than mere concern over the illness. In such instances the nurse should report her observations to the health team.

As mentioned earlier, the manner in which the mother copes with this situation is a result of many factors. Some may fight back at adversity; others who are accustomed to taking flight when faced with stress may be expected to do so again. The nurse can also expect that some mothers, guilt ridden, may attempt to compensate through oversolicitude or else (unable to accept the possibility of being at fault) project their guilt onto the hospital personnel and blame them for everything. In the latter case the nurse might be called on to endure more than one critical tirade. If she remembers to accept it calmly and not to take it personally, she will probably be surprised to discover that the critical parent will end up by warmly praising her competence. The probable reason for this is that the nurse has protected the mother from facing feelings that she could not master.

All behavior, even that which seems bizarre or inappropriate, serves a purpose for the individual who is experiencing a stressful situation. When anxious, he is motivated to seek comfort, or return to former equilibrium. In observing unusual behavior it is easy to conclude erroneously that the person is creating a problem when in reality he is mobilizing his resources and signalling his need for help to solve one.

When Mrs. A. brought Ann into the hospital for cataract extraction, she was nervous and upset and therefore unable to support her child in the early part of her hospitalization. She fled from the ward as soon as Ann's history was taken, without heed to Ann's need for her. When the operation was postponed because Ann developed a respiratory infection, Mrs. A. vented her anger on hospital personnel and on Ann. When she came to visit, she could not tolerate Ann's tears of rebellion. She said that she could not wait to get out of the hospital because, as she expressed it venomously, "It makes me jittery. I can't stay put. The quicker I can get out of here the better."

The nurse tried to find out what was troubling Mrs. A. She discovered that Mrs. A. had cataracts extracted from both eyes when she was 4 years old. She remembered little about hospitalization, but from conversation it seemed evident that she had never made peace with her feelings about her eyes and the treatment she endured. She resented the fact that she had to wear thick glasses and felt she was unattractive in them. She felt guilty because she had produced what she called a "defective" child. After her first child, Billy, was born, she sought medical advice and made sure that his eyes were perfect before she became pregnant again. "I'd never have had another child if I'd known it would have cataracts," she said. When her second child's eyes were found to be imperfect, she felt guilty and angry. Mrs. A.'s brother had also had congenital cataracts, but his children had normal vision. Mrs. A. resented her brother's successful achievement.

After her operation, Ann cried and expressed anger toward her mother when she arrived late for visiting hours. Ann's response to discomfort and disappointment increased Mrs. A.'s guilt and also made her anxious and intolerant of frustration. She reacted with anger and inability to see anyone's problems but her own. It is highly probable that Mrs. A.'s memories of her own painful childhood hospital experiences were revived by her daughter's situation— hence, her anxiety, intolerance and unintentional cruelty. She knew that she was miserable, but she did not know why she acted as she did.

One of the most difficult situations for the nurse in working with parents is dealing with panic induced by one of the most profound of fears—that of the unknown. Many parents have little knowledge of hospitals or of medical matters and therefore appear unreasonable. Knowledge is fundamental to mobilization of coping capacities. The nurse must be prepared to give the most elementary of explanations without seeming patronizing or contemptuous. She must be prepared to counter prejudice based on ignorance or superstition. Some parents may have had a previous unfortunate experience in a hospital and others, because of feelings of helplessness, may react hysterically or aggressively. Since stress and anxiety cause distortions in adaptive capacities and usual behavior, some may have difficulty in dealing with their children and in providing consistent and reasoned guidance. Discipline the mother imposes may consist of fitful and sporadic outbursts of temper interspersed with periods of remorse in which she seeks to obliterate her guilt by overaffectionate demonstration. Such behavior will, of course, affect her child by increasing his anxiety and lessening his self control.

Children's Responses to Stress

A child's responses to stress when ill, hospitalized or handicapped are in many ways qualitatively different from those of his parents. Because of his illness, he has less energy to devote to coping with unfamiliar and frightening experiences. This situation is compounded by the loss of his parents' constant support; and because of his dependence on them, he feels a loss of part of himself. If he is very young, he is still dependent on his mother for control of his actions and responses and without her he feels helpless. The child's ego is still weak and he does not have the defensive and coping strategies available to his parents. Because of his limited experience and immature intellectual capacities, he cannot fully understand what is happening. Misinterpretations and an immature concept of causality increase his stress and anxiety with feelings of guilt and anger. In addition, he feels threatened from within by the impairment of his body functioning.

The major principle underlying effective emotional support is: *Awareness of the feelings of others and readiness to respond to them, so as to strengthen their resources to cope with stress.* The student must gradually acquire the ability to understand the child's point of view toward hospital admission and treatment. She must be able to imagine herself in the place of the child who is listless and passive and know that his behavior is expressive of homesickness, fear of his own anger, loss of his identity or despair at the loss of his mother who means his emotional security. When the student can sense what it may mean to a child to feel abandoned without assurance of acceptance of himself and of his behavior, she will be ready to give to minimize his anxiety and to strengthen his sense of identity. She can then make herself available to him and watch for clues which will further her understanding of him as a person. When he has regained his personal identity and feels trust in her, a change in his behavior will gradually emerge.

The nurse who is able to detect children who are using their energy to cope with anxiety, anger or grief for mothers who have disappeared, will be able to

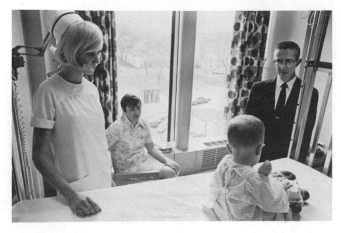

Fig. 2-5. Nurse observing family's interactions at the time of admission to the hospital.

anticipate their needs and prevent the withdrawal from such a dangerous environment. She will learn how to allay the fears that children are unable to express verbally and to find their personal sources of comfort.

INFLUENCING THE COURSE AND OUTCOME OF HOSPITALIZATION

Emotional Climate of the Pediatric Unit

The state of prevailing morale is much more important in a pediatric unit than is its decoration or equipment. The "emotional climate" must be more than superficial friendliness; the composite impression must be a sense of purpose on the part of each member of the staff, of competence and the will to understand

and respect. It is vital that the child and his parents be made aware of this willingness of the staff to exert itself on their behalf, because its absence can engender hopelessness and despair in both the patient and his family.

The nurse's mental and physical health is vital since she is an important part of the environment of a growing, impressionable child and of his parents who have problems of great magnitude. Because children and their parents look to the nurse for comfort, knowledge and strength, she has the power to use herself in ways which can be of immeasurable long range benefit. The nurse's contacts with children and parents must, therefore, communicate understanding, awareness of their particular needs and personal respect.

Adult standards of order and tidiness cannot always be maintained in a pediatric unit although some degree of order is essential for the sake of health and efficiency. Demanding perfection and neatness in a pediatric ward is unrealistic and shows lack of understanding. Children should not be expected to keep their belongings carefully arranged. A nurse who is perpetually tidying up a child's surroundings is communicating that play is not acceptable to her. Learning to put away playthings can become part of preparation for meal and rest periods.

Playthings and mementos of home may have a profound emotional significance to the child which an adult can hardly comprehend. He should have a private place for his cherished possessions and nothing should be discarded without the owner's permission.

A pediatric ward should be flexible enough in its arrangement to permit children to be moved closer to friends or to areas where they can view the activity

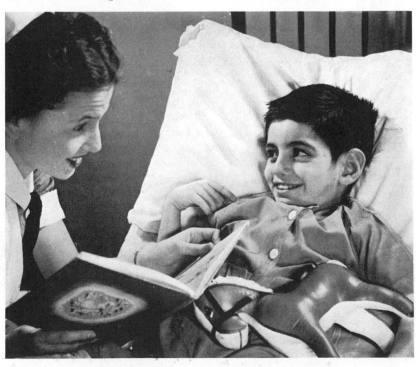

Fig. 2-6. Nurse reading to a child in response to his request for a story.

going on about them. Placement of a child on the ward should be carefully based on assessment of both his psychological and physical needs. Protection from cross-infection must be considered because the seriously ill or debilitated child may be unable to tolerate such an insult. Isolation may need to be imposed to protect others. Infants under 6 months of age should be placed in separate units to protect them from infections that may circulate

Although isolation is unavoidable in certain situations, it must be recognized that it holds dangers through limiting opportunities for sensory stimulation and through exaggerating the effects of separation from the family. Isolation should be regarded as a generally undesirable procedure, imposed only by medical necessity and kept as brief as possible. When unavoidable, the nurse can do much to ameliorate the lack of sensory and psychological stimulation if she understands the child's requirements.

The infant over 6 months of age and the toddler are least able to tolerate isolation because they are most dependent on their mothers. The school-age child is better able to cope with isolation because he has greater inner resources. Nevertheless, even for him, prolonged isolation becomes dreary, boring and anxiety-producing if no provisions are made for play and human companionship.

The grouping of children in a ward should be partly determined by the degree of illness. Acutely ill children, who need quiet and rest, should be separated from convalescent children, who require play and contact with peers. Newly admitted children who are not acutely ill are benefited by contact with children who have become familiar with the hospital environment.

Admission to the Hospital

When the nurse goes into the waiting room, she will find a child and one or both parents, all suffering from varying degrees of anxiety. Both the child and his parents should have been prepared for the experience at the time hospitalization was recommended. Unfortunately, in many instances this will not have been the case.

The manner in which the admitting routine is carried out can lessen anxiety or intensify fear. The nurse should bear in mind that many attitudes toward hospital and medical personnel are formed permanently at the time of admission. Although admissions are routine to her, they are anything but ordinary to the child and his parents. The giving of immediate attention and concern is strengthening and conveys assurance that they are in thoughtful hands.

At the time of admission, the nurse must assume that neither the child nor his parent is knowledgeable regarding procedures. Careful explanations must be made to parents along with assessment of the meaning of this experience for the child. Such appraisal will entail inquiry into the extent of the child's preparation

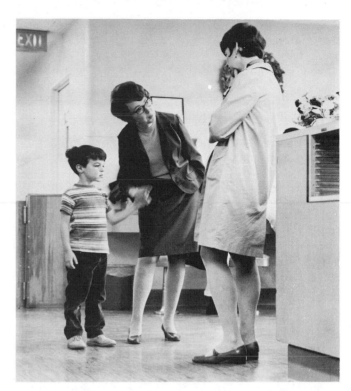

FIG. 2-7. A tour of the unit prior to the day of admission helps to prepare the child and his mother for hospitalization. (Bill Bargagliotti)

and the methods he normally utilizes to cope with apprehensiveness. It can be assumed that because of the young child's close identification with his mother, his mode of managing fearful situations will be similar to hers. Lack of parental preparation will, of course, impose an additional burden on the nurse.

Some children may substitute fantasy for reality because their mothers refuse to accept unpleasant situations. The child of the helpless, anxious mother, on the other hand, may strike out at everything that displeases him because he knows no other way to handle frustrations. Experience has taught him that aggression is profitable and also approved by his parents, and therefore he will use it as a method of overriding the unfamiliar and unpleasant.

Such a situation places a strain on the nurse, but she must keep her temper and exercise the necessary leadership. If the mother attempts to soothe the child with guilty affection, promises to take him home or bribes him to cease crying, the nurse must step in unobtrusively. She will need to win the mother's confidence and let her know diplomatically that they must help the child in learning to face difficulties. Although the mother's efforts at controlling her child are ineffectual, she is of emotional significance to him and he needs her as other children do. Temporary separation is sometimes helpful in assisting both to regain equilibrium.

Sometimes whispering to the child diverts his attention and when he is able to catch the nurse's words he is strengthened, for he has *accomplished* something which lessens his helplessness. He has also received the interest of the nurse and her approval which he has not yet learned to obtain in acceptable ways.

The first approach to the child should be friendly, honest and understanding, yet firm and convey that she will not succumb under hostility. If the child loses control of his behavior, it is wise to sit beside him for a few minutes. Once his emotional equilibrium is re-established and he learns that he has a strong person on whom he can rely, warmly spoken words will further assure him that his interests are being considered. Familiarizing him with his surroundings will support him in dealing with the unknown.

When the nurse is questioning any parent about his child, she must remember that *the child must be protected from hearing what he cannot understand.* He should not be within hearing distance when his personal history, disease or treatment is being discussed. Nor should he hear his mother talk about her feelings regarding his illness or deformity.

If a mother's anxiety is high, she may make derogatory statements within the child's hearing which are frightening to him. To prevent this, information can be obtained and recorded while the child is engaged in the playroom or is being introduced to ward personnel. This information should be readily available for the nurses who are assigned to the child's care. An illustration of a form which facilitates recording of information will be found in the Appendix.

Each nurse caring for the patient must know the history of his disease, its symptomatology and treatment. She must also have information that helps her to understand him as an individual. The nurse admitting the patient can report the observations that she has made regarding his reactions to her, to his mother, ward mates and treatments and the adjustment that he is making to the ward. She can also report the tentative plan of nursing care which she has evolved from the knowledge she has already acquired about him.

The mother's aid should be enlisted in introducing the child to his new environment, because the child is more likely to understand his mother's explanation and also because it allows the mother opportunity to get relief from her tension and any guilt feelings she may have. She must know that the nurse understands the difficulties entailed in this experience and that instant compliance is not expected of her child.

Need for Mother. The child needs his mother's support during admission and early adjustment to his new environment. Allowing the mother to assist in admission procedures proves to her that the nurse wishes to sustain the mother-child relationship and allays fears of losing the child's affection to the nurse. This cooperation also increases the child's security and trust in both, since the mother's acceptance of the nurse may forestall the problem of divided loyalties and he can see the nurse as an extension of his mother rather than a substitute for her. Cooperative admission also allows him to adjust to strangers more slowly and gives the nurse time to observe the mother-child relationship.

Hospital routines must be flexible enough to allow for changes in procedure when they are indicated. When a child is unable to cooperate in some of the admission procedures, force will merely antagonize him. Postponement or modification of the procedure until he has gained confidence in the personnel conveys thoughtful consideration of his wishes and needs.

The child's mother should accompany him to the ward and remain with him until he has related himself to a new world and to the nurse to whom he has been assigned. Parting at the bedside fosters a sense of security in both mother and child; the mother must know where her child has been placed, and the child must be assured that his mother knows where he is in order to lessen his fear of abandonment. As the nurse explains the visiting hours, she can emphasize the child's need for both parents and assist them in anticipating the possible responses which may come at visiting or leave-taking. Many mothers dread parting from their child and hesitate to tell the truth about their leaving. They may fear the child's anger or fail to understand the need for honest explanations. The nurse may need to remind them that truthful preparation for leave-taking is necessary to lessen the child's fear of desertion.

Making Friends with the Child. When a mother and child enter the ward, they should be introduced immediately to the nurse who has been assigned to the child's care. The nurse can assure him that she *is* the person who will care for him in his mother's absence. *He must find through experience that this is true.* When she must leave him, it is her responsibility to inform the child to whom he can turn for help.

It is difficult for an adult to imagine the utter desolation and fear of a newly admitted child, particularly if this is his first hospital experience and previous experiences away from home have traumatized him. There is no sounder way to earn the child's trust and friendship than by relieving his physical and emotional discomfort. He may resist her efforts at first because he wants only his mother and fears that she has abandoned him forever to this stranger. However, if the nurse accepts his behavioral responses to stress, he will begin to see her as a valuable person. She can never become a substitute for his mother, but she can become a real friend if she does nothing which puts him into conflict with his loyalty to the most important person in his life.

A tour about the ward lessens the child's fear and assures him that there is a special place which belongs to him. As the child is being oriented, the nurse can watch for clues as to how he signals his needs. If he can be ambulatory, freedom to explore the ward will strengthen his adaptive capacities. As he senses his nurse's interest, he will gradually reach toward her and indicate ways in which she can relieve his discomfort. He may initially observe her intently and test her reactions to his behavior. The child who discovers that he dares to express what he feels will be fortunate indeed because he will not have to bottle up feelings that are natural during this stage of adjustment to hospitalization.

If the nurse discovers that he has not learned why he is in the hospital, she must explain the reason. Explanation may be required repeatedly before he comprehends.

Hospital routines differ from those he has known before, and the child will watch intently all that happens around him. He will often question incessantly. Because he does not have the ego resources required to overcome helplessness, he needs to be kept informed. Knowing what the nurse is going to do, what is expected of him and what he can anticipate in the immediate future helps him to maintain emotional balance.

When the child requires treatment immediately upon admission, his adjustment will be easier if his nurse is permitted to postpone painful procedures until he begins to trust her. Meanwhile, the nurse can sit beside him quietly until he approaches her. Presenting play materials tells the child that the nurse is a friendly person who understands his need for play. He may need permission to play, but if he is consumed with anxiety, he may be too tense to be diverted. *An inability to play productively is a symptom of acute anxiety and the child must know that he will not be punished for expressing anger or being curious.* Curiosity is a powerful urge—often a response to fear as the child becomes motivated to gain control over that which threatens him.

Billy was 18 months old when he was admitted with suspected cystic fibrosis of the pancreas. When his mother left, he stood in his crib, shook it and went into a rage. He tossed all his toys onto the floor and protested in every way he knew how. When the nurse entered the room he bellowed more loudly and turned his back on her. When the nurse showed her willingness to hold him, he ran into the opposite corner of the crib like a frightened, angry animal. He seemed both panic stricken and furious. The nurse sat quietly by his bedside to give him an opportunity to become familiar with her. Billy's screaming continued for many minutes during which he alternately looked at the nurse and away from her. Then he tore a rubber washer from the cribside and threw it onto the floor. The nurse picked it up and put it back in place. Billy repeated the performance not once but a dozen times. Each time the nurse replaced the washer on the cribside, signifying her acceptance of his anger.

Gradually, Billy's behavior changed somewhat and once he came near to smiling, but he was not without tension by any means. Then the nurse placed a ball on his bed. He

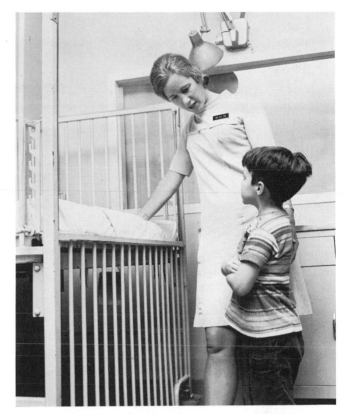

Fig. 2-8. Meeting the people who will care for him and seeing that he will have a place of his own assists the child to feel more secure in a strange environment. Children need to be prepared for the fact that hospital beds may look very different from those they have at home. (Bill Bargagliotti)

used the ball exactly as he had used the washer. Then a pyramid of rings was placed on his bed. Again the nurse watched for clues which would tell her of his needs. Billy began to play with the nurse. He removed the rings from the stick, handed one to the nurse and then held out his hand to have it returned to him. Was this his signal of a need for a give-and-take relationship or was it his way of trying to overcome his fear of separation from his mother? It is interesting to note that this type of play is seen repeatedly in hospitalized children under 3 years of age.

Before long Billy moved closer to the nurse. Soon he scrambled to the edge of the bed and made known his wish to climb onto the nurse's lap. In a few minutes Billy's need for closeness vanished. Or did physical contact with the nurse remind him of his wish for his mother which was too much to bear? He reached for the toy and began to play. Soon he wanted to get back into the crib again.

Later when the nurse said, "Billy, I must go now. I'll be back," she left a child who was a little less anxious than he was when she arrived. Although diverted by other tasks, she watched Billy frequently for signs of anxiety. When he signalled his need for her, she went to him immediately because she wanted him to be *sure* that there was someone nearby who had a personal interest in him. On returning she said, "Billy, I came back. I'll always come back when I tell you I will." A friendly relationship had been established which served to minimize the shock of being separated from his mother.

Billy's ego was not strong enough to adjust constructively to a strange environment without assistance. In addition to his physical health problem he also had the problem of adjusting to separation from his mother. He did have strengths: (1) he was able to express his tempestuous feelings which permitted him to eliminate tension and indicate his need for help; (2) he was able to relate to a stranger when given an opportunity to become familiar with her; (3) he had the capacity to retain trust; and (4) he could play when encouraged.

Billy also had limitations: (1) he had an immature ego which was weakened by physical disease and difficult environmental demands; (2) he could not understand the reason why hospitalization was necessary or why his mother had left the ward; and (3) he was too young to maintain a relationship with his mother *in absentia*.

CARE PLANNING: IDENTIFICATION OF A CHILD'S PROBLEMS AND NEEDS. NURSING DIAGNOSIS

At the beginning of this chapter, emphasis was placed on the development of a science and theory of nursing as a function of direct ministration to patients. In order to progress in this direction, intervention must move from an intuitive and experimental base to one completely conscious, rational and grounded in precise observations and theoretical formulations. Definite goals for nursing care, based on a systematic assessment of the patient's particular needs and problems, must be formulated in order to make possible the evaluation of results of intervention. Careful assessment focuses the attention of the nurse toward furthering nursing goals for the patient rather than centering solely on the physical therapeutic aims of treatment. It also contributes toward elimination of "labeling" or stereotyping of behavior on a foundation of insufficient data. Lastly, the use of scientific methods in studying her patient's physical and psychological responses to disease and his environmental milieu* enhances the nurse's relationship with children and furthers her own learning.

A nursing diagnosis is the process which identifies the patient's problems and particular needs and assesses his resources to assist in decision making as to individual requirements for nursing assistance.

The primary assessment should include all the patient's needs and current problems as far as is possible, both overt and covert, as well as the strengths he possesses in dealing with them. Observational data must be collected systematically with the use of all of the nurse's resources (sense organs, knowledge and problem solving ability) and their meaning then

sought through the application of principles from the biological and behavioral sciences. Interpretations of her observations, based on concepts from these allied disciplines, eventually will become integrated into nursing theory as they affect decisions regarding plans for specific intervention.

The objective for nursing care is derived from this first careful and thorough appraisal of all information available from the above sources. A comprehensive purpose for all nursing care must include the promotion of ego growth and opportunities for intellectual advancement. Immediate goals should include assistance to the child in regaining a state of equilibrium and support for his coping strategies and efforts toward mastery of new experiences. Objectives in care then should include functional and behavioral targets in addition to physical ones. For any particular child the nursing aims must be carefully delineated and specifically stated to allow for evaluation of the child's progress and to determine the effects of nursing intervention. The more specific the goals, and the more the nurse is able to find out about a given child's problems, his strengths and limitations in coping with them (understanding all the while that the effects of disease may produce drastic if temporary changes in his body and his behavior), the better able she is to tailor a plan of care expressly for that individual.

With the formulation of a nursing diagnosis then, decisions can be made as to a course of action, and appropriate methods, resources and personnel needed can be planned in order to meet the identified needs and aims of care. This is in essence, a decision for action. Such a nursing care plan is a step toward nursing therapy and comprehensive nursing care. It also gives direction toward the seeking of additional knowledge since the formulation of a nursing diagnosis is a constant process continuing throughout the hospitalization period or duration of the nurse's contacts with the child and his family. As planned intervention is evaluated for its effectiveness in promoting progress toward the stated goal, and as new information is gathered, both the diagnosis and care plan will be constantly altered and problems restated.

In summary, this identification of patient needs and objectives is the problem solving or research approach toward nursing intervention. It is also the essence of the nursing process and the steps can be briefly outlined: (1) collection of observational and other data, (2) interpretation of the data in order to delineate and assess the problems systematically, (3) formulation of a diagnosis, goals and hypotheses about possible solutions, (4) formulation of plans of nursing care, (5) testing of the hypotheses or action taken, (6) evaluation of the results of care on the child's physical and emotional state and (7) reformulation of plans for nursing care as the child's condition demonstrates that he is moving either forward in the direction of health or backward away from it.

---

* The words *environmental milieu* refer not only to the child's physical environment but also to the persons providing care and visiting him (parents and friends in the ward) and to environmental demands for adjustment such as the staff's expectations, treatments, and separation from home, family and friends.

HELPING THE CHILD DURING HOSPITALIZATION

Factors Affecting Adjustment. A child's adjustment to illness and hospitalization depends on several factors: age, the nature and degree of illness, past experiences, the emotional meaning of his illness to him, his perception of causality and thinking level and the quality of care he receives in the hospital and on his return home.

Of all the influences that are brought to bear on the child's capacity to deal with change, past experiences are the most significant. In the ward there will be children who have not been well fed, others who have had little intelligent discipline, some who have been deceived, and some who are filled with rage and fears which are the outgrowth of disturbed relationships with their parents. However, the majority of children will come from homes where they have been loved. They respect authority because it has been reasonable and has provided them with security. They trust others because they have not been disappointed by their parents. They expect friendliness, protection and care because they are used to these. Such children are the fortunate ones in times of illness but they, too, will be anxious.

Relief from Anxiety. The quality of care the child receives is also significant. The child's first emotional need is for relief of anxiety and it is the nurse's task to learn as much as she can about the possible causation and to plan action toward alleviation. Anxiety has two main origins: that caused by normal developmental crises and that brought about by illness and subsequent hospitalization. Fear of the unknown is especially painful at any age. The child under 3 years of age is predominantly afraid of separation from his mother, of disapproval, physical pain, punishment and his own aggressiveness. In addition to these, preschool children (3-6 years) fear bodily injury. The child over 6 years of age dreads the retaliation of his newly developed conscience as well as the disapproval of his peers.

The adolescent is primarily concerned with the increased intensity of his sexual and aggressive drives and is anxious about his physical and psychological adequacy. Although many of the child's fears are irrational from the adult point of view, this in no way diminishes their severity. To try to explain away irrational fears is useless. The nurse can banish some of his fears by proving through protective, comforting acts that they have no basis in fact; moreover, she can shield the child from disturbing sights and sounds. Every ward should have a room where children can be taken for treatments which are painful or can be misinterpreted by children in the ward. Hospital personnel are all too prone to take for granted occurrences which are shocking to the ordinary individual. If a child sees another child having a paracentesis, for instance, he may well wonder if that will also be done to him. Even if it will not, the sight would be

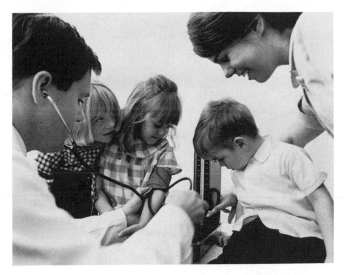

Fig. 2-9. Children are less fearful of medical procedures if equipment and its use is explained to them. Note the boy's interest and absorption in the sphygmomanometer. (George Knight)

upsetting. Likewise, children should be protected from seeing those who are critically ill or dying, and they should be kept from hearing discussions that might arouse fear. Children are keenly sensitive to everything that goes on around them and especially aware of conversations that concern them. When they cannot understand all that is being said, they become anxious just as adults do.

In such cases the nurse's job is to encourage him to express the meaning which the conversation or episode had for him. Probably the child will say nothing directly until the nurse has made him comfortable enough to feel that it is safe to express himself. She should be on the lookout for misinterpretations. For instance, the child may have thought that the treatment was punishment or he may dread the prospect of a treatment he has seen done on another child. The guiding principle in such an instance is to be sensitive to signs of anxiety and to search for their cause.

Preparation for and Support during Treatments. Treatments and procedures which cause unavoidable pain are often necessary to hasten the child's recovery despite possible emotional strain. It is the nurse's task to help the child maintain his trust in the doctor and to promote understanding of the protective value of the treatment. *Children can tolerate discomfort if they are prepared for it, comprehend its real purpose, and receive adequate support.*

Preparation for each step of a painful procedure *before* it is done provides the basis for the maintenance of trust. Without preparation, the child will feel deeply resentful toward all persons concerned, and with good reason.

Some methods for supporting children through

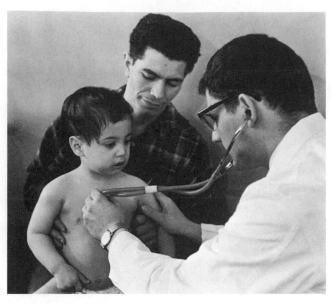

Fig. 2-10. The young child is often better able to cooperate with admitting procedures when one of his parents is able to be with him. (George Knight)

treatments will be discussed in later portions of the text. For all children capable of understanding, the steps in the procedures should be described, they should be allowed choice in method whenever possible and be allowed to perform as much for themselves as feasible. Previous play with unsterilized equipment is often beneficial and the use of a doll to demonstrate what will be done can be valuable. Allowing the child to experiment with the doll, for instance in clipping stitches from a belly band sewn on the doll, will help him to understand that only thread will be cut and removed from the wound. It will also give him ideas of how he can make the process easier for himself and for the doctor. Such preparation is important because it counteracts feelings of helplessness and promotes the sense of participation. It further supports the child's sense of adequacy, his self concept and security through knowledge of coming events. If the child expects pain, he can marshal his resources and with encouragement to express himself, the fear of loss of self control and of disapproval can be relieved.

An approach to the child which communicates the nurse's faith in his power to bear discomfort is strengthening. Most children will try to communicate (perhaps very indirectly) how the nurse can be of help. Because of our cultural expectations of bravery, many children, especially boys over 4 years of age, have a need for self control. Recognition of this need and support in achieving such control bolsters a sense of autonomy.

Steve was a 4 year old hemophiliac who had had 20 admissions to the hospital and 100 blood transfusions and had returned to the outpatient department every 2 weeks for plasma since he was 1 year of age.

On one such occasion Steve began to scream before the procedure had begun. Steve's mother left the room, but she was quickly replaced by a social worker who had befriended him on many previous occasions.

Steve, still crying, said, "Come hold my hand. Tell me the story of the Three Bears. You hold your hand over my mouth while they stick the needle in. Put your hand this way." (He seized the worker's hand and demonstrated how he wanted her to support him in dealing with his fear.)

When the social worker learned what Steve wanted her to do, she withdrew her hand. Steve pulled her hand back to his mouth and insisted that she leave it there. Then he began to ask questions about the story: "She ate it all up, didn't she? She was asleep in the chair when the big bear came. Isn't that right?"

The social worker, her hand over Steve's mouth as he directed, began to tell the story. Meanwhile the doctor began to prepare the area and then inserted the needle. Steve put his hand over the worker's hand to hold it in place over his mouth. "Ow," he shrieked in a muffled voice. Then he tried to turn his head to watch the doctor. The social worker held her hand in place and continued the story. Steve smiled at the worker as she told the story. Then he jumped as the needle was reinserted.

The social worker kept one hand over his mouth and the other on his body, still continuing the story. Steve's body relaxed as he saw the plasma dripping into his vein, and he began to ask questions again. There followed a lively interplay between him and the social worker. The doctor quietly left to bring Steve's mother to him. The mother exclaimed, "I can't believe it's over." (In her own state of anxiety she had been unable to perceive her child's call for help.)

Steve remarked, "I was a good boy. I didn't even cry." Turning toward the worker he said, "When I come again to get plasma, will you hold my mouth again?"

Despite the nurse's efforts, many experiences during hospitalization will be perceived as hostile attacks and provoke anger. If such anger must remain submerged because of fear of disapproval, anxiety and ego-defensive activity will be aroused which may be detrimental to emotional development. The conflict between impulses to retaliate aggressively and the need for love underlies the absolute necessity of play as an opportunity for resolution and assimilation of feelings. If they are quickly repressed, energy needed for growth will be utilized to maintain this defense against anxiety.

Preparations for an Operation. If the child is not acutely ill at the time of admission he may be too easily forgotten by the staff, since he requires no symptomatic treatment. However, the nurse should remember that even a young child will sense that something very unusual is going to happen and will be insecure; while the child old enough to understand the meaning of an operation will probably be acutely anxious over what appears to be an impending ordeal.

The parents should be completely informed of what is to be done. In most instances they will want to know details of preoperative and postoperative procedures. Some parents prefer to be present during the preoperative preparation of the child in order to help him.

Before operation the child must have an opportunity to make friends with the nurse who is to function with his parents in helping him through the oncoming event. Preparation must be gradual, for children can only assimilate one threatening concept at a time. The nurse must be prepared to answer oft-repeated questions. Interrogation is used by many children to signal their failure to assimilate previously given facts and their readiness for further help in becoming prepared for a dreaded event. Observation to see if facts of preparation are digested, denied or misinterpreted is necessary to know the rate at which preparation can be given and what further help the child requires. A 2-year-old will not understand all that he hears, but he will sense the nurse's wish to help. Letting him play at putting a mask on his face or a bandage over his tummy, is understandable to the toddler. Then when he meets the experience he will be more trusting because he knows that the nurse has tried to forewarn him.

If the nurse learns that the child has been prepared for operation by his mother, she should attempt to find out his impressions; often he has misunderstood her explanation. If he has dressed her preparation up with fantasies of his own making, the nurse can correct these misconceptions. Often what he imagines is more gruesome than reality, but, more often than not, the uncomfortable parts of the experience have been minimized by his parents or forgotten by the child himself because he was not ready for the knowledge that he had been given.

The child must be forewarned of discomfort to come, because pain is always harder to bear if it comes as a shock. He must also be helped to realize that his nurse and parents trust his capacity to bear it when it comes and that they will be with him to ease his discomfort. Without assurance that such help will be available, the child probably will react by denying the reality of the forthcoming experience.

To prepare the child for every detail of the experience is practically impossible, since changes in the plan of care often are made at the last minute. Having the mother say something like the following during the evening before operation has proved to be of value in the preparation of many children: "Tim, I think this is the way it's going to be. It may be a little different. You watch and listen carefully to see if I've told you all of the story about having an operation. If I've forgotten a part of it, you remember it and tell me about it when we are together again." Such a statement may be remembered if the child suddenly finds himself confronted with an unexpected threat and may become the means by which his trust is sustained. It is helpful also in that it can prevent delib-

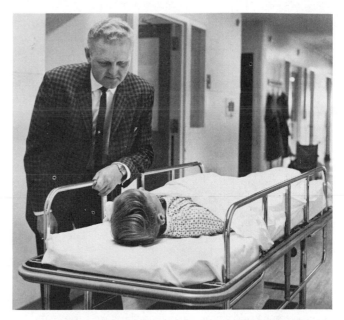

FIG. 2-11. When parents can visit prior to surgery, the child is assured that they know where he is going and that they will be there when he returns. (Bill Bargagliotti)

erate forgetting (repression) of those parts of the experience which were most difficult to bear.

The importance of adequate preparation of a child for operation is shown by the fact that some surgeons will not operate unless convinced that the child is ready to accept this reality. The child who masks his fear by denial needs special help. Whatever the means employed by the child to shut out thoughts that are too painful to think about continuously, the nurse must seek to break through the barrier with the truth even if her words go unheard. Reality must be faced sooner or later, but the nurse should see to it that the child does not have to face it alone.

Sometimes children who use denial as a defense against anxiety cover their fear with aggression and bravado. Vander Veer* cites the case of a boy who entered the doctor's office, drew a pocketknife from his pocket and opened it up. When the doctor asked him what he was doing, he said, "I'm going to cut the doctors before they can cut me." Vander Veer interpreted this behavior as a defense against anxiety over possible injury.

The following is a description of a child's response to an impending operation. This child was capable of verbalizing his feelings but until a nurse came to his rescue he had no support to face what he thought was going to happen. Jim not only needed emotional contact with a person but also a chance to get his irra-

---

* Vander Veer, A. H.: The psychopathology of physical illness and hospital residence *in* Personality Development and Its Implications for Nursing and Nursing Education, p. 65, Springfield, Ill., Dept. of Public Health, 1948.

tional ideas into the open. Helping him to learn the irrationality of his fears was necessary to strengthen his ego so he could face the coming ordeal.

Seven-year-old Jim was left alone in a small room of the operating room suite, following a pneumoencephalogram. He was strapped down to a table and was scheduled for a craniotomy for a brain tumor in half an hour. He was sobbing and his body shook. Perspiration stood out on his forehead and his cheeks were flushed. He knew that he was to have an operation and realized what this meant (he had had one when 3 years old). He also knew that the doctor was going to do something to his head because it had been aching for weeks. His monologue ran somewhat as follows: "I don't want to go to sleep. I don't want a mask. I want to go back to my room. Why isn't my mother here? Don't people around here know I want her here? They are going to cut through the bone aren't they?"

When the nurse found Jim alone in the waiting room, he was in no condition to be anesthetized. She stepped in immediately to be with the child. Fortunately Jim had seen the nurse in the ward and was able to accept her ministrations (some children cannot when they are furious and disillusioned with people). He clutched her hands as she made hers available to him. When she found he could bear bodily contact, she quickly loosened the straps that immobilized him and then replaced her hands near his. As she did so, she said, "I'll not leave you. You'll not be alone when you awaken, either." Then she became silent to give Jim every chance to express himself and also to mobilize her own resources to administer psychological first-aid to Jim. Coming on his plight unprepared unnerved and angered her, and she needed a few minutes to get her feelings under control so that she could concentrate her full attention on Jim.

Jim repeated his questions, and the nurse said, "Of course you're scared about going to sleep and want your mother right here. She'll be with you when you wake up."

J: "How do they do it? How can they take my head apart and put it back together again?"

N: "Jim, I'm going to tell you about it just as carefully as I can. First the doctor will put you to sleep. The stuff he puts on the mask doesn't smell good. Some kids say it stinks. The more deeply you breathe, the quicker you'll go to sleep. You won't feel the operation."

J: "Then what? What's the matter with my head anyway?"

N: "When you're asleep, the doctor cuts through the bone in one part of your head. He does this so he can look inside to see what is making your head ache so much."

J: "How will he know what to do?"

N: "He's taken pictures. Remember when you went to X-ray? He already knows where the spot is that he has to fix. The pictures show the part of your brain that is pressing against your skull and making your head ache. Your doctor knows exactly what to do Jim. He's fixed many children's heads."

J: "Will my head stop hurting then?"

N: "Not right away, Jim. It will ache when you wake up, but your mother will be with you, and nurses and doctors will stay right beside you to help you in every way they can."

J: "Will he put my head together again?"

N: "Indeed he will, Jim. He knows you want to look just as you do now. He fixes the spot that is making your head ache. Then he puts the bone back exactly as he did before. You know how to put pieces into a puzzle don't you? That's the way the doctor puts your head back together again. He puts the bone back where it was. Then he fastens it in place so it'll stay there. Then he'll put a big bandage around it."

J: "How does he do that?"

N: "He winds it around your head. He makes it thick—kind of like a cushion so you'll have something to lie on. You won't feel much like drinking at first, and the doctor knows you'll need water, so you'll have water dripping into a vein of your arm or leg, too. There will be food in the water, too. Holding your arm or leg still will be kind of uncomfortable at first, but you'll get used to it. The doctor will strap it to a board to help you remember to keep it still. Your mother will help you, too."

J: "When will the bandage come off?"

N: "I'm not quite sure, Jim; the doctor will look at it every day, and he'll change it several times before it comes off for good."

J: "Will that hurt?"

N: "Sometimes it will, but you can stand it because a nurse will be there to tell you about it and help you. I'll bet you'll be able to tell her how to move you so it doesn't hurt quite so much."

Tears continued to roll down Jim's cheeks throughout this interchange. His voice shook at times, he wiggled on the table but kept his hands enclosed in the nurse's; gradually he began to relax a little.

N: "Your hair will grow back, Jim, and your skin will heal. You'll be just exactly as you are now—even better because you won't have such a headache."

J: "I want to go back to my room."

N: "I know you do, Jim, but if you did your head wouldn't get fixed. And that just has to be. Boys can't have any fun when their heads ache all the time. Your doctor knows exactly what to do, and I'm going to help you go to sleep."

Relieving the child's fears, reassuring him that he will not be alone in moments of stress takes patience, but this help must be provided not only to minimize his misery but also to ensure smooth recovery in the postoperative period. Until the anesthetist arrived Jim asked and repeated questions similar to those cited above, but as time passed he concentrated more on questions relating to his mother's whereabouts and when she would go to his room. He gradually accepted the idea that the operation had to be. He struggled when the mask was put onto his face, shrieked "Take it off" but continued to cling to the nurse's hands.

Postoperative Support. In the postoperative period the child's primary source of emotional support will come from his parents. However, they must first be adequately prepared for what they will see when their child returns from the operating room. Given the opportunity, most parents inquire about the degree of scarring, especially in such instances as when cardiac surgery is anticipated for a daughter. They should know what treatment measures will be carried out postoperatively.

Observation to detect the point at which the parents feel ready to view their child's wounds and to assist in the provision of care is important. With a little encouragement and help, most mothers rally their forces together quickly to overcome feelings of help-lessness and to be of comfort to their children. Parental participation in care speeds the child's adjustment to changes in his body because his parents' presence and comforting provides reassurance that he is not being punished by either of them.

After operation the child must be given an oppor-tunity to rid himself of the anxiety caused by the experience. One way to do this is to encourage him "to talk out" his feelings on the subject. He may have a highly distorted view of what happened, and an accurate account given by the nurse will go far to banish nameless and irrational fears. Of course, the child's inclination to talk will be determined to a large extent by the interest shown by the nurse and the parents. Those children who are too young to com-municate their thoughts and feelings verbally will be able to express themselves in play, which should be provided as soon as possible.

Play. Activity programs do more than fill the time between visiting hours, which would seem endless to the homesick child if he were left unoccupied and alone. Providing children with play materials tells them that their need for work and play is understood and assures them that although their present situation is often bewildering and painful, they can also find friendliness and consideration. It is through play that young children learn, understand and develop intel-lectually, for until they reach adolescence they need concrete objects to observe and manipulate.

Play helps the sick child regain gradual indepen-dence through enjoyment of group experiences. At first he may wish only to play with his nurse, but as she gives him freedom, he will become less dependent and begin to reach out for experiences with other children. The toddler and preschool child will con-tinue to need the security of the nurse's presence although their need will not be as urgent.

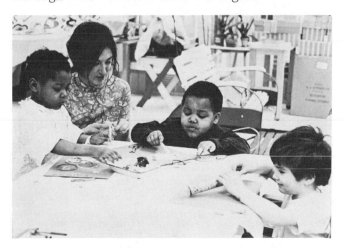

Fig. 2-12. A properly supervised playroom can offer opportunities for learning during convalescence or diagnostic study.

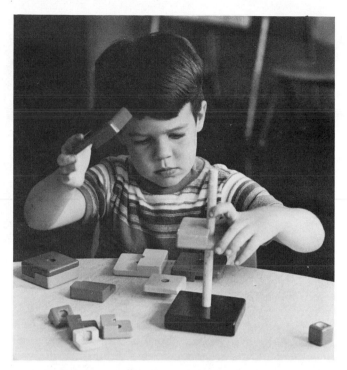

Fig. 2-13. Providing play equipment in the hospital tells the child that his need for play is understood. Wearing his own clothes helps the convalescent child to feel more at home in strange surroundings. (Bill Bargagliotti)

Observations of children at play are valuable in that they reveal progress in mastery of experiences, levels of intellectual functioning, relationships with other children and perceptions of illness and treatment.

Parents are relieved to see their children playing and regaining independence. It also gives them the opportunity to observe the potentials for learning in constructive play.

When the activity program is directed by a play or occupational therapist, nurses should have an oppor-tunity to assist in order to learn methods for encour-aging play interests and to cooperate in promoting a productive activity program for all children on the ward. A playroom is helpful for convalescent chil-dren to avoid interference with the rest needs of the acutely ill and to provide freedom from ward restrictions.

Principles of selection and suggested lists of appro-priate toys and literature for hospitalized children are presented on pages 563-564 of the Appendix. A prop-erly equipped playroom is essential for the many rea-sons cited above and throughout this book.

Dietary Considerations. Mealtime requires that the nurse and dietitian cooperate to provide proper foods in a setting conducive to appetite.

Food from home may be indicated for the child who is not eating. Mother's food is more enjoyable and because of pleasurable associations, keeps the

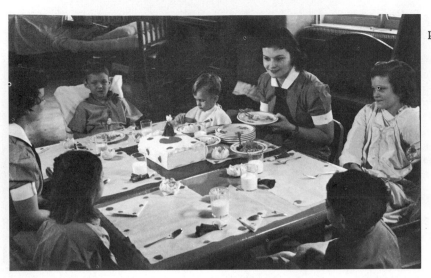

Fig. 2-14. Nurses eating with children to provide a homelike social experience.

child in touch with his mother and reinforces his security.

Self-feeding is difficult for a small or acutely ill child. Otherwise, if the child indicates a wish to be independent at mealtimes, this should be allowed unless all physical effort is forbidden. Enough time devoted to meal periods will give children sufficient help, encouragement and companionship; mealtime should be a happy period.

If the child's appetite is poor, the nurse should investigate his attitude toward food at home. Loss of appetite may be due to illness and hospitalization, or it could be his usual reaction to food.

Many children are prejudiced toward a wide variety of food, and therefore may not receive a well balanced diet. The nurse can help a child overcome such prejudices. Initially, serving only the foods that he likes, she can gradually introduce minute morsels of disliked foods. By commending the smallest sign of cooperation, the nurse conveys understanding that most children have difficulty getting used to new foods, and that she wants to help him learn to eat those he thinks he dislikes.

A small amount, eaten with pleasure, is better than large quantities forced on an unwilling child. *Forced feedings are never justifiable.* Many children express inner conflicts at mealtimes. Forcing food will only increase the need to refuse to eat. Serious cases of refusal to eat (with no physical basis) indicate deep emotional difficulty, and usually require intensive treatment by a psychiatrist or a child-guidance worker.

When a special diet is prescribed, the nurse must help the child to accept it. Feelings of deprivation or rejection will be evoked because what he has been used to is of deep emotional significance to him; allowing a child freedom to complain should help. Children feel understood if they are served the foods they like rather than the less appetizing ones. The nurse and the dietitian can help the school-age child and the adolescent to plan their own menus. If the

child is going home on a special diet, both parents must know the reason for his dietary requirements if only to give him a convincing explanation of the reasons for adhering to it.

All children who are physically able to participate in a group meal period should have the opportunity to do so. Children like eating family style and serving themselves, and a nurse or two can share the meal period with them. More and more hospitals are instituting this form of meal service because both children and nurses profit from it. The children's appetites improve, and the spirit of good-will and comradeship is furthered.

Regaining Independence. A seriously ill child is completely dependent on others and his regression must be accepted. When his physical condition improves, however, he needs encouragement to regain his personality strengths. His efforts to move ahead must be recognized, and although some children may need to be convinced that independent activity is more satisfying than complete dependence, most will struggle to grow out of their former regressive state. At first the child may test his nurse's response to self-assertiveness, but if he discovers that she is willing to help him regain autonomy, his confidence in himself will be quickly restored.*

The introduction of school work during convalescence not only keeps the child abreast of his classmates, but is important in restoring initiative and the satisfaction of accomplishment. Encouraging the child to help in the ward provides opportunities to acquire skills, confidence and recognition. Feeling useful and responsible restores his self-esteem.

---

* See Blake, F.: In quest of hope and autonomy, Nursing Forum *1*:8, 1961, for a description of the way in which a girl reached out for help in reconquering the negative counterparts of the core problems she had solved before she entered the hospital for open-heart surgery. Understanding the way in which healthy children solve core problems in development prepares the nurse to spot readiness for new learning experiences after a period of dependency during acute illness.

Preparation of Parents for Care of Their Children at Home. In addition to help which prepares parents for the particular physical care which the child requires after discharge, they must also be prepared for the changes in behavior which may become manifest at home as a consequence of his recent experience in the hospital. Observation has shown that young children who have been hospitalized frequently reveal symptoms of disturbed relationships with their mothers after they are discharged. Some of them become clinging, demanding and resentful. Others have repressed their feelings and express their hostility indirectly. They withdraw from their mothers and reject their efforts to care for them because they have lost trust in them. Thumb-sucking, night terrors, soiling, enuresis, negativism, eating and speech disturbances and increased aggression are other ways in which the emotional effects of hospitalization may become evident.

CHILDREN WITH SPECIAL PROBLEMS DURING HOSPITALIZATION

The Child from Another Culture

Emphasis has been placed on the importance of the child's early experience as a determinant of later behavior. Children of families with beliefs, values and customs differing from those with which we are familiar in the core culture of middle-class America will exhibit different patterns of behavior when under the stress of illness and hospitalization. The nurse who is working with a child from a culture which varies from her own, needs to have understanding, not only of the values within her own culture, but acceptance and knowledge of the practices within the child's society.

The behavior which the nurse observes is on several levels, and the total is a product both of individual psychological structure and of behavior *shared* by the individual within the child's cultural group. *Culture is that complex set of directives that regulates behavior, including knowledge, patterns for skills, belief systems and goals.* It is a design for living passed down through generations, or a programming of the human mind as it is shared by a society. Culture is fabricated by man to conserve energy and to cope with the exigencies of life as he perceives reality.

Systems of perception are different between cultural groups and therefore the reality perceived by the child may be very different from that seen by the nurse. Cultural variations are *learned* through early experiences in the home and color many later reactions, particularly during stressful occurrences. In order to interpret behavior, the nurse must also give attention to these cultural patterns since they are directly projected into the child's behavior. Some responses often observed on a pediatric ward, such as expressions of aggression and responses to pain and grief, may not have the same meaning in different cultures and subcultures. There are also differing conceptions about health and illness, the causation of illness and the efficacy of treatment. Different methods can also be seen to relieve tension, in denial of sadness, in patterns of spontaniety, restraint, consideration of others and of cooperation with nature. In some cultures, the expected masculine and feminine behavior may be very different for the expression of assertion, achievement, self reliance and compliance. However, behavior and belief are never completely synonymous, so that the nurse should never lose sight of the child's individuality.

Although the nurse may be only marginally conscious of her own cultural background, it nevertheless does give directions for the handling of emotions and for her reactions as well. The *values* within a culture are extremely important as determinants for behavior. Values are those areas of living which have a permeating quality and are of greatest concern to a society. They are things agreed upon as being good, are subjective (located within the person), and although mostly unconscious, have great importance in directing responses to others.

Within our own culture, many values influence our expectations and judgments of ourselves and of others. Some of these may be important in the manner in which we deal with children, such as the value placed on achievement, the importance of work, of "keeping a stiff upper lip," of endurance, fortitude and the control of emotions except under certain circumstances. Unless we become conscious of the values we ourselves hold, we may inadvertently and inappropriately project them onto others in our expectations for their behavior and thus increase anxiety. It is easy to think that the norms of one's own group are right for all people.

The nurse must also be aware of the dangers implicit in stereotyping, or generalizations regarding different people based on insufficient evidence of the individual. Acting on such a generalization can be detrimental to the aims of nursing care. The following brief study illustrates this point.

Running Deer was an American Indian boy of 6 years when he was admitted to a convalescent center for treatment of rheumatoid arthritis. He had formerly lived on an Indian reservation in an isolated, mountainous region with his parents and eight siblings and had never been far from home. He had received little preparation for this hospitalization and initially, although agitated and obviously quite uncomfortable, he was described as "sullen and withdrawn." He tended to be quiet and uncommunicative and complained little, either about pain or of homesickness. However, during this time, he drew many pictures of animals and people in cages and of people hanging from buildings. He was stoical with treatments, exhibiting little discernible anxiety or protest. This behavior was reinforced by some members of the staff, who applauded him as the "brave little Indian," who "kept a stiff upper lip." He had only one obvious source of comfort, a small stuffed elephant he had brought from home and from which he would not be parted.

In addition to his overtly stoical behavior, Running Deer seemed to become more depressed and spoke constantly of his worthless feelings, of being thrown into a garbage can or flushed down the toilet. He spoke of wishing to "kill himself" and of fear of returning home because "he would die" or that "his father might kill him." He often drew pictures of purple mountains under a bright sun. When playing an aggressive marble game, he commented, "Oops, I almost committed suicide. You commit suicide when you don't like yourself." He also spoke frequently about his physical condition, about being "crippled" and of his inability to walk.

Since the distance from home was great, his father was rarely able to visit. When he did, the two sat quietly with arms folded and seldom spoke. Afterwards, Running Deer needed to deny that his father had visited. He did have some relief for his hostility and tension however, in his play. Running Deer became aggressive in this activity, throwing darts, hitting targets and "hunting rabbits."

With frequent visits with a social worker, and with the supportive relationship with a nurse, Running Deer became able to express his anger and aggression directly to people. He became free to weep and began to interact with other children. He no longer spoke of wishing to kill himself or demanded attention from his nurse.

This brief study illustrates several points. Stoicism in the face of pain and distress was valued in the boy's culture as were physical prowess and agility. Conflicts in these areas therefore produced much anxiety and tension. Because of the value placed on control in his society (and in ours), Running Deer was initially restrained from expression of his grief, aggression and hostility at being abandoned by his father with whom he was closely identifying. This hostility became introjected (or taken within himself), resulting in feelings of low self-esteem and self-worth. Reinforcement of the stereotype of the brave Indian was inappropriate in terms of his need, since the emphasis given to this contributed to his inability to experience the natural grief of separation and prevented him from expressing his fear and anger. Although in many cases a child may need support for self-control, acting on a stereotype without further observation may also increase anxiety and worthless feelings because of the child's inability to match this ideal. Running Deer's depression was also deepened because of his self-concept and body image as "crippled" and of his inability to perform those physical feats which were valued by his society as exemplified by his father. He feared his father's rejection because he could not measure up to cultural expectations and values and his behavior gave clues to his anxiety. Such a burden was too much for him to bear; consequently, he "did not like himself" since he felt unable to fulfill these internalized demands.

With understanding and acceptance of his real feelings, Running Deer no longer needed to suppress them and could utilize released energy for reaching out to his environment and for healthy growth. He could express his aggression directly and find relief of his feelings in play. When he returned home, his ego was strengthened to resume the expectations of his society.

Children from homes with cultural expectations differing from our own may have particular difficulty when hospitalized. Many things which we take for granted, such as type of food, language, ways of eating, sleeping and mannerisms, are new and unfamiliar. The hospital environment may be doubly frightening in its strangeness and in its expectations for conformity, and abandonment by parents may be particularly terrifying. Such children need special attention to allow them to communicate their feelings and need particular consideration to discover ways of altering the hospital routine so that they can feel more comfortable. Sometimes special food from home has the dual effect of keeping a tie to parents and of allowing the child to receive foods with which he is more familiar. The importance of support for the child's methods of coping with strangeness and for expressing his anger cannot be overestimated, along with the acceptance and appreciation of his differentness. The nurse must also be aware of her own cultural biases in making judgments about the child's behavior. She can often learn much about a child's background of experience by talking with his parents or reading about the values which are important in his culture.

In working with parents, the nurse must remember that there are also cultural differences as to the value of children and of their role and in beliefs about the value of medical care. She must know that beliefs about illness and treatment are difficult to change by persuasion alone, for beliefs are deep. By demonstrating respect for the parent's values and belief systems, she will support their self-esteem which is necessary before change can be accomplished. The nurse must also respect the rituals which may be practiced in the face of anxiety and uncertainty of outcome in order to relieve tension, for in so doing, she will strengthen the parents in giving emotional aid to their child.

Prolonged hospitalization may cause additional difficulties for the child in identification with his ethnic origins, values and family, and reciprocal distress for his family. The study of Manuel illustrates this point, along with the contrast in his behavior with that of Running Deer, which was partially rooted in the different values within his community of origin.

Manuel, a Spanish-American boy of 8 years had also been frequently hospitalized at the same convalescent center for treatment of rheumatoid arthritis. His early life had been spent with his parents and six siblings in a Mexican community. Although his father was rarely at home, he did insist on the respect of his children and exerted his authority. His mother was often anxious, but loving and spoke Spanish exclusively.

Before his first admission, Manuel was described as cheerful and imaginative although he occasionally exhibited tantrum behavior. With hospitalization, he lost his cheerfulness and demonstrated much aggressive behavior. He displayed anger at the staff with inappropriately morbid and cruel comments. His hostility was expressed with name calling, "making fun" of both adults and children by pointing out their weaker qualities. He remained aloof from peers, though he was greatly competitive with them. He demonstrated resistance to treatments and assumed an extremely aggressive and sadistic attitude, sometimes acting destructively. Unable to relate to others, he became a tyrant, earning the reputation of "the head of the Center Mafia." Because of his behavior, barroom vernacular and disparaging remarks, he was often kept isolated in the hall. This retaliation increased his belligerence and rudeness and he seemed to find satisfaction in seeing others weep.

Yet when a relationship was established with a nurse, Manuel demonstrated his need for understanding, acceptance and affection. Several comments to his nurse were illustrative of his longing for love, though he could not directly ask for care: "Why don't you ever take a boy home? Couldn't you take a boy home for the weekend or longer? If you could take a boy home, would you do it? Would you come here if there were only one boy here?" His feelings about his condition were reflected in such remarks as, "I don't like the word 'crippled.' It's not a nice word. Crippled means you can't walk or walk very good. They're trying to find a cure for arthritis. I won't ever walk—or walk good without limping."

With a relationship of trust, permission and acceptance of his need to express angry feelings, Manuel began to act less destructively to other children on the ward. Permission to have angry feelings was important also to him, for in constant disapproval, his self-esteem was lowered, increasing his frustration and anger. He gained benefits from expressing himself in music and began to improvise musically with a teacher and realize the pure joy of doing a thing for it's own sake. It also gave him a feeling of accomplishment and thereby enhanced his self-esteem.

Because of repeated and lengthy hospitalizations, however, Manuel later had difficulties in readjusting to his family. He had forgotten much of his Spanish and could no longer converse with his mother. This distressed her and contributed to her feelings of loss of control over him. He seemed to reject his Mexican background by refusing to eat Mexican food or to speak Spanish. He often defied his mother and showed his anger by refusing medication or throwing it away. Manuel also suffered from separation from the center to which he had grown accustomed and from the relationships he had formed there.

When Manuel needed to be readmitted, he seemed very uncertain as to who he was, particularly in relation to his ethnic identity, and unsure of what the future held for him in terms of being able to achieve any degree of self-sufficiency. Where originally he had felt a very warm relationship with his family, he now felt isolated from the family group.

Manuel's problems of ethnic identity were also partially the result of weakening identification with his parents brought about by long experiences with a different cultural orientation and values. This illustration underlines the need to find means to sustain a child's tie to his parents and to support his ethnic identity by respect for differing language and customs, by finding ways of keeping these important and viable for him. In addition, Manuel was forced, prematurely by illness and immobilization, to define and identify a future role for himself. His hostility was expressed by oral aggression and stemmed from attempts to make a kind of non-living palatable. There seemed to be little meaning in the future and therefore little meaning to present deprivations.

Manuel's ability to express anger was a strength although his aggression needed to be channeled in order to avoid destructiveness to others. He also needed acceptance of his feelings and permission to express them to feel valued by others and therefore by himself. Manuel had no value inhibitions against such expression of hostility or protest at treatments. Physical aggression was not inhibited in his community of origin; however, value *was* placed on male dominance and on masculinity. Therefore his limitations also caused suffering in terms of his expectations for his future abilities in this direction. Furthermore, in his home community, medical care was sought only in emergencies and hospitals were viewed with suspicion. Manuel therefore had good reason for his distrust, for his fear of what was to happen in the present and for his anxiety for the future.

The Hospitalized Negro Child

The basic reality of color of skin has been an "American dilemma" for the Negro from the time of his earliest interaction with whites. This dilemma has now moved into a stormy present where each member of the majority race can no longer defer facing his own inner convictions and feelings, re-evaluating his assumptions and striving for human understanding. Such understanding is of major importance for the pediatric nurse because of her central importance as the major sources of nurture, comfort and ego support to Negro children when they are vulnerable, under stress and susceptible to lasting psychological damage.

The Negro child who is admitted into a predominantly white, middle class hospital is in a particularly difficult situation. He may perceive this new world as basically hostile, whereas his available coping and defensive strategies may be inadequate to deal with his anxiety. Although in some cases the factor of race may be unimportant in the child's reactions to hospitalization, in other instances it may be an important determining factor in his behavior.

The defenses, ego strength and behavior of the Negro child are partially the product of past experiences within his family and cultural milieu and also a result of encounters with the white race. Many ghetto-bred Negro children may have had a precarious and chaotic early environment because of family mobility, frequent absences of the father, working mother and lack of financial security. They may also have been deprived of the constant warm support, control and guidance necessary for development of firm ego growth. During the period when all children begin to make identification with their parent of the same sex, the Negro boy's efforts at attaining secure sex identity may be troubled, for he is often deprived of a model, or his model may be weak.

In addition, all children at this age must identify with their own racial group. Several studies have demonstrated that children from the age of 3 years perceive differences in skin color and the attendant social role of Negroes and whites. These studies further suggest that by the age of 7, the Negro child can no longer postpone realistic self-identification, although conflict at the very foundation of the ego structure may be precipitated since he must become identified with a race which he has learned often receives discriminatory treatment. With the recent upsurge of racial pride, it is to be hoped that such basic ego conflicts may be reduced in the future.

Many Negro children today, however, may continue to perceive themselves as socially rejected by the prestigious elements of society and thus unworthy of succor and affection. Having no compelling reason for not accepting this officially sanctioned, negative evaluation, they often develop deeply ingrained feelings of inferiority. As they grow older, this sense of inferiority may be intensified by experiences in the wider environment. On school entrance, the lower-class Negro child is often ill prepared to meet the experience successfully. Because of a deprived early environment, he may be intellectually and culturally unready to compete with his classmates. If he fails to learn to read in the first two grades, his negative self-concept is reinforced and the scholastic vicious circle is born which often results in an actual decline of his I.Q. during his school years. Often, because of early experience in assuming adult-like responsibility, precocious separation from the teacher's orbit may occur which is reinforced by his peers. If his parents generally place low value on education, academic achievement may offer little reward, so that loss of ego involvement is accentuated and growth toward ego maturity is retarded. On the other hand, acceptance of traditional American values placed on status and success places him in an untenable position of conflict.

During this time, the child is also building his self-concept through wider situations of social comparison which may reinforce feelings of low self-esteem. From his family, he may learn that white people are dangerous and he must therefore curb displays of aggression, although his experiences have led to resentment of the white race. Although the wish to retaliate may be strong, suppression of hostility and resentment may produce guilt for harboring such feelings along with decreased energy to cope with current problems.

These frustrations during the early years of living may well produce lack of trust in others, which serves to defend against repeated disappointments but also leads to the viewpoint that the world is absolutely hostile. Only a low degree of emotional relatedness is safe in such a world.

The child who has been subjected to prejudice and discrimination is especially vulnerable when ill and hospitalized. Because of his lack of trust, his perception of the hospital and its personnel as harboring aggressive and hostile impulses toward him, his low level of self-esteem and decreased energy available for coping with his experiences, he will need particular care and attention in order to prevent further damage to his developing ego and to support available strengths. Furthermore, in order to deal with the realities of his former life, he may have needed to find mechanisms which defend him against further hurt. Unfortunately, some of these defenses may also retard mastery of the hospitalization experiences. The nurse who is working with a child of any cultural group that is discriminated against must realize that she may be distrusted at first.

Some children may repress their hostility so that it is no longer conscious. Others, by the defense mechanism known as reaction formation, may seem to be exceptionally submissive, compliant, unaggressive and good-natured. Although this may seem welcome, the nurse must not be deceived, for it may be a challenge to her to find ways to really communicate with her patient and to convey her understanding.

Other children may avoid the nurse, withdraw from interaction or isolate themselves from other children on the ward. In doing so, they are communicating their anxiety and distress. On the other hand, some children may respond with aggression and with the hostility they feel, though expression may be indirect and covert. They may give clues to their feelings in behavior which is described as sullen, stubborn or uncommunicative. If the nurse responds with counter-hostility or with rejection, she will lose her opportunity to assist the child to cope with his present difficulties.

The child may also be openly aggressive or demanding, which is his way of testing the nurse's response to him. He may show suspicion and sensitivity and misinterpret her statements as indicative of her prejudice toward him. Although this demands patience, the nurse must find ways for him to express aggression in socially acceptable ways and discover means to give extra attention and consideration, thus communicating that his aggression is acceptable and that he is valued. By careful explanations of hospital routine and of all that is happening and will happen to him, she can help him to feel a sense of control over his environment and thereby decrease his hostility.

The child of a minority group who has learned to defend himself against his hostility by denial will have particular difficulty when in pain. Although most children perceive treatments as hostile, Negro children in particular may view them as aggressive attacks because of their lack of trust and of their perception of the entire environment as basically hostile. A submissive and passive response does not allow for the natural anger which is aroused by a painful treatment, and the energy used for this control is unavailable for more healthy coping and mastery of the experience. In efforts to control fear and rage, the child may quickly lapse into apathy, resignation, withdrawal and depression since he fears that giving vent to his feelings may bring threat of more physical aggression and retaliation. Careful explanations of all steps of a procedure, accompanied by careful listening to determine the meaning the procedure holds for him can be of special benefit. Emotional first aid is particularly important as is encouragement for the mother to be present during particularly stressful procedures. Her presence may provide ego support for the child and counteract some of his fears of the hostile intent of the personnel administering the treatment.

Nurses working with all children of minority groups will want to be introspective regarding their own feelings and attitudes. All children are quickly perceptive to attitudes conveyed in behavior, and children who expect discrimination and have a low level of self-esteem are particularly sensitive to feelings even though the nurse may be unconscious of them.

The nurse can assist such children in other ways. She will need to give thoughtful attention to placement of the child in the ward to provide best available peer support. Liberal visiting hours should be considered to allow frequent contact with the family, which may help to counteract fears of abandonment. Play and occupational therapy can be of particular benefit and careful choice of play equipment can provide socially acceptable outlets for hostility and aggression. Encouragement and approval for productions of the child may increase self-esteem along with the constant demonstration of the nurse's interest.

With awareness of her own feelings, through understanding of the ways the child deals with his problems, and by thoughtful attention toward alleviating unnecessary stress and in support of the child's strengths, the nurse has great opportunities for personal growth and for increasing her effectiveness toward the goals of nursing care.

The Acutely Ill Child

The acutely ill child presents some difficult nursing problems. Often apathetic and too sick to indicate his needs, pain, anxiety and feelings of helplessness inevitably result in regression. If danger is imminent, he and his parents feel it intensely. He must have immediate physical and emotional support because *his survival depends on the energy available to him.* Strength must be communicated to him and even when great haste is paramount to his care, the nurse must remain aware that the child can feel, even though unable to respond overtly. A sensitive little

person who has not yet developed physical or psychological stamina to withstand disease, the child may be desperately ill during the acute phase of an illness. The balance may change quickly.

By learning from his mother his own characteristic way of responding to emotional stress, and those comforts which mean the most to him when he is upset, the nurse receives clues regarding how to help the acutely ill child when he is most threatened. She must be constantly alert to indications of physical distress. Behavioral changes usually precede the point at which the symptom becomes most serious.

The nurse must time her activities, and those of other personnel, so that whenever possible interruption of sleep is prevented. The mother's presence and special items of comfort significant to the child often succeed (where tranquilizers frequently fail) in allowing him to benefit from relaxed sleep.

Many acute illnesses are accompanied by high temperatures which cause irritability, restlessness and loss of sleep. These symptoms impede recovery, and intervention with hydrotherapy or an ice mattress and antipyretic drugs is indicated.

All legitimate measures should be used to reduce the amount of pain a child must endure. In instances where he cannot speak for himself—and this is often the case in acute illness—the nurse must consider the situation from the child's point of view and act on his behalf.

The acutely ill child's lack of appetite or refusal to eat must be accepted and managed so as to encourage cooperation. Appetite loss may result from lessened digestive capacity, or it may be a response to emotional distress. The portions of food should be small, and the child should be fed at shorter intervals and given only those food components which his body requires. Food must look as appealing as possible, and individual likes and dislikes must be considered.

The acutely ill child's need for fluids is urgent; if he is not taking enough to sustain him, fluid and nourishment must be given by gavage or by the intravenous route. Forcing a child to eat probably has more longlasting and damaging psychological effects than the alternatives.

Mothers of seriously ill children are in need of special help. A well-meaning nurse may try to minimize a mother's distress by understating or even denying the seriousness of the illness, but manipulation of the truth gives rise to false hopes and expectations and ultimately undermines the mother's confidence in the staff. It implies a lack of confidence in her ability to care for her child, with the ultimate result of compounding the mother's anxiety. Hospital personnel must recognize the seriousness of the situation and share their concern and understanding with her. Knowing that everything possible is being done, and having an opportunity to talk with someone who can share her burdens will do much to allay her fears, and the child benefits because he will sense her reinforced confidence. *In the care of the acutely ill child, this factor alone may be the decisive one in determining the outcome of the illness.*

The Child with Long-Term Illness and a Poor Prognosis

Working with children in whom the diagnosis carries a grave prognosis is often extremely difficult for the nurse, both personally and professionally. The fact of death has very personal meanings as a factor of prior experience and calls forth deep emotions and feelings which are difficult to face. In addition, the possible or actual death of a patient may imply a professional failure since the profession is dedicated to the prolongation of life. Yet the leaving of life is as important to families as the beginning of it and must be of comparable concern to nurses. In no sphere of nursing are the challenges and opportunities so great, and at no other time are the special skills of the nurse needed more intensely to provide comfort both to the child and to his parents, for both are particularly dependent on the nurse to face the penultimate with them in a knowledgeable and empathic manner.

The inevitability of death has been of great concern to people through the ages and each society has had special ways of dealing with it and prescribed rituals for grieving. In American society, in the Victorian era death was very well known. Nowadays, however, the topic is avoided in every way possible, and is infrequently discussed. The underlying reasons for this difference can be found in the rapid changes in our society and their impact on the value orientations of large segments of our population. The "other-worldliness" and future orientation of our Puritan heritage has given place to emphasis on the present along with a decrease in the dominance of religious concepts as a framework for living. Because of advances in public health measures, death of the young has become more infrequent, although more highly emotionally charged because of the importance of youth and children in our society. In addition, the age of science, although prolonged individual life, has also created a massive new threat to life, that of mass annihilation. The tremendous anxiety raised by such a constant and overwhelming threat to our existence as a nation has required defenses to relieve tensions which are particularly strong.

Such denial and avoidance of the subject of death can also be a protection for the nurse. She has learned the values and attitudes of American culture through her early experiences. In her childhood, her questions may have been met with evasion which implied that this topic should be avoided. She may not have been called upon to face death previous to entering nursing, so that the new and unfamiliar task of providing support when she is herself feeling insecure, sad and drained of energy may be more than she feels capable of undertaking. In addition, the feeling of helplessness to prevent the imminent death of a patient may evoke such a protective measure to relieve the inevitable tension which is aroused.

The child with a poor prognosis, however, is also in a particularly vulnerable position. During the period of socialization, he has also learned through many small encounters that the topic of death and dying is surrounded by a special aura of anxiety. The child, highly valued in our society, has a particular role and must fulfill certain demands of his parents and of his wider environment. From infancy onward, particularly if the child is a boy, he is imbued with the value of mature behavior. It is not considered "manly" to weep and he has heard injunctions to "be a big boy" and to "act his age." This pressure for adult behavior is accompanied by perpetual optimism and hopefulness. Pain and death are given only marginal status in our society. From these many encounters, the child has learned to conform to our cultural norms and to avoid complaints of fear and hopelessness. Perception of those complaints communicated by children are also distorted by adults who receive them in terms of values which have become a firm part of adult personality.

Other of our cultural values accentuate that the child must be self-fulfilling, reach his potential and fulfill the unmet expectancies of his parents. For adults to admit that death will prevent an optimistic future is to admit in various ways that the purpose of life, that of self-fulfillment, is faulty. To the child then, dying and the accompanying fear of death may give him a sense of actually failing his parents. Since all of these cultural attitudes are unconsciously transmitted to the child, both by his parents and by the larger society, the child himself is also inhibited in free expression of concern about death.

During hospitalization, the child with a poor prognosis is extremely sensitive to further reinforcement of our cultural taboo against speaking openly about fears and concerns related to death and dying. Because of the emotional and spatial closeness of the nurse to the hospitalized child, she is a key person in the altered circumstances of his life and has a unique opportunity to give emotional support. On the other hand, since she is also seen as an authority figure by the child, the possibilities are also great for transmitting expectations for "mature" behavior. Therefore, if it is necessary for the nurse to protect herself strongly from reaching empathically to the dying child, the latter's sensitive perceptiveness to the nurse's unconscious communication will prevent him from communicating his possible need for information and comfort to face the unknown.

The Child's Concept of Death. The nurse who is working with children who have been ill for a long time and are old enough to be concerned with the future, may assume that many are anxious about why they have not "gotten well." Many have had some experience with death and may be deeply troubled. The nurse who is engaged in supporting children must have knowledge in addition to compassion and skill in understanding and interpreting verbal and nonverbal clues to the child's fears.

The child's time perspective, logic and reasoning ability change throughout childhood and his current perception of the concept of death may be germane to the focus of his fears. The meaning which the concept holds for him is important in determining his perception of reality. The nurse who is knowledgeable regarding the timing of the dawning realization of cessation of life and of the various possible intrepretations of the concept of death will be in a better position to help the child to whom such personal meanings are of immediate importance.

The mature concept of death is built slowly throughout childhood, both as a result of experiences and as a function of expanding intellectual awareness. The construction of reality is accomplished step by step and concepts of cessation of life are not intelligible to the very young child because his inner mental structures are not sufficiently flexible. The toddler is usually not concerned about death, since he must have reached the "why" stage before there is awareness of function, and therefore of cessation of life. Piaget, in his investigations of mental growth, concluded that in the earliest years, the child presupposes a "maker" such as God or his parents. He is first puzzled by the problem of death; death is inexplicable and a mysterious phenomenon since anything that happens is wished so, by himself or by his parents.

The child's first experience with death (usually of an insect, bird or animal) leads him to equate death with (1) separation, departure or disappearance, (2) sleep and (3) going into a grave, coffin, earth or water. In this first stage, the child may imagine himself to be alive and conscious even in death, and the most painful thing is the separation itself. Usually until after the age of 3 years, death is a mysterious absence and is incomprehensible. The earliest experience with the death of animals may give an early connotation of destruction or violence, or of cessation of life as the result of aggression. The child under 5 years may also have a sense of reversibility around the concept of death, since the separated do return, and since he is unable to comprehend or accept such a reality. There may also be a sense of magic surrounding the concept, and children often believe that the dead are born again.

Children of preschool age think about death more than most adults are willing to admit. The fear of death may begin as early as 3 years as a result of beginning activity of the conscience and guilt formed through the socialization process. Most researchers place the beginning of the fear of death as a realistic problem between the ages of 4 and 6 years in most instances. The first acquaintance with death is crucial to the child since he is exposed for the first time to attitudes toward death of the significant adults around him and his later reactions stem from values of life and death communicated to him at this time.

During the early school years, the child can no longer deny the reality of death but may conceptualize it as gradual or temporary. The distinction between life and death is not complete and while they acknowledge that death exists, they are still unable to accept it as an incontrovertible fact. The quality of time is also still not completely appreciated and therefore the completeness of death may be distorted.

After the age of 8 or 9 years, when the child has a more complete conception of time, number and logic, he begins to realize that his parents are not omnipotent, are powerless to avert death, and that ultimately everyone will die. With an association between the concepts of death, number and age, magical practices may arise in order to alleviate anxiety about death. In the following years, the concept is elaborated with many religious and cultural meanings, and the adult concept of death is reached at approximately 11 to 13 years of age.

Whereas the healthy adolescent lives intensely in the present and personal death is relegated to the distant future which is indefinitely and negatively structured, the adolescent who is chronically ill may be intensely preoccupied with death. Although it is difficult in many cases for adults to accept, this is also often true of much younger children when they are hospitalized, in pain and chronically or terminally ill.

Death Anxiety in Children with Fatal Illness. Although there have been few studies investigating the fears and concerns of children with a poor prognosis on any level, there has been much speculation about this fateful clinical circumstance in the lives of many children. Since specific data have been seriously lacking, professional personnel have been forced to rely on personal and intuitive conclusions and convictions in helping such children face the conclusion of their lives with as much support and comfort as has been possible for nurses and physicians to provide. Despite the tragic and difficult personal and professional meanings involved in ministering to a child and to his parents who are entering such an ultimate experience, the nurse must have knowledge on which to base effective nursing intervention.

Observation of children with a poor prognosis reveals that although few have been given information regarding their illness or prognosis, yet they do indicate fear and anxiety in apathy, depression and withdrawal from their peers and from adults. Available data indicate that such children are much more concerned than adults have been able to see or are willing to admit. Even with children 4 years of age, Bozeman reported that they were "extraordinarily quiet, sometimes apathetic, either alone or in groups, despite the extensive equipment and staff dedicated to their amusement."* Solnit has also reported that in his experience the question of survival has been raised by children of this age.†

Most parents of young children who are fatally ill do not wish their child to be informed as to the nature of his illness and attempt to shield him from this tragic reality and from ever hearing the word "cancer" or "leukemia." Most professional personnel have also assumed an optimistic demeanor of encouraging reassurance and have believed that young children cannot know of their impending death or use denial extensively as a defense against this overwhelming threat.

The entire emotional environment of the child, however, has been drastically altered after such a diagnosis is made. Often the effectiveness of denial for minimizing fear and anxiety may not be complete, since the child is extremely perceptive to altered emotional climates within his home and to the false cheerfulness or evasiveness of those around him. Hackett and Weisman found that the effectiveness of denial was greatly reduced in adult cancer patients where legitimate hope was not present in those caring for the patient.‡ A general apprehensiveness as to the nature of the threat in the interior of his body may not be manifested overtly by the child and fear of death may not be openly expressed. Overt expression of fear of death may be threatening to the child in that he may risk loss of human contact. As previously mentioned, a premium has been placed in our culture on the inhibition of such fear and a frightened child is threatening to adults in that he may present an insoluble problem.

The fear of death from inside the body may be denied and displaced to threat from without. Thus the inner sphere may be changed to an outer sphere of threat so that the environment itself appears to be menacing. Fear of separation or loneliness and fear of mutilation, intrusive procedures and pain may substitute for an underlying general apprehensiveness about survival. Death is the ultimate in loneliness and children may feel most alone in the psychological sense when they feel their parents and the adults around them, on whom they must depend, are keeping something from them. Loneliness may stem from the sense of not being understood. Fear of intrusive procedures may mask an inner threat. These fears and

others may be an outcropping, or objective way of expressing an underlying anxiety. Thus reliance on overt expression of death anxiety may give an incomplete and distorted picture of the actual concerns of the seriously ill child.

Although Knudson and Natterson and Morrissey have reported that children with a poor prognosis are minimally concerned with their own impending death until after the age of 10 years, recent research by Waechter does not support this conclusion. She recently concluded an investigation of death anxiety in children with fatal illness, the variables which affect the amount and quality of expressed anxiety and some dimensions of parental response to the illness. The study was carried out with three groups of hospitalized children (16 children in each group) between the ages of 6 and 10 years of age, with fatal, chronic and brief illness and with a fourth group of normal, well children. These children were matched by age, sex and family background.

A maternal interview elicited information as to the child's previous and current experiences in the home situation and two measures were utilized to measure anxiety expressed by the child. The General Anxiety Scale for Children developed by Sarason and his associates measured expressed anxiety in many areas of living, whereas a projective test, a modification of the Thematic Apperception Test in which stories were requested to eight pictures, measured anxiety specific to current and future body integrity.

The results of the administration of the anxiety scale indicated that children with fatal illness demonstrated significantly greater anxiety than did the other hospitalized groups. The total scores on the projective test also demonstrated that the children with fatal illness expressed significantly more anxiety related to death than did all other children tested.

The children with fatal illness told many more stories containing references to death and loneliness. Their stories also contained a significantly greater number of references to negative affect (fear, sadness, etc.), and more of their stories ended with the death of the main character.

One of the most significant of the findings indicated that children who had had an opportunity to discuss their illness, diagnosis and prognosis expressed less anxiety than did the other children with fatal illness who had not had such an opportunity (correlation = .633, p = .01).

These findings suggest that contrary to the supposition that children below the age of 10 years who have a poor prognosis are not concerned with impending death, these children, although not directly informed as to the nature of their illness, did indicate considerable preoccupation with death in fantasy, feelings of loneliness and isolation. They also suggested a sense of lack of control of the forces impinging on them, along with a sense of incapacity to affect the

* Bozeman, M., Arbach, C., and Sutherland, A.: The adaptation of mothers to the threatened loss of their children through leukemia, Part I, Cancer 8:1, 1955.

† Solnit, A. J., and Green, A.: The pediatric management of the dying child. Part II: The child's reaction to the fear of dying, *in* Solnit, A., and Provence, S. (Eds.): Modern Perspectives in Child Development, New York, pp. 217-228, Internat. Univ. Press. 1963.

‡ Hackett, T., and Weisman, A.: Reactions to the imminence of death, *in* Grosser, G., Wechsler, H., and Greenblatt, M., (Eds.) The Threat of Impending Diaster, Cambridge, Mass., MIT Press, 1964.

inner and outer environment. There was also a great dichotomy seen between the parent's perception of the child's awareness of his prognosis and anxiety surrounding the concept of death expressed by the child. This finding suggests that children *do* perceive the threat through the altered affect in their total environment and from the parent's anxiety communicated in non-verbal ways. It also suggests that adults were perhaps blinded to the child's anxiety because of their own fears and concerns and sense of helplessness related to the diagnosis.

In this sphere too, however, large differences can be seen in the anxiety expressed by individual children and in their methods of coping with it. Children with fatal illness vary greatly in the type of experiences related to treatment, length of time since diagnosis and in their parents' response to the illness. Children with a poor prognosis who are anticipating a major surgical procedure may be acutely anxious in that such surgery is life-threatening in itself. Any surgical process may carry an inherent threat of death. On the other hand, some children with such a prognosis may see minor surgery as therapeutic and anxiety relieving.

Children facing a threat to life may also have other differences in experiences which alter their response to their illness. It is possible that children who have had previous encounters with death in their immediate family circle may show greater concern if they were unsupported through that experience. Children who have had a warm relationship with their parents may also differ in response to their illness from those who have had lesser degrees of warm family support. Although the degree of security gained from a positive relationship with their parents may not reduce specific anxiety related to the possibility of imminent death, it can affect more generalized anxiety in the direction of greater feelings of security relative to the environment in general. The security and faith conveyed to children through religious beliefs can also assist them by supporting their methods of coping with this threat of cessation of life.

Working with patients who are facing death has a heightened significance for pediatric nurses because of the additional poignancy connected with death of the very young. There is a greater sense of loss in that the child will never have the opportunities which we associate with life. The pain of close contact with a child who cannot get well is difficult, and so it seems more comfortable to avoid forming a relationship that can only end in painful separation. Yet such avoidance can result only in utter loneliness for the child at the very time he most needs closeness, and psychological isolation can only lead to heightened anxiety.

To give effective help, however, nurses must also have had experiences which give them a sense of capability and security in working closely with dying children. This sense of competency and empathy can be fostered in the nurse and extended through educational experiences and through thoughtful and organized efforts toward supporting them during and following encounters with death on pediatric wards. Students can gain understanding and support through sharing their experiences with their supervisors and other professional personnel who can be made available to them. If the nurse is able to give of herself to parents and children during such a fateful circumstance, and is supported in her efforts, she will have grown tremendously, both personally and professionally and will have gained the sense of security, empathy and competency which will enable her to meet future experiences with greater equanimity.

Nurses can also keep such children in contact with their peers on the ward as long as they have the energy to profit from the companionship of group experience and from the comfort of individual friendships. Placement on the ward can be an important and effective method for decreasing feelings of isolation.

Efforts designed toward relieving loneliness in children with a poor prognosis may also reduce some of the anger they feel, both in terms of the diagnosis and because "nobody cares." If such anger is internalized, it can result in submission and a sense of hopelessness. Although difficult for the nurse, if she can accept expressions of anger and hostility, they will also prevent repression which further decreases the child's available energy. On the other hand, extreme permissiveness of unacceptable behavior may communicate the nurse's feelings of hopelessness and abandonment.

One of the greatest concerns of the nurse working with fatally ill children is related to effective methods of dealing with the child's questions about his illness. In no other medical circumstance is it so imperative for all professional personnel who are concerned with the child and his parents to communicate feelings, observations and information and cooperatively and continually to plan and evaluate all efforts designed to give emotional and physical support to the child and his parents. In arriving at an individual plan, the wishes of the parents must be respected and the team leadership of the physician responsible for the child's medical care must be supported.

The nurse, however, is an important member of the team and can contribute of her knowledge and of her perceptive observation as to the child's needs as reflected in his behavior. She can evaluate the state of the child's awareness which has been communicated to him through the change in affect which he has encountered. If the child expresses anxiety because his questions have been met with evasiveness, hesitation or embarrassment in those close to him, she may have observed a deepening of the sense of isolation.

Whether to tell or not to tell a child that he has a fatal illness appears to be a meaningless question.

Rather, it seems clear that questions and concerns which are conscious to the child should be dealt with in such a way that the child does not feel further isolated and alienated from his parents and other meaningful adults by a curtain of silence around his most intense fears. "Protection" of the child may result in an aura of secrecy, which in addition to loneliness may arouse hostility, thus increasing the child's burden. Understanding acceptance of the child's fears and conveyance of permission to discuss any aspect of his illness may decrease these feelings of isolation, alienation and the sense that his illness is too terrible to discuss.

In conveying permissiveness to the child for discussion of his concerns, an opportunity is also available to understand and clarify some of the misconceptions the child may hold which can be more fearful than the fact of death itself. Since young children's concepts of death are not complete and because their sense of causality and reasoning are not mature, they may come to frightening convictions related to guilt for past misdeeds, punishment and rejection by their parents or fantasies as to what they will be called upon to bear. Such anxiety-producing and fearful convictions and expectations consume energy and further deplete resources necessary for maintaining important relationships.

Working with Parents of Fatally Ill Children. Assisting parents who are faced with the imminent loss of their child is also a difficult challenge for the nurse, for the threatened or actual loss of a child is one of the most shattering and tragic of experiences. How this contingency is met depends upon the circumstances of the child's illness and the resources of the parents, both personal and environmental. The previous integration of the personality of parents and the closeness of the family circle is clearly reflected during this severe emotional stress.

There is a general consistency in the results of studies related to the observable reactions of parents to the threatened loss of a child with a chronic fatal disease. Following the diagnosis, many parents feel "shocked" or "stunned." Many are unable to hear the fatal implications of the diagnosis or exclude it from consciousness. They may behave in a disbelieving manner, as though the news had not been assimilated. Many mothers report the initial reaction in terms of physical injury to themselves; i.e., "it was a blow in the face."

The manner in which the diagnosis is imparted to parents is of vital importance in determining later attitudes to hospital personnel. If the parents are informed in an abrupt manner or in a way which eliminates any hope, extreme hostility can be aroused which later may be reactivated on any pretext, either realistic or through distortion. Despite all efforts toward gentleness in imparting the tragic news, however, some anger can be expected as a result of parental defenses.

Most parents are usually eager for immediate hospitalization of their child in a frantic attempt to reverse the diagnosis and for immediate treatment which may save the child. For the mother this initial hospitalization is fraught with severe separation anxiety which is communicated to the child and which is related to the threat of permanent separation.

Initially most mothers need to deny the implications of the diagnosis, either by screening the massive threat from their awareness or by extreme efforts to reverse it. This usually does not extend to the fact of the child's illness and many parents feel the need for additional consultations and diagnostic procedures from other physicians of their acquaintance. When the diagnosis is verified both hostility and continued denial, along with a lack of affect, are intensified.

After treatment is instituted and the reality of the situation is acknowledged, most parents feel guilt expressed through such questions as, "What could have caused it?" or "Why did this have to happen?" They often blame themselves for not having recognized early symptoms of the disease, for not appreciating the child to a greater extent before his illness, for failure to protect the child or for some previous wrongdoing or omission on their part. Some may feel and express that they are being punished by divine providence for former sins.

Many parents also need to learn as much as they can about the disease by wide reading or questioning medical staff in the hope of finding some contingency which will prove their child to be an exception to the general rule. Although hope is expressed, it is generally not related to any specific aspect of treatment.

During this time the mother needs to be physically close to her child as much as possible in order to begin to cope with the anxiety of separation and with the guilt she may feel related to the diagnosis. If the child is hospitalized, the mother may feel hostility toward nurses who assume her maternal functions and interrupt her need to give of herself to her child. Anticipatory grief is almost universal and has the function of beginning the emotional separation from the child which is necessary to bear the pain. Although intellectually, parents may no longer expect a cure for the disease to be found in time to save their child, yet they need to continue to hope and are eager for new treatments and efforts designed to prolong life.

As the length of time since diagnosis increases and the disease is seen to progress, most parents experience an increase of anticipatory grief including a preoccupation with thoughts of the ill child, depression, weeping and somatic symptoms including apathy and weakness. This "grief work" is necessary for parents in order to prepare them for final separation. Most parents need to search for an acceptable meaning for this tragic occurrence.

Time seems to stand still for parents during such chronic stress and they call upon all defensive mechanisms and coping strategies available. Former relationships are often found helpful in providing tangible services, to give temporary escape and relief from the awareness of what is to come and for emotional support. Emotional comfort can also be derived from association with parents of other children with the same diagnosis.

The relationship which can be of main support is the marriage itself. The degree to which the partners derive strength and emotional comfort from each other is dependent on the length and stability of the marriage and of the ego capacities of the individuals concerned. Such a shared tragic situation can draw the parents closer together, but this is not always true. Occasionally the father may feel neglected through the excessive amounts of time his wife needs to spend with their child. In such a circumstance, the anxiety of both parents is increased, for the father also feels guilty for harboring such feelings and the comfort to be derived from the marriage relationship is also lessened for both.

The support or additional anxiety which results if there are other children in the home can also be a factor in parental response. Some parents can find comfort in the fact that they will still have a child or children remaining after the death of the ill child and may draw closer to them. However, others may resent the fact that the child who is ill has been singled out for such tragedy or feel additional stress in the necessity of informing them of their sibling's disease and of bearing ensuing grief. If the child is at home during much of his illness, problems in discipline can arise which compound anxiety and feelings of guilt for the entire family.

Many parents may also find great emotional support in religious beliefs from which they derive courage, meaning and faith in the "rightness" of future events, whether for a positive or negative outcome. Religious observances, the ministrations of priest, rabbi, or minister and the prayers of others can convey to parents the sense that their sorrow is shared, that others also care and have faith in their ability to bear their pain.

As the length of time since the diagnosis was made increases, many parents may wish to become involved in the care of other ill children and the intense clinging to their own child may be somewhat lessened as a result of the emotional separation accomplished by the former anticipatory grief work. The parental response to the ultimate death of the child is dependent on the available support and the length of time since the diagnosis was made. If this time is an extended period, the actual death of the child may well be experienced as an anticipated loss at the end of a long sequence of events. The parental response is also related to the psychological significance the child held for his parents, his age and sex, his place in the family circle,

the physical energy available to the parents and other factors previously discussed.

The nurse can be of great assistance to parents through this tragic period of their lives. She can facilitate the mother's presence at her child's bedside whenever possible and thus prevent much misery. Depriving the mother and child of each other when permanent separation is soon to take place is particularly reprehensible. She can avoid assuming details of the child's care which the mother can perform and thus help parents to feel that their value as *parents* is continued despite an overwhelming sense of helplessness. The giving of physical care to the child also facilitates the sense that they are doing everything possible to help him.

On the other hand, during the latter stages of the illness, some mothers do not feel able to assume care and disapproval from others can only heighten their anxiety. Some mothers may feel the need to escape from this tremendous stress or feel incapable of entering their child's room. A non-judgmental attitude and understanding on the part of the nurse if the mother does "run away" can give the additional needed support for her to approach the child physically and emotionally. In this instance, the nurse may also need to help the child to understand the absence of his parents and to provide substitute comfort.

Parents also need to have as much daily information about their child's progress as it is possible for them to understand and to assimilate. Although reports of physical progress are in the medical realm, the nurse can help to keep parents in touch with their physician. She can also discuss with parents the details of the child's day and his activities on the ward while they are absent, for such details can be of tremendous significance to parents anticipating the death of their child.

Many parents may feel a great need to talk about their child or feel heightened anxiety when alone. *Taking time to listen to parents is an important aspect of nursing care.* It further serves to convey to parents that the child is appreciated and understood as an individual, that the nurse who is involved in important and intimate physical and emotional care of their child is aware of his uniqueness as a valued individual and of his great importance to his parents. It has further value for the nurse in that such discussions can provide clues to enhance her understanding of her patient and of his behavior and thus contribute to the effectiveness of her nursing intervention.

In such discussions with parents, the nurse may need to accept hostility directed toward herself, the institution or other medical personnel without retaliating and with understanding of the source of the parent's anger. In most instances, the hostility is not directed toward her personally, but is a result of the total overwhelming circumstances, a displacement of anger, or projection of guilt of which the parents may not be conscious. In other instances, the parent's anger may be justified and give the nurse valuable clues as to how she can assist them and thus indirectly to how she can support their relationship with their child. Although it may seem initially comforting to the nurse, she must also avoid giving reassurances about the survival of the child or premature reassurance to parental feelings of guilt about the illness. Such reassurances may only convey the sense of not being understood and may thereby intensify feelings of hostility.

Nurses can also be supportive to parents by helping them to keep in touch with hospital chaplains, their personal priests or ministers, parents of other children ill with the same disease, or other professional personnel such as social workers or counsellors who can assist them in coping with this experience. In doing so however, nurses should continue the support which only they can give throughout the child's hospitalization.

When the elapsed time since diagnosis has been extensive and hospitalizations have been repetitive, many parents may express the wish to be helpful to other children on the ward. Nurses can make these efforts possible for them, thus supporting parents in their desire to be of assistance to all children. Nurses may also need to understand such changes in parental behavior, and avoid judgmental implications of lesser degrees of parental devotion to their own fatally ill child.

At the time of actual bereavement, all parents need consideration, empathy and emotional support. This is also a time which is very difficult for the nurse who has come to feel for and with her patient. It is natural for the nurse to feel grief at the death of a valued patient, and it is not "unprofessional" to allow the parents to see that she also feels the loss of the relationship. It is to be expected that she will also welcome the emotional support which can be given by her coworkers and supervisor. Yet in order to be supportive to parents, she must not withdraw into her own grief, for this is a time when they greatly need the strength and empathy which she can offer to them. Much of the helping person's strength is in his ability to experience some of the pain of the tragic situation without being overcome by it.

At this time, the parents need privacy and the opportunity to express emotion in their own way. The nurse will need to accept the expressions of sorrow, the sense of loss and the expressions of guilt which may be reactivated at this time. She may also need to accept expressions of disbelief and anger, and indicate a respect for the cultural, religious and social customs of grieving.

The nurse also needs to know that the parents' need to grieve and to weep is important and constructive in assisting them to assimilate the loss that they have sustained. If this is delayed by the need to maintain the morale of others, grief may reappear later with a new bereavement or occurrence which recalls the loss. The nurse can be helpful by her manner of permissiveness and acceptance, by her own support and through facilitating the presence of others who have had a helping relationship with the parents.

SITUATIONS FOR FURTHER STUDY

1. Select a child under 3 years of age who is being admitted to the hospital for a short stay. Observe him daily from the time of admission to the time he has re-adapted to life at home and record what you see, hear, feel and think about. Use the questions which follow to guide you in the study of the child:

A. Describe the behavior of your patient and his mother when you first observed them. How did his mother handle herself in the situation? Do you think it was a stressful one? What makes you think so? What signs of anxiety did the child manifest? How did he handle his anxiety? How did his mother function with him? Describe what you observed about their relationship. How did the mother respond to leaving her child in the ward? Include also how you interacted with the mother and child to further their adjustment to a new situation.

B. What is the child's background of experience within his family?

C. After you have told the child how you will function in his care, sit beside him and observe what he does. How did he respond to you? What were the first things he did after you interpreted your role? How long did it take him to approach you? Describe how he used you during the time you were with him? Do you think that you learned more about him by waiting for him to approach you? What makes you think so? How do you suppose he felt about being in the hospital?

D. What is this child's health problem? What physical support does he require at this stage of his illness? How did you determine his requirements? Describe as much of your interaction with him as you can remember.

E. With what core problem is the child of his age struggling?

F. How does his behavior differ from that observed in a healthy child of his age? What do you think influenced these differences? What are his personality strengths and limitations? What behavior did you observe which helped you to identify his particular needs for emotional support?

G. Using the knowledge that you gained from the above observational study, construct a plan for his care. Include your goals in nursing care.

H. Implement your plan and observe the child's response to it. When physical and behavioral changes occur, record these and indicate the way in which you modified your original plan of care and the reasons why you did so. Include the changes in behavior that occur in relation to you, to treatments, play materials and to activity and indicate the ways in which you think your nursing care has influenced them.

I. Describe the changes that take place in his relationship to his mother and father from day to day. How did you work to help the child to maintain his emotional tie to his mother?

J. At the time of discharge, think through the child's experience and answer the following questions: Was the child's adjustment to the hospital constructive or nonconstructive? On what do you base your conclusions?

K. Visit the child's home after discharge. Use the following questions to guide your study in the home: How did the child and the mother respond to you as a visitor in the home? Describe their behavior toward you. How did the child react on returning home? What changes in behavior did his mother observe? What do you think caused these changes in behavior? How do you think they are influencing the mother-child relationship? How did the mother react to the changes in the behavior that she observed? What did she say and do that indicated her feelings about his behavior?

2. What are the different ways in which parents manifest anxiety? Discuss two of the parents you have observed and describe the behavior that you felt stemmed from anxiety?

3. What are the different ways in which children manifest anxiety?

4. Describe a child under stress whom you cared for. How did he show that he was under stress? How did he cope with it? What did you do to relieve his distress? What results did you have in working with him? How did you evaluate your nursing care?

5. Describe a mother under stress. How did she manifest it? How was she coping with it? What did you do to relieve her anxiety? Discuss your results and cite the way in which you evaluated the help you provided?

6. Orient a newly admitted child to the ward and describe the ways in which he responded to you and to the things he saw. Was he anxious? If so, how did he handle it?

7. Read James Robertson's book (listed in the bibliography) and use the questions which follow to prepare for class discussion: How did reading the book increase your insight into parents' reactions to hospitalization of their child? How has it increased your powers of observation of parents? In what ways did it help you to become more responsive to the needs of parents and children? In what ways did it influence your thinking about visiting hours? Discuss the pros and cons of unrestricted visiting hours? In what ways did it affect your thinking about rooming-in for mothers of young hospitalized children?

8. Do you agree that children should be prepared for treatments? Support your decision with the reasons why you agree or disagree.

9. Describe a situation in which you prepared and supported a child during a painful treatment. Include in your description the method you used and the child's response to it. What criteria did you use in evaluating your work with the child?

10. Prepare a child for operation. Describe your approach, your technic and the child's responses to it. Accompany the child to the operating room and describe his behavior under stress. What elements of support did you use? How did he respond to you, to his parents and to treatment in the immediate postoperative period?

11. Of what value is an activity program in a pediatric ward?

12. Observe one of your patients at play. Describe what you saw, heard and felt. Of what value was this play to him? Was he anxious during play or relaxed and spontaneous? From what observations did you draw your conclusion? What problems did you meet in curtailing your impulse to direct his play? Did you see or hear anything which gave you clues to the meaning which hospitalization and illness had for him? Did this observation period cause you to make a change in your plan of care?

13. To study children and the usefulness of a group meal period, place the ambulatory children at tables for lunch. Group them according to age and eat with them. The questions which follow can be used to guide observation during the meal period: What contributed toward making the meal period successful or unsuccessful? Of what did premeal preparation consist? Did it contribute to the success of the meal period? Describe situations encountered and discuss ways of handling them. Which foods were eaten most readily? Which ones were refused consistently? What comments were made when children were served small servings of food that they disliked? When comments were made, what was your response? How did your servings to individual children vary? What influenced variations in serving? Did the placement of a good eater next to a poor eater bring a change in the acceptance of food by the latter? Was this meal period more successful than the ones served in the traditional tray service style? Why do you think so?

14. Observe a child with poor food habits. Does his physical condition influence his disinterest in food? What is his response when no attention is paid to his unfinished plate of food? What is his response to minute servings of all food except that which you know he particularly relishes? Does he enjoy pouring his own milk and helping himself to "seconds"? Does he eat and drink more when he is given an opportunity to increase his independence? Observe the child when his parents are with him. Do you think their relationship with him influenced the development of his poor

food habits? Talk to the mother to determine her methods of management of meal hours during the period before he entered the hospital. If his food habits improve during the period of hospitalization, what responsibility would you have toward the child and his parents? What would be your approach to the mother? How would you counsel her?

15. What other ways can you think of which might have proved to be more valuable for Jim while he was awaiting a craniotomy?

16. Select a child from another culture, or a culturally deprived child who is being admitted to the hospital. Follow the sequence of questions described in Situation No. 1. In addition, how do you feel that his home experiences influenced his behavior in the hospital? What changes did you make in the usual hospital routine to accommodate for cultural differences? What situations did you feel were particularly stressful? How did the parents respond to the child's hospitalization? What difficulties did you find in caring for the child personally and professionally?

17. What influence do you think hospitalization exerts on intellectual development? How does the level of intellectual development influence responses to hospitalization? How can you support healthy intellectual growth?

18. What changes have occurred in our culture related to death and grieving? What influences in our society have affected these changes? In what ways are such attitudes transmitted to children? How do you feel that they may influence the behavior of a child who is hospitalized with a fatal illness? How do you feel these attitudes may affect the behavior of the professional staff? Do you feel that the behavior of the professional staff affects the level of the child's anxiety? In what ways?

BIBLIOGRAPHY

Alexander, E. E., and Alderstein, A. M.: Studies in the Psychology of Death, in David, H. P., and Brengleman, J. C. (Eds.), Perspectives in Personality Research, New York, Springer, 1960.

Appley, M., and Trumbull, R.: Psychological Stress, N. Y., Appleton, 1967.

Berkowitz, P., and Berkowitz, N.: The Jewish patient in the hospital, Amer. J. Nurs. 67:2335, 1967.

Blake, F.: In quest of hope and autonomy, Nurs. Forum 1:8, 1961.

Bonine, G. N.: Student's reactions to children's deaths, Amer. J. Nurs. 67:1439, 1967.

Bozeman, M., Arbach, C., and Sutherland, A.: The adaptation of mothers to the threatened loss of their children through leukemia, part I, Cancer 8:1, 1955.

Bright, F., and France, Sister M. L.: The nurse and the terminally ill child, Nurs. Outlook 15:39, 1967.

Clark, K., and Clark, M.: Emotional Factors in Racial Identification and Preference in Negro Children, in Grossack, M. M. (Ed.), Mental Health and Segregation, New York, Skinner, 1963.

Cobb, B.: Psychological impact of long term illness and death on the family circle, J. Pediat. 49:746, 1956.

Deutsch, M., Katz, I., and Jensen, A. (Eds.): Social Class, Race, and Psychological Development, New York, Holt, Rinehart & Winston, 1968.

Erickson, Eric: Youth and the life cycle, Children 7:43, 1960.

Erickson, Florence: Play Interviews for Four-Year-Old Hospitalized Children (Monograph), Yellow Springs, Ohio, Antioch Press, 1958.

Erikson, Eric: Childhood and Society, N. Y., Norton, 1963.

Feifel, H.: Death in Farberow, N. (Ed.), Taboo Topics, New York, Atherton, 1963.

Folta, J. R.: The perception of death, Nursing Research 14:232, 1965.

Freud, Anna: The Ego and the Mechanisms of Defense, N. Y., Internat. Univ. Press, 1946.

Friedman, S. B., et al.: Behavioral observation in parents anticipating the death of a child, Pediatrics 32:610, 1963.

Galiardi, D., and Miles, M. S.: Interactions between two mothers of children suffering from incurable cancer, Nurs. Clin. of N. Amer. 4:89, 1969.

Geist, H.: A Child Goes to the Hospital: The Psychological Aspects of a Child Going to the Hospital, Springfield, Ill., Charles C Thomas, 1965.

Gorer, Geoffrey: The Pornography of Death in Stein, M., Vidich, A., and White, D. (Eds.), Identity and Anxiety, Glencoe, Ill., Free Press, 1960.

Grantley, W., and Bernasconi, M.: The concept of death in children, J. Genet. Psychol. 110:71, 1967.

Grosser, C., Wechsler, N., and Greenblatt, M. (Eds.): The Threat of Impending Disaster, Cambridge, Mass., M.I.T. Press, 1964.

Haan, N.: Proposed Model of Ego Functioning, Psychological Monographs, 1963, 77, Whole No. 571.

Hackett, T., and Weisman, A.: Reactions to the Imminence of Death, in Grosser, G., Wechsler, H., and Greenblatt, M. (Eds.), The Threat of Impending Disaster, Cambridge, Mass., M.I.T. Press, 1964.

Haller, J. A., Jr., Talbert, J. L., and Dembro, R. H. (Eds.): The Hospitalized Child and His Family, Baltimore, Johns Hopkins Press, 1967.

Hall, C. S.: A Primer of Freudian Psychology, N. Y., The New American Library of World Literature, Inc., 1954.

Henderson, V.: The nature of nursing, Am. J. Nurs. 64:63, 1964.

Hunt, E. P.: Recent Demographic Trends and Their Effects on Maternal and Child Health Needs and Services, U. S. Dept. of Health, Education and Welfare, Welfare Administration, Children's Bureau, 1966 (Pamphlet).

Hunt, J. McV.: Intelligence and Experience, N. Y., Ronald, 1961.

Hymovich, D. P.: ABC's of pediatric safety, Am. J. Nurs. 66:1768, 1966.

Johnson, D.: A philosophy of nursing, Nurs. Outlook 7:198, 1959.

————: The nature of a science of nursing, Nurs. Outlook 7:291, 1959.

King, J. A.: Parameters relevant to determining the effect of early experience upon adult behavior of animals, Psychol. Bull. 55:46, 1958.

Kneial, C. R.: Thoughtful care for the dying, Am. J. Nurs. 68:550, 1968.

Kubzansky, P., and Leiderman, P. H.: Sensory Deprivation, *in* Solomon, P. (Ed.), Sensory Deprivation, Cambridge, Mass., Harvard, 1961.

Lazarus, R. S.: Psychological Stress and the Coping Process, New York, McGraw-Hill, 1966.

Lindeman, E.: Symptomatology and management of acute grief, Am. J. Psychiat. *101*:144, 1944.

Mahaffy, P. R.: Admission interviews with parents, Am. J. Nurs. *66*:506, 1966.

McCain, R. F.: Nursing by assessment—not intuition, Am. J. Nurs. *65*:82, 1965.

Mead, M.: Understanding cultural patterns, Nurs. Outlook *4*:260, 1956.

Mitchel, M.: The Child's Attitude to Death, New York, Shocken Books, 1967.

Morrisey, J. R.: Death Anxiety in Children with Fatal Illness, *in* Parod, H. (Ed.), Crisis Intervention, Family Service Assoc. of America, New York, 1965.

Mussen, P. H.: Differences between the TAT responses of Negro and white boys, J. Consult. Psychol. *30*:447, 1963.

Natterson, J., and Knudson, A.: Observations concerning fear of death in fatally ill children and their mothers, Psychosom. Med. *22*:456, 1960.

Petrillo, M.: Preventing hospital trauma in pediatric patients, Am. J. Nurs. *68*:1469, 1968.

Pettigrew, T. F.: A Profile of the Negro American, Princeton, N. J., Van Nostrand, 1964.

Pribram, K.: The New Neurology: Memory, Novelty, Thought and Choice, *in* Glaser, G. (Ed.), E.E.G. and Behavior, N. Y., Basic Books, 1963.

Quint, J. C.: The Nurse and the Dying Patient, Macmillan Company, N. Y., 1967.

Richmond, J., and Waisman, H.: Psychological aspects of management of children with malignant disease, Am. J. Dis. Child. *89*:42, 1955.

Robertson, J.: Hospitals and Children: A Parent's Eye-View, New York, Internat. Univ. Press, 1963.

Rothberg, J. S.: Why nursing diagnosis? Am. J. Nurs. *67*: 1040, 1967.

Sarason, S., Davidson, K., Lighthall, F., Waite, R., and Reubush, B.: Anxiety in School Children, Yale University, New York, John Wiley and Sons, 1960.

Scheibel, M., and Scheibel, A.: Some Neural Substrates of Postnatal Development, *in* Hoffman, H., and Hoffman, L. (Eds.), Review of Child Development, Vol. I, New York, Russell Sage Foundation, 1964.

Scott, J. P.: Critical periods in the development of social behavior in puppies, Psychosom. Med. *20*:42, 1958.

Selye, H.: The Stress of Life, New York, McGraw-Hill, 1956.

Solnit, A. J., and Green, A.: The Pediatric Management of the Dying Child, Part II, The Child's Reaction to the Fear of Dying, *in* Solnit, A., and Provence, S. (Eds.), Modern Perspectives of Child Development, New York, International Universities Press, 1963.

Strauss, A., and Glaser, B.: Awareness of Dying, Chicago, Aldine, 1965.

Strauss, A., and Quint, J.: Nursing students, assignments and dying patients, Nurs. Outlook, *12*:24, 1964.

Vander Veer, A. H.: The Psychopathology of Physical Illness and Hospital Residence, *in* Personality Development and Its Implications for Nursing and Nursing Education, Springfield, Ill., Dept. of Public Health, 1948.

Vander Zanden, J. W.: The minority group patient, Nurs. Outlook *12*:57, 1964.

Velazquez, J. M.: Alienation, Am. J. Nurs. *69*:310, 1969.

Vernick, J., and Karon, M.: Who's afraid of death on a leukemia ward? Am. J. Dis. Children *109*:393, 1964.

Verwoerdt, A.: Communication with the Fatally Ill, Springfield, Ill., Charles C Thomas, 1966.

Waechter, E.: Death Anxiety in Children with Fatal Illness, Unpublished Doctoral Dissertation. Stanford University, 1968.

Wagner, B.: Care plans—right, reasonable and reachable, Am. J. Nurs., *69*:986, 1969.

3

Prevention of Disease in Children

Medicine once concerned itself primarily with curing human ills, but in modern times this goal has been broadened to include the prevention of disease and disability. Pediatricians and others concerned with the welfare of children have led this trend during the last half-century by attracting attention to the benefits of preventive medicine and by contributing ideas and scientific discoveries to its rapid advance. The early successes were achieved in the control of infections—diseases which exacted their heaviest tolls among children. Stimulated by the dramatic results of public health measures and prophylactic immunizations in controlling smallpox, diphtheria, typhoid fever and infantile diarrhea, the medical profession has directed an increasing amount of its energies toward the prevention of diseases of all types. Pediatrics always will play a key role in preventive medicine, for "the child is father to the man," and whatever affects the health of children is of great importance to future generations of adults.

Of course, those responsible for the care of children must retain and perfect their curative skills. Fortunately, modern discoveries have simplified the treatment of many diseases. Thus, time and energy can be devoted to forestalling these unfortunate interruptions of normal growth and development. To prepare a proper defense the nature of the enemy must be known.

CHARACTERISTICS OF PEDIATRIC DISEASE

Causes of Death—Mortality

The first obligation of medicine is to preserve life. Thus, a rough measure of its success is the rate at which deaths are occurring in the population under its care. Death rates among children have particular significance, for they exclude those due to the inevitable consequences of aging. Experience has shown that the infant mortality rate (which is described below) provides one of the best indices of the health of a

country or other population unit. Where health hazards are high, the infant mortality rate is high. As medical care and public health measures improve, the infant mortality rate falls. Because of this special significance and because a considerable fraction of all children's deaths occur during infancy, the mortality prior to one year of age will be considered separately from that of later childhood.

In addition to knowing the rate at which deaths are occurring it is desirable to know the cause. Only from this latter information is it possible to evaluate the effectiveness of preventive measures already in force and to identify the directions in which new efforts should be bent. Unfortunately, it is easier to gather reliable figures for mortality rates than to fix the causes of deaths. In the United States where communication is good and enforceable laws provide for the registration of all births and deaths, the rates are highly reliable. Figures for the cause of death are less exact, since even in regions where postmortem studies are usually made, it is not always possible to assign the cause of death accurately.

Infant Mortality. The infant mortality rate is the ratio between the number of deaths of infants less than 1 year of age during any given year and the number of live births occurring in the same year. The rate is usually expressed as the number of deaths per thousand live births. If the infant mortality rate is 65, it means that for every 1,000 live-born infants 65 will die before reaching the age of 1 year. The rate may also be expressed as a percentage, 6.5 per cent in this case.

If the births for any given area are not recorded accurately, the infant mortality rate cannot be computed exactly. It was not until 1933 that all the United States (then 48) required registration of births.

At the beginning of the 20th century the infant mortality rate for those states reporting was approximately 200. In 1930 it had decreased to 64.6, and it continued to fall to 23.1 for 1966. In this latter year the rates for individual states ranged from 16.5 (Nebraska) to 34.6 (Mississippi). Nationwide, the rate for non-white infants in 1966 was 37.0 contrasted to 20.4 for those born to white parents. The difference is attributed mainly to socioeconomic factors rather than to racial differences. On the international scene a similar marked contrast is apparent. The underdeveloped countries of Asia, Africa and Latin America still have infant mortality rates in excess of 50 per thousand live births, whereas most European countries have rates comparable or superior to those in the United States. In 1965 the U.S. was in sixteenth position behind the Scandinavian countries, Canada, Australia, New Zealand, Japan, the U.S.S.R. and several other northern European countries.*

The importance of good medical and nursing care during the neonatal period is emphasized by an examination of the ages at which infant deaths occur during this first year. Between 40 and 50 per cent of infant deaths take place during the first day of life, and nearly 75 per cent occur before the age of one month. It is obvious that programs to further reduce infant mortality must be directed primarily toward this early period of the child's life. The reduction in infant deaths over the past half century has been accomplished mainly in the age group of 1 to 12 months and that significant improvement has been made under the age of 1 month, but almost no improvement has occurred in the death rate during the first day of life.

CAUSES OF INFANT DEATHS. The main causes responsible for infant deaths in the United States during the year 1966 are given in the first column of Table 2. Since it has been pointed out already that more than two thirds of these infants now die before the age of 1 month, it is not surprising to find that 13.3 out of the total 23.3 per thousand live births were due to "diseases of early infancy." Before analyzing further this category which now dominates infant mortality it is

interesting to look back over the first half of the century. Figures for New York City are used for this comparison, since no complete records are available for the country as a whole. In 1905 the total rate was nearly six times that reported for 1958. The great excess of deaths in the former year was due to infections, with diarrhea leading the list and respiratory infections such as pneumonia and bronchitis, pertussis, diphtheria, measles and tuberculosis contributing an important share. It would be easy to assume that the over-all improvement in the prognosis from infections was due to the introduction of antibiotics. But an examination of the figures for 1935, a year in which the very first antibacterial agent was scarcely known, show a tremendous decline in fatal infections. This change must be ascribed to general public health measures which rendered formulas safer and limited the interchange of infectious diseases. To be sure, the discovery of antibiotics has brought about a further reduction in infections, but it would be wrong to give major credit to these new therapeutic agents. Improvements in obstetric and newborn care are reflected in the progressive decrease in deaths due to the diseases of early infancy. Notable is the failure of any real change in the rate due to malformations.

Table 3. Causes of Death in Infants Less Than 28 Days of Age
(Neonatal Mortality in U.S., 1966)

Cause		Rate
Diseases of Early Infancy—Total		14.1
Prematurity Alone	3.7	
Asphyxia and Atelectasis	3.9	
Birth Injury	2.0	
Infections	1.0	
Erythroblastosis	0.4	
Maternal Disease	0.7	
Miscellaneous	2.4	
Congenital Malformations		2.3
All Other Causes		0.8
Total		17.2

Rates are given as deaths per 1,000 live births. Figures from Vital Statistics of the United States, 1966. Washington, D.C., U.S. Dept. of Health, Education and Welfare.

In Table 3 the focus is sharpened to a consideration of deaths occurring during the first four weeks of life. In 1965 these made up 72 per cent of the total infant mortality. Prematurity was the only recorded cause of death in more than a quarter of these infants, and was a secondary factor in several of the other causes assigned to the infant's early demise. Asphyxia, atelectasis, birth injury, infection and erythroblastosis all accounted for significant portions of the mortality rate. Even before one month of age, congenital malformations exact a heavy toll. Birth thus becomes the focal point of danger to the newborn infant. It is small wonder that obstetricians and pediatricians are joining

Table 2. Causes of Infant Mortality

Cause	U.S. Reg. Area 1966	1958	New York City 1935	1905
Diseases of Early Infancy	13.3	12.1	24.0	31.0
Infections—Total	2.8	3.4	15.0	72.0
Respiratory Diseases	(2.4)	(3.1)	(6.5)	(22.0)
Diarrhea	(0.4)	(0.3)	(5.5)	(39.0)
Other	—	—	(3.0)	(11.0)
Malformations	3.4	3.0	4.0	2.0
Miscellaneous and Unknown	3.8	1.7	5.0	15.0
Totals	23.3	20.2	48.0	120.0

Figures are the deaths per 1,000 live births in the area within the year. For the United States Registration Area they are taken from Monthly Vital Statistics Report Vol. 15, No. 13, July 26, 1967. For New York City they are adapted from Holt and McIntosh: Pediatrics, ed. 13, p. 61, New York, Appleton, 1962.

* From Wegman, M. E.: Annual Summary of Vital Statistics— 1966. Pediatrics 40:1035, 1967.

their efforts in programs to study and analyze the reasons behind the causes of death and to establish programs that will improve maternal health and thus make pregnancy and delivery safer.

ASSOCIATED FACTORS. The above analysis of infant mortality is that of the pathologist who tries to assign the immediate cause of death. Many fatalities in the United States could be avoided if all infants were to benefit from the best available care. Some of the elements of this care will be described in following chapters. Sociologists look at infant mortality in a different light, seeking factors that interfere with optimal results. Such economic factors as low family income, poor housing, ignorance and employment of the mother away from home can be shown to have a direct bearing on infant mortality. They interfere with the desire or the ability of parents to obtain adequate care before, during and after delivery of the baby.

Child Mortality. RATES OF DEATH BEYOND INFANCY. After the first year of life the mortality rate decreases very rapidly. Whereas 24.7 infants out of each 1,000 under one year of age in the United States died during 1966, only .93 per 1,000 children between one and four years succumbed, and the older group of five to 14 years had only .42 losses per 1,000. The rates have declined progressively during the last 50 years. As with the infant group, the most dramatic fall has occurred in the rates for younger children. Children in the years just prior to adolescence enjoy the most favorable mortality rates of any age period in the human span.

CAUSES OF CHILD MORTALITY. The important causes of death among children of the United States Registration Area for the year 1966 are listed in Table 4. The rates are given in the same form as those for infants.

A study of the table shows that, with his expanding environment, the preschool child faces a completely new set of hazards. His increased range of locomotion within and outside the home and his natural drives to climb and investigate set the stage for accidents. His movement out of the home environment into neighborhood and later school groups increases his opportunity to pick up infections which are not always controlled

adequately by native resistance or by medical treatment. Those congenital malformations which have permitted temporary survival continue to exact a toll of lives which dwindles during the later years of childhood. In the preschool period the neoplastic diseases (cancer and leukemia) begin to contribute to mortality, gaining slightly in importance among the school-age children. Unlike most of the other causes of death this figure has shown an absolute increase during the last few years. Rheumatic fever appears also as a significantly lethal illness during the school-age period. For both groups, however, accidents are distinctly the most frequent hazard since they produce about one-third of the total deaths.

ASSOCIATED FACTORS. The same sociologic factors that influence infant mortality operate in determining the mortality among preschool children. In the older children accidental death, rheumatic fever and tuberculosis are influenced to a degree, but the differences in rates among privileged and underprivileged children are less striking.

Causes of Illness—Morbidity

What Afflicts Children. The amount and the kind of illness among children is not reflected accurately in the mortality figures. Nearly every child suffers from streptococcal sore throat and chickenpox, but very few of them die of these disorders. Conversely, rabies and leukemia are uncommon, but their victims inevitably enter the mortality tables. An accurate notion of the prevalence of nonfatal diseases in a community is not easy to obtain, for most of them are not reported to a tabulating center. Except for some of the major contagious diseases such as measles, usually it is necessary to rely on the general impressions of those who care for children in hospitals, doctors' offices and clinics.

Pediatrics is general medical practice on patients from birth through adolescence. It is possible for a child to have almost any of the troubles that assail adults. However, the degenerative, neoplastic and metabolic disorders are much less common among the young, while infections, nutritional disorders and problems related to adaptation and growth consume the bulk of pediatric time. As previously intimated, the pediatrician is attuned to the anticipation of serious illness and devotes a high percentage of his time to prevention and to the consideration of incipient or relatively minor disorders. The medical problems of child patients in offices and hospitals are bound to reflect this prophylactic attitude.

How Children's Disease Differs. CONGENITAL ANOMALIES. Defects in the physical formation of the body may be noted at birth or later during the periods of infancy and childhood. In general, the recognition and treatment of such conditions is the responsibility of pediatricians. A few disorders may lie dormant or unrecognized until adult life (polycystic kidneys,

Table 4. Causes of Mortality Among Children in the United States for the Year 1966

Cause	Rate for Ages 1-4	Rate for Ages 5-14
Accidents	.334	.198
Influenza and Pneumonia	.109	.015
Congenital Malformations	.105	.031
Malignancies including Leukemia	.083	.065
Diseases of the Heart	.022	.017
Other Causes	.279	.100
Total	.932	.426

Rates are given in deaths per 1,000 population at the age level. From Vital Statistics of the U.S., 1966, U.S. Dept. of HEW.

Meckel's diverticulum, for example). The severity of anomalous development covers a very wide spectrum from the trivial to the type that does not permit survival for more than a few hours. Improved diagnostic and surgical methods now make it possible to correct or ameliorate many disorders, not only of the heart, but also of the nervous system, the digestive system, the urinary tract and the lungs. Mechanisms responsible for congenital anomalies are discussed in Chapter 11.

DISORDERS OF THE NEWBORN. The special problems of the newborn infant are also unique to pediatrics. Their importance has been indicated on page 51 in the discussion of mortality among infants. More detailed consideration is given in Unit II.

NUTRITIONAL ABNORMALITIES. Rapid growth of the infant makes greater demands on nutrients than does the static state of the adult. Thus, deficiencies are most likely to occur in the infant, less so in the child and least frequently in the adult. Failure in growth is sometimes an indication of a more fundamental disorder of genetic origin.

INFECTIOUS DISEASE. Adults, of course, suffer from infections too, but for children they are particularly frequent and important. Diseases that produce permanent immunity are suffered only once in a lifetime, most commonly during the early years. Respiratory infections which result in only transient immunity are the bane of pediatric practice, presumably because the child is unable to suppress them as readily as the adult who has had a longer experience with them. Exposure to many of these infections is inevitable and to a degree is desirable for the stimulation of immunologic defenses. However, the particularly vulnerable small infant or sick child must be protected in order to avoid serious consequences.

ACCIDENTS AND POISONING have become the main cause of death among children beyond the age of infancy. The child's response to trauma is generally more favorable than that of the adult, due to better tissue resiliency and the more rapid healing which is characteristic of the growing body. The toddler, prodded by his urge to explore and his delight in exploiting newly discovered physical abilities, is particularly prone to burns, scalds, falls and damaging encounters with household appliances. His propensity for putting things into his mouth (and other body orifices) creates problems of foreign-body extraction from ear, nose, esophagus, stomach, larynx, bronchi and vagina that are almost limited to this age period. The common household substances to which he has access are drugs, cleansing agents, insecticides, cosmetics and lead-painted wood or plaster. He may also be poisoned by treatment with drugs such as aspirin, sedatives or tranquilizers used by a physician or parents in a dosage inappropriate to his size. Besides combating the physical and physiologic damage created, the nurse may also have to contend with the remorse, guilt or ignorance of parents who may have been negligent.

NEOPLASMS are not nearly as common during childhood as in adult life. Those that do occur tend to have distinctive features. Leukemia, for instance, is seldom seen in either myelogenous or chronic form but is usually of the acute stem-cell or lymphatic variety. Carcinoma and sarcoma are seen occasionally. The most common tumors of childhood affect the brain, the extensions of the sympathetic nervous system and the kidneys. Many of these appear to be derived from embryologic rests which have grown slowly for a time and then suddenly enlarge under the influence of unknown stimuli. The primitive nature of many of these tumors makes it difficult to recognize them before metastatic or irreparable local growth has occurred.

PSYCHOLOGICAL DISORDERS. Behavior which is judged to be inappropriate for the child's age is an extremely common phenomenon. Many of these disorders are due to unusual intensity or persistence of infantile forms of behavior and correct themselves without long-term effects on the child. Other deviations result in neurotic traits, conduct and behavior disorders, anxiety states and psychosomatic disturbances. The more severe disorders are not common among children, or at least are not frequently recognized. Psychosis is unusual.

SURGICAL PROCEDURES performed on children are directed in a large measure at the correction of congenital malformations and the restoration of tissues injured in accidents. A few disorders such as intussusception and pyloric stenosis are found only in the pediatric age group.

Effects of Disease on the Individual Child

Symptoms. Acute illness in the child usually begins abruptly and dramatically. Before he or his parents recognize that he is sick the onset is announced by a sudden change in disposition or activity. In the early stages of infection a sharp rise in body temperature to 102-104° F. or even higher is common. Other early symptoms seen commonly are refusal of food, vomiting, abdominal pain and diarrheal stools. These do not necessarily give any exact clue to the location of his disease. For example, sometimes tonsillitis is ushered in by abdominal pain and vomiting. Chills are an infrequent counterpart of illness in children. Those who are so disposed may suffer a convulsion during the initial period of rising fever, an alarming event which may appear out of the blue before it is suspected that anything is amiss.

The dramatic onset of acute illnesses understandably stimulates anxiety among parents, particularly when they have had little experience with childhood disease. Often they are rendered temporarily incapable of providing the reassuring support which should be available in order to control the child's own anxiety about his symptoms. Children react differently. Some suffer complete physical and emotional disorganization during illness; others accept it in Spartan fashion. The manner in which a particular child reacts is likely to be repeated during succeeding upsets. This is true not only in respect to his emotional state but also to the sharpness of his febrile rise and the pattern of his associated symptoms.

The younger the child the more labile is his temperature-regulating mechanism. Fevers rise to greater heights than they would in adults with the same disease, and diurnal swings in temperature are characteristic. Usually the child's powers of physical adaptation are good, and he accommodates to fever which would exhaust an adult completely or precipitate delirium. The resilience of the young body is also apparent in the speed with which children recover from acute illnesses. Once temperatures are back to normal, it is common to find the child ready to take up activity where he left off. Those who are caring for him may have a hard time convincing him that full recovery has not yet been achieved.

Physical Effects. Illness places the child's fluid balance in jeopardy. The relatively high water requirements of the infant and the young child are discussed in Chapter 4. When illness strikes, fever, vomiting and diarrhea increase the rate of water loss from the body, and the child's inability or unwillingness to take food may curtail the intake. Serious depletion of body water cannot be permitted, since this has an adverse effect on the progress of the disease itself. Thus, therapeutic measures to prevent dehydration are employed more commonly among sick children than they are among sick adults.

Nutrition always suffers, at least briefly, during acute illness. The effects are more noticeable during the rapid growth of infancy. They are inevitably reflected in irregularities in weight progress and sometimes in temporary cessation of longitudinal growth. Permanent scars of old illness can often be seen in roentgenograms of the bones where dense transverse lines reflect a period of growth failure, and in the enamel of teeth which may show grooves and pits due to the effects of disease which occurred at the time when this portion of the tooth was being formed.

Chronic illness or recurring acute illness may have more serious consequences for nutrition and growth. The mechanism is sometimes obvious in the persistently poor intake of food or the loss of nutriments and minerals through chronic diarrhea. But, in addition, subtle changes in the function of the endocrine organs occur during prolonged inactivity and interfere with the rate of new tissue formation. Chronic major disease may be responsible for growth interferences which are so serious that they result in permanent dwarfing.

Some acute illnesses leave behind permanent defects that saddle the child with a handicap for the rest of his life. For instance, the brain may be irreparably damaged by birth injury, by encephalitis accompanying some of the contagious diseases, by meningitis or by vascular accidents within its substance. Poliomyelitis too often leaves muscular weakness in its wake; rheumatic fever carries the threat of permanent functional damage to the heart; deafness is an occasional sequel of mumps and of protracted infections of the middle ear. Apart from the need to adapt himself to a body which is incomplete in its functional capacity, the child must also be helped to accept and deal with the psychological reactions which his handicap stimulates.

Psychological Effects. The full effects of illness in childhood are by no means reflected by the mortality and morbidity tables. Acute, chronic, crippling or frequently recurring illness can affect the child's psychological development adversely. The normal growth from dependent, egocentric infancy to emotional maturity may receive severe setbacks through the experience of being physically handicapped or ill. The way in which illness or a physical handicap affects the child's personality growth is determined by his parents' attitudes and feelings toward him and his physical condition, and by the quality of care that he receives when hospitalization becomes necessary. A sense of insecurity from the very presence of the illness or the handicap itself cannot help leaving its imprint on the mind of the child. In addition, he may be confronted with hospitalization which results in separation from his parents, an excess of fear-provoking experiences and a dearth of the kind of experiences that he needs for personality growth. Prevention of the traumas that affect the ill child adversely will be discussed in subsequent chapters.

PREVENTIVE MEASURES

Toward the end of the 18th century, Jenner, an English practitioner, introduced the first specific measures for preventing a contagious disease—smallpox vaccination. During the century that followed, preventive medicine focused on the control of contagion, attempting to limit its spread through quarantine and isolation regulations. With the birth of the new science of bacteriology just before the present century began, knowledge of infectious agents advanced rapidly and with it vaccines began to appear which were effective against many of the old-fashioned scourges. In addition to smallpox it is now possible to exert good control over diphtheria, measles, pertussis, typhoid fever and poliomyelitis by this means. Parallel growth in the field of biochemistry and nutrition fostered the development of safe formulas for infants and preparations capable of preventing vitamin-deficiency diseases. In recent decades preventive pediatrics has outgrown the narrower concept of prevention of specific disease and now takes in all measures that are designed to improve the physical health and the psychosocial adjustment of children generally. With this larger goal in view physicians and nurses are extending their responsibilities and now find themselves collaborating with workers in such diverse fields as public health, education, psychology, sociology, research and even genetics and law enforcement. This section surveys briefly the protections which may be placed around the child before and after birth to avoid or ameliorate later troubles. The nurse who understands the implications of these protective devices will be prepared to utilize and to improve the resources of her own community.

Preparation for Birth

Even before his conception, society attempts to shield the child from inadequate parents. In addition to laws which set a minimal age for marriage, many states now require from all applicants for marriage licenses at least a cursory physical examination and blood tests for syphilis. Social, moral and religious forces regulate marriage in a less direct way by setting cultural standards to be met. On occasion, professional advice given by physicians, psychologists, social workers and others who engage in marriage counseling plays a significant role in molding the quality of a marriage relationship. Where undesirable hereditary traits are known to exist in the antecedents of either partner, genetic counseling is useful in evaluating the wisdom of bearing children. (For further discussion, see Chap. 5.)

Perinatal Safeguards

The analysis of infant mortality rates presented in the preceding section emphasizes how birth and its aftermath constitute the most dangerous period of a child's life. Not only the saving of lives but also the saving of cerebral function is at stake. While arguments can be offered to urge the safety and the psychological advantages of home deliveries, the fact remains that infant and maternal mortality rates are lowest where the percentage of babies delivered in hospitals is highest. The concentration of expert professional skills and resources in the hospital setting gives the infant who is destined to have trouble during delivery his best chance of a happy outcome.

Public health and professional organizations are striving continually to render the conditions of delivery as safe as possible for each infant. The quality of obstetric judgment which monitors his birth is often critical to his welfare. State and local health departments, hospitals and certifying boards set standards of professional training which must be met by physicians, nurses and midwives. In many large cities all fetal and neonatal deaths are subjected to critical review by a maternal and child-care panel in an effort to determine the factors responsible for death and to suggest ways in which care could be improved. Rules for asepsis in the delivery room or the home and for the control of infections within hospitals have been promulgated by many interested bodies. Most states have laws which require the prophylactic use of silver nitrate or antibiotics in the eyes of the newborn baby in order to prevent gonorrheal ophthalmia. Detailed consideration of the many ways in which a newborn baby can be protected against mishaps is given in Chapter 5.

The persons who successfully usher the infant into the world have responsibilities which extend beyond the physical care of mother and child. The postpartum period is of crucial importance for each member of the family. Every effort must be expended to help the parents understand their new baby and their new relationship to each other. Parents also require help in becoming adjusted to their parental roles. Care of the family during the postpartum period will be discussed in Chapter 6.

Preventive Measures After Birth

Public Health. At birth the infant becomes a member of a society which assumes a considerable amount of responsibility for the prevention of disease and death among its members. Many of the public health protections from which he profits are discharged so automatically by local and national health agencies that their benefits tend to be overlooked. Disease is rarely transmitted through water, milk or foods because the production of these essentials is carefully policed by community health departments. Sewage and garbage disposal, street cleaning, isolation of contagious disease, investigation of epidemics and inspection of housing are some of the other functions which operate locally to protect the general health. At the state and national level protection is afforded by laws which require licensing of physicians and pharmacists; by the Pure Food and Drug Act which regulates medicines, poisons and the purity of foods; through disaster relief; through programs for the care and the rehabilitation of handicapped children; and through the multiplicity of educational devices used to encourage people to protect their own health and that of their children. Many of these governmental activities are being supplemented by privately financed organizations. The regulation of motor vehicles by state licensing bureaus and by law enforcement agencies should be included as a form of protection which is assuming increasing importance with the rise of street and highway accidents toward the top of the list of causes of death among children.

Parent Education. One of the most important aspects of preventive pediatrics is the education of parents. Until those who have immediate responsibility for children are informed and convinced of the need for protective measures, results will be disappointing.

In the early part of this century efforts were directed toward the reduction of the infant mortality rate, and success was achieved. Education was focused on the provision of a safe milk supply, for much of the infant diarrhea was due to ignorance about the preservation of infant formulas. Prophylaxis against smallpox and diphtheria was soon added as another objective of parent education. Later, the emphasis shifted toward improving the nutrition of infants and children, with specific campaigns against rickets, scurvy and anemia. The results of these efforts are gratifying, for the diseases enumerated have been virtually abolished in communities which have good programs of parent education.

But the task is never finished, for new generations of parents are continually arising to be instructed in the established technics of prevention, and the scope of activity continually broadens. As the task of saving lives and preventing physical disease becomes simpler with modern facilities and a better informed group of parents, more time and energy can be devoted to considerations of physical and psychosocial growth and development and the manner in which they affect the individual child's adjustment to his environment.

PERIODIC EXAMINATION. New parents are usually receptive to the idea of submitting their infants to periodic examinations in order to measure growth and solve feeding problems. Such well-baby visits, if properly conducted, can foster an appreciation of the benefits to be derived from periodic evaluation. The desire to continue will depend in part on the parents' own desire to give the child optimal opportunities for health, but, to an even larger degree, continuation depends on the quality of the help and the sympathetic encouragement that they receive.

During infancy, visits should be fairly frequent, for growth changes are rapid, and a number of aspects of infant care need continual modification. The scope of activity can be enlarged from evaluation of weight and feeding to include the search for incipient disease or abnormality, protection against specific diseases, developmental guidance, accident prevention and mental health measures. As the child grows, the frequency of visits may be decreased from the monthly rate of early infancy, but even at school age an annual visit is desirable. Of course, children with difficulties will have to be seen more frequently. In many communities school health programs attempt to encourage at least minimal health supervision. Programs vary in their extent. Sometimes the parents are requested to submit the results of annual medical examinations made elsewhere; sometimes the school system itself provides a medical staff which makes periodic surveys of the students; sometimes evaluation is restricted to special items such as nutrition, sight, hearing or dental hygiene. The concept of periodic examination which originated in the well-baby clinic has spread to encompass well-child and school health programs and is now taking roots in adult medicine where the benefits of periodic health examinations are becoming appreciated.

Table 5—Recommended Schedule for Active Immunizations in Normal Infants and Children

2 months	DTP plus Trivalent OPV (or OPV Type 1)
3 months	DTP
4 months	DTP plus Trivalent OPV (or OPV Type 3)
6 months	Trivalent OPV (or OPV Type 2)
12 months	Measles Vaccine plus Tuberculin Test
15-18 months	DTP plus Smallpox Vaccine plus Trivalent OPV
4-6 years	DTP plus Trivalent OPV plus Smallpox Vaccination
12-14 years	TD plus Smallpox Vaccine plus Mumps Vaccine

DTP = Diphtheria and Tetanus Toxoids combined with Pertussis Vaccine
OPV = Oral Poliovaccine (Sabin Vaccine)
TD = Diphtheria and Tetanus Toxoids, Adult Type
From American Academy of Pediatrics: Report of the Committee on the Control of Infectious Diseases—1969.

NUTRITION during each period of infancy and childhood is important for general health, not only during the period under consideration, but also for all later periods as well. Good prenatal nutrition produces more vigorous infants. Good infant nutrition gives the baby a better start into childhood. Some of the defects which are discovered later at school (but which may persist through life) may be contracted in infancy and the preschool period, often to a degree which affects the stamina and the learning capacity. Dental caries is as yet an uncontrolled human scourge and is caused in large measure by improper diet.

SPECIFIC PROTECTIVE MEASURES. An important part of the periodic consultation is the protection of the child against the serious infectious diseases which he may encounter in later life. Practices differ somewhat, depending on the health circumstances of the community. Table 5 shows the immunization scheme recommended by the American Academy of Pediatrics as a general guide. With rare exceptions, the child who receives this course of immunizations will be protected against all of the diseases represented.

Injections of DTP should be started early in the course of well-baby visits in order to provide the infant with protection against pertussis, a disease to which he is highly and dangerously susceptible. The basic immunization consists of three doses at least one month apart. Booster injections should be given at around 18 months and 3 years. If significant febrile reactions occur and particularly if the child has a convulsion following a dose of DTP, abandonment or at least modification of the schedule must be considered. The older child should receive booster injections of diphtheria and tetanus toxoids periodically throughout his childhood years.

Immunity to poliomyelitis must be produced against the three different antigenic types of virus. The original killed-virus vaccine of Salk proved quite effective in reducing the incidence of poliomyelitis in this country. It has, however, been largely superseded by the Sabin type of vaccine which consists of attenuated strains of live virus which can be taken by mouth instead of by intramuscular injection. The Sabin vaccine has proved to be equally effective as well as

Fig. 3-1. With adequate preparation of mother and child immunizations can be accomplished with minimum discomfort to all parties. (Parke Davis Co., Detroit, Mich.)

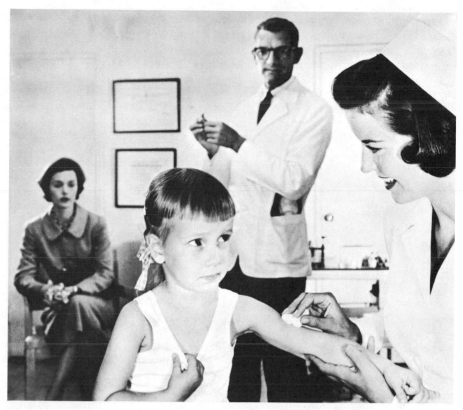

painless and probably provides a longer lasting immunity. When the trivalent type is used, doses should be spaced at intervals of six weeks or longer. Booster doses of the trivalent vaccine are generally advised after an interval of a year in order to make sure that protection against all three types of poliovirus has been acquired. Simultaneous administration of OPV and measles vaccine is not recommended, but OPV and smallpox vaccinations do not conflict.

Vaccination against measles is ordinarily deferred until the infant is about 1 year of age because until this age antibodies transmitted across the placental circulation from the mother are often still present in small amounts. Since the vaccination tries to produce a mild form of the disease following the injection of a live attenuated strain of measles virus, passively transmitted maternal antibody may prevent a proper "take" and adequate active immunity. Two types of live-virus vaccine are in current use—the Edmonston strain, which rather commonly produces a brief febrile disease about a week after administration, and the Schwartz strain, which has been further attenuated and produces a milder type of illness in the recipients. Gamma globulin in small dosage is usually given simultaneously with the Edmonston vaccine in order to minimize the febrile response; it is not considered necessary with the Schwartz strain. Neither vaccine has been followed by the complication of encephalitis, nor will the virus spread contagiously from the vaccinated to the unvaccinated child. A killed-virus vaccine was available until recently but has been with-

drawn because the duration of immunity produced was too brief and because a high incidence of peculiar reactions was observed among children who had received it and subsequently were given live-virus vaccine or acquired natural measles. Its use is now restricted to children who cannot receive the live-virus vaccine because they have malignant disease such as leukemia or lymphoma, or those who are receiving immunosuppresive therapy with steroids or cytotoxic agents.

Although smallpox has been eliminated from the United States and several other areas of the world, routine protection of infants is still advised, preferably between the first and second birthdays. The vaccine is a preparation of live vaccinia virus which must be kept frozen until used since it rapidly loses virulence upon exposure to room temperature. After inoculation by multiple pressures through the superficial skin, a successful "take" will produce a slowly growing area of erythema after four to five days, which reaches maximal size in eight to 14 days, acquires a blister in the center which then breaks and scabs, and usually leaves a recognizable scar after healing is complete. If such a "take" does not occur in the previously unvaccinated individual, it cannot be assumed that he is immune to smallpox. It is more likely that the vaccine used was inactive or that the technic of vaccination was faulty. Another attempt should be made. Individuals who are being revaccinated after a previously successful take will show a milder and more rapidly developing local reaction if their immunity is still present. It is recommended that children be revaccinated about every five years, and at any time when they are preparing for foreign travel. The presence of eczema or other chronic weeping skin eruption in the child or a member of his family is a *contraindication* to smallpox vaccination (p. 343).

In countries with a high prevalence of tuberculosis, infants are vaccinated regularly with BCG (Bacillus of Calmette and Guérin). Like smallpox vaccination, this consists of purposeful infection with a known attenuated strain of the organism in order to produce immunity to the more virulent types. The effectiveness of BCG vaccination appears to be definite among populations which cannot hope to control tuberculosis by isolation and treatment of individual cases. In the United States it is used to protect some infants who must live in environments where tuberculosis is prevalent. Even where the tuberculosis rate is low, routine testing with tuberculin is an important part of well-baby and school health programs in order to discover unrecognized exposure in its early stages and to make early treatment possible. The frequency of such testing is varied, depending upon the prevalence of tuberculosis in the child's environment. A negative tuberculin test should be obtained before measles vaccine is employed in the small infant.

Protection against other diseases is also available. In regions where typhoid fever is prevalent, active protection by the administration of vaccine during the first year of life is desirable. Under special circumstances, active protection against typhus fever, Rocky Mountain spotted fever, mumps and rabies may be desired. Effective treatment with penicillin has made vaccination against scarlet fever obsolete. Vaccines against rubella (German measles) are now available but must be used with careful protection against pregnancy in pubescent girls or women.

In certain instances it is desirable to give a child or an infant temporary protection against a disease to which he has been recently exposed. Immediate but transient protection is available for many infectious diseases through the administration of preparations of convalescent serum or adult blood products. This type of protection is called passive immunization and should not be confused with the previously mentioned immunizations which are designed to give long-lasting protection. Passive protection against measles is desirable for unimmunized infants and children between the ages of 6 months and 3 years when known exposure has taken place. Gamma globulin is the most widely used preparation for this purpose. Convalescent serum is desirable for protection of unimmunized infants who are exposed to whooping cough within the family. Tetanus antitoxin must be given following certain injuries if the child has not been immunized previously.

Of the preparations used for passive protection against disease, those which are manufactured in animals such as the horse or the rabbit carry the disadvantage of serum sickness and the induction of sensitization to animal proteins. Human convalescent serum and gamma globulin do not have this disadvantage.

The Nurse's Role in Preventive Mental Hygiene. The role of the nurse in educational programs for parents and children is expanding with the more comprehensive concept of health which includes the total physical, social and emotional welfare of families. Nurses are now engaged in formal and informal educational programs having as their goal the facilitation of healthy parent-child relationships and the optimal physical and emotional development of children. Nurses are found as discussion group leaders for parents of physically well, chronically ill and handicapped children. They are taking a leading role in the preparation of parents for labor, delivery and parenthood, and in school programs directed toward assisting children in understanding their physical and emotional development and problems.

In many settings which provide health care and guidance, the nurse is assuming increased responsibilities in assisting parents to understand themselves and their children's nature and nurture, and in handling the developmental problems of growth. The nurse is talking with parents in outpatient clinics, in pediatric wards, in public and voluntary health agencies and in the homes of families. Through such contacts with parents, she has the opportunity to detect physical and psychosocial problems in adjustment and to refer families or individuals to appropriate sources of help. "Case-finding" or recognition that a physical or a psychological problem exists is one of the first essentials in the prevention of disease.

Because the nurse spends more time with children than does any other health worker, she can play an important role in identifying danger signals which may forecast unhealthy adjustment unless appropriate medical or psychiatric treatment is provided. It is vitally important that the nurse be able to provide psychological first-aid—another way of referring to emotional support which has as its goal the minimization of anxiety. It is also important that she be prepared to help the disturbed mother to acknowledge her need for help from an expert and to gain an understanding of the way in which the specialist can help her and her child. If emotional disturbances are recognized early and treated by a specialist *before* they develop into fixed patterns of behavior, there is much greater likelihood that the child may be able to overcome the symptoms which block further psychosocial development.

The nurse's role in preventive mental health programs is one which requires keen observation, understanding of one's self and others, a capacity for teamwork and an ability to interpret children's developmental requirements without being judgmental or authoritarian. Functioning in preventive health programs requires preparation to give what Levy calls "anticipatory guidance."

Anticipatory guidance prepares parents 'to understand their children's needs for growth and development. It gives parents understanding of the changes in behavior which are produced with growth and assists them in recognizing their children's readiness for new learning experiences. It also helps to prepare them to help their children to conquer core problems of development.

Providing anticipatory guidance requires understanding of oneself and parents as well as children. The nurse's success in guiding parents depends on her attitudes and feelings toward them as persons. It also depends on her ability to appraise their readiness for guidance and her skill in interpreting knowledge to them. Understanding her own limitations is equally essential, for a nurse's efforts may do more harm than good if she permits herself to become involved too deeply in the complexities of emotional disturbances of parents or children. She can interpret the findings of those who have studied the basic needs of children and parents, utilize her knowledge in her relationships with them, and be alert to symptoms that manifest emotional distress. However, serious disturbances must be left to someone with special training in this area.

Emotionally disturbed parents and children need the help of someone who has special training in the dynamics of human behavior and in the use of therapeutic measures which are required to restore individuals to mental health—a physician, a child-guidance worker, a social worker or a psychiatrist. If the nurse continues to work with the child or the parent after the referral to a specialist has been made, teamwork will further the disturbed individual's return to health.

Other ways in which the nurse can contribute to preventive mental health work will be discussed more fully in the appropriate sections throughout this book.

Within the hospital, the nurse works with children to prevent the detrimental effects of maternal deprivation and to alleviate traumatic experiences. She can also do a great deal to help mothers provide the physical care and guidance that the child needs before returning home, thus preventing further hospitalizations. Mothers of children with special problems of management must have experiences in caring for their children and opportunities for sharing their feelings in order to feel comfortable about taking their children home.

Nurses can also assist mothers who have had prolonged periods of separation from their newborns by keeping them in touch with their babies, thus alleviating separation anxiety and promoting the emotional unity which increases the mother's energy and confidence for mothering.

Nurses can also aid parents after their child's discharge from the hospital by assisting in obtaining the services of a home-maker when needed, by obtaining referrals to community agencies that can give continued support to families, and by keeping the lines of communication open between the hospital and these agencies.

The Nurse's Role in Prevention of Disease in Children. Because of the explosion of scientific knowledge, a changing population, technical advances, increasing specialization and institutionalization of health services, the rise of automation and the widening medical manpower gap, many concerned pediatricians and nurses are re-examining division of responsibilities to assure that children of all ages in America receive adequate and comprehensive well-child care. Technical advances and automation have instigated an intensive analysis of the changing nature of the nurse's role in preventive services. There is increasing concern with the possible depersonalization of patient care, which will intensify the need for nurses skilled in the principles of preventive mental hygiene. Parents are also increasingly better informed and sophisticated regarding the optimum in health care and are demanding increasing excellence in the delivery of health services.

For these reasons, alternative patterns of child health care are now being explored and recommended by both pediatricians and nurses, with a realignment of responsibility for both disciplines and with a critical assessment of functions in child health supervision. The role of the pediatric nurse specialist is receiving increasing attention in preventive pediatric care. More than ever before, the relationship between physicians and nurses must become a closer and more cooperative one; they must work together as professionals to determine division of responsibilities, to identify their potential contributions to the solution of health problems and to further the objectives of preventive care.

Under the Social Security Act, Titles IV and V, programs are being developed to provide for all children the health supervision they will need to assure a good start in life. In addition to the existing state health department services and crippled children's services which are being extended and expanded, federal grants are now available under Title V of the Social Security Act to help reduce the incidence of mental retardation and to help reduce infant and maternal mortality. Nurses are now contributing to preventive care in maternity and infant projects and children and youth projects in many parts of the country. They are also contributing their skills to children in isolated areas and to children with special problems requiring a health team effort. In addition to the above, increasing attention is being given to the furnishing of health care to the lower socioeconomic groups.

THE CHILD HEALTH CONFERENCE

The Purpose of the Conference and Its Personnel

The Child Health Conference is the name commonly given to the clinic which has as its goal the conservation of the well child's health and the promotion of the highest level of physical and psychosocial development which he can attain. It functions primarily for the children who are not directly under the supervision of a physician elsewhere. It may be voluntary in its organization and financial support, or, as it becomes recognized as a necessary public health function, it may be taken over by the tax-supported or official agencies. Child Health Conference service is generally free, but there may be a fee if it is provided by a privately endowed hospital.

Planned health supervision of the child begins with comprehensive prenatal care for the mother and continues throughout childhood. It provides periodic appraisal of the child's health by a pediatrician or a physician who has had experience with mothers and children, immunization (in most instances) and consultation with parents. Recent additions to the available services include new immunization procedures, routine testing for phenylketonuria, testing of urine, sweat tests for cystic fibrosis, expansion of mental health services, and individual and group parent counselling.

Parental guidance during the earliest years of the child's life is especially necessary from the standpoint of prevention and early correction of physical defects and emotional disorders. Before 6 years of age, neurotic tendencies have not become a built-in part of the child's personality structure and, therefore, are modified more easily and with less difficulty for the child and his parents. Thus, every health worker who guides the mother in the care of her young child can play an important role in the ultimate improvement of the health of the community.

The nurse has many functions in the conference. In light of the discussion presented in the foregoing section, many health departments throughout the country are experimenting with the Nursing Child Health Conference, which is a concrete attempt to extend preventive health care and the services of a pediatrician to more children who would otherwise receive little health supervision. In these conferences, nurses are accepting more responsibility for counseling of parents, anticipatory guidance, primary history taking, necessary referrals and assessment of child development. When this type of clinic is in operation, the pediatrician is generally available for consultation and examines the child at periodic intervals.

The nurse has many functions in either type of conference. Although they have long been deflected from patient care by the need to be clinic managers, nurses are now examining and expanding their role in patient care. The nurse is the person who sets the emotional tone and sees that preliminary data such as weight and birth history are gathered for the physician. In doing this she has an opportunity to function as his coworker either before or after the mother has her conference with him. She also supplements his activities by a follow-up conference. Ideally, the mother should see the same doctor and nurse each time she comes for a visit, since once she has come to know them, she feels more comfortable about sharing her problems with them. The worker, too, gains more satisfaction from the experience because she has background knowledge of the family to draw on as she shares an experience with the mother and her child.

The nurse who is in charge of the conference often coordinates the activities of other personnel, guides the experience of students, refers patients and consults with the nutritionist, mental hygiene specialist and dental hygienist.

The nurse who is best known to the family arranges for continuity of services through home visits during her consultation with the mother at the conference. This is valuable to protect the trust and confidence parents have developed in the person who is trying to help them.

The conference is introduced to mothers in many different ways—during prenatal care, in the hospital when the baby is born or by the public health nurse who visits the home. Many parents are not aware of the help that they can get from such a conference. Once a mother has attended a conference in which the personnel have respected her need for self-esteem and provided her with helpful counsel, her use of this resource will expand.

All nurses, especially those who work with mothers of newborns, must know the facilities of the community for well-baby health supervision in order to be able to explain the functions and the values of such services to parents. Mothers of babies who have been ill are especially receptive to suggestions in regard to health supervision, for they are aware of their responsibility in keeping their babies well. Hospital personnel must have a well worked-out plan whereby any baby discharged from the hospital inpatient or outpatient service, who is not going to have the health supervision of a private physician, is referred automatically to the most accessible child health conference in order that health supervision can be continued without interruption.

Conducting the Conference

The waiting room should be attractive, large and comfortable. Because the room is for children as well as adults, space must be provided for them. Small furniture and toys are required. Most preschool children like to move about rather than to sit on their mothers' laps. Toddlers rarely stray far from their mothers. Suitable posters, charts, exhibits and demonstrations can be utilized as teaching devices for waiting parents.

A "play nurse" or a "play teacher" is invaluable in making the waiting period pleasant and profitable for the children and their mothers. It must be remembered that many of the children attending the conference are from homes where there are few play materials and inadequate space for play. A "play nurse" gives mothers an opportunity to take advantage of the educational exhibits and to share experiences with each other. It also gives the nurse opportunities to spot the children who will need extra help through the examination or who are having problems in their relationships with other children. Moreover, the nurse who is well versed in child development has an opportunity to assess the child's developmental level.

A friendly, pleasant atmosphere is more important than elaborate equipment. Mothers must be received in a gracious manner if they are to benefit by the conference and be motivated to return. The hostess, a volunteer or a nurse, must be ready to make mothers and children comfortable, welcome and valued as persons regardless of their social origin. The value of the visit, or even future visits, may depend on this first contact. Therefore, plenty of time must be allowed for collecting the data essential to the health record. To discourage the mother from talking when she first arrives or to jump to conclusions is not only discourteous but also manifests a lack of sensitivity to one of the common ways in which people handle their anxiety in new situations. It also defeats the purpose of the conference. The period in which data are collected is the best time to prove to the mother that the conference is held primarily to benefit her and her family and that the personnel are there to help her to develop her own resources in the care of her children.

Another way to help parents benefit from the conference is to assure them that long waiting periods between consultations do not occur, thus avoiding loss of self-esteem on the part of the parents. Belkin and her associates studied mothers' evaluations of the child health conference and found that the suggestions mothers gave for improvement involved primarily: (1) shorter waiting periods, (2) less indifference to parents, and (3) less crowded conditions. All of these suggestions are concerned with parental feelings of self-worth.

During the nurse's contacts with the mother, she has a splendid opportunity to observe the mother-child relationship as well as the child's physical growth and behavior. During such procedures as weighing or measuring, she has the opportunity to answer the mother's questions, to interpret height and weight tables, and allay the mother's anxiety if her baby deviates slightly from the stated norms.

During conference procedures, the mother may also learn the importance of giving her child emotional

support or learn technics which will assist her, such as reading a thermometer. The mother's questions must be carefully considered, since she will then feel encouraged to ask others when she is perplexed. Some questions can be reflected back to the mother to increase her self-confidence in knowledge she already possesses; others will necessitate giving factual information.

When painful procedures such as immunizations are done, the child who is old enough needs preparation. All children need emotional contact and support for their individual coping strategies.

When a health condition is uncovered that necessitates referral to another agency, the mother must be given the opportunity to share her reactions to the diagnosis and understand the reasons for referral. *It is natural for a mother to be anxious when an abnormality is found, no matter how trivial it may be.* To send a mother home with a worry that could be minimized by knowledge of the problem adds a burden which no busy mother should have to carry.

After the examination, all findings need to be interpreted to the mother. Suggestions can be offered for changes in the baby's physical care, such as diet, and support given to the mother's child-rearing endeavors. Most mothers are now greatly concerned with

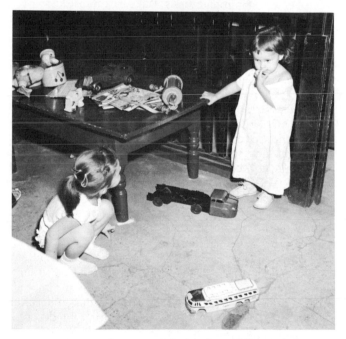

Fig. 3-2. Play materials for the toddler and the pre-school child are necessary to minimize the tensions which are sometimes produced by health examinations. Note the way this two-year-old manifests her uncertainty about the situation. Her tension may have been provoked by fear for her own safety in relation to a child she has not played with before, or it may have arisen because she is anticipating an examination that has frightened her in the past. (Infant Welfare Society of Chicago)

learning healthy child-rearing practices under difficult social situations. Often mothers can be greatly reassured to learn that their child's behavior is not unusual. Other questions which are now giving mothers serious concern involve the broad and difficult problems of family interaction. Here the nurse has many opportunities for bringing her warm and professional capacities to bear upon the problems of families, to provide anticipatory guidance and to prevent more serious emotional problems by detecting early deviations in behavior. Anticipatory guidance also helps the mother's understanding of child development.

In some sections of the country, mothers from other cultures, who speak another language and have different customs and patterns of thinking, may need special consideration. The nurse talking with these mothers needs to be aware of the cultural differences existing between races and of the habits, folklore, beliefs and attitudes which may affect the mother's interpretation of the recommendations. She must phrase her questions so as to be nonthreatening and permissive, and she must not allow her own value system to color her judgments of the beliefs and practices of another culture. When an interpreter is necessary, she must be particularly careful that communication and understanding are not distorted. In the discussion of specific recommendations, the nurse must know, for instance, that local cultural patterns greatly affect infant nutritional practices. Taking these into consideration, she can allow the mother to participate in the dietary planning or discussion of child-rearing practices. The nurse must also be aware of the economic conditions within the family, so that other members of the family are not unnecessarily deprived by the prescription of costly diets or appliances. She must know that long waiting periods in the clinic for a mother who has no one at home to supervise her other children increases the mother's anxiety and hampers her from benefiting from the conference. Often, because of economic restrictions, the urgency of need for medical services must be assessed and plans made to secure care which does not increase the family's financial burden.

The effectiveness of the conference for all mothers will depend to a considerable extent on the willingness of the professional personnel to hear the mother out in full. An inhibited, anxious mother will suffer additional frustration if she is permitted to describe only the superficial aspects of her problems and then is presented with didactic advice which she probably has tried already without success. The approach used to obtain her story is of paramount importance. Mothers who are not yet acquainted with the doctor or the nurse may feel as though they were on trial during their first visit. A general request such as "Tell me about your day with the baby" is preferable to "Are you nursing your baby on a self-demand schedule?," since specific questions often put mothers on the

defensive. The second question implies that the mother probably *should* be nursing in accordance with her baby's demands, whereas the more general request encourages the mother to give all the facts without reservation.

Many a mother may feel guilty over occasional lapses in her affection for her baby or in her dedication to the job of child-rearing. Often such a comment as "I imagine there were times when you wished you might send the baby back to the nursery for care" or "I presume you haven't been able to rest as much as you could before the baby's arrival" will put the mother at ease. Although such remarks may not be welcomed by the occasional mother who is trying to convince herself that she has accepted her new role with unmitigated zeal, the great majority will greet such an acknowledgment with overwhelming relief. At this point the mother will probably be more than willing to discuss aspects of child care which are troubling her.

It is a common tendency for an anxious mother to exaggerate facts. If this occurs, discreet pursuit of details will help discover what is worrying her. If the physician or the nurse accepts her story at face value and suggests corrective measures, he or she will simply reinforce the mother's groundless anxiety. Many of the accounts that mothers give medical personnel are bids for reassurance. If the listener is trapped into agreeing that the condition must be corrected, he increases anxiety rather than lessens it. If he has evidence that proves that nothing abnormal is occurring, his matter-of-fact attitude toward the situation provides the reassurance that the mother is seeking.

As previously mentioned, anticipatory guidance is useful in helping the mother understand that her child's behavior is not unusual and to prepare her for future predictable behavior. Many mothers are concerned about thumbsucking, negativism and masturbation, and the nurse can help the mother think through reasons for their occurrence rather than giving rigid prescriptions, since the basis for the behavior may be very different for different children.

When serious problem behavior is observed, the nurse is expected to provide emotional first-aid, but she must recognize her limitations and be prepared to motivate the parent to accept the help of a specially trained health worker. She can explain the functions of the social worker or child-guidance worker and also can alleviate the fears that arise when a mother recognizes that her child has a problem requiring psychotherapy. The mother who has a disturbed or troubled child usually feels frustrated and incompetent and is often fearful of psychiatric therapy because she expects condemnation from the therapist or from the community in which she lives. In referring a mother to a social worker or to a child-guidance clinic, the nurse must understand these natural feelings. Once a mother learns that therapists in child-guidance clinics are prepared to handle such problems, her fears are often dispelled and she becomes motivated to seek help.

Tact and diplomacy are important in all phases of the Child Health Conference. Many mothers come feeling discouraged, perplexed and fatigued, and a large number of these desire only reassurance and the security of knowing that their judgment is sound. The ultimate goals of the conference can only be realized if the mothers develop their own capacities for mothering and self-direction. Some mothers may have had inadequate mothering in their own childhood and thus have a poor model to follow. In such instances, the nurse can provide information, understanding and guidance which restores self-confidence and resolves perplexity resulting from widely divergent previous advice on child care.

The nurse can also reduce unjustified maternal guilt resulting from the mother's natural irritation with her child. Often the mothers resent their responsibility, feel overburdened and long for their former independence. It is helpful to them to know that adjustment takes time and effort and that others understand that child-rearing, though important, is wearisome and perplexing in a rapidly changing culture where former familiar supports have been withdrawn and child-rearing practices have changed markedly from the time they themselves were children.

At the conclusion of the conference, the health team plans for the future needs of the family. Records should be kept of the child's physical and psychosocial development and of the parents' response to him so that data are available for future reference.

THE FUTURE FOR CHILD HEALTH SUPERVISION

The value of Child Health Conferences has been proved in the reduction of mortality and morbidity rates. Many mothers report their satisfaction with this type of health supervision for their children, when other types may have been unavailable to them.

Many new trends, however, are now under way in the provision of health care. Such trends have been Medicare, Head Start, Comprehensive Maternity and Infant projects, Family Planning, Neighborhood Health Centers, Comprehensive Health Planning, the Public Health Services Amendments of 1966 (Public Law 89-749) and the Child Health Act of 1967.

Many professional people today are greatly concerned about the need for comprehensive health services to meet all the health needs of a family, of which the Child Health Conference is but one. They are considering "one door" health programs, in which the entire family may come for comprehensive health care rather than many kinds of fragmented services. Child health care must be considered in terms of its relationship to the unmet health needs of the total population. Slowly, such services seem to be emerging.

The importance of well-child care has been demonstrated. Now there is need for incorporation of well-child care into more comprehensive family services, better education of the public, favorable legislation and a constant effort toward more effective use of facilities already in existence.

SITUATIONS FOR FURTHER STUDY

1. Why should a nurse know the causes of death and illness in children?

2. What factors have prevented a marked decrease in neonatal mortality rates? How can the nurse function in preventing death in newborns?

3. What are the outstanding causes of disease during childhood?

4. Disease produces different effects on children and adults. What are these differences? How do they influence your attitudes toward pediatric nursing?

5. Use one of your patients to describe the effects of a child's illness on his physical and psychosocial development. Discuss also the ways in which you have planned to minimize the adverse effects of his illness on his potentialities for further growth.

6. Observe a child whom you believe has been affected adversely by illness. Describe his behavior and indicate why you have concluded that his development has been thwarted by his illness. How might retardation in development have been prevented?

7. Describe a situation you have observed which led you to conclude that the child's inner resources had been strengthened by his experience in the hospital. What factors affected the adjustment you consider to be constructive? On what did you base your conclusions?

8. What are the ways in which comprehensive prenatal care can safeguard the mother and the baby physically and emotionally?

9. How can the nurse function in helping mothers to become emotionally united with their infants during the postpartum period? Of what importance is this to the mother?

10. What preventive health measures exist in your community?

11. How does the hospital you are associated with function to protect the health of the family in its community?

12. Observe a mother who was separated from her baby immediately after delivery. Describe her behavior when she meets the baby in the ward. After a period of observation, give her an opportunity to talk with you. Report the content of her conversation and describe the affect which was expressed as she talked with you. How do you think she felt about being separated from her baby, about his illness and about her role as a mother? What leads you to believe she felt as you think she did? What opportunities did you find to help her to feel more comfortable with herself, the baby and with you? Do this daily and report the results of your work and the ways in which

you reacted to the experiences. What parts of the experience made you uncomfortable and which parts increased your satisfaction in working with mothers?

13. In what instances would you deem it necessary to refer a family to a community agency? Cite a situation that you observed which led you to conclude that the family would need further help after the child had been dismissed from the hospital.

14. How is infant health supervision provided in your community?

15. If attendance is falling off in the Child Health Conference, what might be some of the reasons for this?

16. Tony, age 3, cried when his clothes were removed. He also clutched his penis while the doctor was examining his brother. During his examination his face was contorted with fear and he grabbed at his trunks when the doctor started to lower them for a genital examination. After the examination was over he ran to the table to watch the doctor as he examined another child. He looked and then ran back to his mother. He repeated this six times before his mother was ready to help him to get dressed to go home. What do you think provoked Tony's behavior? How would you have functioned had you observed this behavior? When Tony was dressed, his facial expression was vastly different from what it had been previously. His facial muscles were relaxed; he smiled and stopped to play a while before he followed his mother out the door. What do you think caused this marked change in affect? Of what value was this clinic visit to Tony?

17. Describe a conference which you observed between a mother and a nurse. How did the nurse encourage her to talk about her problems? Was she successful? Why? If she failed, what do you think were the reasons? What questions did the mother ask? How did the nurse help the mother?

18. Describe a situation in which you observed a nurse offering anticipatory guidance. Had the mother anticipated the change in behavior that the nurse described? What were her questions concerning it? What feelings did she express? Do you think that the mother received enough insight into the behavior and her feelings concerning it to be able to handle it wisely when it arises?

19. Read David Levy's book—*The Demonstration Clinic*—and report what he calls "the guided listening technic" in working with mothers. Do you agree or disagree with his statement that nurses are often uncomfortable unless they are doing something? On what do you base your decision? How can listening become an active process?

20. If you had listened to an overwrought mother talk of her problems in feeding her baby, what behavior manifestations would lead you to conclude that she had moved toward finding a solution to her problem?

21. What factors would you consider in planning the health supervision of a Mexican-American child, and in discussions with his mother?

22. What trends in our society do you consider important in program planning for comprehensive well-child supervision?

BIBLIOGRAPHY

American Academy of Pediatrics, Council on Pediatric Practice: Standards of Child Health Care, Evanston, Illinois, 1967.

Belkin, M., *et al.*: Mother's utilization of the child health station and evaluation of the child health conference, Am. J. Pub. Health 54:2023, 1964.

Bettelheim, B.: Dialogues with Mothers, Glencoe, Ill., Free Press, 1962.

Connelly, J., Stoeckle, J., Lepper, E., and Farrisey, R.: The physician and the nurse, their interprofessional work in office and hospital ambulatory settings, New Eng. J. Med. 275:765, 1966.

Edelstein, R.: Automation—Its effect on the nurse, Am. J. Nurs. 66:2194, 1966.

Farrisey, R.: Clinic nursing in transition, Am. J. Nurs. 67:305, 1967.

Ford, A., Seacot, M., and Silver, G.: The relative roles of the public health nurse and the physician in prenatal and infant supervision, Am. J. Pub. Health 56:1097, 1966.

Ford, L., and Silver, H.: The expanded role of the nurse in child care, Nurs. Outlook 15:43, 1967.

Ginzberg, E.: Nursing and manpower realities, Nurs. Outlook 15:26, 1967.

Goldman, M., *et al.*: Child health station personnel: a profile, Am. J. Pub. Health 54:1302, 1964.

Gozzi, E.: We plan ahead what to ask, Nurs. Outlook 13:30, 1965.

Hansan, R. C., and Buch, M. J.: Communicating health arguments across cultures, Nurs. Outlook 14:237, 1963.

Holt, L. E., and McIntosh, R.: Pediatrics, ed. 13, New York, Appleton, 1962.

Ingles, T.: A new health worker, Am. J. Nurs. 68:1059, 1968.

Karsch, B., Christian, J., Gozzi, E., and Carlson, P.: Infant care and punishment: a pilot study, Am. J. Pub. Health 55:1880, 1965.

Kissick, W. L.: Effective utilization: the critical factor in health manpower, Am. J. Pub. Health, 58:23, 1968.

Lambertson, E.: Changes in practice require changes in education, Am. J. Nurs. 66:1784, 1966.

Levy, D. M.: The Demonstration Clinic, Springfield, Ill., Charles C Thomas, 1959.

Lewis, E. E., and Resnik, B. A.: Nurse clinics and progressive ambulatory patient care, New Eng. J. Med. 277:1236, 1967.

Little, D.: The nurse specialist, Am. J. Nurs. 67:552, 1967.

Pratt, H.: The doctor's view of the changing nurse-physician relationship, J. Med. Ed. 40:767, 1965.

Schlotfeldt, R.: The nurse's view of the changing nurse-physician relationship, J. Med. Ed. 44:772, 1965.

———: A mandate for nurses and physicians, Am. J. Nurs. 65:102, 1965.

Seacat, M., and Schlachter, L.: Expanded nursing role in prenatal and infant care, Am. J. Nurs. 68:822, 1968.

Siegel, E., Bryson, S.: A redefinition of the role of the public health nurse in child health supervision, Am. J. Pub. Health 53:1015, 1963.

Siegel, E., Dillehoy, R., and Fitzgerald, C.: Role changes within the child health conferences, attitudes and professional preparedness of public health nurses and physicians, Am. J. Pub. Health 55:832, 1965.

Silver, H., and Ford, L.: The pediatric nurse practitioner at Colorado, Am. J. Nurs. 67:1443, 1967.

Silver, H., Ford, L., and Stearly, S.: A program to increase health care for children, the pediatric nurse program, Pediatrics 39:756, 1967.

Simpson, W., and Cosand, M.: Homemaking teachers in public health, Am. J. Pub. Health 57:869, 1967.

Stearly, S., Noordenbos, A., and Courch, V.: Pediatric nurse practitioner, Am. J. Nurs. 67:2083, 1967.

Stine, O. C.: Content and method of health supervision by physicians in child health conferences in Baltimore, 1959, Am. J. Pub. Health 52:1858, 1962.

Tianen, D. A.: Analytic study of the physical findings of the health appraisals of culturally deprived children, Nursing Res. 11:231, 1962.

U. S. Government Printing Office: Services for Children and Families under the Social Security Act, Titles IV and V, 1968.

Wiedenbach, E.: Family nurse practitioner for maternal and child care, Nurs. Outlook 13:1150, 1965.

4

Therapy Related to the Physical Care of the Child

When the procedures used in the care of children are analyzed, certain fundamental principles emerge which are accepted by the personnel of all hospitals. The maintenance of a sterile field may be the basic principle in one procedure, absolute accuracy the essential factor in another, continuous administration of a *specially* ordered intravenous fluid at a *specific rate* of flow may be the requirement in a third. However, the actual performance of the procedures will vary somewhat in different hospitals and in the care of children at different age levels.

The purpose of setting up procedures and working out routines and technics for the care of children is to ensure safety and maximal comfort. Ensuring safety requires adherence to the principles underlying the procedure.

In her care of sick children the pediatric nurse participates in many varieties of treatment. While she rarely has the responsibility for determining the type of therapy to be used or the exact details of dosage, her care of the child will be enhanced if she comprehends the general principles that she is serving and is successful in helping the child to understand and accept them. Some of the medications and technics have rather limited usage and are described with the particular diseases to which they most commonly apply. It is the purpose of the authors in this chapter to consider therapeutic measures which have common application to many kinds of illness in childhood.

In dealing with child patients, the factor of size always must be considered in regulating doses of medicine, amounts of fluid to be administered, and in determining the variations that are necessary in certain technical procedures. With adult patients it is possible to use fairly standard dosages and technics, for the differences in size among patients is not very great. A large fraction of the nurse's adult clientele will weigh between 100 and 200 pounds, and all but the very unusual will be encompassed by the range from 75 to 300 pounds. The maximum discrepancy here is 4-fold. But in her pediatric experience, commonly her patients will range over a 30-fold difference in weight, from 5 to 150 pounds. If we include small premature infants and obese adolescents, the discrepancy may be as much as 100-fold. In some instances dosages may be computed on the basis of age, which is a rough guide. However, in most instances the calculations are more nearly accurate when they are referred to weight. Sometimes a more precise method of comparison through calculation of the surface area of the individual is used. Size differences also dictate variations in certain technical procedures, such as transfusions, where the diameter and the accessibility of veins create special problems in the very small child.

FLUID ADMINISTRATION

Pathophysiology

Water. A continuous supply of water is a more urgent requirement for life than a supply of food. Martyrs have been known to starve themselves for a month or more and still survive, but life will not go on for more than a few days if the body is denied water. The essential processes of the body not only require water for their continuing operation but also they gradually exhaust the internal supply. During healthy existence there is a continuous loss of water in stools and urine, from the evaporation of sweat from the surface of the body and with the air exhaled from the lungs. Disease not only aggravates these losses through such changes as fever, diarrhea, vomiting and increased urine output, but also it may increase the water requirement by speeding up some of the body processes through an increased metabolic rate. At the same time the individual may be unable or unwilling to ingest even his normal quota of fluid. If the process continues, he uses up the reserve fluid stored in his tissues and begins to show the symptoms of dehydration—dry mouth, thick secretions, hollow eyes, loosening skin, concentrated urine and loss of weight.

The child, and more particularly the infant, reaches a stage of dehydration faster than the adult. In part this is due to the fact that he is less able to recognize and satisfy his needs for water, and in part it is because the smaller he is, the greater is the proportional quantity of water in his body and the more rapid is the rate at which it is used. This rapid use of water becomes apparent when we remember that it is not difficult for some adults to get along indefinitely on a pint and a half of fluid per day. Yet the new-born infant, who may weigh only one-twentieth as much, usually cannot manage on much less than a pint of fluid per day.

It is upon cellular processes that the body depends for its vital activities. Although cells differ widely in their appearances, in the functions they serve and in their chemical contents, they have certain general properties in common. Each is surrounded by a semipermeable membrane which ordinarily retains the protein and other large constituents of the cell. Water, oxygen, nutrient materials and certain salts and minerals can enter through this membrane, while the waste products and substances which the cell is designed to produce diffuse out through it into the surrounding space. Cells in general are distinguished chemically from the surrounding tissue fluids by their heavy content of protein and the predominance of potassium and phosphate salts.

INTRACELLULAR WATER. In both adults and infants about 45 per cent of the body weight represents the water contained within these vital units—that is, the intracellular water. To function properly, each cell must be supplied not only with the oxygen and the nutriment that it requires, but its water and salt contents must be kept from varying beyond certain narrow limits. The body tends to defend the integrity of the cells during health and disease.

PLASMA. The fluid portion of the blood (plasma) contains protein which during health remains within the walls of the vessels, and water and mineral salts which can leave the vascular bed freely and enter the surrounding tissues. To function properly the fluid volume of the vascular bed must be kept within certain limits. If it becomes too small due to loss of blood or to extreme dehydration, shock will result; if it becomes too large, the heart may be unable to move it along at the normal rate, and fluid will ooze from the vascular bed to produce edema of the subcutaneous tissues or, more seriously, of the lungs. In health both the adult and the infant have about 5 per cent of their total body weight as plasma or intravascular fluid. In addition to its characteristic content of proteins, the plasma has mineral salts in concentrations which are quite different from those of the intracellular water, since the predominating components are sodium and chloride. As in the case of the intracellular fluid, many mechanisms in the body tend to keep the composition of the plasma within a narrow range.

INTERSTITIAL FLUID. Around the cells and between the blood vessels there is a third type of fluid—the interstitial fluid—which has a composition very similar to that of plasma except that it is practically devoid of protein. Interstitial fluid represents the reservoir within the body which responds most easily to the shifting conditions of disease. When it increases, edema results; during dehydration it is depleted in preference to the plasma or intracellular water supply. Unlike the latter two fluid compartments, its relative magnitude is greater in infants than in adults. The adult carries about 15 per cent of his total body weight as interstitial fluid; the small infant begins life with 25 per cent of his body weight in this form but approaches the adult proportions as he passes beyond the age of 2 years.

Some changes in the fluid content of the body during disease are relatively easy to visualize and understand. The infant with diarrhea and vomiting is obviously losing more fluid than he can take in and suffers a depletion of the interstitial fluid, which gives the typical signs of dehydration. Conversely, the child whose kidneys do not excrete water because of cardiac or renal disease will retain fluid in the interstitial compartment if he continues to take his usual allotment of water and will thus become edematous. However, although water can move freely within the body across the membranes which separate the three fluid compartments, its movements are intimately tied to changes in electrolyte concentrations (particularly sodium) within the body. The mechanisms which regulate the flow of water and electrolytes are still incompletely understood.

Electrolytes. As the body must take in water continually to replace the losses through normal metabolism and excretion, so too it must have access to a continuing supply of minerals, such as sodium, potassium, calcium, magnesium, etc., and of their salts, the chlorides, bicarbonates, phosphates and sulfates. Under normal circumstances there is an ample supply of these materials in the food from which the body can select whatever is necessary to replace losses through metabolism, excretion or normal wear and tear. In the various fluid compartments mentioned above the concentrations of each of these substances (called ions) is kept within definite limits. The kidney plays the most important role in regulating these concentrations, for it has the ability to hoard or discard them selectively, depending on the needs of the moment. (The normal range of plasma constituents is shown in the Appendix, page 558.

In the presence of dehydrating illnesses it must be remembered that loss of water from the intracellular compartment is accompanied by a loss of potassium, and that even though no deficit of this element may be reflected in the blood serum levels, a deficit may exist within the cells which needs correction.

Acid-Base Balance. The relative concentrations of the various ions within the tissue fluids influence the acidity of these fluids. During health the plasma maintains a very constant slightly alkaline reaction. In chemical terms this is measured and expressed by the concentration of hydrogen ions or pH. An exactly neutral fluid has a pH value of 7.0; an acid fluid has a pH value below 7.0 and an alkaline fluid has a value greater than 7.0. The normal range for internal body fluids is from 7.35 to 7.45. (Urine, sweat, saliva and bile are excretions from the internal environment and do not follow the same narrow range.) Life is seriously threatened when the pH value of the plasma falls below 7.0 or rises above 7.7.

In maintaining the acid-base balance of the blood and tissue fluids, the kidneys and the lungs play major roles. The kidney helps to maintain normal equilibrium by its differential excretion of unwanted ions and other substances and by its ability to form ammonia, which greatly enhances its capacity to excrete the acid products of metabolism. The lungs assist in maintaining equilibrium by varying the rate at which carbon dioxide is blown off, hoarding this slightly acid substance when the plasma is getting too alkaline, and blowing it off at a faster rate when the plasma is getting too acid. During health, normal body activities result in the production of an excess of acid substances which must be excreted. Thus the usual productions of the body metabolism (urine, sweat and expired air) are essentially acid in character in order to maintain the balance.

Disease (with a few notable exceptions) tends to aggravate the production of acid substances and places an increased demand on the lungs and the kidneys. This demand must be met if the acid-base balance is to be maintained. Ordinarily, these organs are equal to the task because of their great reserve capacities. When a study of the chemical constituents of the blood reveals that the kidneys and the lungs are being placed under stress but are meeting the challenge successfully and preventing the blood pH from shifting out of the normal range, a condition of compensated acidosis or alkalosis is said to exist. When the stress has become so great that they can no longer prevent the blood pH from descending below 7.35, uncompensated acidosis is present. If the pH rises above 7.45 the condition is called uncompensated alkalosis. (It should be emphasized that in clinical usage the terms acidosis and alkalosis refer to deviations from the normal range of blood pH and are not determined

Table 6. Examples of Acid-Base Disturbance

	pH	CO_2 Content (mEq./L.)*	CO_2 Combining Power (Vols. per 100 ml.)	Chloride (mEq./L.)
Normal infant	7.35-7.45	22	49	98-106
Normal child	Same	25-30	55-65	Same
Mild metabolic acidosis (diarrhea)	7.25	18	40	112
Severe metabolic acidosis (diabetes)	7.10	9	20	95
Mild metabolic alkalosis (pyloric stenosis)	7.50	35	75	90

* This abbreviation is read "milliequivalents per liter." It means that the serum contains so many thousandths of a chemical equivalent in each liter. A chemical equivalent is the combining unit of an ion. In any solution the total number of chemical equivalents of positively charged ions must equal exactly the number of chemical equivalents of negatively charged ions.

$$mEq./L. = \frac{mg./L. \times \text{the valence of the ion}}{\text{the atomic weight of the ion}}$$

It is important not to confuse mEq./L. with mg./L.

by reference to chemical neutrality. Even in severe clinical acidosis with pH values of 7.0 to 7.2 the plasma is still chemically slightly alkaline.)

In clinical pediatrics most of the disturbances of acid-base balance are due to metabolic disorders. Under such circumstances the blood concentration of bicarbonate usually indicates the severity of the process. When facilities for more nearly complete chemical determinations are not available, the values of the CO_2 content or CO_2 combining power of the plasma are commonly used to guide treatment. These levels (which are essentially the same as the plasma or serum bicarbonate) decrease during acidosis so that in a rough way a mild acidosis is usually present when the values are ⅔ of the normal, and a severe acidosis is present when they have fallen to ⅓ normal. In alkalosis the levels rise, and an increase by ¼ ordinarily indicates mild alkalosis; an increase by ½, a severe disturbance. Convenient as these relations are, they do not always indicate the chemical changes accurately. In certain types of acid-base disturbances which originate in respiratory abnormalities, the relationship is actually reversed. For illustration of these statements see Table 6. Additional discussion of acid-base changes will be found with the specific disease entities.

Calories. During the course of disease there is usually an increased need for calories because the metabolic rate has been increased by fever; but, at the same time, several factors commonly conspire to reduce the child's ability to ingest and digest food— vomiting, loss of appetite, weakness, disturbed digestive processes. Consequently, his caloric requirements are usually unmet during the acute stage of an illness, and he must live on reserve stores within his tissues. To an imperfect degree some of his caloric deficit may be met by including calories in the form of glucose in the oral or parenterally administered fluids which are given to combat the more immediate danger of excessive fluid depletion. Calories given in this form also spare body protein and combat the tendency toward the accumulation of some of the organic substances (ketone bodies, acetone and diacetic acid) which play an important part in the causation of acidosis. When fluids can be given only by the parenteral route, the ability to provide calories from glucose or plasma is limited by the amounts of plasma and the concentration of glucose which can be administered safely.

Replacement Therapy

Fluids by Mouth. During many illnesses the loss of fluid and electrolytes is slight, and the child is able to replenish his deficit gradually by taking *fluids by mouth.* The daily amount of fluid required varies with the degree of the disturbance and the size of the child. For infants the daily intake must exceed the normal requirement of 125 ml./Kg. of body weight if they are to catch up. Older children require less per unit of weight, so that intakes of 1,500 to 3,000 ml. per day are ordinarily sufficient. It can be assumed that the electrolytes will be restored if mineral-containing fluids, such as milk, fruit juices and soups, are included as part of the intake. Enough fluid to produce a copious flow of urine is desirable in order to give the kidneys the optimal chance to correct minor changes in the electrolyte composition of the plasma and hence of the interstitial and the intracelluar fluids. If the volume of urine is small, the opportunity for renal correction is handicapped.

Parenteral Administration. When illness is complicated by vomiting, loss of consciousness, refusal to eat, the necessity of resting the gastrointestinal tract or a severe loss of water and electrolytes which requires rapid correction, fluids must be restored by routes other than the oral one. Such *parenteral administration* may be given under the skin, i.e., directly into the interstitial fluid compartment from whence it will be taken up by the blood and distributed in time to the other tissues of the body; or it may be given directly into the vascular system by injection into a vein. A third route which is used occasionally is the injection of fluid into the peritoneal cavity, from whence it is absorbed in a fashion similar to that which follows subcutaneous injection.

Fluids which are to be given parenterally must meet certain requirements. They must be prepared sterilely and must be protected from bacterial contamination until the injection has been completed. Otherwise, the direct insertion of bacteria into one of the fluid spaces may result in local or generalized infection. Parenteral fluids must have a nearly neutral chemical reaction or they will be irritating and painful to the subcutaneous tissues or to the veins into which they are injected. In exceptional circumstances this requirement is broken with respect to intravenous injections,

but it cannot be broken for subcutaneous injections. A third requirement of parenteral fluids is that they have approximately the same osmotic activity as the interstitial fluid (isotonicity). Osmotic activity is the capacity of a fluid to attract water from or dispense water to the surrounding medium. It is determined by the concentration of ions and molecules. An isotonic solution of sodium chloride (commonly called normal saline) is a 0.9 per cent solution; glucose is isotonic in a concentration which lies between 5 and 10 per cent and in practice is used in either of these dilutions. Other fluid mixtures, too, must be constructed so as to meet the requirement of isotonicity in order to avoid undesirable shifts in the distribution of water in the tissues into which they are injected. *Distilled water is never an acceptable fluid for either intravenous or subcutaneous use.* (Given intravenously it may cause hemolysis of the red blood cells which results in a serious or even fatal reaction. Given subcutaneously it is quite painful and may damage the tissues into which it is injected.)

Subcutaneous Infusion (Clysis). When fluids are given by subcutaneous infusion or clysis the total quantity used is adjusted according to the size of the child and his needs. The rate at which the fluid is administered usually is governed by the speed of absorption from the subcutaneous space, the flow being adjusted so that painful swelling of the tissues is avoided. There is little likelihood that too rapid injection of fluid will cause any disturbance other than local discomfort when subcutaneous fluid is used, for the blood stream accepts what it needs at the moment and leaves the remainder unabsorbed. In some instances an enzyme (hyaluronidase) is added to increase the rate of absorption. Under these circumstances the nurse must use great care not to exceed the rate of flow ordered by the physician.

Intravenous Infusion (Transfusion). When fluids are given by intravenous infusion or transfusion the total quantity administered and the rate of injection must be calculated very carefully. Such fluid is passing into a closed space which is distensible only within certain limits; if it is overloaded, it may lead to serious or even fatal embarrassment of the circulation. The normal intravascular space may be visualized as a partially inflated balloon. During a dehydrating illness the balloon collapses somewhat, due to loss of its fluid content. Filling it with fluid to distend it back to normal size is desirable in order to promote good circulation; however, if it is overdistended and tense, the circulation will be hampered, and if pushed to the bursting point life will cease. Fluids which contain only water and nonprotein solutes are relatively safe because they can ooze through the walls of the blood vessels at a fairly rapid rate and relieve the mounting internal pressure if necessary. However, there is a limit to the speed at which they can diffuse out of the vascular bed. For nonprotein-containing fluids it is probably safe to administer 30 ml./Kg. at one time to an infant. When continuous infusion of such materials is being given, the daily volume usually should not exceed 150 ml./Kg./day.

Caution is imperative when protein-containing fluids (blood or plasma) are being used, for these substances cannot ooze out, and whatever increase in distension of the vascular space is produced will remain for a period of hours or days. The hazard is particularly great in infants. As a general rule, it is unwise to give more than 20 ml./Kg. of body weight to an infant in a single dose. It is usually wise to allow 12 to 24 hours to elapse before the procedure is repeated. (The technic of exchange transfusion, which will be described in Chapter 10, involves simultaneous withdrawal of blood so that these rules do not apply to it.)

Selection of the Amount and Kind of Fluids. Clinical circumstances vary so widely that only a brief description can be given here of the general principles used in planning fluid and electrolyte replacement. More detailed discussion is included under the headings of the specific conditions in which it is required.

The physician planning the child's needs for parenteral therapy must think of three general categories:

1. *Maintenance*—the amount of water and electrolytes which will be required per day to substitute for the child's usual intake when he is not ill and is able to consume food and fluid by mouth.

2. *Deficit replacement*—the amount of water and electrolytes lost as a consequence of his illness, which will have to be restored before he can catch up.

3. *Contemporary losses*—the fluid and electrolytes which are being or will be lost during the course of continuing illness from vomiting, diarrhea, through the urine or through body fistulae or nasogastric tube drainage.

Sometimes the situation is simple and only maintenance need be planned, as in the case of a well child who undergoes an operation which temporarily cuts off his oral consumption. More usually, both maintenance and deficit replacement must be planned because some degree of dehydration has followed illness and losses in the interstitial and intracellular water compartments must be met. With severe dehydration there may be additional loss of plasma water to the extent that the child is in or near shock, and immediate expansion of plasma volume is necessary to restore cardiac and renal function. For this latter purpose, the usual electrolyte solutions may have to be supplemented with plasma, plasma substitutes, or transfusions.

Table 7 gives the approximate amounts of water (total fluids) required for maintenance and for the correction of moderately severe dehydration at various ages. Part of the total fluid correction must consist of electrolyte (salt-containing) fluids. Selection of the type of fluid (Table A-2 in the Appendix) depends upon

Table 7. Approximate Fluid Requirements at Different Ages

Age	Maintenance ml./Kg.		Correction of Moderately Severe Dehydration ml./Kg.	
	Total Fluids	Salt Containing	Total Fluids	Salt Containing
Premature	50-70	10-15		
Newborn	80-100	25	150	35
Newborn—1 year	150	35	200	100
1-2 years	100	25	150	75
2-4 years	90	25	120	60
4-10 years	70-50	20-15	100-80	50-40
Over 10 years	40	10	70	30

the doctor's concept of the losses sustained as determined from the patient's history, physical findings and measurements of the chemical constituents of blood and urine. Initially, replacement therapy is usually begun with a solution which simulates diluted interstitial fluid, such as Ringer's solution, lactated Ringer's solution or maintenance electrolyte solution. When the laboratory reports are obtained, more precise calculations of specific needs for sodium, potassium, chloride and the correction of acidosis by the use of bicarbonate or lactate can be carried out and the composition of the fluids administered are changed accordingly. The frequent early change in fluid orders is due not to the fact that the physician cannot make up his mind, but rather to a more precise change in his concept of what is chemically wrong.

Calorie supplements are also desirable to spare body tissues during illness and starvation, but unfortunately they can be supplied only in limited amounts through the intravenous route because of considerations of volume. Glucose in 5 or 10 per cent solution (D/W) is commonly included among the fluids to be given. When starvation is prolonged, some additional calories may be supplied as plasma or as a mixture of amino acids prepared for intravenous use (Amigen).

Nursing Care

Oral Fluids. A skillful nurse can play an important therapeutic role by encouraging the child to accept an adequate amount of fluid by mouth. In doing so she may be able to help him to avoid the discomfort of parenterally administered fluids. She will be more successful if she can adopt an attitude of patient and pleasant encouragement than if she displays demanding exasperation at the child's failure. Too much urging may result only in overfilling the child's stomach and consequent induction of vomiting. In most instances some latitude of choice in the selection of the particular fluid to be given is permitted. Offering the older child a choice or trying the infant on several types of liquid may provide the answer to a problem of obstinate refusal.

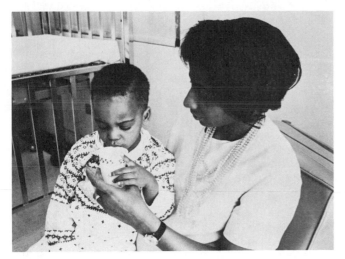

Fig. 4-1. When fluids need to be urged, the nurse or mother will succeed better with relaxed gentle encouragement than by hurried forcing.

Accurate record-keeping is always important in order that the necessity for parenteral fluids can be judged by the physician. Estimates of the volume of vomited fluids should be subtracted from the intake administered. Truth and accuracy in such records promote the best interests of the patient. It is also important to observe the frequency and volume of urine production of a child who is in need of fluid therapy. If urine is being produced freely, it probably means that the kidneys are able to perform their corrective work; if urine is scanty or absent, the fluid intake is probably insufficient.

Venipuncture. Measurement of the chemical constituents of the blood is usually desirable in the presence of important degrees of dehydration. Nurses need to be informed when the fluid and electrolyte balance is in danger, because prompt action is often necessary. Since diarrhea in infants and younger children more often creates fluid imbalance than any other single cause, the nurse must carefully note the fluidity and amount of stools. With acute diarrhea, dehydration and fluid imbalance may develop rapidly, particularly if there has been meager fluid intake. The nurse must therefore be alert to any signs of weight loss, scanty urine volume, dry skin, "furry" tongue or rapid respirations, for these signs may herald impending shock.

With older children the technic of obtaining blood is the same as that used in the adult. However, infants and small children seldom have a vein of adequate size in the antecubital fossa, so that blood must be obtained from the external jugular vein, the internal jugular vein, the femoral vein, or in rare instances from the superior longitudinal sinus. Since failures are frequent, and the risk of reinjection of blood into the vein is a real one, only sterile syringes should be used in venipunctures on infants and small children.

Specific technics for obtaining specimens of blood in infants and young children, for positioning and restraining appear on pages 555-556 of the Appendix.

Subcutaneous Infusion (Clysis). Although this method of parenteral fluid administration is not as frequently utilized as it once was, it continues to be the preferred method in certain circumstances for infants and young children. Several sites are available, but the anterior and lateral aspects of the thighs are generally the most serviceable. The child must be restrained on his back in such a way that he will not be able to reach his legs and remove the needles. For a prolonged procedure, arm and ankle restraints are necessary.

Other places into which the clysis may be given are the pectoral region and the back. Frequently the back is used as a site for single injections of fluid into premature or small infants. It is also sometimes used in older children when the thighs are not accessible. The

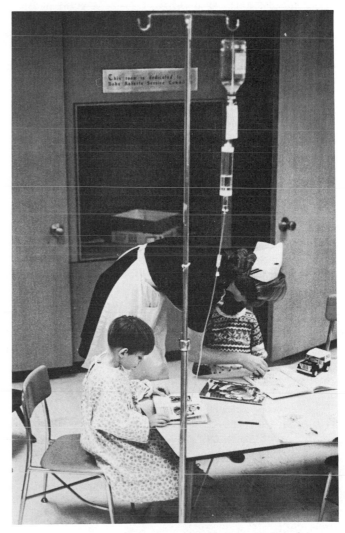

Fig. 4-2. An infusion or transfusion need not interfere with play activities.

equipment to be used for clysis and the procedures to be followed are described on page 560 of the Appendix.

In most hospitals, the nurse is responsible for monitoring the administration of parenteral fluids. She is expected to keep accurate records of intake and output and must be alert to the symptoms of imbalance previously mentioned.

Intravenous Infusion (Transfusion). Any treatment which utilizes a needle is perhaps one of the most frightening of the many unfamiliar experiences of a child in the hospital. The anticipation of pain is a large component of the fear, which is compounded by the equipment necessary for intravenous infusion or transfusion. In addition, children may have many fantasies accompanying this type of intrusion into their bodies which compound the fearful aspects of the experience.

Although children's responses to and management of pain have barely been studied, several aspects have been investigated. It is apparent that several factors are involved in any particular child's response to this type of treatment. Among these are the child's age, his previous experience with needles, his level of ego strength and cognitive functioning and the support he receives throughout the experience.

Certainly, the age of the child is important in his response to intravenous therapy. The small infant has a stimulus barrier which delays his reaction and may reduce his sensitivity to painful stimuli. In addition, his intellectual level and lack of previous experience eliminate the fear and anxiety of anticipation which assail the more mature infant or child. However, this does not mean that the painful experience is unimportant when dealing with an infant, for he *is* quite vulnerable to severe pain or prolonged discomfort and resents the restriction of motor activity. By staying with him and holding him when possible, the nurse can help him to tolerate his discomfort. Perhaps more importantly she will be bolstering his trust in his environment, which is an important ingredient in the development of a healthy ego.

For older children, the meaning attributed to this treatment may be colored not only by their previous real experiences but also by their fantasies. The level of preschool children's reasoning about causality is not mature. They regard their parents as all-powerful and often feel that since the parents have abandoned them to the care of strangers, they undoubtedly wanted to do so and there must be a reason why. The obvious conclusion is that the painful and frightening experience has been imposed upon them because they have been "bad." Some children, because they feel guilty of some wrongdoing that they do not completely understand, may welcome a painful procedure that reduces their guilt.

Because of the above factors, and as previously mentioned in Chapter 2, young children also feel that this type of treatment is a hostile act on the part of the nurse and the physician. Erickson, in her play interviews with preschool children, found that intrusive procedures involving the skin were seen as hostile. Children in the oedipal phase of their emotional development may also imagine such intrusions into their bodies as punishment for masturbation, or may interpret such injury as injury to the genitals.

The unfamiliarity of the child with the equipment necessary for intravenous therapy in most cases is interpreted as a danger much worse than the reality seen by the nurse. Thus the vehemence of the young child's protest may surprise the nurse unless she is aware of the child's possible interpretations.

Although it may not be possible to completely reverse the meaning of this experience to the young child, it is possible to reduce his fear and anxiety and to support his own coping efforts. One way to do this is to prepare the child psychologically for the experience. Vague threats that are not understood, and unexpected stress, are more upsetting than an unpleasant experience which is expected, even to the young child. The timing and depth of explanation must, of course, be geared to the age level of the child. Forewarning children about pain is much more helpful than attempting to assure them that it "won't hurt." Even a young child can prepare himself inwardly and marshal his available coping capacities when a painful procedure is not completely unexpected. If no previous warning is given, the child may fear that even worse things may happen to him later. Giving explanations of what is about to occur also allows the child to express his feelings about them, to communicate his interpretations of them to the nurse, and to develop trust in her. Although the mother's presence is often supporting to the child, the nurse must also understand that the experience of seeing her child receive an intravenous infusion or transfusion can be upsetting and her anxiety may be transferred to the child. However, if the nurse takes the time to explain the reason for the procedure to the parents, their anxiety will also decrease. Some mothers may not wish to be with their child and should not be subjected to further anxiety by the disapproval of the nurse.

Although preparation is more effective for older children, even very young children can benefit from a simple explanation, directed to them. Sexton has stated:

To a child under two years of age, words may mean little; but if these words are directed to the child rather than to the parents and are said in an honest and sincere way, the child will get an idea that something is going to happen that may not be pleasant, but has to happen, and that everything will be done to make it as easy as possible. . . . I believe as early as two years, or even earlier, they can get a feeling of reassurance from the way they are handled and talked to. Sexton, H. M.: Emotional preparation for hospitalization, Amer. Surg. 26:422, 1960, p. 422.

Other ways the nurse can help to relieve the child's tension and anxiety are by controlling the environment as much as possible to avoid unnecessary displays of frightening equipment and, as stated in Chapter 2, by allowing the child freedom of choice as to the manner in which some steps of the procedure are carried out. Staying with the child as much as possible during the infusion or transfusion helps, as does acceptance of his feelings and of his protest. Following the experience, the offering of play activities during which the child can attempt to master the experience may do much to reduce subsequent ill effects on emotional development.

The equipment and procedures necessary for intravenous infusion or transfusion for infants and for older children are described on pages 559-560 of the Appendix.

Collection of Urine Specimens. A urine examination is part of the usual diagnostic procedure for any child admitted to the hospital. It is also often necessary during treatment to measure the rate of excretion of a given medication and the progress of treatment. Alert cooperative older children can be managed in the same way as adults, but special technics are required for infants and toddlers who have not yet acquired bladder control. These are described on pages 556-558 of the Appendix.

For infants, the discomfort involved in collecting a specimen is the necessary restraint. Checking the collecting device frequently so that the specimen can be retrieved before it is spilled or contaminated minimizes the period of annoying restriction of motor activity.

Although catheterization of older children is less often used because it may introduce infection, it may be necessary if urine for culture is desired. Of course, preparation for the procedure is necessary for all children old enough to understand. Cooperation usually can be obtained by showing the child the equipment before it is sterilized, if possible, and explaining the reasons for each step of the procedure. If a prepackaged tray is to be used, it is often possible to allow the child to play with similar equipment, which often helps him to mobilize his resources for cooperating. Practicing deep breathing, which produces relaxation and makes insertion of the catheter easier, also helps the child learn how he can help himself during the actual procedure. A second nurse is desirable, either to support the cooperative child or to help the child who is too young to profit from preparation.

DRUG ADMINISTRATION

General Considerations

It is the physician's responsibility to determine what kind and what amount of drugs are used in the treatment of a child. Determination of the proper dose of

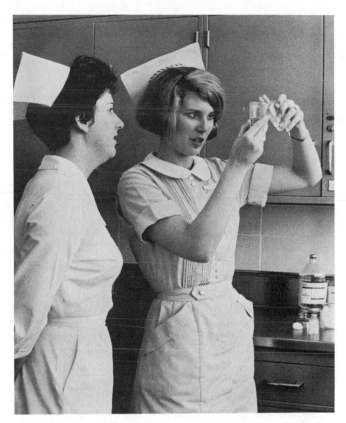

Fig. 4-3. Until the student feels secure in pouring and administering pediatric dosages, she welcomes the help of a more experienced nurse.

drugs is his legal and moral responsibility and is usually converted into a written order so that there is no misunderstanding. Because of the wide range of body sizes of children, drugs must be prescribed according to weight or surface area, or sometimes according to age. The nurse should familiarize herself with the recommended dosages of drugs used on her patients so that she may check the calculations made by the physician. In some instances recommended dosage is contained in the literature supplied in each package of drugs; otherwise, dosages may be obtained from sources such as the Physician's Desk Reference (Medical Economics) or from standard pediatric texts.

Nursing Care. It is impossible to overemphasize the responsibility which the nurse carries when administering drugs to any patient. However, when dealing with a child, that responsibility is especially grave because often the child is unable to communicate verbally signs of distress that indicate overdosage or idiosyncrasy. He has to rely on the nurse's accuracy and on her ability to detect undesirable effects from the drugs that must be reported to the physician.

Since the number of drug forms introduced each year is increasing, and nurses often are given greater responsibility in dispensing and administering medications, the importance of informed observation cannot be overemphasized. There are many sources of information on current drugs, yet no one directory is all inclusive. Some nurses find it helpful to keep a 3×5 index card file with adequate cross references.

Although allergic reactions to drugs are less frequent in children, the nurse must know the common signs and symptoms of drug reaction, such as unexpected rashes, fever or unusual behavior patterns. She should know the potential of the drug she is administering to cause reactions and be informed of the contents of capsules and pills. This could be most important if the child should need the drug again. Emergency equipment necessary for treating drug reactions must be easily accessible and the nurse must be familiar with its use.

The nurse must also promptly record symptoms even if she is not sure of their meaning, and she must check the information on the chart prior to giving medications to be certain that orders have not been recently changed.

When the nurse is familiar with the dosage of a given drug and believes that an order is erroneous, she should always call it to the doctor's attention before administering the drug. The alertness of the nurse may spare her patient a serious episode. It is her primary responsibility to communicate with the physician if she is uncertain about an order. This is especially important in pediatric care because many drugs are not used in standard dosage and must be regulated according to the size of the child. In administering any medication, the nurse should have some general understanding of what the treatment is intended to accomplish and what an appropriate dosage of the drug should be. Some of the drugs commonly used in pediatric practice are considered below. Others will be described in relation to specific diseases.

The nurse also needs to find ways in which to make the unpalatable and the more uncomfortable medications more acceptable to the child. Giving medications in a way that establishes and maintains a constructive relationship with the child is as important psychologically as the drug is important therapeutically.

ORAL MEDICINES. In administering oral medications to an infant, the nurse's chief responsibility lies in getting the prescribed amount into his stomach with the least possible discomfort to him. Many medicines can be made more palatable by mixing them with a small amount of syrup. They can be given from the tip of a small spoon or with a medicine dropper. The baby's head and shoulders should be elevated as a few drops of the medicine are placed well onto his tongue. Giving medicine slowly enough to be swallowed and to prevent choking is a measure of great importance. If too much is given at one time, the infant will spit it out or choke. Choking is uncomfortable and conditions him negatively to the experience of taking medicines.

The nurse's approach in administering medicine to the toddler will be a potent factor in determining his capacity for cooperation. The toddler's nature will be described in Chapter 16. It explains the dynamics which are operating when he says, "No, I don't want to," or attempts to push the medicine away or closes his mouth to avoid the unpleasant. Because medicines are necessary for the child's recovery, the option of taking them or not taking them cannot be left to him. The nurse must help him to know that they *must* be taken but that she understands his dislike of them and his wish to control the situation. Poise, expectancy of cooperation and faith in the child's ability to learn all support the strengths within his personality; they give him the help he needs to make controls a part of himself. At first he may need to be held because he has no inner ability to control himself. After the nurse has helped the child to take the medicine, saying something like the following helps him know that his nurse believes that he can learn to take medicine independently: "Someday you will be able to take your medicine all by yourself. I know you'll learn to do it in a little while." Soon the child will show an interest in holding the glass by himself or in choosing between a spoon, a straw or a glass. With this simple device the medicine often is taken willingly. It is accepted because the fact that he is given a choice indicates to the child a recognition of his struggle to regain the autonomy he had acquired prior to the time he became ill. In the sick child's shaking hand a few drops may be spilled, but the progress made in helping the child to recapture his feelings of self-esteem and power and in developing a constructive relationship with his nurse outweighs any loss of medicine the first time it is given. A good relationship solves the problem in regard to all medicines that are to follow.

Force in giving medicines is never justifiable because it communicates hostility instead of helpfulness. Furthermore, it accomplishes nothing because the child always can have the last word. Usually he can vomit the medicine that has been forced on him—and he will unless he gets support in controlling his drive to remove the unpleasant.

In order to approach the child with the confident expectation that he will take his medicine, the nurse needs faith in the child's capacity to learn to cope with disagreeable things. Gaining this faith comes from *experience* which proves to the nurse that she *can* help children to face reality. Understanding the naturalness of the drive to strike out against unpleasantness with verbal or physical resistance helps the nurse to accept these overt expressions of feeling without becoming anxious about them. Once the nurse has acquired this ability she can continue to build up her self-confidence and her faith in the capacity of children to tolerate frustration of their urge for perpetual pleasure. This takes time, for success does not come instantly.

An interest in learning about the many ways that children have of resisting the unpleasant also helps the nurse to become increasingly more able to take their behavior in stride. She will wait calmly to discover their special ways of reacting and dealing with medicine and will support them with her understanding of their need for help in adapting to the demands of this treatment. The nurse who has confidence in her patient is supportive. The nurse who doubts her competency communicates her uncertainty and weakens the child's capacity to cooperate because she reinforces his anxiety with her own. When sufficient experience has made her a supportive person, the nurse will find that children take in her strength and make it a part of themselves. When the nurse has succeeded in helping a child to accept the unpleasantness involved in taking his medicine, she will notice signs which indicate that his self-esteem has been heightened and his personality has been strengthened through his experience with her. He has become a bigger person in his own eyes, and, in all probability, he will make known his wish to have it recognized by the person who has contributed to his growth.

There is no one absolute technic that can be given to nurses for winning a child's cooperation. Each child manifests his uniqueness at medicine time just as he does at every other time. If the nurse thinks of her patients as persons who are in the process of learning, she will take more understanding into her relationships with children. She will also become motivated to study her patients in order to find ways of teaching which increase each child's capacity to participate in his care.

INJECTED MEDICINES. The psychological principles of giving subcutaneous and intramuscular injections of medicines are the same as those cited for administration of oral medications. The child's need for preparation, support and permission to vent his feelings in relation to painful treatments has been discussed. Intramuscular injections are painful; they are also frightening to the vast majority of children. The sick child's threshold of pain and fear is lower than that of the well child. Therefore, every possible measure must be taken to help him to master his feelings about the experience.

The universal fear of injections among hospitalized children has been very well documented. Gips, in studying how illness experiences are interpreted by hospitalized children, found that at every age, injections ranked first in frequency of mention in discussing treatments. These children also questioned the motivation of the nurses giving the injections, relating the procedure to punishment. The interpretation of painful procedures as hostile has been previously mentioned, but in the case of medications injected into the buttocks, this interpretation is accentuated because this area of the body is frequently associated with punishment.

The first intramuscular injection is of great importance because it patterns the child's feelings and behavior for subsequent treatments. If the child's first experience with intramuscular injections provokes feelings that he cannot handle, his days will be heavily weighted with disruptive feelings, and he will dread medicine time thereafter.

The infant has fewer fears than the preschool child. As mentioned in the preceding section, he is less sensitive to pain because of his stimulus barrier and his anticipatory anxiety is restricted by his lack of experience and cognitive functioning. Levy has interpreted absence of crying in infants before injections as the absence of memory of the pain of prior injections. Although the infants he studied were not hospitalized, he found no anticipatory crying up to the age of 5 months, with an increase at older ages. From 12 to 17 months of age however, there was a sharp increase in anticipatory crying. Kassowitz also found that no children under 6 months of age indicated apprehensiveness prior to the actual pain of injection.

On the other hand, young infants are most perceptive to the anxiety of their mothers. When Campbell investigated the crying of infants prior to receiving an injection, she concluded that infants held by mothers who had received fear-arousing instructions displayed more anxiety. The nurse therefore can lessen the tension both of infants receiving injections and of their mothers by explaining the purpose and method of treatment. If the mother is not present, the nurse can pacify the infant easily after the injection is given by holding and soothing him for a few minutes.

Toddlers and preschool children have the greatest difficulties in accepting prolonged treatments with intramuscular medicinal therapy. Preschool children are in a period when fears are characteristically more numerous, pronounced and difficult to handle. Understanding the reason for intramuscular therapy and for being subjected to pain is impossible at this age level. However, the child can understand that it is medicine that is given in his buttocks or his thigh, and that it will hurt when the needle penetrates his skin. A preschool child can help also by choosing the site of injection if it is a single dose and by cleansing the area if it is accessible to him. The procedure is safer and more comfortable for the child if two nurses are available at the time of injection. When two nurses are available, restraint is usually unnecessary. One nurse can distract and support; the other one can give the injection swiftly and skillfully, thereby lessening anxiety arising during a period of fearful waiting. If the child's tension mounts, and it becomes obvious that he cannot hold himself still, body restraint is necessary for his protection. If it is done with a spirit of helpfulness, the child will recognize that the nurse is providing control that he is unable to supply by himself.

Remaining with the child until his equilibrium becomes re-established assures the child that his feelings and behavior have been accepted. During this period encouragement to vent his feelings is important in protecting his mental health. Providing play materials and encouraging self-directed activity serves to communicate the nurse's acceptance of his individual way of responding to a difficult and painful experience and to make it possible for him to gain some degree of mastery of his feelings.

The school-age child and the adolescent can understand explanations and will become less fearful when they are helped to comprehend the nature of the medicine and the treatment. The nurse's approach should communicate her awareness of the youngster's capacity for control and cooperation. It should also recognize the fact that he probably has a variety of feelings concerning his treatment. Offering him the opportunity to talk about such feelings so that he can discover that they are natural to all youngsters will help him to maintain a healthy concept of himself.

Previous mastery of the technic of giving injections of medicine gives the nurse the confidence and the poise that are required in working with children. The nurse who is skillful and plans her approach to the child thoughtfully can do much to minimize the panic which so often becomes a part of intramuscular treatments.

Since in recent years there have been increasing reports of serious traumatic paralysis in children resulting from intramuscular injections, the nurse must perfect her proficiency and skill, based on sound scientific principles. In very young children, the gluteal area is small and poorly developed and injections into this area may endanger the sciatic nerve. For this reason, many authorities today advocate the lateral or anterior thigh for intramuscular injections for infants and toddlers. For a complete discussion of the recommended sites and the technics to be followed in injecting medications intramuscularly, see pages 560-561 of the Appendix.

PHARMACOLOGIC CONSIDERATIONS

Medical and pharmaceutical research during the past few decades has advanced at such a rapid pace that members of the health team are overwhelmed by the number and variety of products available for treatment of the sick child. Physicians and nurses both are faced with an insurmountable task in learning the real and fancied virtues offered by a myriad of chemical modifications of basic substances obscured by long chemical names and shorter trade names. To keep informed about the potential for good and the possible adverse reactions of the drugs she is administering, the nurse requires repeated access to a source of information such as Shirkey's Pediatric Therapy (Mosby) or the Physician's Desk Reference (Medical Economics). The brief orientation about the common types of drugs

in pediatric usage offered below must be supplemented by reading elsewhere and is amplified in some instances when specific disease entities are considered.

Antibiotics and Chemotherapeutic Agents. Most diseases produced by pathogenic bacteria, some produced by fungi, and a very few produced by viruses are amenable to treatment with these agents. Ideally, the specific organism responsible for the child's infection should be isolated through cultures of blood, spinal fluid, body secretions or excretions or the contents of skin lesions; and the organism so obtained should be tested in the laboratory for its susceptibility to antibiotics or chemotherapeutic agents. Judgment must then be used in weighing the expected advantages of treatment against the possible toxic or allergic effects of the agent or the induction of resistant strains of organisms. In actual practice, however, antibiotics are usually prescribed during important infections before the results of laboratory tests are available. The physician thus makes a preliminary guess concerning the etiology of the disease and the antibiotic most likely to be curative. Unfortunately, this technic is too often used without any laboratory control, particularly for relatively minor illness. Sometimes these agents are justifiably used to prevent the recurrence of infections such as streptococcal sore throat, which triggers episodes of rheumatic fever.

The nurse should be familiar not only with the proper dose of the antibiotics used in patients under her care, but should also be informed about the toxic manifestations known to occur with each of the agents employed. It is within her province to be the first to recognize adverse effects such as rashes, vomiting, diarrhea, jaundice, hematuria, drug fever or changes in behavior which might serve as warnings.

Adrenocortical Steroids. Since the isolation of cortisone from the adrenal cortex and the recognition of its potent influence upon inflammatory, neoplastic, connective tissue and immunologic diseases, many therapeutic applications of this hormone and its derivatives have been found in pediatric practice. These agents may be used with relative impunity for short term relief up to three or four days. However, when their administration must continue for longer periods of time, suppression of the production of cortisone by the child's own adrenals may result, leaving him susceptible to adrenal insufficiency or a severe exacerbation of his original disorder if the steroids are withdrawn too rapidly. Since prolonged use of steroids carries certain definite hazards (growth retardation, demineralization of bone, hypertension, peptic ulcer, loss of potassium and accumulation of sodium, moon face, increased insulin requirements, increased susceptibility to infection), the advantages and disadvantages of such long term therapy must be carefully weighed. Life-threatening situations such as severe acute asthma, anaphylactic reactions, rheumatic carditis and leukemia leave no real choice. But with other disorders such as chronic asthma or eczema, rheumatoid arthritis, allergic reactions, nephrosis and other collagen diseases, mature judgment is required. The uncritical use of the steroid preparations for minor illnesses and complaints is particularly deplorable.

The potency of derivatives of cortisone (prednisone, dexamethasone, triamcinolone, etc.) is usually related to cortisone as a standard of efficacy and dosages are adjusted accordingly. Several derivatives provide lesser effects upon salt retention or more potent effects upon inflammatory reactions than cortisone.

Sedatives, Tranquilizers and Antihistamines. These drugs have the same properties in children as they do in adults. Dosage levels must be carefully checked by the pediatric nurse to be sure that a physician used to prescribing for adults has made an appropriate reduction in the amount prescribed for his smaller pediatric patient. The prevalence of these materials freely in the home provides one of the most common sources of accidental overmedication or poisoning of small children.

Diuretics, Anticonvulsants and Antineoplastic Agents. These drugs are considered under appropriate sections in the following text.

SITUATIONS FOR FURTHER STUDY

1. What understanding does the nurse need when nursing a child who requires intravenous therapy?

2. What observational skills does the nurse require when nursing a child requiring intravenous therapy to replace fluids, calories and electrolytes lost during the acute stages of diarrhea?

3. What are the symptoms of dehydration? Why is dehydration serious for an infant?

4. Describe the ways in which you helped a child to cooperate with you in meeting his oral fluid requirements.

5. Observe an infant of from 1 to 2 years of age and describe his reaction to restraint.

6. How do you imagine a 1-year-old child feels when he is completely immobilized and having fluid administered via a scalp vein? Describe a child for whom you are caring who is receiving fluids via the scalp vein. What substitute satisfactions were you able to provide for him? What was his response to you, his doctor, his mother and the treatments he was receiving?

7. What are the nurse's responsibilities in administering medications?

8. Describe a situation in which you helped a child to cooperate in the process of taking his medicine. What were the factors that helped you to be successful? How did the child respond to his success?

9. Describe a child receiving cortisone therapy. What was his reaction to the drug? How did he respond to the nursing care which he required during the time he was receiving cortisone therapy?

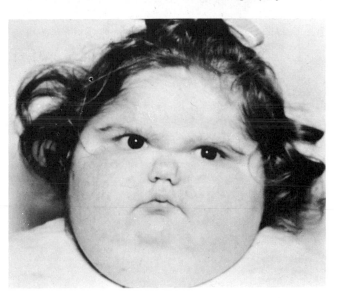

Fig. 4-4. Child with typical moon-face as a result of steroid therapy. (Dr. R. Platou)

BIBLIOGRAPHY

Au, W. Y. W.: Broad spectrum antibiotics, Am. J. Nurs. *64*:105, 1964.

Burgess, R. E.: Fluid and electrolytes, Am. J. Nurs. *65*:90, 1965.

Campbell, E. H.: Effects of Mothers' Anxiety on Infant's Behavior, Unpublished Doctoral Dissertation, Yale University, 1957.

Erickson, F.: Play Interviews for Four-year-old Hospitalized Children, Monogr. Soc. Res. Child Develop. Serial No. 69, Vol. 23, No. 3, 1958.

Frohman, I. P.: The adrenocortico steroids, Am. J. Nurs. *64*:120, 1964.

Gips, C.: How Illness Experiences are Interpreted by Hospitalized Children, Unpublished Doctoral Dissertation, Columbia University, 1956.

Hill, L. F.: Sites for intramuscular injection, J. Pediat. *70*:158, 1967.

Kassowitz, K. W.: Psychodynamic reactions of children to the use of hypodermic needles, Am. J. Dis. Child. *95*:253, 1958.

Kern, M. S.: New ideas about drug systems, Am. J. Nurs. *68*:1251, 1968.

Levy, D. M.: The infant's earliest memory of inoculation: a contribution to public health procedure, J. Genet. Psychol. *96*:3, 1960.

Physician's Desk Reference, ed. 23, Oradell, N. J., Medical Economics, 1969.

Sato, F. F.: New devices for continuous urine collection in pediatrics, Am. J. of Nurs. *69*:804, 1969.

Sexton, H. M.: Emotional preparation for hospitalization, Am. Surg. *26*:422, 1960.

Shaffer, J. H., and Sweet, L. C.: Allergic reactions to drugs, Am. J. Nurs. *65*:100, 1965.

Shirkey, H. C.: Pediatric Therapy, ed. 3, St. Louis, Mosby, 1969.

Unger, D. L.: Non-allergic drug reactions, Am. J. Nurs. 63:64, 1963.

Webb, C.: Tactics to reduce a child's fear of pain, Am. J. Nurs. 66:2698, 1966.

Willig, S.: Drugs, dispensing/administering, Am. J. Nurs. 64:126, 1964.

Wu, R.: Explaining treatments to young children, Am. J. Nurs. 65:71, 1965.

UNIT 2

The Newborn
(Conception to 1 Month)

The newborn period is a time of critical events. The physiologic transition to life outside the uterus subjects the new baby to the greatest mortality risk that he will encounter until he reaches middle age. Defects of genetic or structural make-up must be discovered and evaluated. The rapid rate at which he grows demands careful attention to his nourishment. His ultimate personality development may be strongly influenced by the quality of the emotional climate into which he is born. Particularly, if he is a first-born child, his parents may have to effect a major reorientation of their way of life as they accept him into the family.

In this unit the first four chapters are concerned primarily with the normal newborn. Events prior to his emergence from the delivery room are treated only briefly, for they fall properly in the province of maternity nursing. In the second chapter the infant's view of the world and the world's view of him are considered. Succeeding chapters describe his physical characteristics, nutritional needs and appropriate nursing care. The remaining sections of the unit are concerned with some of the important disorders which the nurse may encounter while working in the nursery for the newborn. These are mainly the consequence of imperfections in the infant's anatomic formation or his failure to adapt satisfactorily to extrauterine life. The nurse's role in providing care to newborns with special health problems is also discussed in this unit.

5

Preparation of the Family;
Nursing Care of the Newborn

PARENT FITNESS

In the United States marriage and the propagation of children are almost entirely a matter of personal responsibility. Most states require serologic tests for syphilis before issuing a marriage license, but otherwise the decision for parenthood is left entirely to the marriage partners. Individuals with family backgrounds marked by inheritable disease can obtain advice about the wisdom of procreating from physicians or from the genetic counseling centers that are appearing in many cities and university centers. Those who have doubts about their psychological fitness for parenthood may consult physicians, mental hygiene clinics or marriage counseling services. Unfortunately, only a very small fraction of the total population is able to avail itself of these professional services.

Babies conceived illegitimately usually create a serious problem for the mother. Among some cultural groups the care of such an infant is assumed frequently by the maternal grandmother who raises the child as her own. More often, moral censure or economic circumstances force the mother to place her child for adoption. Occasionally, legally married women, because of medical necessity, or a surfeit of, or aversion to children, will seek to place their legitimate children in another home.

Adoptions are often a boon to all parties concerned —the mother, the child and the adopting parents. However, certain precautions must be taken if the best interests of the child and the adopting parents are to be served. Ideally, the proceedings should be conducted by an impartial nonprofit agency that is equipped (1) to make proper investigations of the adopting parents, (2) if necessary, to accept guardianship of the child before the legal arrangements are completed and, above all, (3) to preserve the anonymity of the parties involved. Adoptions arranged

without such safeguards may expose the child and his adoptive parents to later harrassment from the natural mother. Legislation governing adoption varies from state to state, and the procedure should be handled by a professional person familiar with the local requirements.

PRENATAL HEALTH SUPERVISION

Once pregnancy has begun, a number of precautionary measures can be invoked to shield both the mother and the child. Unfortunately, the quality of such care varies with socioeconomic circumstances. Comprehensive prenatal care of the mother should include the following: complete medical examination and appraisal of her capacity to adapt to her pregnancy, gynecologic examination, Rh-typing, screening for tuberculosis and syphilis, regulation of diet, protection against certain infectious diseases, and education and support of both parents to help them to adjust to pregnancy, labor, delivery and their parental roles. When physical defects or lack of progress in adjustment to pregnancy are noted, referral to sources of medical and psychological therapy is not only indicated but essential. It is imperative to prevent physical complications and disturbed mother-child relationships in the neonatal period when mutually satisfying experiences are of crucial importance for each person within the family. This is a large program if done properly, but experience has demonstrated that it pays dividends in decreasing maternal and infant mortality and morbidity and in minimizing the problems of child-rearing in the first crucial weeks of life.

Careful physical and laboratory examination of the mother early in pregnancy protects not only her own interests but also those of the fetus. The detection and the prompt treatment of diabetes, anemia, tuberculosis, and cardiac and renal disease has a direct

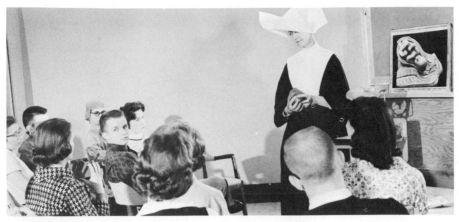

Fig. 5-1. Maternity supervisor conducting a class for expectant parents. (St. Mary's Hospital, Evansville, Indiana)

bearing on infant mortality by decreasing the chances of premature delivery, toxemia and anoxia. Similarly, careful pelvic measurement and periodic gynecologic examination permit accurate planning of the delivery in order to minimize birth trauma and anoxia from mechanical causes. Rh-typing of the mother's blood segregates the negative reactors so that they may have additional tests and be delivered under conditions prepared to handle an infant with erythroblastosis fetalis. States which require all pregnant women to be screened for syphilis can expect almost complete control of the congenital form of the disease, since, when detected during the first half of pregnancy, treatment of the mother can be accomplished before she infects her infant. The detection of tuberculosis in the mother not only permits better protection of her health during pregnancy but also warns of her infectious danger to the infant after his birth. Ideally, screening should be extended to include fathers and others who will be in the child's close environment after his birth.

Vaccination of pregnant women against poliomyelitis is designed to protect them from the extensive paralysis to which they are particularly prone. At the same time the infant is shielded from prenatal or postnatal transfer of the disease from his mother. Rubella with certainty, and perhaps some other infectious diseases, may be responsible for congenital malformation of the fetus when the mother becomes infected during the first three months of the pregnancy. Pregnant women should be shielded from virus infections whenever possible. Gamma globulin or hyperimmune serum may be of some benefit in protecting those who have had a known exposure to rubella. Recently an effective vaccine has been developed which is expected to provide active immunity against rubella and which will be used prior to conception.

Supervision of the food intake of pregnant women is desirable to make sure that sufficient protein and vitamins are being ingested. Severely deficient diets are known to increase the rate of premature delivery, which in turn increases the hazard to the child. Experimentally, it has been possible to produce con-

genital anomalies in the young of pregnant animals deprived of vitamins such as A and riboflavin. Although there is no conclusive proof of a relationship between vitamin deficiency and congenital malformations in man, the supplementation of diets during pregnancy is undoubtedly desirable.

Supportive care during pregnancy is given through group educational programs and within the context of a constructive relationship with a health worker. Education of the prospective parents in the rudiments of obstetrics fosters better cooperation with doctor and nurse, a confident approach to the coming delivery and security in their ability to function as parents. Today the pendulum has swung back from scientific rigidity, and young couples are showing enthusiasm for a return to natural methods of child-bearing and rearing. The increased popularity of educational programs, natural childbirth, breast-feeding, rooming-in and self-regulatory schedules are manifestations of a desire to recapture some of the instinctive emotional forces which have become submerged in the artificiality of scientific medicine.

Classes for expectant parents which are conducted as question-and-answer periods provide a popular device for giving some guidance before difficulties arise. Discussion periods have the advantage of permitting the participants to ventilate their anxieties either directly or vicariously through others who have the same worries. Many parents have said that they accepted with equanimity those aspects of labor and delivery and of their infant's behavior which had been forecast for them in classes for expectant parents. Principles and attitudes which are discussed beforehand are accepted more readily in guidance of the child after birth.

In addition to the group educational program cited above, the expectant mother needs continuity of personal relationship with a health worker who understands the psychology of the reproductive cycle. Continuity of relationship not only gives reassurance but also provides the milieu that is necessary to help the expectant mother with those problems in her personal

FIG. 5-2. When the mother is fully conscious during delivery the husband often can provide emotional support. In a few hospitals there is no regulation against having the father present during delivery. However, individual physicians can deny a couple this privilege if they feel that it is in the best interest of the patient to do so. (St. Mary's Hospital, Evansville, Indiana)

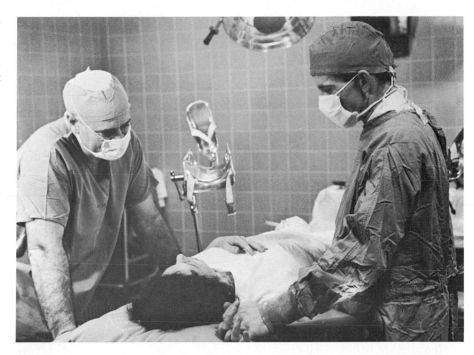

adjustment which cannot be aided in group discussion. Every pregnant woman needs an opportunity to share her feelings, fears and doubts with an understanding person. Many individuals who need the help of an expert will never be detected unless there is continuity in relationship which helps the woman to feel safe enough to disclose her true feelings. Ideally, this relationship should continue throughout the maternity cycle. Under these conditions and with her needs for help understood, the mother can make a healthy adjustment to motherhood.

FETAL GROWTH

The early stages of fetal development are the most remarkable and in some ways the most crucial period of human growth. The new individual starts as a microscopic cell (the fertilized ovum) which in some incredible manner contains the impulse to direct it through a series of carefully controlled subdivisions which mimic the evolutionary history of man and result after 9 months in the emergence of an infant endowed not only with the universal structure of his race but with many of the individual traits of his parents.

When compared with the postnatal growth which we are able to observe, fetal growth takes place at an extraordinarily rapid rate. The adult weighs about 20 times what he did at birth; but the newborn infant weighs about 6 billion times what he did at conception. Within this period he has changed structurally from a single-celled organism to a complex of organ systems which can support life outside his mother's body. During the first eight weeks of the period of gestation growth proceeds at its most frantic pace, and rearrangements are made which bring most of the organ systems close to their final forms. It is during this critical period of organ formation that errors in the sequence of developmental changes are particularly apt to result in malformation or even death of the fetus. Careful prenatal care is designed to maintain an optimal environment for the fetus by shielding the health of his mother.

If the rate of fetal growth were uniform, babies would have identical weights and lengths at birth. But from experience we know that considerable variation occurs. Babies who are born too soon (prematures) are understandably small; those who remain in the uterus too long (postmature) surprisingly do not emerge larger than average. (See Chap. 9 for further discussion.) What then are the influences that account for differences in body size among infants with gestational periods of approximately 40 weeks?

Genetic factors, both racial and individual, account for some of the variation. Mothers of certain ethnic and national groups such as Orientals, Mexicans and Negroes bear infants who tend to be smaller than the average for the United States; those of Dutch, Belgian and German descent are more likely to have babies who are large at birth. Similarly, the body size of individual parents may be mirrored in their offspring from the very beginning.

Nutritional factors also play a role. Mothers with diets that are optimal in calories, protein and vitamins tend to bear larger babies than those on restricted food intakes. It is not always easy to distinguish between the influences of diet and those of race.

The size and the condition of the placenta often appear to determine birth weight, but the reasons for small or diseased placentas are not always clear.

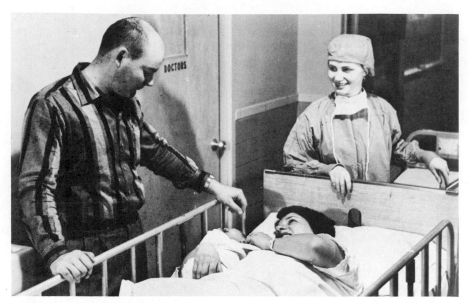

FIG. 5-3. Opportunity for the family to begin functioning as a unit is provided immediately after the baby arrives. (St. Mary's Hospital, Evansville, Indiana)

Some *congenital malformations* interfere with intrauterine growth.

Maternal diabetes is the chief factor which accelerates fetal growth and leads to the birth of infants who are much above the size that would be expected for the gestational age.

PHYSICAL ADJUSTMENTS AND IMMEDIATE CARE AT BIRTH

At the moment of birth the infant is suddenly required to leave the parasitic existence in which his mother supplies all of his physiologic needs and to fend for himself by putting into operation the mechanisms of independent survival which have been developing slowly within his body. The crisis that he faces demands rapid and complex changes. Although most babies complete this transition successfully, the infant mortality rates (Chap. 3) for the first and second days of life show clearly that this is the most dangerous period of childhood.

Prior to birth the infant's connection to his mother through the umbilical cord is literally his "life line." Through the cord circulation he is able to oxygenate his blood, replenish it with the nutriments needed for his growth, and discharge via the placenta and his mother's circulation the waste products of his metabolism. With the severance of the cord at birth, his most immediate necessity is to continue the transport of oxygen to the tissues of his body. If this fails for more than a few minutes, he may suffer important damage, particularly to cells in his brain; if the interruption is prolonged to 20 or 30 minutes, he probably will not survive at all. If the infant is to succeed in this important transition, it is necessary for his brain to respond to the stimuli of birth (especially the falling oxygen concentration of his blood) and, by reflex action, start the muscle movements which make him gasp, cry and eventually breathe. At the same time he must discharge the fluid from the alveoli in his lungs so that air can enter and oxygenate his blood. Simultaneously, his circulation must readjust so that blood which formerly went in large volume through the cord and into the placental circulation is redirected into his own expanding lungs.

The first obligation of the delivery room staff is to see the newborn safely over this hurdle. Usually, it will be sufficient to clear his airway by gently wiping or sucking the excess secretions away from his mouth

Table 8. Apgar Scoring Chart*

Sign	Score		
	0	1	2
Heart rate	Absent	Slow (below 100)	Over 100
Respiratory rate	Absent	Slow, irregular	Good, crying
Muscle tone	Flaccid	Some flexion of extremities	Active motion
Reflex irritability†	No response	Grimace	Cry
Color	Blue, pale	Body pink, extremities blue	Completely pink

* This method is used for evaluating the immediate postnatal adjustment of the new-born baby. The total score of the five signs is 8 to 10 when the initial adjustment is good. Infants with lower scores require special attention. Scores under 4 indicate that the child is seriously depressed. Courtesy of Virginia Apgar, M.D., and Smith Kline & French Laboratories, Philadelphia, Pennsylvania.
† Tested by inserting the tip of a catheter into the nostril.

and nose while he completes the transition to extra-uterine breathing himself. The Apgar scale (Table 8) is useful in making a rapid evaluation of the success and the speed of the infant's initial adjustment. Babies performing normally score 8 to 10 within the first minute after birth. Lower scores which do not improve within the next few minutes are an indication that the infant requires special attention. Some of the reasons for poor adaptation and the methods of handling them are discussed in later chapters of this unit.

Soon after birth the umbilical cord loses its value to the infant because the placenta separates from the internal uterine wall, and the vessels of the umbilical circulation constrict. If the circumstances of delivery will permit it, ligation and cutting of the cord are delayed until vessel pulsation has stopped so that the infant will receive as much of the blood contained in the placenta as possible. Ligation of the cord must be secure to prevent oozing or secondary bleeding, and the stump should be covered with a sterile dressing to avoid infection. When the possibility of an exchange transfusion is entertained, the cord is cut long and kept moist by the application of wet dressings.

At birth the infant leaves an environment which is constantly warmed by his mother's body. Except in hot weather he will lose body heat rapidly unless he is protected. Once separated from his mother he should be placed in a warmed blanket or heated crib if his condition appears satisfactory, and necessary manipulations should be conducted with a minimum of exposure. If resuscitation or other immediate treatment is required, it should be carried out in a place designed to maintain body temperature. A mobile heated unit is often used for transferring the infant to the nursery.

In addition to the immediate adjustments which are monitored by the obstetric staff, the infant will have other transitions to make. He must now ingest his own food and fluids, eliminate his wastes, defend himself against infection and inform the people around him when his requirements are not met. These less urgent adjustments will be considered in more detail in subsequent chapters in this unit.

SITUATIONS FOR FURTHER STUDY

1. What are the principles involved in prenatal health supervision?

2. What are the influences that account for differences in body size among full-term infants? How might size influence a father's view of his son?

3. What physical findings are used to evaluate the newborn's initial adjustment to being born?

4. How would you help a woman who asked you what you thought of adopting a baby?

BIBLIOGRAPHY

Apgar, V.. Proposal for a new method of evaluation of the newborn infant, Current Res. Anesth. & Analg. 32:4, 1953.

Auerbach, A. B.: Parents Learn Through Discussion, N. Y., John Wiley & Sons, Inc., 1968.

Burgess, L. C.: The unmarried father in adoption planning, Children 15:71, 1968.

Daniels, A. M.: Reaching unwed adolescent mothers, Am. J. Nurs. 69:332, 1969.

Davis, M. E., and Rubin, R.: De Lee's Obstetrics for Nurses, ed. 18, Philadelphia, Saunders, 1966.

Fitzpatrick, E., Eastman, W., and Reeder, S. R.: Maternity Nursing (11th ed.), J. B. Lippincott Co., Philadelphia, 1966.

Herzog, E.: Unmarried mothers—the service gap revisited, Children 14:105, 1967.

Milic, A., and Adamsons, K.: Fetal blood sampling, Am. J. Nurs. 68:2149, 1968.

Reed, E. F.: Unmarried mothers who kept their babies, Children 12:118, 1965.

6

The Newborn and His Family

NEUROMUSCULAR ENDOWMENT OF THE NEWBORN

One of the factors that set man apart from the lower animals is the remarkable development of his brain, the organ which not only integrates his sensations, muscle movements and bodily functions but also governs his intellect, emotions and personality. At birth the brain is well advanced structurally. While the body as a whole increases 20-fold before reaching maturity, the brain enlarges only about 4-fold, and most of this growth is completed in early childhood. However, in many respects the brain is functionally primitive at birth. Its ultimate potential will be reached only after years of experience with the world around it. In this chapter we are concerned with the initial endowment of the newborn, his expected behavior and early adjustments to the influence of others.

Sensory Equipment. TOUCH. The infant's first im-

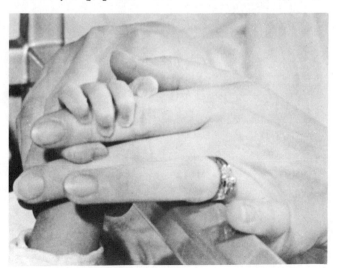

FIG. 6-1. Communication takes place between mother and baby in the grasp reflex. (St. Mary's Hospital, Evansville, Indiana)

pressions of life in this world come to him through the sense of touch. He feels the touch of the attendants at the moment of his birth. He becomes aware of the security of his crib and the comfort of his mother's hands and body long before the world beyond makes any impression on him. Sensitivity is particularly keen about his face where contact of his cheek with a warm object initiates the rooting reflex, and stimulation of his lips produces sucking.

Sensitivity to pain and temperature extremes is present at birth but is not pronounced. During the first week or two the newborn's reaction to painful stimuli is sluggish and delayed. Later he reacts more promptly and violently, but he has little ability to localize the site of his discomfort.

Early knowledge of the people around him is acquired mainly through these tactile sensations which convey to him the feelings of security, pleasure and love. His concept of his mother is gradually built up from the manner in which she handles him. If she is gentle, confident and comforting, he learns to recognize her as a source of solace and pleasure. Through the same mechanisms he may also sense annoyance, anger or anxiety on her part or in others who provide his daily care.

SIGHT. The newborn's eyes are small and deeply set. Although he is quite aware of differences in light intensity and may even follow large moving objects in a vague way, his visual acuity is poor. He cannot focus on objects, for he is farsighted, and the mechanisms for coordinating the movements of his eyes are not yet developed. His pupils respond rather sluggishly to light, but he will blink, squint his eyes or perhaps sneeze when exposed to a bright light. The common notion that bright lights and flash bulbs will injure his vision is unfounded; they merely make him uncomfortable.

HEARING. During the first few days of life the newborn may seem relatively oblivious to noise because his hearing is blurred due to the retention of fluid in the middle ear. Once this fluid has been replaced with air he responds to noise by blinking, starting or crying. However, it will be some weeks before he learns to differentiate sounds and to perceive the directions from which they come.

TASTE AND SMELL. Neither the sense of taste nor the sense of smell is highly developed at birth. Acid and bitter substances placed in the newborn's mouth may evoke reactions of displeasure, and sweet fluids are more readily accepted than bland, but the newborn is relatively indifferent to subtler nuances of flavor.

SENSE OF BODY POSITION. Newborns often show evidence that they prefer to lie in a particular position. In many instances this appears to be related to a position which they maintained in the uterus before birth, during which time some muscles were stretched and others permitted to shorten. Resumption of this posture probably places minimal strain on the structures involved. The newborn also is keenly aware of any disturbances of his equilibrium and reacts to sudden position changes with the Moro or startle reflex.

VISCERAL SENSATIONS. From close observation of newborn babies it seems clear that a good deal of their crying and discomfort arises from sensations within the body itself. When a spell of fretfulness is promptly relieved by food it is reasonable to assume that hunger contractions of the stomach were the source of discomfort. Sometimes burping or vomiting terminates a fussy period, suggesting that overdistention of the stomach was responsible. Many infants fuss and cry for a short period prior to the passage of stool or gas. In this case they undoubtedly feel the preparatory contractions of the large bowel. Other types of internal discomfort undoubtedly lead to crying, but since the newborn cannot communicate with any precision, explanations must remain speculative.

Motor Activity and Reflexes. GENERAL ACTIVITY. The baby at birth has little or no voluntary control over his muscular movements. Most of his activity appears in the form of random movements, mass responses to stimuli and built-in reflexes. Some of these last movements are necessary for his survival, but others appear to be vestiges of movements once useful to his distant forebears in the evolutionary scale.

A hint of the voluntary control that he will achieve later is seen in the unpredictable way in which he looks at and briefly follows large objects which are directly in front of him. This rudimentary eye control is the first in a series of advances that he will make rapidly during the first year (see Chap. 12). Controls appear first in the upper portion of the body and sequentially involve the eyes, the facial muscles, the head and the neck, the arms, the trunk and the legs— the cephalocaudal progression of development.

Newborns differ widely in the number of random movements which they make and in the vigor of their response to stimuli. Some will remain almost immobile during their wakeful periods. Others wriggle, squirm, stretch and turn their heads intermittently or almost continuously. In response to disturbing stimuli the more placid infants gradually become restless, whimper and eventually cry. On the other hand, some react promptly and violently with loud crying and mass flexion or extension of the extremities. At this age the arms and the legs move together when the infant is active, for the ability to control movement of one side of the body or a single extremity separately has not yet been attained.

When lying on the abdomen even a newborn infant may raise his face off the bed momentarily. This should not be taken as evidence of head control, for his muscles are too weak to prevent his head from flopping about helplessly when his body is lifted. Until he is 3 or 4 months of age the persons handling him must take pains to support his head when he is moved about.

REFLEXES. Prominent among the reflexes that are necessary for survival are those associated with nourishment. The *rooting reflex* causes the small infant to turn his head toward a warm object placed against his cheek. Its function is to help him locate his mother's breast when nursing. Those unfamiliar with it misinterpret the infant's behavior when he turns away from the breast toward the hand which is trying to rotate his head in the proper direction. The breast itself must be used as the stimulus. The reflexes of *sucking* and *swallowing* are well developed in all normal infants at term. The *gagging* reflex is also present for the purpose of rejecting material entering the pharynx which is too coarse or irritating to be passed

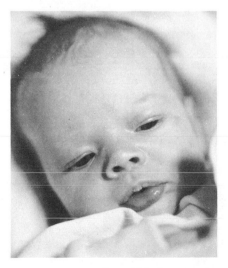

FIG. 6-2. A 10-day-old baby attempting to focus his eyes on an object held directly in front of him.

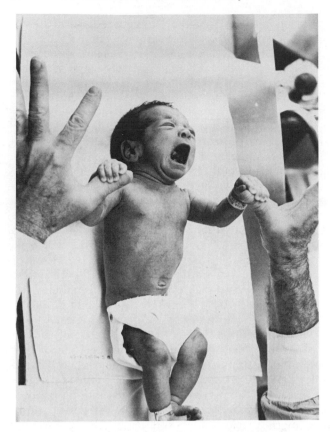

FIG. 6-3. The newborn's grasp reflex is often strong enough to permit his shoulders to be lifted from the bed—occasionally his full weight can be supported.

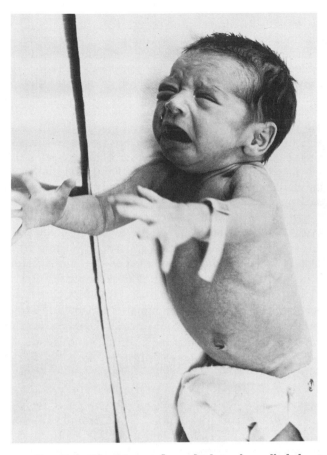

FIG. 6-4. The Moro reflex, which is also called the startle or embracing reflex, is elicited in the newborn by disturbing his equilibrium. In the full response he extends his arms outward with fingers spread and then brings the hands toward each other. The response is accompanied by a cry or other evidence of distress.

on to the esophagus and the stomach. Perhaps *vomiting* should be included as a protective reflex which guards against overdistention of the stomach or the retention of indigestible substances.

Other useful reflexes include *blinking* which protects the cornea from foreign bodies, *sneezing* and *coughing* which keep irritants out of the respiratory tract, and *yawning* which occurs automatically when the infant's rate of respiratory exchange is insufficient to quite meet his needs. *Crying* probably can be regarded as an important reflex, for it attracts the attention of those in his environment to the fact that something is wrong which he is unable to correct by himself.

The functions of the autonomic nervous system are all developed, and, in a sense, these can be considered to be reflex actions.

The presumably vestigial reflexes are the grasping, the Moro (startle) and the postural tonic neck reflexes. In many newborns the *grasp reflex* is so well developed that the infant can almost hang by himself when a rod or a finger is placed in his palms. Of no obvious use to humans today, this strong automatic clutch is almost universal among other young primates who cling to the mother's fur almost continuously until weaned. It is undoubtedly

a holdover from our own more primitive ancestors. The *Moro* or *startle reflex* is elicited by a sudden loud noise or by pounding or jarring the infant's crib or by dropping him a short distance, thus disturbing his equilibrium. The infant immediately extends his arms in a tense, quivering, sustained embrace and usually cries vigorously in fright. The evolutionary function of this reflex is not clear, but it may also be an automatic attempt of the young animal to find and grasp his mother's fur. In contrast, the *tonic neck reflex* is a postural reflex observed chiefly when the infant is relaxed or asleep. In its most characteristic form, the infant, when lying on his back, has his head turned to one side, the arm and the leg on the side toward which he is looking being extended, while the opposite arm and leg are flexed. This arrangement of head and extremities has been called the fencing position. Sometimes, if one turns the baby's head gently in the opposite direction, the position of the extremities can be reversed. Babies often sleep in some modification of this posture, but it usually disappears during waking hours. A similar pattern of coordination is seen among reptiles such as the turtle, suggesting a very ancient origin in the scheme of evolution.

Sleep. A large portion of the small baby's day is occupied in sleeping. For the first few hours following birth he may appear particularly drowsy and unresponsive because of the effects of drugs and anesthetics administered to his mother or from the effects of pressure on his head during passage through the birth canal. By the second or the third day of life he has usually recovered from such temporary depression. The sleep of the newborn is usually neither deep nor continuous. He seems to stay close to the waking level with frequent movements, changes in his respiratory rate and transient periods of wakefulness. Individual differences are seen. Some infants remain in one spot while others may move all over the crib or regularly work themselves into one corner due to repeated kicking with heels or knees. The length of sleeping intervals is also an individual matter which is regulated by hunger as well as other basic physiologic rhythms.

THE NEWBORN'S EMOTIONAL OUTLOOK ON HIS NEW WORLD

Importance of the Mother. The crucial figure in the infant's new world is the mother from whom he has just been separated (although under some circumstances her place must be assumed by others such as the nurse, the father, relatives or others). But for most babies the emotional tone of the outside world is set by the mother. A good many babies are for-

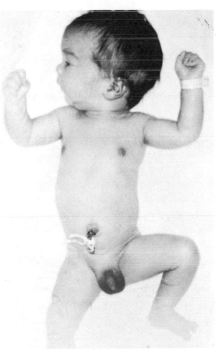

FIG. 6-5. The tonic neck reflex (T.N.R.) position. (Dr. R. Platou)

tunate in having mothers who are able to follow a healthy intuition and quickly create a warm, comfortable environment in which the new baby thrives with minimal problems of adjustment. In such situations there should be a minimal amount of intervention on the part of outsiders. Professional advisors will do well to observe the pleasant result quietly, learning what they can from it and leaving well enough alone. On the other hand, when mothers and babies are less comfortable in their new companionship, the nurse should be prepared to offer practical assistance, and to do so she must have some understanding of the emotional forces at work. The nurse might keep a simple principle in mind: The reduction of a disagreeable (negative) sensation results, not in emotional neutrality, but in an agreeable (positive) sensation. The reverse is true, also. Thus, relief of anxiety promotes confidence; of frustration, satisfaction; of pain, pleasure; of anger, love; and so on.

The Temporary Frustration of Birth. During intrauterine life the fetus enjoyed a comfortable dependence on his mother. He was warm, protected and secure in a close relationship which met his every requirement. The intrauterine environment was presumably free of uncomfortable stimuli such as frustration, pain and anxiety. Instead it supplied all those essentials needed to prepare him for the difficult task of adjusting to extrauterine life.

Physiologically, the healthy full-term infant is prepared for life in the outside world. He has the capacity to breathe by himself, to root for the breast, to suck, swallow and digest his food, and to excrete waste products. With his well-developed nervous system he can signal his needs to others and respond generally to the persons around him.

Even though the newborn is physically equipped for extrauterine life, being born is a hazard for him. Birth is frustrating and threatening because it separates him from the only source of physical and emotional comfort he has known. It thrusts him into a world of new experiences, many of which are anything but pleasant—for example, tracheal suctioning, exposure to bright lights, falling body temperature and the forcible instillation of drops into his eyes. He reacts to delivery as if the new experience were dangerous. It is difficult to believe that all the screaming and the struggling of the first 24 to 36 hours is solely in response to physiologic needs. Close, intimate care given when he cries invariably lessens bodily tension. Thus it seems logical to assume that at least part of his distress is due to the loss of constant physical contact with his mother.

Intuitive mothers supply the desired contact by fondling and cuddling their babies, who soon learn that the missing comfort can be restored on demand. Mothers who are ill, emotionally upset or inhibited either by hospital regulations or by preconceived notions about discipline are more likely to leave their

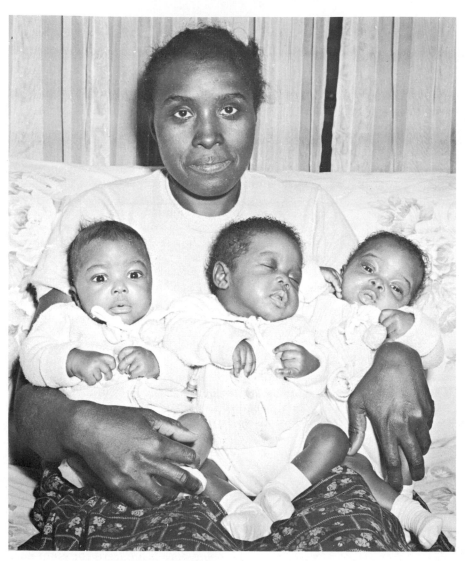

FIG. 6-6. No two babies are alike. Each of these triplets responds differently to being held by his mother while the picture is taken. (Infant Welfare Society of Chicago)

babies frustrated and thus delay the time when they will settle down into a more peaceful state.

A Cry for Help. Besides announcing his distress at loss of contact with his mother the infant will also express discomfort from hunger, fatigue, unsatisfactory body position, abdominal distention, soiled diapers and extremes of body temperature. Because he lacks psychological defenses to handle the frustration and anxiety which these bodily sensations evoke, he quickly becomes physically restless and then uses his main protective weapon—his cry. At first his cry is simply a primitive discharge mechanism, a signal for help which fails to indicate the source of his discomfort. No matter what the stimulus, he wails—as loudly from a minor annoyance as from a strong hunger pain. However, in the course of a few weeks he begins to acquire subtle modulations in his voice which provide clues to the nature of his unhappiness. A responsive mother begins to learn this primitive language and thus becomes increasingly able to meet his needs accurately.

During the early weeks of life the newborn must adjust to a myriad of new experiences so that some periods of fretful crying are inevitable. From his point of view this new world is full of dangers, and his instinctive reaction to them is anxiety. It will take time for his bodily functions to fall into smooth working order and for his senses to handle the stimuli which impinge on them. In order to conquer his constant sense of danger he must have repeated comforting and reassuring experiences. His mother also needs time to become acquainted with his disposition and his own peculiar technics of communicating with her. Experimentation (and, hence, inevitable moments of frustration) will be necessary before a mutually satisfactory schedule of care can be devised. During this period in the early weeks of the child's life it will be the mother who has to yield the major concessions in effecting workable compromises between conflicting desires.

Environmental Factors That Ease Emotional Adjustment. PHYSICAL CARE. The activities associated with the physical care of the newborn have profound emotional significance for him, and their importance cannot be ignored in any discussion of the requirements of healthy personality development. It is easy to see how meticulous attention to his immediate physical requirements for warmth, cleanliness, food, dry diapers and a comfortable position will contribute both to his physical protection and his psychological adjustment. If these procedures are carried out with gentleness and due appreciation for his needs of the moment, the infant cannot help but sense the loving concern of those who are caring for them. Every touch, however received, contributes an impression of the outer world. As the child's nervous system develops, these impressions are integrated into his personality and influence the attitudes that he will form toward other persons and things and toward himself.

Even though the infant cannot appreciate the importance of all physical care measures, they are meant to protect him against traumatic experiences in the future.

ACCEPTANCE OF THE BABY'S UNIQUE PERSONALITY. The newborn is an uncontrolled, dependent, helpless individual who functions on what Freud called the "pleasure principle." He wants what he wants when he wants it, irrespective of the needs of others. To him *want* is a painful and threating experience. He has no resources other than his cry and muscular activity with which to handle the frustration and anxiety which it generates. He cannot satisfy his own desires and has few ways to reject experiences for which he is not ready. His personality is not yet formed. He has powerful pleasure-seeking instinctual drives (which make up the part of him technically called the id), but he can control neither them nor his body. His response to pleasure and pain is automatic. He can only feel; he has no capacity to overcome danger; he is completely helpless and dependent. Others must discover the source of his discomfort in order to restore his physical and emotional equilibrium.

In such respects all newborns are alike, but in other specifics they differ from one another. Constitutional make-up (physical heritage) and temperament vary markedly. Each baby reacts to and deals with discomfort (danger) in his own way. Many newborns make an easy adjustment to neonatal life, but some never seem to relax. Noises, bright lights, handling and sudden changes in position touch off violent crying. Other babies will react to these same stimuli but perhaps not so quickly, frequently or intensely. Similar variations in the need for physical closeness are observed, some neonates requiring a great deal in order to remain happy, while others apparently receive all they need from the process of feeding and a little supplementary cuddling. Soiled diapers, too, evoke varying responses. Some infants cry with every stool and urine passage while others lie or sleep con-

tentedly throughout, giving no indication that they are uncomfortable.

Significant variations in the desire for food and the ability to extract milk from the bottle or the breast are also observed. Some babies appear hungry immediately after birth, while others remain uninterested for several days. It is understandable why some require help in learning to eat. *In utero* no active participation was required; in contrast, after birth, babies must not only find the nipple and suck and swallow but also must contend with the frustration which accompanies the lapse of time between their first hunger pains and the flow of milk. Some babies are able to endure this frustration surprisingly well if a substitute satisfaction such as the motion of a rolling bassinet is provided. Others grow so frantic with impatience that they must be calmed before they can grapple with the task of nursing. The rhythms with which different babies express a need for food are likewise variable. Some are evenly spaced and predictable; others are unevenly spaced but predictable; and some are totally irregular and unpredictable.

The sucking behavior of newborns also differs from one individual to another. Some fasten onto the nipple at once and nurse greedily with full concentration. Such babies resist removal of the nipple for bubbling. Instead of letting go they suck even more fiercely and wail loudly if forcibly separated from their source of comfort. Other infants taste the milk and dally with the nipple before settling down to the task of eating. Still others will rest periodically during the feeding and seem to enjoy the intermissions for bubbling or a change of position. Their need for sucking seems less intense. Attempts to hurry these "resters" through their feedings are fruitless for they only increase tension and ultimately delay the process even further. Such infants are most content when their own slow tempo of nursing is respected.

The newborn requires a long period of dependency with acceptance of his personal idiosyncrasies before he is ready to adapt to those group-sanctioned patterns of behavior which make up the culture into which he was born (for example, the use of a spoon instead of the fingers for eating). The potential for learning to adapt to ever more complex situations is present at birth. It will unfold and develop by itself if the infant is nurtured, stimulated and guided in accordance with his specific pattern of coping with new (probably distressing) experiences. Gradually, he will gain control over his body and will find the inner resources necessary to withstand frustration and to adapt to new customs. But first he must *receive bountifully* from his environment: food, physical attention, love and unconditional acceptance. These are essential not only for physical growth but also for healthy personality development.

THE CULTIVATION OF SECURITY AND TRUST. The newborn must be helped to regain the security that he enjoyed while still a part of his mother's body. Until he can overcome his feelings of helpless inadequacy in the face of this new and unknown world, some of the energy which should be devoted to physical growth will be squandered on emotional reactions of fear and anger. Security is fostered by prompt and skillful response to his distress signals. This principle can be illustrated in the feeding situation. When the baby's needs for food and attention are met consistently and promptly by a mother who enjoys giving, he feels loved and cherished. He begins to associate the pain of hunger which signalled his need with the food which relieved it. At the point at which a connection between hunger and food is made, he begins to gain some degree of mastery over his feelings of helplessness. In his own babyish way he is helping to bring about the satisfaction of his own needs. Thus he gradually acquires confidence in his powers of communication.

The prompt satisfaction of a baby's need for food and comfort does not "spoil" him; rather, it eliminates painful tension. Repeated experiences of fulfillment condition him positively to the feeding process and give him agreeable attitudes toward food. He then becomes more inclined to accept food even when he has not demanded it or even if he is occasionally awakened to receive it. If he learns that his needs are regularly met, he will also learn to accept temporary hunger with less crying and frenzy. As security is developed, his physiologic processes tend to stabilize into a more predictable rhythm of feeding demands followed by periods of restful sleep which lengthen gradually.

The succession of gratifying experiences teaches the infant that he can count on his mother to attend to his needs and assuage his fears. The favorable conditioning he receives toward food is matched by pleasure and trust in the person who does the feeding. After many months of such conditioning the baby probably will have surmounted the first hurdle (trust vs. mistrust) of the socialization process and so will be equipped to move forward toward the solution of other problems. In the meantime each successive new experience which his mother helps him to enjoy will serve to deepen their mutual confidence and affection, besides helping the baby to strengthen the sense of his own identity and preparing the way for the development of close relationships with people other than his mother.

Equally enduring and important influences on the newborn's personality may arise out of repeated *failure* on his mother's part to meet these primary requirements. Deprived of such normal gratifications, he reacts with all the outward manifestations of anger and fear. Even before he learns to recognize his mother as a person he may begin to associate her with his feelings of mistrust, hostility and insecurity. If this most important of the persons in his life fails him in this respect, he will have little foundation on which to build security and faith in others or even belief in himself. Socialization will progress with difficulty, for he will have little incentive either to endure being thwarted or to conform to social custom. In the deep layers of his personality will remain the yearning for satisfaction that he never received and an abiding lack of faith in the future. Since his deprivations occurred at a time when he was not able to understand and the inner resources necessary to cope with such dangers were undeveloped, he may remain a demanding, dissatisfied and insecure individual. Without the basic pleasures and freedom from anxiety which most infants enjoy, his personality will have unhealthy roots, and the steps in subsequent emotional and social development will be difficult to master. Littner comments:

. . . to the degree that his mother can love him and let him love her, and to the degree that he can learn to love her and let her love him . . . to that degree primarily will he be able to be emotionally close to others in later years. Those factors that delay, interfere with or prevent this primary Mother-Child relationship will tend also to decrease his ability to be close to anyone else. Other one-to-one relationships—such as with his father, his brothers, his sisters, his grandparents or the maids—all will contribute, to some extent, to his future ability to relate to others. But even the pattern for these other relationships will be influenced by the nature of his first relationship with the mothering person.*

The Newborn's Cognitive Outlook on His New World. Just as the infant arrives in the outside world with great potential for growth in his emotional repertoire, and in his physical and motor development, so also does he have the inherent potential for tremendous intellectual development, which has great significance to his individual methods of coping with the world. Although at birth the infant's intellectual capacities are completely undifferentiated and he possesses only the ability to respond reflexly, this first period of his life is extremely important to his ultimate level of intellectual accomplishment. Although genetic inheritance imposes limits on the ultimate height of intellectual potential the newborn possesses a vast range of possible achievement, and most people never reach the level of potential intellectual functioning possible at birth.

In the beginning, the infant exists in a state of complete egocentrism, is unable to differentiate himself from his surroundings and responds to others only on a deep body level of sensitivity. Yet from the beginning, originating with such reflexes as sucking and rooting, the infant begins to organize and assimilate his experiences into a cognitive pattern. Individual differences in the newborn's responses to stimulation are also apparent at birth, which have great import

---

* Littner, Ner: Primary Needs of Young Children, p. 1, New York, Child Welfare League of America, Inc., 1959.

FIG. 6-7. Preparation for motherhood begins during the earliest years of a girl's life. (Infant Welfare Society of Chicago)

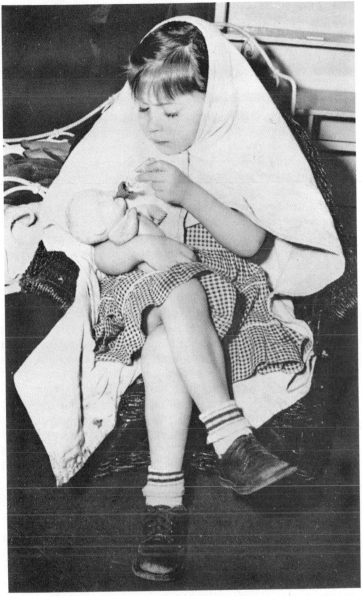

for his later cognitive growth and development and for future learning.

Newborns also have a need for sensory stimulation as well as for abundant rest and sleep. From the many studies now being done with newborn animals, evidence is accumulating that many neural pathways are immature at birth and must be stimulated in order to function adequately, to develop and to become refined. Although infants are unable to focus their eyes on an object at birth, it has been suggested that they can discern patterns within a few hours and need the stimulation of changes in light and shade to develop visual mechanisms which are so important for later perception and learning. They also need tactile and kinesthetic stimulation and variations in the level of sound which surrounds them.

For most newborns, adequate levels of stimulation are soon achieved by the usual activities of care received from a loving mother. Soothing, holding, rocking and changes of position provide skin and kinesthetic sensations; singing and the activities of the home provide differing levels of sound, and visual stimulation is achieved by changing patterns of light and shade as the newborn is moved and carried.

For babies who must remain in a nursery for extended periods of time however, provision must be made for sensory stimulation. Long periods of lying unattended in a crib may well entail sensory deprivation along with emotional deprivation. Experimentation is now being done in providing "rocking-like" movement for premature infants in Isolettes. If the infant is not restricted to an Isolette, nurses can provide sensory stimulation by holding and rocking the newborn while feeding him, by changing his position in space and by other attentions which vary the level of his sensory input.

THE POSTPARTUM PERIOD FROM THE MOTHER'S POINT OF VIEW

The postpartum period is readily recognized as one of emotional instability for mothers. Those engaged in maternity care must learn to accept with equanimity the excesses of enthusiasm, joy, hope, depression and anxiety common to most new mothers. Often the state of mind is difficult to understand because it seems illogical or unrealistic. Many mothers are assailed by a poorly controlled mixture of feelings which include the romantic anticipation of motherhood, anxiety about their capacity to play the new role and the hard facts of practical problems accompanying the new addition to the family. The nurse who understands the factors responsible for emotional instability will find it easier to accept the behavior of the new mother and to present a calm and reassuring approach as she helps her to weather the transition. Only the more common and universal of the endless permutations of maternal attitudes can be considered here. For more detailed discussion the reader is referred to the bibliography.

Development of Emotional Equipment for Motherhood. The capacity for mothering (motherliness) does not become a part of the young woman's character structure the minute her first baby is born. It was engendered during her own infancy through the experience of being loved and protected by her own mother. It grows further through significant personal relationships experienced during childhood and adolescence. During the course of her pregnancy it is likely to be further strengthened by hormonal influences and by her own preoccupation with and planning for the coming event. Of course, mothers who have borne children previously are fortified by personal experience with the mothering process and its pitfalls and rewards.

During the prenatal period important reinforcements in the maternal attitude accrue from the woman's relationship with her husband and the professional persons who are offering support. If she is recognized as an individual with her own specific needs for knowledge, affectionate understanding and relief from anxiety and confusion, she will gain strength for the coming ordeal of labor and the assumption of her new role with its responsibilities. A good program of maternal care is especially important for the primipara. Thus far, continuity of the mother-child relationship has been emphasized as beneficial to the child. Bowlby's summary of the relationship needs of the mother and the child shows that such continuity is equally important to the mother:

. . . the infant and young child should experience a warm, intimate and continuous relationship with his mother (or mother-substitute), in which both find satisfaction and enjoyment. The child needs to feel he is an object of pleasure and pride to his mother; the mother needs to feel an expansion of her own personality in the personality of her child: each needs to feel closely identified with the other. The mothering of a child is not something which can be arranged by roster; it is a live human relationship which alters the characters of both partners. The provision of a proper diet calls for more than calories and vitamins; we need to enjoy our food if it is to do us good. In the same way the provision of mothering cannot be considered in terms of hours per day but only in terms of the enjoyment of each other's company which mother and child obtain.

Such enjoyment and close identification of feeling is only possible for either party if the relationship is continuous. . . . Just as the baby needs to feel that he belongs to his mother, the mother needs to feel that she belongs to her child and it is only when she has the satisfaction of this feeling that it is easy for her to devote herself to him. The provision of constant attention day and night, seven days a week and 365 days in the year, is possible only for a woman who derives profound satisfaction from seeing her child grow from babyhood, through the many phases of childhood, to become an independent man or woman; and knows that it is her care which has made this possible.*

The purpose of the authors in the next section is to suggest some of the ways in which the nurse can function to help the parents after the baby is born.

Sources of Stress During the Neonatal Period. DISILLUSIONMENT. For most women pregnancy eventually becomes a happy state. Abetted by an increase in steroid hormone production, they generally feel healthy and they enthusiastically, almost euphorically, shape an image of the child they are about to bear. The problems which the new child will create tend to be pushed into the background as they bask in the contemplation of their idealized version of motherhood. Birth pricks the bubble of this dream and plunges mothers (from varying altitudes to be sure) down into the world of stark personal reality. Disappointment, anxiety and "postpartum blues" can easily follow when the real baby fails to match the dream baby and the difficulties of motherhood are suddenly brought into the foreground. Part of the function of prenatal preparation is to lessen this disparity between idealistic dreams and probable reality.

DISAPPOINTMENT. Although most women insist that it does not matter to them whether they have a boy or a girl, many actually have a secret preference and so may be disappointed. Some may be displeased to a lesser degree with such characteristics as hair color, eye color, physical features, temperament and size. Of course, imperfections in structure will present a major cause for concern. Such disappointments are usually but not always, temporary. Mothers often admit that they have wished the baby to be different in a certain respect but then added that they have learned to "love him as he is." The nurse can help mothers to overcome disappointment by listening attentively as they express

---

* Bowlby, John: *Maternal Care and Mental Health*, p. 67, Geneva, World Health Organization, Monograph Series No. 2, 1951.

themselves. The opportunity for such confidences with a listener who does not criticize, relieves tension and helps mothers to concentrate on the infant's assets.

SEPARATION. Another commonly expressed feeling is that of "emptiness." Many mothers feel deprived of a portion of themselves when the birth of the baby disrupts the hitherto close physical and psychological union. Part of the maternal instinct is a yearning to restore this contact (we have noted a similar instinct on the baby's part). In many instances there is a period during which the baby, once born, is felt as distant from, or not a real possession of the mother. ("The baby doesn't seem as if he were really mine.") Perhaps this alienation stems in part from the discrepancy between the fancied image of the baby in her womb and the real-life baby with which she is now confronted.

It will take time to re-establish the emotional bond between the mother and the baby, and this period is extremely variable. Many women make the adjustment almost at once. Others may take several days or even weeks before acceptance is complete. Physical difficulties complicating the delivery such as the after-effects of anesthesia, headaches resulting from spinal puncture, and healing episiotomy wounds may delay the re-establishment of emotional unity, for they tend to encourage separation of the mother from the baby until the mother feels more comfortable. A few women never accept the infant and there follows the sad spectacle of a baby growing up in a hostile atmosphere dominated by the rejecting mother. A few such mothers openly admit such feelings toward the infant. More commonly their true attitudes toward the child are buried beneath a frantic attempt to conceal them from themselves and others through guilty overcompensation, which is manifested by excesses of indulgence and anxious concern for the child's welfare.

INSECURITY. In addition to separation, the new mother has many other problems which produce varying degrees of stress. During pregnancy the woman attempts to evaluate her maternal capacities, visualizing in fantasy what it is like to be a mother. However, until she experiences it, she has no real idea of her strengths and weaknesses when faced with the self-sacrifice and the responsibilities entailed in motherhood; nor does she know whether or not the maternal role will be satisfying to her. Even though she has imagined herself in the role of mother and prepared herself for it, the early mothering experiences are often fraught with considerable fear and anxiety ("can I be a good mother and wife?"). She must establish an emotional bond with her baby and learn to trust her capacity for mothering before she can feel at peace with herself and her child. If she has other children, the arrival of the new baby may arouse uncertainty concerning her capacity to succeed in all her intrafamily relationships. Having had previous experience, she realizes the magnitude of her responsibility

to the new baby. She also knows that she will have to help the other members of the family to become accustomed to the new addition.

Changes in the husband-wife relationship are inevitable after the birth of a baby. Husband and wife must learn to share each other with their baby, and their baby with each other. The manner in which each plays the parental role will be subjected to the critical appraisal of the other. The parents are aware of the expectations of their own parents and of their particular social group. Therefore, a new responsibility is required of them: To understand and emotionally support each other not only as mates but also as parents. The success of these parental adjustments will depend on the maturity of the couple and their capacity to accept and understand each other.

DISCOMFORT. While the mother is coping with the aforementioned domestic problems, she also is enduring some real physical discomforts associated with the after-effects of delivery—healing perineum, involuting uterus, engorging breasts and, perhaps, painful nipples. Undoubtedly, the severity of some of these physical symptoms is magnified by the emotional tensions described above, so that it is not difficult to understand why self-concern and self-pity intrude at times and prolong regression. Dependence on others for physical care, pampering and freedom from making decisions is characteristic of women during the period of physical recuperation and adjustment to a new role.

EXHILARATION. These emotional and physical stresses so characteristic of women after delivery may not be at all apparent to the visitor to the maternity ward or the home, who often sees an entirely different picture. The mother may appear to be caught up in an aura of happiness, satisfaction and optimistic planning which usually marks the conclusion of a pregnancy. But the nurse should not be deceived. In more confidential moments with mothers she will find that she must have an appreciation of the conflicting emotional tides that run beneath the exuberant exterior presented to casual visitors.

The Nurse and the Mother. The sympathetic understanding of the nurse who provides her daily care is a tremendous morale booster for a mother who is finding difficulty in adjusting to the after-effects of pregnancy and delivery. The nurse's initial role is to provide physical care and emotional support of the mother (dependency gratification) until she feels physically and emotionally ready to care for herself and her baby. For a time the mother can neither fend for herself in personal care nor manage her baby. Although the system of early ambulation speeds the mother back to full activity, some women nevertheless require a prolonged period of dependency to recuperate physically and regain their prepregnancy level of functioning and independence. If forced too rapidly, such women become resentful and more anxious, and thus the process of adaptation to motherhood is slowed.

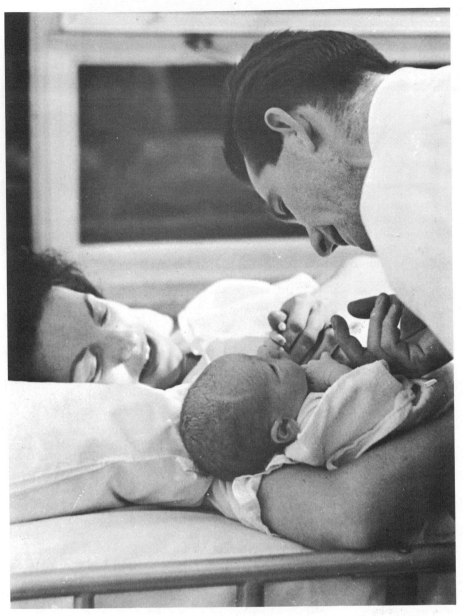

Fig. 6-8. Rooming-in provides advantages for all members of the newly formed family. (St. Mary's Hospital, Evansville, Indiana)

The nurse who respects individual problems is more apt to be accepted as a confidante with whom the mother can discuss her feelings and problems than is the nurse who limits her interest to the mother's physical care. By encouraging the mother to express her worries and resentments the nurse quickly learns what kind of help is most urgently needed. Listening is in itself one of the most important aspects of nursing care. To discuss problems with an interested listener reduces inner tensions and encourages a more realistic view of them. It also promotes self-esteem, for by being attentive, the listener acknowledges the importance of what she has heard.

ROOMING-IN is a physical arrangement of the maternity unit in which the baby is kept by the mother's bed instead of in a nursery. This plan has many advantages, chief among which is that it affords pro-longed close contact for both mother and child. It also makes it possible for the father to visit more frequently and, if he so desires, to have a share in caring for the baby. It gives the mother the maximal opportunity to prove to herself that her offspring is whole, intact and functioning normally. When the interval between delivery and physical contact with the baby is prolonged, the mother tends to worry constantly over his physical state. One short look at the baby in the delivery room is not sufficient; many inspections of the baby are required in most instances. The mother can love and caress him, examine and admire him whenever she chooses without having to worry about the care that he is receiving in a nursery.

Rooming-in has the further advantage of permitting the mother to begin to know her child as an individual very shortly following his birth. This process usually

FIG. 6-9. Note the mothers' interest in watching the nurse bathe the baby. Such demonstrations inspire self-confidence in the mothers. (St. Mary's Hospital, Evansville, Indiana)

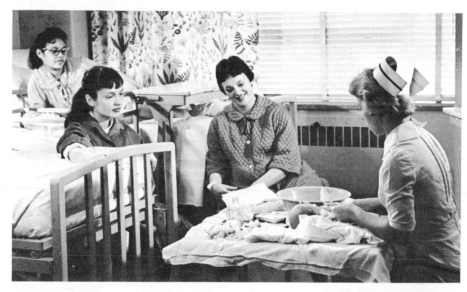

begins with a comparison of his physical features with those she has observed in herself and other members of her family. Gradually she learns in what way he is similar to and different from all other babies; she becomes familiar with the natural characteristics of newborns in general and those of her child in particular. She soon discerns his individual behavior patterns: how he reacts to hunger, physical discomfort and other stimuli. She also learns the means by which he is comforted.

Rooming-in also will bolster the mother's confidence in herself because she can observe and learn from the care measures given by the nurse. During this period the nurse should realize the weight of her responsibility in preparing the new mother for her role. If the nurse is sensitive to the mother's spoken and unspoken appeals for help, many upsetting first experiences in mothering can be prevented.

When mothers and babies room-in together, the maternity nurse is more able to fulfill the role she should properly play—that of a supporting tutor who helps the mother to develop self-confidence. Too often nurses tend to use the nurseries of the maternity ward to gratify their own maternal instincts by "borrowing" the infants without proper recognition of the mother's rights and needs. Sometimes, of course, circumstances prevent this early close relationship of mother and child—for instance, in prematurity or illness. However, in such instances all mothers should have the opportunity to come to know their infants before discharge. Hospitals which are not prepared to offer "rooming-in" may simulate many of its desirable features by liberal interpretation of rules and procedures so that mothers who would like to have extended contact with their infants or who need help in learning to care for them may have it.

DEMONSTRATION AND INTERPRETATION. During the period of dependency immediately after delivery, the nurse must be ready to assume the main responsibility for the care of the infant. But as rapidly as the mother becomes ready to participate in his care she should be encouraged to do so. Unskilled mothers will want help in learning to hold, turn, dress, diaper and bathe the baby. Such help should be offered in a manner which assures the mother that there is nothing complicated or mysterious about the skills required. In the same fashion the nurse's explanation of the infant's behavior and his physical characteristics should be couched in terms which emphasize their normality. For example, if the baby regurgitates and there is no real cause for concern, it is much better to regard it as a common and unimportant nuisance rather than to hint at the possibility of its being a forerunner of pyloric stenosis. If there is cause for concern it is best to acknowledge the presence of the symptom and let the mother know that her doctor is aware of it and will evaluate its significance.

UNDERSTANDING MATERNAL ANXIETY. The several sources of postpartum anxiety have been reviewed previously. Nurses who can listen with sympathetic understanding can shorten this period of anxiety. Recognition that many women must normally go through periods of emotional estrangement from their infants, uncertainty regarding their maternal skills or worry about practical problems at home permits the nurse to offer concrete help in a convincing fashion. When anxieties seem to be unusually prolonged or severe, the physician should be informed of the situation. For the solution of certain practical problems referral to a social worker may be helpful.

FEEDING AT THE BREAST. Of all the mother's ministrations to the new infant, feeding is the one which has the deepest emotional significance to her. In large measure it is through the feeding experience that her confidence is gained or lost. If all goes well, her spirits rise and she is reassured. But if she is unsuccessful by her standards, she is crushed and remorseful.

The mother who wishes to breastfeed her baby will

need help with the new experience. She must be shown how to assume a comfortable position in which she can relax and should be forewarned that the infant's first grasp on the nipple may be painful and that she may feel her uterus contract during the nursing. She must also learn that it is important for the baby to get the nipple and the areola well inside his mouth to prevent irritation and to facilitate sucking. Once she realizes that mothers and babies only gradually become attuned to one another in the nursing process, she will be more inclined to relax and devote more attention to the individual manner in which her baby approaches the breast and uses his rooting reflex to find the nipple.

A hungry baby's interest in the breast and pleasure in sucking affects the mother's whole being. The spontaneous and eager acceptance of the breast does more than stimulate glandular secretion, for it also arouses her love for the baby and increases her confidence in herself as a mother. Thus, from this periodic physical reunion there is a mutual exchange of benefits. The baby receives food, gratification of the sucking instinct and love. The mother finds relief of tension within the breast and the satisfaction of being loved, proving her dependability and gaining a feeling of competence. Benedek has described the dependence of the baby on the mother and the reciprocal need of the mother for satisfactions from the child as a *symbiosis*. Successful feeding serves the needs of the mother and the baby; it re-creates and strengthens the symbiotic relationship that existed prior to delivery.

BOTTLE FEEDING. The mother who decides to bottle-feed her baby needs as much help and encouragement from the nurse as the mother who breast-feeds. She, too, must have the feeling of success to bolster her self-confidence in the maternal role and strengthen her relationship with the infant. The inexperienced mother is disconcerted by the baby's spitting up mucus or regurgitating small amounts of formula, both of which are typical occurrences during the early days. The nurse should show her how and when to "bubble" her infant and how to determine when he has had enough to eat. With the return of physical strength and the growth of self-confidence the mother will gradually be able to attend to forms of care such as bathing, diapering and comforting.

Further discussion of feeding, self-demand schedules, etc., appears in Chapter 8.

THE QUALITY OF NURSING SUPPORT. Helping a mother is more than mechanically teaching the steps of a procedure; it also entails guidance which helps her to achieve fulfillment in her role as a mother. The nurse must be able to relinquish the care of the baby as the mother gains experience and self-confidence. She must also control her impulse to direct, lest the mother rebel at being treated as a child and withdraw because the nurse has failed to credit her with whatever independence she has already achieved. The mother should be encouraged to find her own answers to questions, and where appropriate the soundness of her judgment should be acknowledged. Thus the mother receives professional sanction and emotional strength to surmount the problems she will face alone at home. The knowledge that she acquires of herself and her child will go a long way toward prevention of the panic reactions which many mothers experience when faced with new situations of responsibility.

THE FATHER—THE FORGOTTEN MAN

In attending to the needs of the mother and the baby it is easy to overlook the father as an important participant in the life of the newborn. The traditional notion that rearing children is exclusively the mother's responsibility is obsolete; most fathers wish to be included in the planning for the family at an early stage in maternity care. The absence of a responsible and effective father in the family is recognized as one of the important factors which lead to the rise of delinquency among the young. Fathers should be drawn into the early discussions of the establishment of the family and provided with a significant role in its genesis.

During pregnancy and the postpartum period fathers should be helped to recognize and accept the emotional changes taking place in their wives—instability, dependency, anxiety and uncertainty, all of which increase her need for affection and understanding. They also must learn to accommodate themselves to dislocations in their social and home life created by the last weeks of pregnancy and by the period of the mother's hospitalization, not to mention the problems of financing the maternity care and providing for the new child. If the family has no relative (such as a grandmother) close by, the father will have to plan to take on new duties in the care of the infant and in running the household during the period when his wife is not yet functioning at peak efficiency nor accustomed to her new role of motherhood.

In addition to these specific problems, the father also shares many of the concerns which beset mothers —worry over the normality of the infant, his own ability to function as an adequate parent, and the readjustments which will be necessary within the household.

For these reasons it is desirable to include the father in programs of prenatal instruction and planning for the new baby. Parents' or fathers' classes attempt to clarify the basic facts of labor, delivery and baby care and even to give fathers some practical experience in bathing and dressing a baby and in formula preparation.

Both at the time of delivery and during the newborn period adequate provision should be made to permit the father to take an active part in the welfare of the mother and the baby and to allow his close association with both whenever possible. Early participation in the care of the infant will speed his iden-

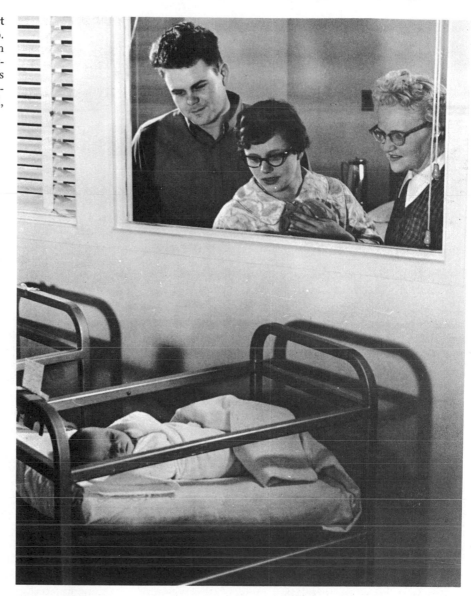

FIG. 6-10. Grandmothers are a part of family-centered maternity care, too. During regular visiting hours when there are visitors other than the husband, the baby is wheeled from his mother's room and placed in an adjoining nursery. (St. Mary's Hospital, Evansville, Indiana)

tification with the baby and diminish feelings of rivalry as the child begins to consume more and more of the mother's time. Early recognition of the father's important part in the new family will help to make the new venture a mutually planned and satisfying one.

EXPANSION OF INTRAFAMILY RELATIONSHIPS

The grandparents-to-be, who probably kept themselves discreetly in the background during the early period of the couple's marriage, become more deeply involved with the new household when a new baby is expected. They not only bring gifts for the newcomer, but they also often feel impelled to impart their own experiences in childbearing and rearing to the expectant parents. Sometimes such advice is a valuable help to the inexperienced couple, sometimes not, depending on a number of factors such as the degree of independence which the couple has achieved from their own parents, the extent to which their

ideas are shared and whether or not it conflicts with the doctor's advice or with the philosophy of child-rearing to which the couple subscribe. This last factor is a classic bone of contention. Philosophies of infant care have changed considerably during the past several decades. Because of the rapid changes in our culture and society, values have also changed and these are transmitted to children through child-rearing practices.

At the time of the grandparent's youth, the nature of the newborn was visualized quite differently from what it is today. At that time the new infant was viewed as endowed at birth with strong and dangerous impulses which needed to be curbed. The mother was therefore advised to wage a relentless battle against her own impulses to "spoil" the baby and to be on a constant lookout for evidences of the child's "sinful nature" such as thumbsucking and later masturbation. Crying was considered to be a bad

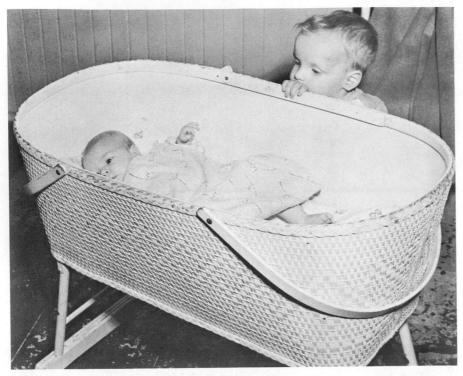

Fig. 6-11. "What's this all about anyway?" (Infant Welfare Society of Chicago)

habit. There was a clearcut distinction made between what was good for the baby and "what he wants."

In a later age, adults began to accept the idea of instinctual gratification for themselves and thus also to pass this concept on to their children in their child-rearing practices. By the 1950's, the nature of the newborn was viewed much differently. Parents were advised by authorities and by popular literature to give their babies plenty of attention, and that their wants for pleasure were legitimate. Under the influence of psychoanalysis, adequate early indulgence was seen as the way to make the baby less demanding as he grew older.

In most respects, this latter view of the newborn continues to be espoused by most child development authorities today. Because the nuclear family is more isolated from their extended family groupings, there is more experimentation with deep biological strivings. Play has been divested of its puritanical association with depravity and parents are urged to "have fun" with their children. Indeed, parents of today often fear that they cannot let go sufficiently to enjoy their infants completely. On the other hand, in recent years, there has been slight reaction toward more emphasis on early development of discipline. This may be due in part to mounting social criticism of the American family as a "pediarchy" in which over-permissive parents are intimidated by their offspring.

Parents are often confused by the varieties of advice they receive and they seek principles to which they can subscribe in guiding their relationship with their children. Often, because they are far from their own parents or feel differently about child-rearing, they turn to professionals for guidance. In addition to the need for knowledge about methods of child-rearing and their effects on later personality development, nurses must be sensitive to the values important to parents and those which they desire to transmit to their children. Nurses also need to know that there is no one correct way for rearing children which holds true for all cultures and societies.

Today, when the period of hospitalization after delivery has been drastically shortened and nurses for home care of mothers and babies are expensive and hard to obtain, the young couple is fortunate indeed if there is a grandmother close by on whom they can depend. If they are comfortable together, she can be of great help to the young mother while she is regaining her strength and learning to combine her old responsibilities with her new ones.

Strengthening relationships with relatives on both sides of the family should begin during the prenatal period. If this task is accomplished successfully before the new baby arrives, the stage is already set for mutually supportive relationships not only during the period when the young people are becoming accustomed to their parental roles but also in the years to come when the newly formed family is comfortably established as an interdependent unit in the larger family circle.

PROBLEMS WITH THE NEXT OLDER CHILD

When a second baby arrives there is inevitably a shift in emotional relationships within the family. The older child must adapt to feelings of displacement as well as he can while his parents make a place for the newborn. On the other hand, parents must also recognize the necessity of safeguarding the older child's status, importance and security within the family. Sometimes, parents are emotionally warmer with their second child than they were with their first. This does not necessarily mean that they love their second child more. It is more likely to reflect the fact that they have become relaxed in their parental roles and, therefore, are able to enjoy their second baby more fully than they did their first.

The firstborn may find this seemingly greater attention for the new baby difficult to accept unless his parents make it plain to him that he is needed, loved and wanted for himself. Parents should understand that anxiety is natural during the period of transition from being the only child to the older one.

During the period of transition it is not unusual for the older child to communicate his need for babying through such regressive acts as wetting himself, demanding milk from a bottle or seeking attention in other ways which were characteristic of him at an earlier age. Some elder children crawl into the baby's crib or try out his carriage in an attempt to communicate their need for more demonstrations of love than they have been receiving. Regressive behavior tends to occur most frequently during periods when the baby is being fed. Scolding the child or ignoring his bids for affection will only make the situation worse. It forces the child to repress his feelings rather than dissipating them harmlessly in the process of coming to terms with a new and permanent family relationship.

Preparation for the coming of the new baby helps the older child to mobilize his resources to cope with a temporary feeling of displacement. However, it will not prevent anxiety, for rivalry is as inevitable as teething. Anxiety is overcome only through repeated experiences which prove that the newcomer has not usurped his place in his parent's affection. Before the baby's birth, he should be told about the changes which will take place in the family and should be assured that the baby will belong to *him* as well as to his parents.

Stories about himself when he was a baby encourage the reliving of early pleasurable experiences with his mother. They also help him to realize that the baby will be small and helpless, unable to play for some time and in need of the kind of infantile care that the older child received when he was younger. It is also appropriate to prepare him for ambivalent feelings (i.e. of both love and hate) toward the baby when it arrives: "There will be times when you will like the baby. There will also be times when you wish he weren't here. He will cry a lot at first, especially when he is hungry. He won't want to wait a minute for his food. You couldn't wait when you were a baby either. At such times you may get mad at the baby and wish he didn't need so much of your mother's

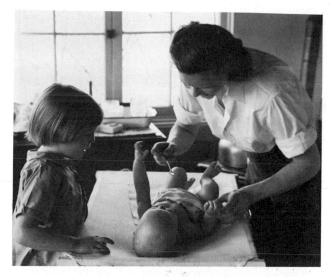

Fig. 6-12. Encouraging the older child's interest in the care of the new baby helps him to find new ways of functioning in the family. (Carol Baldwin)

time." Thus the child is helped to fortify himself against feelings which, while inevitable, should not necessarily leave him helpless and distraught. To try to convince the older child that the arrival of a new baby will be all happiness and bliss gives him no help whatsoever in handling the mixed feelings which are bound to arise. The parent should make an effort to provide special times together when the new baby cannot intrude. Providing opportunities for the older child to take some responsibility in the care of his infant brother or sister is reassuring, especially if he has his mother's helping hand to guide and share the experience with him. The elder child's anxiety will subside when he discovers through experience that he has a special place in his parents' lives that no younger sibling can ever take from him.

PREPARATION FOR CONTINUED CHILD-HEALTH SUPERVISION

Before the family leaves the hospital they should know how community agencies function in providing continued health supervision and guidance for the child. For some parents, particularly when the period of hospitalization is short, the visiting nurse service may be welcome for a short period after the return home. Some mothers are sped out of the hospital before strength and self-confidence are developed. In the absence of helpful relatives nearby, the visiting nurse affords a necessary source of security.

Parents should be urged to see that some form of medical supervision is arranged with a physician or a well-baby clinic so that the necessary immunizations can be given and an evaluation of the infant's progress made. The frequency of such visits varies with the source of care, but in general a first visit should be made within four to six weeks after leaving the maternity unit. The ways in which health supervision can help parents with their problems in child-rearing are discussed in Chapter 3.

SITUATIONS FOR FURTHER STUDY

1. Do you agree or disagree with the statement that birth is frustrating and a threat to the newborn? On what do you base your conclusion? In what specific ways is your behavior in relation to newborns influenced by your conclusion?

2. Describe the behavior of two newborns, showing the ways in which they differ from one another. How was your nursing care influenced by your observation of individual differences?

3. Describe some of the individual differences you have observed in the process of feeding babies from birth to 1 month of age. How was your behavior influenced by your observations? What behavior in the baby gave you the greatest pleasure? What behavior produced feelings of frustration?

4. Trust is considered the foundation on which the personality is built. How does the infant acquire trust? How might illness during the neonatal period prevent the infant from gaining trust? Observe a baby from birth to 1 month in the pediatric ward. How does his disease affect him physically? What basic needs for satisfaction are frustrated as a result of illness and treatment? What are his behavioral responses to this frustration? What have you done to lessen it?

5. What sources of stress have you encountered when giving care to mothers in a maternity ward?

6. What preconceived notions have you encountered which thwarted mothers in meeting their infant's needs?

7. What is the meaning of the words "symbiotic relationship"? What comprises the role of the nurse in helping the mother to re-establish a symbiotic relationship with her baby in the postpartum period?

8. Read Case 1 in David Levy's book, *The Demonstration Clinic,* for an expression of a mother's feelings during the first weeks after her baby was born. What values and disadvantages do you see in encouraging a mother to voice the early feelings she had in relation to her baby? In what other ways might the mother's expression of feeling have been handled?

9. Read Case 2 in *The Demonstration Clinic* and discuss the mother's problems with the baby's grandmother. What do you think accounted for the fact that the mother took further steps in resolving her problems with her mother? How do you explain the fact that the mother's relationship with her baby changed after her experience in the clinic? What purposes do you think the doctor's compliments served?

10. How can knowledge of the importance of success in feeding be used during the period when the mother is first getting acquainted with her baby in the postpartum unit?

11. On the fifth day after delivering a 3-pound pre-mature infant Mrs. J. was ready for discharge. She was dressed and waiting for her husband when the nurse observed that she was perspiring profusely, nervously fingering the chain of her purse and on the point of tears. What would you do in such a situation?

12. Young children often manifest signs of rivalry when a nurse to whom they have grown attached begins to give care to the other children in the unit. What signs of rivalry have you observed in young children? How have you worked to help them handle their feelings?

13. Why is it important for the nurse to know about the intellectual development of infants? What can the nurse do to support this development in an infant who must remain in the nursery for several weeks after delivery?

14. How and why have child-rearing practices changed over the past several decades? Why is it important for the nurse to know about these changes? How can she best help parents who question her about specific practices?

BIBLIOGRAPHY

Aldrich, C. A., and Aldrich, M.: Babies are Human Beings, New York, Macmillan, 1955.

Bellam, G.: The first year of life, Am. J. Nurs. 69:1244, 1969.

Benedek, T.: Psychosomatic implications of the primary unit: mother-child, Am. J. Orthopsychiat. 19:642, 1949.

Bowlby, J.: Maternal Care and Mental Health, Geneva, World Health Organization, 1951.

Brody, S.: Patterns of Mothering, New York, International Universities Press, Inc., 1956.

————: Psychobiological aspects of mothering, Am. J. Orthopsychiat. 26:272, 1956.

Caldwell, B. M., and Richmond, J. B.: The impact of theories of child development, Children 9:73, 1962.

Caplan, G.: The mental hygiene role of the nurse in maternal and child health, Nurs. Outlook 2:14, 1954.

————: Concepts of Mental Health and Consultation, Washington, D. C., U. S. Dept. of Health, Education and Welfare, 1959.

Clark, A.: The adaptation problems and patterns of an expanding family: the neonatal period, Nurs. Forum 5: 92, 1966.

Close, K.: Giving babies a healthy start in life, Children 12:179, 1965.

Dyal, L., and Kahrl, J.: When mothers breast feed, Am. J. Nurs. 67:2555, 1967.

Family Centered Maternity Care, a summary and analysis of the program, Hospital Progress 41:72, 1960.

Family Centered Maternity Care (pamphlet), St. Louis, Mo., The Catholic Hospital Assoc. of the U. S. and Canada, 1960.

Harlow, H. F.: The nature of love, Am. Psychol. 13:673, 1958.

Heinstein, M.: Behavioral Correlates of Breast-Bottle Regimes Under Varying Parent-Infant Relationships, Monographs of the Society for Research in Child Development, Serial No. 88, Vol. 28, No. 4, 1963.

————: Influences of breast feeding on children's behavior, Children *10*:94, 1963.

————: Child Rearing in California, Bureau of Maternal and Child Health, State of California, Dept. of Public Health, 1964.

Hellyer, D.: Your Baby and You, N. Y., Dell, 1966.

Hervada, A. R.: Nursery evaluation of the newborn, Am. J. Nurs. *67*:1669, 1967.

Jenkins, S.: Filial deprivations in parents of children in foster care, Children *14*:8, 1967.

Levy, D.: The Demonstration Clinic, Springfield, Ill., Thomas, 1958.

Littner, N.: Primary Needs of Young Children (pamphlet), N. Y., Child Welfare League of America, Inc., 1959.

McFarland, M., and Reinhart, J. B.: The development of motherliness, Children *6*:12, 1959.

Mead, M.: The changing American family, Children *10*: 173, 1963.

Miller, D. R., and Swanson, G. E.: The Changing American Parent, N. Y., Wiley, 1958.

Richmond, J., and Pollach, G. H.: Psychologic aspects of infant's feedings, J. Am. Dietet. Assn. *29*:656, 1953.

Riker, A. P.: Successful breast feeding, Am. J. Nurs. *60*: 1443, 1960.

Rubin, R.: Basic maternal behavior, Nurs. Outlook, *9*:683, 1961.

————: Puerperal change, Nurs. Outlook *9*:753, 1961.

————: Maternal touch, Nurs. Outlook *11*:828, 1963.

————: Food and feeding—a matrix of relationships, Nurs. Forum *6*:195, 1967.

Sarto, Sister Joseph: Breast feeding—preparation, practice and professional help, Am. J. Nurs. *63*:58, 1963.

Wolfenstein, M.: Trends in infant care, Am. J. Orthopsychiat. *23*:120, 1953.

Wooden, H. E.: Impact of the industrial revolution on hospital maternity care, Nurs. Forum *1*:90, 1961-62.

7

Physical Appraisal and Nursing Care of the Healthy Newborn

To his parents the newborn infant is the culmination of plans, hopes and fears experienced during the long period of gestation. Understandably, parents are likely to be in a state of emotional instability and suppressed excitement during the early days of the infant's life. Relief over the successful conclusion of labor and delivery is soon followed by concern over the normality of their child and over their ability to give him the proper care. Every aspect of his physique and behavior will be subjected to their anxious scrutiny. It is important that those who are assisting with the early care of the infant be able to help parents to become comfortable in the care of their child and to discriminate between aberrations that are of temporary significance and those that may have far-reaching consequences to the infant. In this chapter the discussion treats the relatively normal phenomena of the newborn, leaving to later sections of the unit a consideration of some of the important aberrations that may be present.

EVALUATION OF VITAL FUNCTIONS

Cardiopulmonary Function. Without proper oxygenation of its vital organs the body cannot thrive. Oxygenation is primarily the responsibility of the heart and the lungs. The chief criteria which the nurse can use during her daily observations are the color of the skin and the character of the baby's respirations. Normal skin color varies from a delicate pink to a ruddy red. It is most constant on the trunk and the face. Because the small baby does not circulate blood freely to his extremities, his hands, feet and upper lip are not always reliable indicators of the degree of his tissue oxygenation. During repose they may be dusky or even blue, while, at the same time, his trunk and cheeks are pink. With increased warmth or bodily activity this phenomenon—acrocyanosis—tends to clear. If there is real difficulty in tissue oxy-

genation, crying or increased activity will increase the extent and the depth of cyanosis observed at the periphery. Observation of these changes in the skin of deeply pigmented infants is more difficult. Reliance must be placed on the appearance of mucous membranes or nailbeds. Generalized pallor of the skin may indicate poor cardiac function, or, more commonly, anemia. Its presence should be called to the attention of the physician so that appropriate laboratory studies can be made.

The newborn breathes with shallow, rapid respirations. The rate varies from 30 to 80 per minute, and the rhythm may be irregular. The abdomen usually moves more than the chest, bulging with inspiration and falling with expiration. The excursions of the chest are effortless when the infant is resting; during crying they become slower and deeper. Rapid, labored or grunting respirations indicate imperfect aeration of the lungs, particularly if they are accompanied by retraction of the chest wall during inspiration and by cyanosis of the skin or the mucous membranes. Miller has emphasized that resting respiratory rates which are persistently above 40 per minute indicate abnormal ventilation.

The pulse rate is not easily determined in the newborn. By auscultation of the chest the rate in a healthy infant is found to be from 90 to 160 per minute. Rates which consistently exceed 200 per minute in the absence of crying are probably abnormal.

Blood pressure cannot be measured in the usual fashion in the newborn, but the flush technic gives a fairly reliable approximation of the systolic pressure. The infant's arm (or leg) is elevated, the blood is milked out with a pressure bandage and then retained behind the cuff of a sphygmomanometer applied to the upper portion of the extremity. The cuff is deflated slowly, and the pressure at which color returns to the distal portion of the extremity is noted.

By this method, infants in the first 24 hours of life are found to have systolic blood pressures of 50 to 70 mm. of mercury, which rises in the next few days to 75 to 100 mm. The levels obtained in the leg are usually but not always slightly higher.

Activity and Cry. The amount of activity varies a great deal among newborns. For a period of a few hours to two or three days, many will be quite sleepy and inactive, due presumably to the effects of maternal medication during labor or to the compression of the brain during its passage through the birth canal. Such inactivity need occasion no alarm if the respirations and the color are normal, if the infant arouses at least momentarily on mild stimulation, and if the cry and the sucking reflex are present. After the period of somnolence is over, the newborn still sleeps much of the day, but in a tentative sort of way with spontaneous movements of the extremities, fitful turning and prompt awakening after mild stimulation. In small or slender infants, rapid and vigorous response to mild disturbances may appear during the first few days.

At birth the infant's cry is a welcome sound because it indicates the alert state of his central nervous system. During infancy a deep and vigorous cry continues to give gross reassurance of his physical well being. A change to a weak or poorly sustained effort on adequate stimulation may be an indication of illness or debilitation which requires further investigation. A hoarse cry or one with a high-pitched inspiratory crow should raise the suspicion of an abnormality around the larynx, either congenital or infectious in nature.

Body Temperature. Immediately after birth the infant's body temperature falls to about 96° F., a phenomenon which is now accepted as normal. During the first 12 to 24 hours it climbs gradually to a level between 98° and 99° F. where it stabilizes. Subsequent deviations outside this range may indicate improper temperature of the surrounding environment, insufficient fluid intake, or the onset of illness.

Some infants who are otherwise normal are slow to bring their body temperatures up to the expected levels. In hospital nurseries such babies can be placed in a heated crib or incubator of the kind used in the care of premature infants (Chap. 9). In the home, support of body temperature may be achieved by wrapping the infant in blankets, or, within an enclosed bassinet, by exposure to the heat from an ordinary goosenecked reading lamp. Hot water bottles and electric heating pads must be used with caution and only with a layer of interposed blanket, for the small infant's skin burns readily. Temperatures exceeding 115° F. should be avoided.

After the initial stabilization of body temperature the newborn's clothing must be adjusted to suit the climatic conditions around him. At temperate room heat of 70° to 75° F. most infants will be comfortable in diapers, a light cotton shirt and either a nightgown or a light flannel blanket to prevent excessive cooling during sleep. This amount of clothing may have to be augmented if room temperatures cannot be maintained. However, the usual practice is to dress small infants too heavily, resulting in restlessness or irritation of the skin from excessive perspiration. In testing for bodily comfort, the infant's back or abdomen is a more reliable indication of his body warmth than are his extremities, which normally tend to remain cool. In hot weather, when room temperatures cannot be held below 90° F., even small infants will be comfortable dressed only in diapers if they are guarded against direct breezes from open windows or doors.

THE GASTROINTESTINAL TRACT

The healthy newborn is able to suck and swallow as soon as he has recovered from the immediate effects of delivery. Early feedings should be given cautiously in order to be sure that his reflexes are functioning properly and to prevent overloading of his stomach. Hospital routines differ. In some the infant is placed at the breast almost immediately after delivery to initiate the mutual satisfactions which will develop between the mother and the baby in regard to feeding. In other hospitals, milk feedings are withheld until a brief trial period with sugar water demonstrates the infant's ability to take food satisfactorily.

For reasons that are not entirely clear, many infants suffer from excessive secretions of pharyngeal and gastric mucus during the early days of life. Usually, these can be controlled by gentle wiping or aspiration of the mouth with a bulb syringe. Sometimes there is nausea or even vomiting as well, and it may be desirable to wash the excessive secretions out of the stomach by gastric lavage. Continued accumulation of pharyngeal secretions together with cough and sputtering during the administration of food or fluids is apt to be a sign of atresia of the upper esophagus and should be called to the attention of the physician.

During the early examination and care of the infant, the nurse should make certain that an anus is present and should record the first passage of stool. A continuing record of the number, the type and the amount of stool is an important part of the observation of the newborn. The first stools are composed of meconium, a tarry green material which may be quite viscous. Within two or three days this is replaced by transitional stools (loose, green-black) and later by stools whose consistency depends somewhat on the type of food that the infant is receiving, e.g., breast milk or a formula.

THE GENITOURINARY TRACT

The kidneys are functioning and urine is being formed long before birth. The first passage of urine after birth should be recorded because it proves that urine is being formed and that it has a channel to the outside. The compression of the baby's abdomen during birth may cause him to expel urine at that time, an event that may pass unnoticed. During the first day or two the amount of urine formed is small and occasionally 24 to 36 hours will pass before urination is observed. Until feeding is well established, the urine is likely to be dark yellow in color and may be very dark if the infant is jaundiced.

In male infants the prepuce of the penis is generally long and rather tightly adherent so that the glans cannot be visualized. In some infants the prepuce is partially split and fails to cover the glans entirely—a hooded prepuce. This is often associated with hypospadias, and it is important to search for a meatal opening on the under surface of the glans. The scrotal sac varies considerably in size among newborn infants. Usually, the testes are within the sac, but they may be above it in the inguinal region or even up in the inguinal canals. They migrate readily due to the activity of the cremasteric muscles, and it is often difficult to be sure whether a newborn has two descended testes or not. Commonly, there is a hydrocele (a sac containing watery fluid) present about the testis. Such hydroceles may be large and tense so that they produce a visible mass in the scrotum. Most of them disappear spontaneously during the early months of life, but some are associated with or develop into hernias which contain extruded loops of intestine.

Circumcision is frequently done for religious or cultural reasons. The medical indications for the procedure are debatable, so that the decision should be left to the parents. If the operation is to be performed, it should be completed during the newborn period. Following the operation the raw incision is kept

covered with sterile gauze and petrolatum to prevent infection and adherence to the diapers. Healing usually takes place rapidly so that in two or three days no protection is needed. Since the newborn infant bleeds rather easily, the wound should be watched carefully to make sure that no excessive oozing occurs.

If circumsion is not done, the mother should be instructed in gradual stretching of the prepuce until it can be retracted behind the glans for proper cleansing. She must be warned that if left behind the corona for more than a few seconds, the prepuce may become edematous and be trapped so that it cannot be brought forward easily. This condition is called paraphimosis. If it occurs, she must seek medical assistance in reducing it.

Female infants have prominent labia due to the effects of estrogens produced by the mother during the latter part of pregnancy. A white caseous discharge is usually present in the vagina. Occasionally, the female may discharge small amounts of bloody fluid (pseudomenstruation) as an additional consequence of hormonal stimulation from the mother. Careful inspection of the genitalia is desirable to make sure that the vagina is present and that there is no undue enlargement of the clitoris, a finding which may lead to the early identification of endocrine disturbances.

Both male and female infants may show the effects of maternal estrogen in the blood stream by enlargement of the breasts, which, in some instances, produce small amounts of fluid, often referred to as "witch's milk." The breast enlargement may last as long as four to six weeks after birth. It is of no significance.

THE SKIN

The skin of the newborn varies considerably from one baby to another in respect to its color, texture and general toughness. Many have skin that is poorly supplied with natural oils, making it easily irritated and prone to infection. Hospital routines for initial care differ. Some leave most of the vernix caseosa on at birth to act as a temporary protective vanishing cream. Others bathe the infant completely and then anoint him thoroughly with a bland oil or an ointment with antibacterial properties. Soaps containing hexachlorophene are particularly effective in eliminating skin bacteria. For some infants, water acts as an irritant if applied too frequently. Those whose skin is dry, or parchment-like, or peeling, or those who have cracks and fissures or deep folds which cannot be kept dry, profit from liberal applications of oil and a minimal use of water.

Hyperactive infants may rub off the superficial layers of the skin of heels, toes or ankles unless they are protected with tight blanket swaddling. These are the babies who never seem to relax. They startle to an unusual degree if there is a noise, a sudden bright

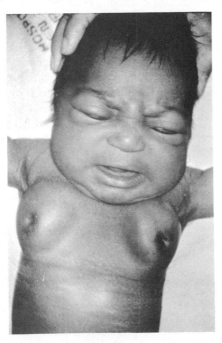

Fig. 7-1. Breast engorgement in the newborn. (Dr. R. Platou)

light or a quick change in position in their crib or while they are being held or carried. During the earliest months of life they are more comfortable if given sponge baths than if suspended in a bathinet or tub. Crying is more fitful than is usual in most babies. This kind of infant will rest best when swaddled in a blanket and held firmly in his favorite position for sleep.

The newborn's nails are thin and pliable and should be kept short in order to prevent the random movements of the extremities from inflicting scratches on the face or the body.

Jaundice. During daily care of the infant a careful search for any sign of jaundice should be made during the early days of life. This examination should be made in strong natural light. The time of its first appearance is of great significance. That which appears during the first 24 hours of life almost surely indicates blood incompatibility between the mother and the baby, a circumstance that requires detailed investigation. Jaundice appears first in the skin as a faint yellow cast over the face or the upper body. As it progresses in intensity, the skin may take on a general yellow color which may deepen to orange. In the later stages, the conjunctivae of the eyes also become pigmented. Jaundice which does not appear until the third or the fourth day of life is usually of limited signifiance and disappears within a few days. The mechanism which produces jaundice is described in Chapter 10.

Mongolian Spots. These irregular areas of greenish-blue pigmentation are concentrated over the lower back. They are present universally in infants of Asian extraction, are frequent among Negroes and the Mediterranean races, and are rarely found on Caucasian infants. They disappear by school age. They have no relation to Down's syndrome.

Pigmented Nevi. Pigmented nevi, or moles, either brown or black in color, may be found at birth. The larger ones may be cosmetically undesirable, but otherwise they have no significance. Large, flat areas of brown pigment are called *café-au-lait* spots.

Cutis Marmorata. This term describes a faint purple marblelike pattern of the skin capillaries in small infants visible during periods of inactivity or chilling. It is a normal phenomenon which is abolished by an increase in the circulation through the skin. The coldness and the occasional blueness of the normal infant's hands and feet have already been described.

Telangiectasia. Telangiectasia or widening of the skin capillaries is extremely common at the nape of the neck, less common over the forehead, the eyelids and along the midline of the scalp and the trunk. These flat, dark-red or purple areas of skin have sharp but irregular borders. Sometimes they are called "stork bites." They fade out but do not disappear entirely as the infant's skin becomes thicker during nor-

mal growth. Occasionally, a similar area of skin will precede the development of a strawberry hemangioma. This is a raised, bright-red collection of small blood vessels which is seldom present at birth but appears during the second or third week of life. Such tumors almost invariably break up and disappear spontaneously before the fourth year of life. No treatment is required.

Forceps Marks. These marks may be identified over the face at the time of birth but invariably disappear within a day or two.

Bruises. After difficult deliveries sometimes bruises are present on the face and the scalp. They are common about the buttocks and the external genitalia of breech-delivered infants. Even large bruises clear up within a few days, leaving no scar.

Milia. Milia are small white lumps about the size of a pinhead, seen usually on the face. They are small collections of the secretions of sebaceous glands trapped beneath the surface of the skin. They eventually establish an opening to the surface and disappear.

Blebs. Sometimes a similar collection of material is found in larger blebs in the skin folds of the neck, the axilla or the groin. They too disappear rapidly once the superficial skin is broken.

Hives. Occasionally, hives are seen on the second or the third day of life. They are small raised white spots surrounded by an area of erythema. They look much like small insect bites. Although they probably are due to some allergic response derived from the mother, they have no known relation to allergy in later life.

THE HEAD AND THE NECK

Pressure applied to the head before and during labor may produce a number of temporary changes which disappear shortly after birth without affecting the infant's welfare.

Molding of the Skull. Molding of the skull with overriding of the bones along the suture lines results when the head is pushed through a tight birth canal. The skulls of most infants delivered by cephalic presentation show some such overlapping of the bones with elongation of the occipital portion of the skull. These irregularities disappear during the early weeks of life. Breech-delivered infants usually have heads that are flattened in the occipital region. Cesarean-delivered infants, of course, have symmetrically round or slightly square heads.

Caput Succedaneum. This is a poorly defined area of edema of the scalp which indicates the first portion of the head to pass through the uterine cervix. A caput usually is gone by the third day.

Craniotabes. This term is used to describe areas of softening of the flat cranial bones. It is most common along the suture edges but sometimes is present in the center of the bone. The condition results from a com-

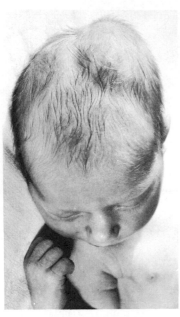

FIG. 7-2. Cephalhematoma of left parietal bone. (Davis, M., and Sheckler, C.: DeLee's Obstetrics for Nurses, Philadelphia, Saunders)

bination of intrauterine pressure and minor disturbances of the mother's calcium metabolism. The areas calcify rapidly after birth and seldom can be identified after two months.

Cephalhematoma. This is a collection of blood beneath the fibrous investment of one of the flat cranial bones, usually the parietal. It is most common in firstborn infants whose heads have been subjected to prolonged compression during labor. Often inconspicuous at first, the swelling enlarges rapidly during the first two or three days, producing a smooth, fluctuant, prominent mass, the margins of which are limited by the edges of the cranial bone involved. Some of the smaller hematomas absorb rapidly. The larger ones

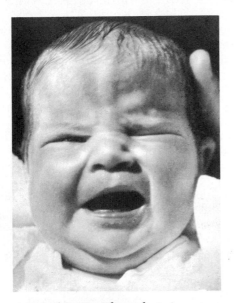

FIG. 7-3. Facial paralysis in a newborn baby, in this instance resulting from a spontaneous delivery.

usually calcify gradually, beginning at the base and eventually converting the swelling into a firm bony lump which remains until it is gradually engulfed by the increased size of the skull. Cephalhematomas produce no outward pressure on the brain and are innocuous except for their peculiar appearance. Aspiration of the contents of the swelling is unwise because of the danger of infection.

Petechiae. Petechiae are tiny hemorrhages into the skin which are sometimes seen sprinkled over the face, scalp and neck. They result from the sudden compression of chest and abdomen during delivery. They clear up within a few days.

Subconjunctival Hemorrhage. This flame-shaped collection of blood on the white portion of the eyeball results from the same mechanism. It usually takes a week or slightly longer to disappear.

Facial Paralysis. This may result from intrauterine pressure on the facial nerve that runs through the cheek. When the infant cries, the paralyzed side of the mouth fails to retract backward and upward as it should. The nerve usually recovers its function during the first six to eight weeks of life. Infrequently, the paralysis is permanent.

Hematoma of the Sternocleidomastoid Muscle. This is a small firm lump in the belly of the muscle which results from tearing of muscle fibers when traction is exerted upon the head (or shoulders in a breech delivery). The lump disappears slowly, and, unless excessive fibrosis takes place during healing, it does not interfere with the function of the muscle.

THE EYES

Chemical Conjunctivitis. Irritation by the silver nitrate instilled into the eyes at birth may result in a chemical conjunctivitis. On the second day of life the eyes are red and swollen shut, with pus exuding from between the lids. If there is any suspicion that the process might be infectious, the pus should be examined for the presence of bacteria. The eyes should be cleansed gently or irrigated with warm saline solution. In spite of the initial severity, the inflammation subsides within a few days, leaving no harmful effects on the eyes.

Obstruction of the Nasolacrymal Duct. This condition may be recognized toward the end of the newborn period by excessive tearing and the accumulation of small amounts of pus in the eye without inflammation of the globe itself. In most instances the duct opens up spontaneously during the first few months of life, requiring no special treatment.

THE MOUTH

Several features of the normal newborn's mouth may occasion unnecessary concern. Frequently, the gums are rough, almost serrated. The frenulum of the upper lip may extend down, partially cleaving the upper gums. Posteriorly, the gums are usually very white.

On either side of the midline of the hard palate a raised white plaque, called an epithelial pearl, may be seen. Concern over tonguetie is usually unjustified. The newborn's tongue is normally short and broad with the frenulum extending out to the tip. It cannot be protruded much beyond the gum margin until its shape is changed by elongating growth in later months.

Thrush. Thrush is a minor infection of the mouth, caused by a fungus which usually is transmitted from the mother's vaginal secretions during birth. The tongue and the mucous membranes are diffusely red and speckled with closely adherent white patches. The infection is easily cured by a few applications of aqueous gentian violet solution or by nystatin suspension (100,000 U./ml.) swabbed over the membranes three or four times a day.

THE UMBILICUS

Granuloma. After the cord separates, healing usually takes place promptly at the navel. Occasionally, a small piece of granulation tissue remains uncovered by epithelium and grows to form a granuloma; the weeping surface produces a chronic discharge. The granulations may be cauterized with a silver nitrate stick which terminates the discharge by drying up the weeping surface.

Umbilical Hernia. This is the result of a defect in the anterior abdominal wall through which a loop of

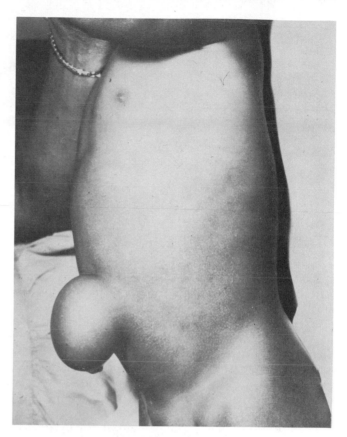

Fig. 7-5. Umbilical hernia in an infant. (Courtesy of Dr. Mark Ravitch)

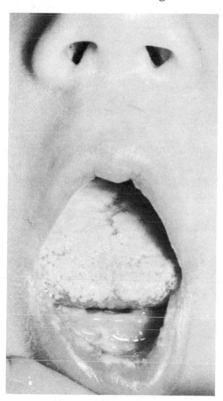

Fig. 7-4. Thrush. (Potter, E. L.: Pathology of the Fetus and the Newborn, Chicago, Yr. Bk. Pub.)

intestine may bulge out under the skin when the infant cries or strains. Although unsightly and often worrisome to the mother, such hernias produce no important symptoms. All but the larger ones close over spontaneously by the second or third year as the abdominal muscles strengthen when the child begins to stand. Application of abdominal binders or adhesive strapping have little effect in hastening the closure of the defect.

THE EXTREMITIES

Before birth the infant's body and extremities must conform to the egglike shape of the mother's uterus. Although it is well known that some infants move about and change position while in the uterus, there are many who are born with muscle shortening and mild positional deformities of the legs and the feet which suggest that they remained cramped in one position. If restored to this fetal position, however bizarre, such infants behave as if they were more comfortable. Babies delivered from cephalic presentations usually have their legs folded up on the abdomen so that passive extension of the thighs and the lower legs is resisted. The upper and the lower legs frequently show outward bowing of the bones which have yielded to the pressure from the muscular

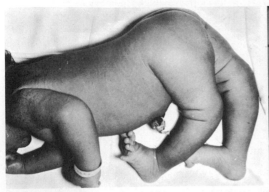
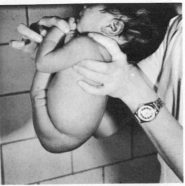

FIG. 7-6. (*Left*) Deformity of legs from intra-uterine breech position. (*Right*) The same baby folded into the ovoid position that he occupied in the uterus. (Dr. R. Platou)

uterine wall. Such bowing is of no significance, for, once the confining pressure has been relieved, the limbs gradually straighten during the course of growth in the next two or three years. The feet also may show signs of unusual intrauterine position, turning too far inward, too far outward or sharply upward. Usually, these deformities involve only the muscular and the ligamentous structures which eventually will adjust by themselves. The extent of the deformity can be determined by ascertaining whether or not the feet can be passively restored (by gentle manipulation) to normal position. The more extreme effects of intrauterine posture are bony dislocation or malformation which requires orthopedic correction. Infants born by breech presentation are more likely to have legs that are stiffly extended rather than flexed at the knee, and there may be a knock-kneed deformity instead of the bow-leg seen in infants delivered from cephalic presentations. These early deformities also improve spontaneously once the uterine pressure has been removed.

The tendency for newborns to lie in the fencing position produced by the tonic neck reflex has been described in the preceding chapter. The response to

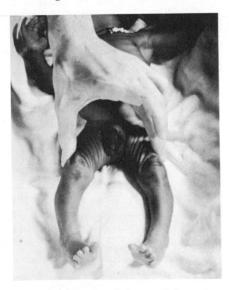

FIG. 7-7. Bowed legs of the newborn. (Dr. R. Platou)

the startle or Moro reflex should be observed both for its presence and its symmetry. Its absence may indicate central nervous system damage; an asymmetrical movement of the arms should arouse suspicion of brachial palsy or a fractured clavicle.

Rudimentary extra digits are not uncommon, particularly among Negro infants in whom the trait is hereditary. The sixth finger usually is a poorly developed phalanx attached to the lateral side of the hand by a thin pedicle of skin. A tight ligature around the pedicle results in atrophy and spontaneous amputation in a few days. Occasionally, extra digits are more completely formed and cannot be removed except by surgical dissection.

The presence of a web between adjacent toes is a relatively common familial anomaly which has no functional or cosmetic importance to the newborn. However, if such webs occur between the fingers, surgical correction must be performed in order to provide free mobility of the digits, but this can be done at a later time.

MEASUREMENT OF THE NEWBORN

At the time of birth it is desirable to record certain measurements to serve as a base line for the evaluation of later growth. Weight can be measured accurately with a reliable balance. The other measurements are less trustworthy unless they are checked and particular attention is paid to making them accurate.

Weight. By custom the birth weight has assumed great importance in describing the newborn infant. It is outranked only by sex in the initial data reported on birth certificates and to inquisitive friends and relatives. Because it can be measured accurately, it is accepted as the best measure of prematurity, but it cannot be accepted as precise (see Chap. 9). Although it is the most convenient index of an infant's size, it may not be a true measure. Conditions within the uterus prior to birth may cause a prenatal gain or loss of weight which disguises his true condition. Many infants are born with excessive fluid in their tissues so that a more reliable weight base line is obtained on the second or third day of life, after this edema has been lost.

The average birth weight of white male infants in America is 7½ pounds (3,400 Gm.). Approximately 80 per cent of such infants will fall within the weight range of 6 pounds, 5 ounces (2,860 Gm.) to 9 pounds, 2 ounces (4,130 Gm.). Newborn infants of Negroes as well as Philippine, Indian and other Asian groups are smaller on the average at birth. Those of the northern European races tend to be larger. Socioeconomic status and birth at high altitude also influence initial weights. In all instances the females tend to be somewhat smaller than the males.

In most nurseries newborns are weighed daily or at least every second day in order to observe weight progress. When the hospital stay is five days or less, the information obtained is of limited significance. Most infants lose weight after birth because they are getting rid of excess fluid stored during fetal life and because they discharge accumulated meconium from the gastrointestinal tract during a period when food and fluid intake is small. Ordinarily, this loss during the first week does not exceed 5 or 10 per cent of the initial weight. Infants who are large at birth (9½ lbs. or over) and those who show obvious puffiness may lose up to 15 per cent of initial weight before consistent gains are initiated. Once the food intake is sufficient and the preliminary drop is over, small babies are expected to gain, on the average, a minimum of 5 oz. (150 Gm.) a week. Breast-fed infants tend to make more modest gains than artificially fed infants, some of whom may gain as much as 12 oz. (480 Gm.) or more a week.

Infants should be weighed on a scale that has been balanced properly. The time of weighing should be approximately the same each day so as to standardize the relationship to feeding and perhaps to stool passage. Proper allowance must be made for pads, diapers or clothing which are weighed with the infant. In general, weighing at home should be discouraged, since it seldom results in reassurance for the mother and is a common source of inaccurate information and unnecessary concern, particularly for the mother who is trying to breast-feed her infant.

Length. Measurement of the newborn's length is difficult because his legs cannot be fully extended easily and because his body must be kept straight during the process. The lower end of the measurement should be taken from the soles of his feet—placed in normal standing position—and not from the tips of his extended toes. Because of these difficulties, the accuracy of length measurements is often questioned. When appropriate care is taken, the average length of American infants is found to be just under 20 inches (50.6 cm.) for boys, with a range of 19 to 21 inches (48 to 53.3 cm.). This includes about 80 per cent of all male newborns. Girls average slightly less.

Head Circumference. The greatest circumference, which includes the brow just above the eyes and the posterior occipital protuberance, is the standard measure of head size. This averages about 14 inches (35 cm.) at birth, but variations of ½ inch (1.2 cm.) or a little more are common. Female infants have slightly smaller heads than males. The measurement is of importance in evaluating the speed of growth of the head when it is necessary to determine whether or not hydrocephalus or microcephaly is present.

PROTECTION AGAINST INFECTION

Before birth the infant is protected from the infectious agents of the outside world by the membranes and the uterus which surround him and by the *biological* defense mechanisms of his mother. Birth precipitates him from this sterile environment into a world teeming with infectious organisms which inevitably lodge on his skin and gain access to his mouth and intestinal tract. His own protective mechanisms, aided by antibodies which have passed across the placenta from his mother's blood into his own, will successfully defend him against the common infectious agents. But, from experience, we know that his general resistance is low and that certain agents have particular virulence for the new baby. Consequently, it is prudent to subject him at first to as few of the infectious agents of the outside world as possible.

The precautions invoked for the protection of the newborn are directed toward two main objectives: (1) to reduce to a minimum the quantity of infectious agents to which he is exposed by maintaining aseptic technic in his physical environment, and (2) to prevent his contact with persons who are themselves infected.

Asepsis is almost as important in the newborn nursery as it is in the surgical operating room. Similar technics are used. The room itself should be enclosed and should have some system of ventilation or air-conditioning in which there is an adequate filtering device. Some nurseries are equipped with ultraviolet lamps which reduce the organisms in the circulating air. The walls should be cleaned periodically and the floors daily, using a wet technic that prevents dispersion of the accumulated dust and lint on which infectious particles travel. The floor is always considered to be contaminated and objects which are dropped must be discarded or sterilized before being used again. Large articles of furniture should be cleansed periodically with appropriate antiseptics. All linen, blankets, clothing, formulas and solutions used in infant care should be freshly clean or, preferably, sterilized. Access to the nursery is usually gained through a scrub room where persons entering are required to put on freshly washed gowns and to undergo a thorough cleansing of hands and arms with careful attention to the nails. Handwashing should be repeated whenever the attendant moves from one infant to another. In modern nurseries each infant has his own set of supplies, including a thermometer, and these items are used on him alone. When it is necessary to remove an infant from his own bassinet to some common facility such as a scale or a treatment table, a clean sheet or a piece of paper should be used as protection. An unavoidable but obvious break in technic occurs when the infant is taken from the nursery to his mother's room.

Even more important than the physical environment which surrounds him are the persons with whom the newborn comes in direct or even remote contact. His introduction to agents capable of making him seriously ill is most often by this route. Persons who have infections of the skin such as boils, carbuncles or paronychia, those suffering from respiratory infections or diarrhea, and those with unexplained fever should be excluded automatically from contact with the infant. The nurse must not only be alert to the importance of such illness in mothers, visitors and nursery personnel but also should conscientiously ask for relief from nursery duties when similarly afflicted herself.

When a transmissible infection appears in a mother in the hospital, her baby must be kept in the nursery until she has recovered completely. If a rooming-in arrangement is in force, the mother and the baby must be removed from the unit. Infants in the nursery who show signs of transmissible illness also must be removed promptly and placed in an isolation nursery.

These protective measures are not carried out so readily for infants born in the home. Fortunately, the hazards are decreased by virtue of the small number of individuals around the infant. The larger the nursery unit, the more people there are who become involved in infant care. This not only opens more avenues through which infection can be introduced, but also subjects a larger number of infants to this risk. For these reasons it is generally good policy to keep the size of nursery units as small as possible and to staff them with persons who do not have duties in other areas of the hospital.

THE NURSE AND THE PARENTS

Any deviation from perfection in the newborn infant, regardless of how transient or common the condition may be, is viewed by parents with anxiety. Unless they are forewarned, parents are greatly concerned about normal newborn characteristics which differ from those of older infants, such as cyanosis of the extremities, molding of the head and enlarged genitalia. Their anxiety will be allayed if they can express their concerns to an understanding individual who is able to acknowledge parental worries while explaining the underlying physiological reasons for the infant's physical appearance or behavior.

When the nurse is in doubt about the medical significance of the physical findings, she should share the parental concern, but should refrain from reassurance or predictions of future difficulty until she can verify them with the physician.

SITUATIONS FOR FURTHER STUDY

1. What observations would you want to make if you were the nurse showing a mother her newborn baby for the first time after delivery?

2. What questions relative to natural physical characteristics of the newborn did mothers in a maternity ward ask you? What physical characteristics seemed to cause them greatest concern?

3. Baby Jones was transferred directly to the pediatric unit from the delivery room because he had a cleft lip. If you were the nurse caring for him and you were notified that his mother planned to visit that day, what would you consider your role to be?

4. If you were giving a newborn his first feeding of glucose water, what observations would be important to make?

5. How would you help a mother who asked you how she should care for her uncircumcised infant's genitalia?

6. How would you help a mother who manifested an unusual amount of concern when she observed her son's engorged breasts?

7. If you observed that the superficial layers of skin on a newborn's heels and ankles had been rubbed off, what plan of nursing care would you institute?

8. How does the body posture of the baby born by breech presentation differ from that of the baby born by cephalic presentation?

9. If on examining a 2-week-old baby in its home you discovered an unhealed, draining umbilicus, what would you do?

10. What is the cause of loss of weight during the first days of a baby's life? Approximately when is birth weight regained?

BIBLIOGRAPHY

Arnold, H. W., Putnam, N. J., Barnard, B. L., Desmond, M. M., and Rudolph, A. J.: The newborn: transition to extra-uterine life, Am. J. Nurs. 65:77, 1965.

Buchanan-Davidson, D. J.: What can we learn from meconium? Am. J. Nurs. 63:112, 1963.

Hervoda, A. R.: Nursery evaluation of the newborn, Am. J. Nurs. 67:1669, 1967.

Keitel, H. G.: Preventing neonatal diaper rash, Am. J. Nurs. 65:124, 1965.

McCaffery, M., and Johnson, D. C.: Crying in the newborn infant, Nursing Science 3:339, 1965.

Miller, H. C.: Clinical evaluation of respiratory function in the newborn, Pediat. Clin. N. Amer., Feb., 1957.

Parmelee, A. H.: Management of the Newborn, ed. 2, Chicago, Year Book Pub., 1959.

Siverman, W. A., and Parke, P. C.: The newborn: keep him warm, Am. J. Nurs. 65:81, 1965.

Smith, C. A.: The Physiology of the Newborn Infant, ed. 3, Springfield, Thomas, 1959.

Thompson, L. R.: Nursery infections: apparent and inapparent, Am. J. Nurs. 65:80, 1965.

American Academy of Pediatrics Committee on Fetus and Newborn: Standards and Recommendations for Hospital Care of Newborn Infants, Full Term and Premature, Evanston, Ill., American Academy of Pediatrics, 1966.

8

Infant Nutrition

BREAST FEEDING

Human milk is considered the ideal food for the young infant despite all advances in the knowledge of artificial feeding. Human milk contains no harmful bacteria, whereas cow's milk must be guarded carefully in this respect. Requiring no modification, human milk contains all the nutritional essentials in adequate, even though minimal, amounts, with the exception of vitamin D and iron. However, it is doubtful whether breast feeding is superior to artificial feeding in survival value for infants in areas where standards of medical care are high and where the infant mortality rate is correspondingly low. In communities where infantile disease is rife and educational opportunities are primitive, human milk is far safer than artificial food.

Successful breast feeding has significance in the formation of a happy mother-child relationship. To the infant it is the natural mode of feeding which satisfies his desires for food, sucking, warmth and closeness to his mother. To the mother it can be a rewarding symbol of the transmission of the love she feels for her child as well as a satisfying contribution to his physical needs. However, not all mothers are physiologically and psychologically able to capitalize on this form of gratification, and for them breast feeding may be contraindicated.

Maternal Contraindications

Illness. A mother with active tuberculosis or with a serious chronic illness, such as heart or kidney disease, usually cannot be subjected to the physical strain of breast feeding her child. Some mental illnesses and physical conditions such as frequent convulsions or uncontrolled insulin reactions make nursing inadvisable because of hazards to the infant. Severe acute illness, communicable disease and major surgical procedures necessitate temporary weaning, during which milk secretion is maintained by periodic emptying of the breasts. Medication of the mother does not usually contraindicate breast feeding. If she receives large doses of drugs such as atropine, opiates, salicylates, sulfonamides, iodides, and some of the antibiotics, small amounts may be transmitted through the milk. Deleterious effects upon the infant are rare.

If the mother has active open tuberculosis, the infant should be completely isolated from her because of the communicability of the infection. If the maternal tuberculosis is active but not transmissible (closed), nursing is generally not advised because of the physical strain on the mother. When tuberculosis is latent or presumably healed, there is no contraindication to breast feeding.

Pregnancy. While the occurrence of pregnancy makes weaning desirable because of the physical strain on the mother, it should be accomplished gradually. Menstruation is *not* an indication for weaning, although during the first day or two the baby may be somewhat disturbed. Birth control pills may diminish milk production in some women.

Mastitis. In the event of the mother developing mastitis, use of the affected breast should be discontinued. If both breasts become inflamed, complete weaning is necessary. Lesser degrees of nipple disorders require management, as discussed on page 115. Inverted, cracked, fissured or painful nipples often can be effectively treated.

Personal Preferences. Personal attitudes, cultural influences, social pressures and psychological needs of the mother are a few of the factors that bear on her choice of feeding method. The establishment of the mother-child relationship may be hindered when a mother who would prefer artificial feeding nurses only because it is strongly recommended.

Infant Contraindications

Local Deformity. An infant with a cleft lip and palate is usually unable to suckle at the breast. Sometimes, when the deformity involves the lip only, an early surgical repair will permit nursing if the mother's supply has been maintained. Obstruction of the nose or marked hypoplasia of the mandible often make it mechanically impossible for an infant to nurse successfully.

Jaundice. Some women excrete pregnanediol in their milk; this is a metabolite of adrenocortical steroids and inhibits the infant's ability to conjugate and hence excrete bilirubin. Such breast-feeding infants may have prolonged jaundice unless the breast feeding is interrupted for a day or two. Rarely does this complication constitute a real indication for termination of the breast feeding.

Prematurity. Whether a premature infant can nurse at the breast depends largely on his initial size. Larger prematures will be strong enough to nurse after a brief period so that the problem of maintaining the mother's supply is not arduous. When nursing is delayed beyond three to four weeks the likelihood of maintaining lactation is diminished.

Illness. Any condition which debilitates the infant interferes with nursing. Acute illnesses may require only a few days of bottle feeding, and a return to the breast is possible. Longer illness or congenital malformations such as cardiac disorders may weaken the infant so as to make nursing too exhausting for him to attempt.

Preparation of the Mother

Psychological. The mother's conscious and unconscious attitudes toward breast feeding have an important bearing on her ability to produce milk. Delivery of milk to the infant will be impeded by maternal worry over the adequacy of her supply or by the necessity for haste in the completion of the feeding.*

During the prenatal period much can be done by those who attend and advise the mother toward creating a positive attitude toward breast feeding. In communities where artificial feeding is manifestly risky it can be urged that the mother nurse her infant. In areas with low infant mortality rates the degree to which a mother should be "sold" on its advantages requires individualized judgment. Nursing cannot honestly be regarded as a medical necessity for such infants, but it can be advised as a procedure which will yield dividends in emotional satisfaction and adjustment for both mother and baby, provided that the mother can relax and allay her fears and doubts. Prenatal advisors can do much to reassure and solve practical problems in advance which may lead some hesitant mothers to give nursing a reasonable trial. The danger of "overselling" lies in the creation of a sense of guilt, defeat or frustration in the mother who does her best to provide milk but fails.

Nutrition and Health. Unfortunately, human milk is not adequate in all instances. Mothers cannot secrete into their milk vitamins which they do not ingest in sufficient amount, and women in poor health or with nutritional deficiencies cannot produce milk of good quality or quantity. Appropriate attention to the health and diet of the mother is conducive to and often essential for successful breast feeding.

The diet of the lactating mother need not differ qualitatively from that which is suitable for her at other times. No food will have an ill effect on the milk if it does not cause a disturbance in the mother. For example, the prejudice against "acid" foods is unfounded.

A mother who is secreting a pint to a quart of milk daily, with an energy value of 300 to 700 calories and adequate protein, minerals and vitamins, must eat at least that many more calories than her customary allowance in order to avoid depleting her own body supplies. Some mothers who because of a restricted diet produce little milk, secrete more when the diet is improved. Too often nutrition is inadequate irrespective of lactation, and during this period it is especially important that all of the essential food materials be included in adequate quantities. Although the milk may contain calcium from maternal body stores (bones), vitamins are absent unless they are ingested regularly by the mother. Allowances recommended during lactation are as follows: 3,000 calories, 100 Gm. of protein, 2 Gm. of calcium, 8,000 units of vitamin A, 1.5 mg. of thiamine, 150 mg. of ascorbic acid, 3 mg. of riboflavin, 15 mg. of niacin and 400 units of vitamin D. To obtain these amounts of nutrients, it is necessary to include in the diet at least 1 quart of milk, preferably more. The daily diet also should contain one or two eggs, one serving of meat and an abundance of fruits and vegetables.

Care of the Nipples. Fissuring, cracking and infection of the nipples is one of the commonest causes of failure early in breast feeding. During pregnancy the breasts should be inspected for adequate protrusion of the nipples. If the nipples are retracted or adherent so that they fail to protrude when pressure is applied to the base, attempts to bring them out can be made by massage, or other means suggested by the physician. Some insurance against blocked alveolar ducts may be obtained by having the mother manually express breast secretions twice a day during the latter weeks of pregnancy. Procedures for toughening nipples are of doubtful value.

Emptying the Breast. MANUAL EXPRESSION. For one who has mastered the technic, the most effective method of emptying the breast is manual expression.

---

* An important connection between nervous tension and the delivery of milk from the breast is embodied in the "let-down" reflex. Stroking of the nipple or the presence of the infant produces reflex contracture of the alveoli of the mammary gland, pushing milk down into the ducts which discharge at the nipple. Fear, excitement, anger and embarrassment may inhibit this reflex and prevent milk present deep in the gland from coming down to the nipple.

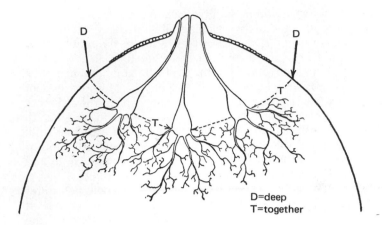

D=deep
T=together

The principle of this method is indicated in Figures 8-1 and 8-2. The thumb and the finger are placed on the opposite sides of and about 1 inch from the nipple, pressed deeply into the breast and then brought toward each other with sufficient pressure to empty the underlying milk sacs. Sometimes better success is attained when the bringing together of the thumb and the finger is followed by a forward motion. There should be no movement of the fingers on the skin; the skin and the fingers should move together. The milk should flow from the nipple in streams, not drops, during the period of pressure. Milk expression is repeated until the breast is empty.

BREAST PUMP. In the cheapest, simplest and most commonly used type of breast pump, negative pressure is obtained by applying the pump with the bulb compressed and then allowing the bulb to expand. The nipple and the areola are drawn into the conical glass with resultant compression of the milk sacs and a consequent flow of milk. The negative pressure must be released by pressure on the bulb to allow the milk sacs to refill and then be reapplied. This process is repeated until the breast is empty. A similar but

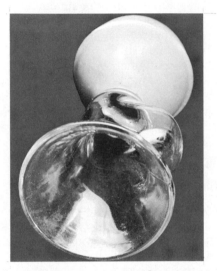

FIG. 8-3. Common type of breast pump.

more efficient method sometimes employed in hospitals uses the same principle of intermittent negative pressure, but the suction is produced by an electrically operated machine pump.

Characteristics of Human Milk

The milk that is secreted during the first few days after the birth of the baby is small in amount and differs from that secreted after lactation is established. Known as colostrum, it is a lemon-yellow color and has a relatively high protein content. Much of the protein consists of globulin which is considered to have biologic and immunologic importance for the infant.

On about the third or the fourth day the amount of secretion increases greatly. The breasts become distended and often tender. A gradual transition takes place in the appearance and composition of the milk. Most of the change occurs within a week or two, and by the end of the first month has been completed. After lactation is established, the milk contains approximately 3.5 to 4 per cent fat, 7.5 per cent

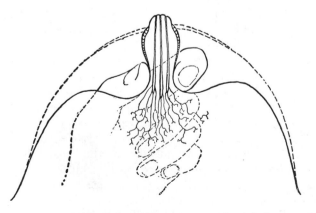

FIG. 8-2. Schematic representation of the manual expression of milk from the breast. (Moore: Nutrition of Mother and Child)

sugar, 1.25 per cent protein and 0.2 per cent mineral salts. It has an energy value of 20 calories to the ounce. The composition remains practically constant throughout the period of lactation. At any one withdrawal the first milk that comes from the breast is low in fat, and the last milk relatively rich in fat. Thus any sample taken for analysis should be an entire breast content. Milk analysis usually gives little information of value in determining the difficulty when a breast-fed baby is not thriving. No validity can be given to the common statement that the milk is weak or watery because of its bluish appearance. This is the normal appearance of human milk because the fat is white in color rather than yellow as that of cow's milk.

Breast milk from lactating mothers who have an excess can be stored. It is usually pasteurized and frozen or canned for future use. Some communities have established breast-milk centers or banks for the collection of surplus milk which can be made available for premature infants or those with special nutritional problems whose mothers cannot supply enough for their needs.

Technic of Breast Feeding

The time at which a newborn infant is first placed at the breast varies in different hospitals. In some, babies are put to breast as soon as the mother and the infant indicate a readiness to be together; in others, babies are not put to breast until six to 12 hours after birth. During the first few days, the infant gets very little from the breast. To supply fluids and a few calories, 5 per cent sugar solution may be offered approximately every three or four hours.

The object of placing the baby at the breast is to stimulate the flow of milk and to establish a mutually enjoyed experience for mother and baby. It is important that the mother be prepared for the fact that the initial grasp of the nipple may be painful and that the baby be awake and ready to participate in nursing. The nurse should remain to help to make feeding a pleasant and comfortable experience for both of them.

Mothers should be aware of the "rooting" reflex which makes the infant turn instinctively toward the warmth of the breast when it is applied to his cheek. He cannot distinguish this from the warmth of fingers which are mistakenly used to try to guide his mouth to the nipple by turning his head. Instead he appears to refuse the breast by turning away from it and toward the warm palm.

Schedule. Regularity in following a feeding schedule occurs in some nurseries for the newborn. In others, more flexibility exists, and babies are taken to their mothers whenever they show a need for closeness or food. At home or under the rooming-in type of hospital care, feeding schedules can be governed by the infant's spontaneous demands for food. By

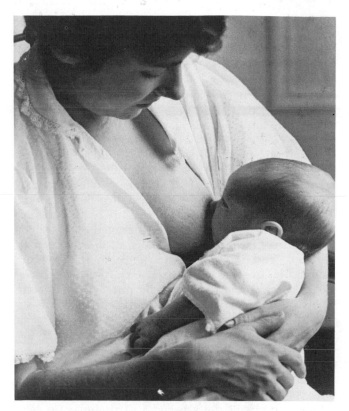

Fig. 8-4. Notice the way this mother holds her baby and concentrates on him. (Ross Laboratories, Columbus, Ohio)

observing the infant, his own pattern of need for food will become apparent. As he grows and matures his shifting requirements will be signaled promptly to his mother.

Feeding a baby when he is hungry encourages the formation of good food habits; it prevents tension and disposes toward positive attitudes about food. When an infant is allowed to cry with hunger because the clock does not indicate the time for feeding, his natural feeding rhythm is upset. The air that he swallows during crying prevents his stomach from filling up and fatigue from crying causes him to fall asleep before his nutritional needs have been satisfied. In a short period he is hungry again; he wakes and cries, and the cycle is repeated.

Many infants who are fed on a self-regulatory schedule select schedules that closely follow the traditional four-hour intervals. Some of the smaller ones or those who are tense or are attempting to make rapid increments in size may require feedings at three-hour or even two-hour intervals for a time. During the third to the seventh day of life a period of constant demand for food is quite common. In most instances, once the mother recovers from the initial period of fatigue and uncertainty about her role as a mother and begins to understand her infant's needs, a regular feeding pattern emerges. The intervals between nursing periods may not be exactly equal—often the period of satisfaction in the late afternoon and the early evening is relatively shorter. During the 24-hour period, few infants will require less than 5 feedings; most desire 6 to 8, and more frequent feeding may be desirable for brief periods. When the latter behavior persists over protracted periods, it may be necessary to inquire into the adequacy of the mother's milk supply.

In most instances, the supply of milk is abundant enough that the infant may obtain sufficient milk from a single breast, and it is desirable to offer alternate breasts at each nursing. By satisfying the infant at one breast, the breast is emptied more thoroughly, and the production of milk is encouraged. When both breasts are given at a single nursing the infant may overfeed, and intestinal disturbance and discomfort may result. In some instances when a four-hour schedule is selected, the baby may be put to both breasts in order to get sufficient milk, and alternate breasts should be offered first.

The average time for an infant to remain at the breast is about 15 minutes. The time depends on the sucking need and the strength of the infant, the amount of milk available and whether or not the breasts are difficult to empty. Some infants will obtain sufficient milk and be satisfied in 10 minutes or less. When there is little milk, in a very few minutes the infant may give up the attempt to obtain it. The only method of determining with certainty whether the infant has obtained a sufficient amount is to weigh him before and after feeding. In general it is unwise to recommend this procedure to the mother, for the information obtained may be inaccurate and it is more likely to create tension than to reassure. If the baby is normally contented and is growing, it can be assumed that his supply of milk is adequate. The flow of milk is much more rapid at the beginning of a feeding; half or more of the total quantity is consumed in the first five minutes, more than a quarter during the next five minutes, and very little after this time. Many infants who remain at the breast for long periods swallow air in considerable amounts and this may lead to vomiting, colic and fretfulness.

Every infant swallows some air during feeding, and he should be held upright and patted on the back until the air is belched. All infants should be so "bubbled" after each feeding and many babies before feeding as well. Occasionally, for young infants it is desirable to allow opportunity for eructation during the course of the feeding.

Difficulties Encountered in Breast Feeding

Overfeeding. Overfeeding of breast milk is an uncommon source of difficulty. Occasionally, a mother may produce so much milk that the infant easily takes more than he can digest properly and vomiting, distention and restlessness may result. Ordinarily, the milk

supply adjusts itself within a few days, and the symptoms subside. Night feeding with the baby sleeping in the mother's bed should be discouraged because of the risks of overfeeding, mutual disturbance of rest and the danger of the mother's rolling onto the infant during sleep.

Underfeeding. The investigation when underfeeding is suspected begins with determination of the amount of milk received by the infant, which is accomplished best by weighing the baby before and after feeding. Since the amount of milk obtained at different feedings may vary, it is well to take the average of several feedings, or better, to determine the actual amount taken over a 24-hour period. The next step is to determine how much milk remains in the breast. If little or none can be obtained, the supply is inadequate. If the supply is adequate, the difficulty may be that the nipples are inverted or small or that the infant is unable to suckle properly. Inverted nipples may be drawn out sufficiently by manipulation or by the suction of a pump. Nipples too small or too much inverted for successful breast feeding seldom are encountered. Feeding the baby by means of a nipple shield may be successful, although there is a tendency for the milk to diminish gradually with this procedure. The infant may be too feeble to suckle; he may nurse for a short time and fall asleep exhausted. A baby with an occluded nose cannot obtain his food satisfactorily; he will grasp the nipple as if hungry, suckle for a brief time and then cry. Many new mothers do not know how to hold the infant in a comfortable position for feeding, or the breast may be allowed to occlude the infant's nares.

The treatment of underfeeding is obvious once the cause is determined. A baby should not be weaned from the breast merely because of insufficient milk but should be given milk from a bottle in addition to that obtained from the breast. Often sufficient milk may be obtained by giving both breasts at each feeding. At the same time, measures such as improving the diet of the mother, helping her to see her need for rest and shortening the feeding interval should be undertaken to increase the supply of milk. If the milk supply increases adequately supplementary feedings may be discontinued.

Inanition or Dehydration Fever. It is appropriate to consider in connection with starvation a condition known as inanition fever. This name is given to a febrile illness occurring in the first five days after birth. The temperature usually does not rise above 102° F., and no evidence of local disease is present. The condition is associated with loss in weight, often rapid, and a persistence of the meconium nature of the stools. The degree of prostration is directly proportionate to the duration of the illness, and its general nature is that of progressive weakness. In the milder forms, there is much crying and restlessness; in the more severe forms, the infant is limp and apathetic, with perhaps a feeble whine. The condition always is associated with dry or nearly dry breasts and always is relieved within a few hours by the administration of food or fluid. The symptoms are due to dehydration. The treatment is to supply fluid primarily and food secondarily, the effect being rapid disappearance of the fever and prostration and recovery of the lost weight.

Mixed Feeding

Mixed feeding means that an infant is fed in part at the breast and in part artificially. This method may be used from necessity because of inadequate supply of milk or as a convenience to the mother in order that she may have liberty for social engagements or be relieved of night nursing. When started early the infant becomes accustomed to the bottle, so that weaning from the breast will be accomplished with fewer difficulties. An older infant who has been fed only at the breast frequently will starve himself seriously rather than take milk in any other manner. If the infant is introduced to the bottle early, it is possible to avoid this difficulty.

When mixed feeding is chosen for the convenience of the mother, usually a bottle feeding is given in place of a single feeding at the breast. When it is employed from necessity, the same plan may be used to a limited extent. However, it is to be remembered that if an infant is fed less than a certain minimum at the breast—usually five feedings—the supply of milk tends to decrease. If it becomes necessary to give considerable amounts of supplemental food, the maternal milk supply is conserved best by having the baby nurse regularly and by giving the necessary amounts of supplemental food immediately after each breast feeding.

ARTIFICIAL FEEDING

When human milk is not available to the infant, a substitute source is required. Because of its availability, cow's milk is the most common basis of infant formulas. Occasionally, the milk of the goat is used, and rarely mare's and ass's milk have been employed. In recent years it has also been found possible to rear an infant without milk by substituting preparations made from vegetable sources. However, well over 90 per cent of artificially fed infants receive some modification of cow's milk. The milk from different breeds and herds of cows varies only in its fat content. In the United States this difference disappears in the processing of milks, since dairies usually reduce the fat content to the minimum required by law. Thus, milk from all sources is essentially of the same composition.

Artificial feeding must be undertaken with the realization that three automatic safety factors of breast milk have been lost: (1) sterility, (2) maximum digestibility, and (3) nearly complete vitamin coverage.

Any scheme of artificial feeding must be designed in such a way as to control these deficiencies insofar as possible.

Control of Bacteria

As he grows, the infant will eventually be able to defend himself against the bacteria which surround him. In the early months of life his immunologic defenses are notoriously poor; it is prudent to shield him against exposure to infectious agents in large numbers or wide variety. A more compelling reason for care in formula preparation is that milk is an ideal medium for the transmission of disase. Pathogens introduced accidentally into a supply may disseminate disease to large numbers of infants or children in a community or in a hospital. The educational value to parents of careful formula instruction should not be overlooked. If properly schooled in this aspect of care, they may extend the principles to other aspects of the infant's hygiene. The age at which sterilizing measures may be relaxed is a matter of varying opinion among physicians and is determined in part by medical and social circumstances. Some insist on careful technic throughout the first year of life or longer; others are willing under good hygienic circumstances to shift infants to pasteurized milk at about 5 or 6 months of age.

Milk taken by the infant from the human breast is sterile except for a trivial number of bacteria from the skin and the surrounding environment. A comparable degree of sterility could be achieved by having the infant nurse directly from the cleansed udder of the cow—a cumbersome procedure which was actually tried around the turn of the century in a frantic attempt to find a safer form of artificial feeding. Obtained from the cow under the cleanest conditions, milk contains from 100 to 1,000 bacteria per cubic milliliter. Since it is an excellent growing medium, these organisms multiply rapidly during any period required for processing and transportation. By the time clean milk reaches the consumer the bacteria have usually increased to 10,000 to 50,000 per cubic milliliter. Milk which is not carefully collected or preserved may have several million bacteria per cubic milliliter. Such milk should be considered unfit for infant feeding. Only Grade A milk should be used for infants, and then its bacterial content must be reduced further.

Partial Bacterial Control. Pasteurization. Shortly after it is obtained from the cow the milk is heated to a temperature of 150° F. for 30 minutes or, by the "flash" method, to a higher temperature for a shorter time. The conditions are sufficient to kill most pathogenic bacteria but do not render the milk sterile. Taste and cream formation are not altered. Following pasteurization the milk must be kept refrigerated in order to hold down the growth of the surviving bacteria. Most health departments require pasteurization of all milk for general sale, but local farms and dairies do not always treat their milk in this fashion. In general, fresh pasteurized milk is deemed suitable for the older infant or child, but it must be sterilized by heat when used in formula preparation.

Methods of Sterilizing Milk. BOILING. In the home the simplest method of sterilizing milk is to bring it to a boil for at least three minutes. Bacteria may also be killed by exposure to steam or by autoclaving the milk at appropriate combinations of temperature, pressure and time.

EVAPORATED MILK. The milk is first reduced to about half its original volume, then sealed in air-tight containers and sterilized by heat. Evaporated milk needs no refrigeration and remains sterile until the can is opened. It is popular in infant feeding because of its safety, low cost and ease of storage and shipment. It is possible to skim the milk partially before evaporation, to homogenize it or to add vitamin D.

DRIED MILK. Raw milk is sprayed into a warm low-pressure chamber or onto hot rollers. Thus, nearly all of the water is extracted, and the powder is collected and sealed in airtight tins. The milk is usually pasteurized before being dried. It may be skimmed or may have carbohydrate added to it before processing. Like evaporated milk, it is sterile and easily kept and packaged.

PROPRIETARY MILKS. Many commercial varieties of sterile canned milk are available either as evaporated liquids or as powders which have been subjected to various chemical modifications to increase digestibility or restore lost vitamins.

Formula Preparation. The exact method used to prepare a formula in the home will depend on the ingredients and on the intellectual and economic status of the parents. Instructions must be precise but tailored to individual circumstances. Whatever the method employed, its objective is to provide a day's supply of formula which is sterile at the conclusion of its preparation and will remain so under refrigeration until each bottle is ready for use. Even though bottles and nipples are going to be sterilized, they should be thoroughly cleansed and well rinsed before use. Detergent soaps must be carefully removed since some of them are poisonous if ingested in significant amount. Once items have been sterilized they should be handled in such a way as to avoid subsequent contamination. Sterilized nipples can be housed in sterile screw-top jars or may be left on the bottles with protective tops or inverted into those which are so designed.

The *terminal method* of sterilization is most likely to result in sterile formula. The ingredients are measured into clean bottles, and the units with their nipples or caps are given a final sterilization in steam. The method has some disadvantages; certain proprietary formulas which contain added vitamins suffer a reduction in the concentration of some of these vita-

Table 9. Approximate Composition of Human and Cow's Milk

	Human	Cow's
Water—per cent	88	88
Energy—calories per ounce	20	20
Protein—grams per cent	1.5	3.4
(Casein)	(0.4)	(2.8)
(Lactalbumin)	(0.8)	(0.4)
Fat—grams per cent	3.8	3.8
Carbohydrate—grams per cent	7.0	4.8
Minerals—grams per cent	0.20	0.72
(Ca)	(0.04)	(0.15)
(P)	(0.02)	(0.15)
(Na)	(0.015)	(0.055)
(K)	(0.055)	(0.150)
(Fe)	(0.0001)	(0.00004)
Vitamin A—International Units per quart	2,000	2,000
Vitamin D—International Units per quart	50-100	3-5
Vitamin C—milligrams per quart	45	20 (raw)
Nicotinic Acid—milligrams per quart	1.7	0.85
Riboflavin—milligrams per quart	0.47	1.6
Thiamine—milligrams per quart	0.05	0.25

mins if terminally sterilized. Under some conditions of temperature and local water supply, a scum may form within the bottles which clogs the nipple holes and interferes with feedings. A simple modification of terminal sterilization makes it applicable to all formulas prepared from liquid proprietary or evaporated milks. The water (with added carbohydrate if ordered) is measured into each bottle, and the units with their nipples, caps, a funnel, forceps and can opener, are steam sterilized and cooled. Then the milk is added directly from the can through the sterile funnel, and the bottles are capped and refrigerated at once.

Chemical Modification of Milk

The major chemical differences between cow's milk and human milk are summarized in Table 9. Both are dilute fluids composed of about 90 per cent water and 10 per cent solid constituents. Their energy values are the same (20 calories per ounce), since the lower content of carbohydrate in cow's milk is exactly compensated by an increase in protein. The minerals are two to three times as plentiful in cow's milk. The natural content of vitamins C and D is low, and the former is usually decreased further by procedures used to sterilize cow's milk.

Historically, the goal in formula preparation has been to achieve a product which simulates breast milk as closely as possible. It is now recognized that infants have a wide range of digestive tolerance, and that exact compliance with this goal is unnecessary for most of them.

Protein. The total concentration of protein in cow's milk is more than twice that in breast milk. However, the quality of the protein differs by virtue of its higher content (85%) of casein and lower content (15%) of lactalbumin. Complete digestion of the protein yields an ample supply of the essential amino acids (those which the body is unable to ·synthesize from other materials).

A major consideration in the modification of cow's milk is the quality of curd formed in the stomach. When milk meets the gastric juice the casein portion is coagulated while the lactalbumin remains in solution. Digestion of the curd depends on its physical qualities—large curds being tough and difficult for the digestive juices to manage; small, flocculent curds yielding more readily. The high concentration of casein in cow's milk favors formation of large curd coagulums and slows digestion, gastric emptying time and later absorption. Thus it is imperative to modify the casein by partial digestion (or denaturation) before it is admitted to the stomach. Historically, this was achieved by diluting and boiling the milk. A similar result is accomplished by evaporation and drying; thus the methods which sterilize are effective in changing casein so that it will form smaller curds. Additional methods of predigestion are treatment of milk with acid or alkali or with a proteolytic enzyme. Homogenization which is primarily directed at breaking the fat into small particles has a modest effect on the character of the resulting curd. Pasteurization is too mild a process to influence the protein significantly. One or more of these processes of protein alteration is invariably used in the construction of infant formulas, whether in the home or during the processing of the milk before sale.

Preparations are available which increase the protein content of formulas. Essentially, these consist of milk to which casein, pretreated with a proteolytic enzyme, has been added (protein milk), or of supplements which consist of casein completely reduced by hydrolysis to its constituent amino acids.

Fat. Although the total content of fat in cow's and human milk is approximately the same, there are differences in the types of fatty acids contained within the fat which render cow's milk somewhat more irritating and less readily digestible. Premature babies and individual full-term infants may require reduction or alteration in the fat of the formula offered. The process of homogenization (forcing milk through a small aperture under high pressure, resulting in dispersion of the fat into very fine globules which remain uniformly suspended in the milk) aids digestion by providing a larger surface area on which the lipases of the intestinal tract can act. Dilution and partial or complete removal of the fat are also used in the modification of formulas.

When the fat content of milk is reduced by partial or complete skimming, its energy value is significantly reduced, since fat supplies 9 calories per gram as contrasted with 4 for proteins and carbohydrates. Thus the formula must be given in larger volume to meet the energy requirements, or it must be fortified by the addition of calories in another form, usually as carbohydrate.

Some commercial preparations remove the fat from cow's milk completely and replace it with another, more digestible type such as olive oil.

Most full-term infants are able to accept the fat of cow's milk in its original concentration. When intolerance of a formula is manifested or during disease, particularly diarrhea, it is common practice to reduce the intake of fat in the infant's formula.

Carbohydrate. The same form of carbohydrate (lactose) is present in both milks, but its concentration is higher in breast milk. Traditionally, it has been the practice to add carbohydrate to formulas of cow's milk in order to reach the same concentration. If dilution or skimming is employed in the formula construction, carbohydrate addition is desirable to increase the energy value and avoid the necessity of feeding unusually large volumes. Some physicians now believe that the addition of carbohydrate to whole or evaporated milk formulas is unnecessary and that infants profit by receiving a higher proportion of their calories in the form of protein.

A great many types of carbohydrate have been used as supplements in the construction of formulas. In addition to simple sugars such as dextrose, levulose and lactose, various residues of starch digestion are employed. Control of intestinal fermentation and of the laxative effect of the formula is imputed to the proper selection of carbohydrate. The importance of this aspect of infant feeding has been overemphasized.

Minerals. In ordinary formula construction no attempt is made to reduce the concentration of minerals, which is two or three times as high in cow's milk as in human milk. Commercially, it is possible to produce milk which is very low in its content of sodium and other minerals. Occasionally, the high mineral content of cow's milk must be considered in feeding prematures or infants with cardiac or renal diseases. The high concentration of phosphorus renders the artificially fed infant somewhat more susceptible to tetany of the newborn. Both human and cow's milk are deficient in iron, which must be obtained from other foods or from therapeutic administration.

Formula Construction

The tasks of prescribing and preparing artificial formulas for infants have been greatly simplified by modern technics of food packaging and by a change in the philosophy of infant feeding. It has been amply demonstrated that most infants thrive on simple milk modifications, and for the few who do not there is now available a multiplicity of canned prepared mixtures. The supervisor of infant feeding usually selects a formula and instructs the parents about the probable limits of intake which will be required to support growth and to avoid digestive disturbances from overeating. The parents are then encouraged to allow the infant to indicate his individual desire in respect to amounts and frequency of feeding within these broad limits. Periodic evaluation by the supervisor is required to judge whether or not the result is satisfactory.

The selection of a formula by a hospital, a clinic or a physician is based on past experience and on the economic circumstances of the clientele. Formulas based on evaporated and dried milks are the most economical. Proprietary preparations are more convenient but more expensive.

Evaporated Milk Formulas. Evaporated milk is popular as a base for formulas because of its low cost, general availability, sterility, and convenience in storage and handling. In the United States, government supervision keeps the more than 400 different brands equivalent in composition so that they may be used interchangeably. For newborn infants evaporated milk is usually diluted with water in a ratio of 1:2 or 2:3. For older infants it is reconstituted to the strength of whole milk by adding an equal volume of water. Although the addition of carbohydrate is traditional, it may be omitted. When sugar is added the concentrations used ordinarily range from 5 to 8 per cent.

Nearly all brands of evaporated milk are fortified by the addition of 400 I.U. of vitamin D to the 13-oz. can. An infant whose daily formula intake includes the contents of a can of evaporated milk will simultaneously receive his quota of vitamin D.

The caloric value of evaporated milk formula depends on its degree of dilution and the amount of carbohydrate added. The weakest dilution ordinarily used (1 part evaporated milk to 2 parts of water) yields about 14 calories per ounce. A dilution of equal parts of evaporated milk and water has about the same energy value as whole milk—21 calories per ounce. Each 1 per cent of added carbohydrate increases the energy value by 1.2 calories per ounce.

Fresh Milk Formulas. When pasteurized milk is used as the basis of a formula it must be boiled in order to modify the curd and to complete sterilization. Soft-curd and enzyme-treated liquid milks require no additional modification of the protein but must be boiled if sterility is desired. For older infants these various fresh milks may be used as they come. Ordinarily, water in amounts not exceeding one third of the volume of milk is added as diluent for young infants. Carbohydrate additions may be made in the customary 5 to 8 per cent strengths. Many fresh milks are fortified by the addition of vitamin D.

Formulas of this type have no particular advantage over evaporated milk. They are more expensive and more cumbersome in preparation. In addition, they require continually fresh supplies of milk and refrigerated storage.

The caloric value of formula prepared from fresh milk is 20 calories per ounce when the original milk is not modified. Dilution reduces the caloric value proportionally; the addition of carbohydrate increases it as noted above.

Dried Milk Formulas. Dried powdered milk is available in canned and sterilized form and can be reconstituted to its original strength by the addition of boiled water. Like the fresh milks it may be diluted or sweetened as desired. Some dried milks are partially skimmed, and others completely skimmed, so that on reconstitution they yield lower caloric values. Dried milk has the advantages of low cost and convenient storage in bulk and is more commonly used as a formula base by institutions than in the home. Vitamin D is not usually added to the powdered milks and must be given as a supplement.

Proprietary Formulas. A variety of commercially prepared formulas are packaged as powders or as liquids which on proper dilution with boiled water provide a "complete" diet for the infant, including an adequate intake of the vitamins required. These preparations are generally satisfactory and convenient but suffer the disadvantage of somewhat increased cost. Special attention is usually given to making the reconstituted mixture resemble breast milk as closely as possible.

Formulas for Prematures. Because of the premature's relative inability to digest and absorb the fat of cow's milk, the most generally used formulas are based on skimmed or partially skimmed milk. The energy value lost by the removal of fat is more than compensated by the addition of carbohydrate, since it is desirable to meet the energy needs of these small infants without having to feed excessive volume. Formulas may consist of half-skimmed milk to which 7 to 10 per cent carbohydrate is added. Another approach is to use evaporated milk in more than the usual dilution and add carbohydrate in similar high percentage. Proprietary milks with low fat content may be used, frequently with addition of carbohydrate. The exact caloric value of such mixtures varies, but it is usually above 20 calories per ounce and may run as high as 27 calories per ounce. Vitamin supplementation is particularly necessary for the premature infant.

Hypoallergenic Formulas. For the infant who is allergic to cow's milk it is necessary to alter or to avoid the protein fraction. When sensitivity is mild, the degree of protein alteration accomplished by evaporation, drying or boiling may be sufficient. More drastic alteration can be accomplished by prolonged heating of cow's milk, which is the basis for some hypoallergenic milks. Avoidance of cow's milk proteins is achieved by using milk from another species of animal such as goat's milk, or through substitution of one of the artificial milks prepared from vegetable proteins such as soybeans or almonds, or a milk which contains protein only in the form of its constituent amino acids. Goat's milk is quite similar to cow's milk and can be obtained in dried or evaporated form and used similarly. It is notorious in its ability to produce anemia and must be supplemented with appropriate hematinics. The milks of vegetable origin have the disadvantages of unpalatable taste and somewhat lower nutritional value but can be used as exclusive sources of protein over long periods.

Vitamin Supplementation

When the type of basic feeding for the infant has been determined it is necessary to be sure that daily vitamin requirements will be met. Only under unusual circumstances will vitamin A be lacking, since both breast and cow's milks contain an adequate concentration. However, when milk is skimmed, much of the vitamin A is removed with the fat component and, unless it is restored or obtained from other foods, the intake may fall below the required 1,500 units per day. Vitamin A in good concentration is present in the fish liver oils which are used to supply vitamin D. It may also be given as carotene, which is a precursor of vitamin A.

A deficiency of members of the B-complex group of vitamins is unlikely, since both breast and cow's milk contains adequate concentrations. However, the optimal intake of many of these substances is not fully determined for infants, and many physicians believe that supplements are desirable if not essential. Individual members of the group may be added as synthetic chemicals or as mixtures in wheat germ or yeast preparations, or they may be obtained through the early addition of other foods to the infant's diet.

Care must be taken to be sure that the minimum of 25 mg. of vitamin C is being consumed. The breast-fed infant will receive most of his allotment if his mother is ingesting a diet well supplied with the vitamin, but the infant whose main food is heated cow's milk will receive little or no vitamin C from this source. Orange and other citrus fruit juices have been the time-honored media for supplying ascorbic acid. One ounce of fresh orange juice or 2 ounces of reconstituted frozen orange juice per day usually will cover the infant's needs. Because infants sometimes dislike or vomit orange juice it has become the more common practice to administer synthetic ascorbic acid in pill or liquid form or as part of a multiple vitamin concentrate. Overdosage with vitamin C is harmless.

Since most of the fresh and evaporated milk and nearly all of the proprietary formulas contain 400 units of vitamin D per quart, it has become debatable whether additional supplements are wise. Because small infants do not take a full quart of formula daily, and because there is no harm in giving two or three times the minimal required dose, it is a widespread practice to supplement. Breast-fed infants and those raised on skimmed milk formulas must be given extra vitamin D. Cod-liver oil has given place to concentrates made from the livers of percomorph fishes. Pre-

matures require higher dosage than full-term infants.

Multiple vitamin concentrates containing at least A, C and D and sometimes B-complex offer an easy way of making certain that the infant's vitamin needs are met. Undoubtedly, there is some economic waste in prescribing these mixtures for all infants no matter what the nature of their formulas, but within reasonable limits, no harm results. Misunderstanding of the function of vitamins occasionally leads to excessive dosage, particularly of vitamin D, in which case appetite and even growth may be hampered by the toxic effects of prolonged overdosage.

Technic of Feeding

In addition to determining the type of mixture to be used for the artificially fed infant, a tentative estimate must be made of the daily quantity which will be required to meet nutritional needs and to satisfy hunger. Most newborn nurseries offer full-time infants 1½ to 2 ounces every four hours. (The feeding of prematures is considered in Chap. 9.) By the time he is ready to leave the nursery, some intimation of each infant's appetite and feeding frequency may be obtained, and parents can be encouraged to permit him some freedom in determining the rate at which he will take the chosen formula. It is desirable to set maximal and minimal daily limits within which framework feeding behavior can be considered normal. After the initial period of adjustment, by the end of a week or 10 days of life, infants will not gain satisfactorily unless they are taking at least 80 calories per kilogram (or 36 per lb.) of body weight. From the infant's weight and the known caloric value of his formula the minimal desired intake can be calculated. Few normal infants will be peacefully satisfied with less than this minimum. At the other extreme are those infants who are very active, fussy or ravenous, due to an unusually strong growth impulse. Parents of such a child will need to know how rapidly and to what lengths they may safely go in making increases in formula in an attempt to appease the child's appetite. With most of the formulas in common use it is permissible to make gradual increases up to 150 calories per kilogram (or 70 per lb.) of body weight or a little more. Infants who consistently demand higher levels of food intake should be watched carefully for evidence of intolerance or should be studied for the possibility of abnormality.

Individualized or "demand" feeding schedules for small infants have been considered previously. Not all physicians subscribe to this approach; some exercise varying degrees of tight control over the times and the amounts of feeding. When dealing with parents of limited intelligence or those who are ritualistic by nature or too upset by anxiety, it is sometimes necessary to issue more didactic instructions. In the authors' experience the prompt accession to the small infant's

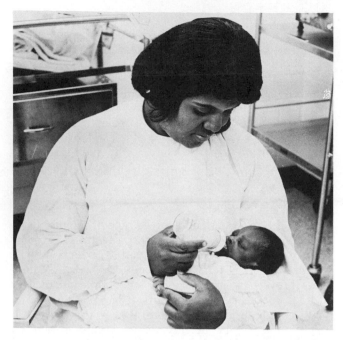

FIG. 8-5. Proper position for feeding the small infant.

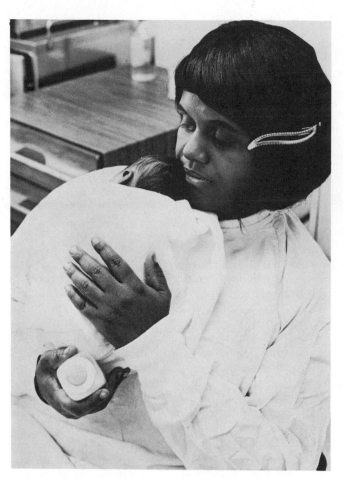

FIG. 8-6. Proper position for "bubbling" after or during feeding.

legitimate demands for food is a most important cornerstone on which to construct a wholesome mother-child relationship, not only in respect to feeding but also as a foundation for mutual confidence and pleasure in other aspects of their future life together.

The temperature of milk warmed to body temperature for feeding is tested by sprinkling a few drops on the inner aspect of the wrist, and the speed of flow observed. When the bottle is turned up, the milk should drop out rapidly but not run in a stream. If the holes are too small, they can be made larger with a hot needle.

The size of the nipple holes must be geared to the type of formula being fed and to the needs of the individual infant. Sick infants with lowered vitality require a nipple with comparatively large holes. The hungry infant who sucks vigorously should be given a nipple with small holes to prevent him from getting his food too rapidly and to provide ample opportunity for sucking.

The baby should be held during feeding as he has need for emotional warmth at feeding time. If holding the baby is contraindicated medically, the bottle should be held throughout the feeding unless the infant wants to hold it himself.

After feeding, the young baby should be "bubbled," cuddled until he is ready for sleep and placed in bed. If he does not seem to be comfortable after being put down to rest, he should be bubbled again. Some babies need to be bubbled before, during and after feeding. It takes time to discover the way of feeding which best meets the individual infant's requirements.

DIGESTIVE DISORDERS

Digestion in Infancy

The digestive equipment of the infant is adequate for its task, but only when the food is appropriately chosen, prepared and administered. The expected rate of growth of the infant is far in excess of that which occurs at any later time. Consequently, in proportion to his size, an infant requires several times as much food as does an adult. Because of the immaturity of the digestive functions, the infant's food must differ from that of the older person in quality as well as in relative quantity. Even with the simple diet that babies customarily receive, the amount of food necessary approaches closely the digestive capacity. Digestive capacity is decreased by illness, particularly by certain common infections, with the result that digestive disturbances are much more common in infancy than at any other age period. Such disturbances, when they occur, are more serious for the infant than for the older person. By them he is deprived of much or all of his food through vomiting, diarrhea and food refusal. When deprived of food, the infant uses his body stores at a much greater rate than an older person, and serious consequences are more quickly evident. In order to prevent or to manage the digestive and nutritional disturbances of infancy, more detailed knowledge and attention are required than for feeding older children or adults.

Gastric Digestion. The important factors in gastric digestion are hydrochloric acid and the enzyme pepsin. Pepsin acts on protein, breaking it down to simpler products, which are further digested later by other enzymes in the intestine. No digestion of sugar or starch occurs in the stomach, and little if any of fat. Hydrochloric acid serves several useful purposes. When in sufficient concentration, it inhibits bacterial growth, activates pepsin, and to some extent influences the pyloric reflexes. The amount of acid present at birth is small, but it increases progressively. It is decreased by any illness and by severe malnutrition. When human milk is ingested, the gastric acidity finally reached is optimal for peptic digestion. Although cow's milk is neither acid nor alkaline, it has the property of binding small amounts of acid without changing its reaction. To bring about the same degree of acidity it is necessary to add three times as much acid to cow's milk as to human milk. Modifications of cow's milk which have proved to be more or less uniformly successful in infant feeding have the common property of requiring relatively small amounts of acid to bring the acidity to a point optimal for peptic digestion, and the production of a fine curd in the stomach.

Soon after the ingestion of milk the casein is precipitated by the enzyme pepsin. Because of the small amount of casein in human milk, the precipitate is divided finely. Unmodified cow's milk, because of the larger amount of casein, gives rise to a large rubbery curd which may resist complete breaking up, and parts of it may be passed eventually in the stool as tough lima-beanlike masses. Cow's milk that has been boiled or has been subjected to heat incident to evaporation or drying gives rise to a curd resembling that of human milk, although somewhat coarser. Milk to which acid has been added in such a manner and quantity as to make a fine curd is better tolerated than either plain boiled or raw milk. The fineness of the curd undoubtedly contributes to the ease of digestion, and this factor is probably of greater importance than the degree of acidity reached in gastric digestion.

Practically no absorption takes place from the stomach. The stomach may be expected to be empty in two to three hours when human milk is fed, and in two and a half to three and a half hours with customary modifications of cow's milk. Emptying of the stomach is delayed by a high proportion of fat in the food and by illness of the infant.

Digestion in Duodenum and Small Intestine. It is in the duodenum and the small intestine that the greater part of digestion is accomplished. Protein that escapes gastric digestion is acted on by the pancreatic secretion, and the resultant products are further broken down into amino acids by an enzyme secreted by the mucous membrane of the intestine. The amino acids are absorbed and either converted to body protein or burned. Fats are changed into soaps and glycerin by pancreatic secretion and bile. These are absorbed from the small intestine to be reconstructed into body fat or burned. Another enzyme of the pancreatic secretion converts starch into sugar. Complex sugars are changed to monosaccharides (dextrose, levulose and galactose) by the secretions of the small intestine before absorption. The ability to digest starch is relatively feeble at birth, but it increases rapidly. If starch is fed in the very early months of life, a portion of it is likely to pass through the intestinal tract unchanged. Usually this does no harm, and only occasionally are fermentative processes set up.

Function of the Large Intestine. The chief function of the large intestine is to absorb water. Though it is capable of absorbing amino acids, salts and simple sugars, it is seldom called on for this purpose. Before reaching the large intestine, practically all the protein and its products will have been digested and absorbed. Sugars reaching the large intestine are fermented quickly by the bacteria present in enormous number. Some soaps remaining from fat digestion pass into the colon, though little or no digestion or absorption takes place.

The period required for food to pass through the gastrointestinal tract varies from eight to 36 hours, depending largely on the degree to which different food substances stimulate peristalsis.

Bacteria are not present in the intestinal tract at birth but gain entrance soon thereafter. They are not present in important numbers until food is given, in the presence of which they multiply greatly. The prevailing type of bacteria depends on the type of food that the baby receives. With human-milk feeding the bacteria are predominantly gram-positive; with formulas of cow's milk they are gram-negative. That one of these two types is more beneficial to the baby than the other has not been shown. Certain bacteria which grow in an alkaline medium are the cause of ammoniacal excoriations of the skin of the diaper region.

Stools

Meconium. Meconium is the term applied to the first stools passed after birth. Meconium consists of partially dried intestinal secretions which have accumulated gradually in the lower tract. It is dark brownish-green in color, semiformed, and is usually passed four to six times daily. About the third day, with the ingestion of food the stools begin to change, and by the fourth or the fifth day they have assumed the characteristics that persist for the subsequent months.

Character of Stools. The character of the stools is determined by the type of food ingested. Normal stools of infants fed on milk are composed of approximately 20 per cent solids, chiefly soaps, and 80 per cent water.

HUMAN MILK. When human milk is fed, stools may be passed only once or twice a day or may occur after every feeding. Characteristically, such stools are unformed but not watery; the color is bright or golden yellow or occasionally light green; the odor is unobjectionably aromatic; the reaction is acid. After the initial adjustment to breast feeding some infants will have soft stools that are passed, only every third or fourth day.

COW'S MILK. When cow's milk is fed in customary formulas, the stools are firmer than those from human milk and are passed less frequently, usually one to three times daily. Although yellow, they seldom have the bright yellow color of the stool from human milk. The reaction is neutral or slightly alkaline, and the odor is more or less foul. A high-sugar, low-protein diet (human milk) tends to cause more frequent stools, which are acid in reaction. A low-sugar, high-protein diet tends to cause the reverse condition.

Color of Stools. The color of stools when milk is the principal food is influenced chiefly by the rate at which the food passes through the intestinal tract. A diarrheal stool usually is green; a soft stool, yellowish; and a firm pasty stool, light yellow or almost white. These variations are due to the fact that the bile pigment in the upper intestine is green, but, after it has remained for some time in the intestinal tract, chemical action changes the green to yellow, and after further stay in the tract the yellow pigment is rendered colorless. When diarrhea occurs, the green bile coloring passes through the intestine so rapidly that it is not changed. A yellow stool, if exposed to the air for some time, often turns green on the surface, due to oxidation. This change of color is of no significance. Cereals, malt preparations or skimmed milk may lead to stools which are less yellow or of brownish color. Certain drugs, such as bismuth and iron, may color the stools black. With atresia of the bile ducts the stools are gray or clay-colored because of the absence of bile (acholic stools).

Mucus, Pus and Blood. A slight amount of mucus may be seen normally in the stools, especially those from breast-fed infants. A larger amount of mucus in the stools of either breast-fed or artificially fed babies is an indication of irritation of the intestinal tract and is often present with diarrhea. Pus does not normally occur in stools and when found, it indicates an inflammation of the intestinal wall (ileocolitis or dysentery). With severe inflammation of the wall of the intestine, blood as well as pus may appear in the stools. The blood may be bright, or, if its source is higher in the intestine, it may be a brownish or black color. It is mixed in streaks in the stool, or the whole stool may be bloody. Bloody stools also occur in association with intussusception. Small streaks of blood occurring on the outside of constipated stools usually mean nothing more than a slight crack or fissure at the anus.

Tarry stools (melena) may occur during the early days of life. It is important to know whether or not the blood being passed is the mother's blood, swallowed by the infant during the course of the delivery. If so, it is inconsequential and does not indicate internal bleeding in the infant himself. A simple chemical test differentiates fetal from adult hemoglobin in the stool and thus indicates from which individual the hemorrhage took place. If fetal hemoglobin is present, the situation is probably more grave, since bleeding into the intestinal tract from some cause such as ulceration, volvulus or hemorrhagic disease must be suspected.

Constipation. Difficult or insufficient stool passage, as an isolated complaint in a baby who is otherwise thriving, often means that normal intestinal behavior has been misinterpreted. Thriving breast-fed infants will commonly have intervals of two or three days between stools which are of perfectly normal consistency. Many infants behave as if in pain prior to passing a soft bowel movement because they feel the strong muscular contractions of the large bowel which precede evacuation. It is erroneous to call such behavior constipation. However, infants receiving diets derived mainly from cow's milk may pass infrequent, hard, dry stools which occasionally split the rectal mucosa while being expelled. This disorder can generally be corrected by augmenting the diet with other foods, particularly laxative fruits such as prunes or apricots. The use of soap sticks, suppositories or small saline enemas can be condoned occasionally, but it is both physiologically and psychologically unwise for the mother or the infant to become habitually dependent on them.

Excessive straining or the passage of stools of small caliber is due in some infants to a minor embryologic defect. In early fetal life the blind end of the hind gut descends within the abdomen to meet the anal dimple which is invaginating from the outside. Normally, these two pouches fuse end-to-end, and the septum between them disappears. Sometimes this process does not go to completion, and a partial constriction of the lower rectum remains about ½ to 1 inch inside the anus. Once discovered it is easily dilated with a finger inserted into the rectum.

Constipation is also a characteristic feature of some organic diseases—intestinal obstruction, pyloric stenosis, congenital megacolon, rectovaginal fistula and starvation.

Diarrhea. Diarrhea implies the passage of an excessive number of stools which are more fluid than normal. It is a potentially serious disturbance in small babies because rapid loss of fluid and electrolytes from the bowel may lead to dehydration and acidosis. However, the significance of loose bowel movements is not always easy to determine. Thriving breast-fed infants may have as many as eight or ten mushy or even fluid stools in a 24-hour period. Among artificially fed infants, one or more liquid yellow stools may be interspersed within a sequence of normal movements. Conversely, a small infant can become rapidly ill from infectious diarrhea before more than one or two suspicious stools have been passed. It is always necessary to consider other aspects of the infant's appearance and behavior in trying to decide the significance of loose stools.

The overenthusiastic use of demand feeding can lead to a mild or moderate diarrhea if the small infant is allowed to take food at a rate which is too rapid for his intestinal digestion. Usually, this mistake can be corrected in a day or so by a brief period of starvation followed by a controlled and graduated intake of food. There will always be some newborns who cannot tolerate the concentration of fat or carbohydrate which is accepted readily by others. The mild diarrhea that ensues can be controlled quickly with appropriate modifications of the formula.

Epidemic Diarrhea of the Newborn. A highly communicable type of diarrhea centering in hospital and newborn nurseries has been recognized with increasing frequency. Originally, the etiology was obscure. Various types of bacteria were implicated, and a virus origin was suspected. More precise methods of investigation have disclosed that many of these epidemics are due to particular strains of the common inhabitant of the intestinal tract—*Escherichia coli.* These pathogenic strains are presumably carried by healthy adults who handle the newborn infant. It is very difficult to identify such individuals by ordinary stool culture methods and to prevent their contact with small infants. Scrupulous technic in the nursery or rooming-in unit and prompt recognition of the epidemic form of the disease followed by rigorous isolation and dispersal of exposed infants are the only preventive measures that can be used. Fortunately, most strains of pathogenic *E. coli* have been found to yield to the antibiotics neomycin and colimycin given by mouth. With this treatment, the previously high rates of mortality among these infants have been reduced considerably. The clinical picture is that of a rapidly advancing toxemia without fever or symptoms other than watery, explosive stools and progressive weight loss. General management is the same as that described in Chapter 14 for other types of diarrhea.

Vomiting

Vomiting is a common symptom in small infants. It occurs both for trivial reasons and as the result of serious disease. The newborn infant in particular must be assisted in clearing the vomitus from his mouth and nose so that it will not be aspirated into his lungs. Special observation is indicated for infants who have shown a tendency to vomit and for all infants for a period after feeding when vomiting is most likely to occur.

Newborns frequently retch and vomit for several hours after birth for reasons which are not entirely clear. Some of them are undoubtedly trying to rid themselves of irritating secretions, amniotic fluid and blood swallowed during the course of delivery. In others the symptoms may be related to mild cerebral damage or the effects of drugs administered to the mother. Occasionally, postnatal vomiting will linger for two or three days and interfere with the establishment of feeding. Lavage of the stomach will often terminate this difficulty. If the infant continues to vomit blood, it is prudent to test the vomitus in order to confirm the fact that it is maternal blood which is being regurgitated. If it is fetal blood, ulceration of or bleeding into the upper intestinal tract must be considered.

Vomiting which occurs immediately after the first attempts to administer fluids or feeding and is accompanied by sputtering, coughing or strangling should be investigated at once for the possibility of esophageal atresia or some abnormality of the swallowing mechanism. The infant may suffer from the repeated aspiration of food if the abnormality is not recognized and treated quickly.

Persistent ejection of vomitus which becomes green in color from regurgitated bile is usually a sign of mechanical obstruction of the intestinal tract and demands careful observation and study. (See Chap. 11.) Vomiting of this kind usually appears within 48 hours after birth.

Infants suffering from any type of infection, intracranial bleeding, hydrocephalus or urinary tract obstructions may vomit repeatedly. Vomiting that progressively increases in frequency, amount and force and is associated with poor weight gain should raise the suspicion of pyloric stenosis, which is discussed in Chapter 13.

A number of trivial causes lead to occasional or even recurrent vomiting in small infants who are learning to adjust to a new method of feeding. Overdistention of the stomach with food or air which is gulped down during the feeding is one of the commonest causes. Careful "bubbling" after feeding will reduce the risk of regurgitation after the infant has been placed in his crib. Some babies almost invariably bring up a small portion of feeding, frequently without apparent effort. The reason seems to lie in a laxity of the cardiac sphincter of the stomach which permits small amounts of the stomach contents to escape back up the esophagus. In some infants the symptom continues for several months until feedings are followed by the assumption of an erect position.

Colic

Infants in the first few months of life who have frequent fits of sudden crying are commonly regarded as suffering from colic. There are many theories about the nature of colic which govern the type of treatment. It is possible that several factors may be responsible and that the behavior observed is merely the response of an immature infant to any of a number of discomforts.

Infants who suffer from colic are generally small at birth (5 to 7 lbs.). They tend to be lean with tense muscles and a nervous system which is easily triggered into a maximal response by the slightest of stimuli. During much of their day such infants are either asleep or violently protesting their discomfort. They do not remain long in the middle ground of quiet, satisfied wakefulness. The symptoms tend to be worse in the early evening and nighttime hours than during the day. The persistence of this type of behavior is variable. In many instances it ceases rather abruptly—often without any particular change in regimen. Such a welcome cessation may come at 3 to 4 weeks or as late as 3 to 4 months. The colloquial designation "three-month colic" suggests the average duration and enforces the suspicion that it is predetermined and not related to treatment.

The behavior of an infant with colic usually suggests paroxysmal abdominal pain due to excessive accumulation of gas in the intestine or the stomach. Crying starts abruptly with loud screams, clenched fists and legs that are drawn up on the abdomen. During the general muscular contraction, gas may be expelled from the anus or may be belched up from the stomach. The traditional efforts to explain and treat colic center around control of the gas production within the intestinal tract.

Excessive air-swallowing often is considered as an important factor. Too-rapid feeding during which the infant gulps down air is blamed. Small nipple holes or a breast that yields little milk can result in vigorous sucking and swallowing efforts which also carry an excessive amount of air into the stomach. Depending on the individual situation, the feeding procedure may need to be altered. Frequent burping of the baby during and after feeding usually is advised. The use of carminatives such as peppermint water and fennel tea to aid in relaxation of the cardiac sphincter of the stomach is a household remedy that generally is not effective. Enemas, suppositories and rectal tubes to relieve distention of the lower bowel are advised sometimes, but the same result usually can be achieved by turning the infant on his abdomen.

The accumulation of gas in the intestine is attributed by some to intestinal indigestion from overfeeding or from excessive use of carbohydrate, which fosters intestinal fermentation and produces gas within the lumen of the bowel. On this basis, various modifications of the amount and the type of formula are made.

Another approach is the attempt to reduce the vigor of intestinal movements by the use of drugs such as antispasmodics, phenobarbital and tranquilizers. The local application of heat by the use of a hotwater bottle also is advocated by some.

Yet another theory holds that colic is largely emotionally conditioned. The fact that many colicky infants are relieved of their distress merely by being held or permitted to suck on a pacifier is cited as evidence that the disturbance may be due to insufficient tensional outlet. Mothers are encouraged to get rest for themselves and to use a pacifier and rocking chair as necessary.

Whatever the importance of these various factors, at the present time it cannot be said that colic has a single etiology or appropriate treatment. The measures that are important for relief of the infant (and his mother) must be worked out by trial and error in each instance.

SITUATIONS FOR FURTHER STUDY

1. If a pregnant woman asked you the advantages of breast feeding, how would you handle her inquiry?

2. If one of your prenatal patients told you that she was unable to make a decision in regard to feeding her baby, how would you help her?

3. Compare the composition of human and cow's milk. How is cow's milk modified to simulate human milk?

4. What principles of feeding an infant do you apply in feeding the babies in the infant unit?

5. How would you help a mother who described symptoms of colic in her month-old baby?

6. What questions would you ask if you were a visiting nurse and a mother told you that her baby had vomited several times?

7. Observe an infant with severe diarrhea. Describe his appearance, symptoms and behavior and outline a plan of nursing care. Observe the infant's responses to you from day to day and record the changes in behavior which occur. How do you account for these changes?

BIBLIOGRAPHY

Cohen, D. J.: The crying newborn's accommodation to the nipple, Child Development 38:89, 1967.

Dyal, L., and Kahrl, J.: When mothers breast feed, Am. J. Nurs. 67:2555, 1967.

Evans, R. T., Thigpen, L. W., and Hamrick, M.: Exploration of factors involved in maternal physiological adaptation to breast feeding, Nurs. Research, 18:28, 1969.

Fomon, S. J.: Infant Nutrition, Philadelphia, Saunders, 1967.

Iffrig, Sister Mary Charitas: Nursing care and success in breast feeding, Nurs. Clin. N. Am. 3:345, 1968.

Ingles, T.: Maria—the hungry baby, Nurs. Forum 5:36, 1966.

Rubin, R.: Food and feeding—a matrix of relationships, Nurs. Forum 6:195, 1967.

Smith, C. A.: Pediatric practice: Human milk and breast feeding, Pediatrics 34:873, 1964.

9

Nursing Care of the Premature, the Postmature and the Dysmature Infant

Between 85 and 90 per cent of live babies are born between 37 and 43 weeks after the mother's last menstrual period and are considered to be full-term. A little less than 10 per cent appear before the 37th week of gestation and are designated as prematures. The problem of rearing these early arrivals has fascinated both the laity and the medical profession throughout the present century and a great deal of research and study has been devoted to working out methods and apparatus to encourage their survival. Many of the problems are understood and adequately handled by modern methods, but the statistics in Chapter 3 show that more than half of the deaths during the first year of life occur among prematures and that the first is the most lethal year of childhood. Only recently has attention been attracted to the 5 per cent of infants who remain in the uterus longer than they should. Their risks, too, are somewhat greater than those of full-term babies. The management of postmaturity is obviously an obstetric rather than a pediatric concern, and discussion will be limited to a description of their characteristic features and some aspects of postnatal care.

PREMATURITY

Definition

A premature infant is one who is born before the conclusion of the normal period of gestation. Ideally, the determination of prematurity should be based on the length of time that elapses between conception and birth. Methods for estimating the date of conception are so notoriously inaccurate that a less debatable standard of classification—the birth weight—has been adopted universally. By international agreement a premature infant is now defined as one which weighs less than 2,500 Gm. (5½ lbs.) at birth. In setting this standard it is admitted that some infants who are actually premature by gestational age (less than 37 weeks) will be classified erroneously as mature and,

conversely, that some infants who are small for reasons other than short gestation periods will be labeled wrongly as premature.

Causes

A physiologic reason for prematurity is apparent in only about half the cases. Abnormal conditions in the mother are the most frequent explanation—toxemia of pregnancy, uterine bleeding, early rupture of the membranes, chronic heart, kidney or thyroid disease, diabetes, syphilis, tuberculosis, acute infections, accidents or abdominal operations. When there is more than one fetus in the uterus, the excessive size causes premature labor approximately three times out of ten. Some varieties of severe malformation of the fetus are responsible for premature labor.

Research to discover other causes of prematurity is urgently needed, for the majority of premature infants are born to women who show no symptoms of physical illness. Studies already disclose the fact that good prenatal care which includes an adequate protein intake decreases the incidence of toxemia and prematurity.

Incidence

Using the criterion of birth weight of less than 2,500 Gm., the incidence of prematurity may vary considerably among different obstetric services depending upon the population group served. Race, socioeconomic status and altitude influence the weights at which full-term infants are born. Caucasian and northern European stocks tend to have large babies; Asiatic and Negro races generally have smaller ones. Poor economic circumstances, even apart from the racial association, probably produce smaller babies. High altitude, i.e., above 10,000 feet, has a marked effect upon birth weights, increasing the percentage of small infants. Thus, individual hospitals may find that their incidence of prematurity ranges from a low of 4 to 5 percent to upper levels of 12 to 15 per cent if based exclusively on birth weight.

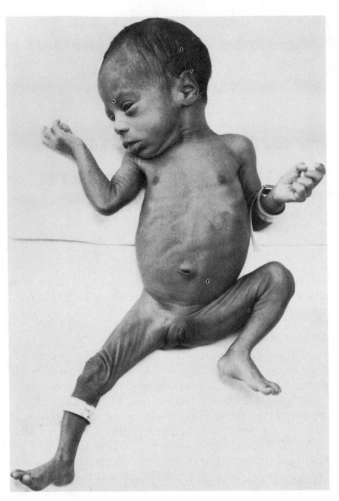

FIG. 9-1. A premature infant, showing the relatively large head, small muscles, loose skin and thin abdominal wall through which loops of intestine may often be seen.

Prevention

The medical profession is attempting to prevent prematurity through improved services to all expectant mothers. Care that protects the infant as well as the mother is being provided for expectant mothers with placenta previa and premature rupture of the membranes. Mothers with placenta previa are hospitalized where bed rest and transfusions can be provided. Instead of inducing labor when membranes rupture spontaneously, some obstetricians are prescribing antibiotics, bed rest and careful perineal care. With special care which includes support to help the woman to adjust to her pregnancy, obstetricians are finding that the pregnancy continues for days and in some instances to term.

Handicaps

It is to be expected that an infant born before he has completed the biologic steps desirable for extrauterine life will have a more difficult time making the adjustment than will the infant who is appropriately mature. This hypothesis is confirmed by mortality figures which show that the premature's chances of failing to survive are 10 to 15 times as great as the risk run by a full-term child. Of all the infant deaths occurring in the first month of life, more than half are in babies who were born prematurely. The handicaps that the premature must surmount in order to survive differ in kind, number and severity, depending on the degree of his immaturity. The smaller the infant is at birth, the more arduous his struggle for survival. After a general survey of the problems that all prematures face and the care that these handicaps necessitate, the characteristics, prognosis and additional nursing care for infants with different degrees of immaturity will be considered in more detail.

Prenatal Disturbance. The same prenatal disturbance that produced the premature birth may constitute a serious handicap. An infant hastily delivered because of his mother's toxemia of pregnancy may be ill from the effects of the maternal disease; one who was extracted because of maternal bleeding may have suffered anoxic damage to the brain. Syphilis in the mother may mean both premature birth and an infection for the infant. Erythroblastosis or severe anomalies may pose insuperable handicaps for the premature infant.

Difficulty in Establishing Respiration. There are many reasons why difficulty in establishing respiration is the most common single cause of death among premature infants. In the very immature infant the fault lies within the lungs themselves, for important structural changes take place during the second half of pregnancy which enlarge the potential air sacs and bring them into closer approximation to the lung capillaries. Failure of this change to proceed to a critical point in the development of the lung accounts for most of the deaths attributed to "previability." In addition, the small premature is handicapped by weakness of the muscles that move his chest wall and by the plasticity of the bony framework which permits it to retract during inspiration, cutting down the effective expansion of the lungs within. Frequently, the stimulation of the respiratory center in the brain is irregular. An added hazard of the first few days is the respiratory distress syndrome or hyaline membrane disease, a peculiar variety of lung disorder which is described in the next chapter. It is primarily a disease of premature infants.

Even when the respiratory apparatus permits survival, symptoms of respiratory difficulty are apparent. The small premature infant is likely to show irregular, periodic breathing interspersed with long moments of apnea. Mild cyanosis is intermittently present.

The administration of oxygen relieves cyanosis and increases the rate and the regularity of respiration in the premature infant. However, its use must be tempered by the realization that oxygen in high concen-

FIG. 9-2. Method of handling a premature baby in an Isolette. (Air Shields, Inc., Hatboro, Pa.)

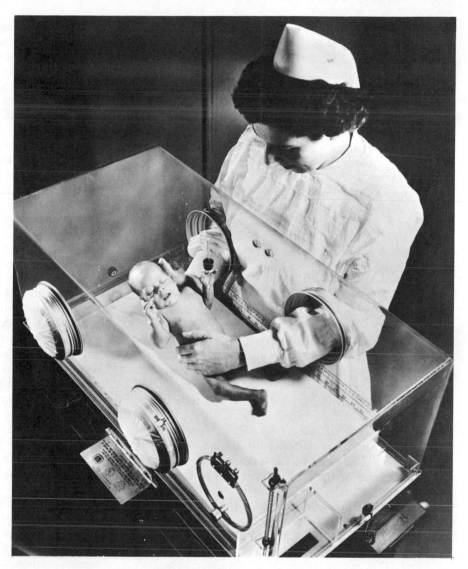

tration in the inspired air is the main cause of retrolental fibroplasia in the premature infant. The former practice of placing all prematures routinely in oxygen until respiratory sufficiency was proved has now given way to cautious administration only when the need is clearly demonstrated by the infant's condition. Since it has been shown that the danger from oxygen mounts rapidly when the concentration rises above 40 to 50 per cent in the inspired air, most premature nurseries require periodic testing of the concentrations in incubators, or use a supply which cannot yield more than 40 per cent. Use of higher concentrations cannot be categorically forbidden but should be regarded as an emergency procedure.

The water content of the atmosphere in the incubator should be kept high for, if the secretions within the bronchial tree are allowed to dry out, they block the exchange of air and produce additional areas of atelectasis. Some nurseries use devices to produce a mist or fog in the incubator, but this procedure cannot be shown to have a significantly better effect than a humidity of 90 per cent or so.

The question of respiratory adequacy usually is settled within the first two or three days of life. If the infant survives this period he may still have some unexpanded areas of lung, but, unless he is handicapped further by infection, the areas of atelectasis will be of decreasing importance to him. As with most other handicaps, the frequency and the severity of atelectasis are greater the less mature the infant is at birth.

Body Temperature. The premature infant has difficulty in regulating his body temperature, for it responds rather promptly to changes in the temperature of the surrounding environment. When placed in cold or drafty surroundings he has trouble conserving his body heat. As a result, his temperature may fall to subnormal levels. The factors that interfere with his efforts to hold or produce body heat are the relatively large surface area in proportion to his body size, the lack of an insulating layer of fat beneath his skin, poor reflex control of his skin capillaries, and the smallness and the inactivity of his muscles—the main source from which body heat is obtained. When the premature is placed in a hot environment, poor control over his skin capillaries and the lack of an adequate sweating mechanism prevent him from losing heat, and his body temperature rises accordingly.

Some type of mechanical incubator is highly desirable if not essential to the small premature infant in order to keep him at a stable temperature and to supply adequately humidified air. Now it is recognized that environmental temperature should be adjusted so that his body temperature ranges between 35.5° and 36.5° C. (96° to 98° F.) rather than attempting to push it up to the accepted normal range for older infants. At such lower levels stability is obtained more easily. The premature nursery should be kept warm (75-80° F.) and free of drafts. In hot climates and seasons, air conditioning is desirable. The humidity of the air should be kept between 55 and 65 per cent. Premature infants dehydrate easily. In humidified nurseries it has been found that initial loss of weight is less, the regaining of birth weight is more rapid, body temperature stabilizes more easily, and the incidence of respiratory infections and gastrointestinal disturbances is lower.

Poor Resistance to Infection. The premature infant's resistance to infection is notoriously poor. He receives less than the usual quantity of protective substances from his mother's blood and is denied the benefits of her early milk (colostrum). In addition, his ability to manufacture his own body proteins, including antibodies, is below par.

Protective measures to prevent infection are imperative because even trivial infections may be devastating to him. The organization of the nursery facilities should be such that prematures are kept in a unit separated from other children and even from the nursery for full-term newborn infants. None but a minimal number of essential personnel should be permitted within the unit. Isolation and aseptic precautions should be observed. The mere suggestion of an infection in one of the personnel should be considered adequate reason for excluding that person from the unit until recovery is complete. Prematures born outside the hospital and those who develop infections should be kept in a separate area. Modern incubators provide additional safeguards within the nursery. Most are so designed that the infant's complete care can be carried out without removing him from the enclosed space of the incubator. It is desirable to sterilize the clothing that comes in direct contact with the infant's skin and also the cotton and oil that are used for cleansing. The nurse needs to be constantly alert to observe symptoms which might indicate the onset of any type of skin, respiratory or gastrointestinal infection. In some nurseries it is standard practice to ad-

minister antibiotics to all small prematures until they have made a promising start and whenever any suspicion of infection arises.

Biochemical Handicaps. The large number of biochemical handicaps of the premature infant arise in part from his extremely rapid growth rate, in part from the immaturity of organs such as the liver and the kidneys, and in part from his failure to linger within the uterus long enough to acquire his full complement of certain essential materials.

The premature infant grows more rapidly than the full-term infant and requires a relatively large amount of food to supply building materials and energy. No other human being grows as rapidly. It is not uncommon for him to double his initial birth weight in the brief span of two months! In order to do this, if calculated in terms of calories per unit of weight, his requirements are from 30 to 50 per cent greater than those of the full-term infant.

The immaturity of the premature infant's digestive and nervous systems complicates the technic of meeting his food requirements. The limited capacity of his stomach must not be exceeded, for vomiting and aspiration of food into his lungs are to be avoided at all costs. The mere ability to suck and to swallow is sometimes lacking or too exhausting for him to perform frequently. Special methods must be used to convey food into his stomach. The ability of his intestinal tract to digest the food brought to it is also limited, particularly in respect to fat which he absorbs poorly. Care must be taken to see that too much is not forced upon him, for, if his tolerance for digestion is exceeded, diarrhea may result.

Immaturity of the liver accounts in part for the premature's poor resistance to infection (he forms antibody protein poorly), for his tendency to bleed (he forms prothrombin poorly), for his tendency to become edematous (his total serum protein concentration is low), and for his susceptibility to jaundice (his liver cannot adequately clear the blood of the pigments which result from the normal postnatal destruction of circulating red blood cells). Immaturity of the kidneys contributes to his limited tolerance for salt, to his tendency to become edematous and to the mild state of acidosis in which the premature normally lives.

The premature infant is born before he has fortified himself with his full quota of vitamins A, C, D and K and of the minerals phosphorus, calcium and iron, yet the rapidity of his immediate postnatal growth demands an unusual supply of these substances. During the last two months of pregnancy the full-term infant draws on his mother for stores of vitamins and minerals and therefore is protected temporarily from the vitamin-deficiency diseases such as rickets, scurvy and hemorrhagic disease of the newborn. Prophylactic quantities of the corresponding vitamins usually are given to the premature in double the dosage recommended for the full-term infant.* Calcium and phosphorus are present in milk in abundance to satisfy the needs of prematures. Iron is not supplied in adequate amounts by most feedings. Even when the diet is supplemented with medicinal iron, utilization is poor during the first six to eight weeks of life. However, it is commonly added in the hope of preventing as far as possible the anemia that regularly develops in the growing premature.

Retrolental Fibroplasia. Since 1940 a disease peculiar to premature infants has been recognized. In its fully developed form retrolental fibroplasia involves both eyes and produces complete or nearly complete blindness due to separation and fibrosis of the retina. For a while it was the chief cause of neonatal blindness until the role of oxygen in its production was discovered through cooperative study in a number of institutions which cared for prematures.

The main peculiarities of the disease are that it apparently did not exist before 1935, that it attacks the most immature infants more frequently than the larger prematures, that its incidence is extremely variable among different populations of prematures, and that its effects are not immediately apparent but are discovered only after weeks or months have elapsed. If the eyes of all premature infants are examined at regular intervals with the aid of an ophthalmoscope, the early pathologic changes may be observed some time before the infant reaches a weight of 1,500 to 1,800 Gm. These consist of dilation of retinal veins, hemorrhage and exudate into the retina and areas of separation of the retina from the inner surface of the eyeball. In some infants these changes regress, but in others there is progressive detachment of the retina until it is brought forward into an irregular, useless fibrotic mass retaining perhaps some light perception but no useful vision. The matted retina can be seen through the pupil as a greenish opacity. Unless routine ophthalmoscopic examination of eyes is made, loss of vision may be easily overlooked in small infants until they are 3 to 4 months of age.

Experimental and clinical study has demonstrated that the main factor in the causation of retrolental fibroplasia is oxygen poisoning. The premature's delicate retinal vessels are unusually susceptible to high concentrations of oxygen and go into spasm, which in turn leads to leakage of blood or serum through their walls. Extensive clinical study has shown that retrolental fibroplasia can be virtually eliminated from premature populations if oxygen is restricted to emergency use and if concentrations are never allowed to exceed 40 per cent. Most nurseries now monitor concentrations in incubators by periodic testing and adjustment of the flow of oxygen, or by valves in incubators which presumably limit the concentrations

---

* Too liberal use of vitamin K prophylactically is now suspected of causing kernicterus in prematures. Vitamin K_1 oxide is preferred in a dosage of 1 or at most 2 mg.

attainable, or by using a mixture of oxygen and nitrogen which makes it impossible to exceed 40 per cent concentration of oxygen. Careless and unnecessary use of oxygen is to be condemned, yet occasions arise when it cannot be withheld if the infant's life is to be saved.

Nursing Care of the Premature

In spite of the many hazards that beset prematurely born infants, 75 to 85 per cent will survive if given adequate care. Better obstetric practices, new medical discoveries and improved mechanical aids are all contributing to better care for these infants. But the benefits of such advances are easily erased if the daily nursing care of the infant is slighted. Many a prematurely born child owes his life in a very real sense to the devotion, skill and judgment of the nurses who administered to his early needs. The requirements of care differ with the initial size of the premature and will be considered separately for each of the main subdivisions by weight.

Prematures of 400 to 1,000 Gm. (14 oz. to 2 lbs. 3 oz.). With good luck and meticulous care about 10 per cent of these infants can be reared. Fetuses of less than 400 Gm. are classified as abortions. They never develop effective respirations and die within a short time after birth. Infants of birth weights between 400 and 1,000 Gm. are called previable and generally are not expected to survive, but some show unusual strength and survive despite their initial handicaps. Infants of such small size are infrequent. They comprise about 0.5 per cent of all live births and about 7 per cent of premature births.

Many external evidences of immaturity are present in this group of premature infants whose gestation period ranges from 20 to 28 weeks and length measures from 28 to 35 cm. (11 to 14 in.). The head is proportionately quite large, with high forehead and small facial features. The eyes are tiny, scarcely visible; the ears are soft and poorly developed; the chin recedes. The extremities are spindly, with tiny muscles and soft rudimentary nails on the fingers and the toes. The skin may be covered with lanugo (fine hair). The subcutaneous tissues are usually full, giving the appearance of plumpness. But if the infant survives a few days the skin hangs loosely on his body, demonstrating that the original appearance was due to edema rather than to subcutaneous fat. Nipples and genitalia are small, and in male infants the testes are often undescended. Activity of the infant is limited to the respiratory efforts, which may be weak and unpredictable. The soft chest wall retracts excessively during inspiration, and the mouth often opens in a gulping fashion. The sucking, swallowing and gag reflexes are usually absent in these very immature infants. They seldom cry. Cyanosis may be present constantly or during periods of prolonged apnea.

The nurse receiving any premature infant must be

wearing a sterile gown, and in addition must have scrubbed her hands and forearms with an antiseptic solution. The first objectives of nursing care are to maintain a stable, appropriate body temperature, to conserve body heat and muscular energy and to support the respiratory effort by the administration of humidified air and oxygen supplemented by stimulation as indicated. After the fluid has been cleared from the respiratory tract, the infant should be placed at once in an incubator, preferably one that has been preheated to 90° to 95° F. Premature infants at this weight level generally have lower rectal temperatures than more mature babies, and a rectal temperature of 95° to 96° F. need not be cause for alarm.

Subsequently, the unclothed infant is placed on his side and should be disturbed as little as possible in order to avoid respiratory distress. Necessary handling in order to aspirate secretions from the nose and for injection of vitamin K and antibiotics must be extremely gentle. All procedures must be carried out inside the incubator. Stimulants or periodic gentle compression of the chest may be required if the respiratory effort fails. Other means of respiratory support are considered in the next chapter.

Constant nursing care during the first 24 hours after birth is essential. The type of respiration, its rate and regularity must be carefully noted. The color and condition of the skin, looking particularly for pallor or cyanosis, must be observed as well as any indication of bleeding from the cord. The activity level of the infant and the strength and frequency of the cry are important indicators of progress. Bowel and bladder function should also be observed as to amount and character of stools and urine. Any noted changes in the infant's condition or abnormal signs must be immediately brought to the pediatrician's attention.

If much mucus is being produced, the infant may be placed in a prone position at intervals and the airways cleared with a sterile catheter. In most hospitals, mechanical aspirators are available; however a simple mouth operated catheter with a mucus trap is effective. Extreme care in inserting the catheter is imperative to avoid injury to the mucous membranes. If cyanosis is extreme, oxygen may be administered directly for resuscitation. However, during this time the oxygen supply to the incubator should be disconnected. Direct administration should be discontinued immediately after recovery in order to avoid unnecessary exposure to high oxygen concentrations, which risk injury to the eyes.

Mechanical incubators have the advantages of maintaining constant and correct levels of heat, oxygen and humidity. They prevent airborne infections, allow for easier observation of the infant and eliminate the need for clothing. However, when such apparatus is not available for the care of a small premature, external heat must be provided by other means. Within the hospital, infant beds can be utilized which have the advantage of easy accessibility and cleaning. They should be deep enough to prevent drafts and to allow for tilting the infant when necessary. Heat can be provided through the use of hot water bottles covered with a flannel washable bag to prevent burns. A thermometer placed between the blankets and the infant and bottles of water at a temperature of from 100° to 105° F. can be used as aids in controlling the temperature. When the water is changed, it should be done at the bedside to avoid a prolonged drop in environmental temperature. The room should be kept at a temperature of 85° to 90° F. The infant's temperature stabilizes more readily when environmental temperature is elevated than when he is heavily clothed and covered with additional blankets. His temperature should be taken every two to three hours until stabilization is acquired. Thereafter, twice daily is sufficient. An electric heating pad can also be used to provide heat, but it has the disadvantages of possible overheating, of electric shock, and risks of cross-infection. Every pad utilized must be covered with a washable cover and rubber sheeting to minimize these dangers and the cot thermometer should be inspected regularly. When an incubator is unavailable, administration of oxygen through a mask is serviceable but gives poor humidification and variable control of concentration.

Administration of food or fluid to these delicate infants may be deferred for a day or two until they have a chance to establish their respirations and to lose the edema fluid with which they were born. Since their power of digestion is very weak and abdominal distention may produce cyanosis, early feedings must be small. Additional fluid may be given by subcutaneous injection or by very carefully controlled intravenous infusion. Glucose solutions are generally preferred to salt-containing fluids, which may result in a return of edema.

Prematures of very low weight are often unable to suck or swallow normally and therefore the first food must frequently be given by gavage. This process of catheter feeding is also least tiring to the infant. Equipment for gavage consists of: a sterile catheter (American No. 8 or French No. 10), a medicine glass containing sterile water, a small pipette or glass syringe barrel, and the prescribed food. The infant is placed on his right side for feeding and the head of the incubator or bed mattress should be raised slightly. It is very important that the catheter tip be placed at the lower end of the esophagus for feeding in order to avoid vomiting or gastric irritation. The distance from the tip of the infant's nose to the lower end of the sternum should be marked on the catheter before it is sterilized. The marked catheter should be connected to the syringe barrel, lubricated with sterile water (not with oil which, if aspirated, can cause lipid pneumonia) and passed into the esophagus through the mouth. The catheter should not be inserted through the nose, because a catheter of this size can easily injure the nasal mucous membranes. When the marked portion of the catheter reaches the lips, the mouth of the syringe barrel is placed in the medicine glass of water to test the position of the catheter. If the tip of the catheter is in the stomach, a few bubbles of air may pass through the tube into the water but will then cease abruptly. The tube is unlikely to enter the larynx and trachea, but, if it should, air will bubble through the water in the glass on each expiration by the baby. In addition, the baby would become cyanotic, and if he were sufficiently vigorous he would have a spasm of coughing at the time the tube was inserted. If this occurs, the catheter must be removed immediately and reinserted.*

After the tube has been placed properly, it should be aspirated and the catheter then compressed tightly to avoid introduction of air into the stomach. The syringe barrel is held stable in one hand and the formula is poured into the barrel until it is full. After the food is poured, the catheter is released, and the barrel may be elevated sufficiently to allow the formula to run slowly into the stomach. The barrel should be refilled if necessary before it becomes empty to avoid unnecessary introduction of air. After all the food has run in, a minute should elapse to be certain the tube is clear and then it can be tightly pinched or bent before it is gently removed. If the catheter is not pinched or carefully and slowly removed, fluid may overflow into the larynx and cause inhalation pneumonia or atelectasis.

Plastic, indwelling nasogastric polyethylene catheters are used for gavage feeding in some institutions. These are usually inserted by the physician and changed every three to five days with alternation of nostrils. They are used to allow for frequent small feedings and to prevent distention and frequent handling of the infant. The method of marking, lubricating, inserting and testing anatomic position is the same as for single gavage feeding except the measurement is made from the tip of the sternum to the lobe of the ear and then forward to the nostril and the tube is inserted through the nose. The plastic, round-tipped catheter is sterilized before insertion and a plastic stopcock may be inserted into the end of it to close the tube when not in use. In some instances, a No. 20 needle may be inserted into the end of the catheter, the hilt serving as an adaptor to receive the syringe barrel for administration of formula. The barrel should be held no higher than 6 to 8 inches above the crib. Care should be taken to prevent air from going into the stomach. Just before all formula has run from the tip of the syringe barrel, a few drops of sterile water should be added to cleanse the cathe-

---

* Another method for determining the proper placement of the catheter tip is to listen over the stomach with a stethoscope for the inrush of air when a small amount is pumped through the catheter with the syringe.

ter of milk. At the completion of the feeding the catheter is again occluded. Compressing the catheter before it is removed is as important when indwelling catheters are used as it is when single gavage feedings are given.

In some nurseries small premature infants are fed through a surgically placed gastrostomy in order to permit safe and early administration of food.

The type of food, amount, frequency and method of feeding are prescribed in accordance with the infant's weight, physical response to ingestion of food and ability to suckle.

There is still difference of opinion as to the best type of milk to use in feeding low weight prematures. Those who advocate breast milk emphasize its superiority in freedom from microorganisms, the digestibility of its fat, its low mineral salt and phosphate content and its effectiveness in preventing enteric infections. In most instances, however, artificial formulas consisting of half-skimmed milk with added salt-free carbohydrate is generally preferred. The first feeding is usually delayed if the condition of the infant warrants. When feeding is begun, the quantity must be restricted to a few cubic milliliters at a time until the infant's capacity is learned. Overloading his stomach must be avoided for a single episode of vomiting and aspiration may prove fatal. Not only is regurgitation to be avoided but also abdominal distention. Distention is a cause of cyanotic attacks because it interferes with respiration, which is chiefly diaphragmatic. Gavage feedings may be given as often as every two hours, but generally longer periods are used to avoid too frequent disturbance. The amounts given are increased gradually until the food intake reaches 120 to 140 calories per kilogram (55 to 65 calories per lb.) of body weight. Water-miscible preparations of vitamins A, B, C and D which may be added to the gavage feedings are available. When the infant begins to suck on the gavage tube, cautious trials may be made with feedings from a dropper.

Feeding with a medicine dropper in low weight prematures should be most carefully done, since their swallowing reflex is generally very poor along with the poor sucking reflex. If it is possible however, such a feeding has the advantage of increasing the infant's pleasure in the feeding process. A medicine glass containing the prescribed feeding should be kept warm throughout the procedure. After the infant's diaper has been changed and the nurse's hands washed thoroughly, the nurse should support his head and shoulders with one hand and open his mouth by applying gentle pressure to the chin. Milk is dropped from a medicine dropper, sheathed in rubber tubing, well back onto the tongue, a drop at a time until the infant's ability to swallow has been ascertained. The feeding should not be hurried or forced. Gentle pressure on the back of the tongue may be used to stimulate swallowing. Care must be taken to make sure that there is no formula left in the baby's mouth at the end of the feeding. The infant may be supported partially erect for a while in order to permit bubbling. After all types of feeding described, the infant should be placed on his right side with his head and thorax elevated slightly in order to facilitate gastric emptying and to prevent regurgitation. Placing a diaper-roll support at his back keeps him in the desired position and may also provide him with feelings similar to those experienced *in utero*. Through a study of 59 prematures, Hasselmeyer* found that larger prematures slept more, cried less and moved about less when rolled-diaper support was used.

During the initial medicine-dropper feedings, the nurse should observe him for signs of fatigue. If the feeding leads to cyanosis and increased lassitude instead of pleasure, resumption of gavage feedings is indicated until he demonstrates increased capacity to participate without fatigue.

The necessary early caution in feeding, combined with the loss of edema fluid, results in a rather sizable loss of weight during the first two weeks. Premature infants usually lose up to 10 per cent of their birth weight, and it may take three to five weeks for the previable infant to regain his initial weight and make a steady daily increment. Three months or more may elapse before such an infant reaches the premature graduation weight of 2,500 Gm.

The prognosis of the previable infant is difficult to estimate because too few of those who survive are observed in follow-up studies. Previable infants who survive generally have rather large heads with narrow faces and slender body habitus. Their early growth and development is likely to be at least three months retarded for their chronologic age. Some of them catch up gradually, and a few at least reach adult life with normal mental competence. The risk of retrolental fibroplasia is a significant one in these small infants. Medicinal iron usually is given at 4 to 6 weeks of age. Administration must be started cautiously in order to avoid vomiting or diarrhea.

Prematures of 1,000 to 1,500 Gm. (2 lbs. 3 oz. to 3 lbs. 5 oz.). Since most of these infants have reached a stage of pulmonary maturity that can support life, the anticipated survival rate is distinctly better—from 40 to 50 per cent. Most of the deaths will occur in the first 48 hours of life from the respiratory distress syndrome (RDS), pulmonary hemorrhage or the effects of anoxia or intracranial injury. The number of infants born with weights in this range is slightly greater than the number of previable infants—a little over 0.5 per cent of total live births and about 10 per cent of all premature births. The gestational age ranges from 28 to 32 weeks, and the infants measure from 35 to 40 cm. (14 to 16 in.) in length.

The physical features are similar to those of the previable infant but less extreme in their divergence from the normal term infant. Periodic and ineffectual respiratory effort is common but not universal. Temperature regulation is poor. The sucking, swallowing and gag reflexes may be present at birth, but gavage feeding is still required as an introductory measure.

The early nursing care is identical with that of the previable infant but is required for a shorter period. Many infants in this group will be able to dispense with gavage feedings and the mechanical incubator within the first weeks of life. Initial weight losses are usually marked, but the food intake can be increased at a more rapid pace, and the birth weight is often regained by 3 to 4 weeks of age, and steady weight progress is made thereafter.

Prematures in this group can tolerate more handling after their initial adjustment to extrauterine life. Generally, infants weighing less than 2,000 Gm. are not exposed to a daily soap and water bath because of the mechanical irritation to delicate skin and risk of chilling. Warmed oil baths may be given every other day, or a warmed solution of 3 per cent hexachlorophene on sterile swabs may be used to clean skin folds. Handling of the baby should always be done before feeding in order to minimize the risk of regurgitation. On alternate days, care may be given only to the head and genitalia, although the entire body can be observed to appraise the general condition.

During the period of adjustment, daily weighing may be eliminated in order to avoid unnecessary handling. Thereafter, exposure should be prevented and care taken to avoid cross-infection. While in a closed incubator, the infant can be weighed in an individual, washable sling. When his condition permits, he may be weighed twice weekly on a scale taken to the side of the incubator or bed. The infant should be covered with a blanket during transfer to the scale, and the scale pan should be covered with a clean sheet of paper. Weight of blanket and clothing are deducted from the total weight.

These infants, too, will bear the marks of their prematurity for many months after birth—large, narrow heads, important degrees of anemia, retardation of growth and development by at least two months. Their chances for eventually having normal mentality and size are fair. The risk of developing retrolental fibroplasia is still significant if oxygen is used heedlessly.

Prematures of 1,500 to 2,000 Gm. (3 lbs. 5 oz. to 4 lbs. 6 oz.). The added maturity greatly improves the rate of survival in this group of infants, so that 75 to 80 per cent may be expected to live. The gestational ages approximate 32 to 35 weeks, and the length at birth varies from 40 to 43 cm. (15½ to 16½ in.). About twice as many infants are born with weights in this range as in the preceding group—somewhat over 1 per cent of total live births and about 20 per cent of all prematures.

* Hasselmeyer, Eileen: Behavior Patterns of Premature Infants, A Nursing Study, Washington, D. C., Division of Nursing, U.S. Public Health Service, 1961.

The physical characteristics of extreme prematurity are less marked. Heads are not as large relatively, edema is less common, and some of the infants show a modest amount of subcutaneous fat. Although initial respiratory difficulty will create a problem for some of them, routine use of high humidity is no longer necessary. The ability to stabilize body temperature is much better, so that most of these infants can be transferred rapidly to a heated crib or an ordinary crib in an evenly warmed room. The sucking, gag and swallowing reflexes are regularly present unless the infant is abnormal in some manner apart from his prematurity. Feeding by gavage is generally unnecessary.

Medicine-dropper feedings may be necessary temporarily for some of these babies, but the majority of them soon indicate their ability and eagerness for sucking activity. The more vigorous infants in this group may be fed from a bottle with a soft rubber nipple after the initial dropper feeding. The nipple should be chosen with care. It should not have holes that are too large or too small. When the nipple holes are too small, the infant becomes unduly fatigued; when they are too large the baby is forced beyond his capacity and is deprived of the pleasure and exercise that sucking supplies.

As soon as the infant's physical condition permits, he should be fed according to his manifest hunger needs and held throughout the feedings. Like the full-term infant, he, too, needs cuddling associated with his feedings. From the moment of birth the nurse should be sensitive to the discomforts and hazards that the prematurely born infant is experiencing, both physically and emotionally. Nursing measures that preserve life and provide gratification should be carried out. He needs a soothing, warm and tranquil environment; he requires interest in him as an individual and care that takes into account his emotional as well as his physical needs. It is possible to gratify an infant when he signals his distress, be it from insufficient sucking, hunger or sheer loneliness and a need for closeness, without exposing him to infection, overfeeding or fatigue.

Within this group steady weight gains are generally established by 2 to 3 weeks of age, and growth and development proceed at a rate that is about one to two months behind the average for the chronologic age. The risk of retrolental fibroplasia is greatly diminished but not entirely absent.

Prematures of 2,000 to 2,500 Gm. (4 lbs. 6 oz. to 5 lbs. 8 oz.). The degree of prematurity is mild in this group of infants, and a proportional reduction in the handicaps permits from 90 to 95 per cent or even more to survive. The bulk of the premature infants falls within this weight range—about 4 per cent of the total births and from 60 to 65 per cent of all the premature births. The gestational ages approximate 35 to 38 weeks, and the infants measure from 43 to 47 cm. (16½ to 18 in.) in length.

Apart from smallness, the physical characteristics and care differ little from those of full-term infants. Slenderness and hyperactivity are common. Mechanical apparatus for the regulation of body temperatures or for the administration of oxygen and humidified air is seldom required. Bottle feeding may be commenced at once, and the infants can be picked up and held during feeding. Some of the larger and more vigorous members of this group can be cared for in the regular nursery or may visit their mothers. Most of them will begin to gain weight steadily after 10 days to 2 weeks. Few of them will have to remain within the confines of the premature nursery for more than a month. Immediate direct breast-feeding is feasible for some of the larger infants; eventual nursing can be carried out for most of them. Mothers should be encouraged to keep their supply of breast milk flowing by regular emptying of the breasts with manual expression or by the use of a breast pump. The main reason for segregating these large prematures from the full-term infants is to shield them from infection and to give them the benefit of skilled assistance in their early feedings.

Growth and development proceed at a pace that is only temporarily behind that of other infants of the same age. Nearly all of them will catch up within the first six months of life. Retrolental fibroplasia is seldom found in infants of this degree of maturity.

Maternal Preparation

Preparing the mother for the care of her prematurely born infant should begin in the immediate postpartum period and continue until she has developed confidence in her ability to understand and meet his needs. To alleviate the mother's anxiety the nurse must be able to understand the emotional problems common to mothers of premature infants. She must also understand and accept her own reactions as she is caring for the infant over an extended period.

The nurse who is responsible for the intimate, daily care of a premature baby is not only vital in maintaining his life, but she also assumes maternal functions to a greater degree than is common for most mature babies. Since the dependency needs of prematures are so great, they demand much of their nurse and thus the possibility of emotional attachment also is much greater. Some nurses may defend themselves against this emotional involvement through mechanical care activities. Others may unconsciously feel distant toward the mother or erect barriers to real understanding of her emotions and needs.

The mother, on the other hand, also has a greater need for empathic understanding and help than do the mothers of full-term babies. She may feel guilty because her baby was born prematurely, particularly if initially he had been unwanted. Because she is unable to handle her baby, she may feel frustrated

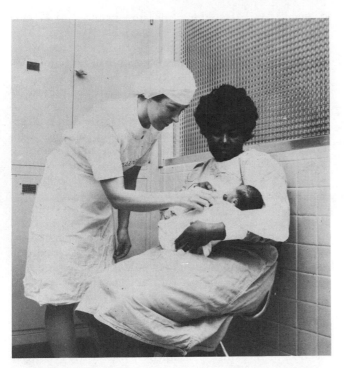

FIG. 9-3. Mothers of premature infants gain confidence and skill in feeding and handling their small charges prior to discharge from the nursery by practicing under the supervision of an experienced nurse.

and doubtful about her ability to be a "good mother." In addition to her anxiety regarding the infant's chance of survival, the complicated equipment and skill necessary for his care may make her feel inadequate and fearful of the future when she must care for him at home. Many mothers resent the nurse who is taking her place as the infant's caretaker and who is more skillful in her handling and care. In addition, as time passes with the infant still in the nursery, she may feel less close to her baby and thus her anxiety may increase.

Because of the hazards to real communication between mother and nurse, more attention and effort must be given to preparing the mother for assuming total care before the baby is to be discharged. The nurse can assist the mother in keeping in touch with her baby by creating opportunities for her to see him, and if possible, to touch him. When reporting on the infant's progress, the nurse can relate incidents of what the baby did during feeding or other activities so that she can learn to know him as an individual. As soon as the baby's condition permits, she should be encouraged to give some care in order to increase her confidence in her mothering ability, and in assuming the responsibilities after he leaves the hospital. The necessity for frequent, cautious feeding, administration of vitamins, avoidance of infection and periodic medical examination can be emphasized in a way that not only ensures protective care of the infant but also

conveys the nurse's confidence in the mother's ability to meet his needs. A practical demonstration with opportunity to practice various aspects of the infant's care and to share her feelings concerning him and his care must be offered to the mother before she takes him home.

Many mothers of prematurely born infants also need the help of the visiting nurse during the period when they are becoming adjusted to their maternal role. Ideally, the nurse should visit the home before the infant leaves the hospital. In such a visit the nurse can attempt to understand the way in which the mother is coping with separation from her baby and with her fears relating to the care he will require when discharged. Also, she can appraise the physical surroundings, available equipment, and the mother's readiness to give her infant care. Such information will assist the nurse in anticipating the kind of support that the mother will need when she begins the care of her baby.

The mother of a premature infant often requires extended counseling and support to alleviate anxiety and to help her to understand his problems and changing needs. Her attitude toward the infant is easily distorted by the anxieties that assail her at various stages of his early life. At first she is concerned about whether he will survive. Then she worries about his prospects for achieving ultimate normal development. At the time of departure from the hospital she is likely to be anxious about the special precautions and requirements of his care and perhaps be dubious about her ability to carry them out as expertly as the nurse. She often believes that he will need the same protective care that he required when he was smaller and one among many in a hospital nursery. Overprotective feelings for the infant may also have been fostered by excessive cautionary advice by professional personnel.

The infant's early behavior at home is not always reassuring, for it is often erratic, and he requires frequent, self-regulated feedings and much more attention and holding than the average full-term infant who has just emerged from the hospital. This is especially true if he has been in a busy nursery and subjected to rigid feeding schedules which have prevented him from acquiring early feelings of trust. Insofar as she can honestly do so, the nurse should offer reassurance and encouragement rather than criticism and hints at additional topics for concern.

Babies who have been isolated in incubators for extended periods of time may also need cautious increments in sensory stimulation, for in addition to the emotional deprivation of isolation during the early weeks of life, they have also necessarily received little tactile and kinesthetic stimulation. This deficit may also be noted in the motor and intellectual development of the infant through the first months of life, and unless understood by the mother, may add to her concern.

After the mother has weathered the first months at home, she will need help to direct her attention to the infant's needs to become gradually prepared for the socialization process. She may need help in recognizing her infant's developing powers and signs of readiness for more stimulation, to begin learning to use his hands for exploration and to develop increasing amounts of independence. Like any other child, he must learn gradually to deal with frustration and to adjust himself to social living. If his mother shields him from such experiences beyond the period when he is ready to learn he is likely to be an unhappy child, poorly prepared to deal with the core problem of the toddler age period.

Certain personality and behavioral characteristics have been observed in infants born prematurely. Investigators have found that children who were born prematurely developed less well than matched controls of normal birth weight, with males being apparently more vulnerable to such impairment. Infants born with birth weights under 1500 Gm. are often retarded intellectually. The proportion of mentally retarded children with higher birth weights (1500-2500 Gm.) is much less, but still significantly higher than that of normal infants. A factor to be considered in these findings is the role played by socioeconomic conditions and the lesser degrees of sensory stimulation received by infants in the lower socioeconomic groups.

Several investigators who have extensively examined children of low birth weight at the preschool or school age period have noted problems of feeding and sleeping, difficulties in mastering bowel and bladder control, negativism, low stress tolerance, diffuseness and difficulty in mobilizing energy, and overdependence. Again the proportion of children of school age considered unsettled or maladjusted increased with decreasing birth weight, with males showing consistently more adverse behavior than females. Other investigators of premature children who have reached school age found poorer performance on many scholastic tests and learning deficits despite adequate intelligence.

These investigators have ascribed the premature behavior syndrome to certain physical and environmental factors. It is possible that prematures, many of whom show early neurological deviations, are more vulnerable to the effects of an impoverished environment. It is also possible that the difficulties these children experience in establishing homeostasis, motility, perceptuo-motor patterning and spatial orientation contributes to the anxiety and overdependence observed later. Some investigators have cited the sensory and emotional deprivation of early incubator isolation as an important factor in later disturbance.

The prematurely born infant's nervous system is less mature than that of the full-term infant so that he is exposed to extrauterine conditions before he is ready. He may well experience more frustration and less gratification than the full-term infant. In addition, he must begin life with the care of many people rather than with the care of one mother who can provide warm, consistent care. Early in life he requires extra protection and care. The necessary early caution in handling her baby, coupled with possible neurological abnormalities, undoubtedly produces tension in the mother, which is transmitted to her infant in a circular reaction. As a result of this early discomfort, many mothers have later difficulties in recognizing their child's signs of readiness for independence and may continue to be rigid or indulgent in their child training practices. They may be overprotective, yet anxious regarding normal developmental achievement so that they communicate expectations for behavior that are beyond their child's capacity. Under such circumstances disturbances in the mother-child relationship are inevitable.

Assisting mothers in observing their infants' individual readiness for new learning experiences helps to prevent the premature behavior syndrome that Shirley & Rothschild describe. The behavior expected should conform to the infant's biologic age rather than to his extrauterine chronologic age. Over-expectancy produces tension within the child; therefore, learning becomes more difficult. Permitting the infant the gratification that comes when his signal of need is met early in life and observing clues that indicate his preparedness for less dependent care and more self-directed activity is the kind of guidance that any young child requires, be he premature, physically handicapped or normal. Both infantilization and unreasonable expectations which demand more than the child can accomplish with satisfaction prevent healthy personality development.

POSTMATURITY

The effects of prolonged residence in the uterus have not been studied as thoroughly as has prematurity. In part this is due to difficulty in recognizing postmaturity with precision, for the birth weight cannot be used as basis of discrimination, and classification depends entirely on the rather unreliable history of the mother's last menstrual period. The generally accepted definition of postmaturity is prolongation of the pregnancy beyond 43 weeks or 300 days. By this standard approximately 5 per cent of liveborn infants are postmature. The mortality rate among them is said to be two or three times as great as among infants born alive at term. There is a sharp increase in the rate of stillbirth in pregnancies carried beyond the 43rd week.

Longitudinal growth slows to a halt at about this time so that no matter how long he is retained in the uterus, the fetus will not generally exceed a length of 23 inches (57.5 cm.). He also begins to lose the downy hair (lanugo) on his body, and the vernix caseosa gradually disappears. Loss of the latter leads to maceration, drying, cracking and peeling of the skin which after birth takes on the appearance of dried parchment. The skin hangs loosely on the infant, suggesting recent weight loss, and the nails grow longer than usual. Postmature infants usually have a good head of hair and look more alert and mature than the ordinary term infant. Most of them suffer little from their delayed birth and rapidly assume the appearance of their fellow newborns. However, some will show more severe evidence of declining function of the placenta as a source of nutriment. The "placental insufficiency syndrome" or "dysmaturity" is easily confused with postmaturity. It is described in the next section.

DYSMATURITY—PLACENTAL INSUFFICIENCY

Strictly speaking, the term dysmaturity includes all examples of birth taking place at times and weights removed from the normal expectation. However, in practice premature infants who are born with weights commensurate with their gestational ages, and postmature infants are not included. The infants of diabetic mothers who are born with weights in excess of that expected for gestational age should also be regarded as dysmature, but they cannot be said to suffer from placental insufficiency (Chap. 10).

Recently the term "small-for-dates" has been used to classify those infants whose birth weights fall significantly below the average for their gestational ages. In such instances it is presumed that poor placental circulation is responsible if there is no abnormality intrinsic within the infant to explain the small size. The phenomenon is not infrequent in twins where discrepancies of 500-1,000 Gm. in the birth weights may be observed. The smaller twin is almost invariably attached to a smaller placenta or shares an inferior segment of a joined placenta. The consequences of this type of dysmaturity are an increase in the hazard of intrauterine death, a greater incidence of hypoglycemia shortly after birth, and a slightly higher risk of anomalous development. These infants require careful observation during the first few days; thereafter they may progress at a faster rate than those of similar weights. The features observed in postmature infants are often present in dysmature or placentally insufficient infants.

SITUATIONS FOR FURTHER STUDY

1. From observation of a prematurely born infant weighing 800 to 1,000 Gm., list the characteristics that differentiate him from a full-term infant. As a result of these physiologic characteristics, what are his needs for nursing care? How would his nursing care differ from that required by a premature infant weighing 2,000 Gm.?

2. Study mortality rate statistics of infants born prematurely. At what period of life do most deaths occur? By what measures could this rate be reduced?

3. How do you imagine a mother would feel giving birth to a premature baby? What are the various ways in which she might react to separation from her baby? Select a mother of a premature infant and observe her behavior as you help her to learn methods of caring for her baby before she takes him home. Provide her with an opportunity to talk about her feelings and write a report of the understanding that you acquired during the experience.

4. Read Hasselmeyer's study and be prepared to discuss her findings relative to the use of back support in the care of premature infants. How does knowledge of the premature infant's behavior aid you in providing nursing care?

5. Read the case material presented by Owens to learn the effects of premature birth on two families. Contrast the parents' emotional responses to crisis and think of ways in which nurses might have been of greater help to the Smith family.

6. What special nursing care would a mother require during labor and in the process of delivering a premature infant?

BIBLIOGRAPHY

American Academy of Pediatrics Committee on Fetus and Newborn: Standards and Recommendations for Hospital Care of Newborn Infants, Full Term and Premature, Evanston, Ill., American Academy of Pediatrics, 1966.

Bascola, Elini, *et al.*: Perinatal and environmental factors in late neurogenic sequelae, I. Infants having birth weights under 1500 grams, Am. J. Dis. Child. *112*:359, 1966.

————: Perinatal and environmental factors in later neurogenic sequelae, II. Infants having birth weights from 1500 to 2500 grams, Am. J. Dis. Child. *112*:369, 1966.

Battaglia, F. C., and Lubchenco, L. O.: A practical classification of newborn infants by weight and gestational age, J. Pediat. *71*:159, 1967.

Blake, F. G.: Role of the Nurse in the Care of Newborn Infants Who Deviate from Normality *in* The Child, His Parents and the Nurse, pp. 87-102, Philadelphia, Lippincott, 1954.

Braine, M. D., Heimer, C., Wortis, H., and Freedman, A. M.: Factors associated with impairment of the early development of prematures, Monographs of the Soc. for Res. in Child Dev. *31*:1, 1966.

Bruce, S. J.: Reactions of nurses and mothers to stillbirth, Nurs. Outlook *10*:88, 1962.

Callon, H. F.: The premature infant's nurse, Am. J. Nurs. *63*:103, 1963.

Clifford, S. H.: Postmaturity—with placental dysfunction, J. Pediat. *44*:1, 1954.

Crosse, V. M.: The Premature Baby, ed. 6, Boston, Little, 1966.

de Hirsch, K., Jansy, J. J., and Langford, W.: Predicting Reading Failure, New York, Harper and Row, 1966.

Drillien, C.: The Growth and Development of the Prematurely Born Infant, Edinburgh and London, E. and S. Livingston Ltd., 1964.

Egge, O. W.: Follow-up care of the premature baby, Am. J. Nurs. *58*:231, 1958.

Ghash, S., and Daga, S.: Comparison of gestational age and weight as standards of prematurity, J. Pediat. *71*:173, 1967.

Hasselmeyer, E.: Behavior Patterns of Premature Infants, a Nursing Study, Washington, Public Health Rep. 840, Dept. of Documents, U. S. Gov't Printing Office, 1961.

Hasselmeyer, E., de la Puente, J., Lundeen, E., and Morrison, M.: A weight chart for premature infants, Nursing Res. *12*:222, 1963.

Lanman, J. T.: Dysmaturity, *in* The Biological Basis of Pediatric Practice, pp. 1521-1528, R. E. Cooke (ed.), New York, McGraw-Hill, 1968.

Lundeen, G. C., and Kunstadter, R. H.: Care of the Premature Infant, Philadelphia, Lippincott, 1958.

McDonald, A.: Children of Very Low Birth Weight, Spastics Society Medical Education and Information Unit in Association with William Heinemann Medical Books Ltd., Grange Press, Southwick, Sussex, 1967.

Medovy, H.: New parameters in neonatal growth, cell number and cell size, J. Pediat. *71*:459, 1967.

National Society for the Prevention of Blindness: Retrolental fibroplasia still a problem, Nurs. Outlook *8*:549, 1960.

Owens, Charlotte: Parents' response to premature birth, Am. J. Nurs. *60*:1113, 1960.

Patz, A.: The role of oxygen in retrolental fibroplasia, Pediatrics *19*:504, 1957.

Prugh, D. G.: Emotional problems of the premature infant's parents, Nurs. Outlook *1*:461, 1953.

Rothschild, B. F.: Incubator isolation as a possible factor to the high incidence of emotional disturbances among prematurely born persons, Psychological Abstracts, *42*:52, 1968.

Shirley, Mary: A behavior syndrome characterizing prematurely born children, Child Develop. *10*:115, 1939.

Silverman, W. A.: Dunham's Premature Infants: A Manual for Physicians, ed. 3, N. Y., Harper, 1961.

Warkany, J., Monroe, B. B., and Sutherland, B. S.: Intrauterine growth retardation, Am. J. Dis. Child. *102*: 249, 1961.

Wortis, H., and Freedman, A. M.: The contributions of social environment to the development of premature children, Am. J. Orthopsychiat. *35*:57, 1965.

Yerushalmy, J.: The classification of newborn infants by birth weight and gestational age, J. Pediat. *71*:164, 1967.

10

Nursing Care of the Newborn With Disease

During the neonatal period a number of serious disturbances are encountered which do not occur during any other age period. Some of these relate to events that have taken place during intrauterine life, some are defects in transition to independent existence, and some are disorders which also may occur later in life but which have special implications when they afflict the newborn. Many of these disturbances are brief, critical periods of illness which have no lasting effect on the infant's welfare. Others are the early stages of lifelong handicaps.

Anoxia. Anoxia occurs when the oxygen supply to the infant's vital organs, the brain in particular, is seriously reduced. It may occur before birth if the mother suffers from some severe illness, such as extreme anemia, heart failure, shock or pneumonia, which prevents her circulation from supplying the placenta with adequate amounts of oxygenated blood. It may occur also from compression of the umbilical cord within the uterus, or from premature separation of the placenta from the inner wall of the uterus (*abruptio placentae*). Anoxia is a serious circumstance to the infant, and when it is recognized, steps usually are taken to deliver him rapidly. At birth the infant is limp and unresponsive, and measures to support him are of vital importance. He has difficulty establishing his respirations and maintaining his body temperature. External warmth, oxygen and resuscitative measures are required. Infants may recover quickly and completely from brief periods of anoxia, but, after prolonged lack of oxygen, the brain is damaged to such an extent that respiration either cannot be established at all or can be maintained for only a few hours after birth. It is believed that some of the central nervous system disturbances that appear in later life (cerebral palsy, mental retardation, etc.) are the aftermath of nonfatal periods of anoxia experienced during or just prior to birth.

Anoxia suffered before or during birth also can re-

sult in filling the lungs with undesirable debris that hampers their early expansion, a complication which Schaffer has called the "massive aspiration syndrome." Three things happen when the oxygen supply to the fetus is compromised before birth. He becomes restless, moves about more actively and churns up the amniotic fluid with its normal sediment of vernix, lanugo hairs and desquamated cells from the skin surface. He is likely also to move his bowels under stress and further contaminate the fluid with meconium. Finally, the reflexes which make him breathe are stimulated prematurely so that he draws amniotic fluid with its suspended particles into his lungs. Here the fluid portion is absorbed by his pulmonary circulation, but the solid particles are strained out and remain lodged in the alveoli and the small tubes that lead to them. The cellular portion of the debris causes mechanical obstruction; the meconium is irritating and may cause inflammatory swelling of the mucosa of the bronchial tree. Should the mother's membranes be ruptured and the amniotic fluid be infected by organisms from the vaginal secretions, the possibility of pneumonia is added to the infant's other pulmonary difficulties.

RESPIRATORY FAILURE (ASPHYXIA)

Initiation of Respiration in the Normal Infant

Once the newborn infant is separated from his mother he takes over the responsibility for oxygenating his blood through the activity of his own lungs. Under optimal circumstances the baby is born with a small amount of thin fluid in his respiratory passages. Perhaps even before his body is delivered, the stimulus of chilling or manipulation, or the chemical changes taking place in his blood as the flow from the placenta is diminished, will activate the respiratory center in his brain. Thus a series of reflex muscular activities is set in motion, and they cause him to gasp and emit a cry—a most welcome sound in the delivery room!

During the first few cries, most of the amniotic fluid in his lungs is expelled, and the air sacs become distended with air. Thus, oxygen is brought in contact with the lung capillaries. Adjustments are made in the fetal blood circulation which send a larger proportion of blood through the lungs. The respiratory center in the brain gives periodic signals that remind him to breathe, and within a few seconds the infant is ready to oxygenate his own tissues and participate in his own survival.

Causes of Asphyxia

Taking over the responsibility for oxygenating his own blood through the activity of his own lungs is a critical step for the newborn infant, for if he fails to discharge this duty within a matter of a few minutes, he will either die or suffer irreparable damage. Infants who have difficulty in making this transition are said to suffer from asphyxia. The term is admittedly a broad one that encompasses respiratory failure from a number of causes. The asphyxiated infant presents an emergency that must be dealt with before there is time for more than a cursory examination. Frequently, the exact reason for this difficulty is not immediately apparent.

The normal sequence of events cited above may be impeded if (1) the respiratory movements are adequate but the air passages are obstructed, (2) the respiratory center fails to emit the proper signals to the muscles that move the chest and the diaphragm, (3) the respiratory movements and the airways are adequate but intrinsic factors in the lungs or the chest interfere with proper expansion of the lungs, or (4) respiratory movements, airway, lungs and chest are all normal but oxygenation of the blood is incomplete because of an abnormality of the heart or its major vessels.

Obstruction of the Air Passages. In actual practice attention is first directed to the infant's *airway.* Even before the first breath is taken, the secretions of the mouth and the nose should be sucked out gently to prevent their being drawn back into the lungs. Thick mucus may block branches of the bronchial tree and prevent full expansion of the lungs. Inhaled meconium is an even worse offender, since it is very irritating and difficult to remove. During suction of the mouth the infant should be held inverted to promote drainage from the trachea. If these measures are deemed insufficient to clear the airway, an operator skilled in the use of the tracheal catheter or the infant bronchoscope should be called to deal with the secretions below the larynx. On rare occasions the airway may be blocked by congenital abnormalities of the larynx or by compression of the trachea by an anomalous structure within the chest.

Inactivity of the Respiratory Center. This condition is the most hazardous aspect of asphyxia. Under normal conditions, a fall in the oxygen content of the blood triggers the center to send out its signals. But the center may fail to respond if the oxygen concentration falls too low or if it is already damaged by prenatal anoxia, intracranial injury or the injudicious administration of sedatives or anesthetics to the mother during the course of delivery.

If the infant has made no effort to breathe during the first minute after birth, resuscitative measures are begun. Frequently, a torpid respiratory center can be aroused by physical stimulation of the infant's skin through rubbing, slapping or blowing on it. Usually, oxygen is administered so that the maximal benefit will be derived from any respiratory effort, no matter how feeble. If a tracheal catheter is in place, oxygen can be carried directly into the lungs. Caution is needed in regulating the pressure so that the delicate lungs are not damaged by overdistention. Similar care must be exercised if any of the methods of artificial insufflation are used, i.e., mouth-to-mouth breathing, inflation of the lungs through an intratracheal catheter or by mechanical respirator.

Respiratory activity is sometimes stimulated with drugs designed to combat the effects of narcotics or anesthetics administered to the mother. Caffeine sodium benzoate in an intramuscular dose of 0.5 ml. is the most dependable. If morphine or one of its derivatives such as Demerol is responsible, Nalline hydrochloride or Lorfan can be used intravenously for their specific antagonistic effects. Central nervous system stimulants such as Metrazol, Coramine, strychnine and picrotoxin are now considered too dangerous for use in the newborn. When the cause of feeble respirations is anoxia or intracranial injury or abnormality, drugs are less likely to be effective.

Intrinsic Disorders of the Lung. ATELECTASIS. Among the intrinsic disorders of the lung which produce asphyxia is atelectasis. This term indicates that areas of the lung are collapsed without air in the alveoli (air sacs) and consequently are useless for respiratory exchange. At birth the lungs are normally collapsed and devoid of air, but with the first breath many air sacs inflate, and with each succeeding breath more areas are opened until expansion is complete. Atelectasis may be due to the initial failure of the air sacs to open up. This in turn may depend on incomplete development of the lung, feeble respiratory movements or blockage by mucus in the small ducts leading to the air sacs. The anterior and superior portions of the lung open most easily so that atelectatic areas usually are found posteriorly at the base of the lung.

Atelectasis also is fostered by the aspiration of amniotic debris and meconium prior to or during delivery. The mechanism has been described above in the section on anoxia. Meconium in the upper air passages should be removed as rapidly as possible. However, the main damage is caused by debris that is so far down in the branches of the bronchial tree that it cannot be removed even with a bronchoscope.

The symptoms depend on the extent of the collapse. Small areas of atelectasis are often discovered accidentally when a chest roentgenogram is taken for some other purpose. No discernible symptoms may be present. Moderate degrees of atelectasis produce mild cyanosis but little distress. When extensive portions of the lung are involved there is cyanosis, labored or grunting respirations, weakness and, ultimately, exhaustion. Treatment consists of continuous administration of oxygen and saturation of the inspired air with water vapor. Oxygen is given so that those areas of lung that are open will have the maximal effect in oxygenating the blood passing through. The moist atmosphere is desirable in order to liquefy secretions and make it easier for the infant to cough them up. Frequent changes of position offer the best opportunity for the collapsed areas to open. Since there is danger that the inactive portions of the lung will become infected secondarily, some type of antibiotic is often administered.

THE RESPIRATORY DISTRESS SYNDROME OR HYALINE MEMBRANE DISEASE. The respiratory distress syndrome (RDS) is the most lethal pulmonary disturbance in newborn nurseries. It is a peculiar variety of atelectasis intensive study of which for two decades has failed to produce uniform opinion as to pathogenesis or appropriate treatment. The *clinical features* of RDS are fairly well defined. The disorder occurs almost exclusively in prematurely born or caesarian delivered infants, or in those whose mothers have diabetes. Within 12 hours after birth, affected infants show a progressive increase in the rate and difficulty of their respirations. Expiratory grunting, flaring nostrils and retraction of the suprasternal and intercostal spaces with mild cyanosis are characteristic of the early stages of the disease. Later, gasping, cyanosis which is not relieved by oxygen and finally apneic episodes with complete exhaustion herald the more severe phases of the disorder. Spontaneous recovery usually begins before 48 hours of age, whereas most deaths occur before 72 hours of age. Chest roentgenograms show a general decrease in aeration of the lungs with a diffuse pattern of finely stippled infiltration, usually called reticulogranular infiltrate. Blood chemical determinations reveal a decrease in oxygen saturation (p_aO_2) and an increased retention of CO_2 (pCO_2) with acidosis and an increase in the level of serum potassium.

The *pathophysiology* of this syndrome has not yet been finally agreed upon by the numerous investigators who have studied it. Currently, the most widely held view is that the disorder begins from a reduction in the rate of blood flow through the pulmonary circulation leading to stasis of blood in the capillaries of the lungs, exudation of serum into the alveoli, and the production of the characteristic hyaline deposits seen in sections of postmortem lung. A decrease in the amount of surfactant (or wetting agent) normally present in lungs has also been demonstrated and presumably results in greater tendency for the alveolar walls to adhere. Secondarily, hypoxia, acidosis and other biochemical changes interact to aggravate the disturbed pulmonary ventilation.

Treatment is directed at supporting ventilation of the lungs and the provision of an atmosphere rich enough in oxygen to control cyanosis. The intravenous administration of glucose and bicarbonate to provide calories and correct the acidosis is usually part of the therapy. Infants should be disturbed as little as possible. Digitalization is advocated by some. If they can be tided over the first 48 hours without resort to mechanically assisted respiration, most infants will recover. For those who require the more extreme measures, the prognosis is poor.

INTERSTITIAL EMPHYSEMA AND PNEUMOTHORAX. Interstitial emphysema results when air is admitted into the space between the air sacs from a tear in the lining of one of them. If a large amount of air becomes trapped in this way, there will be insufficient room within the chest to permit expansion of the alveoli. Pneumothorax in the newborn is an extension of the process just mentioned. Air passes into the pleural space and collapses the lung, rendering it temporarily inefficient. Tension in the chest sometimes mounts progressively because of a valvelike mechanism that permits air to be drawn into the chest with inspiration while preventing its discharge. In such cases needle aspiration of the chest will give dramatic relief. However, if the situation persists, the insertion of a chest tube and the application of suction may be required.

MALFORMATION OF LUNGS OR CHEST. A number of congenital defects of lungs or chest may be encountered. While fortunately rare, it is imperative to recognize them quickly. All or a portion of one lung may be absent (agenesis), sometimes with surprisingly little inconvenience to the newborn. A defect in the diaphragm (diaphragmatic hernia or eventration) which permits the intestines and other abdominal organs to push into the thoracic cavity can often be corrected surgically if it is recognized before irreversible respiratory failure occurs. Small or large cysts may be present at birth and, because of the volume of dead gas that they contain, encroach on and interfere with the function of the adjacent normal lung.

CONGENITAL MALFORMATION OF HEART AND GREAT VESSELS. A comprehensive discussion of congenital heart defects will be found in Chapter 22. The most severe abnormalities are not compatible with life for more than a few hours and produce intense cyanosis and respiratory distress in the newborn. Less severe defects permit survival with varying symptoms and degrees of incapacitation or, in some cases, no distress at all.

Nursing Care

The nurse is a most important factor in the care of infants with respiratory failure, for on her powers of observation and ready availability depend the recognition of the onset of trouble and changes in its severity. Since respiratory distress tends to occur among infants who have suffered anoxia, who are premature or delivered by cesarean section, or whose mothers have diabetes or other complications of pregnancy, it is incumbent on the nursery attendants to watch closely for early symptoms so that appropriate supportive measures can be introduced. The important indices that must be monitored are skin color, muscle tone, rate and character of respirations (flaring alae nasi, grunting, retractions of the chest wall), vigor and depth of cry, the infant's response to handling and the degree of his apprehensiveness. Unfortunately, it takes experience and judgment before these signs can be interpreted accurately. However, the nurse is in a better position for continuous observation than is the physician. She must transmit her observations promptly if she is suspicious of a turn for the worse.

The baby with respiratory distress needs a nurse who can institute supportive measures immediately and watch him with undivided attention. Aspiration of gastric contents to prevent their inhalation and suctioning to keep the airway free of secretions are emergency measures. Oxygen, humidity and warmth must be provided constantly during the period of distress and be kept at a *constant level*. Administration of fluids at the designated rate is very important during the first few days, since by the end of that time either death or definite improvement with signs of hunger is likely to occur. Infants who continue to have respiratory difficulty after this period need to be fed by gavage. Handling should be gentle and reduced to a minimum to avoid stimulation they cannot tolerate. Preventing distention is important, for it impedes normal expansion of the lung. Observing the infant's response to change in position helps the nurse to discover the position in which he breathes most easily and is less cyanotic. Prevention of infection is an important part of the nursing care, for the addition of otherwise trivial disease may prove to be fatal to an infant who is already desperately ill.

BIRTH INJURIES

Intracranial Injury

This is the most common and serious form of birth trauma. Since the head is the largest portion of the infant body which must traverse the birth canal, it is most likely to be damaged when delivery is difficult. Sudden, violent alterations in the shape of the skull, such as occur with precipitate delivery or difficult forceps or breech extractions, are more likely to result in injury than is the gradual molding of a slowly progressing labor. Temporary or permanent damage

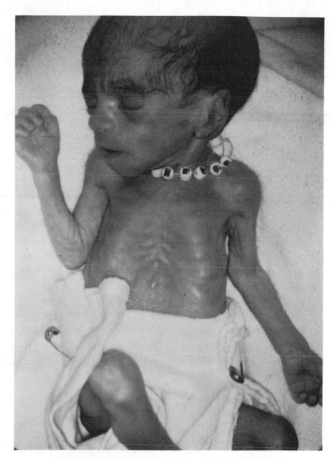

Fig. 10-1. Sternal retraction in a premature infant. (Dr. R. Platou)

is suffered by various portions of the brain if their blood supply is compromised by edema or hemorrhage from large blood vessels that have torn or have burst in response to the unusual stresses. Large hemorrhages occur most commonly from the veins coursing in the membrane that separates the two halves of the brain (*falx cerebri*) or in the membrane that divides the cerebellum from the cerebrum (*tentorium cerebelli*). In premature infants the delicate vessels of the choroid plexus may burst, resulting in a hemorrhage into the ventricular system of the brain.

Following intracranial injury, the infant is abnormally sleepy, difficult to arouse, does not demonstrate the Moro reflex and may be unable to suck or swallow. If intracranial pressure is high, his respirations are slow, irregular and periodic; his heart beats slowly; his fontanel bulges; and his eyes turn inward. There may be generalized spasticity of the muscles with backward arching of the head and the neck and extension of the legs. Evidence of irritation of the cerebral cortex may be present in the form of generalized convulsions or convulsive twitchings of muscle groups. The body temperature may be elevated or may hover at subnormal levels. In mild cases the symptoms are limited to general listlessness, poor appetite and occasional vomiting.

The prognosis following intracranial injury varies considerably, depending on the extent and location of the damage. When large or vital areas of the brain are affected, the immediate mortality is high, and infants who survive are likely to show spastic paralysis or mental retardation in later years. When the brain damage is less extensive, recovery may ensue with reasonably normal mental development. Neurologic complications, such as hemiplegia, convergent strabismus or convulsive attacks, may appear later. In some cases recovery is complete without any residua.

Treatment is unsatisfactory, for there is seldom opportunity to stop the bleeding or control the increased pressure within the skull. While waiting for the symptoms to subside spontaneously, general supportive measures are used. If there are convulsions, phenobarbital is indicated. Vitamin K usually is given to minimize bleeding. Unresponsive infants are not fed or handled more than necessary, and measures to supply warmth or decrease elevated temperature are instituted. Sometimes it is possible to relieve intracranial pressure by withdrawing bloody fluid from the spinal canal or from the surface of the brain by tapping the dura at the lateral edge of the fontanel. The latter procedure may be repeated effectively if the bleeding has become localized to a walled-off area over the surface of the brain (subdural hematoma). The best management of intracranial injury is to prevent it through judicious obstetric management of the mother. Under ideal circumstances it is possible to reduce the infant deaths from this cause to less than 1 per thousand liveborn babies.

Fractures

Sometimes fractures occur during birth. The clavicle suffers most frequently. It is broken by direct pressure of the finger during extraction of the shoulder. No special management is required, for this bone heals rapidly with the formation of a callus but without producing much pain or disability. Occasionally, linear fractures of the skull are discovered in infants whose birth has not been unusually difficult. Unless there is associated intracranial hemorrhage, or depression of a fragment which presses on the brain, such cracks are of trivial importance and heal quickly. Rarely, the humerus is broken during efforts to sweep the arm down over the face during breech delivery; or the femur may be fractured during version and extraction. Breaks of an extremity are usually apparent from the abnormal angulation that they produce. They heal well when immobilized in corrected position.

Brachial Palsy

This is a partial paralysis of one arm which results from excessive stretching of the nerve fibers that run from the neck through the shoulder and toward the arm. The trauma is produced by the forcible pulling of the shoulder away from the head during obstetric maneuvers. The most common type of paralysis involves the muscles of the upper arm and spares those of the hand and fingers. The arm is held at the side with elbow extended and hand rotated inward. In mild cases when the injury is the result of stretching of nerve fibers that have not broken, recovery is rapid and may be complete within three weeks. More commonly, the fibers are stretched to such an extent that they break within their sheaths. Recovery from paralysis then depends on the regeneration of nerves which are guided back to the appropriate muscles by the intact sheaths. Regeneration usually takes from two to three months. During the waiting period, the muscles of the shoulder should be manipulated gently and given massage to prevent contractures from forming. Failure of recovery to take place within three months probably indicates that the nerve roots have been torn loose from their connections with the spinal cord and that recovery will not occur unless the pathways can be restored surgically—a very difficult feat.

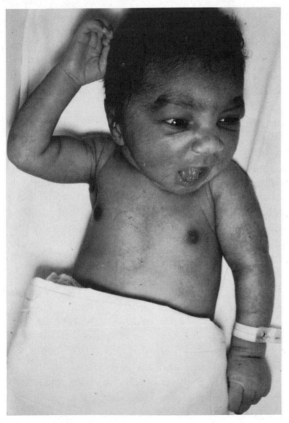

Fig. 10-2. Brachial paralysis. Note the position of the left arm which is held close to the body and rotated inward. (Dr. R. Platou)

FIG. 10-3. Diagram of the mechanism of jaundice. The spleen (and other portions of the reticuloendothelial system) break up the hemoglobin of worn-out or abnormal red blood cells and release into the cirulation unconjugated or indirect bilirubin (O). When brought to the liver most of the indirect bilirubin (O) is transformed by enzyme action into direct bilirubin (—) which is water-soluble and able to pass through the filter and into the bile ducts and the intestines for excretion. Some of this excreted bilirubin is reabsorbed from the intestine, carried to the liver and re-excreted.

If the liver enzymes are unable to cope with the amount of indirect bilirubin (O) brought to them, some of it may be passed along into the general circulation where it may, if of sufficient amount, color the body tissues and result in the symptom of jaundice. The direct bilirubin (—) formed in the liver also may fail to be excreted if the bile ducts are obstructed or if there is diffuse liver disease. It, too, may circulate in the blood if it is not being excreted. Unlike the indirect bilirubin, direct bilirubin can be excreted by the kidney.

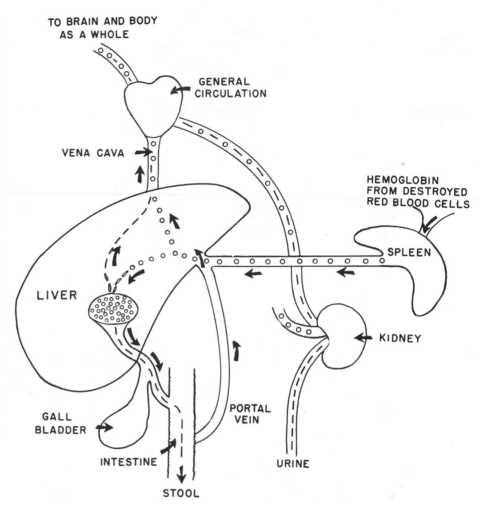

JAUNDICE

Normal Physiology

Jaundice is a common symptom during the newborn period. In the majority of infants it is a normal phenomenon, but, in an important minority, it indicates serious disease. Jaundice results from an interference with the disposal of pigments formed in the breakdown of hemoglobin. The physiologic mechanisms are complex and cannot be treated fully here. Figure 10-3 is an oversimplified scheme which attempts to present a picture of the main transformations involved and the manner in which hepatic abnormalities produce jaundice.

The story begins with the spleen, which is the most discrete but not the sole portion of the reticuloendothelial system. Blood brought to it from the general circulation contains hemoglobin from fragments of worn-out normal red blood cells, from congenitally defective cells which are unusually friable, or from red cells which have been destroyed by the action of toxins, hemolytic antibodies or other mechanisms. The spleen breaks up such hemoglobin, releasing protein and iron for re-use by the body and converting the porphyrin residue into a yellow pigment, bilirubin. In its initial form bilirubin is not very soluble in water. It travels in the blood stream loosely bound to albumin. Although it can diffuse into and stain body tistues, it avoids excretion by the liver and kidney. In this original form it is known as indirect or unconjugated bilirubin. It is represented in the diagram by small circles.

From the spleen (or other portions of the reticuloendothelial system) indirect bilirubin is carried to the liver by the bloodstream. Here the liver cells, through the mediation of certain enzymes (glucuronyl transferase, UDPG dehydrogenase), attach glucuronide to the bilirubin molecule which converts it into direct or conjugated bilirubin (represented by the broken line in the diagram) and makes it more water soluble so that it can be excreted by the liver into the biliary passages or by the kidney into the urine. In the properly functioning liver most of the indirect bilirubin brought to it is converted quickly into the direct form and is filtered out of the bloodstream into the bile ducts. In the normal adult or the older child

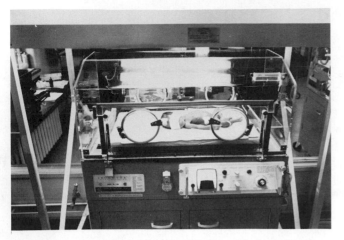

Fig. 10-4. The bililamp. Infants with high levels of indirect bilirubin are exposed to blue light which converts the pigment into less toxic compounds as it circulates through the skin capillaries. Either term infants in bassinets, or prematures in isolettes may be placed naked under the lamp during most of the day. The eyes are shielded to prevent corneal irritation.

small amounts of both types of bilirubin may pass back into the general circulation through the vena cava. Their concentration in serum is measured by the van den Bergh test. Indirect bilirubin is normally present in a concentration of less than 1 mg./100 ml. of serum; direct bilirubin in less than 0.3 mg. per cent.

Direct bilirubin, which has passed through the liver filter into the bile capillaries, moves into the larger bile ducts, hepatic duct, gallbladder, common duct and eventually the duodenal portion of the intestine. Here chemical activity of bacteria converts it into new forms of pigment—urobilin, stercobilin, biliverdin—which are responsible for the various hues of normal stool. Quantitative chemical determination of the amount of such fecal pigments excreted daily yields important information about the rate at which red blood cells are being destroyed in the body.

Not indicated in the diagram but of diagnostic importance is the subsequent course of urobilin which, in part, is reabsorbed from the intestinal tract and carried by the portal vein to the liver. Here, after slight modification, it is both re-excreted by the liver and passed on into the bloodstream, whence it reaches the kidney and appears in the urine. Absence of urobilin derivatives in the urine indicates a complete blockage of the bile-duct system.

Physiologic Jaundice (Icterus) of the Newborn

If carefully observed, nearly two thirds of newborn infants will show some yellow coloration of the skin or the bulbar conjunctiva during the first week of life. Clinical jaundice usually means that the level of bilirubin in the blood has risen to at least 2 to 3 mg.

per cent. Two main factors are believed to be responsible for this event in the presumably normal newborn. (1) There is a sudden increase in the rate of destruction of red cells shortly after birth. This is confirmed by the rapid changes in the red blood cell count of newborn infants which starts at high levels, averaging 6 million/cu. mm. on the first day of life, and falls to an average of 5 million/cu. mm. by the age of 2 weeks. It is presumed that for a time the small baby destroys his red cells faster than his immature liver can clear away the waste products. (2) Recent studies have shown that in many newborns the liver cells are relatively deficient in the enzymes necessary to convert indirect bilirubin to direct bilirubin so that the former compound accumulates in the blood while awaiting its turn for conversion and excretion. This enzyme deficiency is particularly prevalent in premature infants.

Physiologic jaundice does not appear before the end of the second day of life. *In utero* the infant was able to get rid of indirect bilirubin via the placenta and his mother's circulation. It takes two or three days from the time this route of excretion is cut off before he accumulates enough in his blood to seep out and stain his tissues. The duration and intensity of the jaundice are quite variable. In most infants the activity of the liver enzymes picks up after a few days, and the blood is promptly cleared of pigment. At this time the nurse may notice a sudden darkening of the urine as the conjugated bilirubin is also excreted by the kidneys. Occasionally, jaundice for which no other explanation can be found will last for two or three weeks, and the blood levels of bilirubin will rise toward the 18 to 20 mg. per cent level, beyond which lies hyperbilirubinemia.

Simple physiologic jaundice requires no special management. The main concern of the medical staff should be directed toward making certain that none of the other causes of newborn jaundice is present. Accurate determination of the time of onset is particularly important, for erythroblastosis must be suspected when jaundice is observed within the first 36 hours of life. The jaundiced infant also should be watched carefully for evidence of illness or infection of any kind. Pale stools in the presence of jaundice suggest an obstruction of the bile-duct system.

Hyperbilirubinemia and Kernicterus

Hyperbilirubinemia of the newborn occurs when the level of indirect bilirubin in the blood reaches 20 mg. per cent. This arbitrary dividing line is selected because extensive studies of infants with jaundice due to erythroblastosis have shown consistently that little or no brain damage occurs in infants whose bilirubin levels are kept below 20 mg. per cent. In contrast, those whose levels rise above this run a risk which mounts with the concentration (at 30-40 mg. per cent, 7 babies out of 10 will be damaged).

Prematurity and hemolytic disease of the newborn (erythroblastosis) are the common causes of hyperbilirubinemia. The latter is discussed in the next section, along with the technic for its management—exchange transfusion. In this country opinions differ concerning the necessity of controlling the late rise of bilirubin levels in premature infants. Excessive hemolysis and brain damage are fostered in these immature infants by the administration of high doses of vitamin K or the use of Gantrisin (sulfisoxazole).

Recently it has been found that exposure of infants who are developing jaundice to light in the blue end of the spectrum during most of the day will depress the level to which the blood bilirubin rises. This method is likely to be more effective among prematures without blood incompatibility than among infants who may be suffering from erythroblastosis. Special equipment is needed and the infant's eyes must be shielded during the treatment.

Kernicterus occurs when cells of the central nervous system, particularly those in the basal ganglia, are damaged by excessive levels of indirect bilirubin in the blood. In erythroblastosis the symptoms usually begin on the third or fourth day of life and consist of convulsions and spasticity. Many of the afflicted infants die. Those who survive generally are seriously affected, suffering mental deficiency and persistent spasticity and convulsive diathesis.

Hemolytic Disease of the Newborn (Erythroblastosis Fetalis)

When a pregnant woman carries an infant whose red blood cells contain antigens inherited from the father which differ from those on her own red blood cells, she may become sensitized. Several families of red-cell antigens are known, and their passage from the parents to the child follows predictable laws of inheritance. The infant receives half of his complement of antigens from his mother's endowment and half from his father's. The most important sets are the Rh antigens (also designated by the letters C, D, E and c, d, e) and the well-known blood-group antigens A and B. Rarely, hemolytic disease is produced by antigens of other groups (Kell, Duffy) by the same kind of mechanism.

The mere existence of a difference in blood types between the mother and the developing fetus is not in itself sufficient to cause hemolytic disease. The mother must be adequately exposed to the antigen and must be capable of forming antibodies in sufficient quantity to flow back across the placenta and destroy a significant number of fetal red cells. The means by which fetal antigen enters the mother's body is presumed to be through small leaks in the placental circulation which permit admixture of the baby's blood with the mother's. Fortunately, not all women exposed to foreign antigen from the fetus are capable of responding with the production of anti-

bodies. Occasionally, however, a woman is sensitized long before pregnancy by transfusion or injection of improperly matched blood.

Rh Sensitization. Nearly all persons of the Asiatic and Negro races are Rh positive and incapable of being sensitized. Among Caucasians, however, approximately 15 per cent are Rh negative, meaning that their red cells contain only the antigens designated by the small letters c, d and e. By Rh-typing all pregnant women it is possible to identify those few who may become sensitized. If the husbands are typed as well, some will be found to be Rh negative, thus eliminating the possibility of Rh sensitization, since all children of the union will also be Rh negative.

Experience has shown that Rh-negative women almost never have trouble with the first Rh-positive infant which they bear. Usually, the process of sensitization proceeds so slowly during the first such pregnancy that the infant is born before his mother's body can produce antibodies in sufficiently high titer to create discernible disease. (This rule does not hold if the mother was sensitized by improper transfusion prior to her first pregnancy.) However, once her body has learned how to produce antibodies, it does so with greater speed during subsequent pregnancies with an Rh-positive child. If the mother is being stimulated by her fetus, the antibodies will appear in her blood in increasing amounts during the latter half of pregnancy. By repeated tests of maternal blood it is often possible to know in advance of delivery which women are going to have erythroblastotic infants and to make appropriate preparations.

It should be emphasized that most Rh-negative women never become sensitized even though they bear several Rh-positive infants. The popular misconception that every Rh-negative woman is threatened with erythroblastotic babies is far from true. However, once a mother has produced an infant with the disease, there is a strong probability that subsequently Rh-positive babies will also be affected.

The first sensitization of an Rh-negative mother probably occurs at the end of a pregnancy. It is now possible to stop this from occurring by treating previously unsensitized mothers with an anti-Rh gamma globulin (Rhogam) immediately after the birth of each Rh-positive infant.

PATHOGENESIS. The anti-Rh antibodies produced by the mother cross back through the placental circulation into the fetal bloodstream and attach themselves to the Rh-positive cells. Some of the antibodies are capable of agglutinating the infant's red cells, thus causing them to be strained out of the circulation and destroyed prematurely by the infant's spleen and reticuloendothelial system. Fetal anemia and jaundice may result. The bone marrow and other foci of blood production in liver and spleen attempt to compensate for the too rapid destruction of red cells by pushing new cells into the circulation before they

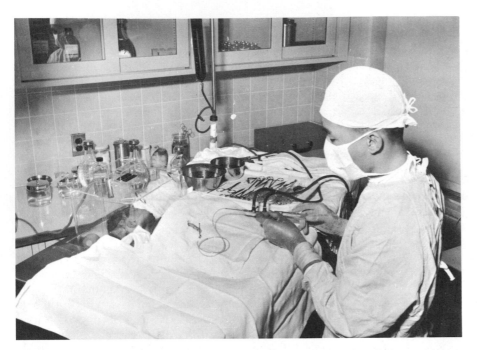

FIG. 10-5. Equipment for exchange transfusion. The infant lies in an oxygen hood with the long umbilical cord protruding onto the sterile field. The plastic catheter is inserted into the umbilical vein of the cord. The operator removes blood into the syringe, ejects it through one tube, refills the syringe from the reservoir of Rh-negative blood and injects it into the infant. This sequence is repeated until approximately 500 ml. of blood has been withdrawn and replaced.

are completely mature. These nucleated cells (erythroblasts) are found in the peripheral blood of the affected newborn in abnormal quantities and are responsible for the original name of the disease—erythroblastosis fetalis. If anemia progresses in spite of these efforts, the function of the vital organs is affected, and the infant may be born with edema due to poor protein formation, may suffer cardiac failure, or may even be stillborn. During intrauterine life the indirect bilirubin which results from rapid detruction of red cells does not collect in the infant's blood because the placenta carries off most of the excess. However, once he is born, the level of bilirubin rises rapidly, without the lag in time characteristic of physiologic icterus.

SYMPTOMS. The cardinal symptoms of erythroblastosis are jaundice and anemia, which are present at birth or appear during the first 36 hours. *Any infant found to be jaundiced on the first or second day of life should be brought to the doctor's attention because he requires thorough investigation.* In severe cases the mother delivers a stillborn fetus or one suffering from *hydrops fetalis,* which is characterized by extensive edema, marked anemia, jaundice, and enlargement of the liver and spleen. Similar findings of lesser intensity are present in infants afflicted with milder forms of the disease. If no treatment is given, both anemia and jaundice are likely to increase in severity during the first few days of life. Sometimes hemorrhages into the skin are present, and occasionally a fatal pulmonary hemorrhage occurs on the fourth day.

Infants who are severely jaundiced run the risk of serious damage to the brain (kernicterus). The symptoms of this complication appear from the third day on and consist of vomiting, spasticity, convulsions and inability to feed. Kernicterus is often fatal shortly

after its appearance. Survivors may suffer from mental retardation with spastic paralysis or have nerve deafness.

Mild forms of erythroblastosis produce no symptoms except slight jaundice and anemia—indeed, cases may be overlooked entirely unless special laboratory tests are performed. The effect of the antibodies obtained from the mother is temporary. If the infant survives the tenth day of life without evidence of complications, his outlook is good. Except for anemia which is corrected easily by transfusion, erythroblastotic infants suffer no additional consequences of the disease after this time.

DIAGNOSIS. When there is clinical suspicion of hemolytic disease, immediate laboratory confirmation should be sought. If not already known, the mother's Rh type should be determined, and a test made for anti-Rh antibody in her blood. The father's blood type is sometimes helpful in identifying the discrepancy between mother and baby. In the presence of high antibody titres or with a previous history of severely affected infants, the *in utero* progress of disease in the infant may be followed by amniocentesis and measurement of the pigment levels in the amniotic fluid. Intrauterine transfusions have been successfully administered to severely affected infants.

After birth, blood should be obtained from the infant for Rh and ABO typing, for hemoglobin and red cell level to evaluate the severity of anemia, for bilirubin determination to establish a base line for subsequent rises, and to search for nucleated red blood cells and the presence of damaging antibodies (Coombs' test). If the diagnosis is confirmed by such studies, the course and severity of the condition must be followed carefully, not only by observation of the infant but also by repeated determinations of the level of hemoglobin and indirect bilirubin in the blood.

TREATMENT. The treatment of erythroblastosis consists in the transfusion of Rh-negative blood to combat the anemia. The Rh-negative cells will persist in the infant's circulation, since they are unaffected by the antibodies received from the mother. While repeated simple transfusions are often effective, the more elaborate technic of exchange transfusion is to be preferred. Through a catheter inserted into the umbilical or some other large vein, small amounts of the infant's blood are withdrawn, and an equal amount of the Rh-negative donor's blood is injected. The procedure is continued until most of the circulating blood of the infant has been replaced. This technic not only provides new red cells, but also removes the harmful maternal antibodies and the products of the destruction of the infant's red cells which produce jaundice. Even moribund infants are sometimes salvaged by the prompt application of this treatment.

Exchange transfusion requires considerable preparation and is frequently an emergency procedure. Hence, it is desirable that the birth of an erythroblastotic infant be anticipated so that preparations may be made in advance. This can be done if all pregnant women are Rh-typed, and if Rh antibodies are sought periodically during pregnancy in the blood of those who might be expected to produce an erythroblastotic baby.

NURSING CARE. The nursing care of an infant with erythoblastosis consists of careful observations and supportive measures which provide protection during the period when he is receiving medical treatment. She must also observe carefully for warning signs of impending kernicterus which include decreased responsiveness, a less vigorous cry, the loss of the Moro reflex and opisthotonos. Severe edema should be promptly reported, since it may signal congestive heart failure.

Babies born with erythroblastosis frequently require measures to combat shock. When the birth of an infant with erythroblastosis is anticipated, an incubator and oxygen should be in readiness to maintain the infant's temperature and to combat cyanosis. These babies are lethargic, because of generalized weakness and anemia. Frequent change in position prevents atelectasis and intercurrent infections.

Usually the infant's strength to suckle is greatly reduced, indicating a need for a method of feeding that will conserve his energy. A nipple with enlarged holes or a medicine dropper may be required for feeding a weakened infant. With all methods of feeding, patience in feeding slowly enough to prevent aspiration is necessary.

In caring for an infant with erythroblastosis, the nurse must be constantly on the alert to detect untoward symptoms. She must not only assist with the replacement transfusion but she must also observe the infant's response during the procedure and in the period after it is completed.

Any nurse caring for newborn infants should also remember that any baby may develop erythroblastosis, and that jaundice during the first 36 hours indicates erythroblastosis rather than infection. Frequent inspection of babies' scleras and general body color, in natural light, is important in the admission nursery to detect early jaundice which should be called to the attention of the physician.

Hemolytic Disease Due to AB Incompatibility. Mothers of blood group O may have infants with hemolytic disease if the latter's blood type is A, or less commonly, B. Although the basic mechanisms and management are the same as those for Rh sensitization, there are a few important differences.

The anti-A (or anti-B) antibodies occur naturally in individuals who do not have the corresponding antigens on their red cells. For this reason it is possible for a mother to bear an affected baby with her first pregnancy, since she is already able to produce the damaging antibody. The baby's presence in her uterus may stimulate an increase in the titer of her natural antibody. The disease in the infant is usually not as severe as that produced by the Rh antigens, and there is a greater tendency for the bilirubin levels to crest under 20 mg. per cent so that exchange transfusion is not needed. Consequently, the incidence of serious complications, particularly kernicterus, is small. The direct Coombs' test on the infant's blood is usually negative, even in the presence of disease. For reasons which are not clear it is unusual for a mother to have more than one infant with erythroblastosis due to AB incompatibility.

Other Causes of Newborn Jaundice

Any of the infections discussed in the next section may be associated with jaundice during the early days of life. Congenital malformations of the bile ducts produce late appearing jaundice with acholic stools (see Chap. 13). Rarely, disorders such as galactosemia, familial nonhemolytic jaundice and familial hemolytic icterus are found to be responsible for the symptom.

Some women excrete in their breast milk a product of adrenal steroid metabolism (pregnanediol) which interferes with the development of the normal enzymes which conjugate bilirubin and make it available for excretion. Infants of such mothers may remain jaundiced for days or weeks while nursing. Usually the level of bilirubin is not dangerously high. It will drop if breast feeding is interrupted for 48 hours and will not ascend again when the breast is again used.

INFECTIONS OF THE NEWBORN PERIOD

During the latter portion of the pregnancy the mother transmits to her infant antibodies against some of the infectious diseases to which she has become immune. Passive immunity of this sort protects the infant for a variable time after birth—about six months in the case of measles, probably less than three months for chickenpox, and not at all for whooping cough. Unfortunately, such a protective mechanism exists for only a few diseases, and the newborn remains highly susceptible to most of the infectious ills of man. In fact, he may even become infected by those bacteria that normally dwell in his intestines (colon bacilli) or on his skin (staphylococci). The special measures designed to shield him from infection have been discussed earlier in this unit. When these safeguards fail, the character of the ensuing infection has special implications for the newborn.

Bacterial Infections

Sepsis. Sepsis occurs when bacteria gain access to and multiply in the bloodstream. Thus, organisms are transported to all parts of the body and may set up secondary areas of infection almost anywhere. The portal of invasion is not always apparent. Sometimes the route passes from an infected umbilicus through the umbilical vessels to the liver and thence to the general circulation. At other times invasion appears to take place through normal skin or through the mucous membrane of the intestinal or the respiratory tract.

The symptoms of sepsis are not uniform. In some cases there is a dramatic rise in temperature, rapid weight loss, convulsions, jaundice and hemorrhagic phenomena. Abscesses appear in the skin, or pus is coughed up from the lungs. To an experienced eye, the nature of the disease is obvious at once. In other cases the onset is insidious. The temperature may remain normal or fall to subnormal levels. Sudden weight loss in spite of a reasonable food intake may be the only warning of trouble. Usually, those caring for the infant sense that something is amiss, but the true state of affairs may not be uncovered until a systematic search for infection is made by taking cultures of the blood, urine, spinal fluid and secretions of the nose and throat.

In all cases cultures are most important, for treatment rests mainly on the use of antibiotics, the rational use of which depends on isolating the invading bacterium and determining its sensitivity to the drugs that are available. In addition to specific antibacterial therapy, transfusions and oxygen are commonly needed.

The prognosis of sepsis depends to a great extent on the speed of recognition of the disease and the accuracy of antibiotic administration. Even with good care the mortality is high. If meningitis occurs, complications such as hydrocephalus, convulsions or mental retardation must be feared as sequels, even when a bacteriologic cure is obtained.

Pneumonia. Pneumonia in the newborn is always a serious disease. The added burden of infection is frequently more than the lungs can tolerate, for even in the healthy newborn they are tenuously prepared for their new function of respiration. Furthermore, the bacteria responsible for pneumonia of the newborn are less likely to respond to the common antibiotics. Instead of pneumococci and streptococci, the infant is more likely to be infected by staphylococci, colon bacilli or other varieties of intestinal organisms. Pneumonia occasionally begins before birth when there is premature rupture of the membranes with infection of the amniotic fluid. When present at birth it is difficult to differentiate from atelectasis.

Epidemic Diarrhea. Epidemic bacterial diarrhea due to pathogenic strains of *E. coli* has been described in Chapter 8.

Staphylococcal Infections. Unusually virulent and antibiotic-resistant strains of staphylococci may be carried unwittingly into the newborn or premature nursery by personnel who have become contaminated in other areas of the hospital. Prevention and control of the dissemination of these organisms is hampered by a number of practical difficulties. The persons guilty of transporting them to the nursery are difficult to identify because they can carry them not only via trivial skin infections but also as a component of their nasopharyngeal bacterial flora, unattended by signs or symptoms of illness. The organisms are difficult to recognize, since they must be separated from the more common varieties of staphylococci through the special technic of bacteriophage typing. Even when discovered to be present in a nursery they do not necessarily create illness among the infants. An additional mysterious virulence factor appears to be necessary to initiate an epidemic. Another practical difficulty lies in the short residence of the newborn within the nursery, which often means that he is discharged before the evidences of his infection become apparent. Thus, although the nursery may not appear to be infected, it serves as a focus for the dissemination of infection which breaks out later in the infants' homes. Babies who become infected may have skin lesions (impetigo, furunculosis), conjunctivitis, infected umbilical cords, osteomyelitis, pneumonia or bloodstream infections. Closure of the infected nursery is sometimes required.

Tetanus. Tetanus of the newborn is practically unknown in the United States but still occurs in countries where hygienic care of the umbilicus is so poor that tetanus spores may gain access to and grow in its recesses. The disease is described in Chapter 19.

Gonorrheal Conjunctivitis. Gonorrheal conjunctivitis (ophthalmia neonatorum) is losing its importance as a cause of congenital blindness, partly because of the impact of state laws that require prophylactic treatment of all infants at birth and partly owing to the advent of penicillin which provides an effective cure of the infection in both mother and child. The disease is acquired during birth by contamination of the infant's eyes with the infected secretions of the mother's vagina. The symptoms are similar to those of chemical conjunctivitis of the newborn but become evident on the second or third day of life rather than in the first 12 to 24 hours. Prompt differentiation is important, for a delay in the treatment of gonorrheal conjunctivitis may permit ulceration and scarring of the cornea. False security sometimes arises from the knowledge that silver nitrate presumably has been instilled immediately after delivery while the infant was still in the birth-room. However, the technic of instillation of the drops into the eyes of a newborn infant is sufficiently difficult that drops sometimes fail to get into the sacs. When the disease is suspected, smears and cultures of the pus should be made, but treatment usually is initiated before the laboratory results are known. Penicillin given by injection and by direct instillation into the conjunctival sacs at frequent intervals results in prompt healing.

Tuberculosis. Tuberculosis is practically unknown during the newborn period, but it must be kept in mind as a disease to which the small infant is highly susceptible. It is hazardous for him to go home into an environment in which he will come in contact with someone harboring an active form of tuberculosis. Special efforts should be made to see that not only his mother but all other members of his family as well are free from the disease. When this is impossible vaccination with BCG should be considered. (See Chap. 19.)

Nonbacterial Infections of the Newborn

Viral, protozoal and spirochetal infections of the mother may be transferred to the infant before or immediately after birth. Although of serious consequence to the newborn, transmission of these diseases is fortunately rare. Formerly, infection with the *Treponema pallida* of *syphilis* was a relatively common occurrence, but since serologic testing of mothers both before marriage and during pregnancy has become universal in this country, congenital syphilis has almost disappeared. It is described briefly in Chapter 14.

Two diseases which are inapparent in the mother cause serious generalized infections, which resemble both sepsis and hemolytic disease of the newborn. One of these diseases is *cytomegalic inclusion disease* caused by the virus of salivary gland disease; the other is *toxoplasmosis* which is caused by a protozoan organism, *Toxoplasma gondii.* In each case the mothers are unaware of their own infection. At or shortly after birth the infant is found to be jaundiced, febrile and anemic and to have a large liver and spleen. Hemorrhages may be present in the skin. The diseases are frequently fatal within the newborn period, and in-

fants who do recover usually suffer damage to the brain or the eyes. Roentgenograms of the skull may show calcification of the damaged areas. Mental retardation or hydrocephalus is a common sequel. Laboratory studies can be used to differentiate between the two conditions. The virus of cytomegalic inclusion disease may be recovered from the urine or the spinal fluid, or cells containing characteristic inclusion bodies may be passed in the urine. No effective treatment is known. Toxoplasmosis can be identified by antibody studies of the blood of mother and infant. Some improvement may be expected from the administration of sulfadiazine and Daraprim. In either disease the excessive accumulation of indirect-reacting bilirubin in the blood should be treated by exchange transfusion; anemia by simple transfusion.

Rubella infection of the mother during the first trimester of her pregnancy may have serious and long-lasting consequences for the infant. Unfortunately, many women are not sure whether they have had the disease and acquired immunity. Furthermore, it is possible for the pregnant woman to contract infection with the virus without showing obvious manifestations of disease. It is hoped that a preventive vaccine will soon be available that will protect potential mothers from this damaging virus infection. The dangers to the infant are greatest when maternal infection takes place early in pregnancy. After 12 weeks of pregnancy, the risk to the infant rapidly disappears.

Infants who are infected *in utero* may show a variety of congenital abnormalities which include microcephaly, cataracts and microphthalmos, congenital malformations of the heart, purpura, deafness, encephalitis and bone defects visible by X-ray. Such infants may remain infectious for long periods, excreting rubella virus in urine and stool for periods up to a year after birth, thus serving as a potential hazard to susceptible nurses or other attendants who are in the early stages of pregnancy.

The *herpes simplex* virus also is capable of causing widespread infection in newborn infants. It is usually transmitted from a mother who either has trivial fever blisters or no symptoms at all. A mother infected with *Coxsackie viruses* usually has symptoms of respiratory illness. If transferred to her infant the ensuing disease is apt to be fatal, since this virus often attacks the myocardium of the newborn, producing severe and often fatal myocarditis. No specific treatment is available for either of these viral infections.

Inclusion blenorrhea is a mild but chronic infection of the conjunctiva contracted during birth from contamination with maternal vaginal secretions. In the adult the disease is an asymptomatic venereal infection. The virus is not affected by silver nitrate treatment of the eyes, and after five or six days, infected infants show a granular inflammation of the inner surface of the eyelids with some associated discharge.

Typical inclusion bodies may be found in scrapings from the palpebral conjunctiva. The disease does not harm the eyes permanently, but the inflammation may persist for several weeks unless treated with sulfonamide ointments.

MISCELLANEOUS DISTURBANCES OF THE NEWBORN

Hemorrhagic Disease of the Newborn

This is a condition in which spontaneous bleeding occurs during the first week of life. Hemorrhages may occur into the skin, from the orifices of the body, or from the umbilicus. Blood passed in the stool is called *melena*. Large hemorrhages or very numerous small ones occasionally threaten life by the loss of blood.

The disturbance is due to a failure of the blood to clot properly, which in turn is caused by an insufficient production of prothrombin, one of the main activators of the clotting mechanism. The body requires vitamin K in order to manufacture prothrombin. Before birth the infant obtains vitamin K from his mother; after birth it comes from his food or from the synthetic activity of the bacteria which invade his intestinal tract shortly after birth. All infants have relatively low levels of prothrombin in the blood during the first few days of life. Premature infants and full-term infants whose mothers have not provided them with adequate amounts of vitamin K may suffer decreases of prothrombin to such low levels that hemorrhage occurs.

Treatment consists in supplying vitamin K_1 oxide by intramuscular injection, following which the infant begins to produce prothrombin at an adequate rate within an hour or two. In severe cases where significant blood loss has occurred, transfusion is desirable to supply red blood cells and to correct the prothrombin deficiency at once.

Anemia in the Newborn

In addition to the anemia which results from hemolytic disease and infection, the newborn infant may have low levels of hemoglobin and red blood cells because of blood loss prior to or at birth. Only rarely does the gross vaginal bleeding of abruptio placentae or placenta praevia include significant amounts from the fetal portion of the circulation. The loss is almost entirely of maternal blood. Hemorrhage from the fetal portion of the placenta may occur occasionally if marginal veins rupture or if the placenta is torn or incised during the course of the delivery. A more subtle form of hemorrhage takes place when abnormal channels within the placenta permit significant quantities of fetal blood to flow into the maternal circulation. The shared placentas of twins (or triplets) are sometimes connected in such a way that one infant pumps blood into the other, making himself anemic and his mate polycythemic.

Uncomplicated anemia may be suspected when pallor, restlessness, weakness or tachycardia is present. In extreme situations there may be evidence of heart failure. Treatment consists in the prompt administration of properly crossmatched blood.

The anemia which follows premature birth is discussed in Chapter 12.

Infants of Diabetic Mothers

Diabetes in the mother increases the hazard to her infant, especially if the disease is of long duration or poorly controlled. Infants of diabetic mothers usually are oversized for their gestational ages, edematous, plethoric and bothered by excessive secretions of mucus from pharynx and stomach. Careful observation and repeated gastric aspiration may be necessary to prevent interference with respirations. Those who have been delivered by caesarian section run an increased risk of the respiratory distress syndrome. The incidence of congenital malformations is somewhat higher among infants born to mothers with diabetes.

Hypoglycemia, which is considered in the next section, is often present for a day or two. Increased insulin-like activity can be demonstrated in the serum of such infants.

Hypoglycemia

Hypoglycemia in the newborn infant may manifest itself by increased irritability which in the extreme instance goes on to convulsions and coma. It may also produce listlessness, inactivity, apnea and cyanosis. The newborn normally has a rather low blood sugar level (40-60 mg. per cent) and may fail to show any symptoms even if the level falls lower. Symptomatic hypoglycemia is potentially serious for the newborn because if not successfully treated it may produce brain damage. Particularly careful observation and measurements of blood glucose are usually indicated for babies of diabetic mothers, for those born with weights that are disproportionately low for their gestational ages, and for those with a history of previous infants in the family who have suffered from hypoglycemia or died of unknown causes. Treatment consists of the immediate intravenous injection of 50 per cent glucose in small dosage followed by an infusion of 10 per cent glucose. Glucagon and, less frequently, epinephrine or ephedrine may also be of assistance in raising the blood level of glucose.

Hypocalcemia

Because of poor parathyroid or renal function, newborns may occasionally have hypocalcemic tetany. Symptomatically they are irritable and may have convulsions. Blood calcium levels are normally quite low in the newborn as compared to the older infant, but levels below 8 mg. per cent are considered significant. Treatment consists of the slow intravenous injection of calcium gluconate for immediate relief followed by calcium chloride by mouth.

SITUATIONS FOR FURTHER STUDY

1. What happens when the fetus's oxygen supply is compromised before delivery? What physical signs would signal an infant's need for special care in the nursery?

2. What factors seem to predispose to the development of respiratory distress or pulmonary failure in the newborn?

3. What symptoms spell respiratory distress in the newborn?

4. What would you look for as you changed the position of an infant with respiratory distress?

5. When does physiologic jaundice appear? What mechanisms produce it?

6. What symptoms in a baby with erythroblastosis would alert you to the fact that his condition was worsening?

7. What help could you give a young woman who told you that she was anticipating marriage and was worried because she had discovered recently that she was Rh negative?

8. What physical characteristics of the newborn make pneumonia a hazard?

9. What symptoms in a baby of a diabetic mother would alert you to his need for medical assistance?

BIBLIOGRAPHY

Avery, M. E.: The Lung and Its Disorders in the Newborn Infant, Philadelphia, Saunders, 1964.

Buchanan-Davidson, D. J.: Erythroblastosis neonatorum, Am. J. Nurs. 64:110, 1964.

Cornblath, M., and Schwartz, R.: Disorders of Carbohydrate Metabolism in Infancy, Philadelphia, Saunders, 1966.

Hardy, J.: Rubella and its aftermath, Children 16:90, 1969.

Lin-Fu, J.: New hope for babies of Rh negative mothers, Children 16:23, 1969.

Pringle, J. A.: Respiratory distress unit, Am. J. Nurs. 68:2370, 1968.

Shaffer, A. J.: Disease of the Newborn, Philadelphia, Saunders, 1965.

Weller, T. H., Alford, C. A., Jr., and Neva, F. A.: Changing epidemiologic concepts of rubella with particular reference to the unique characteristics of the congenital infection, Yale J. Biol. Med. 37:455, 1965.

11

Nursing Care of the Newborn With Congenital Malformations and Hereditary Diseases

The care of a congenitally malformed child presents the nurse with several challenges. The physical aspects of nursing care are likely to be not only complex and demanding, but frustrating and discouraging as well. These emotional aspects of nursing care are trying. Until the nurse becomes aware of her feelings toward the child and the parents and learns to deal with them appropriately, the initial experiences with malformed infants will create tensions and conflicts. The inexperienced nurse will find that a discussion of her feelings with an instructor or head nurse will help her to face and handle them with increasing comfort.

In addition to managing her own emotions, the nurse must also work with the disappointed parents whose attitudes toward the malformed child commonly need to be converted from hopeless despair to a constructive, realistic plan for salvaging his assets. To face the latter challenge the nurse should know the prognosis of the deformity, the degree to which it can be modified by treatment, and the steps that will be necessary either to eliminate the defect or to help parents and child toward an optimal disposition of his life.

This chapter will consider only defects which are apparent at birth or soon afterward. It cannot hope to cover the infinite variety of known deformities but will present the peculiar problems of some of the more common abnormalities. Information about malformations which evade discovery until later infancy or childhood will be discussed in sections appropriate to the age at which they are most frequently uncovered.

INCIDENCE

Anomalies cover such a wide range of severity from the fatal to the trivial that an exact statement of incidence depends on what changes are included within the definition. At one extreme it is possible to say that almost every infant has some anomaly such as a pigmented mole, facial asymmetry or slight webbing of the toes. At the other extreme the definition may be limited to defects which seriously interfere with function of the body; roughly 1 per cent of newborns will be found to be thus afflicted. More exact are the figures for malformations which result in death during the first year of life. As detailed in Chapter 3, approximately 1 out of 7 or 8 of the deaths which go to make up the infant mortality rate can be attributed to anomalous development. Over the years this incidence has not changed much because measures for preventing malformations are not very effective. In contrast, the surgical technics for correcting or ameliorating those anomalies which are compatible with life have been greatly improved in recent years so that this aspect of pediatric care is assuming increasing importance.

ETIOLOGY

Genetic Factors

Some malformations are determined when fertilization of the ovum takes place. The genetic material of the ovum itself or of the sperm which fertilizes it may be such that it will direct the growth of the new individual along aberrant lines. The science of genetics studies the way in which traits, both normal and abnormal, are transmitted from parent to child through the activities of the genes.* Some of the anomalies of man are known to follow the same rules of transmission as those established for animals by research and experimentation. Such hereditary or genetically transmitted malformations are identified by their occurrence in other members of the child's family. Those which are passed along by a dominant type of inheritance are relatively easy to identify, but those with a recessive mode of transmission may appear too infrequently to permit adequate study (see Table 10). It should be noted that a given abnormality such as cleft palate can at times be the result of genetic factors and at other times be due to influences on the fetus developing *in utero* which have no hereditary basis.

Mutations. The causes of abnormal gene development are not entirely understood, but from experiments with lower forms of life, it seems clear that exposure to various types of high energy radiation is an important factor. A fundamental change in the structure of a gene, resulting in the transmission of a trait different from that normally carried by the gene, is known as a mutation. It is presumed that mutations are taking place by chance at a slow rate among many fertile human beings. Presumably, some of the conversions or mutations within sperm cells and ova are due to inescapable radiation which everyone receives from sources such as outer space (cosmic rays) or the small amount of radioactive isotopes present in the elements of the earth, the food we eat and even in the substance of our bodies. Although factors other than radiation may be responsible for mutations, present-day concern is focused on reducing this hazard to a minimum by keeping diagnostic and therapeutic radiation (x-rays, radium, isotopes) to a minimum, by shielding us from industrial sources, including radioactive waste in our communities. As far as we know, most genetic mutations result in the appearance of undesirable traits, but we cannot reject the possibility that they also pave the way for improvements in the quality of the race. The hazards of radiation are difficult to assess quantitatively. Some radiation is inevitable, more is probably undesirable, but at what point does it become genetically hazardous? Opinions among experts differ widely on the amount of radiation to which man can be exposed safely. The correct answer may not be revealed until the mutations produced today appear in the next or following generations.

---

* Genes are the basic units which determine the transmission of characteristics from one generation to another. In general they direct the formation of proteins in the newly developing cells. Among the proteins being formed are enzymes which control various aspects of metabolism. Lack of a necessary specific enzyme will result in a disorder known as an inborn error of metabolism, which is considered in a subsequent section. For fuller discussion of genetic principles the reader must consult a textbook on the subject.

Table 10. Genetic Inheritance*

Mode of Inheritance	Mother Genes	Mother Abnormality	Father Genes	Father Abnormality	Children Genes	Children Abnormality	Per cent of Offspring
Normal	M M / O O	None	F F / O O	None	M F / O O	None	100
Dominant	M M / O O	None	F f / O ●	Present	M F / O O	None	50
					M f / O ●	Present	50
Recessive	M M / O O	None	F f / O ●	Carrier	M F / O O	None	50
					M f / O ●	Carrier	50
Recessive	M m / O ●	Carrier	F f / O ●	Carrier	M F / O O	None	25
					M f / O O	Carrier	25 } 50
					m F / O O	Carrier	25 }
					m f / ● ●	Present	25

* To visualize the main modes of inheritance, each gene must be thought of as having two parts. Individuals who are completely normal with respect to the characteristic which a particular gene determines are normal in both parts of the gene pair (OO). When an abnormality which is transmitted by dominant inheritance is present, the individual is abnormal in one half of his corresponding gene pair (O ●). Thus, a dominant trait is expressed in bodily abnormality when only half of the genes involved are faulty. If the recessive mode of inheritance is involved, both halves of the gene pair must be defective (● ●) before the trait appears. If only one half of a recessive gene pair is defective (O ●) the individual's body is normal with respect to the trait, but he retains the capability of passing the abnormal gene on to his children. Such a person is said to be a carrier of the abnormal gene in question. He may also be called a heterozygote.

At the time of fertilization of the ovum, the newly formed individual must obtain each of his gene pairs by selecting one half from the corresponding gene pair of his father and one half from that of his mother. Normal genes are represented here by capital letters and abnormal genes by small letters. The possible combinations are not affected if the gene constitution of the father (who appears here as the villain) and the mother are reversed.

The less common matings such as dominant Mm × Ff, or matings between individuals, one of whom has only abnormal gene components (homozygote), are not included here.

Hereditary Inborn Errors of Metabolism. Although inborn errors of metabolism do not produce symptoms apparent at birth, they are important to our understanding of the origin of congenital abnormalities. Some are relatively common disorders (sicklemia for example), but most are rare conditions (galactosemia, Gaucher's disease, phenylketonuria) in which an enzyme necessary for the completion of a biochemical reaction within the body is congenitally missing. A rapidly increasing number of such disorders is being discovered, most of which have a recessive mode of inheritance. This means that to be affected by the disease, a child must receive a pair of abnormal genes —one from his father and the other from his mother. The parents who themselves carry the abnormal gene in single dosage are not affected with the disease. However, the children resulting from such a marriage will have 1 chance in 4 of receiving the double dose of the gene and manifesting the disease. Sickle cell

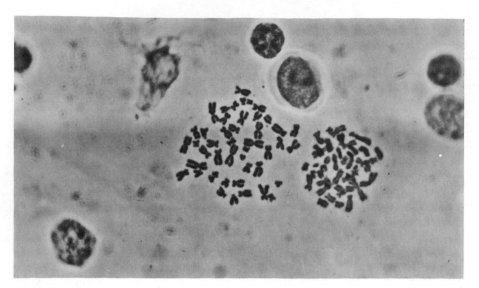

Fig. 11-1. The chromosomes of two dividing human cells are shown. In the upper group it is possible to count the 46 individual chromosomes and to see that 2 of each kind are present. By enlarging the photograph the individual chromosomes may be cut out and matched in pairs and the identification of each can then be made. (Dr. James L. Burks)

anemia is a good illustration. About 10 per cent of American Negroes have an abnormal gene which causes them to manufacture chemically abnormal S-hemoglobin in their red blood cells. When present in single dosage the gene does them no harm, for only a relatively small fraction of their hemoglobin is S-hemoglobin. Its presence can be recognized by electrophoretic tests on hemoglobin obtained from their red cells or by a simpler test of the red cells themselves for the sickling trait. However, when two individuals who have the asymptomatic sickle trait produce children, about one fourth of the offspring will receive two abnormal genes and in consequence will produce such a large proportion of S-hemoglobin that the symptoms of sickle cell anemia will result. While 10 per cent of Negroes carry the abnormal gene, only about 0.25 per cent have it in double dosage and suffer from sickle cell anemia. It can be understood that abnormal genes which are less frequent in the population as a whole will produce disease with corresponding rarity. The rarity itself makes study difficult. It is possible that many disorders whose origin we do not now understand will eventually be found to depend on the conjunction of two rare recessive genes.

A partial list of the disorders which fall in this category is given here. Fuller treatment of several of these entities will be found elsewhere in the book.

Hemophilia A
Christmas disease (Hemophilia B)
Agammaglobulinemia
Wilson's disease
Sickle cell anemia
Thalassemia
Congenital spherocytic anemia
Phenylketonuria
Hurler's disease (gargoylism)
Marfan's syndrome (arachnodactyly)
Glycogen storage disease

Xanthomatosis
Galactosemia
Adrenogenital syndrome
Some types of cretinism
Niemann-Pick disease
Gaucher's disease
Tay-Sachs' disease
Porphyria
Cystic fibrosis of the pancreas
Idiopathic hypoglycemia

Chromosomal Abnormalities. Thus far the consideration of heredity has been concerned entirely with the genes. Genes are so small that they cannot be seen by present microscopic technics. They are known entirely by what they do. In all animals (and plants too) the genes are known to be grouped into larger aggregates called chromosomes. The chromosomes are large enough to be readily visible within cell nuclei under the microscope, and the process of their division during cell reproduction has been studied extensively. Each animal species has a characteristic number of chromosomes which can be distinguished and labeled individually. Experiments on lower animals have shown that a given gene is always found within the same chromosome and never elsewhere. Furthermore, the exact position of the genes within the chromosomes of some species has been mapped carefully. As yet this information is not available for human chromosomes, but it is assumed that particular genes belong to a specific chromosome and have a definite position within its structure.

Only within the past few years has it become possible to make accurate counts and establish a classification of the chromosomes of human cells. An erroneous impression that the normal number was 48 has been corrected as superior technics have been developed. Actually, there are 23 pairs or 46 chromosomes. The pairs numbered 1 through 22 each contain a set of identical chromosomes, while the 23rd pair, which determines the sex of the individual, consists of two large X-chromosomes in the normal female, and one large X-chromosome and a smaller Y-chromosome in the normal male. At least one of the inborn errors of metabolism (hemophilia A) is due to defective genes in the sex chromosome pair, since it occurs only in males (see Chap. 21). Actually in such sex linkage the defect is within the X-chromosome. Since the male has only one X, and since that is defective, he is homozygous for the abnormality and it is expressed as the disease. The female, having two X-chromosomes, will be heterozygous and only a carrier unless both of her X-chromosomes are abnormal.

Just before fertilization both ovum and sperm undergo a reduction division in which the cell separates into two parts each of which normally contains one member of each chromosome pair (haploid). Sometimes this division is faulty so that both members of one chromosome pair get into one of the haploid units (non-disjunction) while the other has none of that pair. If such a defective haploid ovum joins with a normal haploid sperm, or vice versa, a new organism may be formed which has either an excessive number of chromosomes (47) or a deficient number (45). When 47 chromosomes are present, *trisomy* is the term applied to the defect because there are three of one of the chromosomes. The known instances produce a number of somatic abnormalities, usually including some defect in intelligence. Gonadal dysgenesis is the only well known clinical condition in which the chromosomal number is reduced to 45 by the absence of one of the sex chromosomes. More complicated disturbances of chromosomal number can also occur but are relatively uncommon and usually afflict the sex chromosomes primarily. Individuals who possess two populations of cells which have differing numbers of chromosomes are known as mosaics. They may show clinical findings which are intermediate between the normal and abnormal constitutions represented by the two populations of cells.

Three *trisomies* will be considered later in the text—trisomy 21 (Down's syndrome), trisomy 13-15, and trisomy 18. A trisomy of the sex chromosomes, Klinefelter's syndrome, is usually not discoverable until the child is approaching puberty.

Intrauterine Environmental Effects

The construction of the human body begins at conception with the division of the fertilized ovum, first into two cells, then into four, eight, and so on until the process has been repeated an estimated 44 times by the conclusion of the 40-week period of gestation. Along the way the dividing cells differentiate into the many types found in the completed body and group themselves into masses and layers which form the organ systems. These latter undergo a predetermined sequence of changes in shape through the development of curves, bulges, ridges, tubes, projections and

tunnels as they progress toward their final anatomic form. Simultaneously, the whole growing mass of protoplasm migrates into the fallopian tube, traverses it rapidly and fixes itself to the wall of the uterus. Here it develops a placenta through which it eventually acquires nourishment by way of the maternal circulation. During later growth the fetus distends the uterus so that it occupies a large fraction of the maternal abdominal cavity. Malformations arise when the expected changes in this complicated assembly-line fail to take place in proper sequence or to the

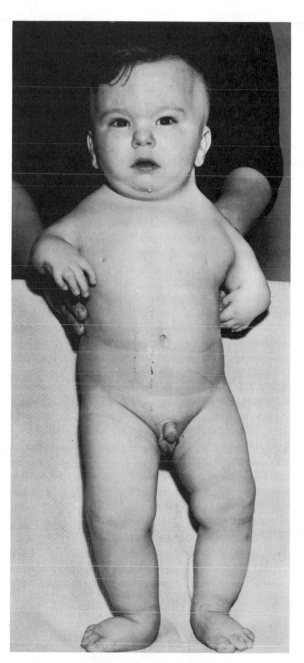

Fig. 11-2. Infant with phocomelia, or seal arms. This is the type of skeletal abnormality attributed to the use of thalidomide during early pregnancy.

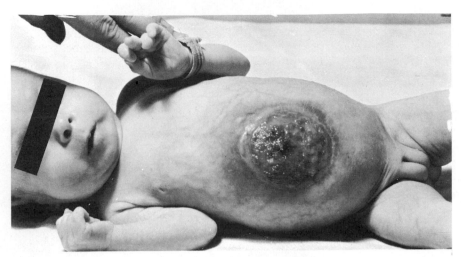

FIG. 11-3. Omphalocele.

proper extent. Interferences at any stage may affect the final form of a portion or even of the whole of the body. It is small wonder that malformations occur; it is the miracle of reproduction that the intricate changes follow the blueprint exactly in more than 9 out of 10 gestations.

The first 12 weeks of fetal development are a crucial period in which the major organ systems of the body complete the transformation into their final shapes, albeit not their final sizes. Any interference with growth during this "organogenetic" period may result in permanent deformity of the organ or part involved.

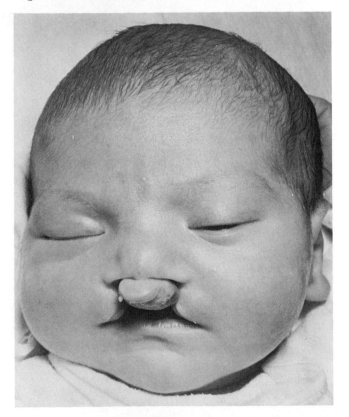

FIG. 11-4. Bilateral cleft lip. (Dr. H. P. Jenkins)

In experimental work with animals it has been shown that various types of disturbance of the mother during the corresponding period of gestation can be used to produce anomalies in the young. Deprivation of oxygen or of certain vitamins, administration of hormones, drugs, poisons, anti-metabolites and cortisone or exposure to irradiation from radium or roentgen rays are among the methods used to interfere with the normal development of animal fetuses. In man it has been suspected that similar influences on the pregnant woman might be responsible for anomalies, but only a few such examples have been definitely established. Exposure to radium, roentgen rays and the atomic bomb have resulted in the delivery of infants with abnormalities of the brain. Maternal infection with rubella is generally accepted as being responsible for a combination of defects of the eye, the heart and the brain. Infants who are subjected to the hormonal disturbances of a mother who has diabetes during pregnancy suffer a distinctly greater incidence of congenital malformations. In Europe a tragically large number of babies were born with absence or maldevelopment of extremities before it was discovered that a new analgesic, Thalidomide, given to mothers during pregnancy was at fault and the drug was banished.

In the latter two thirds of pregnancy the adverse effects on the fetus are better understood. Disease of the mother may be transferred to him (syphilis, toxoplasmosis and, rarely, other infections). Antithyroid drugs given to the mother may result in her child having a goiter at birth. Erythroblastosis is the effect of abnormal antibodies in the mother on the red blood cells of the child. In fact, the mechanisms of many of these defects are now so well understood that we no longer regard them as congenital malformations. During the last few months of pregnancy some infants appear to remain in one position and, in consequence, suffer pressure effects from the uterus or from bony prominences of the maternal skeleton. Positional anomalies of feet, legs, jaw and face are explained in

FIG. 11-5. (*Left*) Incomplete unilateral cleft. (*Right*) Unilateral cleft repair. (Dr. H. P. Jenkins)

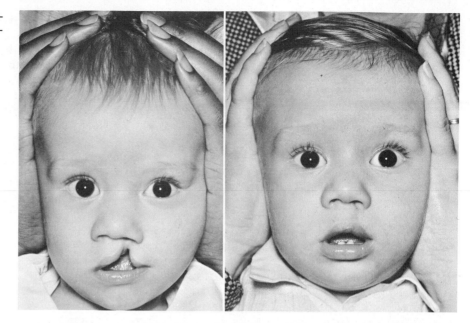

this fashion. The reason why certain infants fail to change position is not understood.

Prevention of malformations is largely an unrealized hope. Careful supervision of maternal diets in pregnancy, exact regulation of diabetes, and shielding of mothers insofar as possible from infectious disease and from radiant energy probably prevents some malformations, but it must be admitted that our understanding of the mechanism of malformation is too inexact as yet to permit the prevention of more than a small percentage.

DIGESTIVE TRACT

Omphalocele

Omphalocele is a rare but important anomaly in which the contents of the abdominal cavity protrude into the root of the umbilical cord or through a defect in the skin of the anterior abdominal wall. The protruding mass may be small in size or large enough to contain much of the intestines and the liver. It is covered with a delicate membrane rather than skin. Immediate surgical repair is necessary before the sac ruptures and infection is introduced into the abdominal cavity. In about half of the instances of omphalocele, other congenital defects are present. Surgical repair is made difficult by the small size of the abdominal cavity which may make it almost impossible to mobilize enough skin to cover the defect. This problem and the presence of other anomalies lead to a high postoperative mortality.

Cleft Lip and Palate

The deformity of cleft lip (harelip) or cleft palate or both combined results from failure of growth and union of the bony and the soft tissue structures on one or both sides of the midline of the palate and the upper jaw. The failure in union may be on one or both sides of the lip alone, or it may extend backward into the upper jaw and even through into the nasal cavity. The defect of the posterior palate is a failure of midline closure which may occur alone or in conjunction with clefts in the lip or the anterior palate. These anomalies are fairly common, occurring once in 500 to 1,000 newborns. In some families there is a clear hereditary transmission. In other instances no etiologic basis is known. Sometimes isolated defects of the palate are associated with very marked hypoplasia of the lower jaw (Pierre Robin syndrome), suggesting that the palate has been prevented from closing by backward pressure of the tongue and the jaw due to intrauterine anteflexion of the head on the chest.

Plan of Treatment. The general plan of treatment and the prospective outcome depend on the extent and combination of the deformities. Surgical repair of the lip and the upper maxilla usually is performed within the first few weeks of life. Where only the lip is involved, the result of early operation (sometimes performed within the first 12 hours after birth) may be final and satisfactory. Involvement of the maxilla usually foreshadows irregularities in later dentition and perhaps some abnormality of growth. Defects of the palate are more difficult to handle, and their correction usually is deferred until at least the second year and often later in order to take advantage of changes which occur with growth. Cleft palates usually foreshadow speech difficulties and may be attended by recurrent infections of the upper respiratory tract and the middle ear. When it is deemed advisable to postpone surgical repair of the palate, prosthetic speech appliances are fitted so that speech development can approximate the normal. Prostheses are used after the deciduous teeth have fully erupted and the child has developed emotionally to the point where he can accept the use of the speech appliance. Prostheses have been used for children as young as 2½ years. Sometimes speech proceeds normally without benefit of formal speech training. However, in most instances speech therapy is imperative. Sometimes prostheses are used as interim devices before the palate is repaired or when the palate is repaired in two or more stages. When the deformity is too severe for adequate plastic repair, prosthetic speech appliances are used as a permanent means of speech rehabilitation. As the child grows, the appliance must be modified.

An important aspect of the initial management is the problem of dealing with the disappointment and anxieties of the parents. Considerable justified reassurance can be given when the defect is confined to the lip. If the palate is also involved, parents usually can be assured that much improvement is to be expected but that it will take time, skillful judgment and care, and patience on their parts to help the child adjust to his deformity and to assume a normal place in the community.

The optimal management of a child with a cleft palate requires coordinated efforts of the pediatrician, plastic surgeon, dentist, speech therapist, social worker and nurse. In large metropolitan areas and in State Crippled Children's programs there is an increasing tendency to provide cleft palate clinics where the several specialists can work jointly with easy consultation among themselves. When such facilities are available to an infant with cleft palate, early referral even within the first few weeks of life is desirable so that changes taking place with growth can be observed and appropriate plans for ultimate corrective measures can be made accordingly.

Nursing Care of the Infant with a Cleft Lip. Immediate nursing care of the infant born with a cleft lip does not differ substantially from that of other infants except for the necessary alterations in feeding procedures. Most infants with a defect of the lip are unable to breast feed and many may have difficulty in bottle feeding. If bottle feeding is possible, it has the advantage of allowing the infant to obtain gratification through sucking and of making the feeding process more comfortable for the mother if she is to take him home for a period of time before repair of the lip is planned. A trial with a bottle should be made using a nipple larger and softer than is customary. A "lamb's nipple" often serves well in that it is longer and softer. If the infant is unable to manage a nipple, feeding can be accomplished with the use of a sterile, rubber-tipped medicine dropper or with a 10 cc. Asepto syringe with a bulb and a 1½ inch rubber catheter extension. In order to facilitate swallowing, holding the infant in a semi-upright position is often helpful. Frequent bubbling is necessary to prevent regurgitation because of the tendency to swallow excessive amounts of air. Following the feeding, the tissue around the cleft should be cleansed gently with a dropperful of sterile water in order to prevent crusting. If surgery is planned after a period of weight gain, the mother must be acquainted with the method of feeding before discharge and have sufficient practice so that she feels comfortable with the technic.

After admission for lip surgery, the infant should be fed with a rubber-tipped medicine dropper or Asepto syringe in order to accustom him to the postoperative method of feeding. The rubber tip is inserted into the corner of the mouth to prevent interference with the suture line and the formula is placed on top of the tongue to facilitate swallowing. Feeding should be given slowly and at a rate suitable to the capacity of the individual infant, with the milk mixture kept warm continually throughout the procedure.

The nurse should observe the infant for signs of respiratory or gastrointestinal disease during the preoperative period, for it is imperative that surgery be performed when the infant is in the best possible physical condition. Protective isolation precautions are helpful in preventing cross-infection. Arm restraint is necessary immediately after the operation, and the effect is less distressing to the infant if he has become accustomed to it before. If the infant is old enough to turn himself onto his abdomen and face, a jacket restraint to keep him on his side or back will also be necessary.

After operative repair of the lip, the infant needs observation and meticulous care. Clear liquids may be given as soon as he reacts fully and is able to swallow. Formula feeding may be resumed from three to 12 hours postoperatively. The infant is held upright and is fed slowly and carefully with frequent bubbling to prevent regurgitation and aspiration of formula. The catheter tip of the syringe or dropper is placed in the side of the mouth and care should be taken to avoid catching internal sutures. After feeding, the serosanguineous drainage and formula must be removed carefully with a gauze swab dipped in saline or hydrogen peroxide to prevent crusting and excessive scar formation. In some hospitals, the sutures may be kept covered with an antibiotic ointment applied after feeding. If swabbing is the method of choice, a tray containing sterile swabs, hydrogen peroxide or saline, forceps in alcohol and a paper bag should be available at the bedside. Careful and frequent cleansing of the entire suture line is the responsibility of the nurse. Should there be sloughing of the sutures, the vermilion border of the lip becomes uneven, and additional repair makes a good cosmetic effect impossible.

Postoperatively, the infant is positioned on his back or tilted slightly to one side to facilitate drainage and prevent aspiration. After feeding he should be placed on his side to prevent aspiration of any regurgitated milk or mucus that may accumulate. Support with a rolled bed pad will be necessary to keep him in this position. A sterile bulb syringe should be in readiness to aspirate mucus from the mouth.

Arm and body restraints should be in readiness for application immediately after his return to the ward. Tongue-depressor arm restraints will prevent the infant from getting his hands to his mouth but will not prevent him from rubbing his face with his upper arms. For this reason, the cuffs should be pinned securely to the shirt. Periodically, he should be given relief from his restraint. His arms should be massaged and exercised one at a time. Restraints should not be removed for weighing, nor should both be removed at one time during the morning bath. The infant's position should be changed frequently to prevent both hypostatic pneumonia and discomfort. Crying causes tension on the suture line. His need for emotional satisfactions are no different from the normal infant. The infant who has had a surgical repair of the lip cannot suckle; therefore, he needs extra cuddling to keep him free from anxiety and tension.

During the first 48 hours after operation, difficulty in breathing may be encountered. When bilateral clefts have been repaired, the infant must become accustomed to nasal breathing, a type not required before. In some instances a sterile airway made of a small piece of ¼-inch rubber tubing is sutured to the corner of the infant's mouth before he leaves the operating room. If no airway has been inserted and difficult breathing is observed, downward pressure on the chin to open the mouth will bring relief. If a Logan bow has been applied to prevent suture tension, care should be taken to keep the adhesive strapping dry and clean. Moisture loosens it, and then its effectiveness is negligible.

Sutures are generally removed by the physician at any time after the fourth postoperative day until the wound is entirely healed. If the sutures are removed early, the Logan bow is left in place, restraints are continued and the infant may be discharged. Bottle feedings may be resumed from a few weeks to a month after the surgery. In some instances, if the infant also has a cleft of the palate, the Asepto technique may be continued until after palate surgery. If the mother still has breast milk, she should be encouraged to maintain her supply during the period in which the infant is having surgical repair. The use of pumped milk during the postoperative period is an added advantage to the infant.

When a cleft lip has been repaired successfully in a baby who has an associated cleft palate, the improved appearance usually has a remarkable psychological effect on the parents. It gives them hope and helps the mother to face the future care that the infant with cleft palate requires. Before the infant leaves the hospital, the mother should have had experience in

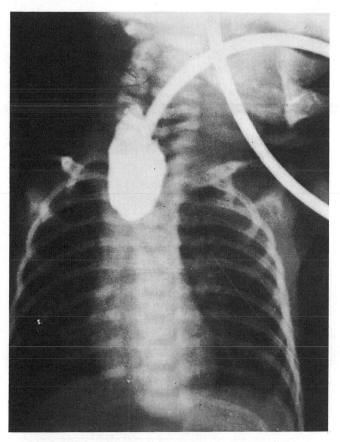

FIG. 11-6. Chest X-ray of a newborn with the common type of esophageal atresia. The contrast media is seen filling a blind pouch high in the neck. None has entered the lower esophagus, stomach or bronchi.

feeding her baby and should be taught how to prevent respiratory infections. Many infants with cleft palates can learn to suckle from a bottle if the nipple bulb is soft and long, and if the holes are large enough. If the usual method of feeding can be used, the mother is less inclined to feel that her child is abnormal. These babies require slow feeding to prevent excessive air swallowing and regurgitation. Holding them in a sitting position with the head and chest tilted slightly backward facilitates swallowing without aspiration.

Obstruction of the Intestinal Tract

Atresia of the Esophagus. Failure of the embryonic development of the esophagus to result in a continuous tube connecting the pharynx with the stomach is a serious but uncommon congenital malformation. Several variations of this condition are known. The most common one consists of a blind pouch at the upper end of the esophagus and an errant lower segment which runs upward from the stomach and opens through a fistula into the trachea near its bifurcation. At birth, air enters the stomach by way of the trachea, the fistula and the lower segment of the esophagus.

Attempts to swallow liquids or even the normal secretions of the mouth, result in rapid filling of the blind pouch and overflow of liquid into larynx and trachea. The infant chokes, coughs and turns blue whenever attempts are made to feed him. Unless the situation is corrected quickly, he will contract bronchitis or pneumonia from the repeated aspiration of food and secretions. Rarely, the esophagus is fully open but communicates with the trachea by an abnormal fistula. The same symptoms result, and the treatment is identical.

Atresia of the esophagus should be suspected when an infant has excessive mucus, particularly if he coughs, sputters and becomes cyanotic after eating. Diagnosis of atresia is made from stoppage of a catheter at the site of atresia or it is revealed on roentgenogram with iodized oil in the esophagus; barium never should be used for this purpose because of the danger of pneumonia from its aspiration.

As soon as atresia of the esophagus is suspected, the infant should be placed in a supine position with his head and shoulders elevated no less than 30 degrees. This position is important in preventing gastric secretions from rising up into the distal esophagus and into the tracheobronchial tree through the fistula.

TREATMENT. Only prompt surgical treatment offers hope of correcting the defect and saving life. Surgical treatment consists of ligation of the fistula and end-to-end anastomosis of the upper and the lower segments of the esophagus. This procedure is successful in some instances. Occasionally, a stricture develops subsequently at the site of anastomosis; the stricture usually is overcome satisfactorily by dilatation. In a few instances anastomosis is not possible at the primary operation because of shortness of the lower segment or the wide separation of the two segments. In such cases the fistula is ligated, the upper segment of the esophagus is brought to the surface, and gastrostomy is done. Subsequent feeding is by way of the gastrostomy. Three to 12 months later, a portion of the colon is brought into the chest and used to join the upper normal portion of the esophagus to the stomach.

Nursing Care in Atresia of the Esophagus. After birth the infant is placed immediately into a heated, humidified crib or Isolette and the mouth and pharynx are suctioned to remove secretions. An atmosphere of high humidity liquefies the thick mucus which characteristically accumulates in the respiratory tract. Careful observation to detect the need for nasopharyngeal aspiration is imperative to prevent aspiration pneumonia which can be rapidly fatal. If the infant is to be transported to another hospital, saliva must first be suctioned from the upper esophageal pouch and the head and thorax of the infant should be elevated approximately 20 degrees.

Preoperatively, antibiotics and parenteral fluids are invariably administered. If a gastrostomy is done, the tube must be kept open by injection of 2 to 4 cc. of air through the tubing. Suction or irrigation is contraindicated to avoid pull on the stomach wall or regurgitation. The upper esophageal pouch should be kept free of secretions by suctioning. An indwelling nasal catheter may be placed by the physician and changed daily since it is easily occluded by mucus. The infant's head and thorax are kept elevated 30 degrees and handling is kept to a minimum.

Postoperatively, the infant is returned immediately to the heated and humidified Isolette. It is the responsibility of the nurse to observe the vital signs carefully, to turn the infant periodically and to keep the airway clear of secretions by suctioning the oropharyngeal area with a sterile No. 8 or 10 French soft rubber catheter. If respiratory distress is noted despite suctioning, the physician should be notified immediately.

The time at which feedings are begun and the manner in which they are given depend on the operation performed and the condition of the baby. Feedings may be given by mouth, through a tube into the esophagus or through a gastrostomy tube.

If the esophagus has been brought to the surface, the exposed portion should be protected by a sterilized gauze dressing held securely in place by a knit binder of the type used as an abdominal binder. After the first few months, when salivary glands become more active, frequent change of dressing is necessary. Saline solution should be used to cleanse the area, and the surrounding skin should be kept scrupulously clean. Frequent change of position is desirable to help prevent respiratory infection.

If gastrostomy has been done, feedings are begun after gastric secretions are noted to pass readily into the duodenum. Feedings are usually started with small amounts of 5 per cent glucose water introduced into the gastrostomy tubing by means of a syringe barrel or special drip apparatus. During this time the infant must be watched closely for signs of regurgitation. When the glucose water is tolerated and the fluid passes readily into the duodenum, warmed formula feeding may be instituted. Before compression of the gastrostomy tube is released, a funnel or syringe barrel should be attached and partially filled with the formula. The funnel must always contain fluid to prevent air from entering the stomach. Elevation of the funnel should be sufficient to allow the food to run in slowly. When the milk is at the level of the end of the funnel, the tube should be folded onto itself and compressed with a rubber band or a clamp. While the milk is running into the stomach, the infant may be given a pacifier to suck. The pacifier provides normal sucking activity, exercises the muscles of the jaw and relaxes the musculature. When opportunity for sucking is not provided, the infant will suck his fists to satisfy his needs. It has been observed that unless the infant is comfortable and happy, the formula fails to run into the stomach. When the feeding is completed, the infant should be picked up for a period of attention. Normal babies have pleasure associated with their feedings. Babies with gastrostomies usually require long periods of hospitalization and unless attention is paid to their psychological needs, they do not thrive.

The skin around the gastrostomy tube should be kept clean and protected with a mild protective ointment. The adhesive strips that hold the tube in place should not adhere to the gauze dressings that encircle the tube.

Oral feedings are usually not begun until approximately two weeks postoperatively. If 5 per cent glucose water is tolerated without difficulty, small amounts of formula are offered by bottle. The gastrostomy tube is usually removed when the infant tolerates complete oral feedings well.

Because of the necessity for lengthy hospitalization and specialized care and equipment, many parents welcome the financial assistance offered by community agencies or the State Crippled Children's Services and such referral plans should be made early whenever indicated. Referral to a community or state agency also provides for continuity of care through continued home visits by community nurses which are supportive to parents during the first postoperative year while the infant is susceptible to pulmonary infections or stricture at the site of anastomosis.

Atresia of the Duodenum. Strictly speaking, this term should be applied to the failure of the duodenum to open into a continuous tube, connecting the stomach with the upper small intestine. Also, it is used to describe obstruction in the duodenum due to valves or diaphragms within the lumen or from bands, kinks and abnormal pressure from without. The symptoms of all these conditions begin immediately after birth and consist of persistent nausea with vomiting of bile-stained fluid. Diagnosis may be confirmed by x-ray examination, which will show that neither air nor barium passes out of the duodenum. Treatment is by surgical relief through release of the obstructing mechanism or by an anastomosis which bypasses the area of atresia.

Atresia of the Small Intestine. Single or multiple regions of the small intestine which have failed to canalize properly in their development are not very uncommon. The symptoms and treatment are like those of duodenal atresia. The lower they are along the course of the intestinal tract, the later the symptoms will occur and the greater the accompanying degree of abdominal distention.

Meconium Ileus. Obstruction of the small intestine during the first few days of life may occur because of the presence of meconium which is so viscid that it cannot flow through the ileocecal valve. The symptoms are the same as those of anatomic abnormality of the small intestine, and relief must be sought through prompt surgical intervention. The true nature of the obstruction can sometimes be suspected from the

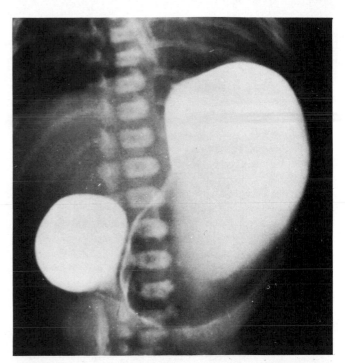

Fig. 11-7. Abdominal X-ray of a newborn infant with congenital atresia of the duodenum. The swallowed barium shows the characteristic "double bubble" sign with a large collection in the stomach and a smaller one in the duodenum. Barium does not pass beyond the duodenum, and there is no gas in the lower bowel.

roentgen appearance of loops of intestine. At operation the surgeon has a difficult task. Often a large portion of the small bowel is impacted with meconium of the consistency of chewing gum. The bowel must be opened and the obstructing contents cleared from, at least, the proximal segment. Irrigation with solutions containing proteolytic enzymes is usually successful. It may be possible also to clear the lower segment of the intestine by the same procedure, thus restoring the continuity of the bowel. If the lower segment cannot be cleared at operation, an enterostomy is done and the irrigation is continued postoperatively.

Meconium ileus is invariably associated with cystic fibrosis of the pancreas (Chap. 13), the other symptoms of which can be expected to appear later during infancy.

Volvulus. Early in fetal life a large portion of the intestinal tract lies in the umbilical sac outside the abdomen and in a position reversed from that which is normal later; that is, the ascending colon is on the left. With continued fetal development the intestine gradually is withdrawn into the abdomen with concurrent rotation to the newly and permanently normal position. After withdrawal and rotation, the mesentery attaches to the posterior wall of the abdomen, and the transverse colon becomes attached to the stomach by the gastrocolic ligament.

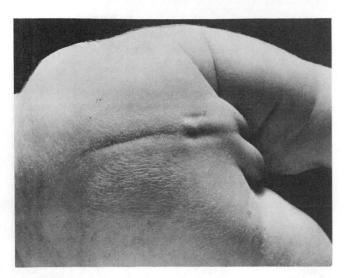

FIG. 11-8. Imperforate anus. (Potter, E. L.: Pathology of the Fetus and the Newborn, Chicago, Year Book Pub.)

In a few instances, rotation of the bowel is faulty, in that it is incomplete or absent. In such circumstances, the mesentery cannot attach in the normal places or in the normal manner. The abnormal attachment may give rise to peritoneal bands which subsequently may cause obstruction by pressure on the bowel at some point or by entangling a loop of bowel. A bowel with incomplete mesenteric attachment is not well anchored and at any time may become twisted in such a manner as to cause obstruction and to cut off the blood supply to a portion of itself. Volvulus is the term applied when obstruction occurs from twisting of the intestine. Volvulus from abnormal rotation may occur at any time in the first few years but is much more common in early infancy. The only treatment is prompt surgical attention, with cutting of constricting bands or with the untwisting of a twisted intestinal loop. Often some anchoring of unattached bowel is indicated.

Atresia of the Rectum and the Anus. Abnormal development of the lower intestinal tract may be apparent on inspection of the infant if no anal opening is found or if the initial attempt to take the baby's temperature reveals a shallow blind pouch instead of a normal anus. At other times the failure of the infant to produce meconium and the progressive distention of his abdomen lead to the discovery of an incomplete canalization of the rectum in spite of an externally normally anus.

In the normal embryologic development of the lower bowel, a blind pouch within the abdomen descends toward the perineum and meets another pouch which is invaginating the skin in the region of the anus. The ends of the two pouches fuse, and the septum between them breaks through to form a continuous passageway. The mildest form of atresia is that in which the development is complete, except for the disappearance of the membrane between the two pouches. This situation is relieved easily by splitting the membrane with a small knife introduced into the anus. Even if the two pouches have not quite met, the surgeon may be able to join them from below and make a proper anastomosis at once. The opening must be dilated periodically for several months afterward to prevent its constriction during scar-tissue formation. More serious abnormalities result when the internal blind pouch lies at some distance from the skin of the perineum or aberrantly joins the vagina, the urethra or a fistulous opening into the perineum. Often primary union cannot be undertaken in these circumstances, and a temporary colostomy is necessary until a later, more extensive operation can be performed.

Diaphragmatic Hernia

Congenital defects in the diaphragm allow intestines, spleen or liver to invade the pleural cavity through the abnormal opening. Infants with this defect may appear normal at birth but have increasing respiratory distress as the collapsed intestines begin to fill with swallowed air. The heart and lungs are thus compressed into the opposite side of the chest, and ventilation rapidly becomes inadequate. The con-

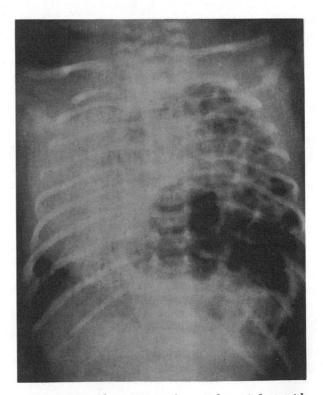

FIG. 11-9. Chest X-ray of a newborn infant with a diaphragmatic hernia. The left chest is filled with dilated loops of intestine which displace the heart and mediastinum into the right chest.

dition can be distinguished from other causes of neonatal respiratory distress by roentgen demonstration of loops of intestine in the chest cavity. Immediate operation is necessary to repair the diaphragmatic defect and permit adequate expansion of the lungs. Difficulty may be encountered in restoring the viscera to their proper position, since the development of the abdominal cavity may also be incomplete. Surprisingly, a diaphragmatic hernia may pass unrecognized or may produce only minimal symptoms for several years. Once discovered, operation is still the preferred treatment.

GENITOURINARY TRACT

The Kidneys

Anomalous formation of the upper urinary tract is common and is found in approximately 10 per cent of all autopsies performed on children. Many of the malformations are of no consequence to the child, but when they result in stasis of urine flow, they are prone to become chronically infected or to produce pain from obstruction. Such conditions as hydronephrosis, double kidney or ureter, dilated ureters and hypoplastic kidneys are identified only during the course of urologic examination in the search for a focus of urinary tract infection. This subject and its management are considered in Chapter 14.

On occasion renal anomalies are discovered during the newborn period. *Renal agenesis* which implies total failure of the kidney to develop is unimportant when it is unilateral, but fatal to the infant within a few hours after birth if the condition is bilateral. Infants with this disorder have a characteristic facial appearance with low-set ears and widely spaced oriental eyes. Treatment is impossible even when the condition is recognized at once. Severe degrees of polycystic kidney may produce early renal failure and abdominal enlargement. The condition is due to a failure of the kidney tubules to make normal connection with the developing glomeruli. The number and size of the fluid-filled cysts which result determine the effect upon kidney function. Although serious malformation of this type leads to early death, milder degrees may pass unrecognized until adult life. No treatment is effective.

The Bladder

Exstrophy of the Bladder. This condition is caused by failure of union between the two sides of the lower abdomen, a failure which produces a fissure in the midline from umbilicus to genitalia. The defect includes the abdominal wall, the anterior wall of the bladder, the symphysis pubis and the urethra. The posterior and the lateral surfaces of the bladder are exposed, and the ureteral outlets are visible. The condition is more common in boys than in girls. In boys, usually a groove is present in the anterior sur-

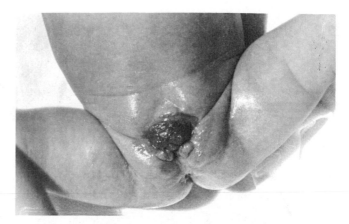

Fig. 11-10. Exstrophy of the bladder.

face of the penis; in girls the clitoris is divided, and the labia may be separated. Other congenital malformations may be associated.

Treatment consists of operative removal of the bladder, the ureters first having been transplanted to the colon. A suitable age for the operation is 3 to 4 years after the child has acquired bowel control and can learn to hold urine within his rectum.

Nursing Care in Exstrophy of the Bladder. The nursing care of the newborn with exstrophy of the bladder differs from that of other newborns only in that the bladder area must be protected from trauma and from irritation. Diapers should be changed frequently and the infant should become accustomed to sleeping on his back or side. The bladder area can be kept clean by washing with a mild soap and water and further protected by a sterile gauze covering to which a mild ointment has been applied. The nurse caring for the infant must also be alert to any signs of infection which should be reported immediately to the physician.

Bladder Neck Obstruction. Congenital valvelike folds in the posterior urethra or bladder neck may seriously hamper passage of urine through the male urethra and lead to enlargement of the bladder, hydronephrosis and progressive loss of renal function. The difficulty is often present even before birth, but it takes an alert observer to recognize that a small male infant is not voiding a sufficiently forceful stream. Prompt urologic examination and relief of the destructive back pressure on the kidneys may save the child from a lifetime of crippling disease.

Hypospadias. Hypospadias is a malformation in which the urethra opens on the under surface of the penis proximal to the usual site. Minor degrees of hypospadias are very common and require no treatment. When the urethral opening is on the shaft of the penis or at its base, surgical correction will ultimately be required. It is deferred until after infancy and sometimes until puberty when advantage may be taken of the full growth of the structures.

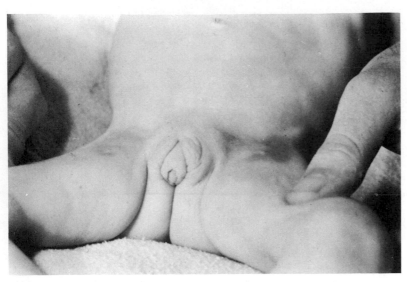

Fig. 11-11. Adrenogenital syndrome. (Dr. R. Platou)

Epispadias. A much less common anomaly is epispadias in which the urethra opens on the dorsal surface of the penis. It likewise is corrected surgically when the defect is pronounced.

Undescended Testis (Cryptorchidism). The testes, which originate within the abdominal cavity, have usually descended into the scrotum by the time the infant is born. Absence of one or both is not necessarily a cause for immediate concern, since late descent often takes place during infancy or early childhood. The management of undescended testis is presented in more detail in Chapter 29.

The Female Genitalia

Malformations of the female genitalia are so infrequent that no extensive discussion is warranted. With anal atresia in the female there may be an abnormal entrance of the rectum into the vagina so that meconium escapes through it. An imperforate hymen may lead to accumulation of secretions with the formation of a mass which is visible bulging out between the labia. Simple incision permits discharge of the retained contents.

Pseudohermaphroditism. When structural abnormalities of the genitalia of the newborn are discovered, prompt study is indicated. Many varieties of genital configuration intermediate between the male and the female may occur. One of the most common aberrations—the adrenogenital syndrome—is due to the masculinizing effect of cortical adrenal hormones on the developing female genitalia, resulting in enlargement of the clitoris and sometimes in sequestration of the vaginal opening. A congenital hereditary deficiency of enzymes necessary for the proper fabrication of hydrocortisone (or other hormones) in the adrenal gland results in excessive stimulation of the gland by the pituitary. Instead of producing the desired steroid hormones the adrenal responds by overproduction of androgenic hormones. The infant suffers

from masculinization (virilization) so that female genitalia deviate toward the male type, while the male infant may soon show precocious sexual development. Later in life growth is stimulated, and the maturation of the skeleton is accelerated. The excessive production of virilizing substances can be confirmed by measuring the rate of excretion of 17-ketosteroids in the urine. Abnormal urinary steroids may also be present. If the enzymatic defect is severe, it interferes not only with the production of hydrocortisone but also with the production of adrenal steroids which regulate the metabolism of certain electrolytes. In the latter form low levels of sodium and chloride, associated with high levels of potassium, are found in the blood. Treatment with cortisone can be expected to correct the excessive excretion of androgens and prevent the abnormal masculinization which otherwise would occur early in childhood. If electrolyte disturbance is also present, desoxycorticosterone and salt are usually indicated. Dosage is regulated by periodic determination of urinary 17-hydroxy-ketosteroid levels and of blood electrolytes.

Not all abnormalities of the genitalia are associated with the "adrenogenital syndrome" described above. However, it is equally important to attempt to arrive rapidly at a decision concerning the infant's proper sex through hormonal and anatomic studies, for it is psychologically very disturbing to both child and parents when uncertainty exists or when attempts are made to shift the child's way of life from one sex to the other after the period of infancy.

RESPIRATORY TRACT

Congenital Laryngeal Stridor

Congenital laryngeal stridor is a noise produced on inspiration because of obstruction to air flow. It can be due to any of several laryngeal conditions, all of which are the result of immaturity of the larynx or persistence of fetal characteristics. The larynx may be

Fig. 11-12. Myelomeningocele. (Dr. R. Platou)

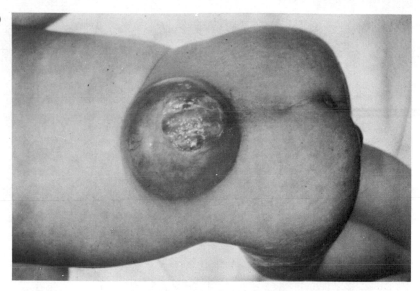

soft and collapsible, large tissue folds may be present between the larynx and the epiglottis, the epiglottis may be soft and flaccid. In any of these conditions the parts are brought together on inspiration to cause obstruction and noise; they are pushed apart on expiration, and no symptoms are present. During inspiration the soft parts of the chest also are pulled in.

The noisy breathing appears in the first few days after birth and persists from 1 to 2 years, by which time the larynx has grown and matured sufficiently to permit normal breathing. The stridor is worse during periods of crying and excitement. At such times cyanosis is likely to appear. During quiescent periods no cyanosis is present, and the baby appears to be in no distress. Rarely, if at all, is congenital stridor dangerous to life, though there are occasions when the appearance and behavior of the baby are alarming to the parents. By means of laryngoscopy the diagnosis can be confirmed, and a more serious abnormality excluded. No treatment is indicated.

THE SKIN

Disorders of the skin that have a congenital or hereditary basis are numerous and diverse in characteristics. In Chapter 7 some of the more common aberrations seen in the newborn infant are described, and the significance to the child is indicated. Individual variations in the pigmentation, the texture, the reactivity to stimuli and the degree of oiliness of the skin are so great as to defy comprehensive description. The more serious congenital disturbances are too rare to warrant inclusion in a short text, and the reader should consult one of the treatises on dermatology for a full description and illustrations.

CARDIOVASCULAR SYSTEM

Congenital malformations of the heart are considered in Chapter 22. Some of the functionally more severe malformations produce symptoms during the newborn period and demand prompt diagnostic study and, in some instances, early surgical correction (e.g., severe coarctation of the aorta, transposition of the great vessels, large patency of the ductus arteriosus). Clinical manifestations which may lead to the recognition of severe malformations in the newborn are cyanosis and dyspnea which is not attributable to pulmonary disorder, tachycardia, weak peripheral pulses, enlarging liver. Cardiac failure is seldom accompanied by edema in the newborn.

CENTRAL NERVOUS SYSTEM

Spina Bifida

Spina bifida is a malformation of the spine in which the posterior portion of the bony canal containing the spinal cord is completely or partially lacking because of failure of the vertebral laminae to develop or to fuse. Some degree of this defect is relatively common, especially in the lumbar region. When it exists without associated changes in the cord or the meninges, it is known as spina bifida occulta and, being symptomless, it is not discovered unless sought by x-ray examination.

A more serious condition is a protrusion of the cord and its membranes (myelomeningocele) or the cord membranes alone (meningocele) through the defect to form an external cystic tumor, which is present at birth. The tumor is rounded, fluctuating, more or less compressible, and contains cerebrospinal fluid. It is commonly about the size of half of a small orange and most frequently is located in the lumbar or sacral region. The wall of a meningocele is made up of spinal membranes and skin. In a myelomeningocele a portion of the spinal cord is spread out and embedded in the cyst wall. Commonly, the condition is associated with increased pressure of the cerebrospinal

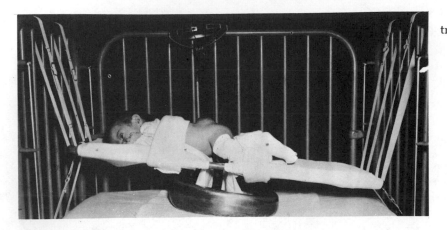

Fig. 11-13. A baby with spina bifida, illustrating also a method of care on a frame.

fluid, so that the tumor tends to increase in size, the wall becoming thinner. With continued enlargement the tumor may rupture spontaneously, or more commonly it is the seat of ulcerations, often perforating, consequent on the poor blood supply. Rupture or ulcerative perforation usually leads to meningitis. Spina bifida with meningocele causes no symptoms. If the cord is included in the cyst wall, urinary and fecal incontinence and paralysis of the legs are likely to result.

Prognosis. When the sac contains no nerve elements (simple meningocele) surgical removal with reinforcement of the tissues over the defect may provide a complete recovery. In some instances, however, the removal of the sac is followed by the development of a communicating hydrocephalus which must be treated by shunting procedures (see Chap. 13). Surgical correction of myelomeningocele in which nervous elements are involved in the tumor not only carries the risk of postoperative hydrocephalus but there may also be rectal or bladder paralysis with spasticity and deformity of the legs. Even without operation hydrocephalus may develop.

Treatment. Surgical excision of meningoceles and myelomeningoceles is usually performed soon after birth if the sac is unruptured and the infant does not have meningitis. Even when the ultimate prognosis for a good functional result is poor, nursing care of the infant can be greatly simplified by making a closure of the posterior lesion. At a later date the problems associated with bladder paralysis must be considered.

Nursing Care. When the covering over the tumor is very thin, the surface must be kept clean and protected from pressure. In the period preceding operation, nursing measures to prevent or clear infection must be carried out. Placement on an infant Bradford frame facilitates care, exposes the tumor and prevents pressure on it. To keep the infant in position over the frame opening, ankle and chest restraint is necessary. Diapers folded as cravats can be placed around the chest and also around one ankle, under the frame and

over the other ankle. To prevent deformity, a small pillow made of abdominal pads should be placed under the lower portion of the legs to keep toes and feet from pressing into the hard surface of the frame.

When the spinal cord is included in the tumor wall, urine and feces are excreted constantly. Therefore, care to prevent excoriations around the perineum becomes necessary. Folded diapers under abdomen and the legs, over the edge and into a receptacle beneath the frame opening protect the frame covers and permit easy change to keep the infant dry. Cleansing the perineum and the groins with oil each time the diapers are changed will keep the skin in good condition.

When an infant is kept in this position for long periods of time, attention to the skin of face and knees becomes imperative if excoriation is to be prevented. If paralysis of the lower extremities is present, abrasion of the knees does not occur frequently, but if the infant's motor development is normal, frequent knee movement may cause skin irritation. Stockings prevent skin irritation in many instances. Good care of the knees and the skin of the face with applications of zinc-oxide ointment to the tip of the nose, the chin and the cheeks will prevent abrasions.

Various methods to prevent or to clear infection of the tumor mass may be used. Cleanliness with exposure to light may be all that is necessary. Alcohol, antibiotic or petrolatum gauze dressings may be desired. If used, they should be changed frequently enough to keep them sterile and the area free of exudate.

During the preoperative period the infant should be held for feedings. It gives him needed position change and affection and facilitates feeding and bubbling. The infant should be handled gently, for the tumor area is sensitive. The tumor should be covered with a sterile towel, and the infant held in such a way that pressure on the area can be eliminated. Observation as to his weight and his behavior before and after feedings will serve as a guide to his need for food. An optimal nutritional state is neces-

FIG. 11-14. Newborn baby showing the facial characteristics of Down's syndrome. (Potter, E.: Pathology of the Fetus and the Newborn, Chicago, Year Book.)

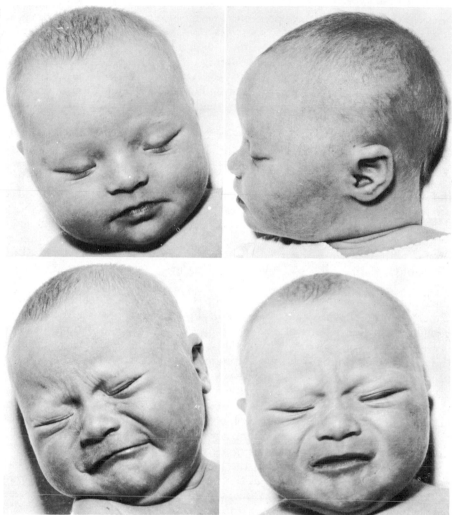

sary before surgical intervention, and more frequent feedings may be necessary to satisfy his needs.

The sac may be excised, or the meninges may be folded in to preserve the absorbing surface of the sac before the skin is closed over them. In either type of operation the principles of postoperative care remain the same. In the period immediately after operation, symptoms of shock should be watched for, and appropriate treatment given if they occur. The dressing must be kept clean and free from feces, and the prone position must be maintained by the same method used in the preoperative period. No covering directly over the infant should be used, as it will become soiled.

If the infant's temperature is subnormal, a light should be placed over the infant, and the bed should be covered with blankets, encasing the child in a heated unit. When the infant's temperature is subnormal and unstable, care in an incubator may be indicated. Temperature of the incubator should be regulated according to the individual needs of the infant.

Nursing measures used preoperatively should be con-

tinued, with the exception of the position used to feed the infant. Until sutures are removed, the baby should be fed on his frame, which is now hung so that his head is from 3 to 5 inches lower than his body. The chest restraint can be loosened, and the infant may be turned slightly to make feeding less difficult for him. The same method should be used to bathe the undersurface of his body.

During the postoperative period, observation as to whether or not the head circumference is increasing guides the physician and the nurse in the type of advice that the parents will need on the baby's discharge from the hospital. Many times, operation is performed in the neonatal period. Therefore, the mother will require help in understanding the total needs of her child. The infant has been born with an anomaly: the development of wholesome attitudes toward it can be influenced by the nurse.

Down's Syndrome (Mongolism)

One group of mentally defective children usually can be recognized at birth by virtue of the associated physical defects which they present. The facial characteristics simulate those of persons of Oriental races, hence the name. The face is round, with close-set eyes which slant upward at their lateral extremities. Epicanthus is usually present. The head is small in circumference and grows at an abnormally slow rate. It is flattened in the anteroposterior diameter. Posteriorly, the infant has a flat occiput with a broad and pudgy neck. Anteriorly, the nose is flat, and the cavities of the nasopharynx and mouth are shallow in the anteroposterior diameter. The tongue is often large and constantly protruded. There may be marbling of the irides of the eyes (Brushfield's spots). The muscles are lax, and the joints are loose, so that hyperextension is possible with the assumption of bizarre postures without apparent discomfort. The hands are usually broad, with short and incurved fifth fingers and abnormalities of the creases of the palm. The great toe often is separated from its neighbor by a wider space than normal through which runs a deep skin crease. Other abnormalities may include umbilical hernia and congenital malformations of the heart.

Down's syndrome occurs with greatest frequency in the children of women who are approaching the end of their child-bearing period. Such a child is very often the product of the last pregnancy possible for the mother. In a minority of the cases, the affected child occurs first in the sequence of pregnancies of a young woman. Under these circumstances the subsequent children are almost always normal. Rarely, Down's syndrome may appear in the middle of a succession of pregnancies or twice in the same family.

The most common form of Down's syndrome, i.e., that which occurs in infants born to older women, is usually associated with trisomy of chromosome 21, giving a total number of 47 chromosomes. A smaller number of subjects, particularly those born to younger women, have an abnormality of the 21 chromosome known as translocation. In this instance, the total number of chromosomes is the normal 46, but there has been an interchange of a portion of another chromosome with chromosome 21. In some instances this latter situation increases the hazard to the mother of bearing a subsequent child with the defect.

These children develop slowly. Their ultimate intellectual level is somewhat variable but cannot be expected to exceed that of 7-8 years. When the family is prepared to accept the child's limitations, he can be successfully raised at home with attendance at a special school and ultimately may be able to be employed at jobs which do not require a high degree of intelligence. When the family circumstances are less accepting, such children are often happier in foster homes, institutions or colonies which are specially adapted to their needs. Prognosis for health and longevity is below normal even when cardiac abnormalities are not present, for children with Down's syndrome suffer more severely from the common infections of childhood and even in later life have a shorter life expectancy.

Trisomy 18

Less common than Down's syndrome is a constellation of abnormalities associated with nondisjunction of a chromosome in Group E (16-18). These infants are usually born to parents over the age of 30 and are of low birth weight for their gestational age. Low-set abnormal ears, micrognathia, flexion contractures and overlapping of fingers, congenital heart defects and rocker bottom feet may be present in varying combinations. The infants are usually mentally retarded and have a poor prognosis for life even when the abnormalities are corrected.

Trisomy 13-15

Fortunately even rarer in occurrence is trisomy of a D-group chromosome which shares some of the clinical features of trisomy 18 but in addition generally includes abnormalities of the forebrain, nose, eyes (microphthalmia) or face (harelip, cleft palate). Prognosis for survival is very poor since most of these infants die before reaching 1 year of age.

The Congenital Rubella Syndrome

Mothers who become infected with rubella (German measles) virus during the first 12 weeks of pregnancy may transmit it to their developing infants with unfortunate consequences. Intrauterine infection of the infant may result in perversion of the development of organ systems to produce one or more of the following defects: microcephaly, microphthalmos, cataracts, deafness, congenital cardiac defects, congenital purpura and hemolytic anemia, mental retardation and failure to thrive. Some of these infants may continue to be infected with the virus and serve as a hazard

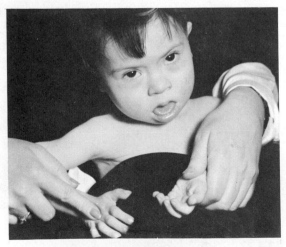

FIG. 11-15. A 2-year-old infant showing the facial characteristics of Down's syndrome which are now defined more clearly than in the newborn.

to their caretakers. The management of such infants will depend upon the particular variety of abnormalities which is discovered.

Amyotonia Congenita

Two forms of this disorder are recognized; both may be observed in the same family. The outstanding feature is generalized weakness of muscles without loss of intelligence. In the congenital form (Oppenheim), weakness is present from birth and prevents the child from learning to hold up his head, to sit or to make any forceful voluntary movements. Because of his difficulty in coughing and clearing his respiratory passages he eventually succumbs to aspiration pneumonia, usually within the first two years of life. Nursing care can prolong life by attention to his accumulating pharyngeal secretions, but any illness is likely to be fatal. In the acquired (Werdnig-Hoffman) type of the disorder, early development for most of the first year may be normal but is followed by progressive weakness which terminates fatally for the same reasons. Whether or not there is a real distinction between these two disorders is debated.

Phenylketonuria (PKU, Phenylpyruvic Oligophrenia)

Although the symptoms of PKU are not apparent during the newborn period, the fact that early diagnosis and treatment can prevent some of the mental deficiency which would otherwise be expected, has led to routine testing of infants (legally demanded in some states) before discharge from the nursery. The disorder, which occurs about once in 10,000 births, is a recessively transmitted inborn error of metabolism. The lack of an enzyme (phenylalanine hydroxylase) prevents the proper metabolism of phenylalanine which is one of the common amino acids in proteins. This substance accumulates in the blood of affected infants who have had a day or two of full milk feedings. Routine determinations of the phenylalanine blood level will then identify infants with abnormally high levels who must be further investigated for PKU. The mental deficiency—usually severe—which appears later in infancy may be wholly or partially prevented if the child is placed on a diet in which the intake of phenylalanine is restricted. Unfortunately, the diet is expensive, not very palatable and must be carefully monitored by expert laboratory control.

Untreated, most infants with the genetic defect will show signs of mental retardation before the age of 2 years. Convulsions and eczema are common. Most subjects are blonde and blue-eyed because the metabolic defect also interferes with the normal development of pigment. After the newborn period, the untreated infant excretes in his urine the products of incomplete metabolism of phenylalanine where they may be recognized by diagnostic testing with ferric chloride or the impregnated paper, Phenistix. Unless the abnormality is suspected before 6 months, irreparable damage may have occurred. Diet therapy is probably useless after the age of 2 years.

ORGANS OF SPECIAL SENSE

The Eyes

Retrolental Fibroplasia. This disorder of prematures was the most common cause of blindness among infants. It is actually a postnatal disorder resulting from the toxic effect of oxygen rather than an anomaly and is discussed in Chapter 9.

Glaucoma. Glaucoma may occur in the newborn because of a congenital structural defect in the eye which prevents proper absorption of the aqueous humor. The eye becomes tense and enlarged and, if the condition is not relieved surgically, vision may decrease slowly. The condition should be suspected when the eye of the newborn, particularly the cornea, appears to be too large.

The Ears

Minor variations in the formation of the external ear are very common among newborn infants. These usually consist of supernumerary projections of skin with or without cartilage beneath, projections which are easily removed surgically when they are large enough to be unsightly. Less common is an anomaly in which the external auditory meatus fails to canalize and the underlying bony portion of the ear is imperfectly developed. When this anomaly is unilateral it presents mainly a cosmetic problem, since hearing will be adequate from the other, normal ear. However, if the defect is bilateral, the infant will have defective hearing, and measures will have to be instituted to perform a plastic repair and establish a connection with the bony internal ear if function is present.

MUSCULOSKELETAL SYSTEM

Generalized disorders of bone which later will result in dwarfed stature and other deformities are seldom apparent at birth. In *achondroplasia* a generalized defect is present which interferes with growth in length of the long bones and the trunk. Such newborns can be recognized by the unusual shortness of the upper segments of their arms and legs and by a characteristically squared shape of the skull. *Cleidocranial dysostosis* is a combination of faulty growth in the membranous bones of the skull and a partial or complete absence of the clavicles. The latter defect permits the infant to bring the tips of the shoulders together anteriorly. There is also an unusually large anterior fontanel. Both of these disorders limit the final size of the child, achondroplasia markedly and cleidocranial dysostosis only moderately. There is no particular association with mental deficiency.

Osteogenesis imperfecta is a rare disorder in which the bones are unusually brittle so that normal intra-

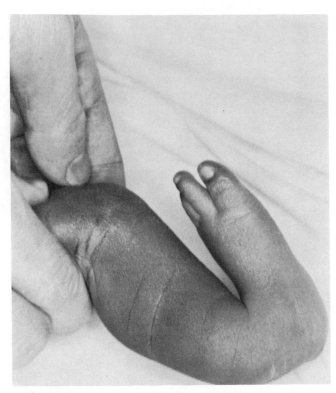

FIG. 11-16. Club foot resulting from severe distortion of the developing extremity during intrauterine growth.

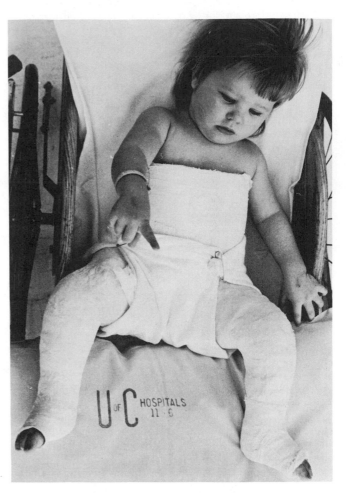

FIG. 11-17. Child in double hip spica cast for correction of congenital dislocation of the hips.

uterine or postnatal pressures produce fractures of extremities or ribs. Although these fractures heal rapidly, they are sometimes so numerous and accompanied by so much displacement of the fragments that the child is seriously malformed and stunted in growth if he survives.

Polydactyly

Well formed extra fingers and toes are not very common. They require no treatment. Rudimentary sixth fingers attached to the fifth finger by a narrow isthmus of skin (postminimi) are not at all uncommon, particularly among Negroes where they may appear as a dominantly transmitted familial trait. They are easily removed by ligature of the skin isthmus.

Intrauterine Positional Deformities

In a preceding chapter the common consequences of intrauterine pressure have been noted which tend to correct themselves spontaneously once the external pressure has been removed following birth. Occasionally the consequences of intrauterine displacement are more severe and require more active correction.

Clubfoot or *talipes equinovarus* is an extension and inversion of the foot severe enough to displace tarsal bones so that the foot cannot be passively restored to

normal position. It may occur alone or in association with other anomalies of the spine or central nervous system, or when there has been a deficiency of amniotic fluid during pregnancy. Soon after birth the feet are manipulated into correcting position and held there by the application of plaster boots. In severe cases several changes of cast may be necessary to complete the correction.

Congenital dislocation of the hip should be looked for at birth although the findings may not be immediately apparent. The disorder is betrayed by an asymmetry of the buttocks and thigh creases of the newborn with lifting of the leg on the affected side. The infant's hip on the dislocated side will not abduct completely or may do so with an audible click if forced. X-rays of the pelvis will reveal lateral displacement of the upper end of the femur and poor development of the acetabulum on that side. Treatment consists in maintaining abduction of the hips during the early months of life, usually by the application of a cast or insertion of a bar apparatus to keep the knees apart. The disorder is much more common in female infants than in males. Full correction depends upon early discovery and treatment.

Torticollis is an abnormal shortening of the sternomastoid muscle which causes the infant or child to keep the head cocked to one side and prevents full rotation of the chin toward each shoulder. In most instances the dysfunction is temporary, due either to muscle shortening from intrauterine position or to trauma of the sternomastoid muscle following a breech delivery with pulling upon the shoulder. Such torticollis clears spontaneously as the infant grows. In a few instances there will be shortening of the muscle because it is replaced by a fibrous band. Deformity will then persist until operative measures are undertaken to lengthen the fibrous cord.

THE ROLE OF THE NURSE IN GENETIC COUNSELING

The tremendous increase in knowledge related to the transmission of genetic characteristics and the improvement in technics of investigation have important consequences and implications for the nurse who is a part of the team dealing with parents of children with inborn errors of structure or metabolism. Since the general population is becoming ever more knowledgeable regarding genetic transmission, nurses of today can expect to be questioned by patients, their families and friends regarding inheritable characteristics. These questions are often of great concern to parents and the information given may direct their course of action. In other instances, the early diagnosis and treatment of inheritable disease may be crucial to the welfare of the family and their plans for the future. The nurse in the hospital and in the community has a vital role in case finding and in anticipatory guidance.

The actual process of advising parents regarding the possibilities of transmitting defective genes to their children is the responsibility of the physician or geneticist. However, the nurse may be called upon to assist in gathering information from which to prepare a family pedigree or statistical graphs and charts. It is often the nurse who assists in clarifying the information given by the geneticist, corrects misinterpretations and deals with the family's feelings about their problems. The revelation of a defective gene pattern is often emotionally upsetting to parents and may activate deep feelings of parental inadequacy, a sense of guilt and great concern related to future pregnancies.

The nurse is also often responsible for interpreting the function of the clinic to parents, for coordination of appointments, for collection of specimens and for reinforcing the information given by the geneticist. She is important in follow-up contacts with the family and in acting as a continuing liaison between the clinic and the family.

In order to enrich her care of patients and their families, the nurse should have knowledge of genetic theory and principles and acquire understanding of the methods utilized in studying genetic transmission. She must also acquire skill in counseling technics so that she can be in a better position to direct families with genetic disabilities to available resources. Through knowledge of the meaning which inheritable disease may hold for parents, she will enhance her therapeutic effectiveness by the understanding and empathy which she can extend to them.

EARLY PLANS FOR THE CHILD WITH A HANDICAP

When a congenital defect is discovered in a newborn infant the physician in charge has the unpleasant responsibility of relating the news to the parents. Parental response is greatly influenced by their previous life experiences and by the manner in which personnel of the helping professions respond to them and to the distressing event.

Parents of children born with malformations are faced with painful, anxiety provoking problems which they must resolve constructively before they can achieve the emotional equilibrium which is of importance in their own lives and in the lives of their children. Most parents feel physical and psychic shock when first confronted with such news, for all parents hope for a perfect child. Many parents also report initial feelings of inadequacy, shame, guilt, disappointment, anger, grief and confusion. Feelings of confusion often stem from a lack of understanding of the genesis and nature of the disability and of its treatment.

Too often the natural tendency to delay notification or to conceal the extent of the defect in order to protect parents has unfortunate long range consequences. During the anxious period of waiting, the mother's fears and fantasies may be far worse than the reality of the situation. Delay also creates an aura of mystery about the defect and either confirms the parents' guilty suspicions that they are somehow responsible for the outcome or points an unjustifiably accusing finger at the obstetrician who delivered the infant. Discussion of the infant's disability at the earliest possible time with both parents in a straightforward manner maintains trust in both physician and nurse which can have important consequences for long range treatment plans. The support and professional advice which they will require are better accepted from a person who has been completely honest with them from the start than from one who has practiced deception, however well-meant.

The nurse has many opportunities to help shape the attitudes of parents toward their defective children. She can be of great assistance during the period of initial shock by remaining with parents, by listening and accepting the released feelings without probing and when indicated, by respecting the need for solitude. After the discussion by the physician, she can clarify and reinforce with direct and accurate information that which may have been unheard or misinterpreted during severe stress.

Since the parents provide the environment in which the child will develop, their feelings about him are crucial to his adjustment.

Guilt feelings must be dispelled not only for the parents' comfort but also to prevent them from rearing the child in a too compassionate or too permissive way which fails to develop his character assets and leaves him poorly prepared to compete in the outer world. Excessive parental guilt may also have a devastating effect on her normal children if the mother does penance by devoting herself exclusively to the abnormal offspring.

The attitude which parents adopt toward the handicapped child will also influence his acceptance by friends, relatives and other members of the community. Frank acceptance of the defect as a misfortune which requires him to modify his way of life but does not necessarily bar him from all constructive and satisfying pursuits is a healthy entrée into the life of the community and the school. Details concerning the nurse's functions in relation to the handicapped child and his parents are discussed in Chapter 29.

Mary was born with an abnormal, fingerless hand which her parents were able to accept in a healthy fashion. No attempt was made to conceal the deformity. Relatives, friends and neighbors soon satisfied their curiosity about the *hand* and accepted the *child* as the attractive person she was. When Mary entered nursery school she held out her hand for all to see, explaining that this was the way she was born. After due inspection the children's curiosity was appeased, and she promptly became a "normal" member of the group.

Chronic handicaps frequently require special facilities for prolonged medical care and training. Most states recognize the excessive financial drain which this imposes on the average family and provide free clinics and hospital care through a division of services to crippled or handicapped children. Other community organizations provide similar or supplementary services. States also provide institutions for the permanent placement of those children whose handicaps are too severe to permit their continued care at home. The nurse should familiarize herself with the resources of her local community and learn the methods by which referral to them can be made.

SITUATIONS FOR FURTHER STUDY

1. During the course of caring for a baby with a congenital anomaly, observe his parents and report your findings and reactions to the experience. Read pages 87 to 105 in Blake: *The Child, His Parents and the Nurse* as a basis for thinking through your experience with the parents of your patient. Discuss the section you read in terms of your own feelings while reading it and in relation to what you observed. Describe the ways you think your patient's parents are handling their disappointment. What help were you able to give them?

2. If you had cared for a 1 to 4-week-old infant with a cleft lip and palate during the period after repair of the lip, what would you include in preparing the mother for his care at home? What observations would you want to make before you began to teach her how to feed her baby?

3. In feeding a newborn baby, what observations would lead you to believe that the baby had an atresia of the esophagus?

4. If atresia of the esophagus was suspected, what position would you keep the infant in and why?

5. What elements of postoperative nursing care are of primary significance in the care of an infant with atresia of the esophagus?

BIBLIOGRAPHY

Atkinson, H. C.: Care of the child with cleft lip and palate, Am. J. Nurs. 67:1889, 1967.

Blake, F. G.: The Child, His Parents and the Nurse, p. 87, Philadelphia, Lippincott, 1954.

Bonine, G. N.: The myelodyplastic child: hospital and home care, Am. J. Nurs. 69:541, 1969.

Brantl, V., and Esslinger, P.: Genetics—implications for the nursing curriculum, Nursing Forum 1:90, 1962.

Bright, F.: The pediatric nurse and parental anxiety, Nursing Forum 4:30, 1965.

Brodie, B., and Von Haam, J.: Children born with adrenogenital syndrome, Am. J. Nurs. 67:1018, 1967.

Campbell, M.: Principles of Urology, Philadelphia, Saunders, 1957.

Emergency Surgery of the Newborn, Clin. Symposia, Vol. II, No. 2, 1959.

Forbes, N. P.: The nurse and genetic counseling, Nurs. Clin. North America 1:679, 1966.

Ford, F. R.: Diseases of the Nervous System in Infancy and Childhood, ed. 5, Springfield, Ill., Thomas, 1966.

Gross, R. E.: Surgery of Infancy and Childhood, Philadelphia, Saunders, 1964.

Kallmans, J.: The child with cleft lip and palate (the mother in the maternity unit), Am. J. Nurs. 65:120, 1965.

Keogh, B., and Legeay, C.: Recoil from the diagnosis of mental retardation, Am. J. Nurs. 66:778, 1966.

Kuszaj, J., and Wirch, B.: Nursing care of the patient with cleft lip and palate, Nurs. Clin. North America 2:483, 1967.

Lis, E. F.: The Child with Cleft Lip and Palate *in* Michal-Smith, H.: Management of the Handicapped Child, p. 147, New York, Grune, 1957.

Martin, L. W., Gilmore, A., Peckham, J., and Baumer, J.: Nursing care of infants with esophageal anomalies, Am. J. Nurs. 66:11, 2463, 1966.

————: Care of the infant with exstrophy of the bladder, Nurs. Clin. North America 2:573, 1967.

McDermott, M. M.: The child with cleft lip and palate—on the pediatric ward, Am. J. Nurs. *65*:122, 1965.

Owens, C.: Parents reactions to defective babies, Am. J. Nurs. *64*:83, 1964.

Pidgeon, V.: The infant with congenital heart disease, Am. J. Nurs. *67*:290, 1967.

Potter, E. L.: Pathology of the Fetus and Infant, ed. 2, Chicago, Year Book Pub., 1961.

Ragsdale, N., and Koch, R.: Phenylketonuria, Am. J. Nurs. *64*:90, 1964.

Ripley, I. L.: The child with cleft lip and palate through his years of growth, Am. J. Nurs. *65*:124, 1965.

Roberts, J. A. F.: An Introduction to Medical Genetics, N. Y., Oxford University Press, 1967.

Stein, C.: Principles of Human Genetics (2nd ed.), W. H. Freeman and Co., San Francisco, 1960.

Valsomis, N. W., and Valsomis, M. P.: The child with Tay-Sachs disease, Am. J. Nurs. *63*:9497, 1963.

Von Schilling, K. C.: The birth of a defective child, Nurs. Forum *7*:424, 1968.

UNIT 3

The Infant (1 Month to 1 Year)

The first year of life is characterized by very rapid change. Growth will never again be so dramatic; the initial weight is trebled, and the height is increased by 50 per cent. Relatively large quantities of food are required to support such growth so that intakes that are a third or even half the caloric value of the mother's diet may be seen. Vitamins are more essential than at any other period of life. Athletic prowess moves from the stage of helpless waving to early self-feeding and a start at locomotion. Even more fascinat-ing to the parents are the conversion of the infant from an animated mass of protoplasm to an individual whose personality shows responsiveness, humor and inquisitiveness.

The troubles of the first year are largely those of feeding regulation and the effects of previously un-recognized congenital and hereditary disorders. In-fections are relatively scarce because of limited social contacts, but when they do appear, the threat to well-being is usually significant.

12

Growth, Development and Care During the First Year

PHYSICAL GROWTH

The tremendous speed of fetal growth begins to slow down after birth and continues to decelerate until it stops completely when adulthood is reached. Using average weight as an example, this trend can be visualized by remembering that in the last part of pregnancy it takes about two months for the fetus to double his weight; after birth the first doubling requires five months and the second about 25 months. This pace will never be approached in later life.

Even during infancy there are rather wide variations in initial size and speed of postnatal growth. To interpret measurements it is necessary to know not only the average figures for a particular age but to have some standard for the allowable deviation from this average. This information can be obtained from any of several tables which have been compiled. A better view is obtained when the infant's measurements are plotted on a growth chart such as the Iowa forms from which at a glance the relation of his height and weight to the average can be seen. By periodic addition of new plots a graph of his progress is obtained. Since girls grow a little more slowly than boys, a separate chart is provided for each sex. The middle line is the average figure for height or weight at each age. The line above it bounds the 16th percentile and the line below it the 84th percentile. This statement means that infants whose measurements fall above the top line stand with the tallest or the heaviest 16 per cent of their age-mates; those below the bottom line are included among the shortest or the lightest 16 per cent. Thus, 68 per cent (two thirds of all infants) will fall somewhere between the top and bottom lines of the chart. (In statistical terminology the top line is designated as + 1 standard deviation and the bottom line as − 1 standard deviation from the average.)

Height

Changes in height are more difficult to measure accurately and consequently are less popular as an index of growth than are the changes in weight. However, growth in length is a more consistent attribute of the infant and should be taken into account in any interpretation of weight changes. From the growth charts it will be seen that the average infant increases his length by 50 per cent during the first year (from 20 to 30 inches). It will also be seen that two-thirds of the infants stay within about 1 inch of the average. The height curves obtained during this first year are likely to be erratic because of difficulties in making accurate measurements. At later ages this aspect of growth becomes a reliable guide to changes in body size.

Several unusual forms of height progress during the first year still fall within the realm of normal phenomena. Infants born prematurely start well below the normal curves, but many of them will catch up before their first birthdays. Conversely, infants of diabetic mothers may begin with lengths longer than average and then make slow gains until they have found their true positions in the curve, perhaps at average or even below. Some infants, short at birth, are impelled by a strong growth impulse which may speed the height curve from below the bottom line up into the top 16 per cent in less than a year. Such behavior suggests that intrauterine growth was impeded by unknown factors and that with postnatal access to sufficient food the infant's true genetic endowment becomes revealed.

In general the successive height measurements of an infant will gradually produce a curve which runs parallel to the lines on the growth chart. Such a curve may be accepted as an indicator of his inherent body size. Upward shifts of its direction can be accepted with equanimity, but a progressive and persistent downward deflection probably means disease or abnormality which, if not already apparent, demands further investigation.

For the first half-year the baby appears to do most of his growing in the region of his head and trunk. Later his legs begin to stretch out, straightening gradually as they lengthen. But even when he begins to stand at the end of the first year they will seem disproportionately short and are likely to be bowed.

Weight

The rate of weight gain during the first year is rapid in the normal infant. During the early weeks gains approximate an ounce a day in artificially fed infants, somewhat less in breast-fed infants. Of course, this pace must diminish gradually. If it were maintained indefinitely, as mothers sometimes expect, the average child would weigh over 30 pounds by the end of the year and 60 pounds by the end of 2 years. Even with the gradual decline in weight increments most infants

will double their birth weights before 5 months of age and will approximately treble them in a year's time. The initial growth surge is generally accompanied by a good appetite and an obvious accumulation of fat so that many infants become quite chubby. Rather frequently the spurt in growth and its accompanying appetite tapers off between 6 and 9 months of age and a distinct drop in food consumption is noted. From this point on, further accumulation of fat gives way to the construction of larger muscles and bones as the cuddly baby begins to change into the more dynamic toddler.

The weight curves on growth charts are subject to more variation than the height curves. Although the majority will pursue courses within the normal limits depicted, the number of exceptions is greater. The same special circumstances enumerated above for height create similar aberrations in the weight curves. In addition, weight curves respond very rapidly to changes in diet and to disease. Loss of weight or

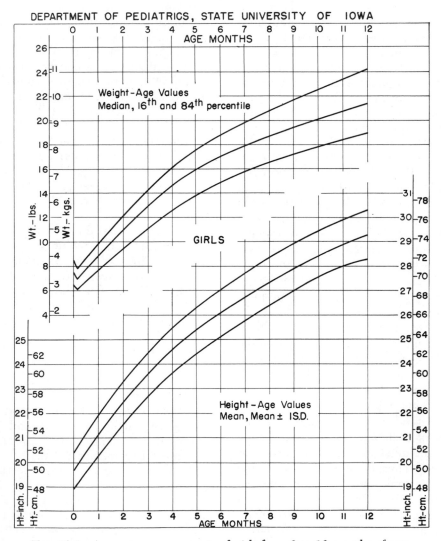

FIG. 12-1. Average measurements of girls from 0 to 12 months of age.

failure to gain is a transient phenomenon in many acute illnesses, recovery from which is accompanied by rapid restoration of the curve to its previous level. Chronic illness is usually reflected in a sharp and persistent downward deflection.

Changes in Body Components During the First Year

As growth (increase in size) and development (increase of functional capacity) of the body as a whole proceeds, the component parts of which it is made do not all advance at the same rate. Details of the changes taking place are too numerous for description here, but some of the more significant relationships will be mentioned.

The Head. Skull growth advances almost as rapidly as total body growth during the first year. It is determined mainly by the rate at which the brain expands. The latter is progressing rapidly toward its final adult size and will be two thirds of the way toward its goal

by the end of the first year, whereas total body weight will be less than one quarter of the ultimate adult figure. The changes in function which accompany brain growth are discussed with neuromuscular and psychosocial development (p. 196).

This rapid expansion of the brain is possible because the newborn infant's skull is fashioned from separate bones which do not unite permanently until brain growth is complete. The cracks between adjacent bones can be palpated at birth and in two areas there is a hiatus large enough to admit a finger tip—the anterior and posterior fontanels. By the age of 2 months the posterior fontanel has usually closed so that it can no longer be felt. The anterior fontanel persists with considerable variation in size among different babies. The smaller fontanels begin to disappear by the time the baby is 9 or 10 months of age; larger ones remain open and palpable until well into the second year. The base of these fontanels is composed of a very tough membrane (the dura mater), so that

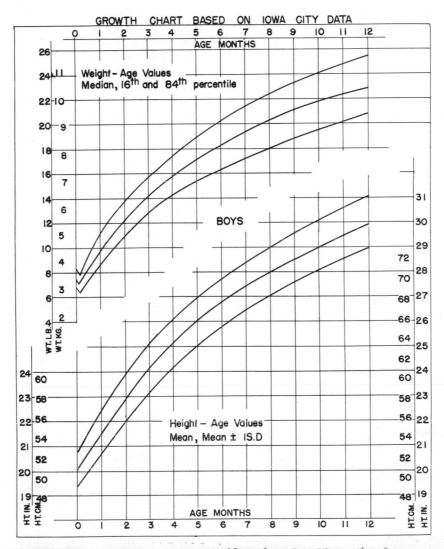

Fig. 12-2. Average measurements of boys from 0 to 12 months of age.

there is no substance to the common fallacy that this area must not be touched for fear of injuring the brain beneath.

The circumference of the head increases from an average of 35 cm. (13¾ in.) at birth to 47 cm. (18 in.) at 1 year. Normal infants infrequently differ by more than 1½ cm. (½ in.) from the average at each age period. Too rapid growth should lead to the suspicion of abnormal expansion of the brain (hydrocephalus) or the intracranial contents (subdural hematoma). Insufficient growth usually means defective development of the brain (microcephaly).

The small infant's bones are relatively soft and pliable so that if he sleeps in one favored position, the dependent region of his skull may become visibly flattened. No harm to the brain results, and the asymmetry produced will gradually be corrected by later growth in the size of the skull after the infant begins to spend a significant portion of his day with head erect.

Occasionally, but rarely, infants are born with teeth. Because of the danger of aspiration if they become loosened, such useless rudiments should be extracted. Normal eruption of teeth seldom begins before 4 to 5 months of age. Almost invariably the two lower central incisors appear first, followed after an interval by the four upper incisors and then the two lower lateral incisors. The time of first eruption is quite variable. A significant number of babies erupt no teeth until toward the end of the first year. Traditionally, teething has been blamed for fever, irritability and digestive disturbances in small infants. Although some infants are undoubtedly made uncomfortable by the process, teething should not be used as a convenient explanation of illness until more significant disease has been ruled out.

At birth the infant's lower jaw is rather markedly recessed so that the maxilla juts out over it. Growth of the two structures is more rapid in the mandible. By the end of the first year many babies have developed prominent chins, and the discrepancy between the biting surfaces of the anterior jaws has decreased.

The Chest. Growth of the chest is also rapid during infancy. The circumference at the nipple line is slightly less than that of the head at birth. It generally catches up at around 5 to 7 months of age and normally exceeds head circumference thereafter. The lungs increase in size more rapidly than the other thoracic contents permitting them to ventilate more efficiently. In consequence there is a slight decrease in the rate of respiration to around 30 per minute. The heart grows in size, but less rapidly than the thorax so that its radiologic appearance at the end of 1 year is smaller than that seen at birth. The pulse rate remains quite labile during infancy and ranges from 80 to 160 per minute depending on extraneous circumstances. Blood pressures are difficult to obtain but are approximately 85/60 mm. Hg.

The Abdomen. No significant development of abdominal muscles takes place during the first year, and the healthy infant continues to be pot-bellied when sitting or standing. The liver grows in proportion to the total body and can still be felt during this first year. In a certain fraction of infants who have no abnormality the tip of the spleen is also felt. Kidney function, which is reduced at birth, improves during the year and approaches adult performance by the first birthday. The external genitalia retain their infantile appearance. Because of the loss of stimulation by maternal hormones they may actually appear less prominent than at birth.

Osseous Development. The changes in height which have been noted are reflections of the growth of the long bones and the spine. In addition to its increase in size, the skeletal system is also maturing. During growth all the bones are first formed in cartilage which gradually changes into bone. Before birth the central portion of all the larger bones has already undergone this transition, but the ends of major bones and the smaller bones such as the carpal and the tarsal bones are still cartilaginous. As the body grows, the appearance of new centers of ossification and the enlargement and extension of others can be followed by taking roentgenograms of various portions of the skeleton. Bone is visible on a roentgen film; cartilage is not. The pattern of appearance is sufficiently regular to make it possible for the radiologist to use standard charts and state the "bone age" of a given child. If this matches the chronologic age, the skeleton is maturing at the expected rate. Significant variations from normal are found with certain diseases such as cretinism and the adrenogenital syndrome.

During the first year the number of ossified tarsal bones increases from 2 to 4 and the number of carpal bones from 0 to 2. Changes take place in the ossification of other bones, but these are the ones most generally used to assess bone age.

Skin and Hair. The skin gradually loses its propensity to peel and secretes more lubricating sebum as the baby passes through his first year. The skin acquires some toughness, but in many infants it continues to react easily to topical irritants. The sweat glands, which are dormant at birth, begin to secrete after the first or second month and assist the infant in regulating his body temperature when the external environment is too hot. During the second half year many infants acquire a yellow sheen due to excess carotene circulating in the blood. This is a normal phenomenon for the age and is distinguished from jaundice by the absence of scleral pigmentation.

Many babies are born with areas of fine down on the skin; this is the persistence of the lanugo hair of fetal life. It usually is shed during the first year. The hair on the head is replaced by a new growth. Marked differences among individual infants are seen in the manner and speed of shedding. One common pattern is loss of the top hair and the persistence of a peripheral ring of long locks, giving the infant a certain resemblance to a tonsured friar. New hair appears as a uniform downy growth beneath. By the end of the first year mothers should be preparing themselves psychologically for the first haircut if the child is a boy.

The Blood. During the first year of life there are pronounced shifts in the quantities of the cellular elements which circulate in the peripheral blood. In order to interpret properly the results of blood counts made on patients, the nurse must be aware of the expected normal changes. The high levels of red cells and hemoglobin of the newborn infant decline rapidly during the early weeks until they reach a low point at about 4 months of age and then rise slowly, reaching the usual adult levels only late in childhood. White blood cell counts are high during the early weeks, and although average total counts decline toward adult levels at the end of the first year, considerable lability remains so that elevation of the leukocytes in an infant must be interpreted with caution. The differential blood count, which enumerates the various types of white cells, normally shows a heavy preponderance of lymphocytes and monocytes during infancy. Eosinophils may also be found with somewhat greater frequency than in the older individual. The platelets change little in quantity. A summary of these values is given in Table 11.

Table 11. Normal Blood Values During the First Year

	Birth	12 wks.	6 mos.	1 yr.
Red Cells (millions/cu.mm.)	4.5–5.5	3.5–4.5	4.0–4.5	4.3–4.7
Hemoglobin (gm./100 ml.)	15.5–18.5	10–12	11–13	12–13.5
White Cells (average/cu.mm.)	20,000	12,000	12,000	11,000
Platelets (average/cu.mm.)	350,000	300,000	300,000	300,000

The Lymphatic System. In early infancy the lymphatic glands are small and difficult to see or feel In response to infection of the local area which they drain, rapid increase in size may bring them into prominence as they form antibodies in defense of the local tissues. By the age of 1 year many infants have acquired general or localized hypertrophy of lymph glands. Once enlarged the nodes do not shrink to their original size even though the infection has been controlled. The tonsils, which are really specialized lymph nodes, are likewise small at birth and very difficult to see. As respiratory infections occur they enlarge progressively. The adenoids are not visible but follow a similar course of hypertrophy in response to nasal infection.

NUTRITIONAL REQUIREMENTS OF INFANCY

General Considerations

In Chapter 8 the practical aspects of early nutrition were considered without much attention to the underlying reasons. In this section the theory of nutrition will be discussed, and some of the penalties which ensue after neglect of its principles will be outlined. Many of the remarks are applicable to all ages, but they have particular importance for the infant whose rapid growth and skimpy stores make him especially vulnerable to nutritional disease. The disorders which arise from insufficient supply of each type of nutriment are included in this section.

The human body requires a continuing supply of oxygen, water and food to support its vital functions.

Oxygen is the most critical of these imports, for the body has no reserve on which to draw. During health the supply is monitored by reflex control of respiration which operates automatically no matter what the state of consciousness. If the intake is interrupted for more than a few minutes, the oxidative chemical reactions which drive the body machinery come to a halt, and life ebbs rapidly. Hence disease or accident which threatens the oxygen supply is an immediate medical emergency.

Deprivation of fluid can be tolerated for a few days while the body draws on its reserves. But the continuance of water loss from skin and lungs and through the urine and stools eventually concentrates the body fluids and seriously impedes its vital chemical reactions. Thirst assures an adequate water intake when the accessible supply is unlimited and when losses from the body are not excessive.

During complete starvation the body may survive for two or three weeks or even longer by consuming its normal nutrient reserves and its own tissues. In health and with a plentiful supply, hunger forces a sufficient quantitative intake of food and to some degree guides the selection of types of food. Unlike oxygen and water, which are simple chemical substances and subserve straightforward functions within the body, food is a broad category enclosing a very wide variety of substances needed by the body as fuel to provide energy, and as building blocks to repair old tissues and to fabricate the new ones required by growth.

The science of nutrition is concerned with determining the amounts of the various food components —protein, carbohydrate, fat, vitamins and minerals— which are required not merely to support life but also to provide the best opportunity for growth and the maintenance of health. For many of the dietary constituents *minimum* levels of intake have been determined with some accuracy. It is usually more difficult to fix *optimum* levels; consequently, authorities are not always in agreement when recommending goals in dietary construction. To supplement knowledge of requirements, the nutritionist must be skilled in making foods attractive and acceptable.

Water

Approximately 70 per cent of the body weight is water. It is the basic constituent of the cells in which the important chemical reactions take place, of the interstitial fluid which lies between the cells, of the transport fluids such as blood, lymph and spinal fluid, and of the various excretions from the body—sweat, urine, bile and intestinal juices. Under usual conditions of climate and physical activity an adult gets along with about a quart of fluid per day. But a small infant, only one twentieth of the adult's weight, will need one third as much. The reason lies in the greater speed of the infant's metabolism. Consequently, his fluid requirements parallel his heat production or oxygen consumption which are considered in the next section.

The older child can be expected to cover his modest water needs (30 to 50 ml./Kg./day) by satisfying his thirst. He obtains fluid not only from the liquid components of his diet but also from the significant water content of many foods which we commonly regard as "solid." Technics for assuring an adequate fluid intake during illness are considered in Chapter 4.

In infancy the rate of water turnover within the body is much more rapid; from 100 to 150 ml./Kg. of weight must be ingested each day in order to keep pace with normal fluid losses. Both the natural and the artificial sources of food for the infant are very dilute liquids so that his water needs are usually satisfied if he is being fed properly. But since the infant is unable to go after water when he becomes thirsty, closer supervision of his intake is essential. An uncertain breast milk supply, hot weather, fever, or losses in the stool or by vomiting can lead to dehydration much more rapidly than in the adult or even in the older child. In practice it is usually sufficient to offer water once or twice a day during health and to permit the infant's thirst to decide whether or not he is in arrears. The effects and treatment of severe water deprivation (dehydration) are discussed under Diarrhea in Chapter 14.

Energy

Like any machine the body must have a source of energy in order to perform its work. Food serves two purposes: (1) it provides fuel which is burned in the body, consuming oxygen in the process and liberating energy and heat, and (2) it provides chemical substances needed in the construction of new tissues. Both purposes must be considered in determining requirements or in planning or evaluating diets. In practice it is simplest to begin by considering the total amount of fuel or energy needed per day. Then the proportion of different types of fuel (protein, carbohydrate and fat) within the total amount is determined.

Finally, a check is made to be sure that the necessary vitamins and minerals are included.

The energy content of foods is rated in calories; i.e., the amount of heat they will produce when burned in the body. A large calorie (the unit employed in metabolic work) is defined as the amount of heat necessary to raise 1 liter of water by 1° C. By experimental methods it can be shown that carbohydrates and proteins when burned in the body yield on the average about 4 calories per gram; whereas fat provides about 9 calories per gram.

The speed at which the body uses energy is called the metabolic rate. It can be determined directly by measuring the amount of heat given off from the body. If 1,500 calories are given off per day, an equivalent amount of fuel will have to be ingested as food in order to provide this amount of energy. In clinical practice it is less cumbersome to measure the amount of oxygen used in the combustion, a figure which necessarily parallels exactly the rate of heat production. This can be done by determining the amount of oxygen extracted from the air which goes into and out of the lungs during a standard period of time. Metabolic measurements of this kind are made under standardized conditions called the *basal state*. Ideally, this is a state of minimum body work in which the subject should be in good health, rested, relaxed, not digesting food and performing no unnecessary muscular work. Such conditions are obviously difficult to obtain when working with infants or small children, but a number of patient investigators have been able to determine fairly accurately the basal requirements of children and even of premature infants.

Basal energy requirements are proportionately high during the early months of life (55 to 60 calories/Kg. of body weight per day) and taper off gradually to approximately half this level at maturity. In addition to this fuel which is required for the minimum housekeeping activities of the body, energy is needed for muscular contraction, for growth, for the work of digesting food (specific dynamic activity) and to cover an inevitable loss in the stools. Individual infants and children vary considerably both in the speed at which they grow and in the amount of physical activity they perform. Consequently, it is difficult to make precise predictions of the total amount of fuel that a given child will require. Few infants will remain satisfied and grow on less than 80 calories/Kg./day; most of them require from 100 to 120; and a few rapidly growing or very active babies may burn up 150 or more.

General Malnutrition—Starvation. When an inadequate intake of calories is continued for any length of time, malnutrition appears. In its more extreme forms this condition of infant starvation is known as marasmus, atrophy, or athrepsia. It may arise because of poverty, insufficient food supply, or ignorance of food requirements, or in association with disease in which there is vomiting, diarrhea, prolonged therapeutic underfeeding or an abnormality of absorption. In areas where there is careful supervision of infant health, malnutrition is disappearing rapidly. But in many parts of the world it remains a serious problem, being due to factors of ignorance, neglect and poverty.

When sufficient energy is not forthcoming from the ingested food, the infant begins to use up the substance of his own body. His fat depots in the skin and subcutaneous tissues go first, leaving his skin loose and paper thin. When the fat of the buttocks is used up, the skin in this area sags like a pair of trousers that are too large. The sucking pads in the cheeks are the last depot to be used up, so that the hollow-cheeked pinched face which results should be taken as a warning of serious weight loss. The fat within the orbits is also consumed, and the eyes sink deeper into the skull. The bony parts of the skeleton become more prominent and the hands clawlike. When body growth pauses, the head may continue to grow, reaching a size that is disproportionately large.

Starvation is also accompanied by loss of function of various organs. Consumption of plasma proteins as well as the other body proteins leads to reduction in the levels within the circulating blood and may be associated with a reduction in blood volume or with edema. Peripheral circulation is slowed, pulse and blood pressure decline and body temperature falls to subnormal levels as the general metabolism fails.

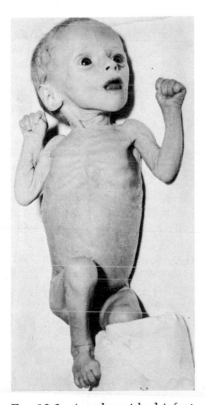

FIG. 12-3. A malnourished infant.

Eventually the infant may have sudden episodes of syncope which can terminate in death.

As starvation progresses, the resistance to infection is lowered so that it is often complicated by respiratory disease, urinary tract infection, furunculosis or thrush. The infection in turn may interfere with food digestion initiating a vicious cycle. Either constipation or a mucoid "starvation" diarrhea may be present. Deficiency of one or more vitamins may accompany the general malnutrition, and iron deficiency anemia is a regular component. As activity and peripheral circulation decrease, the skin becomes vulnerable to bedsores at points of pressure.

Treatment includes correction of dehydration, if present, and general support through frequent small transfusions. Feedings must be introduced cautiously, for the ability to handle food is limited. If too much is offered at first, the infant may begin to have diarrhea and lose rather than gain. Dilute, easily digested foods are begun first, and the intake is gradually increased according to tolerance. Eventually it may be necessary to offer as much as 200 to 250 calories/Kg. of actual body weight before recovery begins. Infections must be treated vigorously and a liberal intake of vitamins maintained.

NURSING CARE. Nursing care is directed toward the maintenance of body temperature by a heat lamp or incubator and by appropriate clothing. Care of the skin is most important to guard against decubitus ulcers. Abundant emotional warmth and attention in the form of extra cuddling, meeting sucking needs and holding are essential adjuncts to the physical care being rendered.

Foods

Protein. Protein is an essential part of all living cells. As the cells function, protein is used up and needs to be replaced. Additional supplies are demanded by growth. A growing child requires more protein in proportion to size than one who has stopped growing.

PROTEIN REQUIREMENT OF THE INFANT. Estimates of the protein requirement of the infant have been based largely on the amounts of protein received when infants are breast-fed and thriving. In these circumstances the amount of protein ingested is from 2 to 2.5 Gm. daily for each Kg. of body weight. When human milk is unavailable, cow's milk is the customary substitute. It is a widely accepted concept that cow's-milk protein is biologically inferior to human-milk protein because of the difference in relative proportions of essential amino acids. On the basis that it may be inferior by approximately 20 per cent, the protein requirement when cow's milk is fed is from 2.5 to 3 Gm. for each Kg. When cow's milk is fed to infants in customary quantities, the protein intake is at least 3.5 Gm. for each Kg., sometimes as much as 4.5 Gm. The excess over the theoretic requirement is well utilized

Table 12. Summary of Chief Minerals of the Body

Mineral	Symbol	Normal Blood Concentration	Normal Daily Infant Intake	Remarks
			Electrolytes	
Sodium	Na	135–145 mEq./L.	1 gm. +	Low levels from excessive sweating, diarrhea, adrenal insufficiency. Produce muscle cramps and poor renal function.
Potassium	K	3.5–6 mEq./L.	1 gm. +	Low levels in diarrhea, steroid therapy, burns and recovery from diabetes. Produce weakness and cardiac irregularities.
Chloride	Cl	95–105 mEq./L.	2 gm. +	Low levels from sweating, vomiting, diarrhea. Contribute to electrolyte disturbances, alkalosis.
Calcium	Ca	5–6 mEq./L. (10–12 mg. %)	0.5–1.0 gm.	Low values in rickets and tetany result in muscle irritability or convulsions.
Phosphorus	P	2.5–4 mEq./L. (4.5–7 mg. %)	1.5 gm.	Low values in rickets. Closely associated with calcium metabolism.
			Nonelectrolytes	
Iron	Fe	50–100 micrograms %	6 mg.	Chronic lack results in anemia due to poor hemoglobin formation.
Copper	Cu			Needed in minute amount to aid hemoglobin synthesis. Deficiency rare.
Iodine	I	6–8 micrograms % (as PBI)	50 micrograms	Absence from food leads to goiter or cretinism.
Fluorine	F			Minute concentration in drinking water reduces dental caries. A necessary constituent of teeth.

mEq. = milliequivalent or 1/1000 of a chemical equivalent (see p. 68).
microgram = 1/1000 of a milligram.
PBI = protein-bound iodine.

and produces increased growth. Infants tolerate well any amount of protein that it is possible to give them as undiluted milk provided that some means has been used to adapt it to their digestion. Sometimes, when babies are allergic to cow's milk, vegetable preparations, such as soybean "milk," are used in substitution. Soybean protein is complete, but a much larger quantity must be fed in order that all essential amino acids be present in sufficient amount. The amount of soybean protein fed is commonly 50 per cent more than that of cow's milk.

Fats. Fats consist of a chemical combination of glycerin and fatty acids. They differ from each other by reason of the differences in the fatty acids. Certain fatty acids (linoleic and arachidonic) have been found to be essential for some animals. Some infants deprived of these fatty acids suffer changes in the skin. No specific quantitative fat requirement can be set. The chief nutritional function of fat in the diet is to supply energy, and in this respect it can be replaced completely by carbohydrate. However, certain fats are highly desirable in the diet because they contain fat-soluble vitamins which are essential, though these vitamins may be supplied by special preparations if necessary. Fats are desirable also because they furnish considerably more energy for each unit of weight than protein or carbohydrate, thus conserving the functions of digestion and absorption and distributing the burden of energy production among a greater number of body functions. Also, fats contribute materially to the palatability of the diet, and without them insufficient total food is likely to be ingested if the amount is left to choice.

Carbohydrate. The chief function of carbohydrate is to supply energy. It is an essential constituent of the body. Carbohydrate becomes available through the breakdown of protein and, to some extent, of fat. While it is theoretically possible to derive sufficient carbohydrate from these sources, it is much more practical to consider that a carbohydrate requirement exists. A certain amount of energy must be derived from sources other than fat in order to spare fat combustion. The capacity of the body to burn fat completely is limited. When the energy requirements demand that an excessive amount of fat be consumed, ketone bodies are formed which in excessive amount may create acidosis. In the usual diet, the amount of carbohydrate taken in is far in excess of this minimum, and it is seldom necessary to worry about the carbohydrate requirement. When carbohydrate is consumed, as it frequently is, in amounts which exceed immediate energy needs, it is stored in the body as fat.

Minerals

A number of minerals are essential constituents of the body and necessary for growth and the conduct of vital processes. With a few exceptions (notably iron) these elements are consumed in sufficient quantity with all infant diets, being present in milk in concentrations which are adequate to meet daily needs so long as hunger is appeased. Under the special circumstances of disease or unusual dietary conditions, the body stores may be depleted and the function of a particular mineral may then be revealed by its deficiency. Table 12 summarizes the main facts about the biologically important minerals.

Two types of anemia occur during infancy which are primarily the result of insufficient intake of iron. Their mechanisms and management are quite similar.

Hypochromic or Iron-Deficiency Anemia. The most common form of anemia in infants is that which develops from a failure of the child to take in enough iron in his diet to supply building material for the new hemoglobin which he needs for his expanding size. The anemia is characterized by a relatively normal production of red blood cells. The cells are smaller than normal and very deficient in hemoglobin content, so that each may contain less than half the normal quantity. This type of anemia is called hypochromic or microcytic. It occurs between the ages of 9 months and 2½ years. Almost invariably the infant has developed an inordinate fondness for milk, consuming 1 or 2 quarts per day and refusing most other foods. In spite of rather severe degrees of anemia, there is little interference with activity. The child is usually pale, irritable and obstinate about his refusal of solid foods. Treatment consists of the addition of one of the iron preparations to his daily milk ration. This usually produces a rapid improvement in anemia and at the same time increases the appetite for foods other than milk so that gradually the child can be encouraged to accept a diet which is better balanced nutritionally. Restoration of normal blood values can be expected in 4 to 8 weeks' time. If the anemia is so severe that the circulation is embarrassed or if the child is otherwise ill, it may be necessary to effect a more rapid correction by transfusion.

Anemia of Prematurity. At the time of his birth the premature infant usually has average normal values of hemoglobin and red cells. Likewise, he has a store of iron from his mother which is appropriate for his small size. However, since he grows at a very rapid rate during the first few months of life and since his diet contains very little iron, his bone marrow is frequently unable to keep pace with the demands for new blood cells, particularly with the demand for more hemoglobin. In consequence, an exaggerated decline of the red blood cell count and of the hemoglobin level of the blood takes place. This is similar to the fall in values suffered by the full-term infant but is more exaggerated in degree. The smaller the premature at the time of his birth, the more severe his anemia is likely to become during these first few months.

Usually, iron is given to prematures routinely in an attempt to prevent or to lessen the degree of fall in hemoglobin. Success in this type of therapy is not always achieved, for it now seems to be true that the premature is not able to absorb and utilize iron very well for the first 6 to 8 weeks of his life. Usually the hemoglobin can be permitted to fall as low as from 6 to 8 Gm. per cent. A more marked degree of anemia may demand transfusion. Iron preparations for intramuscular use are now available which can be administered early during prematurity. None of the other mineral deficiencies occurs with any recognized frequency. Imperfect calcium absorption is in part responsible for the defects in rickets which is included in the discussion of vitamin D.

Vitamins

Vitamins are accessory food substances required by the body in quite small amounts to guide certain metabolic processes. They are organic chemicals of known structure, most of which can now be synthesized in the laboratory. However, they cannot be synthesized by the human body and consequently must be ingested already formed in the food. The body is able to store most of them so that reserves are available. In contrast to the more immediately essential nutrients, deprivation of vitamins must be prolonged before symptoms appear. Complete oxygen lack is lethal in a matter of minutes; water, in days; food, in weeks; but vitamins, only after months. This is due in part to the presence of body stores which must be exhausted before symptoms appear and in part to the fact that life can go on fairly well in spite of the presence of a vitamin deficiency. The rapid growth of infancy not only increases vitamin requirements but also speeds depletion of vital stores. Hence, most of the deficiency diseases are likely to be found during infancy rather than at later periods of life.

Detailed knowledge of vitamin function has permitted almost complete abolition of the corresponding deficiency diseases among properly tended infants. This goal has been reached through a combination of public education in well-baby clinics, by production of relatively cheap and almost universally acceptable preparations of the vitamins, and in some instances by prophylactic addition of vitamins in appropriate concentration to milk and proprietary baby formulas. Unfortunately, not all infants are protected by such community safeguards. In the United States examples of deficiency still appear and in countries where educational and economic standards are less favorable the conditions described may be more widespread. The virtues of vitamins have been inflated by promotional technics to a point where many infants, children and adults now receive unnecessarily large quantities in a misguided attempt to ward off disease or produce a condition of superhealth. The evidence that more than minimum requirements of vitamins has any additional salutary effect is scanty except in the presence of a few diseases. In most instances the practice of overdosage is not harmful apart from the economic waste, but toxic effects may appear after prolonged overuse of some of them. In this section standard requirements of the more important vitamins are considered together with the symptoms of deprivation and overdosage.

Vitamin A. SOURCES. Included under the term "vitamin A" are both the ultimate form of the vitamin itself and the carotenoid pigments which are its precursors (provitamins). In animals and in man the liver transforms carotene substances derived from the ingestion of leafy and yellow vegetables into vitamin A and stores the excess within its substance. Both animals and man may also obtain the final form of vitamin A from the liver (or liver extracts) of fish or other animals which are part of the diet. Both forms of the vitamin are absorbed with the fat of the diet. Neither is affected by the usual cooking procedures.

REQUIREMENTS. The vitamin A requirement varies with the size or weight of the body. The requirement of the young infant is met easily by the content of either human or cow's milk.

Customary additions to the milk diet as the infant becomes older increase the intake to maintain it at a fully adequate level. In fact, at all ages any reasonably good diet supplies adequate vitamin A without resort to special preparations of this material. Important deficiency of intake occurs only with diets which depart markedly from a satisfactory pattern. Even with a good intake of vitamin A, deficiency may arise from poor utilization. Utilization becomes markedly impaired by illness, particularly acute infection. The allowance of vitamin A recommended has been set at 2,000 to 2,500 I.U. (International Units) per day for infants. It rises gradually to 5,000 I.U. for adolescents.

DEFICIENCY. Since vitamin A is widely distributed in the fat of animal meats and milks and in the carotene component of vegetables, deficiency occurs only under the unusual circumstances of a very limited diet or of imperfect absorption. Infants fed on skimmed milk products, or older children receiving little except starchy foods are potential victims. Diseases such as the malabsorption syndromes in which fat absorption is impaired may also be accompanied by clinical evidence of avitaminosis.

TOXICITY. Overdosage of vitamin A in amounts which accumulate to several hundred thousand units within a few weeks may result in a combination of symptoms which include loss of appetite, poor weight gain and itching of the skin. Examination may also show enlargement of the liver and increased thickening of the cortex of the long bones visible on a roentgenogram.

Vitamin B Complex. Vitamin B complex includes thiamine (B_1), riboflavin (B_2 or G), niacin (nicotinic acid) and many other components. These substances are found in the same foods, though the proportion of each to the others varies in different foods. Deficiency of only one B vitamin is rare, but often one may be more deficient than others. Thiamine, riboflavin and niacin, and probably other members of the complex, are components of enzymes necessary for cell respiration.

THIAMINE. Thiamine is necessary for normal appetite and gastrointestinal function and for successful lactation. Impairment of growth may result from poor appetite. Thiamine has been synthesized on a commercial scale and is available abundantly in crystalline form. In nature it is found in important amounts in whole grain cereals, peanuts, yeast and lean meat, especially pork and liver. It is found in smaller amounts in many foods, including milk, eggs, vegetables and fruits. It has been added in small amounts to enriched flour and bread. Despite its fairly wide distribution, it is the B component which is most likely to be deficient in the average diet. It is easily destroyed by heat; the usual cooking processes result in an average loss of 25 per cent or more. It is water-soluble and often is discarded with the water of cooking. Thiamine is necessary for the combustion of carbohydrate, and the requirement is proportional to the nonfat calories of the diet. Recommended allowances vary from 0.4 mg. in the first year to 1.5 mg. at 15 years for average diets, or 0.05 mg. for each 100 calories of the diet.

Older children with thiamine deficiency may have localized or generalized muscle weakness, loss of tendon reflexes and neurotic manifestations.

No toxic effects from overdosage with thiamine are known.

RIBOFLAVIN. Riboflavin is necessary for growth, and probably also for successful lactation. Riboflavin is a yellow pigment, stable to the heat of cooking but destroyed by exposure to light. The best source in the daily diet is milk. The customary milk formula supplies the requirement of the infant, and a quart of milk supplies most, if not all, of the requirement of the child. Riboflavin is present in important amounts also in liver, egg yolk, meat, whole-grain cereals and green vegetables, but the requirement is not likely to be met from these sources without the inclusion of milk in the diet. The appropriate allowance for riboflavin is approximately 50 per cent greater than that for thiamine, namely 0.6 mg. in the first year, increasing to 2.0 mg. at 15 years.

NIACIN (NICOTINIC ACID). Niacin deficiency causes pellagra. This vitamin exists commercially both as the acid and as its amide. No common food is a rich source of this material, but liver, lean meat, eggs, whole-grain cereals, enriched bread, wheat germ and yeast have it in important amounts. The amount in milk is small, both human and cow's, being approximately 1 mg. to the liter. However, it is well established that the dietary requirement for niacin decreases when milk is contained in the diet, presumably because of bacterial synthesis in the intestine. The appropriate allowance of niacin is ten times that of thiamine in all age groups. The material is stable to usual food handling.

OTHER B-COMPLEX FACTORS. Other B-complex factors exist which are known to be essential for experimental animals and presumably are important in human nutrition. Folic acid under ordinary circumstances is produced in the intestine by the bacteria that dwell therein. After heavy antibiotic therapy this source of supply may be cut off because the bacteria are destroyed. Folic acid normally requires an adequate amount of vitamin C to convert it into folinic acid (citrovorum factor) which in turn is essential in the formation of nucleic acids. Disturbance of this complicated chain of chemical events may result in megaloblastic anemia because of inadequate formation of red blood cell protein. Pyridoxine (B_6) is also essential in human metabolism but can be lacking from the average diet only under very special circumstances. A few instances of convulsions in infants have been traced to its destruction during the preparation of commercial canned milk formulas. The remaining members of the B-complex are choline, biotin, inositol and pantothenic acid. Their essentiality in human nutrition has not been proved. The incompleteness of our knowledge about the details of vitamin requirements emphasizes the wisdom of depending on a mixed diet for nutritional essentials rather than on special preparations of the known vitamins.

Vitamin C (Ascorbic Acid). SOURCES. Ascorbic acid, a relatively simple chemical compound, can be synthesized by many of the lower animals but not by man. It is a necessary component of all living cells and in the human body is required for the normal growth of connective tissue and capillaries. In its absence the cement substance between the cells is defective, capillaries leak readily, and wounds fail to heal.

Ascorbic acid is present in many fruits and vegetables, particularly the citrus fruits such as oranges, lemons, limes and grapefruit. Freshly squeezed juice of these fruits is the most reliable source, but canned frozen juices are also satisfactory if used soon after thawing. Tomatoes, potatoes and other growing and sprouting vegetables are also a good source. However, cooking destroys a considerable portion of the vitamin as do alkalies such as bicarbonate of soda, or exposure to the air for long periods of time. The breast milk of women is an adequate source if the maternal diet is good. From 20 to 75 mg. per quart of breast milk is the usual concentration. Cow's milk

is an unreliable source because the initial concentration is 20 mg. per quart or less, and the heating to which it is subjected in pasteurization, evaporation or boiling for purposes of storage or formula preparation reduces the quantity of vitamin C to a third or half of the original level.

REQUIREMENTS. The small infant requires 20 mg. per day to maintain saturation of his body stores. Usually at least 30 mg. per day is allowed. For the older child the requirement rises progressively to about 80 to 100 mg. at 15 years. Overdosage is non-

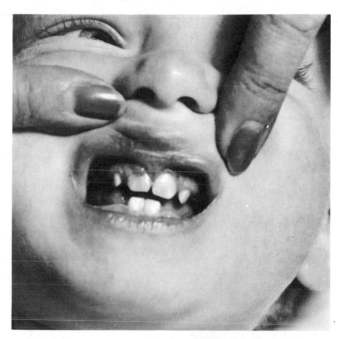

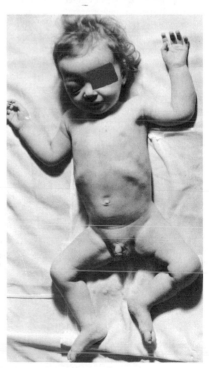

FIG. 12-4. Scurvy. *Upper,* characteristic gum changes. *Lower,* characteristic posture of an infant with scurvy and periorbital hemorrhage.

toxic, and the synthetic vitamin is quite inexpensive. Excesses are excreted in the urine.

SCURVY (VITAMIN-C DEFICIENCY). Scurvy is rare in children and adults. In infancy, the diet is much more limited, and it is chiefly at this period that scurvy may occur if the mother does not ensure that the artificially fed baby has orange juice or some equivalent source of ascorbic acid.

In its early stages, preceding the clinical signs by which it may be recognized, scurvy is characterized by indisposition, fretfulness, pallor, diminished appetite and failing nutrition.

The hemorrhages of scurvy occur through the capillaries because of loss of cement substance between the cells of the capillary walls and because of arrested growth of connective tissue and its collagen-supporting structure. They are not caused by any change in the blood. Hemorrhage may occur in many places. Blood may appear in the urine or the stool. Small hemorrhages may appear within the skin, the appearance often resembling a bruise. Hemorrhage occurs in the gums and is usually limited to the site of erupted teeth. The gums become dark and swollen and bleed easily. Their appearance is strikingly suggestive, almost diagnostic, of scurvy.

The characteristic hemorrhages are in the long bones and are subperiosteal. They start at the growing end of the bone and strip off the periosteum, producing subperiosteal hematomas.

One of the characteristics of scurvy is pain and tenderness of the extremities, especially of the legs. The baby resents handling, the legs are not moved voluntarily, paralysis is simulated, and the thighs and the legs are held flexed with outward rotation of the hips.

Scurvy responds quickly to ascorbic acid, whether given in crystalline form or as foods naturally containing this material. The pain and acute symptoms are relieved within a few days. A longer period is required to recover from anemia and nutritional and bone changes. For the first few days of treatment, from 100 to 200 mg. of ascorbic acid may be given daily in divided doses. Subsequently, the normal allowance is sufficient.

Vitamin D. SOURCES. Vitamin D can be produced in the body by the action of ultraviolet light on cholesterol in the skin. In this way children from underdeveloped countries can manufacture enough to meet their needs if they have a daily exposure to the midday sun lasting about 15 minutes. The child from Western countries can obtain the same effect on a beach in summer or from a shorter exposure to a mercury vapor lamp indoors in the winter. However, civilized living in temperate climates is likely to interfere with the natural formation of vitamin D in adequate amounts. The ultraviolet rays, which have waves less than 320 millimicrons in length, are filtered out by ordinary window glass and by atmospheric conditions such as clouds, smog and the oblique passage

of light from the sun through the earth's atmosphere. Adequate exposure of the child's skin is further hampered by clothing and by the fact that he spends much time indoors, particularly during the cold seasons. Consequently, it is unwise to rely on the automatic production of vitamin D in the skin, and adequate amounts must be supplied with the diet.

Vitamin D is present in ordinary foods in unimportant quantities only. It occurs in small amounts in milk, butter and egg yolk. Liver is a good source, the liver oils of fish being the richest natural source. Vitamin D is prepared artificially by irradiation of cholesterol, an animal product, or ergosterol, a vegetable product. Activated ergosterol, when purified to contain only vitamin D, is known as calciferol. Inconclusive evidence indicates that activated cholesterol and naturally occurring vitamin D may be somewhat superior to activated ergosterol in effectiveness for humans, but the difference, if any, is small. Vitamin D is relatively stable and resists destruction in the various processes of cooking food. Vitamin D may be stored to some extent, chiefly in the liver.

The function of vitamin D is to improve and regulate the utilization of calcium and phosphorus of the diet. Vitamin D deficiency is known to lead to rickets and tetany in the infant and to osteomalacia in the adult. It leads also to subnormal mineralization of teeth and bones in the growing child, even though rickets may not be clinically evident.

REQUIREMENTS. Except for children who are consistently exposed to the sun, vitamin D should be offered regularly as part of the diet. The speed of growth and consequently of bone formation determines to a considerable degree how much vitamin D is required. For this reason the infant's small body must have between 400 and 800 units per day, the same amount required by the much larger body of the adolescent or adult. Premature infants who grow at the most rapid rate of all require from 800 to 1,200 units per day. Originally, vitamin D was given as cod-liver oil in a dose of 1 or 2 teaspoonfuls per day. The large volume and the objectionable smell have been overcome by preparing concentrates of other fish-liver oils with approximately 100 times the vitamin D content of cod-liver oil. These and synthetic preparations of vitamin D have largely replaced the old-fashioned vehicle. Vitamin D can also be added to milk in amounts which almost completely satisfy the child's daily requirement. In the United States most large dairies so fortify the fresh milk they produce, and nearly all brands of evaporated milk contain 400 units in each reconstituted quart. When practically all the available milk is fortified, rickets disappears. A common practice in infant feeding is to give fortified milk and, as an additional precaution, a vitamin D supplement. Although overdosage of vitamin D may interfere with appetite and result in abnormalities of the calcium metabolism of the body,

Fig. 12-5. Very marked active rickets, showing enlargement of the head from "bossing," a marked "rosary," enlarged epiphyses and inability to stand or sit.

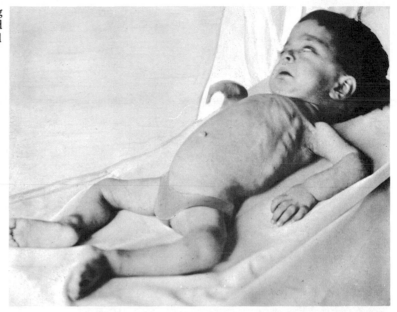

these toxic symptoms generally appear only when intakes of 5 to 10 times the minimum daily requirements are maintained consistently for several weeks.

Rickets (vitamin-D deficiency) can occur only when growth is active. The counterpart of rickets in those fully grown is osteomalacia. The more rapid the growth the more likely is rickets to develop. The most rapid growth occurs in infancy, and it is almost exclusively among infants that rickets occurs as a deficiency disease.

Rickets is more common in artificially fed than in breast-fed babies. It occurs chiefly in the temperate zones, where babies may have long periods without sunshine. It is more common in dark-skinned races because some of the ultraviolet rays are filtered out by the pigment. Rickets is not common in the tropics, even in dark-skinned races with the poorest of diets. Rickets is seasonal. It begins to be active when babies are more closely housed for the winter. Its activity is at its height in the northern hemisphere in March and subsides as babies are allowed sunshine again in the spring.

The disturbance of calcium and phosphorus metabolism is evidenced by poor retention of these materials by the body, by abnormal blood levels of calcium, phosphorus and phosphatase, and by faulty mineralization of bones. Normally, the blood of an infant contains from 10 to 12 mg. of calcium and from 5 to 7 mg. of phosphorus for each 100 ml. of serum. When rickets is present and active, the blood calcium may be expected to be from 9 to 10 mg., and the phosphorus less than 4 mg. for each 100 ml. When the product of the calcium and the phosphorus values is less than 30, rickets is present and active. Phosphatase is an enzyme which increases in the blood in proportion to the severity of the rickets.

The growth in length of the long bones takes place

in the shaft at its junction with the epiphysis. This area of growth change is the metaphysis. The normal process of increase is by growth of cartilage cells (osteoid tissue) and mineralization of these cells at such a rate that only a thin layer of osteoid tissue is present. In rickets, the deposit of calcium and phos-

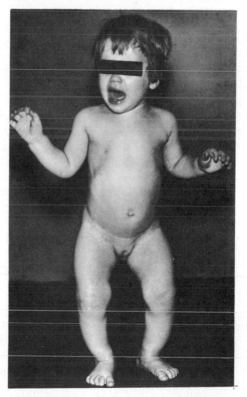

Fig. 12-6. This 18-month-old child shows the effects of rickets: bowed legs, large wrists and large skull with prominent bosses.

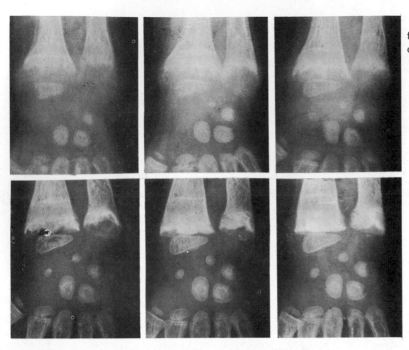

FIG. 12-7. Various stages in the healing of active rickets. Note the progressive increase of calcification.

phate in the newly grown cartilage is deficient. The roentgenogram shows a raggedly calcified bone end. The osteoid tissue continues to grow, producing enlargement of the end of the bone by overgrowth or a mushrooming effect of pressure on soft tissue. Enlargement of the bone end becomes apparent on inspection and palpation. This same process produces small knobs at the junction of the ribs with the cartilage near the sternum. Because of their distribution, these enlargements have been designated collectively a rachitic rosary.

The shafts of the long bones eventually become soft from lack of mineral, and they may bend according to the direction in which stress is put on them. The pull of the diaphragm on the softened ribs, particularly when combined with nasal obstruction, causes deformities of the chest, the most common of which is depression of the ribs at the line of attachment of the diaphragm (Harrison's groove). Softening of the spine may result in scoliosis or kyphosis. The bones of the skull sometimes become sufficiently soft to permit indentation by the finger as though they were made of stiff parchment. This condition, craniotabes, occurs chiefly in the occipital bones of young infants. Sometimes overgrowth occurs on the parietal and frontal bones of the skull, producing bosses and giving to the skull a somewhat square shape. Rickets causes delay in eruption of teeth and in closing of the fontanel. Whatever the bone changes may be as a result of rickets, they tend to occur similarly and equally on the two sides of the body.

Muscles as well as bones suffer in rickets. As rickets advances, the muscles show a general weakness and loss of tone. Because of these changes, sitting, standing and walking are delayed, or the baby may retro-

gress in these acts if they were already established. The abdominal wall is relaxed, and the abdomen protrudes when the child is erect. Constipation may result from loss of muscle strength. Ligaments about joints may become lax and permit unusual mobility. Sometimes the spleen is enlarged by simple hyperplasia, and the liver may be increased in size.

The diagnosis of active rickets is made by finding the characteristic changes in roentgenograms of bones or abnormal blood levels of calcium and phosphorus, or both. Also, blood phosphatase is increased above the normal.

Rickets is not a direct cause of death, though it may be a contributing factor by predisposing to other diseases. With rare exceptions, rickets subsides, even without treatment, by the time the period of infancy has passed, because growth is not so rapid, and the child can get more sunshine under his own power. The deformities of rickets may persist. There is considerable tendency for moderate deformities to disappear in the period from 2 to 5 years of age. Severe deformities remain unless corrected by operative or mechanical means. Some deformities, such as those of the chest, are not easily amenable to corrective procedures.

The treatment of rickets consists primarily of the administration of vitamin D. The larger the dosage the more quickly the healing process begins. Since the baby is not ill and no emergency exists, moderate rather than massive dosage is preferable. Vitamin D in the amount of from 1,500 to 3,000 units daily may be expected to produce evidence of recovery in the blood in about a week, and in the bones in approximately two weeks. Concentrated preparations may be preferred to low-potency oils because of the bulk of

Table 13. Summary of Dietary Requirements of the First Year

Substance	Requirement of 1-Month-old Infant Wt. = 4.0 Kg.	Requirement of 12-Month-old Infant Wt. = 10 Kg.	Volume of Milk to Give Daily Quota			
			At 1 Month		At 12 Months	
			Breast Milk	Raw Cow's Milk	Breast Milk	Raw Cow's Milk
Water	150 ml./Kg. = 600 ml.	130 ml./Kg. = 1,300 ml.	30 oz.	30 oz.	65 oz.	65 oz.
Energy	110 cal./Kg. = 440 cal.	100 cal./Kg. = 1,000 cal.	22 oz.	22 oz.	50 oz.	50 oz.
Protein	3 Gm./Kg. = 12 Gm.	3 Gm./Kg. = 30 Gm.	27 oz.	9 oz.	68 oz.	23 oz.
Calcium	0.25 Gm.	1.0 Gm.	20 oz.	5 oz.	80 oz.	20 oz.
Iron	6 mg.	same	200 oz.	500 oz.		
Vitamin A	2000 U.	same	32 oz.	32 oz.		
Thiamine	0.4 mg.	same	*250 oz.	50 oz.		
Riboflavin	0.6 mg.	same	40 oz.	12 oz.		
Niacin	6 mg.	same	*100 oz.	200 oz.	(more if processed)	
Vitamin C	30 mg.	same	20 oz.	45 oz.		
Vitamin D	400 U.	same	*150 oz.	300 oz.		

* The apparent deficiency of breast milk in these substances is not borne out by the occurrence of clinical deficiency in totally breast-fed infants. In the case of niacin, a milk diet decreases the theoretic requirement so that the figure given is probably too high. Breast milk contains calcium and phosphorus in optimal ratio, thus lowering vitamin D requirements, but rickets does occur in some breast-fed infants. The discrepancy for thiamine is not adequately explained.

oil required for the larger doses. In any case, a large dosage serves a useful purpose only until the healing process has well begun; thereafter a maintenance dose of from 300 to 400 units daily is adequate. Except for correction of existing dietary faults, no other treatment is necessary in most instances.

In a few instances, corrective appliances may be desirable during the healing stage of rickets and subsequently. These appliances would be for the correction of deformity such as bowlegs or knock knees. Operative correction of deformity, if necessary, is deferred until the rickets has healed completely.

Vitamin E (tocopherol). Vitamin E deficiency in animal experimentation leads to sterility in both sexes, and when females have received only minimum amounts their young have muscular dysfunction similar to muscular dystrophy of the human. It is believed that vitamin E may be necessary for muscle development. Satisfactory evidence of deficiency in the human has not been presented. Vitamin E has a distribution so wide that any mixed diet contains an abundance.

Vitamin K. Vitamin K as found naturally in food is a fat-soluble material, chemically a naphthoquinone which has been given the name *menadione*. Other and synthetic derivatives of naphthoquinone have vitamin K activity, and some are water-soluble.

Vitamin K is necessary for the liver to use in its manufacture of prothrombin, which in turn is essential to the blood clotting mechanism. Vitamin K is sometimes deficient in the newborn infant or the premature. Symptoms are those of spontaneous bleeding, and control is achieved by administering certain synthetic quinones which provide the basic material necessary for the synthesis of prothrombin. Intestinal bacteria and a wide variety of foods provide sufficient vitamin K in later infancy and childhood so that the disorder is encountered only under peculiar circumstances. Liver disease may render the body unable to synthesize prothrombin; then replacement therapy is required via transfusions. On occasion, heavy antibiotic dosage may sterilize the intestinal tract to a point where vitamin K-producing bacteria are no longer present. Salicylate therapy over long periods of time may interfere with the synthesis of vitamin K. In the newborn period from 1 to 2 mg. of a synthetic preparation such as Synkavite, Hykinone or menadione is sufficient to correct hemorrhagic disease. For older children, from 5 to 10 mg. per day should be given while the conditions which interfere with prothrombin formation persist.

Infant Diets

The basic nutritional requirements and some of their changes during the first year are summarized in Table 13. Since milk is the major item of the infant's diet, calculations are appended to show how much of either breast or raw cow's milk would have to be consumed to meet the theoretic daily requirements. Examination of the third column discloses that a nursing mother able to produce the reasonable quantity of 30 oz. of milk per day will comfortably cover all the needs of her infant except for iron, the B-complex vitamins and probably vitamin D. Thus, at this age breast feeding alone is nutritionally sufficient. But if no supplements are added, the infant who is almost a year of age approaches inadequacies of water, energy, protein and calcium unless his mother is able to improve her milk production by nearly 100 per cent. Furthermore, the cumulative effects of low iron intake over a whole year will exhaust his antenatal store and render him anemic; likewise, the marginal vitamin D consumption will lead to rickets unless he has adequate exposure to ultraviolet light from the sun. Less clear-cut, but possibly significant, is his need for more of the B-complex vitamins. The infant fed on a modification of cow's milk has little difficulty meeting his requirements of protein and calcium (6th column) but will suffer marked deficiency of iron, vitamin C and vitamin D before the year is out. Hence, early supplementation of the milk diet is somewhat more important for an artificially fed infant than it is for a breast-fed infant.

In practice all infants are offered water and a vitamin preparation which contains at least their requirements for vitamins C and D. Many proprietary infant formulas now contain these additives. The amount of vitamin D in fortified whole or evaporated milk is probably marginally sufficient to prevent rickets, but infants are commonly given more for insurance. The addition of other foods such as cereal, strained fruits, vegetables, eggs and meats varies greatly with individual physicians, mothers and infants. Many babies will accept such supplements before the first month is over although they may be awkward at getting solid material over the top of the tongue back into the pharynx where it will be carried by reflex action into the stomach. Until they acquire this skill the foods offered should be well diluted with formula or milk in order to make them almost liquid in consistency. Although survival does not depend on the addition of these new foods, it is wise both nutritionally and psychologically to establish them as part of the infant diet before the age of 3 to 4 months—nutritionally, in order to supply organic iron and additional vitamins and roughage; psychologically, because many infants begin to resist new foods around the age of 6 months.

Practices differ in respect to the age at which un-modified cow's milk can be added to the diet. Some physicians feel that for reasons of sterility and ease of digestibility, only properly prepared formula should be used during the first year. A more liberal attitude considers modification unnecessary after about 5 months of age. This latter view must be conditioned by the sanitary practices of the individual family.

NEUROMUSCULAR AND PSYCHOSOCIAL GROWTH AND DEVELOPMENT

Accompanying the rapid changes in body size which mark the physical growth pattern of the first year are equally remarkable and exciting developments in the infant's ability to handle his body and to communicate with the physical and social world around him. So many aspects are changing simultaneously that each three-month period will be described separately.

Some facets of developmental progress are primarily reflections of the maturation of the central nervous system which permits increasing sensitivity and analysis of the stimuli coming from the environment and provides ever better control of muscular movements and their integration. The infant achieves control of his body from above downward—the cephalocaudal pattern of development. It should also be noted that there is a rather wide range of ages at which individual infants arrive at the different mileposts. The *sequence* in which the new skills are acquired is much more regular than the age. For other aspects of development, too, a similar allowance for individual variation must be made, and statements about what is true for the *average* infant cannot apply literally to each specific infant. Neuromuscular progress is most readily charted, but it is inextricably entwined with

Growth, Development and Care During the First Year

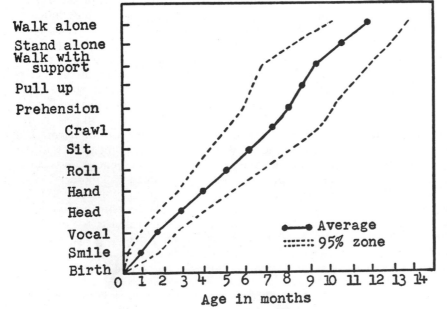

Fig. 12-8. A developmental graph for the first year, showing the average age for the beginning of the achievements selected and the zone in which 95 per cent of the infants' developmental graphs fell. (Aldrich and Norval: J. Pediat. *29:*304)

social and emotional adjustment. The infant progresses not only by virtue of that learning which is amassed through repeated contacts and consistent responses from the physical environment but also from the social stimulation and emotional satisfactions contributed by the persons around him. Separation of his development into its motor, sensory, adaptive, social and emotional components is convenient for description but is rather artificial.

From 1 to 3 Months

The infant at the beginning of this period has most of the characteristics of the newborn, but he is infinitely more stable physiologically. His heart beat is steadier and his respiratory rate more regular. His body temperature does not fluctuate as readily. Muscle tonus is considerably improved. Although the young infant is protected from perceiving environmental stimuli for the first months of life by a stimulus barrier, he does react to internal states of discomfort and to strong external stimulation. His emotional response however is limited to tension states, which if unrelieved increase to a panic reaction. When frustrated by hunger or discomfort, he arches his back, extends and flexes his extremities and breathes rapidly or shallowly. There may be a change of skin color with disintegration of coordination and increase in total activity. Individual differences can be seen very early in the strength of noxious stimuli which produce tension and in response to comforting. There is also great individual difference in aggressive responses, in temperament and in total activity patterns.

By the age of 2 months his capacities and behavior begin to show significant changes. At first his posture tends toward the tonic neck position (TNR) with limbs extended on the side toward which his head is turned and flexed on the opposite side. His Moro response is still brisk, and stimuli of any sort tend to evoke mass undifferentiated responses. By 3 months the frequency of the TNR position and the vigor of the Moro response are rapidly diminishing. The baby is more likely to be found with his arms and legs in bilaterally symmetric positions and to use them simultaneously, but not separately. Differentiation of motor responses occurs with increasing maturation of the nervous system. Although the infant's responses merge in a smooth way from one action to another, there is also increasing independence in the use of extremities after several months.

From a prone position he will now be able to raise his head and peer around steadily and perhaps can even get his chest up off the bed. When held erect his head no longer flops forward on his chest but is held under fairly good control by the muscles of his neck. Hands which previously waved as clenched fists begin to open and serve as outlets for his curiosity. They play with each other and begin to bat out at objects which they seldom reach. Articles which were placed

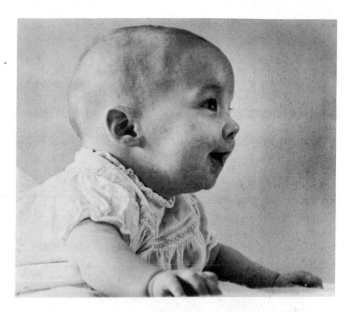

FIG. 12-9. At 3 months the baby can raise her chest from the bed and take an active interest in events in her environment. (Carol Baldwin)

in the hand at 1 month of age were dropped at once; now they are retained for brief periods of inspection.

Although infants in the first 15 weeks appear to have an indefinite vacant stare directed only at things which happen to be in the direct line of vision, they do give indications of pattern discrimination and response to contour with a definite change at about 2 months. There is clear preference for more pattern complexity as measured by the length of attention. *Perception,* however, implies contact with the environment and appears later with inquisitive pursuit of interesting objects, even when they are at the periphery of the visual field. It is only after experience in the framework of a close mother-child relationship that environmental stimuli begin to take on meaning. Much learning must take place before the infant is able to perceive objects, to recognize them and to discriminate their attributes.

Social responses begin to appear after several months: a communicative smile, animated response to the appearance of a face, perhaps even a vague and ill-defined recognition of the mother. The voice changes from inarticulate noises to responsive coos. The cry which was previously used indiscriminately for any type of distress begins to have more meaning and is used for attention as well as relief. Tears which were infrequent at 1 month of age are copious by 3 months.

The First Prize—A Smile. The very young infant makes facial movements which are fondly interpreted as smiles; in reality they are reflex or automatic movements which lack the quality of a social response. By the age of 6 to 8 weeks, however, the smile takes on

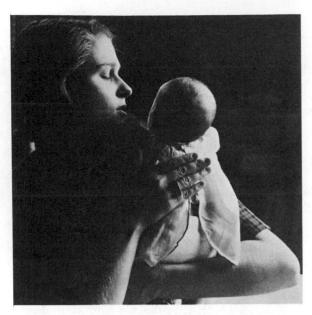

Fig. 12-10. The first relationship with her mother is the basis for all later social relationships. (Carol Baldwin)

a new quality which betokens the infant's capacity to respond to human love and care.

The first real smile usually appears in the third month and marks a developmental milestone. It indicates that memory traces have been laid down and the beginning of thought processes in that the infant can now recognize the human face. This capacity is still limited however, and does not indicate recognition of the face as a person since the smile ceases when the head is turned to profile.

Even though the smile is used indiscriminately in response to any comforting face, it acquires great significance for his mother for it is the first outgoing, giving, appreciative manifestation that her care is satisfactory. The first smile is associated with gratification in that it is a response to the memory of the mother's face while receiving the breast or bottle. The difference in the timing of the appearance of the first smile can greatly influence the emotional climate of the mother-child relationship.

Some mothers fully enjoy the early helpless period when the infant's complete dependence stimulates the full flow of their protective nurturant feelings. The gratification that they derive from such close identification with the baby is sufficient. Other mothers who are uncertain of their maternal capacities are less fortunate and remain troubled because the baby's communications of discomfort are threatening. For them the fact that the baby reacts to comforting by dropping off into blissful sleep is not sufficient reassurance of the adequacy of his care. They need more tangible evidence. The appearance of a responsive smile is a welcome boost to their confidence and provides a new

impetus to identify more closely with the infant and cope with his ever-changing behavior.

Perceiving and Responding. During the first few weeks the baby responds only reflexively and the cerebral cortex is little involved in control. He does not yet have the perceptual and social abilities which he will need for life in the physical and personal world around him. The acquisition of these powers is greatly influenced by the stimulation which he receives from those charged with his care. It must be adapted to his ability to respond. Either overstimulation or neglect will impede his progress.

Both maturation and learning are involved in development. That set of behaviors which occurs in sequential pattern for all individuals is mainly maturational and yet are influenced by experience. The effects of experience and maturation are additive in even the most basic of behaviors.

In the beginning, cues from the environment stimulate a deep body sensitivity and the baby responds only in terms of internal need. Although the sensory organs receive external stimuli, they do not have meaning and are therefore not actually consciously perceived at this early stage. He is generally uninterested in the world about him, although he derives satisfaction from the feeding situation, receives pleasurable stimulation through his skin from cuddling, rocking and tender fondling and enjoys his mother's voice as she talks to him.

Stimulation of the sense organs, however, is necessary for development of perception in each modality, and deprivation of such stimulation can result in a deficit in efficiency of use in any specific organ of sense. Such early deprivation may have reverberations in regard to particular cues the baby will need for later learning from experience.

From an early ability to differentiate figure from ground, the baby must learn to know objects by coordinating different experiences with the same object. A new dimension is added when he gains control of the 12 small muscles which move his eyes so that he can "take in" visually. He now begins to lie quietly staring at his mother's face, at bright lights and moving objects. His rapt absorption does not mean that he perceives these objects clearly, for the development of the nerve cells in his brain is not yet sufficiently advanced to give him a clear picture. But his enjoyment and need of visual stimulation are attested by the pleasure he shows during its reception and by his unhappy wails when his "visual hunger" is no longer satisfied.

With the ability to follow objects and lights visually, the infant also begins to have the ability to coordinate stimulation to several sense organs; noises heard direct visual attention and objects within the visual fields are grasped. Repeated stimulation also begins to evoke perceptual recognition as memory traces are laid down. Now when the bottle approaches, the infant begins to make sucking movements suggesting expectation and he may show signs of recognizing a familiar toy. At this stage, however, objects have no permanence as attested by the fact that he makes no search for the toy that has disappeared from his visual field.

Out of this beginning of perceptual recognition and response grow the rudiments of social relationships. Although he is not yet able to act independently to evoke response in others, he will soon be caught up in the mutually rewarding interchanges of a social relationship from which each partner derives pleasure, satisfaction and increasing self-esteem. From the first relationship with the mother, the baby will learn to expand his emotional attachments to other people and experience the interchange of pleasure and esteem which is the foundation for a lifetime of rich social relationships.

The infant's requirements for stimulation must be carefully observed so that the amount preferred maximizes his potential for intellectual growth without causing undue fatigue. If stimulation is excessive or his energy is reduced by illness, he must protest or withdraw from the environment. In the case of illness, internal stimuli consume much of his energy so that he has less to invest in mental growth. Nursing and diagnostic procedures should be carefully timed to provide uninterrupted periods of rest.

Even during illness, however, too little stimulation can be injurious, for it produces apathy, arrest and regression of intellectual growth and a turning in on the self for pleasurable satisfactions. When the infant shows signs of responding to the environment, it is an important nursing responsibility to provide sensory stimulation in amounts which he can assimilate. If the infant must remain in the hospital for long periods of care, such sensory stimulation is imperative to support healthy mental development and to maintain contact with and interest in the environment. If such stimulation is not provided, some infants may develop bizarre bodily movements such as head-rolling, or body-rocking—technics of self-stimulation which have become more interesting and satisfying to them than their contacts with the outside world. Psychologically they are on the level of the newborn. Their bodies and body needs have remained the focus of their interest. Having received little pleasure from persons, they are unable to enjoy the world outside themselves.

Sucking—A Legitimate Instinctual Urge. Some mothers or nurses who are overjoyed when an infant sucks well at feeding time will illogically become upset and frown on the same instinctual urge if it is displayed between meals. The need for sucking is at its height during the first 3 to 4 months of life when the baby must depend on someone else to satisfy it. A few small infants learn how to get their thumbs and fingers into their mouths, but, since they have poor control over body position, such self-satisfaction is not dependable. If the infant's need for sucking is so intense that it is not satisfied during the feeding period, he becomes frustrated. Contrary to what many mothers and nurses believe, a frustration such as this intensifies the urge to suck rather than lessening it. Thus, attempts to "train" a baby not to suck are likely to backfire by making his fingers all the more desirable. When the infant's neuromuscular development progresses to the point where he can direct his hands to go where he wants them to, it is likely that he will resort to thumb-sucking to make up for any unsatisfied longing he may have had.

Attempts to prevent abnormal prolongation of thumb-sucking really begin at birth and extend through this period of greatest sucking need. If the baby is given ample opportunity to suck, his need will gradually taper off and will disappear during the latter half of the first year when he finds many new uses for his hands through which he can discharge his tensions and derive substitute pleasures. The infantile behavior pattern is readily released as the normal sequence of events gives him increased mastery of himself and of the world around him.

Levy's observations in well-baby clinics and in the course of experiments with puppies support the theory that thumb-sucking occurs because the baby has not satisfied his sucking needs during feeding. Levy found that babies on a 3-hour schedule sucked their thumbs less than babies on a 4-hour schedule. The length of time at nursing was also a factor. Those babies who nursed for only 10 minutes at each feeding were more prone to suck their thumbs than were babies who nursed for 20 minutes or more. In his experiments with puppies, Dr. Levy discovered that those which were taken off the breast after a few nursing experiences and raised with a medicine dropper sucked their own and each other's paws and skin. The behavior of these frustrated puppies resembled that of babies who have not had sufficient sucking at feeding time.

The sucking requirements of individual infants are quite variable. Many have their needs easily filled by breast or bottle feeding. Others with a stronger sucking urge struggle to get their hands to their faces and root around for something to nuzzle or suck. This is the signal to examine the feeding situation. The time to forestall thumb-sucking is *before* the baby has worked out his own substitute for the nipple. If one waits until later it becomes harder to get him to release the new-found pleasure after a long period of frustration. Breast-fed infants should be allowed to dally with the feeding if the mother's nipples are in satisfactory condition. Even if no additional milk is obtained, the sucking satisfaction is important. If the baby is bottle fed, the physical characteristics of the nipples in use should be investigated. Old nipples softened by repeated boiling and with artificially enlarged holes will deliver milk rapidly and promote efficient completion of the feeding, but they may not allow the infant an adequate period of sucking. New nipples with smaller holes will slow the rate of feeding and prolong the period of sucking.

Pacifiers, Pro and Con. Another technic for increasing the sucking activity of the small infant is the use of pacifiers. Many still consider them repulsive and worry lest the infants be encouraged to continue their use into the second and third years. However, many physicians believe that they serve a useful purpose in the treatment of colic and the prevention of thumb-sucking. Few babies become thumb-suckers when pacifiers are used liberally during waking hours when small infants are restlessly trying to get something into their mouths. However, if pacifiers are used during sleep, the baby may become accustomed to dropping off with something in his mouth and will eventually be ·unable to fall asleep unless he has his pacifier or bottle. Under these circumstances, of course, the period of dependency is prolonged. Spock favors "pacifier sucking" over thumb-sucking for several reasons. The use of the pacifier will be given up before the use of the thumb. The pacifier is less readily available than the thumb so that the infant is more easily diverted to other activities and interests which will supply extraneous pleasure and the satisfaction of learning. Pacifiers are not as likely to contribute to the deformation of the child's upper jaw and cause his teeth to protrude.

Many parents become concerned about thumb-sucking because they fear permanent deformity of the child's jaw. Studies have shown that thumb-sucking may be a cause of malocclusion in the deciduous teeth, but that this malformation tends to correct itself if the habit is given up before 5 years of age. However, persistence in the habit beyond that age tends to make the malformation permanent.

Prolonged thumb-sucking in a child who is apathetic and shows little interest in the world outside himself is a sign of insecurity; it is a symptom which indicates that the child's life and living are not as emotionally satisfying as they should be. The child may be in need of toys or playmates to prevent boredom, or perhaps help in learning to play and socialize with other children. Or he may feel emotionally isolated from his mother or nurse and afraid of making his need for closeness known. Finding the cause of his discomfort and eliminating it is the only intervention which is valuable for the child. Nagging, scolding or shaming merely serves to heighten his need for comfort. He not only has to make up for the twinges of pain he feels over being reprimanded or frowned on, but he also has more need to depend on his thumb.

The Spoonfeeding Debate. Debates about the optimal time to start an infant on foods offered from a spoon cannot be settled by arbitrary pronouncements. There are too many individual variables to be considered. Fortunately, from the nutritional point of view there is a span of several months during which the resolution of such problems may be achieved before the infant is seriously deprived of desirable roughage, iron and accessory vitamins. Factors other than nutrient value which must be taken into account include the infant's neuromuscular adaptation, his appetite and his sucking drive; the quality of the relationship between feeder and fed; and the social pressure of competition, suggestions, criticisms and professional advice which bear down on the mother (or the nurse).

The average baby acquires the necessary muscular control to accept cereal and fruit willingly by 2½ to 3 months of age; vegetables at 4 to 4½ months; and meats and soups at 5½ to 6 months. However, mature or hungry babies can, with a minimum of schooling, learn to take these substances 2 or even 3 months before the ages stated. Their ability to digest such food is seldom a factor, for it has been demonstrated that newborn or even premature infants can safely manage such foods if they are properly puréed. How necessary nutritionally or desirable psychologically such feeding is remains an unsettled question which requires individual solution.

Regardless of the age at which solid foods are introduced, new mothers (and inexperienced nurses) should be forewarned of the pitfalls that may occur in the process of encouraging a baby to accept new items in the diet. They should realize that *all* babies at first act as though they dislike solids. Some of this behavior is probably due to surprise at the taste and feel of the new foods. Actually the feeder's conclusion is more often due to a misinterpretation of the movements of the baby's tongue. He is attacking the solids in the same way he would milk, but the protrusion of his tongue during the sucking sequence makes it look as though he were attempting to push the food out of his mouth. It is easy for the inexperienced feeder to lose patience and become angry, frustrated or anxious. The result may be forced feeding or resigned defeat. Neither is a good solution to the problem for either the feeder or the fed. Forced feeding leaves the mother feeling inadequate or angry at herself or the baby. The baby cannot help but "catch" the feelings of the adult and may begin to associate the food with them so that subsequent experiences are tension-ridden rather than a gratifying learning experience. Thus mealtime may be converted into a battle of wills which can disrupt a previously pleasant relationship between mother (or nurse) and infant. Abandoning the attempt to introduce the new foods is not a proper solution to the problem either. It leaves the feeder in defeat. A short period of respite from the new foods is apropos, but indefinite postponement only courts nutritional deprivation and solidifies the infant's resistance to change. Repeated gentle persuasion or a shift to a different variety of food will almost always succeed in broaching the initial resistance.

When solid foods are first introduced a hungry baby *expects* milk and *wants* to suck. He may be surprised and disappointed at the taste and feel and wail his displeasure as the food pours out over his chin. Milk responded automatically to his sucking movements and slid back into his pharynx and down his throat without effort. But now he has a new problem. He must learn how to convey the lumpy or pasty material up over the top of his tongue so that it will fall back within reach of the swallowing muscles without stimulating his gagging or cough reflexes. Such a maneuver must be learned, and in the meantime the baby should have the support of a feeder who is prepared to see him through this new experience in a calm and relaxed fashion without introducing the tension of anxiety or frustration which will only aggravate the baby's own disappointment. It may be too much to expect him to accept this new experience with enthusiasm unless his hunger has been at least partially assuaged by some milk from bottle or breast. Eventually he will learn that solids also relieve his hunger, and he may not oppose the idea of beginning his meal with them. The learning process can also be speeded by offering his new foods well diluted with milk in order to make them easier for him to handle mechanically. A small-bowled demitasse spoon will fit the contours of his mouth much better than an adult teaspoon. The type of food offered can also facilitate learning. Many doctors advise starting with fruit because this is universally enjoyed. Once fruit has been established as a desired food, the manipulation of the tongue for other foods is likely to improve. Admixtures of desired fruit and less welcome vegetables or meat may also help to smooth the introduction of new articles into the diet. As soon as the appetite becomes enthusiastic for a variety of new substances, the offerings may be adjusted to conform with the usual food pattern of the household meals—cereal, egg and fruit for breakfast; soups, vegetables, meat and puddings at the midday meal, and a supper adjusted to the individual appetite. During this period of infancy the acceptance of foods is often at its best. It is wise to take advantage of a cosmopolitan appetite and familiarize the infant with as wide a variety of foods as possible. During the second half of the first year he is likely to become more finicky and refuse those foods which have not yet been included in his eating experience.

During the first 6 months of life allowance must be made for some day-by-day variation in food requirements. Unless there are other signs of ill health, periodic deviation from the usually accepted meals need not arouse concern. Growth produces a changing pattern in the requirements not only for sleep but for satisfaction of appetite. The interval between feedings gradually lengthens as more is consumed at each sitting.

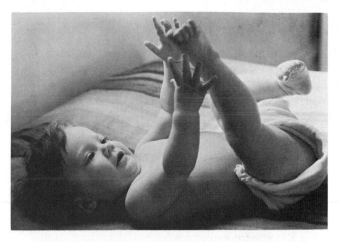

Fig. 12-11. During the first year of life the baby makes important strides in separating himself from his environment and in learning the boundaries of his own body. (Carol Baldwin)

Babies whose individual patterns are respected will usually place themselves on a four-meal-a-day schedule by 4 to 5 months and will shift to a three-meal day sooner than infants who are raised according to a prescribed schedule.

From 3 to 6 Months

This period is marked by explorations into the erect posture, increased facility of the hands, mouth exploration and a growing discrimination in the social sphere. Two of the early reflexes finally disappear during the 5th and 6th months—the TNR position and the Moro response. When pulled up from the supine position the infant's head no longer lags but instead flexes eagerly forward to see where it is going. At the beginning of the period he will enjoy sitting up well-supported, and then toward the end of it he can manage for a short time by himself if propped forward on his arms. When held in the standing position he progresses from an ability to push down with his feet and bear a portion of his weight to a good active bounce or sustained stand. Increasingly his hands reach out for objects, at first only for those within his immediate reach; later, as his binocular vision improves, he goes after things beyond his reach—and with good aim. More and more objects (including his feet) are carried from hand to mouth for tactile exploration. By 6 months he is beginning to show some exuberance and shakes and bangs rattles or other objects which he is holding. He may even begin to transfer them from one hand to another toward the end of the period. He also begins to use his hands singly rather than simultaneously. He can roll over all the way and has learned how to hitch himself backward when sitting. The drooling which began at 3 to 4 months and which his mother took as a sign of impending teething may at last be followed by the eruption of a lower incisor or two. Socially he has become more exuberantly playful but also more touchy and discriminating.

Growth in Perceptual and Intellectual Capacity. This three month period is marked by rapid growth in sensorimotor development under optimum environmental conditions. Visually directed reaching and visual attentiveness herald the beginning of self-initiated intentionality. The infant is now interested in affecting the environment to achieve his aims. He has grown remarkably in his ability to perceive and recognize objects and people, is now capable of adopting the attitude of experimentation and of anticipating the consequences of his own acts. When presented with an unfamiliar object, he may exhibit not only interest, but also lively astonishment. In the beginning of this period, however, when grasping the new object he does not yet attempt to find out in what way it is new but uses it in the same way that is customary for him with familiar objects.

The beginnings of intentionality are usually first seen in attempts to prolong or repeat some interesting phenomenon in the environment. If a small toy is swung in front of the infant's eyes and stopped, he may shake his legs or arms or vocalize in an attempt to regain the interesting swinging motion.

Recognition of familiar objects ushers in the response to strangeness. However, if the new object is not too

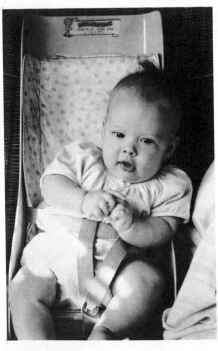

FIG. 12-12. At 3 months short periods of sitting up provide a variety of stimuli. Note the way this baby spots things with her eyes and grasps them with her hands. (Mr. and Mrs. Gene Birchfield)

strange and frightening, he explores it visually and orally and encompasses it into his widening world of recognized objects. During this period, environmental variety and stimulation of the sense organs is of great importance in supporting rapid intellectual development.

The infant is now also capable of coordinating different visual impressions of an object and to recognize it when it is presented to him in another way. He is also learning to differentiate incidental characteristics of an object from those that are essential; he is beginning to be able to recognize his mother when she is dressed differently or puts on glasses.

During the latter portion of this three-month period an important milestone is reached in the baby's construction of reality. Objects begin to acquire permanence beyond his own immediate perception of them. If he drops a toy, he will now search for it for a brief period of time. Although in the beginning the search may be only visual and limited to objects he himself holds, it is active and self-initiated.

The infant's perception of sounds is now also becoming increasingly discriminatory and he shows signs of intentionality and initiative in this sphere also. He becomes aware of the sounds he himself makes and gives indications of interest in them by stopping or reproducing them. Babbling is pleasurable, not only in tension release, but in a sense of mastery in that he is now capable of providing his own sensory stimulation.

Growth in Emotional and Adaptive Capacity. With available surplus energy, the infant's interest in his mother heightens and he rewards bountifully with smiles and playfulness during their experiences together. His father and siblings, too, become more important as they contribute to the expansion of his interests outside himself. So affable, lovable and loving is the baby at this stage of his development that he easily approximates the image his mother probably created in fantasy during her pregnancy.

Signs of the baby's increasing trust and security become manifest during this age period. He can now wait a short while from the first awareness of hunger pains until he makes an imperious demand for food. This power to postpone gratification and handle stress will increase progressively during the first year of life. Some babies acquire this adaptive capacity at a rapid rate, others are slower to develop such inner resources. But all healthy babies will progress gradually in this direction. The speed of adaptation depends on an interaction between the baby's previous experience of consistently given care and the emergence of new skills provided by his developing nervous system.

The baby whose needs have been met promptly during the early months of life does not panic in fear that food and love will not be forthcoming; he trusts. Consequently, he is freed from worry and frustration

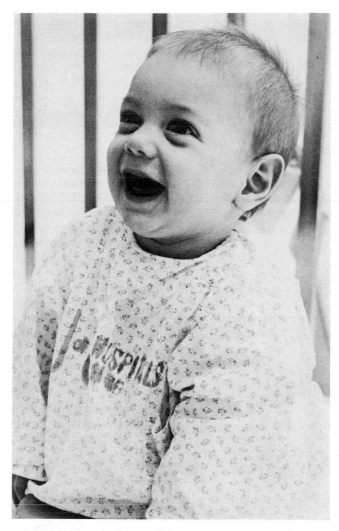

FIG. 12-13. At 6 months the infant sits well and responds to social stimulation with enthusiastic laughter.

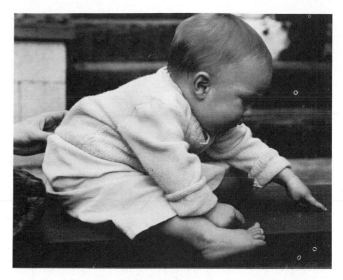

FIG. 12-14. At 9 to 10 months of age the infant can probe with his index finger. (Carol Baldwin)

and instead can devote energy to further self-discovery and socialization. He finds that his ability to wait until his mother is ready to minister to his needs is rewarded by smiles, pleasant-sounding words and an extra hug. This in turn motivates him toward additional experiments in socialization.

As his control of his muscles improves, he acquires new skills and experiences the joy of independent activity which in turn provides adequate substitute satisfactions while he is waiting for his mother to care for him.

The periods of maternal care become playful interludes of socialization. By this age the baby has become so accustomed to the routine procedures of his care that he awaits them with happy expectation, showing his anticipation of pleasure in his behavior. His face lights up, his respirations accelerate and he moves his body toward his mother as she prepares for a feeding. She in turn chats more freely with him

because she is more confident in her ministrations and has observed that he now is more inclined to play. She begins to add many extras to the care procedures just as nurses do when a baby begins to recuperate from his illness. She allows time for visiting as she responds to his innuendoes of coos, gurgles, bubbles and even a well-developed laugh. She recognizes the pleasure that he gains from exercise in the tub and permits time for extra joyous splashes. She permits him to explore her hands, head and chest, his own body and the equipment she uses. Whereas he used to "take in" objects only with his eyes, this is no longer sufficient stimulation. He must pick them up for further exploration with his hands and if possible, put them into his mouth for a complete investigation. Such extras not only provide experiences which lead to a more relaxed mother-child relationship, but also enable the baby to begin to differentiate between his own body and the things of the outside world. In this way the concept of self begins to form.

Through such experiences awareness of self is acquired, and the ego or the "I" of the personality begins to develop. This part of the personality mediates between the instinctual urges (the id) and the demands of the outer world. Later the ego will also have to take into account the demands of the conscience (super ego) which becomes an important part of the personality during the late preschool years.

The ego helps the child to endure increasingly larger doses of frustration, many of which arise from a conflict between his instinctual urges and his mother's expectations. During the first 6 months he does not completely differentiate himself from the outer world, nor does he recognize his mother as a person separate from himself. She is only the aspect of his environment from which he receives his greatest pleasure. She represents to him "the outer world." But the myriad impressions of his outer world which he has been storing up since birth will very shortly

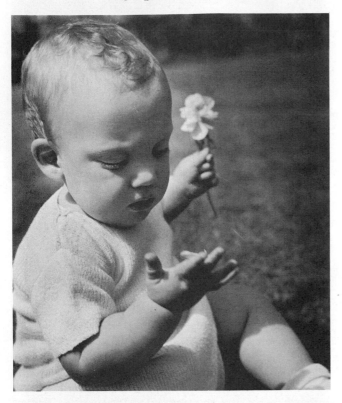

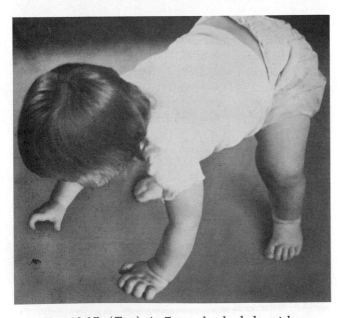

Fig. 12-15. (*Top*) At 7 months the baby picks up an object by placing his palm over it and drawing his fingers around it. (Carol Baldwin) (*Bottom*) At 10 months she is able to pick up small objects with her thumb and index finger.

lead him to discover the difference between this personality—his mother—and the rest of his environment. When he makes this discovery in the coming months, his mother's expectations will become of utmost importance to him. With her help he will learn how to adapt the new capacities of his mind and body to the cultural patterns of his family. Thus his ego grows, and he identifies himself as a separate person.

6 to 9 Months

During this period the infant is improving previously acquired skills. Sitting becomes steadier; he rolls over adeptly; the bouncing stand becomes a steady stand if he has some support. His hand-eye coordination is improving so that he makes few errors in reaching for objects. In the use of a single hand he advances by learning how to release objects at will, watching the effects of gravity on them. He also develops the ability to probe with his index finger and learns to change his method of grasping so that small objects are held with index finger and thumb rather than being scooped with the whole hand. He learns to hold his own bottle and to feed himself with his fingers. His locomotion improves to a crawl in which he at first drags his tummy on the floor and later masters the art of creeping on all fours with his abdomen clear. During the creeping stage he is likely to play with his toes and, if a boy, may begin to tug at his penis and scrotum. This latter behavior will be viewed with alarm by the mother unless she has been forewarned that it is a natural phase of bodily exploration.

Coming to Terms With Reality. The infant's beginning awareness of the environment as separate from himself grows apace during this period. Recognition of the existence of objects outside himself is shown by the active exploratory search for lost objects outside his perceptual field. By 9 months of age, he may turn over a cushion to look for a hidden object, though his conception of the object continues to lack unity: to him the object may have several identities and reside in several places.

During this growing realization of "what is me" and "what is not me" through the manipulation of objects, the infant also begins to acquire a rudimentary sense of space and depth. He shows appreciation for what is within his grasp and what is far away for him to reach. When placed on a table, he indicates fear of the edges, though he must be watched carefully, for he is now exploring actively and can move himself toward objects of interest. Although the sense of time is still vague, there is a dawning appreciation of sequences of events as his ability to remember for brief periods of time becomes more clear.

The beginning of imitation (and of later identification) which is destined to play such an important role in emotional development is now emerging with growing playfulness. In attempts to recapture a plea-

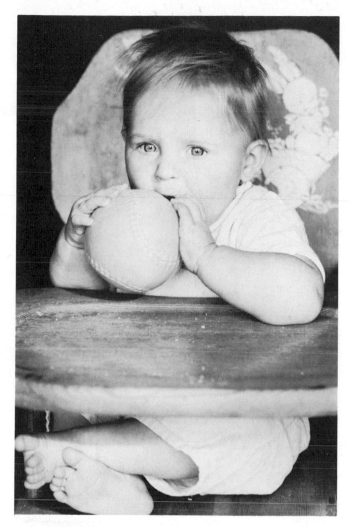

FIG. 12-16. Through manipulation and tasting of objects the baby comes to terms with reality. (Carol Baldwin)

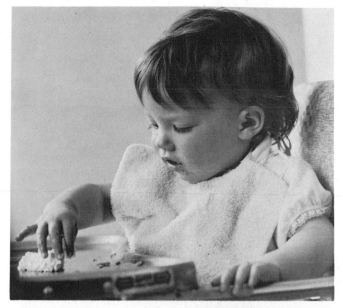

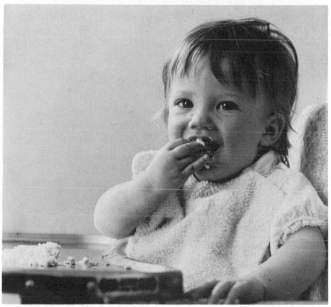

FIG. 12-17. Enjoyment in eating is increased when the baby is permitted to finger feed himself, even though his face becomes smeared. (Carol Baldwin)

surable act on the part of another, such as singing or whistling, the infant may make imitative efforts. Such goal-directed action also indicates the beginning of a sense of causality, though still rudimentary, and of the differentiation of means from end in intentionality. This can be demonstrated by placing an obstacle between an infant and a desired toy; in order to obtain the toy, he will push away the obstacle.

With growing interaction with his environment, the infant now shows a lively interest and curiosity about his new world. The novel can be absorbing, and play for the sheer pleasure of the activity is of increasing importance.

Oral Aggressiveness. With the beginnings of a sense of self, the baby no longer passively receives his environment, but actively meets it, grasps it and attempts to incorporate it by biting and mouthing. He tackles his problems aggressively and is determined about his actions. This new aggressiveness is not hostile, but

is constructive and directed toward the eventual learning of technics of self-sufficient living which will be necessary at a later age.

This period of aggressive activity may be distressing to the mother who places a high premium on tidiness or values passive dependence. Attempts at preventing mouthing or biting merely set the stage for rebellion, for the impulse is intense. Biting relieves uncomfortable gum tension and provides information by which the infant differentiates himself from the environment. Frustration for both mother and baby can be avoided by provision of chewable objects.

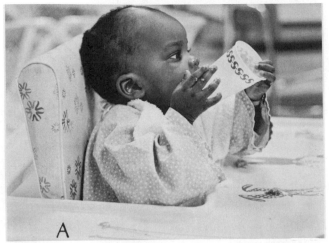

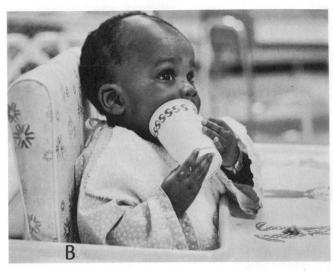

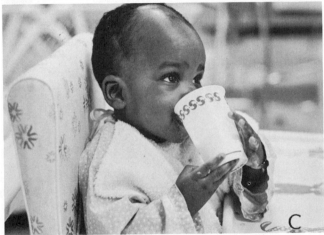

Fig. 12-18. *A*, Exploration of cup feeding—trial. *B*, Exploration of cup feeding—error. *C*, Exploration of cup feeding—success.

Dietary Changes—From Soup to Steak. The process of introducing chewy foods is simple if the infant's interest is exploited during the biting stage. Foods such as zweibach, teething biscuits, toast and celery will be welcomed and a shift to chopped foods can be instituted. He may initially spit out foods that he is sampling, but will gradually discover the pleasure of chewing. Much of this chewing will be done with his gums, and even before his teeth are fully erupted, he can make the transition to table foods.

Fingers Were Made Before Forks. Permission for the baby to use his hands in feeding himself facilitates acceptance of new foods and supports learning about his environment with all of his senses. Placing bite-sized pieces of food within his reach encourages such research. He may initially investigate the food orally, remove it from his mouth to study it visually or smear it over his tray, but if his mother can tolerate his play with food, it will encourage an important step in the process of self-feeding. The early stages, during which food is smeared on the face, hair, clothing and floor can be a trial to mothers who value cleanliness and table manners, but it is an important activity for the baby and if thwarted, will cause rebellion and decrease his opportunities for learning.

The permission to satisfy desires for exploration with food encourages curiosity and strivings toward independence and is a natural prelude to the use of cup and spoon. Skills acquired from finger-feeding are easily transferred to the mealtime tools. However, the infant will need time to study the implements, to investigate them and to play with them before using them to convey food to his mouth. He should not be hurried, for when he has investigated them thoroughly, he will be ready to imitate his parents and siblings in their use of the implements. If allowed free exploration, mastery in the use of the cup is usually achieved by the end of the first year and skill with the spoon before the middle of the second year.

Increased Attachment to Mother. The second half of the first year, the infant is no longer promiscuous in his passive acceptance of attention from other people; he is becoming increasingly selective, active and demanding of his mother's attention. He may now show anxiety when confronted by strangers, reject their advances and protest when his mother leaves his visual field. This rejection of others may be distressing to mothers and seem like regression in social responsiveness. Such a change in behavior, however, is a sign of normal development and of intellectual and emotional growth. It indicates that he has made great progress in differentiating himself from his mother, he begins to recognize her as a separate person and to realize his need for her. Where formerly the satisfaction of his bodily needs was more important than the person who served him, he now indicates awareness of the importance of his mother for her own sake. Her mere presence is pleasurable and loss of her, even for a moment, is a threat to which he reacts violently. The routines of going to bed may no longer be pleasurable because of his fear of separation and his daytime clinging and shyness of strangers may increase and persist in varying degrees throughout the toddler stage of development.

Children at this stage must be given time to observe strangers and to initiate new relationships. Abrupt approach by others usually provokes a negative response, but if they are given time, they will usually initiate investigative advances. If the mother is present (obviating the fear of losing her) the baby will be less fearful. Nurses who are first assigned to the care of a baby of this age will improve their chances for establishing a relationship if they arrange for time with mother and baby.

This manifestation of growth in the intellectual and emotional spheres has been termed "eight month anxiety" and considered the earliest manifestation of anxiety proper—a prototype for all later anxiety.* It indicates that the infant has differentiated a sense of *feeling*, memory for previous pleasure and unpleasure, advancement in perception and object relations and ego function on a higher plane than formerly. With recognition of the mother as separate from himself, the groundwork is laid for later identification.

The manner in which this critical period of development is handled is of great importance for further intellectual and emotional growth. Mothers may need reassurance of its normalcy and support in their efforts to understand their infants' reactions and to tolerate the discomfort and embarrassment resulting from this behavior. With such understanding, the mother can assist her infant in collection of his internal resources and controls which will eventually permit him to master separations for brief periods of time, though such inner strengths are not well developed until he is over 3 years of age.

Such support in strengthening of the infant's ego depends on the degree of his attachment to his mother and his interest in pleasing her. In circumstances and cultures where the mother-infant relationship is less close, lesser degrees of anxiety on separation will be noted. It is through the growing drive to please his mother that he will gradually learn to overcome infantile impulses, tolerate frustration and redirect aggression into socially approved and satisfying channels. As he grows in independence he will be increasingly able to welcome broader social experiences. By three years of age most children can make a comfortable adjustment to nursery or play school if their mothers are close by during the period of acquaintance with the new environment and with those in charge.

The Effects of Prolonged Maternal Deprivation. The damaging effect of prolonged lack of adequate mothering to the infant during this critical period of psychosocial and intellectual development has been a

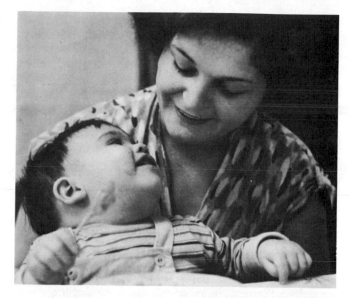

FIG. 12-19. The baby's relationship with his mother is strengthened when he is permitted to do those things he is capable of doing. (Infant Welfare Society of Chicago)

subject of great interest and of many significant studies. In 1948, John Bowlby studied the needs of infants separated from their families.† The results of his investigation stimulated much following research as to the conditions under which developmental retardation can occur.

Differences of opinion about the results of many of these studies stem from varying viewpoints and theories of child development and from attendant convictions regarding the important factors in the child's environment which affect developmental progress. Such studies are beset with methodologic difficulties which result in different interpretations of results. Confusion also arises from inexactness of terminology and from the complexity of circumstances usually associated with separation of the infant from his mother. The overwhelming majority of studies, however, point up the damaging effects to the infant in motor, intellectual and emotional development which result from separation from the mother during the early years of life.

The term "maternal deprivation" is used to denote circumstances during which an infant is deprived of the opportunity of forming an initial tie with a mother figure, it also implies deprivation of the mother figure after a meaningful tie has been formed. Deprivation of mothering may also occur without physical separation whenever the mother is emotionally or physically incapable of providing continuity of loving care and security for the child. The extent of intellectual, motor and psychological damage sustained under all condi-

* Spitz, Rene A.: The First Year of Life, Int. Universities Press, N.Y., 1965.

† Bowlby, John: Maternal Care and Mental Health, Geneva, World Health Organization, Monograph Series #2, 1951.

tions depends on the degree of emotional and sensory deprivation experienced, the stage of development of the child when it occurs, constitutional determinants, the quality of the relationship with the mother prior to separation and the concomitant accessory circumstances during the period of separation. The longer the separation and the more inadequate the substitute mothering and intellectual stimulation, the worse are the results.

A study by Spitz and Wolf was one of the earliest of research observations of infants separated from their mothers between the ages of 6 and 8 months. All of these infants had had healthy relationships with their mothers and were later given little substitute mothering or stimulation. Within a brief period of time, they became progressively more apprehensive, withdrawn, anorexic, grief stricken and unresponsive to play materials or to people who approached them. These symptoms were accompanied by physical deterioration, a drop in developmental quotient and progression in severity of the disturbance to the point of death. Spitz and Wolf termed this syndrome "anaclitic depression" and concluded that unless the separated infant was returned to his mother within five months, irreparable damage would occur.[*] They later hypothesized that recovery may be possible if the infants are reunited with their mothers within three months.

This pioneering study which provided needed clinical data was followed by much definitive and statistical investigation during the following two decades and many of the variables and relationships are now being clarified. During a study of the behavioral development of infants in several institutions in Iran, Dennis found extreme motor retardation among children who received paucity of handling. He concluded that the retardation was due to restrictions of specific kinds of learning opportunities.[†] Other studies also indicated that those separated infants who were provided with adequate mother substitutes and stimulation did not show the extremes in developmental retardation. Another factor found to be highly significant was the quality of the mother-infant relationship prior to separation. Among those infants who had tenuous ties with a mother figure, less overt emotional disturbance was noted, although overall developmental progress was retarded.

Bakwin found important effects on children of an even younger age from deprivation of maternal care. His observations are summarized as follows:

Infants under 6 months of age who have been in an institution for some time present a well-defined picture. The outstanding features are listlessness, emaciation and pallor, relative immobility, quietness, unresponsiveness to stimuli like a smile or a coo, indifferent appetite, failure to gain weight properly despite diets which, in the home, are entirely adequate, frequent stools, poor sleep, an appearance of unhappiness, proneness to febrile episodes, absence of sucking habits.[‡]

Studies by Yarrow and Goodwin[§] also indicate that reactions to separation from the mother may occur as early as 3 months of age, while disturbances of social responsiveness, excessive clinging or rejection of a substitute mother may occur increasingly after the infant is 6 months of age. These findings suggest the importance of the total environmental alterations usually involved with separation, including patterns of social and sensory stimulation which the infant had previously received.

Such findings emphasize that separation from the mother during the period when the child's dependence on her for both emotional and intellectual growth is greatest can damage personality development, retard intellectual progress and may cripple potentials for forming and maintaining later relationships. Vulnerability to such maternal deprivation decreases to some extent after the age of 3 to 5 years. The child who has had continuity of warm maternal care prior to this age has begun to acquire inner resources that help him to adapt to situations of moderate stress. After the age of 3 to 5 years most emotionally healthy children can maintain a relationship with their mothers *in absentia*, if they are prepared for the experience, if their main care is served by persons who understand their physical and psychological needs and if they are able to keep in touch with their mothers by frequent visiting.

Such findings also emphasize the desirability of making it possible for mothers to room-in with their sick children or to visit them as much as possible. Also implied is the young child's need for continuity of relationship with a nurse who can accept his responses to loss when he is separated from his mother and who can provide emotional gratification and necessary sensory stimulation.

The section below is concerned primarily with guidance of mothers who have babies at home. However, many of the suggestions advanced will also be useful to the nurse in the hospital as she serves as an extension of the mother when the latter is away from the ward. When a nurse repeatedly succeeds in alleviating a baby's physical and emotional distress, she may find that his anxiety on separation from her is even more intense than that displayed when he first lost his mother on the day of admission to the hospital.

* Spitz, Rene and Wolf, K. M.: Anaclitic depression: an inquiry into the genesis of psychiatric conditions in early childhood, *in* The Psychoanalytic Study of the Child, 2:213, New York, Int. U. Press, 1947.

† Dennis, Wayne: Causes of Retardation among institutional children: Iran, J. Genet. Psychol. *96,* 47, 1960.

‡ Bakwin, Harry: Emotional deprivation of infants, J. Pediat. 35:512, 1949.

§ Yarrow, L. J. and Goodwin, M. S.: Effects of change in mother figure during infancy on personality and development, Progress Report, 1963. Family and Child Services, Washington, D.C.

Having lived through one separation, the threat of a second loss of a person upon whom he has become dependent is terrifying.

Maternal Attitudes Toward Separation Anxiety. The skill which a mother can exert in helping her infant to sustain his trust during this period of his life is of great importance.

If she can give him both adequate reassurance to relieve his anxiety when separated from her, and freedom to develop his own independence, his trust in himself and others will be reaffirmed, making him more capable of solving the problems of later childhood and adult life. Lacking such assets he may not be able to reach his full potential in intellectual development or deal adequately with the interpersonal relationships which he must face.

The infant's first step in overcoming separation anxiety is to acquire the concept that his mother exists in substance even though he cannot see her at the moment. This is no easy hurdle for the small baby, but the concept must be grasped and integrated into his personality before he can bring his anxiety under control. Many months of exploration backed by warm maternal reassurance are needed before success is achieved. Many of the problems of bedtime and night-waking are related to the infant's struggle to master this concept.

Much of the infant's play during these months is more than random activity directed toward learning to crawl, walk and manipulate objects. Repeatedly he can be seen to search for solutions to the problem of disappearance and return of the important persons in his life—his father and siblings to a degree, but primarily the main object of his love, his mother. He devises innumerable games and repeats them again and again in his effort to master the fear of her loss and to gain trust in her return. He plays peek-a-boo with diapers, towels, shower curtains and clothing. With a solemn countenance he covers his face and then bursts into gales of laughter when he removes the drape and brings his mother back into view. He shuts and opens doors repeatedly, following the same principle. He revels in hiding things in paper bags, boxes and purses and then finding them again. One of his favorite pastimes is playing hiding games with his mother. Invariably the rediscovery of the object is the part of the game which evokes the most pleasurable response. Thus, through his own powers he learns to control the disappearance and reappearance of the objects and begins to overcome his anxiety. Through his own creation of games he converts what might be a frightening situation of real life into a joyful, fear-releasing pastime.

The mother can help the baby to understand that her absence does not indicate that she is completely gone out of his life if she provides support when he needs it and continues to be in range of vision or voice until he builds up sufficient tolerance

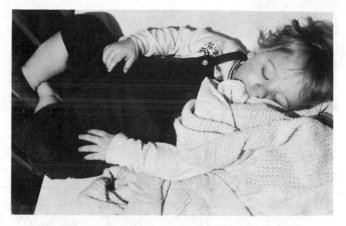

Fig. 12-20. Close contact with a "security blanket" decreases separation anxiety and fosters peaceful sleep.

to permit separation. He must have freedom to reach her when he needs reassurance and freedom to depart when he feels more powerful. Infants who are confined to a bed or playpen for hours on end have insufficient opportunity to do either. The infant who is confident of being able to go to his mother when necessary can enjoy much more liberty to explore the world about him and otherwise acquire increased independence. As he builds up confidence he voluntarily prolongs the periods of separation and begins to accept care from other familiar persons, provided that he is in surroundings that he has already explored.

Failure to give the infant opportunities to develop his own methods of dealing with anxiety is just as depriving as too much separation. "Spoiling" results when the mother is so frightened by her infant's changing behavior that she feels obliged to stay with him and pacify him constantly. The infant's fear of separation then becomes reinforced, and he derives no encouragement to move on to the next stage of development.

Fear of separation becomes most intense at bedtime and frequently produces a trying end to a difficult day. Often it is most convenient for the mother to settle the disturbance by yielding to the infant's demands for rocking, food or even companionship in bed. However, settling him down by such methods has the disadvantage that it tends to acknowledge that his fear of separation is justified and gives him no aid in dealing with it. It is preferable for the mother to take a sympathetic but firm attitude which permits him to express his displeasure but insists that there is nothing to be feared from bed, the dark or separation. If necessary the child can be held in his usual sleeping position until he calms down. Caressing him or singing to him while he is held may help to communicate that the restraint is offered as help rather than as punishment. If such assistance is pleasant but firm it may take many minutes or even an hour at first,

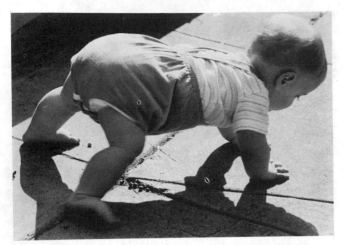

FIG. 12-21. At 10 months the baby delights in moving about on all fours. (Carol Baldwin)

but on subsequent evenings as the infant becomes convinced of the outcome, the time interval is likely to shorten.

If the mother can be available to the infant when he first wakens, he will eventually anticipate this pleasure and the sleep period will be associated with the *return* of his mother rather than her disappearance. It is rewarding when the child's behavior changes to indicate that he is no longer afraid of going to bed and that he has accepted the mother's controls and reassurance which help him to relax by himself.

Night-waking is another manifestation of separation anxiety which requires judicious handling. The first step is to test the child's ability to control his anxiety by himself. Many times the crying will subside without intervention of parents. However, if it persists and indicates that the infant is terrified, reassurance and comfort must be given. Often a familiar voice and a gentle pat will suffice to get him back to sleep. Sometimes it is necessary to remove wet diapers. Taking the child out of bed is generally contraindicated unless he is in a panic or is ill. Particularly unfortunate is the practice of taking the child into bed with one or both parents. This solves nothing. It only makes the night-waking more attractive to the child, who persistently converts it into a nuisance for the parents. It becomes a detour in the infant's progress toward independence.

9 to 12 Months

During the last part of his first year the infant begins the last stage in his transformation from the sessile helplessness of the newborn to self-propulsion with all its attendant privileges and dangers. He no longer likes to lie down unless he is exhausted, but spends his day sitting or moving around on all fours. By 10 months he is standing with help and may even be pulling himself up into that position unaided. By a year he is likely to be standing alone and beginning to walk with his mother's help or by moving along furniture. As he adopts the erect posture, his straight back acquires the normal lumbar curve. His mother also begins to see him from a new angle. The previously unnoticed bowing of his legs and turning of his feet become items of concern in spite of the fact that they are normal for the infant who is just learning to walk. Toward the first birthday the baby may master the trick of getting down from the standing position to a sit without an uncomfortable thump. The

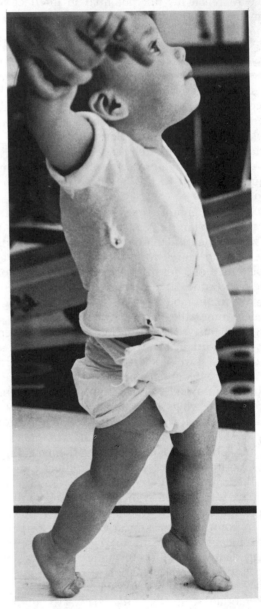

FIG. 12-22. At 12 months, or even earlier, the first enthusiastic efforts in walking are made on tip toe and require assistance in maintaining balance.

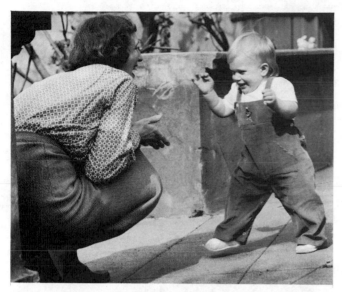

FIG. 12-23. Illustrating the joy aroused in learning to walk and the pleasure the baby gets when his accomplishments make his mother proud of him. (Carol Baldwin)

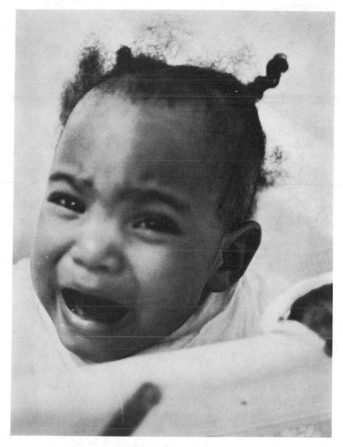

FIG. 12-24. The year-old child who is learning to walk finds long periods of confinement to the playpen frustrating.

use of the hands is more skillful so that he can pick up the tiniest of objects and, unfortunately, potentially dangerous foreign bodies that do not belong in his mouth. His language comprehension has improved so that he recognizes his own name, responds to the word "No" and may also obey his mother occasionally. He also begins to cooperate in getting dressed by raising a foot for a stocking, for example.

On the Go. At this age, the baby experiences a powerful, relentless urge to control his body and get it into the upright position. Nothing deters the normal infant from practice which will eventually lead to the skills of walking and climbing. He accepts bruises, bumps and frightening objects which he pulls over on himself but returns to the effort. He may get into precarious positions; far from deterring him, these accidents seem to spur him on to renewed efforts.

Each new skill in locomotion increases his independence and confronts him with new challenges and dangers. His energy is derived from a compelling biologic urge toward the pursuit of newly acquired goals since he is no longer solely interested in the satisfaction of bodily needs. When he succeeds in achieving a goal, he experiences joy, not only of the activity itself, but also of mastering his fear of it.

Babies and toddlers vigorously resent confinement in playpens, high chairs or beds. Even when ill or hospitalized, unless seriously debilitated, their drive toward mastery of their bodies and world continues. In some cases, this drive may be accentuated in an attempt to overcome the fears associated with removal from home and with the fear-provoking atmosphere of the hospital. The unfamiliar sights and sounds and the painful procedures to which they are subjected give rise to fears which cry out for mastery through exploration of danger. Thus children who must be restrained or isolated during illness are thwarted in pursuit of personal goals and can be expected to react aggressively. Although treatments and tests must be performed, permission should also be granted for protest and for whatever freedom is safe within the hospital environment.

Are Restrictions Necessary? As the baby becomes capable of locomotion and of exploration of his new world, his relationship with his mother is likely to be threatened if he is constantly thwarted. A wise and understanding mother or nurse will respect the baby's need for exercise and freedom to experience his world and satisfy his curiosity. Although dangerous and valuable objects must be removed from his reach, such control should be done in a consistent and understanding manner in order to assist the child to learn self-restraint and to endure frustration.

Prolonged confinement in playpens may protect the decor of the home and keep the child within range of constant surveillance, but it also limits learning opportunities and depresses curiosity. It further suggests to the child that his mother is restrictive and

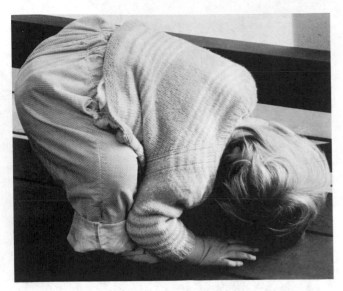

FIG. 12-25. Toward the end of the first year of life, babies enjoy and learn from observing the world from different viewpoints. (Carol Baldwin)

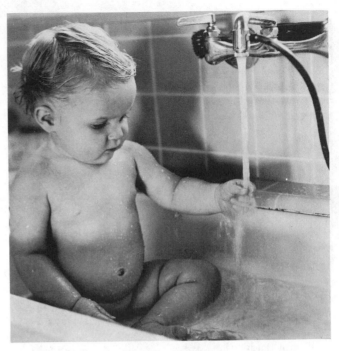

FIG. 12-26. During her bath, the baby enjoys learning some of the characteristics of running water. (Carol Baldwin)

dominating in her control and fosters rebellion and conflict between his dual urges toward exploration and toward maintaining his mother's approval.

Curiosity and Learning. Close to the end of the first year, the child makes tremendous strides in learning due to his new ability to approach objects of interest and to view them from various angles, spurred on by his intense curiosity. He has a growing interest in novelty, in manipulation and a fascination with the movements he can produce. He is ceaseless in his efforts to learn all he can about his new sphere, and any object he encounters stimulates him to use all of his sense organs in the manipulation. He feels, pushes, pulls, overturns, tastes, bites, smells and tests each object to see if it will produce a sound. Banging thrills him both because of the noise it produces and because it makes him feel powerful. Any new object is fascinating and he is not easily diverted from his learning. As Fraiberg says:

The baby is in love with the world he has discovered through his mother's love, and he behaves like those intoxicated lovers in song and verse who find that the whole world has been transformed through love and the most common objects are infused with beauty [and therefore greatly desired].*

Motivated by an insatiable curiosity, the child's elaboration of reality becomes sharper and his relationship with the environment is ever changing. Through interest in objects, in dropping and throwing them, space, time and causality begin to have more objectivity. Manipulation of objects leads to discovery

* Fraiberg, Selma: The Magic Years, Charles Scribner's Sons p. 55, N.Y., 1959.

of their properties and of their continued existence when removed from sight. The variety and richness of objects available to him stimulates a heightened curiosity and the drive to experience and to assimilate ever new and expanded aspects of his environment. It is through this relationship that the stimulation received during the first years of life has an enduring effect upon later developmental progress.

With the freedom to manipulate objects, the child now begins to evidence signs of active experimentation. He will attempt various approaches in drawing an object within range of his reach and eliminate unsuccessful methods. With each experimentation, discovery of the correct procedure becomes more rapid.

This attitude of experimentation also extends to the now rapidly expanding sphere of speech development. From the age of 6 to 7 months, the infant has been babbling and playing with sounds. At approximately the age of 9 months he can respond to speech and simple commands. From that time he begins to imitate sounds and at the age of 11 to 12 months, pseudo-words appear. Experimentation with pseudo-words is of consuming interest and pleasure as he is rewarded by the response he receives from his mother, father and siblings. These pseudo-words usually consist initially of a consonant with one vowel (ba, da, ma) but they are the forerunners of later jargon and eventual reliable use of language.

The Weaning Process. During the period of early infancy, emphasis has been placed on the necessity to satisfy bodily needs and to provide pleasure in order to engender trust which will be needed to overcome the inevitable obstacles in future development. During the latter part of the first year, however, the environment and culture begin to exert demands on the infant. One of the first of these is the weaning process. The principles involved have general application to other aspects of the infant's developmental growth.

Prolonged continuation of permissiveness can be damaging in that it does not promote independence or the learning of tolerance for frustration. It is important to assist the child to dispense with infantile behavior and to achieve increasing independence when readiness is demonstrated.

The propitious moment of readiness is individual, and although guidelines can be given, the mother or nurse will need to be sensitive to the individual child's behavior in order to recognize the signs of readiness to dispense with former comforts and to find pleasure in new achievements. Judgment is necessary to avoid undue fostering of dependence or premature expectations for more mature behavior. If the child's resistance to a new demand is intense, the issue should be dropped for a time rather than insisting upon submissive defeat.

PREPARATION FOR WEANING. With increasing mastery of his body and of independent activity, the child will show signs of readiness for weaning by shortening the nursing time, by struggling when held or by seeking to hold the bottle himself. At this time introduction to cup feeding may be rewarding as an acquisition of a new skill which merits mother's approval. With gradual practice, the cup will become an acceptable substitute for the bottle or breast.

WEANING SHOULD BE GRADUAL. As the infant demonstrates his ability and willingness to receive increasing amounts of milk from the cup, the bottle or the breast can gradually be eliminated, feeding by feeding. The process must not be hurried to the point where milk intake is insufficient or the baby shows resentment at being denied sucking on the nipple. Usually the evening feedings are the most difficult to shift because the infant is tired and more in need of his old-fashioned sucking comforts. However, not all babies retain the evening bottle longest. Some need a bottle to get them started on the new day.

The speed of weaning must be suited to a particular infant's indications and not forced according to an arbitrary schedule. If the process is gradual and pleasant, many babies will be able to achieve exclusive use of a cup by the end of the first year and retain the sense of adventure and pleasure in progress and mastery. In some, however, the sucking impulse is so strong that they are not willing to forego a bedtime bottle until well into the second year. Gradual substitution of an alternative method of gratification will usually help them to give up this symbol of a happy past.

Once weaning is achieved in a satisfactory manner, it marks the decline of the earliest stage of psychosocial development, characterized by complete dependence, impulsive demands and the need for oral gratification and physical closeness to the mother.

PREVENTING TRAUMA DURING ILLNESS. During illness the infant has a decreased store of energy with which to approach new feeding experiences. For the breast-fed baby, the separation necessitated by hospitalization is particularly painful, since he not only loses his mother but must in addition learn a new method of feeding. Whenever possible the mother should be encouraged to remain with her breast-fed infant during the crisis of illness. When this cannot be done, substitute, consistent mothering is imperative to help him to adapt to his new surroundings, foods and method of feeding.

Illnesses which prohibit the use of oral feedings arouse anxiety in the small infant and he requires additional mothering. Unless contraindicated by the physical condition, the use of a pacifier is desirable as a partial substitute for the missing oral gratification. The danger of air-swallowing from the use of a pacifier is greatly overemphasized. As a matter of fact, the frustrated infant who is screaming his displeasure is much more likely to gulp large quantities of air into his stomach than is the infant who is quietly nursing a pacifier.

During illness the infant who has already made progress toward cup feeding may retrogress temporarily and show his desire to suck again by turning away from proffered cup feedings. Until he begins to recover physically, his request for bottle feedings should be honored. During convalescence his readiness to resume the weaning process can be gently tested periodically. Such progress is best fostered by the same nurse rather than by a series of nurses. Only with continuity of care is the infant likely to have a sufficient incentive for growth.

SITUATIONS FOR FURTHER STUDY

1. Why is an infant's proportionate need for water intake greater than that of the older child?

2. What is the infant's daily water requirement? His daily basal energy requirement?

3. Why is protein so essential in the infant's diet? What is his protein requirement?

4. What changes must be made in the infant's diet before he is 4 months of age and why are they necessary?

5. How do early feeding experiences affect appetite?

6. Babies are often in hospitals for many months during the period when they would normally be introduced to junior and table foods. Yet they are kept on "baby soft" diets which customarily consist of puréed foods. If you were caring for a 10-month-old

baby with a tuberculous gland of the groin, how would you go about helping him to make the transition from a baby soft to a "regular" or "house" diet? Select a baby in the ward who needs a change in his dietary regimen and record your experiences in helping him to become accustomed to you and the food you present.

7. If you were a public health nurse and encountered a lower-class English-speaking mother who had given her 6-month-old baby nothing but breast feedings and vitamins, how would you react? If she said she had offered rice and sweet potatoes at 4 months and "he didn't like them," how would you proceed from there? What values might she have to which you could appeal in motivating her to see her baby's need for supplements in his diet?

8. After providing daily periods of nursing care to a 1-year-old baby begin to contrast his response to your leave-taking now with that observed when you first began caring for him. Record the changes that you note in his behavior from day to day and discuss your methods of handling them.

9. John was 11 months old when he was admitted to the hospital for repair of an inguinal hernia. What behavior would you expect to see in the hours immediately following his mother's leave-taking on the day of admission to the hospital? What nursing care would you anticipate that he needed? How do you imagine he would respond to his mother when she arrived on the following day? If John is her only child, what help would you give his mother so that she would be able to supply the warmth he needs to maintain his trust in her?

10. Read the case of Carol on pages 79-83 in Fraiberg, *The Magic Years*, to learn the cause of her sleep problem and the way in which her mother helped her to overcome her fear. What did you learn that can be applied in the provision of nursing care to hospitalized infants? Study an infant between 9 and 12 months who repeatedly awakens from naps shrieking and is difficult to pacify. Record your observations of his behavior on several such occasions and discuss any change that you noted in his response to you and the things that you did to help him reestablish his equilibrium.

11. Read the case of Barbara in *The Magic Years*, pages 89-91. What was the purpose of Barbara's behavior in the playroom? How did she communicate her problem? How had she acquired rigid inhibition of her impulses to explore? Does this case help you to see the connection between freedom to explore and success in learning at school? What were the results of Barbara's rearing on her intellectual and emotional growth? What principles of guiding the exploring baby does Fraiberg advance? On what theory of child development does she base her recommendation? What did you learn from reading which can be applied in the nursing care of hospitalized infants?

12. Read the article by McDowell. What do you think of the statement: "In many cases thumbsuckers seem to be born not made." On what findings did the writer base her statement? What findings does the author give concerning the effects of thumbsucking in the production of a faulty bite? How might a dentist aid a child in becoming interested in overcoming thumb-sucking?

13. Read the article by Bernath. How does she explain the fact that it is hard to spoil a baby? Discuss the ways in which you agree and disagree with the author. Mrs. Jones brought 1-year-old Gina into the outpatient clinic one week after she had been hospitalized with pneumonia for two weeks. After greeting the clinic nurses she said, "Gina is so different from what she was before she was sick. I think the nurses spoiled her." If Mrs. Jones had said this to you and you had been the nurse who had cared for her during the day hours, how do you think you might have felt? What might have caused the change in Gina's behavior? How would you have handled this situation with the mother? If you tried to hold Gina and she clung more tightly to her mother, how do you imagine you would respond? What do you think this behavior indicates?

14. Mrs. Hayes, mother of 7-month-old Regi, was upset because his appetite was declining considerably. She said she felt tied down and was considering returning to work. "He gets my mind upset," she said as she put her hands at her temples and looked as if she felt unusually anxious. During the first six months of her baby's life, she was generally composed and seemed to take the care of her baby in her stride. Now, however, she was obviously upset to the extent that she contemplated taking flight from some of her responsibilities. What might have been the cause of this change in feeling about mothering? How would you handle such a situation if you were a public health nurse?

15. Place an 8-month-old baby in a "baby tender" and put a series of toys before him and observe his behavior with each one. Record each gesture he used from the time you were in the process of placing the toy beside him and the time you put it within the box beside you. List the different gestures he used in examining it.

BIBLIOGRAPHY

Bakwin, H.: Emotional deprivation in infants, J. Pediat. 35: 512, 1949.

Bernath, M.: Babies are hard to spoil, Parents' Magazine 37:48, 1962.

Bettleheim, B.: The Children of the Dream, Macmillan Co., Collier-Macmillan, Canada Ltd., Toronto, Ontario, 1969.

Bowlby, J.: Maternal Care and Mental Health, Geneva, World Health Organization, 1951.

————: Separation anxiety, Internat. J. Psycho-Analysis *41*:89, 1960.

————: Grief and mourning in infancy and early childhood, The Psychoanalytic Study of the Child *15*:9, 1960.

————: Separation anxiety: A critical review of the literature, J. Child Psychol. & Psychiat. *1*:251, 1960.

Bronson, G.: The development of fear in man and other animals, Child Dev. *39*:409, 1968.

Casler, L.: Maternal Deprivation: A Critical Review of the Literature, Monogr. Soc. Res. Child Development, 1961, No. 26.

Dennis, W.: Causes of retardation among institutionalized children: Iran, J. Genet. Psychol. *96*:47, 1960.

Eichorn, Dorothy: Biological Correlates of Behavior, *in* Child Psychology, Stevenson, H. (ed.), Univ. Chicago Press, 1963.

Erikson, E. H.: Childhood and Society, New York, W. W. Norton Co., 1963.

Fraiberg, S.: The Magic Years, New York, Charles Scribner's Sons, 1959.

Goldberg, S., and Lewis, M.: Play behavior in the year-old infant: early sex differences, Child Dev. *40*:21, 1969.

Hunt, J. McV.: Intelligence and Experience, N. Y., Ronald, 1961.

Josselyn, I. M.: The Happy Child, New York, Random, 1955.

Kidd, A. H., and Rivoire, J. (eds.): Perceptual Development in Children, N. Y., Internat. Univ. Press, 1966.

Kohen-Raz, R.: Mental and motor development of Kibbutz, institutionalized, and home-reared infants in Isarel, Child Dev. *39*:488, 1968.

Levy, D. M.: Experiments on the sucking reflex and social behavior of dogs, Am. J. Orthopsychiat. *4*:203, 1934.

McDowell, M. S.: Don't worry about thumbsucking, Parents' Magazine *35*:50, 1960.

McGrade, B.: Newborn activity and emotional response at eight months, Child Dev. *39*:1246, 1968.

Moss, H., and Robson, K.: Maternal influences in early social visual behavior, Child Dev. *39*:401, 1968.

Piaget, J.: The Origins of Intelligence in Children, N. Y., Internat. Univ. Press, 1965.

Provence, S., and Ritto, S.: Effects of Deprivation on Institutionalized Infants: Disturbances in Development of Relationship to Inanimate Objects *in* Psychoanalytic Study of the Child, Vol. 16, p. 189, New York, Internat. Univ. Press, 1961.

————: Infants in Institutions, Internat. Univ. Press, N. Y., 1962.

Public Health Papers, No. 14: Deprivation of Maternal Care, A Reassessment of its Effects, World Health Organization, Geneva, 1962.

Recommended dietary allowances, Seventh Revised Edition, 1968. Food and Nutrition Board, National Academy of Sciences, National Research Council, Pub. No. 1694, Washington, D. C.

Rheingold, H. L.: The Effect of Environmental Stimulation Upon Social and Exploratory Behavior in the Human Infant, *in* B. M. Foss (ed.), Determinants of Infant Behavior, N. Y., Wiley, 1961, p. 143-177.

Ribble, M.: The Rights of Infants, New York, Columbia, 1943.

Robson, K., Pedersen, F., and Moss, H.: Developmental observations of diadic gazing in relation to the fear of strangers and social approach behavior, Child Development *40*:619, 1969.

Schaeffer, H. R., and Callendar, W. M.: Psychological effects of hospitalization in infancy, Pediatrics *24*:528, 1959.

Spitz, R.: Anxiety in infancy: A study of its manifestations in the first year of life, Internat. J. Psycho-Analysis *21*:138, 1950.

————: The First Year of Life, N. Y., Internat. Univ. Press, 1965.

————: and Wolf, K. M.: Hospitalism: An Inquiry into the Genesis of Psychiatric Conditions in Early Childhood *in* Psychoanalytic Study of the Child, Vol. 1, New York, Basic Books, Inc., 1945.

Stern, G., and Caldwell, B.: A factor analytic study of the mother-infant dyad, Child Development *40*:163, 1969.

Taylor, A.: Deprived infants: potential for affective adjustment, American Journal of Orthopsychiatry, *38*:825, 1968.

Todd, G., and Palmer, B.: Social reinforcement of infant babbling, Child Dev. *39*:591, 1968.

Tryon, A.: Thumb-sucking and manifest anxiety: a note, Child Dev. *39*:1159, 1968.

Werner, H.: Comparative Psychology of Mental Development, N. Y., Internat. Univ. Press, 1964.

White, B. L., and Held, R.: Plasticity of Sensorimotor Development in the Human Infant, *in* The Causes of Behavior II, Rosenblith, J., and Allinsmith, W. (eds.), Boston, Allyn and Bacon, Inc., 1966.

Whiting, J., and Landauer, T., and Jones, T.: Infantile immunization and adult stature, *39*:59, 1968.

Yarrow, L. J.: Separation from Parents During Early Childhood, *in* Review of Child Development Research, Vol. I, Russell Sage Foundation, N. Y., 1964.

————: and Goodwin, M. S.: Effects of Change of Mother Figure During Infancy on Personality Development, Progress Report, 1963, Family and Child Services, Washington, D. C.

13

Nursing Care of the Infant With Congenital Malformations and Hereditary Disorders

Errors of fetal development that are apparent at birth or create clinical disturbances that require early treatment have been considered in Unit II. Structural aberrations which, although present at birth, cannot be recognized or confirmed until later in the first year are described in this chapter, as are examples of hereditary conditions in which the abnormal genes pervert metabolic processes and gradually lead to clinically recognizable disease. Even at the conclusion of infancy the revelation of congenital and hereditary disease is incomplete, for some malformations (of the heart and the genitourinary tract, for example) are not discovered until the adult years. Similarly, although clearly heritable, diabetes rarely appears during infancy.

Detailed discussion of some of the infantile anomalies and hereditary disorders is postponed to later chapters, where comprehensive consideration is given to the general principles of diagnosis and treatment.

THE GASTROINTESTINAL TRACT

Congenital Hypertrophic Pyloric Stenosis

Hypertrophic pyloric stenosis is commonly classified as a congenital abnormality of the intestinal tract. It is considered here because its late onset places it outside the newborn period and makes it a constant topic of concern whenever an infant's early adjustment is marred by chronic vomiting.

Symptoms. Vomiting is the outstanding symptom. It seldom begins earlier than 2 or 3 weeks or later than 2 months of age. It progresses gradually in frequency and force until most of the ingested food is expelled, often in a projectile manner which carries it over the side of the bed. The vomitus is never bile-stained but may contain mucus or streaks of blood.

The stools usually decrease in size and number. Chronic loss of food results in a decline in the infant's rate of gain in weight until progress ceases and then reverses. The infants are uniformly hungry and chronically so, being willing to eat immediately after vomiting. Dehydration follows the weight loss and may reach life-threatening proportions. Unlike most other types of dehydration, it is associated with alkalosis of the body fluids rather than acidosis. The infants have no fever except during dehydration or intercurrent infection. Pain is not obvious apart from the discomfort of chronic hunger. An observant attendant will often notice upper abdominal distention after feeding within which peristaltic waves can be seen to sweep across the abdomen from left to right, reversing themselves just prior to or during vomiting.

Pyloric stenosis is about three times as common in male infants as it is in females. It appears to involve first-born children primarily and tends to recur within certain families, suggesting a hereditary background. Its incidence among Caucasian infants has been reported as high as 1 in 150 liveborn males. It is uncommon in Negroes.

Pathophysiology. The symptoms are readily understood from the findings at operation or at autopsy. The pyloric canal—the channel through the distal, muscular end of the stomach which conducts food into the duodenum—is greatly narrowed by a combination of muscular hypertrophy, muscular spasm and edema of the mucous membrane within the canal. Behind the obstructed channel the wall of the stomach is thickened owing to hypertrophy caused by its efforts to force material through the narrowed channel. This hypertrophy accounts for the visible abdominal waves and for the ability of the stomach to propel vomitus out of the mouth with some force.

Fig. 13-1. Showing peristaltic waves of pyloric stenosis.

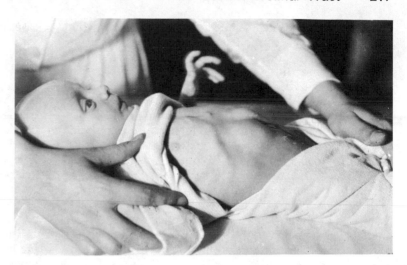

The inability of food to pass readily through the pylorus into the duodenum accounts for the decline in weight and the decrease in volume of stool. Little or no food absorption occurs from the stomach, but some water may be taken up before passage into the duodenum. Thus the malnutrition of these infants is usually more severe than the dehydration. The fluid being lost from the body in the vomitus is primarily acid in character because of the hydrochloric acid in gastric juice. The deficit of acid ions can be compensated by kidneys and lungs for a time, but beyond a certain point the reaction of the blood plasma shifts into the alkaline range.

Diagnosis. The diagnosis can be suspected from the history which is usually typical in respect to the age of onset, the character of the vomiting and its progressive course. In addition, the infants have a characteristic hungry, pinched, anxious facies which experienced nurses soon learn to identify. Observation of peristaltic abdominal waves is possible in advanced cases, and a skilled clinician can frequently feel the hypertrophied pyloric muscle through the abdominal wall. Changes in the chemical anatomy of the blood will often demonstrate the loss of chloride and help to indicate the severity of the disturbance. Final proof of the diagnosis may be obtained by roentgen examination with barium. Enlargement of the stomach, delay in passage of the barium into the duodenum, a narrowed, elongated and curved pyloric canal, and bulging of the hypertrophied pyloric muscle into the antrum of the stomach are findings which support the clinical impression. In early or mild cases the roentgen findings may not support the clinical diagnosis, and it is presumed that the chief obstructing mechanism is spasm rather than hypertrophy of the pyloric muscle. Infants whose troubles simulate pyloric stenosis but are not regarded as having the fully developed disorder are often said to have *pylorospasm,* an entity of somewhat vague definition which occupies the middle ground between normality and true pyloric stenosis.

Treatment. Treatment varies with the severity of the disease and the concept of its pathogenesis. Medical management can be tried where the diagnosis is uncertain or the symptoms relatively mild. In Europe there is greater enthusiasm for medical management of the severely affected infants than in the United States, where the prompt termination of symptoms and excellent prognosis from skillful surgical correction wield greater influence in the decision. Medical management, even when successful, is likely to be a prolonged and inconvenient process. It is not usually undertaken in successfully breast-fed infants or in those whose disease has carried them into obvious dehydration, chemical imbalance or significant malnutrition. In the latter case the hazard of temporizing with medical management may convert the infant into an increasingly poorer operative risk.

The symptoms of pyloric stenosis tend to decrease after the age of 3 or 4 months. If an infant has been

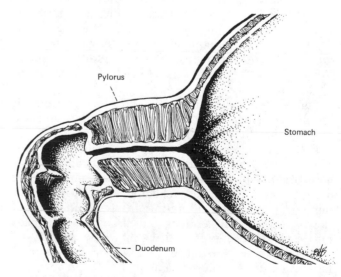

Fig. 13-2. Showing hypertrophied circular muscle of the pylorus in pyloric stenosis.

treated with some success up to this age, usually medical treatment is continued. As time passes, little diminution of hypertrophy occurs, but the lumen enlarges with growth.

MEDICAL TREATMENT. Several or all of the following procedures may be employed: gastric lavage, refeeding, the use of thickened feedings and the administration of cholinergic blocking agents to relax pyloric muscle spasm.

Drugs which may be effective if the degree of obstruction is mild are atropine, methantheline bromide (Banthine), methscopolamine bromide and sedatives. The cholinergic blocking agents should be used in very small dosage with cautious progressive increase until toxic symptoms are observed such as flushing or tachycardia. The dosage should then be reduced to eliminate the side effects.

Medical management should not be attempted in infants who are seriously dehydrated or malnourished since failure to succeed will render the child a poorer operative risk ultimately.

SURGICAL TREATMENT. The Fredet-Ramstedt operation in which the surgeon makes a longitudinal incision in the pyloric muscle down to but not through the mucosa, is the operation of choice. In skilled hands it is rapid and almost always curative. It permits the pyloric canal to gape because of the interruption of the circular muscle fibers. Care must be taken that all the fibers are divided from the stomach antrum to the beginning of the duodenum. The surgeon must also be careful not to open into the thin-walled duodenum and spill its contents into the peritoneal cavity.

Preoperative preparation is directed first at restoring the infant's hydration and correcting electrolyte abnormalities. Mildly affected infants may be operated upon at once if such disturbances are absent. The typical electrolyte abnormalities include low values for chloride and potassium and an increase in pH and CO_2 content of the blood, denoting an alkalosis. Usually, adequate intravenous fluid replacement with salt-containing fluids and additional potassium chloride will correct these defects within 12 to 48 hours.

Immediately before operation the infant's stomach should be lavaged and the gavage tube left in place to keep the stomach deflated for the surgeon.

Following operation, intravenous fluids are continued at first and small feedings with water or glucose are begun during the first day if no vomiting occurs. On a graduated schedule which varies with different institutions, dilute formula is introduced and slowly increased in amount and strength. Full feedings can usually be reached within a few days.

Preoperative Nursing Care. Gastric lavage in a baby is carried out in the same manner as in an adult, with a few minor differences. The infant may be recumbent or held in the lap of an assistant. In either case, restraint by wrapping in a sheet usually is necessary. A catheter (size 10 or 12 French) connected to a syringe by 2 feet of rubber tubing is moistened in sterile water and passed rapidly into the stomach. Passage into the larynx is practically impossible. If by chance the catheter should go into the larynx or the trachea, breathing would stop, and cyanosis from suspended respiration would develop rapidly. As evidence that the tube is in the stomach, the infant is able to breathe (not through the tube), and usually gastric contents will appear in the syringe. In infants, when the tube has been inserted 9 inches from gums or teeth it reaches well into the stomach. Coughing, gagging and redness of the face caused by passage of the tube cease quickly if the tube is held without motion. After siphoning off the stomach contents, an amount of fluid somewhat less than the gastric capacity is allowed to run in. An initial failure to flow, caused by a column of air in the tube, can be corrected by "milking" the tube gently.

The stomach is emptied by lowering syringe and tube below the level of the child. The process is repeated until the water returns clear. Usually from a pint to a quart of fluid is required. Suitable amounts for each washing are: 1 week, 1 ounce; 1 month, 2 ounces; 6 months or more, 4 to 6 ounces. For removal, the tube is pinched tightly in order that fluid may not leak into the pharynx and cause choking. Gastric lavage is seldom required more than twice daily. The fluid commonly used for lavage is either sterile water or normal saline.

Atropine is a toxic drug when given in overdosage. It should be diluted with water and given with a medicine dropper. When the dosage has been increased cautiously until flushing occurs, the flushing appears soon after the drug has been given and disappears after a short time. The effect is transitory and harmless. The flushing is the most obvious sign that the tolerance without harmful effect has been reached. In some instances, atropine in a flushing dose causes moderate fever. High fever should be reported.

A thickened feeding should be so thick that it will not drop from an inverted spoon. A baby may be fed with a spoon, or the food may be placed in a large "Hygeia" nipple, the tip of which has been cut off so as to leave a large hole. The nipple is placed in the infant's mouth, and the food is pressed into the end of the nipple by a spoon or a tongue blade.

When unthickened feedings are ordered, the formula should be given with such care that the likelihood of vomiting is decreased. Infants with pyloric stenosis tend to suck their hands and get a great deal of air into the stomach. Bubbling before and frequently during feeding is necessary. The baby should be fed slowly and should be held in an almost upright position to lessen vomiting.

Charting accurately the approximate amount vomited, the type and color and its relation to feeding aids in diagnosis. Refeeding the infant an equivalent of the amount vomited should be done when it is directed.

Impairment of nutrition causes lowered · resistance to infection, and every means possible should be used to prevent the infant from developing intercurrent infection. Technic to protect the baby from infections should be carried out. Position should be changed frequently. If the infant has a lowered body temperature, extra warmth should be added to keep his temperature stable and in a normal range. Lamps attached to a bed cradle can be placed over the infant to provide this additional warmth. Supportive treatment, such as blood transfusions and fluids administered parenterally, is given the infant to supplement his food and fluid intake. Urine output should be noted, and accurate charting of the stools is important.

Postoperative Nursing Care. When the infant returns from the operating room, he should be placed on his side with back support to prevent aspiration of vomitus. Additional warmth will be needed to prevent shock. The quality of the pulse, the type of respiration, and the color of the infant's skin should be noted frequently. If shock occurs, the foot of the bed should be elevated, and additional warmth should be supplied. Position change should be done gently to prevent vomiting.

Customs differ as to when the first feedings are given after operation. If the pyloric mucosa has not been punctured at operation, no strong contraindication exists to feeding small amounts soon after operation when a local anesthetic has been used or as soon as recovery occurs from general anesthesia. However, peristalsis is impaired by the operation, and some vomiting is usual when food is given early. Because of impaired peristalsis and resultant vomiting, some physicians leave a nasal tube in the stomach for 24 hours and defer feeding for the same length of time, maintaining body fluids by parenteral administration. While the nasal tube is in place, the infant's arms should be restrained to prevent removal of the tube. When feedings are resumed, they are ordered in small amounts. Hunger is observed soon after operation. To prevent vomiting from hurried feedings, the food should be given by medicine dropper. If vomiting occurs, it is best to feed the baby in bed with his head slightly elevated. When the feedings are increased and tolerance is noted, they may be given by nipple and bottle, with the infant in the nurse's lap where he can be cuddled and bubbled more effectively. The amount of food is increased as the infant shows a readiness to take larger amounts. His behavior before and after feeding is a guide in determining his needs.

If the infant received breast feedings prior to operation, the feeding of human milk should be resumed subsequent to operation. At first, he can be fed expressed milk in order to regulate the quantity, but within 2 or 3 days he can be placed directly at the breast and allowed to suckle until he is satisfied. During the period when the milk is being expressed, the breasts should be emptied completely in order to maintain the supply.

Until the stitches have been removed, the dressing must be kept clean. Applying the diaper low, below the dressing, prevents wound contamination.

Chalasia

Regurgitation of feedings occurs rather commonly during the first year of life. In most infants it is infrequent and ascribable to abdominal compression, coughing or the eructation of a gas bubble from the stomach. Some infants, however, habitually bring up a portion of most of their feedings without active vomiting or signs of distress. In most of them weight gain is satisfactory and the symptom is more nuisance than a real cause for concern. Barium examination of the esophagus usually shows that the sphincter muscle at the cardiac end of the stomach is lax and readily permits swallowed formula to slop back into the lower esophagus from the stomach. Babies who are progressing well in other respects need no special treatment, although mothers have to be reassured that the symptom is unimportant and that it will abate later when the child adopts the erect position. Occasionally, however, the loss of food is sufficient to interfere with normal weight gain and special measures must be taken. These consist of thickening the formula with cereal and maintaining the infant in an erect posture for an hour or two after feeding by strapping him in an infant seat or similar apparatus. When weight gain is not satisfactory, careful barium study should be made to be sure that the baby does not have a hiatus hernia or congenitally short esophagus—conditions which may require surgical relief.

Obstruction of the Bile Ducts

Pathophysiology. Postnatal, non-obstructive jaundice due to hemolytic anemia or failure of the infant to conjugate bilirubin, is discussed in Chapter 11. When jaundice progresses beyond the newborn period and is accompanied by dark urine and light stools, obstruction of the bile ducts should be suspected. If a significant fraction of the bilirubin circulating in the blood serum is of the direct-reacting or conjugated variety, the suspicion is confirmed. Such findings indicate that the fault lies not in the overproduction of bilirubin or in the inability to conjugate it, but rather in the inability of the liver to excrete it through the bile duct system (hepatic duct, gallbladder, common duct) into the intestines. It is usually difficult, but unfortunately crucial, to determine whether the obstruction is being produced by hepatitis (with inflammation and swelling of the smaller branches of the ducts or damage to liver cells, either of which may eventually subside spontaneously) or whether there is a congenital failure of the duct system to develop properly and maintain its patency. Short of surgical exploration, the differentiation cannot be made with certainty. Some diagnostic aid is obtained from study of blood enzymes (phosphatase, SGOT, SGPT), by measurements of the intestinal excretion of radioactive Rose Bengal and by percutaneous liver biopsy.

Treatment. If the obstruction is due to hepatitis, anesthesia is contraindicated since it will diminish the chances of spontaneous cure. Yet if the obstruction is due to anatomic abnormality of the ducts, there is a small chance (probably less than 10 per cent) that an anastamosis can be made between the intestine and a portion of the bile duct system. If the obstruction does not clear spontaneously or respond to surgical maneuvers, the liver becomes cirrhotic and eventually loses its various functions. Death may occur between 1 and 3 years of age, or is occasionally postponed longer.

Symptomatic treatment requires a diet low in fat and high in carbohydrate. Vitamin K is usually given to prevent hemorrhages due to insufficient production of prothrombin.

Nursing Care. During the period of observation and diagnosis, the color and amount of stools should be noted and their description should be charted accurately.

If an anastomosis is done, shock preventive measures should be instituted postoperatively, and frequent inspection of the abdominal wound should be made to check for bleeding.

Careful observation should also be maintained to check for distention and its presence reported to the surgeon. If gastric suction is continued, elbow restraints will be necessary to prevent the infant from

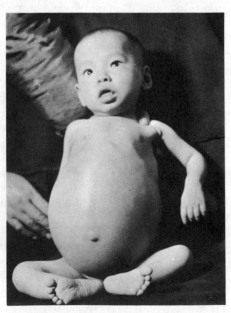

Fig. 13-3. A baby with Hirschsprung's disease.

removing the tube, and irrigation with small amounts of warm saline will keep the tube patent.

Until adequate feeding can be resumed, fluids are administered parenterally. When feedings are begun, they should be given slowly from a medicine dropper. These infants may be picked up for feeding and bubbling, but it must be done with care.

Meckel's Diverticulum

Aproximately 2 to 3 per cent of all children have a vestigial remnant of the omphalomesenteric duct remaining as a small pouch off the ileum about 18 inches from its junction with the colon. Usually this structure, called a Meckel's diverticulum, gives no symptoms. In some children there is aberrantly placed gastric mucous membrane within the pouch which secretes acid gastric juice. This juice is irritating to the wall of the ileum and may produce ulceration and bleeding. The usual symptoms are painless passage of tarry or grossly bloody stools. Diagnosis is made from suspicion when no other explanation of the bleeding can be found, but it cannot be confirmed without an exploratory abdominal operation. Surgical removal of the diverticulum is simple and curative. The postoperative care is the same as that for any abdominal operation.

Megacolon

Pathophysiology. Megacolon is most commonly a primary congenital abnormality (Hirschsprung's disease). The essential lesion is partial obstruction in the distal portion of the colon, which causes obstinate constipation, enlargement of the abdomen and dilatation and hypertrophy of the colon. When the bowel is examined at operation or at autopsy no gross explanation for the obstruction can be found. The fault appears to lie in an abnormality of the innervation of the intrinsic musculature of the bowel wall, which under normal circumstances, produces the coordinated peristaltic movements that propel feces and gas downward toward the anus. In Hirschsprung's disease one or more segments of the colon do not participate properly in coordinated peristaltic activity, either because the essential ganglion cells are absent from the muscles or because there is a disturbance of the balance between the activities of the sympathetic and the parasympathetic nerve fibers. Stool reaching such an area is not passed along normally, and the bowel proximal to it eventually hypertrophies in its attempt to force the accumulating mass through the malfunctioning segment of bowel. Often such an area can be identified by a small barium enema and careful study of the activity of the area between the rectum and the sigmoid colon.

Megacolon may also occur as a disorder secondary to anatomic (rectal stricture or rectovaginal fistula with a small opening) and psychogenic obstruction. Of course, in these instances successful treatment will depend on the ability to provide an adequate channel by surgical measures or to correct the emotional disturbance that leads to spastic withholding of stool.

Symptoms. The symptoms of megacolon· are manifest early in infancy. Constipation that persists in spite of treatment, and progressive enlargement of the abdomen are the first symptoms. Periodically, the distention may be so great as to cause discomfort, vomiting and interference with respirations. The absorption of toxic materials retained in the bowel may produce nausea, lethargy or even collapse when the obstipation has been prolonged. Unless close attention is given to bowel evacuation, the accumulation of dry fecal masses may lead to inflammation or even ulceration of the bowel so that once the obstruction is relieved, diarrhea ensues. The effort of the colon to pass the fecal mass along is often apparent by peristaltic activity which is visible through the abdominal wall. Malnutrition may be present as a consequence of vomiting or food refusal. In some of the milder cases spontaneous recovery may take place. Children who continue with the disorder unrelieved may have a serious social problem because of inability to control the escape of gas under pressure. An occasional child who reaches adolescence will learn how to evacuate his bowel successfully by the use of his abdominal muscles.

Diagnosis. Diagnosis is seldom difficult. The combination of gross enlargement of the abdomen, visible peristalsis and obstinate constipation with passage of stools of excessive size is regularly present in all cases. A roentgen study of the colon is indicated in order to confirm the diagnosis and identify, if possible, the main area of disturbed peristalsis. This procedure should be undertaken cautiously in instances where the obstruction can be identified as anatomic or functional in the lower rectum, for the addition of barium to the retained fecal mass above such an obstruction may turn a partial intestinal obstruction into a complete one.

Treatment and Nursing Care. These may be considered under three general headings—emergency relief of fecal impaction, long-term medical management and surgical treatment.

EMERGENCY RELIEF OF FECAL IMPACTION. Intestinal obstruction from fecal impaction requires prompt relief. Various types of enemas are used to soften the impacted mass and increase the effectiveness of bowel contractions. Because of the large size of the colon, the enemas are only partially returned. It is possible to produce water intoxication in these patients if excessive amounts are run in without being recovered. Normal saline solution is probably safer to use than plain water. In neglected cases the danger of perforating a colonic ulcer must be considered. Digital removal of stool from the rectum is often the safest and most effective method of relieving fecal impactions.

LONG-TERM MEDICAL MANAGEMENT. Long-term med-

ical management may be sucessful in keeping the child in good health and maintaining an adequate rate of colonic evacuation. An attempt is made to keep the stools soft by offering a low-residue diet or by the continuous administration of mineral oil. Mild laxatives may be given periodically. Many children will require regular cleansing of the colon with enemas or colonic irrigations administered through a large tube passed well up into the descending colon. Drugs that alter the activity of the sympathetic and the parasympathetic nervous systems are sometimes useful in effecting more or less regular bowel evacuations. These include Prostigmin, Urecholine, atropine, Syntropan, Mecholyl Chloride and others. Dosage must be initiated cautiously, for all of these drugs have toxic effects that must be recognized promptly. Children who can be managed successfully by medical treatment require careful attention to general hygiene and diet.

SURGICAL TREATMENTS. A number of surgical approaches may be considered when medical management is deemed unsatisfactory. The practice of sectioning the sympathetic nerve connections to the colon has not given very satisfactory results, since constipation usually is ameliorated but not cured. In cases where an area of constriction can be demonstrated by barium enema, sometimes a complete cure may be effected by removal of the constricted area and anastomosis of the bowel. The procedure offers the best chance of a completely satisfactory cure. Usually it is not undertaken in children under the age of 2. When medical management is failing, and the preferred surgical approach cannot be done, colostomy or even complete resection of the colon may be performed. The specific elements of the child's postoperative care will depend on the type of procedure that is done.

PROCEDURE FOR CLEANSING ENEMA FOR AN INFANT. The equipment consists of an irrigating can and pole, rubber tubing, glass connector, stopcock, catheter (No. 10 to 12 French), lubricant, waterproof material and towel, rubber-covered pillow, bedpan and cover, kidney basin, enema solution (105° F.) and oiled cotton for cleansing after the enema has been expelled. For a soapsuds enema, 2 drams of soap jelly to a pint of water is used; for a saline enema, 1 dram of salt to a pint. When giving a cleansing enema to an infant, not more than 300 ml. of solution should be used unless specific instructions have been given. After protecting the bed with the waterproof material and towel and removing the diaper, the pillow is placed under the infant's back. Since retention of fluid is impossible for the infant, the bedpan padded with a diaper is placed under the buttocks. After the catheter is lubricated and the air is expelled, it is inserted from 2 to 4 inches into the rectum. Hanging the can not higher than 18 inches above the infant's hips allows the fluid to run in slowly. When the tube has been

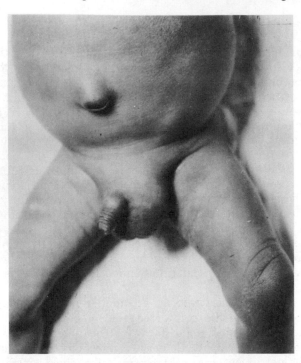

Fig. 13-4. Left indirect inguinal hernia in an infant distending the scrotal sac. (Courtesy of Dr. Mark Ravitch)

removed, the abdomen may be massaged gently until the solution has been expelled, if there are no contraindications. After expulsion, the buttocks should be cleansed and the diaper reapplied. In charting the procedure, the results should be noted.

PROCEDURE FOR AN OIL-RETENTION ENEMA. The equipment consists of a funnel, rubber tubing, glass connector, catheter (No. 10 to 12 French), lubricant, bedpan and vegetable oil, from 60 to 150 ml., at 100° F. In some instances it may be necessary to inject the oil slowly into the rectum with a syringe. Pressure over the anus or adhesive strapping will prevent the oil from being expelled. After the oil has been retained for 30 minutes, a cleansing enema should be given.

Intestinal Hernia

A hernia of the intestine is the protrusion of a part of the bowel through an abnormal opening in the containing walls of the abdomen. Hernia may be either congenital or acquired. The majority of acquired hernias in childhood arise from congenital abnormalities. The management of a hernia in a young child is the same whether congenital or acquired and no further distinction between these two types need be made. The most frequent locations for hernia are at the umbilicus and through the inguinal canals. Hernias through the diaphragm are uncommon, and those at other sites are rare.

Umbilical Hernia. Umbilical hernia consists of a protrusion of a portion of the intestine or omentum through the umbilical ring, producing a bulge under the skin at the navel. The size of the tumor varies but seldom exceeds that of a golf ball. Umbilical hernias are usually not apparent at birth but appear within the early months of life and enlarge during the acts of crying or straining. They are reduced easily, and strangulation is practically unknown. All but the largest hernias will heal spontaneously at least by the time the child begins to develop strong abdominal muscles—between 3 and 4 years of age. The traditional treatment of strapping or binding the abdomen of such an infant is generally unnecessary, although it improves the cosmetic appearance. Hernias that are large and fail to close spontaneously may be repaired surgically in later childhood.

Inguinal Hernia. In the male the testis descends from the abdominal cavity into the scrotum, carrying with it the parietal peritoneum, thus forming a tube from abdomen to scrotum. Normally, this tube closes completely. When it has failed to close partially or completely, descent of the intestine into it is possible, thus producing hernia. In girls, the round ligament extends from the uterus through the inguinal canal to its attachment in the abdominal wall. In fetal life, the ligaments are surrounded by a peritoneal process which later obliterates. Weakness of the tissues about the round ligament, together with increased abdominal pressure, sometimes permits inguinal hernias in girls. However, about 90 per cent of the inguinal hernias of children occur in the male. An inguinal hernia in an infant causes no symptoms unless it becomes strangulated, and this event is uncommon. Strangulation results when a portion of bowel becomes so tightly caught in the hernial sac that its blood supply is cut off. Severe symptoms of pain, intestinal obstruction and inability to reduce the mass occur. If unrelieved, gangrene of the bowel will result. Immediate operation is mandatory.

Usually, an inguinal hernia is reduced easily. When the inguinal rings are small, reduction cannot be accomplished by pressure alone on the herniated bowel, because the hernia then mushrooms against the external inguinal ring. In addition to moderate pressure, it is necessary to make lateral pressure on the bowel with the fingers at the base of the mass in order to elongate the bowel at this point. Sometimes reduction is made easier by having the child lie with the buttocks elevated.

Hernias in female infants frequently contain an ovary or even the uterus. Because of the hazard to the circulation to these organs, surgical repair should be done promptly. In the male, repair of inguinal hernias which do not strangulate may be deferred, but the operation is sufficiently benign to encourage early closure of the defect. Some surgeons automati-

Fig. 13-5. *A*) Infant of 1 year, showing moderate malnutrition from cystic fibrosis of the pancreas.

B) The same infant at 2 years of age, showing congestive heart failure as a result of pulmonary fibrosis.

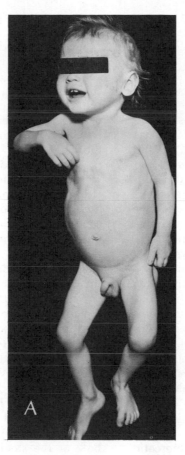

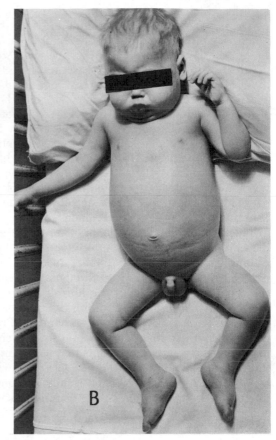

cally explore both sides since there is a high probability of eventual bilateral involvement.

If the hernia can be kept constantly reduced by means of a truss, the defect in the abdominal wall will close in many instances. Use of a truss for a year or more may be necessary. If the truss fails to hold the hernia or to permit ultimate cure, surgical repair is indicated. Even the youngest of infants stands a hernia operation well if he is in good condition.

When a hernia is corrected surgically, the postoperative care is directed at keeping the wound clean until healing has taken place. Diapers are left open to prevent wound contamination. Infants may be picked up for feedings and to relieve distress. Older children may be permitted activity as soon as they feel able to play. Unless bowel resection is required, feedings can be resumed a few hours after operation.

Disaccharidase Deficiency

Congenital defects in the enzymes of the intestinal mucosa which are responsible for the breakdown of the double sugars of the diet (disaccharides) are now recognized as occasional causes of low-grade persistent diarrhea with poor weight gain in infants. Careful diagnostic study of such infants can pinpoint the offending sugar and lead to amelioration of symptoms by eliminating it from the infant's diet.

Cystic Fibrosis of the Pancreas——Mucoviscidosis

This disorder is a generalized affliction of several portions of the body. Its onset is usually recognized during infancy through its effects on the digestive tract. Attention used to be focused on the pathologic changes of the pancreas and the lack of pancreatic secretions which determined the nutritional defect. Later investigations have emphasized the hereditary nature of the disease and its widespread effects on secretions of glands in the intestine, bronchial mucosa and skin.

Etiology and Pathogenesis. The condition is inherited and is transmitted as a recessive trait. Thus each parent must be an unaffected carrier of a defective gene. A double complement of this gene appears in one fourth of their offspring and results in the full-blown disease. It is estimated that between 2 and 6 per cent of the white race are carriers and that the disease will appear in between 1:1,000 and 1:2,000 newborns. The gene is rare in Negroes and absent from the Mongoloid races.

Practically all children with the genetic defect have abnormally high concentrations of sodium, potassium and chloride in the secretions produced by their sweat glands. This portion of the disorder is of minor consequence except in hot weather when they may suffer excessive salt depletion. Of greater clinical significance are the changes produced in the excretions of the pancreas, the intestinal glands and the bronchial mucus-secreting glands. The degree of involvement of these different structures varies somewhat, so that individuals with the general disease may be affected in different ways and with different degrees of severity. Thus meconium ileus (see Chap. 11) may be present at birth when the viscosity of the secretions of the intestinal tract is so marked that the gummy intestinal contents cannot pass through. Obstruction of the ducts of the pancreas by thick secretions blocks the egress of important digestive enzymes produced within the gland and leads to abnormality of stools and nutritional failure. Most important of all is the effect of abnormally thick bronchial mucus within the lungs in blocking off small segments of lung and encouraging chronic infection and fibrotic changes. Symptoms of this complication may appear in early infancy or may be delayed until later childhood. Treatment of the digestive aspects of cystic fibrosis is effective, but methods available for controlling the pulmonary complications are likely to be temporary. Progressive changes in the lungs lead to fibrosis, which in turn may interfere with circulation of blood through the lungs and result in heart failure. Children who die of cystic fibrosis of the pancreas usually succumb to the immediate or the remote effects of pulmonary disease.

Symptoms. The symptoms of meconium ileus are described in Chapter 11.

Symptoms which indicate insufficiency of pancreatic enzymes are insidious in their onset but usually are discovered before the age of 6 months. The stools tend to be large in volume, mushy but not usually watery. They have an offensive odor, and when the diet contains much fat some of it comes through undigested. The infant's appetite is usually good, if not ravenous; yet, in spite of a normal food intake, his weight increases at an abnormally slow rate.

Pulmonary symptoms may arise spontaneously or after an acute respiratory infection. They consist of a chronic cough and obstructive bronchitis. Infants may escape this complication but during later childhood are prone to show evidence of increasing emphysema and patches of atelectasis on chest roentgenogram and chronic or recurring bronchitis on physical examination. In the later stages of pulmonary disease clubbing of the fingers and chronic cyanosis appear, and when fibrosis of the lungs is taking place the heart enlarges and the child becomes dyspneic and edematous.

Diagnosis. The diagnosis is usually suspected in infancy from the clinical picture of lowgrade diarrhea, good appetite, failure to gain weight and cough. It may be confirmed by demonstrating the absence of normal concentrations of trypsin in the secretions obtained by drainage of the duodenum. Measurement of the concentration of sodium and chloride in the sweat now offers the preferred means of supporting the diagnosis.

Several methods are used to determine the concentration of electrolytes in the sweat. One utilizes paper and agar impregnated with silver salts which change color on contact with sweat of high chloride concentration. These methods are subject to error and are used mainly as screening devices. Positive results must be checked by more accurate chemical methods. For the latter, sweat is collected in plastic bags tied over the hand or bandages applied to the skin and covered with plastic. The areas of skin application must be clean and uncontaminated with urine or with secretions of axillary or inguinal sweat glands. The chloride concentration of the sweat obtained offers the clearest distinction between normal (less than 60 mEq./L.) and abnormal. Sodium and potassium are also elevated in cystic fibrosis of the pancreas, but here the distinction is often not as clear cut.

Iontophoresis of the skin with pilocarpine has largely replaced the above methods of collecting sweat. Modern apparatus is available which makes direct readings of electrolyte sweat concentrations by measuring conductance of the fluid obtained.

Treatment. When diagnosis is established during infancy several dietary measures should be invoked. Poor absorption leads to wastage of dietary fat in the stools. Skimmed or 2 per cent fat milk, or a formula low in fat content is generally preferred to reduce the bulk of the stool and to steer the major food intake toward proteins and carbohydrates. Total caloric intake should usually be increased to 150-200/Kg./day if the infant has sufficient appetite. Vitamins are usually given as the water-miscible variety since A, D and K are poorly absorbed as fats. Double the usual dosage is recommended. To compensate for the lack of pancreatic juice, substitution therapy with pancreatic enzymes is desirable. Panteric granules, Viokase and Cotazym are the preparations commonly used. The amounts are individualized according to the effect upon the stools. These preparations should not be added to warm or hot food since their activity will be destroyed.

The child with obstructive respiratory disease requires continuous care, either in the hospital or at home, directed toward loosening his sticky secretions and permitting better aeration of his alveoli. During the night and the resting portions of his day he may live in a mist tent designed to carry fine droplets of water to the deeper recesses of his respiratory passages. The mist is best supplied by a nebulizer which divides the water into very small droplets. Propylene glycol is added to stabilize the dispersion of the water in air and a compressor is used to force the mixture through a small nozzle. Periodically during the day intermittent positive pressure breathing treatments can be administered to the older child who is able to cooperate. This inhalation treatment, which attempts to dislodge plugs of thick mucus by forcing air behind them, may also be used to carry bronchodilating solutions such as isoproterenol or phenylephrine into the smaller bronchioles. After such local therapy, dislodging of the plugs may be aided by postural drainage with the assistance of a skilled physical therapist administering clapping or vibration to the chest wall.

Infants with cystic fibrosis should be zealously protected from respiratory infections within the household or hospital. The use of prophylactic antibiotics, however, is not generally advised. If respiratory infection does occur, it should be treated promptly and vigorously.

Nursing Care. When an infant is hospitalized because of pulmonary infection, tent aerosol therapy may be used to thin mucous secretions and to administer medication through inhalation. Oxygen is generally not used unless specifically indicated. The tent should be cooled to keep the temperature below 80° F. and frequent checks should be made to verify that adequate mist is maintained. Since the solutions used for aerosol therapy may easily clog the tent equipment, parts should be washed and rinsed thoroughly after each use.

Infants with cystic fibrosis need meticulous nursing care. They should be bathed frequently with special attention to skin folds in order to prevent irritation. Diapers should be checked and changed frequently to prevent odors. The character and color of stools should be accurately noted and charted.

Because of their vigorous appetite, these infants should be fed promptly with the recommended dietary modifications. Medications must be given with meals and can be added to cold foods until the child is able to take them in capsule form. When out of the tent, these infants can be held for procedures and for feeding and bubbling and the cuddling they require.

In order to prevent further respiratory infections, strenuous efforts must be maintained to prevent cross contamination. Reverse isolation technics are sometimes recommended.

When the infant has been admitted for diagnostic procedures, the nurse can be helpful to parents confronted with the implications of the illness for the first time. As well as the myriad of feelings associated with the transmission of a genetic defect to their child, these parents may be overwhelmed by the regimen of care which will be necessary in the years ahead. In addition to the support which she can provide by empathic listening and by conveying understanding and acceptance of the meaning of the diagnosis to the parents, it is often her responsibility to assist them by clarifying information relating to the disease processes and in learning the complex technics required in treatment. Since such treatment plans are long range and often financially draining, she can also be helpful by directing or supporting referrals to the hospital social worker or to community agencies who can continue the necessary support and assistance after the infant is discharged.

THE NERVOUS SYSTEM

Structural or functional disturbances of the central nervous system occur in bewildering numbers. Their complexities can be understood only with an extensive knowledge of the anatomy and physiology of the nervous system. In this and later sections it is possible to mention only a few representative types. For more detailed consideration, the reader is referred to the bibliography.

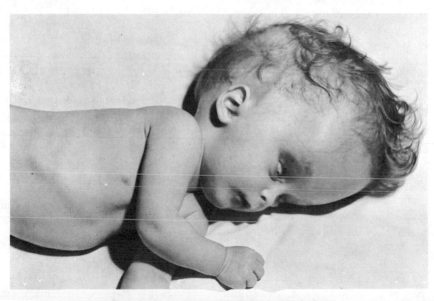

FIG. 13-6. An infant with hydrocephalus.

Hydrocephalus

Hydrocephalus is a condition in which the normal circulation of spinal fluid is impeded, resulting in pressure deformity of the brain and progressive enlargement of the head. It is most often due to anomalous development of the brain or spinal cord but also may be seen as a result of infection of the meninges, trauma to the head or subdural hematoma.

Pathophysiology. Cerebrospinal fluid is produced in a network of veins known as the choroid plexus which hangs into each of the lateral ventricles. Fluid passes from this point of origin through the foramina of Monro, the aqueduct of Sylvius, the 4th ventricle and the foramina of Luschka and Magendie out into the subarachnoid space at the base of the brain. From here it diffuses down around the spinal cord and up over the outer convexity of the brain. It is reabsorbed by the arachnoid villae of the dural sinuses and, to a minor extent, by other veins of the covering membranes of brain and cord. Ordinarily, the rate of production of fluid is equal to the rate of reabsorption, but, if fluid is produced faster than it can be absorbed, pressure develops within the skull. Some varieties of congenital hydrocephalus are caused by blockade somewhere along the chain of foramina and ducts between the choroid plexus and the subarachnoid space. The resulting enlargement is mainly in the ventricular system of the brain. Dye, such as phenolphthalein, injected into a lateral ventricle fails to appear in the spinal fluid because it cannot get out of the ventricular system. This variety is known as non-communicating hydrocephalus. Another type, communicating hydrocephalus, permits free flow of dye through the ventricular and subarachnoid systems. It is presumed to be due either to excessive production of spinal fluid or to imperfect absorption from the regions of the arachnoid villae. This type follows or accompanies myelomeningocele. In some cases of spina bifida the medulla oblongata and part of the cerebellum are pulled down into the foramen magnum because of firm attachment of the cord and its meninges at the site of the bony defect. Further growth in the length of the bony spinal cord aggravates the herniation (Arnold-Chiari deformity) and prevents the proper flow of spinal fluid up to the outside surface of the brain.

Symptoms. The progressive accumulation of unabsorbed fluid distends the ventricles and causes the head to enlarge and the brain cortex to become thin. With continued enlargement of the head the skull sutures separate. The infant becomes increasingly helpless, first because of inability to support the large head, later because of damage to the brain and because of malnutrition which always accompanies severe degrees of hydrocephalus. During the late stages, pressure sores are frequent unless most carefully avoided by changes of position and protecting pads.

Death finally occurs from either progressive malnutrition or intercurrent infection.

Diagnosis. The head may be larger than normal at birth, but more often no change is noticed until several weeks of age. The finding that the head is larger than normal is strongly suggestive of hydrocephalus. Question as to diagnosis arises only in the early stages when the head size is not greatly in excess of normal. The diagnosis can be made certain by pneumoencephalogram (skull roentgenogram taken after the spinal fluid in the ventricles has been replaced with air), which shows the dilated ventricles. Increase in head size of an inch or more a month is also good evidence of hydrocephalus.

Treatment. In a few instances, hydrocephalus undergoes spontaneous arrest, a balance between secretion and absorption having been reached by some means. When the hydrocephalus is of moderate degree, it is well to defer radical surgical treatment until the rate of head growth can be determined. Operation may be unnecessary.

Since the cause of hydrocephalus is entirely mechanical, not much is to be expected of any but mechanical treatment. Surgical treatment offers the only hope of cure. Procedures which are used include: (1) removal or destruction of the choroid plexus to decrease the production of spinal fluid, (2) shunting operations which attempt to lead off the accumulated fluids through artificial openings in the ventricular system or through catheters to absorbing areas such as veins, the peritoneal cavity or the ureter, and (3) removal of a portion of the occipital bone and the vertebral lamina in the presence of the Arnold-Chiari deformity to provide decompression and improve the circulation of spinal fluid.

Nursing Care. Preoperatively, the chief nursing problems are concerned with the maintenance of nutrition and the prevention of pressure sores on the head. Babies with hydrocephalus often have increasing nutritional failure as the hydrocephalus progresses. It is important to arrange feeding schedules which avoid vomiting and at the same time permit an adequate intake of food.

As the head increases in size the baby becomes more helpless. He cannot hold up his head to assume a sitting position and ultimately cannot move the head much while lying in bed. The head must be moved for him, and this must be done often enough to prevent pressure sores. Special care of the scalp and the use of a soft pillow are measures suggested. Unless the head is enormous and heavy, holding the infant for feedings will relieve pressure for short periods.

After operation, the temperature, pulse and respiration rate should be observed every 15 minutes until the child is fully conscious. In children over 2 years of age blood pressure readings should also be taken. Subsequently, until the vital signs become stabilized, they should be taken hourly. During the first day the nursing measures must be adapted to the child's vital signs. With marked rises in temperature, cooling measures must be taken. Fluids are given parenterally and suctioning may be required.

Postoperatively, the infant should be positioned on the unwounded side to prevent pressure on the shunt valve. To prevent pressure on the ear, cotton should be placed behind and over the ear before bandaging. When intravenous fluid therapy is discontinued, the infant may be held for feeding, but the position on the unwounded side should be continued until healing of the wound site is complete.

If a catheter has been inserted into a ureter during surgery, the position of the child postoperatively is based on measurement of fluid that is draining through the catheter and by observation of the anterior fontanel. A child with a ventriculo-ureteral shunt usually has a depressed fontanel after the operation. When the anterior fontanel is depressed, the child should be kept flat in bed or with his head lowered slightly. Children in whom there is a lumbar subarachnoid-ureteral shunt often have slower drainage of cerebrospinal fluid into the urinary tract. In them, the anterior fontanel shows no signs of depression during the first postoperative day. When the anterior fontanel appears to be normal, the child is kept flat or with his head elevated to a moderate degree. Whether the child's head is kept elevated or lowered, he should be turned at 2-hour intervals to prevent development of pressure areas and hypostatic pneumonia.

Because salt and fluids are lost by drainage of cerebrospinal fluid, total intake and output measurements must be done with the greatest accuracy as a basis for determining parenteral electrolyte replacement. In most instances 24-hour urine collection is essential.

Small amounts of fluids are given orally (generally 5 per cent dextrose and saline) as soon as the child reacts fully. Formula is introduced gradually, followed by solid foods according to the child's age and tolerance. Additional salt is usually added to the diet to replace that lost through spinal fluid drainage. The child can be held for feeding, bubbling and cuddling after the fourth postoperative day.

It is the responsibility of the nurse to report promptly any symptoms of vomiting, signs of infection, abdominal distention, symptoms of dehydration or bulging of the anterior fontanel. It is also her responsibility to assist the mother to become acquainted with such signs and with methods for preventing illness which is a great threat to the infant who has had a ventricular or subarachnoid shunt. This teaching must be done carefully to ensure caution but without instilling abnormal fears which prevent the mother from following her intuitive feelings of motherliness. These babies can be handled as other babies are. The only significant differences are those cited above.

Seizures (Convulsive Disorders)

The term "seizures" is used to encompass a number of varieties of episodic disturbance of brain function. Most seizures are accompanied by loss of consciousness; many of them, by abnormal muscle tone. They cannot be regarded as a specific disease, for they appear in association with a variety of known and unknown brain disorders. Some of these latter are postnatal infections and metabolic and traumatic disturbances. However, the large majority of convulsions occur in patients who present additional signs that imply a congenital abnormality of brain function.

Seizures create two general types of medical problems—the management of an acute convulsion and the study and control of recurring attacks.

Single Convulsions. Symptoms. Convulsions usually are sudden in onset, though in some instances their imminence may be suspected by the general behavior of the child. In a typical case, the entire body becomes stiff and consciousness is lost. More or less skin pallor is present. The eyes tend to be fixed in some one position, perhaps rolled up or crossed. As a part of the general tonic state, the head is held backward, the back is more or less arched, the arms are flexed, and the hands are clenched. Immediately after the general stiffening of the body, twitching or clonic movements occur. These may be generalized in the beginning or may start in one part and extend to all parts of the body. The clonic movements consist chiefly of quick, jerking to-and-fro movements of the extremities and similar spasmodic movements of the muscles of the face. The spasm includes the muscles of respiration, so that breathing is irregular and ineffectual, and cyanosis results. Inability to swallow saliva may produce frothing at the mouth and rattling in the throat. The pulse becomes weak and often irregular. Convulsions may be very brief or may last a half hour or more. Usually, after a few minutes the convulsive movements become weaker and finally cease. The body relaxes, and consciousness returns. If the convulsion is severe, the child may remain somewhat stuporous, and at times certain parts appear to be paralyzed temporarily.

A convulsion may not be repeated or it may recur in a few minutes or hours. In some cases, convulsions may recur frequently over a period of several days. All are not so severe as the preceding description indicates. They may be lacking in several of the described features and may be of very short duration. In some instances, convulsions may involve only part of the body; in other instances of repeated convulsions, one part may be affected during one convulsion and other parts during other convulsions. Partial involvement of the body in this manner is not necessarily evidence of a localized intracranial lesion.

Etiology and Prognosis. A convulsion is a symptom of an underlying disorder and not itself a disease.

The prognosis both for life and for the patient's mental and neurologic future depends on the setting in which the convulsion occurs. Often the significance of an acute convulsion can be determined only in the light of future developments.

Febrile Convulsions. Some infants and young children have convulsions at the onset of infectious diseases when the temperature is beginning to rise. These are commonly but somewhat inexactly called "febrile convulsions." The phenomenon is analogous to the chill that takes place in adults under similar circumstances of disease, but it depends on the individual susceptibility of the patient to convulse. The infection itself may be trivial; a rapidly rising or excessively high fever triggers the convulsion without necessarily implying that the disease is a serious one. Children who have such a tendency ordinarily lose it as they grow older, so that febrile convulsions generally are not observed in children beyond the age of 4 or 5. Such convulsions are alarming but rarely fatal. When they are occasional, brief and limited to the period of early childhood and feverish illnesses, they probably have no adverse effect on the child's ultimate development.

Infection of the Central Nervous System. In the presence of fever, an acute convulsion sometimes announces the presence of infection of the central nervous system. Meningitis, encephalitis, rabies, cerebral sinus thrombosis and brain abscess are examples. The prognosis will depend on the kind of infection and the adequacy of treatment that can be marshaled to combat it.

Increased Intracranial Pressure. Acute convulsions may be seen associated with increased intracranial pressure from causes other than infection—subdural hematoma, brain tumor, uremia, lead encephalopathy. Here the immediate prognosis for life and the later prognosis for complete recovery of function are relatively poor.

Toxic and Metabolic Disorders. Many toxic and metabolic disorders can be listed as causes of acute convulsions. Kernicterus in association with erythroblastosis of the newborn, rachitic or parathyroid tetany, hypoglycemia, asphyxia and inhalation anesthesia, alkalosis, hypertension and prolonged treatment with steroids are some of the disturbances with which convulsions may be associated. Prognosis depends on the ability to recognize the precipitating disorder and bring it under control.

No Associated Disturbance. Many acute convulsions have no associated disturbance. Some of them represent the first in a series of recurring episodes which are considered in Chapter 28.

TREATMENT. Most acute convulsions are the unexpected harbinger of an illness. The majority are brief and self-limited and subside spontaneously, no matter what is done. When they are brought to medical attention, immediate sedation usually is indicated to ensure their termination. Many drugs have been used in the past, but the safest and easiest to administer is sodium phenobarbital by subcutaneous injection. Doses from ½ to 1½ grains may be used, depending on the size of the infant. If the fever is high, the use of a tepid bath or sponging to reduce the temperature gradually is rational. Aspirin or acetaminophen may be given to forestall future hyperpyresis.

If simple measures fail to terminate the convulsion within a period of ½ to 1 hour, rectal anesthesia with Avertin may be employed. A search for associated disease requiring independent treatment always is indicated, whether the convulsion ceases spontaneously or not.

NURSING CARE. Protection of the child from injury is one of the first considerations during a convulsion. Regardless of age, a crib bed is essential. If the convulsions are severe, the crib sides should be padded. Inspection should be made of the child's toys to remove those that might produce injury during a seizure. To prevent suffocation, soft pillows should not be allowed. A padded tongue depressor should be in readiness to place between the teeth to prevent biting of the tongue. If convulsions produce increased secretion from the pharynx, a suction set should be kept in readiness. In some instances, oxygen may be necessary for extreme respiratory difficulty produced by muscular incoordination.

There is nothing that a nurse can do to stop a convulsion; her duty lies in observing and recording it in all its detail and in protecting the child from injury. In describing the movements, the term "twitching" should be used when the movements are clonic or jerking and "contraction" when the child holds himself in a tonic or a contracted and stiffened state. A record of the following should be made: behavior state preceding onset; length of the seizure in minutes; the site where the twitching or the contraction began and the parts of the body involved; eye movements and pupillary changes; types of movement; degree of perspiration; incontinence before, during or after the seizure; pulse and respiration rates; posture of the body; color; secretions from the mouth; the first and the last areas to relax; behavior at the end of the convulsion. If the child is old enough to talk, the state of consciousness can be observed. Degree of memory for recent events, type of speech and amount of coordination are observations that are needed to detect the extent of cerebral dysfunction produced by the seizure. After the convulsion the child should be placed in bed if he is not already there. Usually he will sleep for long periods, the time depending on the severity of the seizure.

After one convulsion the child should be protected by continuing administration of sedatives until the danger of recurrence seems to be past.

Lightning Major Convulsions (Infantile Myoclonic Seizures). A type of recurring seizure sometimes seen in infants during the first or second year of life consists of frequently repeated rapid forward ducking of the head with simultaneous flexion of the arms and the legs. The duration is often so brief that the significance of the attacks is not recognized. They tend to occur in bursts and may recur as often as several hundred times in a day. A characteristic electroencephalographic pattern is found with disorganized high peaks and slow waves (hypsarrythmia). Treatment has been notoriously difficult, as the seizures usually fail to respond to the ordinary anticonvulsants. More ominously, the persistence of the attacks is frequently followed by mental deficiency. Recently, some therapeutic success is reported from the combined use of anticonvulsants and ACTH or cortisone.

ABERRANT NEUROMUSCULAR DEVELOPMENT

The expected sequence in neuromuscular development during the first year has been described in some detail at the beginning of this unit. Significant lag in progress is most often an intimation of mental deficiency with or without associated systemic disease. Divergence which shows up definitely during infancy is likely to mean moderately severe restriction of eventual mental capacity. Therefore, it is most important to be certain that neuromuscular deviations are real before conveying such suspicions to the parents. The medical personnel responsible for an infant who appears to be abnormal must on the one hand avoid false prognostication, while on the other hand carrying out their moral obligation to share the truth about the infant with his family. Few situations are so prone to strain the relationship between parents and physician or parents and nurse.

Not all developmental failures are *necessarily* associated with mental retardation. For this reason the motor and sensory defects are considered separately. They may be associated with either normal or abnormal mental capacity.

The General Problem of Mental Deficiency

Etiology. Mental deficiency occurs in association with so many different clinical conditions of both known and unknown etiology that classification is hampered by the great complexity of names and terms. Although some types are associated with obvious gross malformation of the brain, the more important structural defect lies in the congenital lack of brain cells or the later destruction of cells originally present. It is simplest to think in terms of general factors that can destroy or interfere with the function of brain cells. Current knowledge indicates that in most cases mental retardation is due to factors which operated before birth or during the process of delivery. The examples listed below follow a scheme devised by Yannet*:

---

* Yannet, Herman: *In* Nelson's Textbook of Pediatrics, ed. 8, p. 1233, Philadelphia, Saunders, 1964.

I. Prenatal
  A. Genetically determined
    1. Familial or subcultural
    2. Phenylketonuria
    3. Galactosemia
    4. Cerebral lipidoses (Tay-Sachs, Niemann-Pick)
    5. Cerebral degenerative diseases (Schilder's)
    6. Gargoylism (Hurler's)
    7. Cranial anomalies (microcephaly, craniostenosis, hydrocephalus)
    8. Congenital ectodermoses (tuberous sclerosis, cerebral angiomatosis)
    9. Hereditary cerebral maldevelopment, not classifiable
    10. Chromosomal aberrations (Down's syndrome, Klinefelter's syndrome)
  B. Prenatal, of known cause
    1. Infection (syphilis, rubella, toxoplasmosis, cytomegalic inclusion disease)
    2. Fetal irradiation
    3. Kernicterus (Rh, ABO, nonspecific hyperbilirubinemia)
    4. Cretinism
  C. Prenatal, of unknown or indefinite cause, not classifiable
    1. Associated with placental abnormalities; toxemias of pregnancies; prematurity; nutritional deficiencies; anoxia; poisoning; trauma
II. Natal
  A. Birth injuries (direct trauma, hemorrhage, anoxia)
III. Postnatal
  A. Cerebral infections (meningitis, encephalitis, abscess)
  B. Cerebral trauma
  C. Poisoning (lead, CO)
  D. Cerebrovascular accidents (occlusions and hemorrhages)
  E. Postimmunization encephalopathies (pertussis, smallpox)

Symptoms. The cardinal symptom of mental deficiency is failure to reach the normal developmental milestones at the appropriate age. The appearance of symptoms depends in large measure on the severity of the defect. A few types, such as Down's syndrome and microcephaly, are identifiable at birth owing to the presence of characteristic physical defects. However, usually the disorder is not suspected during the early months of life unless the defect is quite severe. The first inkling of abnormality comes with delay in reaching, sitting, standing and walking. Slowness to talk and difficulty in self-feeding and toilet training appear later. The infant's behavior may be very placid,

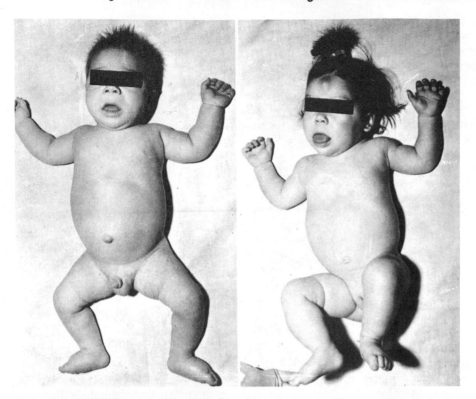

FIG. 13-7. Two infant cretins, showing characteristic facies, large tongues and trunks which are long in proportion to the extremities.

so that he is regarded as a "good" baby, or he may present the opposite extreme of restlessness, hyperactivity, irritability and sleep disturbances. Drooling of saliva is common. Convulsions, feeding difficulties and spasticity of muscles are sometimes the first indications of defective development.

When the defect is of lesser severity the child may pass through infancy and the preschool years without showing obvious symptoms. The difficulty may become apparent only when he attempts to cope with the abstract concepts of his school work (see Chaps. 25 and 28).

Diagnosis. As indicated above, only the more severe grades of mental deficiency can be diagnosed with confidence in infancy. Caution is necessary in the interpretation of delay in motor performance, for there is a wide variation from the average among intellectually normal children. It is important to be sure that delay in motor achievement is not due to associated physical disability, to the effects of chronic illness or to severe malnutrition. Poor hearing or vision may complicate the diagnosis by hampering the development of normal skills in an otherwise competent child.

Formal testing of intellectual development before the age of 1 year depends mainly on the accurate observation of the infant's use of sensory and motor skills. Interpretation of results is not as reliable as with intelligence estimates made on the older child. The most commonly used test is the Catell infant intelligence scale.

Prognosis and Management. Those forms of mental deficiency that are discovered in infancy through char-

acteristics other than the delay in neuromuscular development (Down's syndrome, microcephaly, cretinism) are often associated with a fair prognosis for mental growth. But those in which discovery depends primarily on failure of early development are, in general, fated to be severe. The earlier retardation becomes apparent, the poorer is the ultimate prognosis.

Only a few forms of mental retardation are associated with treatable conditions; cretinism, phenylketonuria, galactosemia, and convulsions due to hypoglycemia comprise a fairly complete list. It is imperative that these types be recognized as early as possible, for delay in treatment may sacrifice a portion of the infant's potential for mental growth.

The physical care of most mentally retarded infants presents no unusual problems. They merely retain their infantile behavior for a longer time. Exceptions are those in whom frequent convulsions, excessive vomiting or interminable crying accompany the defect. The major problems in management arise from the impact which the infant's condition and its implied prognosis have on his parents. Some parents react with unwillingness to accept the diagnosis and visit a number of physicians in the hope of finding one who will give a more favorable opinion. Some are overwhelmed with guilt, feeling that the infant's handicap must in some way be due to their own past misdemeanors. Such parents find institutionalization of the child hard to accept and too often martyrize themselves to his detailed care with the idea of making restitution for the wrong that they fancy they have done him. Unhappily, this attitude may result in neglect of normal children in the family. Still other parents react with grief, frustration or outright disgust to the shattering of the ambitions that they had held for the baby. Planning for the child must take cognizance not only of such varieties of parental reaction but also economic circumstances, and the availability in the community of special schools, clinics and institutions. For the seriously afflicted child the ultimate objective is custodial care. For the one with greater potential, a constructive program should be devised to capitalize on whatever assets the child has and to train him for productive and self-satisfying activities.

Systemic Disorders With Associated Mental Retardation

Hypothyroidism (Cretinism). Cretinism is the condition produced by complete absence of thyroid secretion from birth. Cretinism occurs only sporadically in this country but is found endemically in goitrous regions of other countries. Sporadic cretinism is associated with congenital absence of the thyroid gland or with an inability of the gland to make thyroid hormone. The mother of the cretin is presumably normal. Cretins develop normally up to the time of birth because of the availability of the mother's thyroid secretion. The effects of lack of thyroid make their appearance gradually. The characteristic physical features do not appear for a period of from 2 to 4 months, although certain chemical changes in the blood characteristic of hypothyroidism can be detected earlier if examination is made.

Once the condition of cretinism has developed fully it is distinctive and unmistakable, although the inexperienced often confuse it with Down's syndrome. These children are conspicuously backward mentally and have characteristic physical abnormalities. The facial features are heavy and almost pathognomonic, although an adequate word picture of them is scarcely possible. They lack the slanted eyes and the epicanthic folds of the child with Down's syndrome. The tongue protrudes from the mouth; the voice or the cry is hoarse. Two cardinal symptoms of cretinism are absence of sweating and obstinate constipation. The skin is dry, and often the hair is coarse. Generally, growth in length is greatly retarded, the retardation showing itself chiefly in the short extremities. Because of slow bone development, the fontanel remains open far beyond the normal closing time. Roentgen examination of the bones discloses that the ossification centers appropriate for the chronologic age have failed to appear. Tooth eruption is delayed. The poor muscle tone leads to protrusion of the abdomen, and often there is an umbilical hernia.

In addition to the clinical appearance and behavior of the child, various laboratory tests may assist in confirming the suspicion that thyroid function is depressed. Radioactive iodine given by mouth fails to reach a normal concentration in the thyroid gland, as determined by the Geiger counter. Chemical examination of the blood shows an abnormally low level of iodine which is bound to protein (PBI or BEI). Direct measurement of thyroid hormones T-3 and T-4 also gives lower values. Blood lipids may be abnormally high. More cumbersome but useful are tests of basal metabolism and creatine excretion in the urine, both of which give low values in hypothyroidism.

The prognosis in cretinism depends on how early and how effectively treatment is given. If an adequate amount of thyroid is given very early, the physical growth will proceed in a normal manner, and the mental development will tend to be relatively normal. It is seldom that mental development is fully satisfactory, even when the best methods of treatment are instituted early in infancy.

The treatment consists of the administration of dried thyroid gland by mouth. The amount of thyroid should be the maximum that can be taken without symptoms of overdosage. A cretin infant will require from 0.5 to 1.5 grains daily. The original dose should be smaller, and then the amount should be increased to tolerance. The diet should be complete and should include ample vitamin D. Without vitamin D, rickets is very likely to develop because of the very rapid rate at which the bone will grow when thyroid is first given. The symptoms of overdosage of thyroid are

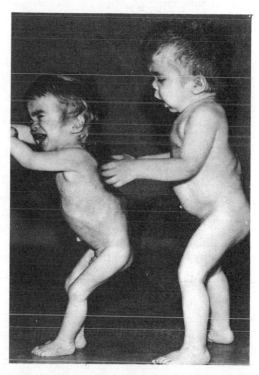

Fig. 13-8. Two children in the same family, showing the typical features of Hurler's syndrome (gargoylism). (Buchanan, D. N.: *In* Grulee, C. G., and Eley, R. C.: The Child in Health and Disease, Baltimore, Williams & Wilkins)

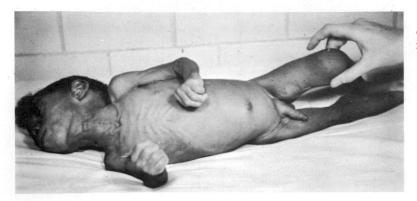

FIG. 13-9. Spastic paralysis. Note the retraction of the head, the arching of the back and the clenching of the fists. (Dr. R. Platou)

the same as those of hyperthyroidism; notably, vomiting, diarrhea, irritability, fever, rapid pulse and weight loss.

Tay-Sachs Disease (Amaurotic Familial Idiocy). This disorder affects infants, usually of Jewish ancestry, and leads to arrested and then regressing mental development around the age of 6 months. Characteristic changes are visible in the fundus of the eye. The degenerative changes progress so rapidly that life seldom is spared for more than a year after the diagnosis is made. In Tay-Sachs disease, lipid degeneration is observed mainly in the central nervous system.

Niemann-Pick Disease. This is closely related to Tay-Sachs disease but attended by additional widespread deposition of lipid substances in organs such as the spleen, liver, lungs and lymph nodes.

Gaucher's Disease. This is another form of lipoid storage disease. In its usual form it affects adults and older children without threat to life or mentality. When seen during infancy, severe mental retardation occurs.

Hurler's Syndrome (Gargoylism, Lipochondrodystrophy). In this hereditary disorder there are widespread changes in the body due to abnormal deposits in the brain, spleen, liver, bone marrow and the cornea of the eyes. It is recognized easily by the gradual appearance of facial features and body characteristics which are almost identical in all affected children. The appearance is much like that of the Duchess in the popular illustrations of *Alice in Wonderland*. Mental retardation is usually definite but moderate, and the disease often permits the child to survive for a number of years.

Hurler's syndrome is due to the recessive transmission of a defect in the metabolism of connective tissue which leads to the accumulation of abnormal products in the soft tissue and the growing bones. This is accompanied by the excretion of a characteristic chemical in the urine. No method is currently known for controlling the defect.

Phenylketonuria (Phenylpyruvic Oligophrenia). See Chapter 11.

Galactosemia is a recessively inherited metabolic defect in which the enzyme that converts galactose to glucose in the liver is missing. Accumulation of galactose in the body gradually leads to enlargement of the liver and spleen, cirrhosis, cataracts and mental retardation. The diagnosis is confirmed by the chemical demonstration of an excess of galactose in the blood or, more simply, by finding it in the urine from which it is normally absent. Since galactose is a component of milk sugar (lactose), it is highly important to discover the defect early and change the infant to a diet free of lactose before irreversible damage has occurred in the liver and brain.

Motor Disabilities of Cerebral Origin (Cerebral Palsies)

"Cerebral palsy" is the term commonly but unwisely used as a comprehensive diagnostic one for children who have difficulty with voluntary muscle control. It erroneously implies that such children suffer from a specific disease entity which has some uniformity of etiology, symptomatology, prognosis or therapy. Such is not the case. On the one hand, the use of an all-inclusive label may unnecessarily stigmatize the child who has a mild disability and a good prognosis; on the other hand, it may encourage the parents of a hopelessly disabled child to pursue the chimera of recovery because of the knowledge that others with the same diagnosis have improved under treatment or have made a good adjustment in society.

Etiology. In a few children with motor disability the etiologic mechanism is clear and not subject to debate. In such children the symptoms begin after a specific postnatal illness. The most common cause is encephalitis, either primary or as a complication of one of the contagious diseases. Other precursors of motor disability are brain damage due to lead poisoning or to severe febrile illness, such as pneumonia, complications of meningitis, head injury, and kernicterus, the cerebral complication of erythroblastosis fetalis.

However, more numerous than these are the instances of motor defect in which natal or prenatal disturbances are thought to be at fault. There is considerable disagreement concerning the relative importance of abnormal brain development during fetal life and the potentially damaging mechanisms of birth—

narcosis, anoxia, trauma and hemorrhage. The presumptive mechanism may be apparent in certain children, but it is necessary to admit that in a great many the relative importance of prenatal and natal factors cannot be designated.

Clinical Manifestations. SPASTICITY. The most frequent manifestation of motor disability is spasticity. In this condition the voluntary muscles lose their normal fluidity and respond with difficulty to either the voluntary efforts of the child or the passive efforts of the examiner to alter their position. Abnormally strong tonus of certain muscle groups keeps the extremities and other portions of the body in characteristic attitudes which are altered jerkily by voluntary efforts. Spasticity is most often apparent in the lower extremities, where it tends to point the toes and cross the legs. In the arms it usually produces some clenching of the fist, flexion of the forearm and adduction of the upper arm against the chest wall. In severely affected children there may be an involvement of the muscles of the trunk which keep the back arched and the head extended.

All degrees of severity of the symptoms are observed. Severe generalized spasticity results in a rigid, physically helpless child. Very mild degrees may not be apparent to casual observation and can be detected only by a careful neurologic examination. In some instances spasticity may be limited to one side of the body or to one extremity. The eye muscles may participate with the production of a convergent strabismus. In severely affected infants and children, swallowing may be difficult or impossible, owing to the involvement of muscles of the face, tongue, jaws and pharynx.

WEAKNESS. Localized and diffuse weakness of muscles often is mixed in with the more obvious symptoms of spasticity. In some children the signs of brain damage are exclusively those of general or local weakness without associated spasticity.

INVOLUNTARY MOVEMENTS. Several varieties of involuntary movement may be seen, usually in conjunction with other manifestations of brain damage.

Chorea consists of quick, brief movements of a localized portion of the body, most commonly an arm or the face.

Athetosis is a slow, prolonged, writhing movement of the extremities.

Frequently, the athetosis is combined with chorea, and the resulting motions are designated as *choreo-athetosis.*

A persistent vibration of an extremity is called a *tremor.*

ASSOCIATED DISTURBANCES. Children with motor disability frequently have the additional problems of convulsions or mental retardation or behavior disturbances. These aspects are probably a concomitant of the brain damage which has produced the motor disturbance and the parents' reactions to it. They are of varying importance to individual children and have no necessary relationship to the severity of the motor disturbance. A child with severe choreo-athetosis may have normal or even superior intelligence; one with mild spasticity may be severely retarded. Their management must be considered in relation to the child's total problem and his and his family's response to it.

Diagnosis. Motor disability of cerebral origin may be recognized shortly after birth when the symptoms are severe. The early appearance of afebrile convulsions, feeding difficulties or spasticity in the first few months of life may raise the suspicion of brain damage which is confirmed by the subsequent failure of the child to follow the normal pattern of motor development. Except for the milder and the localized varieties of motor disability, all manifestations, such as spasticity, weakness and involuntary movement, interfere with the achievement of sitting, walking, talking, feeding and other coordinated muscle activities. Often it is the failure in such performance that first attracts attention to the possibility of brain damage. While the presence of motor disability is an adequate explanation for developmental failure, it does not necessarily imply that the more complex functions of the brain are damaged. It is imperative to evaluate the intellectual capacity of the child separately in order to guide his management. This is often a very difficult task, because the motor disability may hamper his ability to communicate and vitiates many of the performances required by the standard intelligence tests.

Treatment and Nursing Care. No form of therapy can be expected to restore the cerebral defect. Appropriate management must be based on a realistic appraisal of the individual child's assets and ultimate potentialities. If convulsions are present they should be controlled by the measures discussed in a preceding section.

In the period of infancy, the child with cerebral palsy may show difficulty in sucking, swallowing and learning to eat solid foods. A hyperactive gag reflex often initiates vomiting. The whole body tightens up, and when feedings are not given slowly enough, vomiting and aspiration may result. Gradually, he will need to be taught to eat solid foods. At first, swallowing them will produce difficulties, but patience and calmness when they are refused, spit out or vomited eventually will help him to learn to eat them.

Respiratory difficulties and body spasticity in early life are not uncommon. The changes in respiration may be due to mucus or to the cerebral lesion. Often, the infant lies with his back arched, and spasticity may make movement difficult. Frequent change of position lessens his irritability and discomfort.

In the management of the child with cerebral palsy, one of the first objectives is the prevention of contractures. If contractures develop or seem to be imminent, the baby should be provided with corrective splints. For most babies these may be worn only at night. A back support or a corset may be needed to enable the baby to sit. Leg splints usually are used in the daytime if the Achilles group of muscles go into spasm whenever the baby is placed on his feet.

During this early period in the child's life, the parents will require help to accept the child and to gain security in their ability to satisfy his needs. To accomplish this the strengths within the family and the community must be utilized to the fullest. Concentration on the child's assets is not enough. More important is recognition of the family's real problems, their feelings about them and their capacities to shoulder responsibility for the education and the socialization of their child. They will need strong professional support and understanding to make independent decisions relating to plans for his care. They will also need help to discover the community resources which are available to them and to find ways to meet the particular needs of their child.

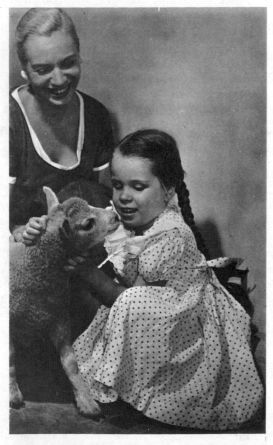

Fig. 13-10. This blind child has learned to explore her environment through her other senses. Aided by appropriate stimulation and permission from her mother to try things independently, she is able to attend school and participate in the full program with sighted children. (From Miriam Norris)

Sensory Defects

Recognition of Visual Defects. The analysis and the correction of visual defects constitute a highly technical specialty which can be performed only by those with special training. When there is obvious deformity or abnormal movement of the eyes the infant usually is brought quickly under the care of such a specialist. But in many instances the visual defect is a subtle one which is discovered only through the astute observations of parents, nurses or physicians. In some instances early discovery and proper management are essential to preserve bilateral vision; in other instances it is necessary to prevent later problems of social and educational adjustment. Most of the visual defects that are not grossly apparent depend on errors of refraction in one or both eyes. A few are due to abnormal development or disease of the retina and its vascular or nervous supply.

Visual defects in infants may easily go unnoticed for several weeks or months. Early suspicions may be aroused after the infant has reached the age of 2 months if he fails to observe objects or to follow them with his eyes or to blink when they are brought close to his eyes. During the second half of the first year the child's failure to locate distant objects and his propensity for bringing things very close to his face for inspection may lead to the suspicion that he has severe myopia.

An infant who has a severe refractive error may begin to squint. More importantly, he may begin to favor his better eye and slowly lose the vision in the other eye because of disuse. Unless the poor vision in the defective eye is discovered early and efforts are made to correct it or to encourage the child to use the eye some of the time, its vision may be lost irretrievably.

Psychological Considerations. Minor or correctable visual defects seldom create important problems of adjustment. Glasses have become so common among young children that the average child soon accepts the fact that he must wear them and makes an easy adjustment.

The parents of infants who are discovered to have serious visual defects or total blindness nearly always require help in adjusting to the handicap suffered by the child, in understanding the normal aspects of his individual development, in recognizing the cues that signal his need for new learning experiences and in seeing the child's urgent need to learn in his own natural way. After a five-year study of preschool blind children, Norris, Spaulding and Brodie concluded that blind children, including those with retrolental fibroplasia, have the potentialities to grow up into independent, trusting, self-respecting, free-functioning individuals who can be compared favorably with healthy sighted children.

Deafness. Complete deafness may go unrecognized

until after the first year when the child's failure to begin to speak and to relate himself normally to his parents and other children stimulates further investigation. Loss of hearing should be suspected during infancy if the baby fails to blink at loud noises. The etiology may be congenital defects of the internal ear or the auditory nerves. Erythroblastosis, mumps, meningitis and recurring infections of the middle ear are afflictions of infancy that may be followed by loss of hearing. Treatment is generally deferred until the child is old enough to cooperate with the technics of lip-reading and the acceptance of special apparatus to improve his hearing. The subject is considered further in Chapter 28.

THE CARDIOVASCULAR SYSTEM

Congenital abnormalities of the heart and the great blood vessels are discussed in Chapter 22 where basic aspects of anatomy, physiology, diagnosis and treatment are considered. The problems of cardiovascular defects are encountered in all age groups from newborn to adulthood. The more severe the functional disturbance, the earlier clinical symptoms appear. Some of the malformations permit survival for only a few hours or days. Those of slightly lesser functional severity interfere with growth during the first year or precipitate heart failure. Others may be clinically silent for a number of years. Medical and nursing care is directed at bringing the baby into optimal condition to withstand the hazards of surgical correction of his defect if such drastic treatment is both possible and warranted.

THE GENITOURINARY TRACT

Except for those anomalies which are externally visible, congenital malformations remain clinically silent until infection or obstruction of the urinary stream attracts attention to their presence. Infection is by far the most common signal of their presence. This is discussed in the next chapter.

THE HEMATOPOIETIC SYSTEM

Hereditary abnormalities of the blood produce various types of anemia and one coagulation defect—hemophilia. Although frequently identified in the first year, their more characteristic features tend to appear later and, consequently, discussion of these abnormalities is deferred to Chapter 21.

SITUATIONS FOR FURTHER STUDY

1. How does understanding of the mechanism that produces pyloric stenosis influence your nursing care of the baby with this disorder?

2. What stressful situations would you anticipate encountering in working with parents of children with cystic fibrosis? Discuss these and your feeling about them. How would you plan nursing intervention in order to be of assistance to parents? What agencies are available in your community to help parents with long range planning for necessary treatment and financial assistance? What are the necessary procedures for referral to a community or state agency?

3. Describe the screening technics now used in your hospital to detect phenylketonuria. What facilities are available in your community and state for case finding and follow-up of families who have children with this disease?

4. How would you outline the responsibilities of the nurse in the care of infants with cerebral palsy? What anticipatory guidance would you give to parents? What assistance can be given to parents of children with cerebral palsy through your state agency for the care of handicapped children?

5. Study the article by Legeay and Keogh regarding the impact of mental retardation on family life. What defenses would you expect parents to use when confronted with such a diagnosis for their child? What influence might the birth of a retarded child have on the other family members? What values in our society make it difficult for parents to accept such a diagnosis? What information must the nurse have who is working with parents of a mentally retarded child? What plans for nursing intervention would you make to assist parents through the crisis of institutionalization?

6. Read the article by Boyd and discuss the stages through which parents pass in adjusting to the birth of a mentally deficient child. In what ways could a nurse function during stages I and II?

7. How would you anticipate that the development of a blind infant might differ from that of a child with normal vision? What anticipatory guidance would the parents require to assist the infant to develop optimally? What sensory stimulation would you suggest to replace visual exploration?

BIBLIOGRAPHY

Basara, S.: The behavioral patterns of the perceptually handicapped child, Nursing Forum 5:24, 1966.
Bonine, G.: The myelodysplastic child: Hospital and home care, Am. J. Nurs. 69:541, 1969.
Boyd, Dan: Three stages in the growth of a parent of a mentally retarded child, Am. J. Ment. Defic. 55:608, 1951.
Burgess, L.: Morale boosting in cystic fibrosis, Am. J. Nurs. 69:322, 1969.
Centerwall, W. R., Centerwall, S. A., Arman, V., and Mann, L. B.: Phenylketonuria. II. Results of treatment of infants and young children, J. Pediat. 59:102, 1961.
Cohen, N., and Baker, G.: Jean's story, Nurs. Outlook *11*: 721, 1963.
Fackler, E.: The crisis of institutionalizing a retarded child, Am. J. Nurs. 68:1508, 1968.
Ford, F. R.: Diseases of the Nervous System in Infancy, Childhood and Adolescence, ed. 5, Springfield, Ill., Thomas, 1966.
Frankenburg, W., and Dodds, J.: The Denver Developmental Screening Test, J. Pediat. *71*:181, 1967.

French, E. L., and Scott, J. C.: The Child in the Shadows: A Manual for Parents of Retarded Children, Philadelphia, Lippincott, 1960.

Hall, Elizabeth, and Johnson, Gertrude: They turn to nurses, Am. J. Nurs. *61*:60, 1961.

Hill, M., Shurtleff, D., Chapman, W., and Ansell, J.: The myelodysplastic child: Bowel and bladder control, Am. J. Nurs. *69*:545, 1969.

Johnson, M., and Fassett, B.: Bronchopulmonary hygiene in cystic fibrosis, Am. J. Nurs. *69*:320, 1969.

Jubenville, C. P.: Day care centers for severely retarded children, Nurs. Outlook *8*:371, 1960.

Keogh, B., and Legeay, C.: Recoil from the diagnosis of mental retardation, Am. J. Nurs. *66*:778, 1966.

Legeay, C., and Keogh, B.: Impact of mental retardation on family life, Am. J. Nurs. *66*:1062, 1966.

Livingston, S.: Living with epileptic seizures, J. Pediat. *59*:128, 1961.

Lynn, H. B.: The mechanism of pyloric stenosis and its relationship to preoperative preparation, A.M.A. Arch. Surg. *81*:453, 1960.

Milio, N.: Family-centered care for cystic fibrosis, Nurs. Outlook *11*:718, 1963.

Paine, R.: Hydrocephalus, Pediat. Clin. N. Amer. *14*:779, 1967.

Ragsdale, Nancy, and Koch, Richard: Phenylketonuria, Am. J. Nurs. *64*:90, 1964.

Schwab, L., Collison, C. B., and Frank, M. P.: Cystic fibrosis, Am. J. Nurs. *63*:62, 1963.

Swenson, O., and Davidson, F. Z.: Similarities of mechanical intestinal obstruction and aganglionic megacolon in the newborn infant, New Eng. J. Med. *262*:64, 1960.

Yannet, Herman: Mental Deficiency *in* Nelson, W. E. (ed.): Textbook of Pediatrics, ed. 8, Philadelphia, Saunders, 1964.

14

Nursing Care of the Infant With Infection

CONGENITAL SYPHILIS

Congenital syphilis disappears rapidly when prenatal medical supervision is good. In the United States it has practically vanished in regions where serologic tests on the blood of all pregnant women are required.

Etiology

Syphilis is caused by the motile spirillum *Treponema pallidum,* which is ordinarily transmitted as a venereal infection. During recent infection the spirochetes circulate in the bloodstream from time to time. A pregnant woman in this stage of the disease may transmit spirochetes to her fetus. If a severe infection of the placenta occurs, abortion or stillbirth of the baby may result. With lesser degrees of infection or when the transmission occurs late in pregnancy, a live-born infected infant may result. Many such infants show no clinical manifestations of disease despite positive serologic evidence. Others may be born with obvious infection or, more likely, will develop symptoms between 3 and 8 weeks of age. Adequate treatment of the mother during pregnancy can prevent the passage of disease to the fetus or effect an *in utero* cure if transmission has occurred already.

Symptoms

Syphilis is capable of producing many different lesions but never do all of them occur in one infant. Therefore, the average or typical case cannot be described.

Of the various lesions, rhinitis ("snuffles") is the most frequent.

Skin eruptions of the copper-colored macular variety seen in the secondary stage of acquired syphilis occur in a high proportion of cases. The palms and soles become reddened and thickened, with later desquamation. This same type of inflammation may occur in the skin about the mouth. When it does, it is accom-

panied by fissures that radiate in all directions from the mouth. Untreated, these fissures tend to remain for a long period and finally to heal with permanent scarring. The radiating scars are known as rhagades and are considered as pathognomonic of a former syphilitic infection.

Syphilitic inflammation at the ends of the long bones may be severe enough to cause pain which inhibits voluntary motion. This pseudoparalysis of syphilis occurs almost exclusively in the first 6 months of life.

Neurosyphilis. Syphilitic infection of the central nervous system occurs in approximately one third of all syphilitic infants. The diagnosis is made by examination of the cerebrospinal fluid.

Syphilis of the eye is relatively uncommon in infancy, although in the older child it is the most com-

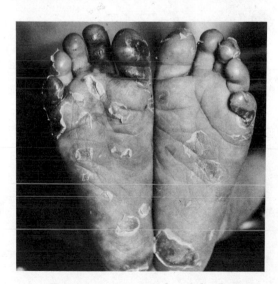

Fig. 14-1. Congenital syphilis showing shiny erythema and desquamation of feet before treatment.

237

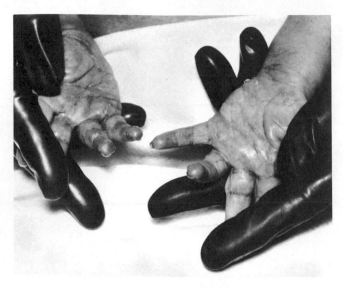

FIG. 14-2. Congenital syphilis showing shiny erythema and desquamation of hands after treatment.

mon of all lesions. A high proportion of babies with syphilis have enlargement of the spleen, and approximately one third have fever in some degree during the acute stages, but this usually is not high.

Late Manifestations. The symptoms that appear in early infancy correspond to the secondary stages of adult syphilis. If the infection goes untreated, the child may show the effects of his chronic disease in a great variety of ways in later years. During the 2nd and 3rd years condylomata, mucous patches and gummata may

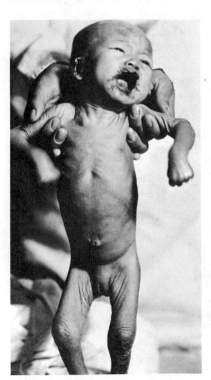

FIG. 14-3. Illustrating some of the skin manifestations of syphilis.

be found. The truly late manifestations emerge in the school-age child. The incisor teeth of the second dentition may be peg shaped and notched (Hutchinson's teeth), and crumbled deformation of the cusps of molar teeth may be observed. Nerve deafness and interstitial keratitis are found. The central nervous system may suffer extensive destruction, producing optic atrophy, pupillary abnormalities, tabes, paralysis and dementia. Thickening of the periosteum of the long bones and chronic effusion into and destruction of joints, particularly the knees, are other late manifestations. All of these unfortunate consequences can be avoided if the diagnosis is made early and treatment is carried out.

Diagnosis

From some of the early lesions such as nasal discharges and open skin ulcers it is possible to detect living spirochetes under the microscope. (Such material is potentially contagious so that it is prudent to observe good isolation technic including the use of gloves.) Usually, however, diagnosis depends primarily upon the demonstration of a positive serologic test for syphilis (STS). It must be remembered that the antibodies which react in most of such tests can be transmitted across the placenta from mother to baby prior to birth. If the baby shows no clinical manifestations of syphilis and the mother's serologic reaction is positive, it is possible that the positive serologic reaction of the infant merely reflects transmitted antibody and not disease. When this is the case, such antibodies disappear rapidly within the first 3 to 4 months. The Treponema pallidum inhibition test (TPI) is probably a more conclusive method of differentiating real infection from passively transmitted antibody, but the test is difficult to perform and many laboratories are not equipped to do it.

Treatment

The older methods of treatment with heavy metal injections have been superseded completely by penicillin given in a dose of 100,000 to 1,000,000 units per kilogram of body weight over a period of 3 to 5 days. With the possible exception of spirochetes which have long been entrenched in the central nervous system, this treatment can be expected to kill all the organisms present in the body. Of course, it cannot be counted on to undo the scars of previous damage. Although the need for additional therapy is remote, generally it is agreed that children should be kept under surveillance for one to two years after treatment. Reversal of the blood serologic reaction from positive to negative occurs in all but a small fraction of cases. The broad-spectrum antibiotics are generally effective against the spirochete of syphilis when penicillin sensitivity makes its use inadvisable.

THE CONTAGIOUS DISEASES

The traditional contagious diseases infrequently affect infants. During the early months they enjoy varying degrees of protection from passively transmitted antibodies from their immune mothers. A more important factor is the relative isolation in which they live, permitting them to escape contact with persons who are infectious. When special circumstances—usually the presence of an infected sibling in the household—result in exposure, small infants can acquire any of the contagious diseases. The severity varies with the different infections and with the age and the immune status of the infant. Usually, rubella and mumps create only minor illness. Measles and diphtheria are rarely seen before 6 to 9 months of age but may be quite serious if they occur. Chickenpox and poliomyelitis can appear at almost any period of the first year and are apt to be relatively severe. Because they are particularly hazardous for the infant, pertussis, exanthem subitum and streptococcal infections are discussed in this and the succeeding section. More information about the other forms of contagion may be found in Chapters 18 and 19.

Pertussis (Whooping Cough)

Pertussis is described with the diseases of infancy because it carries the greatest risk of morbidity and mortality in this age group. Receiving *no* passive protection from his mother, even though she has had the disease or been immunized, the small infant is at once vulnerable to exposure from older children in the family, neighborhood, hospital or clinic.

Pathophysiology. Whooping cough is caused by a gram-negative bacillus, *Hemophilus pertussis,* discovered by Bordet and Gengou. It invades the whole respiratory tree in susceptible individuals, producing at first a catarrhal inflammation with outpouring of mucus from the nasopharynx and bronchi. Large numbers of the organisms invade the walls of the bronchial tree where extensive lymphocytic invasion suggests the source of the chronic irritation and explains the exaggeration of the bronchial markings which can be seen by x-ray. Usually the disease is afebrile, its drastic symptoms depending more upon the mechanical discomfort and secondary consequences of the extreme cough than upon toxicity. However, the debilitated mucosa is sometimes invaded by other bacterial agents and a damaging form of pneumonia may ensue which has the capacity to lead to permanent scarring and deformity of the bronchial tree.

Typical Symptomatology of the Older Infant and Child. The incubation period varies between 7 and 14 days. The disease begins as an ordinary bronchitis with only slight fever and little or no prostration. The cough becomes increasingly severe and finally assumes the peculiar paroxysmal nature characteristic of pertussis. The early stage is known as the catarrhal stage.

Its duration is about a week but it may vary from 2 days to 2 weeks. The stage of severe cough is known as the paroxysmal or spasmodic stage. The duration of this stage also is variable but is usually from 2 to 3 weeks.

The typical paroxysm of pertussis consists of a series of explosive coughs rapidly repeated on a single expiration with no time for a breath between them. When the breath is expired to such an extent that no more coughing is possible, there is a rapid intake of air, and the coughing continues. This procedure may be repeated three or four or even more times.

Each inspiration during the paroxysm is accompanied by a peculiar crowing sound or whoop. The sound is produced by a spasm of the glottis. A severe paroxysm is a serious and terrifying ordeal for the child. Due to inability to breathe over such a long period, there is a feeling of impending suffocation. At first the face becomes red because of the coughing effort. As the attack progresses, the face becomes darker in color, the eyes and the veins of the neck become prominent, the tongue protrudes with each cough, and tears, saliva and perspiration flow freely. The paroxysm continues until the mucus which was the immediate exciting cause is dislodged. Toward the end of the paroxysm this mass of ropy mucus may be expelled a considerable distance from the mouth. Vomiting is frequent immediately after a paroxysm, often making the nutrition of the child a serious problem. The paroxysms vary in number, from only a few up to 50 or 60 in 24 hours.

Unless the child suffers from loss of sleep because of frequent cough and from loss of food by vomiting, he passes through the paroxysmal stage with unimpaired nutrition and in apparent good health. In the absence of complications there is no fever. As in other infectious diseases, pertussis occurs with varying degrees of severity. Sometimes the paroxysms are infrequent and mild, and no doubt there are many instances of pertussis infection in which the symptoms are so mild that the condition is not diagnosed.

Symptomatology of the Small Infant. Before the age of 3 to 4 months infants do not show either the catarrhal stage of the disease or the characteristic whoop. Instead, coughing paroxysms are likely to be replaced with apneic spells in which the small infant is unable to raise the thick, obstructing mucus from his lungs owing either to fatigue or to the less efficient cough mechanism. Unless continuous vigilance is taken, the small infant may fail to resume breathing during such a spell and die of suffocation.

Dehydration and weight loss from starvation are more likely to occur in the small infant if his coughing spells are followed by vomiting. Immediate refeeding after a vomited meal will usually maintain hydration and nutrition.

Complications. Interstitial bronchopneumonia is the most frequent and serious complication of pertussis apart from the smothering episodes described above. The mortality from pneumonia is highest in the small infants. Due to the increased pressure within the veins of the head and neck during the forced expiration of the cough, hemorrhages may occur as petechiae in the skin, epistaxis, subconjunctival hemorrhage and rarely intracranial hemorrhage. Except for the latter, these hemorrhagic manifestations are not serious. Inguinal hernia and rectal prolapse may occasionally follow the increased abdominal pressure experienced during repeated paroxysms.

A rare but serious complication is encephalopathy with convulsions, coma and residual brain damage.

Diagnosis. When the characteristic whoop followed by vomiting is present, the clinical diagnosis is easily made. At this stage there is usually a marked increase in the number and percentage of small lymphocytes in the peripheral blood. Laboratory confirmation of the diagnosis depends upon the demonstration of the *H. pertussis* in the mucus brought up from deep in the lungs. Unfortunately, many laboratories have difficulty in making the isolation with assurance.

Treatment. Children or infants with pertussis should be isolated from susceptible persons for a period of 2 to 3 weeks after the onset of the paroxysmal stage during which they are still expelling organisms. Unfortunately their degree of contagiousness is probably even higher during the catarrhal stage of the disease before it is recognized as pertussis.

For the older child whose risk of serious consequences is relatively small, treatment consists mainly of measures to relieve his cough and maintain nutrition. Cough medicines and sedatives have but a limited effect upon the cough. If isolation in his own back yard can be enforced, these children are often more comfortable out of doors in good weather. As with infants, refeeding after a paroxysm with vomiting is a useful technic because the cough is usually inhibited for a time immediately after the paroxysm.

For the infant with a less favorable prognosis, antibiotics and hyperimmune serum or gamma globulin preparations prepared against the specific organism are generally used. Chloramphenicol, ampicillin, streptomycin and the tetracyclines have all been used with some doubt about their efficacy. Proof of the effectiveness of the preparations providing specific immune substances is also debatable. However, most clinicians feel that some benefit is derived from them. A moist atmosphere is generally soothing to the infant, but it should be so arranged that the very important aspect of nursing vigilance is not obstructed.

Prevention. Since the introduction of active immunization against pertussis, the incidence has fallen progressively and the mortality, particularly among small infants, has almost disappeared. Where public health programs fail to reach a high percentage of the child population, however, the disease still prevails and constitutes a threat to the small infant. When exposure of an infant is known to have occurred, administration of hyperimmune serum or gamma globulin should be given as soon as possible.

Exanthem Subitum (Roseola Infantum)

Exanthem subitum is a benign, presumably infectious, disease of infancy and early childhood characterized by fever of from 3 to 5 days' duration which terminates by crisis and a morbilliform eruption which appears as the temperature declines.

Etiology. The causative agent has not been identified but probably is a virus. Although direct communicability is not evident and no epidemics have been reported, sporadic cases tend to occur in a community at approximately the same time. The disease occurs predominantly in infancy and nearly always under 3 years of age, though a few cases in older persons have been reported.

SYMPTOMS AND COMPLICATIONS. The onset is abrupt, with fever which rises to between 102° and 105° F. in a few hours. Accompanying the fever may be a moderate amount of restlessness, fretfulness, irritability and food refusal, but these are not constant. Despite the high fever, the child does not appear to be toxic and even may be playful and apparently comfortable. On examination, no abnormality other than fever may be noted. One constant characteristic of the disease is leukopenia, with relative increase in lymphocytes. In different cases the white count varies from 2,500 to 7,000, and the proportion of lymphocytes is between 75 and 85 per cent.

A few children present slight redness of the throat. In some groups of cases reported, moderate enlargement of the superficial glands of the neck has been present; in other groups, this has been absent. The glandular enlargement, if present, appears on the second or third day. The fever continues for approximately 4 days, with some tendency to slight morning remissions. The fever ends usually by crisis, and at the same time the characteristic eruption appears. With the cessation of fever and appearance of the eruption, any previous indisposition disappears, and the child seems to be as well as ever.

The *eruption* is macular or at times slightly maculopapular. The early individual lesions are pink or pale red and about 3 mm. in diameter. They tend to increase in size and to coalesce, in this respect resembling measles. The color disappears on pressure. As the lesion becomes older, it tends to fade at the center and irregularly acquires a slightly bluish color, similar to some lesions of erythema multiforme. No unanimity exists in published reports as to the site of first appearance of the eruption, and one is led to the conclusion that no uniformity exists. Regardless of where it begins, it spreads rapidly to its maximal extent and when fully out is most extensive and prominent on the trunk or perhaps the trunk and neck, and the lesions are relatively sparse on the face and extremities. Usually the eruption reaches its height in 24 hours or less and disappears in another 24 hours or more. Either no desquamation, or at most a very faint branny desquamation, follows.

No complications or fatalities ever have been reported.

Isolation. Isolation is not required. Any transmissibility that the disease may have probably is terminated by the time the rash appears and the diagnosis is made.

Diagnosis and Treatment. The diagnosis cannot be made with certainty before the eruption appears. After it appears, the diagnosis presents no difficulty. The two diseases with which it might be confused are measles and rubella. It does not have the catarrhal symptoms or the Koplik's spots of measles. High prodomal fever is absent in rubella.

No treatment is needed.

RESPIRATORY INFECTIONS

General Considerations

To some extent—as in the case of the contagious diseases—small infants are protected against respiratory infections by the sheltered life that they lead. Instead of the numerous people whom the school-age child meets, members of his immediate family are the only vectors of infection for the infant. It is apparent that the larger the family and the more crowded the living conditions the less complete his isolation will be.

The complicated question of etiology is discussed in Chapter 18 to which the reader is referred for details. In a general way, infants are more susceptible than adults or older children to infection by the common agents. In fact, others in the family may not be aware that they are carrying the infectious agent to the infant, since they themselves suffer no symptoms. Little or no protective immunity is passed from the mother to the infant through the placental circulation. However, infants nursing at the breast seem to have relatively good resistance against infections to which they are exposed.

An important handicap for small infants is the size of the various tubular structures of the respiratory passages—particularly the eustachian tubes, larynx and bronchi. Serious obstruction is much more likely to occur in these small tubes than in the larger structures of the older individual. This fact alone accounts for many of the complications and the increased mortality rates from respiratory disease in infants.

The Upper Respiratory Tract

Nasopharyngitis

The common form of upper respiratory infection is known by many names—cold, rhinitis, coryza, virus infection. Most of these start as virus infections which create a catarrhal inflammation of the membranes of the nose and throat, and sometimes the conjunctiva.

The symptoms that result are nasal discharge, sneezing, cough, restlessness and loss of appetite. Usually, fever is absent, but in some instances the onset is more dramatic with significant or even marked elevation in temperature, vomiting or diarrhea, and perhaps a convulsion.

For the mildly afflicted infant his illness is annoying mainly because it obstructs his nose, interfering with breathing and feeding. If it remains uncomplicated, the upper respiratory infection may run a course of 3 to 10 days during which the secretions from the nose become thicker and gradually disappear. Cough often lingers for several days after obvious discharges have disappeared. Treatment consists of the instillation of drops into the nose in order to shrink nasal membranes and alleviate breathing difficulty as much as possible. Liquid secretions should be wiped or sucked away and a few drops of nasal decongestant such as 0.25 per cent Neo-Synephrine instilled. If this is done a short time before feeding, it produces a temporary airway which allows the infant to breathe more comfortably while feeding. Since thick secretions are difficult for him to expel, a well humidified atmosphere is desirable.

When infections are accompanied by high fever, a search for complicating bacterial invasion or otitis media should be made. If either is proved to be present or is strongly suspected, antibiotic therapy usually should be added to the symptomatic measures just described.

Retropharyngeal Abscess

A retropharyngeal abscess arises from suppuration in the lymph glands back of the posterior pharyngeal wall. Infection in these glands is preceded by infection elsewhere in the upper respiratory tract. Often the primary infection is a common cold. Retropharyngeal glands are present at birth and tend to atrophy and disappear after a few years. For this reason, retropharyngeal abscess occurs most frequently under 3 years of age.

Symptoms. As the abscess develops, the infant becomes restless and is found to have fever, which, though variable, is often high. Prostration frequently is out of proportion to the obvious physical findings. Swallowing is painful, and attempts to swallow may give rise to choking. Sometimes the taking of food is impossible. The head may be held retracted toward the affected side, the abscess usually having a unilateral origin. A swelling may be visible externally on the affected side. When the swelling in the pharynx increases sufficiently, obstruction to breathing occurs, and stridor and dyspnea result. Respiratory obstruction may be great enough to threaten life unless relieved promptly.

Diagnosis. Examination of the throat is difficult because of the small size of the infant, difficulty in opening the mouth, and the presence of frothy mucus in the pharynx. The presence of swelling is determined by palpation. It may have a boggy feeling, and sometimes fluctuation will be observed. The use of a laryngoscope usually is of considerable assistance in the diagnosis because of the better opportunity for adequate inspection.

Treatment. Retropharyngeal abscesses should be incised without anesthesia and with the infant's head lower than his chest so that the pus released will not obstruct his airway. The operator, in any event, must be prepared for sudden respiratory arrest which occurs with some frequency. After the pus is released and the pharynx suctioned, the incision is usually spread to permit free drainage. Antibiotics, usually penicillin, should be continued or started since retropharyngeal abscess is always bacterial in origin and most often due to beta hemolytic streptococcal infection.

Otitis Media

Pathogenesis. The middle ear is a small air-containing cavity interposed between the drum, which separates it from the external ear, and the inner ear, which is set into the temporal bone and contains the organs of hearing and equilibrium. The ear drum is a sensitive curtain hung between the air of the external and the middle ear. It transmits the minute changes of pressure created by the sound waves through a chain of small bones (the ossicles) to the oval window of the inner ear. The middle ear communicates through a long narrow channel (eustachian tube) with the pharynx. During health the eustachian tube is closed most of the time by its external muscular coating but opens briefly during the acts of swallowing, yawning and crying to permit rapid equalization of air pressure between the middle ear and the pharynx. (Except during violent nose-blowing, the pressure in the pharynx is automatically the same as that of the air on the external surface of the ear drum.) The symptoms of mild pain in the ear and blurred hearing which are experienced during air travel are due to imperfect equalization of air pressures on the two sides of the drum. The middle ear also communicates with the mastoid antrum and its ramified system of air cells within the temporal bone.

Infection of the middle ear almost invariably arises from the pharynx by way of the eustachian tube. Consequently, the bacteria usually involved are the same ones responsible for pharyngitis and tonsillitis—hemolytic streptococci, pneumococci and influenza bacilli. A wide variety of other organisms may be implicated under the special circumstances of specific diseases, such as diphtheria and tuberculosis, or during debilitating illness or prolonged treatment with antibiotics which sometimes changes the flora of the respiratory tract. Viral infections do not produce suppurative otitis. They may be responsible for transient serous otitis or for inflammation of the drum alone—myringitis.

The mechanical changes that occur during otitis media usually begin with obstruction of the mouth of the eustachian tube due to swelling of the mucous membrane. Complete or partial obstruction prevents air exchange between the pharynx and the middle ear, and the air within the middle ear is slowly absorbed. The ear drum bulges inward due to the unopposed external air pressure, and tension of the drum results in pain and blurring of hearing. If the obstruction persists, the air in the middle ear is replaced by fluid which may produce outward bulging of the drum. If the fluid is not infected, the process is called catarrhal otitis media. When infection has spread up the tube to the middle ear the accumulation of fluid is more rapid, and the drum bulges outward tensely, becomes exquisitely painful and not infrequently ruptures, permitting the accumulation of pus in the middle ear to discharge into the external canal.

Infants are more prone to middle ear infection than are older children or adults. The eustachian tube is shorter, wider and straighter in the infant so that infected material is carried more readily from the pharynx to the middle ear. Infected adenoid masses in the vicinity of the mouth of the eustachian tube are often responsible for recurring blockage of the tube or otitis media.

Symptoms. The child who is old enough to communicate complains of pain in the ear and blurred hearing. The severity of the pain depends upon the rapidity with which fluid accumulates in the middle ear. Fever, headache and vomiting are also present in variable degree. Smaller children and infants cannot localize their symptoms. The source of their fever, irritability, discomfort and vomiting may be disclosed only through otoscopic examination. In small infants there may be convulsions, diarrhea, refusal of food and rolling of the head from side to side.

Complications. With almost any acute inflammation of the middle ear there is some extension of the infection into the mastoid antrum and air cells. When treatment is delayed or ineffectual, mastoiditis may occur. From the mastoid area there may be spread of the infection to the venous sinuses within the skull (sinus thrombosis and septicemia) or to the meninges (meningitis) or to the brain (brain abscess). These complications are now rare, since the antibiotics have made treatment simple and usually successful.

Prevention. The prevention of otitis depends on the rapid and accurate treatment of pharyngitis and tonsillitis in most instances. Some children who are unusually prone to otitis media benefit from the removal of hypertrophied or infected adenoid tissue.

Treatment and Nursing Care. Antibiotics are indicated to combat the infection. At the beginning of treatment the appropriate drug may not be known, because the bacteria responsible for the infection have not yet been determined. Penicillin is effective in most instances and usually is given initially. One of the tetracycline antibiotics or sulfonamides may be used when the response to penicillin is inadequate or when bacteriologic study indicates that they will be more effective.

Often symptomatic relief of pain may be obtained by giving nose drops to shrink the nasal mucous membranes and promote drainage from the blocked eustachian tube. Neo-Synephrine (0.25%) or ephedrine (2%) may be used every 2 or 3 hours until relief is obtained. Sometimes drops containing phenol and glycerine are instilled into the external ear. Their effect is variable, and they have the disadvantage of preventing accurate observation of changes in the ear drum. Occasionally, when the drum is extremely tense, incision (myringotomy) may be indicated to relieve pain and promote drainage. Aspirin and sedation with the barbiturate drugs will give temporary relief of pain until the other measures have had time to take effect.

NURSING CARE. When there is drainage from the middle ear, the ear canal must be kept clean. The nurse's hands should be washed thoroughly before cleansing the canal to prevent mixed infection of the middle ear. Sterilized cotton should be made into pledgets and used to cleanse the canal of all drainage. Hydrogen peroxide is useful in preventing the exudate from caking. In cleansing the ear canal of the young child, the ear lobe should be pulled down and back to straighten the canal; in the older child, the ear lobe should be pulled up and back. Ear wicks should be small and inserted lightly; packing them in tightly prevents free drainage and may cause extension of the infection into the mastoid process. When drainage is profuse, zinc oxide ointment or petrolatum should be applied to the external auricle to prevent excoriation of the skin.

Adenoid Hypertrophy

Lymphatic tissue comparable to the visible tonsillar masses in the pharynx is present in the nasopharynx, deep in the nose and above the soft palate. This tissue, the pharyngeal tonsil, is visible only with special instruments but, if hypertrophied, may be felt with a finger in the posterior pharynx. When hypertrophied it is referred to as adenoids. Normally, it serves as part of the body's defense against upper respiratory infection. In some infants it outgrows this usefulness and produces such severe obstruction to nasal breathing that deformity of the chest and the face begin to appear. In severe instances nutrition may suffer. The enlargement can result from congenitally excessive growth but is probably more often due to the response to chronic infection with bacteria or viruses. Adenovirus infection is known to last for long periods within this lymphoid mass. Although adenoidectomy is generally undesirable in small infants, curettage of the mass may be necessary if severe nasal obstruction is present.

Croup

Croup is a general term for inflammations of the larynx that cause hoarseness, barking cough or obstruction to breathing, or combinations of these. The term *membranous croup* has been used as a synonym of laryngeal diphtheria. In many young children, catarrhal inflammation of the larynx causes spasmodic contraction of the larynx, which results in respiratory difficulty. It is known by a variety of names: for example, catarrhal croup, spasmodic croup and spasmodic laryngitis. Croup of this sort tends to recur in the same child during respiratory infection of whatever etiology until the child outgrows his propensity to have laryngeal spasm by 3 to 4 years of age.

Some croup is now known to be of viral etiology—due to one of the para-influenza viruses or occasionally the respiratory syncytial virus. Under these circumstances, the degree of laryngeal obstruction is more constant than that described below and the element of spasm based upon anxiety is less marked. Viral croup is usually limited to a single episode in any one child.

Symptoms. Croup is a generally mild infection, of low communicability, occurring chiefly in children under 5 years of age and characterized by occasional acute episodes of laryngeal spasm. It is associated with little, and often no, fever. There is a laryngeal cough, hard and barking, usually spoken of as "croupy." Attacks of spasm of the larynx occur chiefly and often only at night. They may last from half an hour to between 2 and 3 hours. They may recur once or twice the same night. The attacks recur on the second night, and often on the third, after which time spontaneous recovery from the affection occurs. Except for hoarseness and occasional croupy cough, the child seems to be completely well between the attacks of spasm.

During a spasmodic attack, there is very difficult inspiration and an inspiratory stridor. Expiration is little disturbed, and there is no expiratory stridor. The child sits up in bed, brings the accessory muscles of respiration into use, and on inspiration there is retraction of the soft tissues above the clavicle and between the ribs and retraction of the ribs at the attachment of the diaphragm. In a severe attack, the whole picture is very alarming because of the appearance of impending asphyxia. However, croup rarely is fatal.

Diagnosis. The diagnosis of croup usually is not difficult. Diphtheria may be excluded if no membrane is found on examination of the larynx. The obstruction due to diphtheria is both inspiratory and expiratory; it gradually increases in severity and does not occur in spasmodic attacks, although occasionally in diphtheria, spasm is superimposed on the typical clinical picture. Streptococcic laryngitis may cause swelling and membrane formation which give symptoms similar to those described for diphtheria.

Treatment and Nursing Care. Treatment and nursing care of a child with croup are directed chiefly

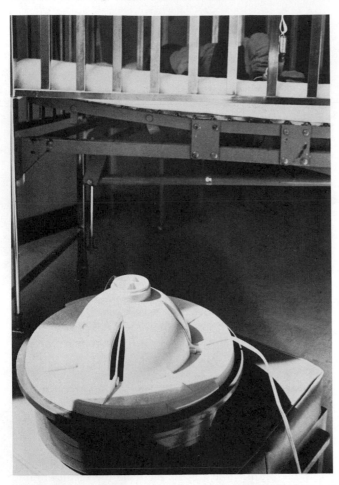

Fig. 14-4. Room humidifier which moistens the air by mechanical dispersion of water vapor.

toward relief of laryngeal spasm. Breathing warm moist air often gives complete relief. Various volatile drugs, such as benzoin, may be employed along with "steam," but the essential part, and usually the only necessary part, of the inhalation is the water vapor. Various methods may be used to supply moist air. The most commonplace is a "croup tent" kept filled with moist air by a humidifier. Croup tents may be made by draping a sheet and a bath blanket over the crib. The outlet of the humidifier should point upward and away from the child to prevent the outflowing moisture from dropping onto him. Of course, care in keeping his clothing and bed dry is essential.

Several antispasmodic drugs are useful in preventing or relieving muscle spasm of the larynx. Syrup of ipecac (½ teaspoonful) is sometimes given to infants every 15 minutes until emesis occurs, or until 3 doses have been ingested. Administration in subemetic doses may be useful in preventing an attack.

The larynx of the infant and the young child is relatively smaller than that of the older child. It is more flexible and susceptible to spasm, and when infection of the larynx is present, respiratory difficulty may be-

come marked and prostrating. In caring for the child with croup, the nurse should be constantly alert for a rise in pulse and respiration rates, sternal retraction, flaring nostrils and increased restlessness. If cyanosis develops and the child becomes increasingly prostrated from labored breathing, tracheotomy may be indicated. For such children constant nursing care is required.

Coughing, laryngeal spasms and enclosure within a tent are frightening to an infant or child. Whenever possible the mother or a nurse should be in constant attendance not only to observe for respiratory distress and cyanosis but also to provide the child with the comfort of emotional closeness to a protective person. Holding the baby closely during coughing helps to prevent fear which probably is a factor in producing symptoms that make tracheotomy necessary.

The Lower Respiratory Passages

Acute Bronchitis

Etiology and Symptoms. Acute bronchitis is one of the common illnesses of infancy and childhood. It is somewhat more frequent before 2 or 3 years of age than after. It may be primary or secondary. When primary, it has much the same causes as the common cold; when secondary, it is a complication of other diseases.

The mild and common variety of acute bronchitis usually has a gradual onset. For the first 2 or 3 days the temperature may be from 100° to 102° F., after which time it becomes approximately normal. Prostration is not great and is of short duration. The appetite is decreased. During the first few days the cough is dry and nonproductive. Auscultation of the chest reveals rales which are variously described as dry, sonorous and whistling. Moisture gradually appears in the bronchi, and after a few days the rales become bubbling. The cough becomes looser and productive. Cough is often started by change in position. It is increased in the morning on awakening and on first lying down at night. The cough is variable in severity in different cases. In some instances, repeated paroxysms of cough disturb sleep through the night. In the average infant, bronchitis may be expected to last from 7 to 10 days.

In the more severe type of bronchitis the smaller bronchi are affected. This type is more common in infants than in older children. The rales are smaller, and fever and prostration are greater than in cases of bronchitis of the larger tubes. Pneumonia is much more likely to result. The cough is tight, and dyspnea and cyanosis may be present. In infants, diarrhea and vomiting are common.

In many instances, bronchitis in infancy and early childhood is associated with asthmatic symptoms. In these cases, wheezing respiration is prominent, and difficulty in getting sufficient air into and out of the lungs may be experienced. The asthma disappears along with the symptoms of bronchitis.

Treatment. For the ordinary attack of mild bronchitis, the only treatment needed is inhalation of warm, moist air. If respiratory exchange is seriously compromised, oxygen may have to be added. When the disease is due to specific bacterial infection, the appropriate antibiotic may shorten the course of the symptoms. Mild sedation may be used for restlessness. Cough medicines are seldom effective as long as the inflammatory reaction persists.

Nursing Care. Decrease in appetite can be expected throughout the illness and particularly during the febrile period. Adequate hydration may be further compromised by vomiting and diarrhea, which are frequent in infants and small children during the onset of a respiratory infection, and because of the difficulty in sucking due to clogging of the nasal passages. Clear fluids should be offered frequently during the child's waking periods to prevent the necessity for parenteral therapy.

If difficulty in breathing continues despite inhalation therapy, the nasal passages may be cleared of obstruction by gentle removal of accumulated mucus with a nasal aspirator. Closure of the opposite nostril during the procedure is indicated to reduce the possibility of pushing mucus into the sinus. If a catheter is used for suctioning, it should be introduced gently while pinched off and negative pressure should be just sufficient to remove secretions.

It is the responsiblity of the nurse to observe any changes in the child's condition and to report them promptly and accurately. Symptoms such as increase in heart rate, temperature, rate of respiration, restlessness, pallor or cyanosis should be brought immediately to the physician's attention since such symptoms may indicate increasing obstruction of the respiratory tract.

Bronchiolitis (Obstructive Bronchitis, Capillary Bronchitis, RS Virus Infection)

Pathophysiology. This clinical entity has from time immemorial plagued small infants during the winter and spring months, often appearing in epidemic form. Modern technics of viral isolation have now demonstrated that the majority of cases are associated with infection by the respiratory syncytial virus (RS) and a smaller number with para-influenza viruses. The RS virus is widespread among population groups studied, since 80 to 90 per cent of children of school age have specific antibody in their blood sera. The newborn infant acquires antibody by transplacental passage from his mother, but such substances give him no protection from the disease. It is now thought that immunity depends upon the acquisition of locally operative antibody contained in the 19S fraction of gamma globulin, which is too large to pass across the placenta and has to be actively manufactured by the child in response to exposure to RS virus.

The infant who becomes infected probably gets the virus from an asymptomatic or mildly affected older carrier who is immune. The RS virus produces a generalized inflammation of the respiratory mucosa which may be limited to the upper respiratory passages or may spread downward through the bronchial tree and even into the pulmonary alveoli. Swelling of the cells lining the bronchi together with the production of thick, sticky mucus lead to partial and complete blockade of the smaller passageways. Air becomes trapped behind the partially obstructed radicles, since it can be pulled in during inspiration but cannot be expelled because the narrowed passages collapse during expiration. If obstruction is complete, the air is absorbed and areas of atelectasis or consolidation distal to the point of obstruction may occur. In general the total lung volume of the infant is increased by the predominating process, which is air-trapping.

Symptoms. Bronchiolitis may be preceded by rhinitis and cough, but for some reason almost never is associated with otitis media and rather infrequently with croup. Fever is often absent but may be present if the involvement of the lungs is extensive. As the process progresses into the lungs, the respiratory rate increases and the infant has to work harder to effect an adequate exchange of air. The chest becomes overdistended and the inspiratory effort is labored, with retraction of the chest wall. A hacking, non-productive cough is usually present. The infant becomes restless and has little tolerance for feeding because it interferes with his efforts to breathe. Severe disease is associated with an increasing degree of tachypnea, chest retractions, cyanosis, restlessness, tachycardia and eventually exhaustion with apneic spells.

Chest x-rays confirm the clinical impression of overinflated lungs and in some instances reveal patches of atelectasis or pneumonic consolidation. Leukocytosis may be present.

Although bronchiolitis is always a worrisome illness, the prognosis for survival is relatively good. Deaths are uncommon and usually limited to infants who have some other defect such as Down's syndrome or unrelated debilitating disease. After a day or two of severe obstruction, the respiratory secretions usually begin to liquefy and the acute inflammation decreases, permitting the infant a better air exchange. However, after the crisis has passed, the symptoms of cough, rales in the chest and milder degrees of dyspnea may persist for a week or ten days. Recurrence of symptoms in the same or a subsequent year happens in a small fraction of the infants.

Treatment. The primary aims of treatment are to improve the infant's air exchange and conserve his energies during what is likely to be a self-limited disease. Feedings can be omitted or reduced to amounts which he can take without undue tiring. Hydration may have to be maintained by intravenous infusion if the disorder is unusually protracted, but usually this is not necessary.

Moist air in a Croupette or other humidifying device is usually given in the hope of promoting the liquefaction of bronchial secretions so that they can be expelled more easily during coughing. Sedation is probably unnecessary in the mildly afflicted infant and unwise in the one who is exerting every effort to maintain an adequate air exchange. In severely afflicted infants, oxygen may be required to relieve cyanosis, but it must be well humidified or it will aggravate the mechanical problem by drying out the mucus in the small tubes.

Antibiotics are frequently given to infants who appear dangerously ill, but they seldom have any dramatic effect and there is no theoretic reason why they should influence the progress of the disorder. Steroids (oral prednisone or intravenous hydrocortisone) are often used in an attempt to decrease the extent of the bronchial inflammatory reaction and possibly to relieve bronchospasm. Opinions differ about the effectiveness of such agents.

Nursing Care. General procedures for removal of secretions in nasal passages are the same as described above. Since an infant has great difficulty in breathing through his mouth, the importance of removal of accumulated mucus is obvious. Changes in position from side to side may aid in drainage of the lower passages. If an infant indicates substantial breathing difficulties, he may be placed in an elevated position or in an infant seat within the Croupette. If oxygen is being administered, the nurse should observe the infant and small child carefully for symptoms of respiratory irritation, substernal soreness or sore throat. She should also check the oxygen equipment frequently to determine that no more than the prescribed concentration of oxygen is being delivered.

Acute Laryngotracheobronchitis

Etiology. The causative organism varies and sometimes cannot be determined. At times, hemolytic streptococci, influenza bacilli and pneumococci appear to be responsible, but frequently no bacteria other than those normally expected in the pharynx can be isolated. Infection with a virus has been suspected and recently proved. The disease appears to depend more on the low resistance of the individual child than on the specific infecting agent. It is much more common in infancy and early childhood than at later ages.

Symptoms. The symptoms depend in part on the severity of the infection, but in larger measure on the character of the exudate. The temperature tends to be high. The inflamed tissues are edematous, but the edema does not cause special difficulty except as it may affect the vocal cords and the region immediately below them and produce obstruction to respiration. In all instances the inflammatory exudate is a major cause of symptoms. It is so thick and viscous that it cannot be coughed up. The normal reflex for cough is incited by movement of foreign material in the respiratory tract. If the material is too thick to move, no cough occurs. Thus the cough reflex may be abolished. Respiratory obstruction may occur from accumulation of the exudate. A large bronchus may become plugged so that atelectasis of the part of the lung supplied by the bronchus results. Air passing partial obstruction causes stridor. Dyspnea and cyanosis also result from respiratory obstruction. The mortality is high. Death may be due to respiratory obstruction, secondary pneumonia, general sepsis or exhaustion.

Treatment. Immediate treatment includes full dosage with one of the broad-spectrum antibiotics such as ampicillin, tetracycline or chloramphenicol and placement of the child in an atmosphere saturated with water vapor. How much additional treatment is given will depend on individual circumstances and often requires astute clinical judgment. The administration of oxygen may give immediate relief of cyanosis and dyspnea, but unless the oxygen is well humidified, ultimately it may aggravate the disease by drying out the thick secretions and making it more difficult for the child to cough them up from the respiratory tract. When obstruction at the larynx is severe, tracheotomy must be done. Sometimes the decision to do a tracheotomy is delayed too long; at other times the tracheotomy increases the inspissation of mucus in the bronchial tree and leads to generalized obstruction of bronchioles. Sedatives must be used with caution, and atropine derivatives are contraindicated. When the child is struggling to maintain his respirations, food and oral fluids should be avoided and hydration preserved through infusions.

Nursing Care. Careful observation is essential in all cases of acute laryngotracheobronchitis. A close watch must be kept for evidence of increasing respiratory obstruction or fatigue. Increasing cyanosis, restlessness, tachycardia or pyrexia are danger signals which should be called to the attention of the physician. If a tracheotomy has been done, the care of the patient is similar to that described in the Appendix. Even when the tube is in place, continued watchfulness must be maintained to detect evidence of obstruction at the end of the tube or deeper in the branches of the bronchial tree. Adept attention to the patient's emotional and physical needs without disturbing him unnecessarily is an important factor in maintaining comfort and preserving his trust and strength.

Pneumonia (Pneumonitis)

Pneumonia or pneumonitis is an inflammation of the lung. It may be caused by any pyogenic bacterium or, in some instances, by a virus. It may occur as a primary disease or it may be a secondary or complicating infection in association with some other illness. As a primary infection with pneumococci, the inflammation may be massive in one lobe of a lung and involve all the alveoli of the lobe. In such case the disease is designated as lobar pneumonia. Pneumonia may be disseminated in various parts of the lungs, not be confined to a lobe or not involve a whole lobe completely, and in such cases the disease is designated as lobular pneumonia or bronchopneumonia.

Anoxia produces cyanosis, dyspnea and cerebral symptoms, including delirium and inability to sleep. These symptoms increase as anoxia increases. Anoxia is also a cause of failure of circulation.

Pneumonia occurring as a complication of some other illness is called secondary pneumonia and is of the lobular pneumonic or bronchopneumonic type.

Pneumococcal Pneumonia. As a primary disease pneumonia is likely to appear suddenly, without warning, or with only mild preceding symptoms, such as those accompanying a common cold.

Primary pneumonia of infants is a disseminated inflammation in the lungs. Lobar pneumonia is seldom observed in the first year, but it occurs with increasing frequency with advancing age.

SYMPTOMS. The onset of pneumococcal pneumonia in infancy is likely to be sudden, with fever and prostration. Vomiting is frequent, and convulsions may occur at the onset. The temperature is high and usually irregular, with fluctuations of from 3° to 4° F. The respirations are rapid, from 60 to 70 or more to the minute, and associated with effort and with retraction of the soft parts of the chest on inspiration. The alae of the nose move laterally with each inspiration. The pulse rate increases to 160 or more and is likely to be irregular. Cough is frequent, persistent and annoying. Moderate diarrhea usually is present. Leukocytosis is high (20,000 to 50,000). Blood culture occasionally grows the pneumococcus. In the milder illnesses and without chemotherapy, improvement occurs in approximately a week. In the more severe illnesses, improvement, if it occurs, may not be observed for as much as two weeks or longer.

DIAGNOSIS. The correct diagnosis is often suspected by an experienced person merely from observation of the infant's respiratory behavior. Physical examination of the chest discloses areas of moist rales in the involved portions of lung. When the patches of consolidation are large enough there may be typical changes in the quality of the breath sounds heard through a stethoscope. Roentgen examination is frequently conclusive, but if the consolidated areas are small, interpretation of the shadows which they cast is sometimes difficult. The etiologic diagnosis is important as a guide to proper antibiotic therapy. Cultures of the nose, the throat, or sputum when it is available, always should be made. Blood cultures may yield the invading organism in some instances. Once isolated, the organism should be tested for sensitivity to the various antibiotics in order to speed selection of the most effective drug.

COMPLICATIONS AND PROGNOSIS. Otitis media and fibrinous pleurisy are common complications of pneumonia; usually they are not serious and they respond to the treatment being given for the pneumonia itself. Rarely, an infant develops meningitis, peritonitis or empyema. These serious complications increase the mortality of the disease and require special measures of treatment as described in the sections that deal with them.

Primary pneumonia of infancy is a serious disease if it remains untreated or is treated inadequately. Before modern antibiotic treatment was available the mortality rates ranged as high as 30 to 50 per cent. The outlook is very much better today, but pneumonia in the small infant is not a disease to be regarded lightly.

TREATMENT AND NURSING CARE. The cases of primary pneumonia in infancy that are caused by pneumococci respond promptly to penicillin, which should be given intramuscularly in full dosage. Other types of antibiotic may be necessary when the pneumonia is shown to be due to other organisms. Ordinarily, if treatment is effective the infant's temperature will approach normal levels within 24 hours. A delay in response beyond 48 hours should raise the suspicion that the wrong antibiotic has been selected. Immediate testing of the sensitivity of organisms isolated from infants with pneumonia will greatly assist in directing the choice of drug.

Oxygen with high humidity is administered when there is cyanosis or other evidence of anoxia. The Croupette provides an environment of high humidity and oxygen without overheating the baby. The plastic canopy makes it possible to observe the infant from any direction. The chamber of ice at the back is useful during periods when the infant's temperature is elevated. The jar which is used for distilled water must be thoroughly cleansed each time it is refilled to prevent the accumulation of a film of dirt on the plastic filter and the sides of the jar. Cleansing of the atomizer tip and the filter should be done with a toothbrush under running water. It must be remembered that the Croupette does not take the place of crib sides, which must be pulled to the top and fastened securely when the baby is left alone.

In large measure the nursing care of the infant with pneumonia is symptomatic and geared to his individual requirements. He requires rest and relief of his physical and psychological discomforts. Nursing procedures should be organized in such a way as to disturb the infant as little as possible. Frequently, feedings are omitted until the expected improvement from antibiotic therapy has taken place. Usually, fluids are administered by mouth when possible, by infusion when necessary. Feedings must be given cautiously because they tend to aggravate coughing and produce fatigue.

The infant's position may influence his comfort to some extent. He may be more comfortable in a semierect posture or when lying with the affected lung

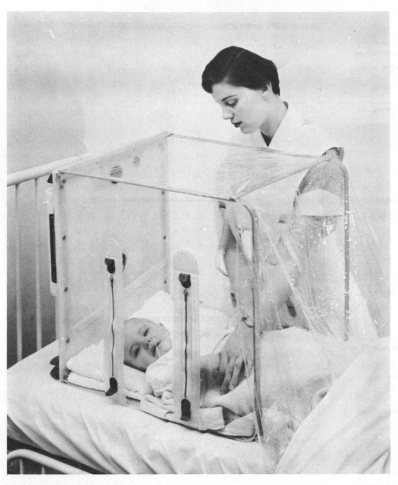

FIG. 14-5. Illustrating care of a baby in a Croupette. (Air-Shields, Inc., Hatboro, Pa.)

down. He should be kept off his back because of proneness to vomiting and the danger of aspiration. A suction machine should always be available because of the ever present hazard of aspiration.

Abdominal distention from paralytic ileus is a common and distressing aspect of pneumonia in infants. It is both painful and embarrassing to the respiratory effort and should be relieved by small enemas or suppositories.

Temperatures up to 104° F. usually require no special measures for their control. Excessive fever is most readily controlled by placing the child on a cool water mattress. Since pneumonia is a communicable disease, isolation technics must be used.

Staphylococcal Pneumonia. Staphylococcal pneumonia is mainly a disease of small infants. Occasionally, it is seen as a complication of staphylococcal bacteremia in the older child or the adult. The disease is characterized by a tendency to form multiple abscesses throughout the lungs. Even in small infants the contents of these abscesses may be apparent in purulent sputum or vomitus. Abscesses that form on the surface of the lung often create an empyema or pneumothorax by discharging their contents into the pleural cavity and at the same time establishing a communication between the pleural cavity and the bron-

chial tree. The diagnosis is made by culture of sputum and by the discovery of characteristic abscess shadows in the roentgenogram of the chest. Treatment is complicated by the fact that increasing numbers of staphylococci are becoming resistant to the older antibiotic drugs such as penicillin. The sensitivity of each individual strain of staphylococcus must be tested in order to guide treatment.

Strains of staphylococci from the outside community are usually sensitive to penicillin, which should be used in full dosage. Strains acquired within hospitals are more likely to be resistant to this agent and require the use of methicillin or oxacillin. For patients sensitive to penicillin, a wide range of agents are available—erythromycin, cephalothin, tetracyclines and others—which must be selected according to laboratory indications. When empyema is present, the mechanical principles described in the next section should be used. Untreated staphylococcal pneumonia is almost universally fatal. Even with early and adequate treatment by antibiotic drugs the mortality is likely to approach 25 per cent. Small infants may die before the nature of the disease is recognized.

Secondary Bacterial Pneumonia (Bronchopneumonia, Lobular Pneumonia). Secondary pneumonia (lobular or bronchopneumonia) is similar in many respects to primary pneumonia of infants. It may occur at any age as a complication of any acute illness. It is a more frequent complication in infancy than in late childhood.

SYMPTOMS. The onset of secondary pneumonia is usually gradual, with subsequent increase in the severity of the illness. The degree of fever varies with the severity of the illness and the general condition of the child. In general, it tends to be high and irregular or intermittent. Prostration is present. The symptoms and signs are the same as those described for primary pneumonia of infants. Clinically, secondary pneumonia differs from primary pneumonia chiefly in its persistence and its relatively bad prognosis. Many of the victims are already weak and poorly nourished from the effects of a protracted illness or from convalescence following a surgical procedure. Their resistance is consequently poor. The type of secondary pneumonia which follows acute contagious diseases, such as pertussis, measles and influenza, may respond adequately to antibiotic therapy but may invade the structure of the lung to set the stage for bronchiectasis. The bacterial etiology of secondary pneumonia is often mixed or composed of organisms which are less easily influenced by the available antibiotics.

TREATMENT AND NURSING CARE. The same measures are required as in the case of primary pneumonia. Some prevention of secondary pneumonia is possible if its occurrence is anticipated. Chronically ill or immobile patients should be isolated from contact with respiratory infections among the patients around them. They should have their positions changed frequently to avoid imperfect ventilation of portions of the lung. Sometimes prophylactic administration of antibiotics is warranted when the risk of secondary pneumonia is great.

Pleurisy and Empyema

Pleurisy is an inflammation of the lining membrane of the thoracic cavity and the external surface of the lungs. It is a common part of pneumonia and accounts for the pain that is felt by the patient. In its early stages pleurisy is dry or fibrinous, but progression during untreated pneumonia may lead to the collection of fluid or pus within the chest cavity. In conditions other than pneumonia, an effusion of *sterile* fluid may take place. This is seen in heart failure, nephrosis, early tuberculosis and pulmonary metastasis.

An accumulation of purulent exudate within the chest cavity is known as empyema. In childhood it occurs most frequently as a complication of staphylococcal pneumonia. Organisms enter the pleural space from a small abscess on the surface of the lung and rapidly produce a generalized infection of the adjacent cavity. Since the small abscesses in staphylococcal pneumonia frequently connect with a bronchus, a fistula results which allows air to enter the infected pleural cavity from the trachea and creates a pyopneu-

mothorax. Often this complication is already present when the first chest roentgenogram is obtained.

Diagnosis. The diagnosis of empyema or pyopneumothorax depends on the appearance of the lungs in the roentgenogram. The organisms in the contaminating pus must be determined for proper control of therapy. This is done by needle aspiration of the chest (thoracentesis). From cultures of the material obtained the bacterial etiology and the antibiotic sensitivity of the invading organisms can be determined.

Treatment and Nursing Care. *Thoracentesis* may be done for diagnosis, for relief of dyspnea caused by pressure of fluid, for the obtaining of exudate for culture or for the instilling of penicillin into the pleural cavity. Sterile equipment required for thoracentesis consists of: 50-ml. syringe, 2-ml. syringe, hypodermic needles, 3-way stopcock with short piece of rubber tubing attached, aspirating needles, procaine 1 per cent, curved clamp, lumbar puncture drape sheet, cotton balls, small gauze squares, graduated receptacle, gloves and medication as ordered by the physician. Unsterile equipment consists of a skin preparation tray, culture media, test tubes and adhesive plaster. Epinephrine should be ready for use in case of need.

One of several positions may be required for successful thoracentesis. If the patient is a baby, he should be placed on his unaffected side in a semirecumbent position. If the patient is of preschool age or older, the doctor will probably want him to be in a sitting position with his arms and trunk brought forward over an over-bed table with a pillow on it for comfort. One nurse will be required to hold the child in the desired position, prepare him for the procedure, give him emotional support and observe his response to treatment. A second nurse will be needed to assist with the skin preparation and to collect specimens of aspirated fluid. During the procedure the nurse should watch for changes in the child's respiration and pulse rates, for changes in his color and for any increase in coughing.

After the treatment the child should be kept warm and observed for changes in his general condition. Charting should include a description and the amount of the aspirated fluid, the amount and the kind of medication instilled, any symptoms of shock or syncope and the child's physical and psychological response to the treatment.

Pneumococcal or streptococcal empyema is treated by the administration of antibiotics and by periodic withdrawal of pus from the chest. Penicillin in saline solution may be instilled into the chest cavity to hasten the eradication of infection. Most empyemas caused by these organisms respond readily to this simple management.

If the empyema persists or the infecting organisms are staphylococci, surgical drainage is indicated. Early in the course of the disease this is usually done by inserting a rubber catheter between the ribs. A Y-tube is attached to the catheter, and then tubing is attached to both arms of the Y-tube. One piece of this tubing is connected to a fluid-sealed syphon bottle placed below the level of the bed. The other piece is attached to an irrigating bottle of sterile fluid hung above the level of the child's head. With each expiration the irrigating fluid is pushed out of the pleural cavity, establishing a closed-irrigation system to facilitate drainage and encourage expansion of the lung. Frequent changes in position are important for adequate drainage. Care must also be taken to make sure that the connections are reinforced with adhesive tape and that there are never at any time any kinks in or pressure on the tubing.

After the surfaces of the lung have become adherent to the chest wall, empyema is frequently treated by open drainage through a rib resection without suction apparatus. When this method of treatment is used, the skin around the tube must be kept scrupulously clean to prevent excoriation. Frequent change of dressings is indicated.

Usually, infants with staphylococcal empyema are desperately ill and often require such physical supports as oxygen, extra humidity and intravenous fluid therapy. Sometimes additional warmth supplied by an incubator is also necessary.

DIARRHEA

Diarrhea is a common symptom among infants and is particularly important because of the resulting fluid loss which threatens the relatively unstable water balance of the human young. Like vomiting, it has multiple causes. In a small minority of instances the reason for diarrhea is obvious or can be inferred from other events taking place around or within the infant. Usually its exact basis is unknown. It either remains obscure or is not clarified by laboratory study until after the crucial period of illness has passed. Thus the practical management of diarrhea is a symptomatic approach which attempts to correct the physiologic changes from moment to moment, while keeping a wary eye open for specific etiologic agents which may require appropriate antibiotic attack.

Pathophysiology

Diarrhea results from an increase in the rate of peristalsis which carries the intestinal contents along so rapidly that they are expelled before the large intestine has had time to reabsorb water in the usual way. A change in the color of the stools also depends on rapid passage of material through the tract. Bile pigment which enters high up in the duodenum is ordinarily changed by the chemical action of the intestinal contents from green through yellow to brown. If passage through the intestinal canal is too rapid, this reaction is not completed by the time the stool emerges.

Minor degrees of diarrhea are sometimes ascribed to noninfectious factors such as the mechanical and chemical irritation resulting from bulky or undigested food, antibiotics or drugs, allergic response to specific items of diet, increased irritability due to nervous tension, or as a nonspecific effect of any illness which depresses the tolerance for food. This variety of diarrhea can be prevented only through a knowledge of the individual infant's idiosyncrasies and avoidance of foods and drugs known to upset him.

Practically all of the serious diarrhea and many of the milder afflictions are associated with or directly due to infection. Past experience has demonstrated the urgency of handling infants with diarrhea as though they had a disease which could be readily transmitted to others either by direct contact or by contamination from their stools. Some of the bacterial agents responsible for diarrhea are well known and can be isolated by culture of the stools. These include the dysentery group of organisms (Shiga, Flexner, Sonne and other types), the typhoid bacillus and the salmonella group of related bacteria. In recent years certain antigenic types of colon bacilli (enteropathic *E. coli*) have been added to this list as a definite cause of epidemic diarrhea, particularly among newborn infants. Other bacteria such as staphylococci, pseudomonas and proteus organisms have often been suspected as specific causes of infantile diarrhea, but their guilt has been more difficult to fix with certainty. The epidemiologic characteristics of old-fashioned "summer diarrhea" from which incriminating bacteria could not be cultivated have for a long time placed it under the suspicion of being a virus infection. Proof of this etiology has been obtained on infrequent occasions. Diarrhea has also been attributed to "toxic effects." Some theories have regarded it as being analogous to food poisoning and due to the action of soluble toxins from bacterial growth accumulating in contaminated and poorly refrigerated formula. Other theories have blamed changes which take place within the infant's body during the course of infections of the nose, the throat and particularly the ears and the mastoids. It is quite likely that each of these theories offers the correct explanation for some cases of diarrhea.

Prevention

The prevention of diarrhea which is caused by a communicable infection is achieved through careful formula preparation, isolation of sick infants and general public health improvements in safeguarding milk, water supplies and sewage and in the control of insect vectors. Where these measures and standards of personal hygiene are of dubious quality it becomes increasingly important to encourage breast feeding of small infants, for the incidence and the severity of diarrhea are much lower among breast-fed infants.

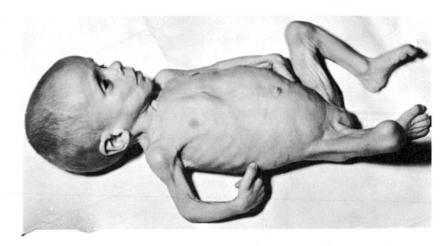

Fig. 14-6. Dehydration, showing loose skin and sunken eyes.

Mild Diarrhea

Diarrhea which is not severe enough to produce significant dehydration or acidosis may be classified as mild. The distinction is admittedly arbitrary, and all gradations will be found in practice between that described here as mild, and that considered later as severe. In mild diarrhea the infant may appear quite well except for an increase in the frequency and fluidity of his stools. Sometimes there is irritability, loss of appetite or disturbance of sleep. Infrequent vomiting and lesser degrees of fever may also occur. Treatment consists of a decrease in food intake, particularly with reduction of carbohydrate and fat in the formula, and of an increase in water intake to compensate for fluid loss. Unsweetened boiled milk or boiled skimmed milk or even brief starvation for 12 to 24 hours is usually employed. If there is no vomiting, water or a balanced salt solution is given by mouth in amounts to meet the normal fluid requirements plus the estimated loss in the stools. Mild diarrhea usually responds to such changes within 2 to 3 days so that the usual feeding schedule can be gradually resumed. Occasionally, a mild diarrhea is associated with prolonged intolerance for fat, and the infant must be kept on a low fat formula for several weeks in order to prevent recurrence of symptoms. Kaolin products and pectin or scraped apple have been used to speed the resumption of normal stools in mild diarrheas, but the wisdom of their usage is debatable. Diarrhea which remains mild is a nuisance but not a serious disease.

Severe Diarrhea

Symptoms. Diarrhea may progress from a mild to a severe illness within a matter of hours or over the course of several days. As the frequency and volume of stools increases the infant becomes more restless and fretful. Stool passage may become painful, partly due to griping and partly due to the tenderness of the skin in the diaper area which rapidly becomes inflamed or even ulcerated from the irritation of constant moisture and the acid stools. In dysentery the stools may become bloody or contain gross pus. In any type of diarrhea there may be mucus present. Vomiting may interfere with attempts to assuage the infant's thirst.

Between the lack of food and the loss of fluid the infant begins to lose weight progressively. The mucous membranes of the mouth become dry and cracked. The skin dries and loses its normal elasticity so that it does not snap back into place when pinched up into a fold and then released. The fontanel and the eyes become sunken, and the face adopts a pinched and anxious look at first, followed later by impassivity with eyes half-closed. The urine becomes scanty in amount and dark in color. Fever may appear if it has not already been present as part of an infection. These are the main signs and symptoms of dehydration.

With significant degrees of dehydration there may be changes in the respirations which betoken acidosis. These consist of an increase in depth of respiration with a sighing quality often present. The rate may be slowed or accelerated. Grayish color of the skin and cold extremities in spite of an elevated body temperature indicate sluggishness of the peripheral circulation and impending shock due to decreased plasma volume.

Severe diarrhea sometimes begins quite abruptly with high fever, listlessness, extreme toxicity and convulsions or coma. The onset may be so sudden that little warning of the disease is available. Liquid stool may accumulate within the intestinal tract and not be expelled until after the toxic symptoms begin. The prognosis in diarrhea with this type of onset is particularly serious, and such infants constitute a therapeutic emergency.

Metabolic Alterations. The principles of water and electrolyte balance and fluid administration are presented in Chapter 4. During severe diarrhea the loss in weight is due primarily to loss of water from the body, which in turn is chiefly intercellular water (interstitial fluid). This compartment of the body fluids is used up first, and its loss accounts for the symptoms of sunken fontanel and eyes and loss of skin elasticity. The body is not able to maintain the plasma volume indefinitely, and when water loss becomes severe there is also shrinkage in plasma volume which accounts for hemoconcentration, for poor peripheral circulation and for the small volume of urine. The water of the body cells themselves (intracellular water) is also lost, but the changes are more subtle and less easily recognized clinically. Loss of vigor and dulling of the sensorium are probably external manifestations of the loss of intracellular water.

The losses sustained are not merely losses of water, however, for the electrolytes of the body fluids invariably accompany them. Restoration of water to the body must be combined with a restoration of the lost electrolytes as well. Usually in diarrhea a number of factors conspire to produce acidosis. The liquid stools carry off a disproportionate amount of basic electrolytes. The normal products of metabolism are acid, and when starvation and fever are present the quantities produced are increased. When the blood flow to the kidney is decreased by shrinking plasma volume, the excretion of these products is hampered. For a time the kidney is able to select an excess of acid radicals for excretion and thus tends to correct the acid-base balance in the blood. Similarly, the lungs, by hyperventilation, blow off more carbon dioxide than usual in an attempt to increase the excretion of carbonic acid. But eventually these measures become insufficient, and the pH of the blood begins to change from its normal range of 7.35 to 7.45 downward toward 7.0, the level which is barely compatible with survival.

When dehydration has progressed to the point where intracellular water is being lost, the body loses potassium from within the cells. Unless special care is taken to replace potassium during treatment, the function of cells such as those of the myocardium and other muscles may be impaired by falling concentrations of this important element. Excessive potassium administration must also be feared, since high blood levels are equally dangerous.

The losses of both water and the individual chemical substances do not always follow the same pattern. It has been discovered that a few infants lose more water than electrolytes during diarrhea and have inordinately high levels of sodium and other ions in the blood. Such infants are likely to show evidence of central nervous system impairment, such as coma or convulsions, and suffer an unusually high mortality rate.

Treatment. ACIDOSIS AND DEHYDRATION. In diarrhea of any severity the most urgent aspect of treatment is relief of acidosis and dehydration. Ideally, these procedures should be guided by repeated determinations of blood components such as hemoglobin, hematocrit, carbon dioxide content (or combining power), pH, sodium, chloride, potassium and nonprotein nitrogen. If the recent weights of the infant before he became ill are known, the present figure provides an important measure of the quantity of water lost. The other measurements assist in computing the relative losses of water and electrolytes and in judging the level of kidney function.

Infants who appear moribund at the time of admission are often given a sizable injection of physiologic saline or Ringer's solution into the peritoneal cavity in order to initiate rehydration rapidly. Continuous intravenous infusion is always advisable when severe diarrhea is present, for the poor condition of the circulation makes absorption from the subcutaneous spaces slow and unreliable. The mechanical problem in establishing a continuous infusion in a small infant in circulatory collapse is often great. When success has been attained the flow through this lifeline must be regarded as precious, for its failure endangers the infant's survival. The physician must determine the desired type of solution and the rate of dosage; but the nurse has an important part in policing the flow to make sure that it is running at the predetermined rate and must keep accurate track of the amounts infused.

Many schemes are used for estimating fluid and electrolyte losses and for restoring deficits (see Appendix for an example). Isotonic solutions of glucose, sodium chloride and the more complicated salt mixtures are generally used as the main basis for restoring water. If plasma volume can be bolstered to the point where kidney function improves progressively, the natural mechanisms for correcting acidosis begin to operate again. More rapid correction of acidosis is often accomplished by injecting calculated amounts of sodium bicarbonate or ⅙ molar sodium lactate solution. After urine flow is established, solutions containing potassium, such as Darrow's solution, are usually added in order to permit this substance to re-enter the cells which are undergoing hydration. In anemic or starved infants plasma or transfusions are used as supportive measures. Once the major electrolyte defects have been corrected and vomiting has ceased, the intake of water and salt can be gradually shifted over from the intravenous or subcutaneous route to the oral one.

MANAGEMENT OF FEEDING. In addition to correcting the deficits already suffered, it is imperative to prevent additional ones from being incurred through the persistence of diarrhea or vomiting. A preliminary period of starvation is always advisable in severe diarrhea. The length of this period must be determined by changes in the clinical condition and the extent of the diarrhea. Usually at least 24 to 48 hours' rest must be given to the intestinal tract and in severe instances the starvation may be prolonged to as long as a week. When feedings are resumed, water, glucose or balanced salt solution is offered first to test the irritability of the tract. If this is tolerated, small amounts of dilute skimmed milk, lactic acid milk or breast milk are tried, and the amounts and the strength of the feedings are increased at a rate judged slow enough to prevent recurrence of the symptoms. During prolonged periods of starvation the intake may be augmented by the use of parenteral vitamin solutions, by plasma, transfusions, or intravenous amino acid mixtures.

OTHER ASPECTS OF TREATMENT. If high fever is present it should be controlled by the use of a cold water mattress in order to forestall convulsions. Sedatives are usually avoided in these desperately ill infants because they may be dangerous and may confuse the clinical indications of progress. In the presence of upper respiratory infection, antibiotics should be given to bring the associated disease under control as rapidly as possible. Direct attack on the etiologic agent causing the diarrhea will have to depend on the results of laboratory studies of the stools. When specific infection with dysentery or salmonella organisms is suspected, the use of sulfonamides, tetracyclines, ampicillin, or chloramphenicol is rational. Neomycin or colimycin given orally is generally effective against pathogenic strains of *E. coli* and some of the other agents implicated in infantile diarrhea. Neomycin is too toxic for parenteral administration.

NURSING CARE. In addition to her important responsibilities in monitoring the parenteral fluids, the nurse has several challenges in caring for the infant with severe diarrhea. Strict isolation technic must be maintained in order to protect other infants in the ward. Hands should be washed carefully, and stools and diapers disposed of in appropriate containers. Charting must be accurate, especially of the number and the description of the stools and the frequency of urination. At the beginning of the treatment, nursing maneuvers are often obstructed by the necessity for maintaining a particular position of the infant in order to keep his intravenous fluids running. While changes of position are desirable to prevent respiratory complications, the position of the needle in the vein must be safeguarded.

In the endeavor to prevent redness and excoriation of the buttocks, the diapers should be changed frequently, and the buttocks and the genitalia cleansed with oil on cotton. If redness or excoriation should appear, a further protection against the acid stool is afforded by a bland ointment or paste.

Often it may be desirable to avoid contact of the skin with the stool to a greater degree and to have the affected skin exposed to warm air and light to promote healing. Keeping the infant on his abdomen gives the greatest exposure, but care must be taken to prevent irritation of the skin of the knees, toes and chin, and, above all, the danger of suffocation. The equipment to be used for exposure to light depends on what is available and to some extent on the season of the year. A bed cradle with a lamp attached in the dome serves well, or the lamp may be attached to the side of the crib. The lamp should be equipped with a 25-watt bulb, protected by a shade or a wire cage and adjusted 12 inches from the infant's body. These precautions are to prevent overheating and skin burns.

After cleansing the buttocks and the genitalia, the infant should be placed comfortably on his abdomen or on his side, with back support. A sheet can be used to cover the frame.

Judicious use of mothering procedures, such as the pacifier, stroking and holding the infant, are important elements of nursing while the baby is ill and convalescent.

MENINGITIS

Bacterial infection of the meninges can occur at any age, but the common forms are seen with greatest frequency in infants and young children. Diagnosis is both more difficult in the very young, who can give no subjective help, and more imperative because the longer treatment is neglected the greater the likelihood that irreparable damage to the brain will occur.

Before antibiotics appeared there were almost no recoveries from meningitis except for the variety caused by the meningococcus. Today the outlook is very much more hopeful provided treatment is prompt and accurate.

Tuberculous Meningitis

Etiology. Tuberculous meningitis is caused by the tubercle bacillus (*Mycobacterium tuberculosis*), which gains access to the meninges from a focus elsewhere in the body. The disease may occur in association with a generalized miliary tuberculous infection, in which case the symptoms of miliary tuberculosis elsewhere are likely to be masked by those of meningitis. It often occurs also when symptoms and signs of tuberculosis elsewhere are not manifest and when a careful examination reveals perhaps nothing more than a hilus gland infection. Thus, tuberculous meningitis may appear in a child who previously had had apparently excellent health and nutrition. Tuberculous meningitis may occur at any age, but it is encountered with the greatest frequency under 5 years of age.

Symptoms. The onset is gradual and insidious in most instances and is manifest by some variety of change in behavior. These changes vary with the person and probably are brought about chiefly by increased intracranial pressure caused by an increased amount of cerebrospinal fluid. The child is likely to become cross and irritable. The play habits and reactions to associates change. Drowsiness and mental dullness are common. Because of the increased intracranial pressure, vomiting, anorexia and constipation are frequent, especially in infants, and headache becomes a complaint of older children. The temperature during this period is elevated only slightly. These symptoms of the early stage do not give very definite indication of the cause of the difficulty, but after perhaps a week, sometimes longer, the symptoms become more severe and point more definitely to their intracranial origin.

Drowsiness and headache increase. Hyperesthesia

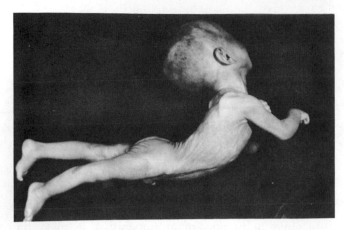

FIG. 14-7. Opisthotonos position in a baby with meningitis.

appears, and the child prefers to remain undisturbed. Intolerance of noises and bright lights frequently develops. In some cases, the child screams intermittently. The reflexes are increased, the pupils are of normal size or small, the neck is stiff, the head is held back, and very often the extremities also are held rigidly. Convulsions sometimes occur. This period of more severe illness has been called the irritative stage. Gradually, the illness goes through a transition into what is known as the paralytic stage. The stupor becomes more marked and continuous and eventually becomes so deep that the child cannot be aroused. Respiration becomes irregular. The pupils are large and fixed. The reflexes diminish until they no longer can be elicited. Various paralyses, often transitory, may be noted. Muscle movements are chiefly automatic and not purposeful. General muscular relaxation increases. Death occurs either quietly in deep coma or in a few instances with terminal convulsions. At the very end, the temperature, which has been relatively low throughout the illness, rises rapidly to a high point.

Diagnosis. A positive tuberculin skin test or the demonstration of pulmonary lesions by x-ray of the chest may raise the suspicion of tuberculous disease. The spinal fluid is usually under increased pressure, is opalescent but not grossly purulent and contains a few to several hundred lymphocytes. The protein is increased and the sugar decreased. Confusion with aseptic or viral meningitis occurs. Tubercle bacilli may be present in the fluid but are hard to find on direct smear. Cultures or animal inoculations will eventually show positive results, but several days or weeks must elapse before the results are known.

Prognosis. Before the discovery of streptomycin, tuberculous meningitis was almost invariably fatal. Today the outlook depends upon prompt recognition and adequate treatment. Under favorable circumstances, nearly all patients will recover and most will do so without residual damage. When treatment is started after coma has appeared, the mortality is likely to be 25 per cent or greater and residual damage frequent. Since the disease is more difficult to recognize in the infant, later diagnosis is to be expected and consequently the final prognosis is not as good.

Treatment. When the diagnosis is established or seriously suspected, intensive treatment is indicated with two or three antituberculous agents. Streptomycin by injection is used at the start in a dosage of 20-40 mg./Kg./day and is usually continued for several weeks after clinical improvement is apparent. Isoniazid hydrazide (INH) in dosage of 20-30 mg./Kg./day is the cornerstone of therapy which is usually continued for at least a year after apparent clinical recovery. It may be given by mouth if the patient's condition permits, otherwise intramuscularly or intravenously. Unlike the adult, pyridoxine deficiency is not observed in children during the administration of INH. Para-aminosalicyclic acid (PAS) is usually added to the regimen in a dosage of 300 mg./Kg./day and may be continued as long as the INH. It has the disadvantage of being relatively expensive and requiring consumption of a large bulk of drug. A newer agent, ethionamide, has been used extensively in Europe but at the present time has not been cleared for other than experimental use in children in the United States.

Because tuberculous meningitis has a strong tendency to produce adhesions between the membranes lining the central nervous system and thus interfere with proper circulation of spinal fluid, steroids are usually administered at the start of therapy to prevent such adhesive arachnoiditis. Prednisone in a dosage of 1 mg./Kg./day usually proves adequate and superior to other measures such as the intrathecal injection of enzyme preparations, or antibiotics.

Meningococcal Meningitis (Epidemic Meningitis, Cerebrospinal Fever, Spotted Fever)

Etiology. Meningococcal meningitis is caused by the diplococcus, *Neisseria intracellularis* or *meningococcus*. This organism gains entrance to the body by way of the nose and throat and during the early stage of the disease may be cultured from this locality and from the blood. Therefore, the disease is naturally transmissible. Great variation is shown at times in the ease and the frequency of transmission. Most of the time meningococcal meningitis exists as an occasional sporadic disease, but at other times it becomes widely epidemic. In approximately three-fourths of all cases, this disease occurs in children under 10 years of age and in nearly half of them, in children under 5.

Symptoms. As with other infectious diseases, this one has its abortive, mild, severe and malignant forms. The symptoms of only the common form are here described.

After a short incubation period, usually less than a week, prodromal symptoms lasting a day or two may appear. More commonly the onset is sudden, with vomiting, prostration, headache, pain in the neck, back and legs, and frequently convulsions. Although present, fever seldom is high. The head is bent backward, and the neck and the back are held rigidly. A position of marked episthotonos may be assumed. The child prefers to be undisturbed, and movement causes much discomfort. Delirium is common. Stupor and coma appear in the more severe illnesses but are not so common in those of ordinary severity. Fretfulness and irritability may alternate with periods of drowsiness or stupor. Bulging of the anterior fontanel is common in the infant and may be the first evidence of disease.

In older children, but less often in infants, a characteristic skin eruption is usually present, consisting of purpuric spots which may vary from pinhead size to large ecchymoses. Such an eruption is found almost exclusively in association with meningococcus infections and, when present, thus gives a strong clue to the etiology of meningitis. In a small percentage of cases the eruption becomes rapidly extensive and is associated with great toxicity and shock which may rapidly progress to a fatal termination. In this, the Waterhouse-Friderichsen syndrome, hemorrhage into the adrenal glands is usually found at autopsy.

Diagnosis. The etiologic diagnosis of this or any other variety of meningitis is extremely important in order to direct antibiotic therapy effectively. Lumbar puncture reveals that the spinal fluid is under increased pressure. It may be clear in the early stages of illness, but becomes turbulent later on. The protein content is increased and the glucose decreased. By direct smear and bacterial staining, meningococci can often be identified if a careful search is made. Culture of the fluid must be carefully handled since the organisms die off rapidly after exposure to air or extremes of temperature. When skin lesions are present, the meningococci may be found in smears made directly from a scraped lesion.

Prognosis. Except for neglected cases in which complications such as adhesive arachnoiditis have already developed, and those with the Waterhouse-Friderichsen syndrome, full recovery is usually expected when appropriate therapy is instituted. Strains of meningococci which resist sulfadiazine have begun to enter some communities and make the hazard of inexact treatment a real one.

Treatment. Sulfadiazine given intravenously at a rate of 100 mg./Kg. of body wt./day to older infants and children is the most generally effective antibiotic. Infants under 2 months of age should receive half the dose. Because of the possibility of sulfonamide-resistant strains, penicillin or chloramphenicol may be added until the sensitivity of the organism has been determined. Ampicillin and Gantrisin have also been used but their effectiveness has not been as thoroughly determined.

Influenza Bacillus Meningitis

Except during times when epidemic meningococcal meningitis is present, influenza bacillus meningitis is the most common form of purulent infection of the meninges in children.

Etiology. The disease is caused by the *Hemophilus influenzae*, a gram-negative rod which differs markedly in size and shape under various circumstances of cultivation. The same organism causes respiratory infections among children and in particular is responsible for a severe variety of croup.

Symptoms. The early symptoms are similar to those of meningococcal meningitis except that the purpuric rash is absent. In infants the onset is likely to be insidious, with unexplained fever, vomiting, lassitude or peculiar cry or behavior as the presenting complaints. In older children the disturbance advances rapidly toward stupor or coma with the usual evidences of meningitis.

Prognosis. Before the discovery of antibiotics, the fatality rate from influenza meningitis was nearly 100 per cent. Prompt diagnosis and treatment now permits survival of 80 to 90 per cent of the victims. Delayed or inadequate treatment carries an increasing hazard of neurologic sequelae, even if life is spared. Despite optimal treatment, some of the afflicted infants fail to make a complete recovery.

Treatment. Since 1940 a number of substances have been discovered that are capable of curing children suffering from influenza meningitis. Sulfadiazine, streptomycin, chlortetracycline, oxytetracycline, tetracycline, chloramphenicol, and ampicillin are included in the list. Because of the propensity of the influenza bacillus to acquire resistance to many of these agents before treatment can be completed, it has been considered prudent to use at least two of the substances simultaneously. Streptomycin is toxic to the 8th cranial nerve and does not enter the spinal fluid rapidly. The preferred method of treatment at the present time is full dosage of sulfadiazine and either ampicillin or chloramphenicol in addition. At the beginning of treatment these substances usually have to be given by parenteral routes—intramuscularly or intravenously—because of vomiting or coma. Once improvement begins, they may be given orally. Treatment must be continued until repeated spinal fluid cultures have been shown to be free of influenza bacilli.

In infants treatment which has apparently been successful may be complicated after a few days by the reappearance of fever and vomiting. A search must then be made for loculated collections of fluid beneath the dura and over the surface of the brain. These must be evacuated by needle aspiration through the infant's open suture lines, or by burr holes in the skull of the older child. Usually they can be cleared up by repeated aspiration so that more extensive neurosurgical procedures are not required.

Other Types of Bacterial Meningitis

Any one of several varieties of bacteria may cause a purulent type of meningitis similar to meningococcal meningitis. The more common varieties of organism are the pneumococcus, the streptococcus, the staphylococcus and the organisms which normally inhabit the intestinal tract. Without specific treatment the outcome is uniformly fatal. The bacteria usually enter the meninges by way of the blood stream, except when there is direct extension from an infected mastoid or cranial sinus cavity. The onset is usually sudden, and the symptoms include vomiting, convulsions and stiffness of the neck with eventual stupor and coma.

Pneumococcal Meningitis. This disorder is seen most frequently in small infants as a complication of pneumonia, otitis media or mastoiditis. Unless it is treated promptly it is rapidly fatal. The symptoms are similar to those of other types of meningitis. Rapid recognition of the disease is usually possible, for the pneumococci are found in large numbers in the spinal fluid and are identified easily by microscopic examination. Treatment consists of heavy dosage with penicillin and sulfadiazine administered by a parenteral route at first and continued until the patient has had sterile spinal fluid for at least a week, since this variety of meningitis is prone to recur if treatment is stopped too soon. Chloramphenicol and ampicillin are also effective. The results of treatment depend on the speed of recognition of the disease. When full treatment is begun within the first few hours of symptoms, recovery may occur in as many as 75 per cent of the children affected. Infants may have subdural effusions and are more prone than older subjects to suffer brain damage.

Streptococcal Meningitis. During hemolytic streptococcus infections the meninges are invaded in rare instances. The symptoms and the management of this variety of meningitis are almost identical with those of pneumococcal meningitis.

Staphylococcal Meningitis. This organism may gain entrance to the spinal fluid from trauma to the skull, from erosion of the sac of a myelomeningocele or in the course of a bloodstream infection with the staphylococcus. The symptoms and the diagnosis of staphylococcal meningitis are similar to those described previously. Treatment is complicated by the fact that the staphylococci present in the environment are not uniformly sensitive to any one antibiotic. It is essential to test each strain, as it is isolated from the patient, for its sensitivity to all the available antibiotics. This procedure takes a day or two to complete in the laboratory. Hence, it is desirable to treat with more than one antibiotic from the start until the best agent can be identified accurately. In general, the newer the antibiotic, the less likely is the staphylococcus to be resistant to it. Penicillin is effective against many of the strains of staphylococcus at the present writing and should be used in conjunction with another substance, such as ampicillin or cephalothin.

Intestinal Organisms. In small infants, in chronically debilitated children and in those who have wound infections following neurosurgical procedures, meningitis may occur due to a wide variety of organisms which ordinarily are found in the intestinal tract —colon bacilli, proteus, pseudomonas, salmonella, *Streptococcus faecalis*, for example. The meningitis so produced tends to be a relatively low-grade chronic process. Treatment depends on identification of the organism (or organisms, for sometimes mixed infections are found) and laboratory determination of the most appropriate antibiotic, as in the case of staphylococcal meningitis. The difficulty of suspecting and recognizing meningitis in the newborn infant has been discussed in Chapter 10.

Unknown Organisms. Rather frequently, the precise etiology of meningitis is not determined owing to preceding antibiotic therapy or technical laboratory difficulties. Under such circumstances, combined treatment with sulfadiazine, penicillin and chloramphenicol can be expected to cover the most frequent possibilities— i.e., meningococcal, *H. influenzae* and pneumococcal meningitis.

Nursing Care of Children with Meningitis:

Children with meningitis may present a variety of degrees of prostration and illness according to the stage of the disease. In the early stages, vomiting, anorexia or constipation may need nursing attention. Depending on the general condition of the child, food may be given by gavage, or if vomiting is severe, it may be administered parenterally. Fecal retention should be anticipated and when it occurs, should be brought to the attention of the physician, although it does not have the major importance that urinary retention does.

During the stage of irritability, children with meningitis are hyperesthetic and prefer to remain undisturbed as much as possible. Special attention should be given toward reducing general noise level around the child with avoidance of sudden loud noises. Subdued lighting should be maintained except when treatment procedures are necessary. General handling of the child should be kept at a minimum, although his psychological needs must be kept in mind. Sitting quietly beside the child and speaking in a low, well modulated tone of voice will help in reducing his anxiety.

During later stages of the disease, one may have to deal with convulsions, delirium, stupor, cyanosis and urinary retention. The management of convulsions has been previously discussed. If administration of oxygen is required to alleviate cyanosis, the necessary precautionary measures must be taken and the child observed closely for respiratory distress.

When stupor is present, special attention is required

for food and fluid intake. The nurse should also keep records that are suitable for the prompt detection of urinary retention, which may require catheterization.

The child with early stages of meningitis may be irritable and restless, but if the disease is fulminating, his movements are limited and he lies on one side, his back arched in the position of opisthotonos. Good skin care and frequent turning will lessen the incidence of complicating upper respiratory infection and pressure sores about the ears and over the hips. The use of a cold water mattress may be necessary to control high temperature and to make the child more comfortable. If fever is present and orally administered fluids are not tolerated, special mouth care is indicated. If the meningitis is severe, suction apparatus and stimulants should be on hand for emergency use.

During convalescence, return of function of the extremities should be observed, and when it occurs it should be recorded. During this period too, behavior that might indicate complicating brain abnormality, deafness or, in the infant, symptoms of developing hydrocephalus should be noted.

The procedure to be followed for lumbar punctures which are done for diagnostic purposes and to determine the progress of the disease, to give medication intrathecally and to relieve pressure symptoms is described in the Appendix.

Viral (Aseptic) Meningitis

A number of virus infections produce symptoms similar to those of meningitis and spinal fluid like that found in tuberculous meningitis. Examples are mumps, poliomyelitis, the enteroviruses and the arborviruses. These entities are discussed more fully elsewhere. Sometimes the findings in an early bacterial meningitis are difficult to distinguish from those of aseptic meningitis. If the wrong conclusion is reached, antibiotic treatment may be delayed to the detriment of the child.

INFECTION OF THE GENITOURINARY TRACT (PYURIA)

A number of terms are employed to designate the presence of infection within the urinary apparatus. Pyelonephritis implies that the inflammation is primarily in the kidney parenchyma; pyelitis indicates the pelvis of the kidney; ureteritis, the ureter; cystitis, the bladder. The more indefinite term "pyuria" is preferable, for infection within the tract usually is not confined to a single location, nor is it possible always to localize the major site exactly.

Pathophysiology

Pyuria is more common in infants than in older children and more common in girls than in boys. Intestinal bacilli are the infecting organisms in from 75 to 80 per cent of the cases; streptococci and staphylococci in most of the remainder. The infecting bacteria may reach the urinary tract by way of the blood or from below by ascent from the exterior. Some controversy exists as to which of these routes is the more common. A widely held view is that staphylococci and streptococci reach the urinary tract by way of the blood, with the primary infection in the kidney, and that infections with intestinal organisms are chiefly of the ascending type. The wearing of diapers and the relatively short urethra of the female are sufficient to account for the greater frequency of the disease in babies and in girls.

Obstruction in the urinary tract plays a highly important role in urinary infection. Once infection has occured, obstruction aggravates the condition and is an important factor in making the infection severe and chronic. Most often, in childhood the obstruction is produced by some congenital malformation, seldom by stone. A relationship exists between urinary infection and infections of the upper respiratory tract and gastrointestinal disturbances, particularly diarrhea.

Symptoms

The symptoms of pyuria are extremely varied. In the infant and the young child they are not localizing. In the older child they may simulate those of appendicitis, meningitis, pneumonia or other febrile illnesses. Fever is almost always present with acute attacks and frequently is marked by rapid fluctuations, with chills or convulsions during the rising portion of the fever curve. Leukocytosis is generally present.

With chronic pyuria or pyuria which persists beyond the initial attack, the systemic manifestations of fever, chills and general malaise are usually milder or completely lacking, in spite of severe infection.

Unlike older children, the newborn infant is affected with equal frequency in the two sexes. It is assumed that such infections are the result of blood-borne bacteria. In the older infant or child, pyuria in the male is much less common than in the female, and its occurrence almost invariably means the presence of some anatomic or functional malformation of the urinary tract.

Diagnosis

The clue to diagnosis lies in the discovery of pus on microscopic examination of the urine. Pus must be present in abnormal amount, and there must be assurance that it did not come from preputial or vaginal secretions. When there is doubt, a "clean catch" or a catheterized specimen of urine is required. The latter procedures have the advantage of permitting accurate culture of the urine in order to identify the bacterium responsible and to test its sensitivity to various chemotherapeutic and antibiotic agents. For procedures relating to the collection of sterile and clean specimens of urine see the Appendix.

Prognosis

The prognosis of uncomplicated pyuria is good. In many cases in which no obstruction or urinary retention exists, the pyuria and the bacilluria will cease spontaneously or with little treatment, when associated parenteral infection or gastrointestinal disturbance has subsided. The cases of most troublesome and persistent infection are those in which obstruction exists. Obstruction alone leads ultimately to kidney failure. When infection is present in addition, kidney failure is hastened.

Treatment

Control of pyuria requires the elimination of the infecting organisms from the urinary tract. Sulfonamides are highly satisfactory in the treatment of most acute attacks; sulfadiazine and Gantrisin have the greatest popularity. Furadantin is also effective. Because these substances are concentrated by the kidney, an effective level in the urine can be obtained with moderate doses. In some instances the infecting organism is not readily susceptible to these substances or has acquired resistance to them. Then rational treatment must be guided by isolating the infecting bacteria and testing its sensitivity to the many antibiotic agents that are now available. In long-standing or recurrent pyuria, bacteria of the Proteus and the Pseudomonas families may be encountered. These organisms not infrequently defy the most carefully planned antibiotic attack.

With the exception of the initial attack of simple pyuria in girls, all cases should be studied carefully for the presence of abnormalities of the anatomy or the physiology of the urinary tract so that, whenever feasible, situations that produce stasis of urine can be corrected in the hope of forestalling future episodes of pyuria. Such studies usually begin with an x-ray visualization of the upper urinary tract by intravenous pyelography. An opaque dye such as Renografin is injected into the blood stream of the child after a period of partial dehydration, and roentgenograms of the abdomen are taken at intervals thereafter. Usually, the outline of kidneys and ureters can be discovered by this method, and some indication of the excretory power of each kidney can be obtained. The lower portion of the urinary tract may be visualized by a voiding cysto-urethrogram. This procedure involves the injection of an opaque dye into the bladder through a catheter in the urethra. Then x-ray films are taken which demonstrate the size and shape of the bladder and during voiding may reveal posterior urethral obstruction or reflux of dye into the ureters if their orifices are abnormally patulous. A satisfactory understanding of the abnormality sometimes requires the additional information provided by cystoscopy with retrograde pyelography. Direct visualization of the bladder and urethra is possible; urine may be collected from the two kidneys independently for study, and better x-ray visualization of the ureters and the kidney pelves can be made when catheters are passed up into the upper portions of the tract. Unfortunately, the procedure of cystoscopy is painful and upsetting to

male children and usually cannot be done without a general anesthetic.

SKIN INFECTIONS

Impetigo Contagiosa

Impetigo contagiosa is a skin disease caused by an infection that invades the superficial layers of the skin. The infection tends to spread from one area to another on the affected person. It is transferred easily to other persons by direct or indirect contact. Both streptococci and staphylococci are causative agents.

The individual lesion varies in size from 3 mm. to 3 cm. or more. It appears first as a vesicle located superficially in the skin, with a loose and often wrinkled, rather than a tense and distended, top. Soon purulent material can be seen through the skin covering. The skin immediately surrounding the lesions shows no change from the normal. The pustule ruptures easily, and the exudate over the lesion tends to dry and form a crust. The crust eventually falls off, leaving an area slightly reddened. Soon all trace of the presence of

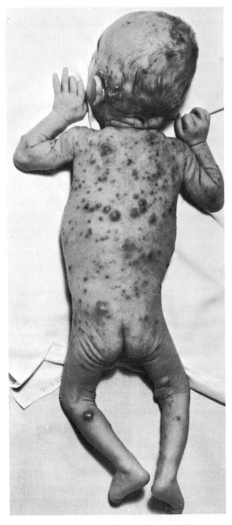

FIG. 14-8. Furunculosis or pyoderma.

the lesion disappears. The individual lesion runs its course in a week or two, but the disease has no uniform duration. Because of continued auto-inoculation, it may persist for many weeks.

The number of lesions on the body varies greatly, the total number depending on the amount of reinoculation from earlier lesions. Exposed parts (hands and face) are chiefly affected, but the lesions may be in any location, especially in babies. Symptoms of consequence are rarely associated with the disease. In a few cases of severe impetigo, acute hemorrhagic nephritis has occurred as a complication. When the infection occurs in the newborn, the lesions usually are large blisters, and often the condition is designated as pemphigus neonatorum.

The treatment consists of removal of the crusts and the tops of bullous lesions and the application of some germicide. The crusts may be removed by washing gently with warm saline solution.

Antibiotic ointments are usually quite effective. Preparations containing bacitracin, polymyxin, chlortetracycline, erythromycin and neomycin are employed commonly. Ointments containing sulfonamides and penicillin are generally less effective and are more likely to result in sensitization of the child. The ointment should be applied at least twice daily to areas where it cannot be protected by dressings from being rubbed off. When local therapy is not effective within a few days, it may be necessary to give an appropriate antibiotic systemically. If the impetigo is superimposed on scabies or pediculosis, the underlying condition also should be treated.

Furunculosis

Symptoms. Furunculosis is a condition in which multiple small abscesses or boils are present in the skin. While a furuncle may occur at any age, multiple lesions, constituting furunculosis, occur chiefly in infants and especially in infants who are malnourished. The furuncles are caused by pyogenic bacteria, chiefly staphylococci, which gain entrance to the skin by way of the hair follicles. They are most common about the head but may occur in any location and may be generalized.

Symptoms of furunculosis in a baby are few or lacking. Little or no fever is present in most instances. No doubt, furunculosis produces some constitutional effects, but such effects are vague and usually undetectable.

Nursing Care. In the management of skin disease, meticulous cleanliness is important. The hair should be shaved around any lesions on the scalp, and that area should be cleansed with green-soap or hexachlorophene solution several times daily. Incision is indicated only after the furuncle has pointed. In some instances, it may be desirable to hasten maturation of the lesions by the use of hot compresses. Draining furuncles should be covered in order to prevent spread of the infection. The dressing should be changed frequently enough to keep the drainage from the surrounding area. Elbow restraints may be necessary to prevent the infant from removing the dressing and transplanting the infection to other areas of the skin. Application of an antibiotic ointment may assist in destroying the infecting organisms as they emerge in the contents of the boil. Systemic treatment is often desirable. The selection of the antibiotic to be used can be made best by isolation of the infecting organism from the pus expressed from within the furuncle and determination of the sensitivities of the particular agent recovered. Staphylococci in particular have become resistant to many of the commonly used antibiotics.

Modification of the diet to exclude as much carbohydrate as possible seems to aid in healing the lesions. Yeast or other preparations containing vitamin B complex are also useful.

CONGENITAL AGAMMAGLOBULINEMIA AND DYSGAMMAGLOBULINEMIA

Some infants and children suffer from repeated and severe infections with bacterial agents because of abnormalities in their immunologic mechanisms. Technics for the study of immunity have recently enlarged our understanding of the intricacies of the process and led to the identification of a variety of new syndromes, most of which are fortunately rare. Three varieties of gamma globulin are now recognized: γ-G, γ-A, and γ-M. During fetal life there is a relatively free transfer of γ-G globulin from mother to baby so that at birth the infant acquires a store of such antibodies which will temporarily protect him against some infections—mainly those due to viruses—for a few weeks or months. He must make his own γ-A and γ-M globulins immediately after birth and his own γ-G globulin within three to four months after birth if he is to acquire adequate protection.

Congenital agammaglobulinemia (Bruton's disease) occurs only in males because it is a sex-linked recessively transmitted disease like hemophilia. All three of the gamma globulins are made in very small amount by affected boys. Measurements of their total serum gamma globulin show levels of less than 300 mg. per cent instead of the normal of 800-1,200 mg. per cent. Administration of gamma globulin derived from pooled blood plasma will keep the child free of severe infections if his level can be kept around 300 mg. per cent by giving monthly or bi-monthly injections.

A more severe type of agammaglobulinemia (Swiss) affects infants and is associated with an additional lack of lymphocytes and lymphoid-forming tissue, particularly the thymus gland. Such infants usually die within the first 2 years of life.

Dysgammaglobulinemia denotes imperfect production of one or more of the varieties of gamma globulins or an overproduction of abnormal gamma globulins associated with poor resistance to infection. Examples are the Wiskott-Aldrich syndrome and the ataxia-telangiectasia syndrome. Pediatric texts should be consulted for further details.

UNEXPECTED SUDDEN DEATH—CRIB DEATH

During the first 4 to 5 months of life a significant number of infants die suddenly for no obvious reason. Although such incidents are more common in infants raised under poor socioeconomic circumstances, they are also seen in families of all walks of life. Usually the infant is described as having been free of any evidence of illness and having been put to sleep after receiving a feeding only to be found dead in his crib or baby carriage within the next few hours. Careful autopsy studies fail to disclose the basis for death although a sudden, overwhelming infection is suspected. It is important to remember that most of these deaths are clearly not due to parental negligence.

SITUATIONS FOR FURTHER STUDY

1. If you visited a home where a 6-month-old infant had not yet been immunized against whooping cough, how would you react and what approach would you use in motivating the parents to recognize their child's need for protection?

2. If during a home visit you discovered a 3-month-old baby with a respiratory infection, what symptoms would lead you to suggest that the mother take him to a hospital? If the symptoms were mild, what help in the provision of nursing care would you give the mother?

3. Observe a baby with severe croup and enumerate the physical signs that manifest fear. Could you detect any change in the symptoms during periods when you were in close physical contact with him and when you were observing him from a distance?

4. What observations would you make while caring for a baby with staphylococcal pneumonia?

5. If you were a public health nurse visiting the home of a 3-month-old baby who had had repeated episodes of diarrhea, what steps would you take in attacking the problem of prevention?

6. What symptoms in a 1-year-old baby would lead you to suspect that the baby had an infection of the urinary tract?

BIBLIOGRAPHY

Alexander, H. E., Pertussis, *in* Cooke, R. E. (ed.): The Biologic Basis of Pediatric Practice, ed. 1, p. 743, N. Y., McGraw-Hill, 1968.

Flatter, P. A.: Hazards of oxygen therapy, Am. J. Nurs. *68*: 80, 1968.

Geis, D. P., and Lambertz, S. E.: Acute respiratory infections in young children, Am. J. Nurs. *68*:294, 1968.

Gregg, M. B.: Communicable disease trends in the United States, Am. J. Nurs. *68*:88, 1968.

Kendig, E. L., Jr. (ed.): Disorders of Respiratory Tract in Children, Philadelphia, Saunders, 1967.

Larsen, G. I.: What Every Nurse Should Know About Congenital Syphilis, Nurs. Outlook, Vol. 13, 52, 1965.

Levesque, L. A.: Nurse's role in croup management, Hospital Top. *39*:66, Nov. 1961.

Lewis, B. J., and Gunn, I. P.: Tracheostomy, oxygen administration and expiratory air flow resistance, Nurs. Research *13*:301, 1964.

Moffet, H., Shulenberger, H., and Burkholder, E.: Epidemiology and etiology of severe infantile diarrhea, J. Pediat. *72*:1, 1968.

Nelson, W. E. (ed.): Textbook of Pediatrics, ed. 9, Philadelphia, Saunders, 1969.

Parrott, R. H., and Chanock, R. M.: Respiratory Viruses, *in* Cooke, R. E. (ed.): The Biologic Basis of Pediatric Practice, ed. 1, p. 657, McGraw-Hill, New York, 1968.

Rodman, T.: Management of tracheobronchial secretions, Am. J. Nurs. *66*:2474, 1966.

Ross Laboratories, Nursing Education Series, No. 16: Exanthematous Diseases of Infants and Children, Columbus, Ohio, May, 1967.

Thomas, J. M., and Ulpis, E. B.: A seasonal hazard—laryngotracheobronchitis, Amer. J. Nurs. *61*:52, 1961.

Top, F. H.: Communicable and Infectious Diseases, ed. 6, St. Louis, Mosby, 1968.

Totman, L. E., and Lehlman, R. H.: Tracheostomy care, Am. J. Nurs. *64*:96, 1964.

Valdés-Dapena, M.: Sudden and unexpected death in infants: The scope of our ignorance, Pediat. Clin. N. Amer. *10*:693, 1963.

Wright, F. H., and Beem, M. O.: Management of acute viral bronchiolitis in infancy, Pediatrics *35*:334, 1965.

15

Nursing Care of Infants With Other Disorders

SKIN DISEASES DUE TO PHYSICAL AND CHEMICAL AGENTS

Reaction to Body Excretions

Miliaria. Miliaria (miliaria rubra, "prickly heat") is the result of inflammation about the sweat glands in association with sweating from any cause, whether summer heat, excessive clothing or febrile illness. It is common in babies. It is manifested by a bright red papular rash. Some of the lesions may be topped by a small vesicle; others may become pustular. The rash tends to be most prominent about the neck and the body folds.

Treatment includes management of hygiene to avoid sweating. Frequent bathing without soap is useful. Some simple dusting powder should be applied to the affected areas. The occasional use of calamine lotion is helpful, especially if itching is present.

Intertrigo. This inflammation of the skin occurs in body folds where moisture accumulates and two moist surfaces remain in contact. It is more common in obese infants. The infant's skin reacts more easily to irritation than does the skin of the older person. In infants, intertrigo may occur in the axilla, between the upper parts of the thighs, in the folds of the groin and the neck and in any other location where two skin surfaces come together. The affected skin is red and sometimes more or less raw from the loss of the outermost layer of skin. Intertrigo may be both prevented and treated by keeping the skin dry and clean in the body folds. Exposure of the affected areas to permit complete evaporation of moisture is desirable whenever possible. Clothing should be light and porous, and any material, such as plastic or rubber diaper coverings, which holds in moisture must be avoided until the lesions heal. In some cases the intertrigo becomes infected secondarily by skin bacteria or

fungi. Application of mild antiseptics, antibiotics or fungicides may be necessary.

Diaper Rashes. In infancy, irritation or excoriation of the skin beneath the diapers is a common annoyance. In addition to the irritant effect of moisture from sweat and urine, there may be the burning erythema produced by organic acids in the stool or by ammonia that results from bacterial decomposition of the urine.

Diarrheal stools contain large amounts of organic acids which may result in a chemical burn of the skin if allowed to remain in contact with it for any appreciable length of time. The lesions produced have a characteristic distribution that conforms to the area of soiling by the stool. Dermatitis from this cause clears up when the diarrhea is brought under control. Prompt cleansing of the skin, preferably with a bland oil, helps to prevent this form of diaper rash. Protection against the next stool may be given by spreading a layer of protective ointment over the affected area. A number of proprietary preparations are available for this purpose.

Diaper irritation from urine generally is due to the formation of ammonia by bacterial action on the urea normally present as a constituent of urine. The bacillus responsible is a common inhabitant of the intestinal tract, particularly of the artificially fed infant. Since it readily contaminates the perineum and the buttocks of the infant, it has easy access to urine in the wet diaper unless this is replaced rapidly by a dry one. The distribution of ammonia dermatitis corresponds to the spread of urine—mainly over the buttocks in an infant who habitually sleeps on his back, and over the anterior abdominal wall in an infant who sleeps face down.

ULCERATION OF THE URINARY MEATUS. This is a common disorder of circumcised male infants and probably depends on the same general mechanism. It may occur even without an associated diaper rash. A small ulcer is produced at or just within the opening of the urinary meatus at the tip of the penis. A small crust forms over this ulcer, which is washed away easily by the stream of urine, producing pain and the appearance of a small drop of blood on the diaper. If the crust remains firmly attached, the urinary stream may be diverted to one side, or occasionally the opening will be blocked temporarily.

Treatment of ammonia dermatitis consists in thorough drying of the affected parts by persistent exposure to the air and by application of bland oils and protective ointments. Creams and lotions containing steroids, antibiotics or iodochlorhydroxyquin may accelerate the healing process. Prevention may be achieved by measures designed to interfere with the growth of the bacteria that produce ammonia. Diapers may be given a final rinse in 1:5,000 mercuric chloride solution or one of the proprietary antiseptics prepared for this purpose. Whichever substance is used, the diaper should be hung up wet so that the antiseptic can remain in the diaper in good concentration.

Seborrheic Dermatitis. In the common form of this disorder, surface lipids, scales, serum and dirt accumulate into yellowish crusts on the scalp in infants and, if neglected, may become thick, irritated or secondarily infected. Periodic removal of crusts and scales with a soap and water shampoo or the application of a bland oil is sufficient for mild accumulations. Ointments containing salicylic acid or sulfur are useful in removing heavy scales. The tendency toward seborrheic dermatitis of the scalp usually decreases when the infant reaches a year of age. Occasionally other parts of the body are affected.

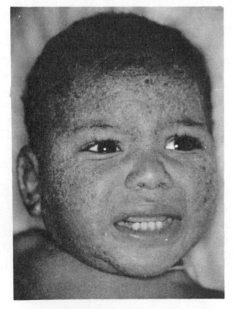

Fig. 15-1. Eczema in an 11-month-old baby. (Dr. R. Platou)

Exogenous Irritants

A very large number of substances are capable of stimulating a sensitivity reaction after repeated contact with the skin. Infants and young children are generally more likely to acquire such sensitization because of their relatively thin skins. In its mild form this contact dermatitis or allergic dermatitis appears as an area of redness with mild itching. In a more severe form it may result in swelling or even blistering. The main problem in treatment is to discover the offending substance and prevent further contact with it. Bleaches and detergent soaps used in laundering clothing or diapers are perhaps the most common sources of trouble today. Occasionally, such items as rubber pants or sheeting, plastic substances, cosmetics, adhesive gum, nail polish, iodine, or dyes from clothing are found to be responsible.

ECZEMA

Eczema is a dermatitis caused by internal or external irritants. It has definite characteristics that distinguish it from the dermatitis of bacterial inflammation, and it tends to run a chronic course with periods of remission and exacerbation. Eczema occurs at all ages, but it is considerably more frequent in infancy than at any later time. In the majority of cases, the eczema appears before 6 months of age, though seldom in the first month.

Manifestations

Eczema of infancy differs from that occurring later in its greater severity and in the distribution and the general nature of the lesions. The common type of infantile eczema occurs most often in fat or well nourished babies. The lesions are most severe on the face, but they may appear also on the scalp, the forearms, the legs and the trunk. In the early stages and in exacerbations, the superficial epithelium is lost and the skin surface is raw and oozing. The exudate tends to dry, forming crusts. The skin is not thickened.

A less common type, more frequent in malnourished babies, is characterized by a reddened, thickened, scaly skin. The lesions of this type may appear anywhere on the body. This latter type is most common in older children, except that it is more likely to be limited to the body folds, especially at the elbows and the knees.

Infantile eczema is accompanied by considerable itching or burning, and, as a consequence, the baby, if permitted, will rub or scratch most of the time, thus aggravating the condition markedly. Remissions and exacerbations of the eczema occur at irregular intervals. Eczema usually is much worse in winter and better in summer, often disappearing entirely in the warm months only to recur in the fall. In the majority of instances, the skin heals between 1 and 2 years of age, and the eczema does not recur. In some infants the lesions change gradually into those of neurodermatitis which continues into later childhood.

Etiology

The cause of infantile eczema cannot be stated definitely. That allergy is a large factor in many instances is an acceptable belief, but any claim that it is the cause in all cases is not supportable by the evidence at hand. Approximately three fourths of the older babies with eczema have positive reactions to various proteins when applied to the skin by customary testing methods. Babies in the first half year, especially those under 4 months, seldom present good evidence of skin sensitivity to test proteins, even though the eczema may be caused by these proteins. The food proteins to which infants most commonly are found to be sensitive are egg white; various cereals, especially wheat; cow's milk; fruit, especially apple and orange; and potato.

Even though a considerable proportion of babies with eczema have positive skin reactions to test proteins, only about one third or fewer will obtain relief when removal of the supposedly offending protein from the diet is the only therapeutic measure employed. Factors other than allergy seem to play an important role. The skin of the infant is more sensitive and delicate than that of the child and reacts to milder stimuli. A large factor in the increased sensitivity of the infant is the large water content of the body, in which the skin shares. This explains why eczema is aggravated by the trauma of rubbing and scratching, by local infections which are acquired so easily in the affected areas of skin, and by sudden marked changes in temperature such as those to which the baby is exposed when taken outdoors in winter.

Infants with eczema are prone to infections both of the skin itself and of the respiratory tract. Hospitalization carries a certain risk to the infant by placing him close to others who are infected. Isolation procedures are thus desirable for protection, though often undesirable for psychological reasons. *The eczematous infant must be kept away from children who have recently been vaccinated against smallpox and must not be vaccinated himself,* for the vaccinia virus can diffusely infect his weeping skin and produce serious or fatal disease. Individuals with herpes virus infections or streptococcal or pneumococcal infections are also a potential hazard. The debilitated eczematous infant does not fare well with severe respiratory disease, particularly pneumonia.

Nursing Care

Ideally, the infant with eczema should be restrained only when absolutely necessary to prevent scratching and infection. These infants often substitute scratching for the more usual crying. Since restraints inevitably increase frustration and result in a greater need to scratch, caution should be exercised and restraints applied only if the benefits outweigh these disadvantages. If a nurse can be with the baby, she can follow his cues, provide satisfaction according to his needs and thus decrease frustration and scratching. A warm, continuous relationship with a nurse who recognizes the baby's need to express his feelings overtly is thus particularly important for the baby hospitalized with eczema.

Restraint. When constant attendance is not possible, cuffs that prevent flexion at the elbows are of assistance, but usually the arms must be held with additional restraint to prevent rubbing of the face with the upper arms. They must be adjusted securely because the baby's discomfort and desire for activity drive him to find methods of freeing himself. On the other hand, particularly during hot weather, the restraints must not be applied too tightly since the infant is susceptible to heat and pressure. They should also be applied gently to minimize feelings of anger at being restrained.

A good type of elbow cuff is one splinted with tongue blades. For young infants, the tongue blades are cut to about 4 inches in length. In order to retain the cuff securely, the shirt sleeves should be folded over the lower end of the cuff and pinned to it. Ankle restraints are necessary if eczema is present on the legs. When the weather is warm or when the infant tends to perspire profusely, it is advisable to eliminate the use of the shirt. To keep the cuff restraints in position, a 4-inch strip of old linen can be brought across the shoulders and down the arms and then pinned back over the cuff.

Fingernails and toenails must be cut short. If necessary, gloves or stockings can be put on the hands and pinned to the cuffs to minimize scratching.

Protection by Pliofilm. When an infant tends to rub his face on his shoulders, a bib of Pliofilm prevents excoriations. Such a bib may be made of an 8-inch square of Pliofilm with tabs of adhesive and tape at the corners for pinning it into position. In some institutions, Pliofilm covers over the head of the mattress have been used with excellent results. When the Pliofilm bib and mattress covers are used, the infant can be turned from side to side and on his abdomen without danger of increasing the severity of the lesions. Changes in position are important in the prevention of respiratory infection, a complication to which the infant with eczema is very susceptible.

Local Application. The selection of appropriate dermatologic remedies and their meticulous application are useful in all cases of eczema and, in addition to other general measures discussed, are sufficient in many instances to bring about recovery without recourse to radical dietary changes. If the skin is moderately infected when the baby comes under care, an antibiotic ointment, such as bacitracin or neomycin, may be used until the infection has disappeared. Systematic use of antibiotics may be necessary to control severe infection. In instances of more severe infection, or if the baby is scratching, cool wet packs of normal saline or Burow's solution serve better than an ointment to relieve itching. These dressings should be left open rather than being wrapped with plastic, to prevent irritation and heating. If the skin is not infected or if the infection has been treated effectively, a protective or soothing ointment is indicated. Such an ointment may be 2 per cent Ichthyol or Lassar's paste. If satisfactory improvement is not obtained with the soothing ointment, a stimulating ointment, such as 6 per cent tar ointment or carbonis detergens cream is indicated, but only after the protective ointment has failed. When tar ointment is used, exposure to the sun should be avoided because the ointment contains a photosensitizing fraction that produces skin irritation as a result of exposure to sunshine.

Ointments containing hydrocortisone or related adrenal steroids are useful in controlling the inflammatory reaction. The ointment may be applied sparingly 3 to 4 times daily, but systemic use of these hormones is to be avoided.

Applying the ointment with long strokes has been found to produce a more soothing effect. After application, the area should be bandaged with old, soft sheeting, secured with 2-inch elastic bandage.

In order to ensure satisfactory retention of ointments or wet dressings applied to the face, it may be necessary to use a mask. A mask is prepared by cutting holes in a piece of old linen or cotton stocking, the holes corresponding in shape and location to the eyes, nose and mouth. The mask should be large enough to go around the head and should be held in position with attached tapes. Binding and friction must be avoided when adjusting the mask.

Cleansing the Skin. Oil applied by means of cotton, or water to which sodium bicarbonate and starch have been added is used for cleansing. The use of soap is not advisable. When ointments are being used, it is customary to cleanse the skin once daily or less frequently. Cleansing should be done gently without rubbing. If itching is intense and restraint is being used, only one extremity at a time can be released for cleansing.

Sometimes a colloidal bath is desired. In preparation, an infant-sized tub is filled with water at 95° F., and ¼ cup each of soluble starch and sodium bicarbonate is mixed in thoroughly. Floating toys should be at hand to divert the infant's attention and prevent scratching during the procedure. A diaper should be placed in the bottom of the tub to prevent the baby from slipping, and a firm hold is necessary to prevent the child from feeling insecure in the tub. During the time the infant is in the tub (15 to 20 minutes), the washcloth should be used to pour water over the infant's head and body. Rubbing the skin may produce a paroxysm of itching.

Diet. Usually it is not possible at the first examination to determine whether or not infantile eczema has an allergic basis. When special dietary measures are not instituted at the beginning of treatment, they may be employed if response to local treatment is not definite and prompt. More than half the babies with eczema will respond to local treatment without dietary change. If the eczema is dependent on allergy to foods, the offending foods should be omitted from the diet, while at the same time the diet should be kept "complete."

One good method of management is to use what is known as an elimination diet. This is accomplished by starting with a simple basic diet which is hypoallergenic to the extent that improvement in the eczema is permitted. Then one food at a time is added to determine the infant's reaction to each new substance. In such a scheme, new foods should be introduced in small amounts. The diet and the skin changes should be charted in full in order to determine the foods to which the baby is sensitive.

The chief article of the basic diet should be some form of milk or milk substitute. Prolonged or high heating of protein alters its character in such a way that it is less allergenic, often sufficiently so that babies who are sensitive to the raw protein can take the cooked protein without disturbance. It is the alteration produced by heat that gives to evaporated and dried milk a considerable degree of usefulness in the management of babies with allergic eczema. Babies sensitive to cow's milk often are able to take goat's milk. Synthetic milks are commercially available. Some of these are prepared from soybeans, and one is prepared from hydrolyzed casein. Regardless of which of these foods may be chosen, the formula must be supplemented by vitamins C and D and perhaps other essentials, depending on the food chosen. In the dietary management of babies with eczema, foods should be eliminated because of adverse reactions to feeding, not on the basis of skin tests.

Prevention

The most satisfactory management for eczema is prevention of skin lesions in infants suspected of being susceptible. General cleanliness is of great importance and mothers should be instructed to bathe the infant frequently with a bland soap. Thorough rinsing and gentle drying are necessary to prevent skin irritation. Heavy oils should not be applied unless the infant's skin is excessively dry. Special attention should also be given to skin folds, with frequent drying of perspiration. The skin should be cleansed immediately and gently dried after drooling, regurgitation or elimination.

Eczema is rarely completely dependent on sensitivity to foods but often is aggravated by either internal or external environmental irritants. Feathers, wool, kapok and certain dusts may irritate the skin. Cotton clothing and bedding seem to be the least irritating.

Stuffed toys may contain allergenic factors and should be carefully selected.

Immediate attention should be given to any indications of heat rash or skin irritation. Linens coming in contact with the body should be thoroughly rinsed to remove all skin irritants. Exposure to extremes of heat and sunlight should also be avoided.

Psychological Aspects

Emotional factors may also play a part in producing eczema. Many investigators who have studied children with eczema have found emotional disturbances in the mother-child relationship. If the mother is uncomfortable in the care of her child or finds his responses frustrating and unrewarding due to her previous experiences, she will communicate her anxiety to her infant. The infant may respond to deficiencies in the mothering he receives not only by distortions in healthy emotional development, but by somatic symptoms.

Dunbar concluded that a climate with "smother love" was the characteristic emotional climate to which the child with eczema was subjected. She felt that many of these children experienced conflict between their desire for affection and their fear lest they be hurt if they sought it. Other investigators found these children overprotected and recipients of domineering love. Overcompensation for negative feelings toward the child may result in such excessive protection and restrictiveness. Some investigators believed that a frustrated need for love was one of the dynamic factors operating to produce the condition.

Because of the factor of emotional determinants, the infant hospitalized with eczema needs a nurse who is knowledgeable and sensitive to the behavioral cues he gives in respect to his emotional needs. He requires cuddling and should be held for feeding just as a healthy child is. This gives him kinesthetic stimulation and the affection he needs for normal intellectual and emotional growth. Time of feeding should be gauged by his need for food. Awakening a sleepy baby with eczema increases his frustration and need to scratch.

Frustration and tension may be relieved by providing additional sucking through the use of a pacifier, particularly if restraints are necessary. Additional satisfaction may also be achieved through a continuous, nonsmothering type of interpersonal relationship with his nurse and through sensory stimulation which is carefully provided in accordance with his readiness.

In preventing scratching, the nurse must remember that her patient needs the same satisfactions and opportunities for learning as the healthy infant. He needs freedom for self-directed play and opportunities to develop his mind and body. Restraints should be removed each time the infant is fed, and his arms and legs should be exercised. If he is old enough to be interested in self-feeding, his interest in learning should be encouraged. As soon as the skin lesions show sufficient improvement, all the restraints should be removed and the infant allowed to move about and play freely under close supervision. Toys suited to his individual needs should be introduced. Diversion prevents scratching and gives the infant needed experience with play materials.

When caring for a child with eczema, the nurse must also direct her interest to the needs of the mother. The nurse needs to reflect not only on her own feelings toward the child with eczema but also on her reactions to his mother. Mothers of babies with eczema are often unusually fearful and see the baby's condition as evidence of their failure to fulfill the mother role. Some tend to handle the baby less than do mothers of normal infants, and the manner of handling is usually less gentle. Others overstimulate the baby with excessive handling. Some hesitate to restrain and to restrict the baby's diet because it frustrates their deep need to overprotect. Many mothers fear that their infants are afflicted with a chronic disease that may produce scars and prevent normal development.

The mothers of babies with eczema need help before they assume complete charge of their infants. Encouraging the mother to talk about her feelings toward her child and the amount of care he requires not only meets her need to share her burden with another person but also gives the nurse increased understanding of her as a person. If the nurse knows of the mother's fears, she can help her gain increased mastery of them. Detailed instructions and demonstrations of care are important, but they are not enough to ensure continuity of nursing care for the baby. Experience can verify this statement. It is not unusual to see recurrences very soon after the baby has been discharged. They can be minimized if the mother has opportunities to take care of her baby in the presence of an understanding nurse. During such experiences, the nurse should direct her interest to the mother. Supporting her through experiences which are fear provoking builds up the mother's self-confidence, increases her feelings of self-esteem and frees energy for the building of a warmer relationship with her child. The nurse can help the mother to find ways to restrict scratching and thus minimize her feelings of guilt and provide her child with opportunities to use his extremities in play. She can also increase her hope and clarify any misconceptions that she is harboring.

Nervous mannerisms are seen frequently in children with eczema. The long periods of restriction with constant frustrations tend to produce emotional instability, insecurity, aggression, extroversion, restlessness and an unusual drive to dominate. Parental anxiety is often reflected in their behavior. When frustrated in play, these children not uncommonly revert to scratching, even though their skin shows little or no irritation. According to some studies, such children show superior mental ability. If this is true, it is not surprising

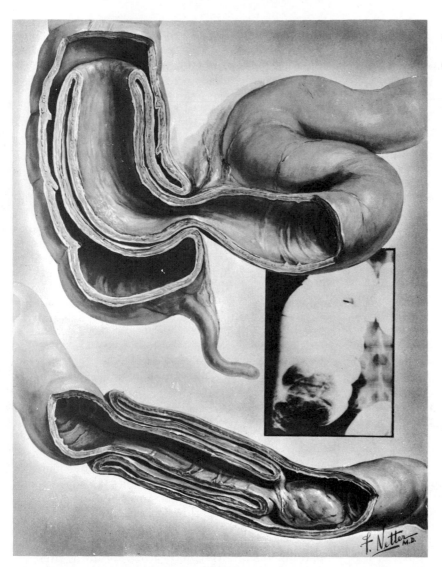

Fig. 15-2. Intussusception. (*Top*) Ileo-colic variety. (*Inset*) Roentgen appearance. (*Bottom*) Ileoileal variety. (Ciba Collection of Medical Illustrations)

that they are eager to investigate their environment when freed from the limiting and infuriating restraints. To prevent these nervous mannerisms, the nurse must understand the problems of the mother and help her to feel the need to give her child more independence in play and in learning to do things for himself.

INTUSSUSCEPTION

Intussusception is the invagination of a segment of the bowel into the portion immediately distal to it. It probably is caused by hyperactive peristalsis in the proximal portion of the bowel with relative inactivity of the distal segment. Although it may occur at any level of the small or the large intestine, nearly always it is discovered at the junction of the ileum and the colon. As the bowel invaginates it carries along its mesentery. The blood supply is cut off, as it is pulled into the tightening ring, and if the condition continues, the bowel will become gangrenous. Death may result if the condition is not recognized and corrected. Most of those who develop intussusception are infants, and usually they are robust boys who have been thriving.

Symptoms

The disease may begin suddenly with a shriek of pain and rapidly appearing symptoms of intestinal obstruction—vomiting, constipation, abdominal pain and eventually prostration and shock. At times the origin of symptoms is more insidious, with indefinite discomfort, poor appetite and unexplained vomiting. Despite the constipation characteristic of obstruction, small bloody stools containing mucus and little or no fecal matter may be passed. The tumor mass that results from intussusception may be palpated through the abdominal wall or may be detected with the finger on rectal examination if it has progressed far enough down the colon.

Treatment

Intussusception requires immediate relief, for the mortality rises sharply with increasing duration of symptoms. In rare instances the intussusception will reduce spontaneously, but this is not an outcome that can be awaited with safety. In many instances the barium enema given to confirm the diagnosis can safely be made to exert enough retrograde pressure to reduce the telescoped bowel, and the fluoroscopic examination or films will demonstrate that complete relief has been achieved. However, if relief cannot be demonstrated after a reasonable trial, prompt surgical exploration is indicated in order to reduce the intussusception before irreversible gangrene of the bowel has occurred. In the latter instance, resection of bowel is necessary—a procedure which is poorly tolerated by a seriously ill infant.

Nursing Care

The postoperative symptomatic care of the infant is not unlike that given after other types of abdominal operation. If simple reduction of the bowel is accomplished, feedings may be started shortly after peristaltic activity is audible in the abdomen. If resection of gangrenous bowel is necessary, constant gastric suction and parenteral administration of fluids are required for several days. During this period an infant may find some measure of solace in being permitted to suck on a pacifier or a nipple, and in being held.

RECTAL PROLAPSE

Sometimes a distinction is made between anal and rectal prolapse. In anal prolapse, the mucous membrane immediately proximal to the anus is extruded. In rectal prolapse the large tumor is composed also of bowel wall. A combination of relaxed sphincter, large hard stools and straining at stool is likely to cause moderate prolapse in otherwise normal children. Rectal prolapse is associated with weakness of the muscles of the pelvic floor. Any condition such as severe malnutrition, hypothyroidism and cystic fibrosis of the pancreas, which brings about muscle weakness, is thus a predisposing cause. The immediate cause is straining, due either to diarrhea or to constipation. It occurs only at defecation and is common in only the first 2 or 3 years.

The prolapsed part of the rectum should be replaced and, as far as possible, kept replaced constantly. During defecation, the buttocks should be held firmly, either manually or with the use of adhesive strips. A tight pad or bandage may be used. Constipation or diarrhea should be managed in such a way that straining is avoided. Usually no other measures are necessary. Operative treatment is unsatisfactory.

SPASMUS NUTANS (NODDING SPASM)

This queer affliction is confined to infants and runs a self-limited course of a few months. Its cause is unknown, and it has been seen with decreasing frequency in recent years. The manifestations consist of a peculiar shaking of the head from side to side or up and down, together with nystagmoid movements of the eyes and a tendency to cock the head on one side when looking at objects. No treatment is known or necessary.

LYMPHANGIOMA (CYSTIC HYGROMA)

The main lymphatic channel from the intestine, the thoracic duct, empties into a branch of the subclavian vein in the left side of the neck. Errors in the formation of lymphatic and venous structures in this region are not uncommon. A variety of swellings in the lower face, the neck and the upper thorax or the back are

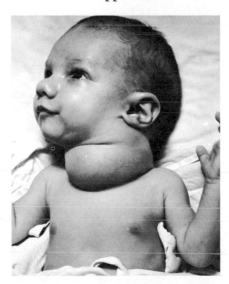

FIG. 15-4. Cystic hygroma in a 2-month-old infant. (From Dr. H. P. Jenkins)

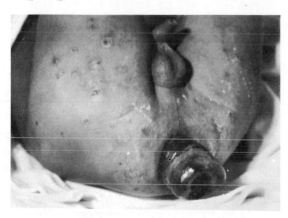

FIG. 15-3. Prolapse of the rectum, with beginning gangrene of the distal ½ inch of mucosa.

attributable to such faulty development of the lymphatics. Most common are diffuse soft, indefinite swellings which have no palpable elements within them. Such diffuse lymphangiomas are not amendable to surgical removal and must either be left alone or treated with some type of radiation. The latter procedure carries the risk of interference with growth of the bones of the face and is usually avoided unless the disfigurement is severe. Fortunately, some diffuse lymphangiomas will regress spontaneously if left alone.

Some lymphangiomas are composed of a series of palpable cysts in addition to the diffuse surrounding swelling. These cysts may contain only a clear fluid—lymph—or may be partially filled with blood due to their connections with the veins of the neck and the shoulder. In some instances it is possible and advantageous for the surgeon to remove the main mass of such a tumor and improve the child's appearance. Unfortunately, the extent of the cysts cannot always be anticipated, and remnants may be left behind which will continue to fill with fluid.

INFANTILE CORTICAL HYPEROSTOSIS (CAFFEY'S DISEASE)

This disorder of unknown etiology appears in infancy, lasts a few months and then disappears completely without leaving any residua. The changes consist in thickening of the cortical surfaces of bones and are more obvious in radiologic examinations than in clinical appearance. The mandible, clavicles, ribs, and bones of the arms and legs are most commonly involved. Symptoms include visible deformity of the jaw, the clavicle or an extremity, with low-grade fever, irritability and local soft-tissue tenderness and swelling. The condition sometimes must be distinguished from mumps, from osteomyelitis and from congenital syphilis.

RETICULOENDOTHELIOSIS

Disease of the reticuloendothelial system may result in widespread involvement of bones, skin, lymph nodes, spleen and liver or may be confined to one or a few localized lesions in such tissues. The name *Letterer-Siwe disease* is applied to a rapidly advancing diffuse form of reticuloendotheliosis which is seen occasionally in infants and small children. A diffuse skin rash and seborrhea of the scalp often initiate the symptoms and are followed by enlargement of liver, spleen and lymph nodes with progressive wasting. Recently, some dramatic relief has been obtained through the use of ACTH, steroids and antimetabolites. *Eosinophilic granuloma* is a localized lesion of bone which is usually discovered incidentally in roentgenograms taken for some other purpose. Roentgen-ray irradiation therapy or surgical excision may be curative. Between these two extremes lies the *Hand-Christian-Schüller syndrome.* This disorder is characterized by multiple lesions of the skull and the long bones which, in its classic form, produces diabetes insipidus and protrusion of the eye. Therapy is not entirely predictable, but some improvement usually results from the use of ACTH or irradiation therapy.

NEOPLASMS

Children and even infants may suffer from neoplasms of practically any of the types seen in the adult. The incidence of malignancy is very low except for leukemia, brain tumors, Wilms' tumor and neuroblastoma of the adrenal. Other varieties are rarely observed. Leukemia is discussed in Chapter 21, brain tumor in Chapter 24.

Neuroblastoma of the Adrenal

This tumor affects infants or young children. It arises from sympathetic nervous system tissue, usually of the adrenal gland but sometimes from ganglia elsewhere in the body. It tends to spread quickly and widely so that recognition of its presence is often achieved by discovery of the metastases rather than the original tumor. In addition to a local tumor in the adrenal region, enlargement of the liver or multiple metastases in the bones may be the presenting symptoms. In the latter form it can be confused with leukemia or with rheumatic fever because of the diffuse pains in the extremities. Diagnosis is accomplished by finding microscopic metastases in the bone marrow or by examination of tumor material removed at operation. Treatment consists of removal of the major tumor and treatment of the metastases by irradiation or with nitrogen mustard, ACTH or one of the antimetabolites used in leukemia. The prognosis is generally poor but not invariably so.

Wilms' Tumor

Wilms' tumor is one of the most frequent types of neoplasm seen among children. It is an adenosarcoma arising from fetal rests in the kidney, i.e., from abnormal bits of tissue which are left behind during early embryonic life and which have the capacity to begin unrestrained cancerous growth after the child is born. For this reason, Wilms' tumor is seen mainly in the first year of life and almost exclusively during the first 5 years. It appears as a mass in the kidney region which is discovered accidentally by the parent or the examining physician. Usually the mass has reached considerable size by the time it is discovered. Since the tumor has a strong predilection to extend locally through the kidney capsule or the renal vein and to disseminate to other parts of the body by the blood stream, prompt recognition is imperative. The diagnosis usually can be confirmed by intravenous pyelography, which shows displacement and distortion of the pelvis of the kidney.

Treatment consists of prompt surgical removal of the tumor, followed or preceded by x-ray treatment to the area about it. Additional treatment with actinomycin-D has accomplished a very significant decrease in the mortality rate and has even permitted successful treatment of metastatic lesions in the lungs. The prognosis is generally quite good for children under the age of 2 years, but even for older victims, an optimistic outcome can now be foreseen.

Nursing Care of Wilms' Tumor and Neuroblastoma

Infants with neoplasms need the same sensitive attention to their physical, intellectual and emotional needs as do other infants. In addition, they require knowledgeable and skillful nursing care which can improve their chances for survival.

Prior to surgery, 24 hour urine specimens are usually collected. The technics for this procedure are discussed in the Appendix.

Postoperatively, gastric suction may be required to prevent distention or vomiting. It is the responsibility of the nurse to check the equipment frequently for adequate functioning and meticulously to measure and record the infant's intake and output, since parenteral replacement of fluids and electrolytes may be required. If necessary, the tube can be irrigated with one-half isotonic saline solution. It is also her responsibility to observe her patient frequently for any symptoms of shock or change in general condition as indicated by the vital signs. If the progress of the infant is satisfactory, the gastric tube may be removed within 48 hours and oral feedings begun with small amounts of clear liquids.

If chemotherapy is used, some degree of nausea and vomiting can be expected. The nurse should also be alert for signs of soreness of the mouth and tongue, for dermatitis or loss of hair. She should observe the oral cavity frequently and promptly report ulceration since this may be a first sign of toxicity. To minimize vomiting, fluids must be carefully selected although increase in total intake is usually prescribed. Careful charting of number, character and consistency of stools is important as an indication of individual reaction to the particular drug used in treatment.

Careful observation and attention to the patient's skin is necessary when either radiation or chemotherapy is utilized. Frequent bathing is indicated if there is excessive perspiration or to remove the residuals of elimination. The skin should be dried thoroughly but gently. If the skin becomes reddened, cornstarch or a bland ointment may be applied to reduce irritation.

The nurse caring for an infant with neuroblastoma or Wilms' tumor will need to deal not only with her own emotions and reactions to the diagnosis, but also with those of the parents. Although the prognosis is no longer uniformly pessimistic, such a diagnosis invariably raises acute anxiety and fear as to the eventual outcome. The nurse must face and accept her own feelings in order to be able to understand parental anxiety and to be of help to parents. The subject of parental reactions to a poor prognosis for their child is discussed in Chapter 2.

TRAUMA

Infants under the age of 1 year are seldom responsible for their own accidents, but are likely to be the victims of falls when left improperly attended. Head injury is the most common and upsetting result of such falls. If the infant is not rendered unconscious by the fall, local ecchymosis of the scalp is likely to be the only consequence. In an occasional instance, a linear skull fracture will result which can be discovered only by taking a skull x-ray. If there is no depression of the fragments, no particular therapy is required. Depressed fragments should be elevated by the neurosurgeon to prevent irritation of the brain beneath. Automobile accidents and falls from high places may of course result in fractures of extremities or internal injuries.

Subdural Hematoma

Pathophysiology. The brain is covered by a delicate filmy membrane which encloses the surrounding layer of cerebrospinal fluid. This membrane is known as the pia-arachnoid. Bleeding into the space which it encloses is called subarachnoid hemorrhage, and the blood usually is found circulating freely in the spinal fluid. Between the arachnoid and the tough membrane (dura mater) which lines the inner surface of the skull, there is a potential space (subdural space) which is normally empty because the arachnoid is in close apposition to the dura. Under certain conditions such as trauma or some form of hemorrhagic disorder, bleeding from small vessels may occur into the subdural space. The extent of the bleeding is limited by the pressure required to push away the brain in order to make room for the clot. Once formed, the clot usually liquefies. Its high protein content tends to draw more fluid into the space within the membrane that surrounds the clot. Thus, a slowly enlarging space-occupying mass exists within the rigid confines of the skull and creates an increase in the intracranial pressure.

Subdural hematoma in older children is almost always the result of trauma. In infants it often is found in the absence of any obvious trauma other than the more or less normal events of birth and early infancy. It is more likely to be found in poorly nourished infants or those with bleeding tendencies. However, this is not exclusively the case, for it also is seen in otherwise healthy infants.

Symptoms. The bleeding usually takes place rather slowly, so that the symptoms appear insidiously. Abnormal enlargement of the head, slow developmental progress, irritability, convulsions, vomiting and poor weight gain may be present. In many of the infants, hemorrhages are seen in the eyegrounds, and some

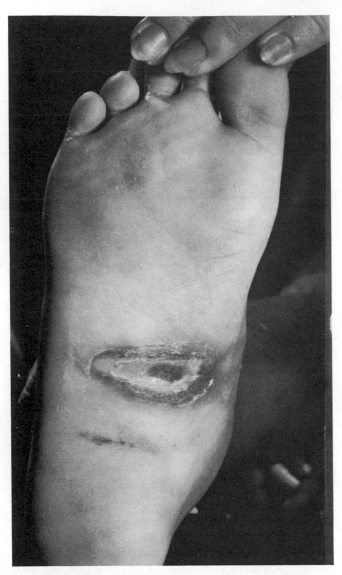

FIG. 15-5. The battered child syndrome. One of numerous lesions inflicted upon an older child by her guardians. This burn was obviously the result of the application of heated metal to the soles of the feet.

degree of swelling of the optic nerve head betrays the presence of an increase in intracranial pressure. Occasionally, the bleeding takes place rapidly, and the child passes into a state of shock, coma or uncontrolled convulsions.

Diagnosis

Diagnosis is suspected from the enlargement of the head and from the symptomatology. The finding of hemorrhages in the eyegrounds of an infant is almost certain to mean the presence of a subdural hematoma. Confirmation of the clinical suspicion is obtained by inserting a needle through the dura of the skull and withdrawing yellow, chocolate or bloody fluid from the liquefied clot. In infants with open suture lines,

such taps are performed easily between the margins of two separated cranial bones. In older children, exploratory burr holes must be made by the neurosurgeon.

Treatment and Nursing Care

Subdural hematoma is primarily a neurosurgical problem. In older children a craniotomy has to be done, and the clot and its surrounding membrane must be removed. In infants often the same procedure is indicated, but in some instances repeated aspirations through the dura will effect a cure without the need for a craniotomy. Postoperative nursing care is similar to that which is employed after brain tumor operations. It should be emphasized that early recognition and prompt treatment of the disorder are necessary to permit normal growth of the brain during infancy. When the diagnosis is overlooked and treatment is delayed too long, permanent damage to the brain and irreversible mental deficiency result.

THE BATTERED CHILD

During the past decade there has been a growing concern over the number of infants and children being seen in hospitals and physicians' offices with evidences of trauma or willful neglect from caretakers or parents. Purposely administered bruises, fractures, burns and beatings with ropes and belts are the common forms of trauma observed. Both starvation and emotional deprivation by sequestering the infant or child are forms of purposeful neglect.

Such children are obviously the victims of emotionally disturbed adults who, because of aberrations in their own personalities are unable to control their sadistic impulses against one or more of their own children. Sometimes the attackers themselves bring the child for medical assistance, concocting a story to cover their act. At other times, neighbors become suspicious and enlist the investigation of the legal authorities.

The immediate care of such children is usually a surgical matter of diagnosis and correction where necessary. But more important to the child is the recognition of the true source of his trauma, for if he is returned unprotected to his home, it is very likely that a future attack upon him will occur and that he will again be harmed or even killed.

Several states now have laws requiring the reporting of suspected battering of children to a designated agency and provide immunity from legal suit to the physician or nurse making the report. However, it is too often difficult to either persuade the battering parent to accept psychiatric help for himself, or to persuade a court to protect the child from further abuse by removing him from the custody of his disturbed parents.

Role of the Nurse in Failure to Thrive and Physical Abuse

The line between infants who fail to thrive and those who are neglected or physically abused is often a fine one. The underlying causative factor in each of these instances is a basic disturbance or distortion of varying degrees of severity in the mother-child relationship.

The development of motherliness on which the infant and small child is dependent for health, progress and survival begins in the early childhood of the mother herself. Unless she has had those experiences of love and mothering which result in the ability and desire to give of herself to her own child in adulthood, she will have difficulty with a relationship which entails the complete dependency of her partner, in reliving a difficult period of her own early life and consequently will find the later relationship unrewarding, threatening and frustrating. Feelings of inadequacy and guilt in her mother role compound these problems. In addition, in our society, a large number of factors are influential in the quality of motherliness demonstrated, including social and financial problems, the amount of support received from the marital partner, the mother's available physical energy and other stressful family circumstances. When the emotional progress toward maturity of either of the parents has been fraught with more severe problems and difficulties, the risk of physical neglect or actual abuse of their child becomes more acute.

Although the challenges involved in the nursing care of an infant who has failed to progress physically, intellectually and emotionally are great, the rewards can be equally satisfying. In no medical circumstance is the importance of understanding and skillful nursing care so pronounced. Since these children have not experienced a warm, satisfying relationship with their mothers, their needs are intense. However, for the same reasons, they have little ability, interest or hope in forming the important therapeutic relationship with the nurse. Many such infants have received little stimulation during their lives and thus may be developmentally retarded and incurious about their physical and emotional environment. Because of insufficiency of love, they may be unattractive, unresponsive and stiff when held or cuddled. On the other hand, they show little of the normal fear of strangers or distress when left alone, but may lie or sit lethargically in their cribs or cry continually in a manner which suggests little hope of comforting.

Such infants require continuity of nursing care from a nurse who is knowledgeable about child development, who is understanding and accepting of the child's unresponsiveness and who has a large supply of patience. They need warm, personal and loving care from a nurse who can respond to their needs and signals of distress. In addition to satisfying urgent needs for emotional gratification, the nurse must also be alert to opportunities for sensory stimulation. Holding and cuddling and walking the infant also provides tactile and kinesthetic stimulation, change in position and variety in the visual field. Talking and singing to the baby is also supportive to the development of cooing and vocalization. Carefully selected toys, presented when the infant demonstrates readiness, may also provide needed sensory stimulation.

The importance of working with mothers of infants who have failed to thrive cannot be overstated. Understanding and support must also extend to mothers who will resume the care of their child. A judgmental attitude on the part of the professional team attempting to assist mothers will merely increase feelings of inadequacy, guilt and resentment and will ensure the mother's flight from a helping relationship. If the nurse, physician or social worker is able to form an accepting relationship with the mother, the circle of tension may be broken and the mother helped to establish a healthier and more satisfying relationship with her infant, while discovering his characteristics, progress and needs as a separate individual.

In those instances where the parents have seriously neglected their child or intentionally abused him, psychiatric help will usually be required along with protective measures for the child. Almost all cases of intentional physical trauma inflicted by parents involve severe interpersonal conflict between the parents and complex and long standing personality damage. Although frank psychosis is rare, most parents of such children who come to medical attention are themselves unable to form any meaningful relationship, and are absorbed in their personal problems and frustrations. Violent, compulsive and explosive behavior toward their dependent children is symptomatic of inadequate controls and communicates a basic feeling that the world is hostile. In order to uncover the meaning which the abused child holds for them and to protect other children in the home who may be recipients of abuse if the present selected child is removed, a long term relationship with the parents is necessary. Such a therapeutic relationship must be undertaken by a trained professional—psychiatrist, psychologist or social caseworker. In addition, such an effort requires community and team effort and commitment and a program of public education in order to progress beyond legal prosecution and toward humane rehabilitation.

The nurse, however, has important responsibility in case finding and in follow-up of families by virtue of her closeness to them spatially and psychologically. When an abused child is admitted to the hospital, the nurse may be the first to observe him closely and to interview the parents. She must be aware of the possibility of parent administered trauma and when suspicious, allow the parents to talk freely without attempting to obtain admission of their implication in the injury. Danger signs to which she should be alert include a lack of concern about the injury, diagnosis and prognosis, vagueness as to the circumstances of the injury, indefiniteness regarding visiting plans or lack of questioning as to length of hospitalization. Allowing the parents to discuss their own problems and concerns may reveal important information which may be of later help to the physician, psychiatrist or social worker.

The nurse in the community is in a key position to detect instances of possible child neglect or abuse. Through her work in homes, well-baby clinics, outpatient departments, emergency rooms, day care centers and schools she may gain information and insight about actual or potential danger to children and thus contribute substantially toward prevention of severe physical damage. Through her work with mothers prenatally and after delivery, she can be alert to early signs of disturbance in the mother-child relationship, clues as to maternal emotional immaturity or postpartum crises which have the potential for physical or developmental trauma to children. If recognized early, extreme deterioration in parent-child relationships may be prevented through provision of services to families during this prime intervention period. Through collaboration with social agencies, public health and public welfare services, nurses are also in a strategic position to help in the amelioration of social ills which contribute to the high incidence of physical, emotional and intellectual damage to the children of our society.

SITUATIONS FOR FURTHER STUDY

1. What help could you provide a mother whose baby had a severe diaper rash?

2. What symptoms would make you worry about the possibilities of intussusception in an 18-month-old infant?

3. Study an infant with eczema and describe his behavior when he shows signs of frustration. How might his frustration be prevented? Plan his care to prevent it and record your observations of change in behavior and in the condition of his skin.

4. Study a mother of a baby with eczema during the period you were assigned to his care. What did she talk about? How did she use you in solving her problems? What specific help did you provide? How did she respond to your suggestions?

5. What problems would you anticipate in the care of a child who has failed to thrive? What principles would you incorporate in a nursing care plan? What background knowledge would be helpful in planning and carrying out nursing intervention? How might you approach the mother in order to form a helping relationship?

6. Study the reactions toward hospitalization of a child who has been physically abused. How do they differ from those of children with a warm, supportive relationship with their parents? What are your responsibilities as a nurse to this child and to his parents?

BIBLIOGRAPHY

Bass, L. W., Sieber, W. K., and Girdany, B. R.: The treatment of ileocolic intussusception, J. Pediat. 55:42, 1959.

Burgin, L. B.: Emotion as an "allergen," Pediat. Clin. N. Amer. 6:657, 1959.

Dunbar, H. F.: Mind and Body: Psychosomatic Medicine, p. 190, N. Y., Random House, 1949.

Elmer, E.: Children in Jeopardy: A Study of Abused Minors and Their Families, Pittsburgh, University of Pittsburgh Press, 1967.

Elmer, E., and Gregg, G.: Developmental characteristics of abused children, Pediatrics 40:596, 1967.

Goldman, L.: Prevention and treatment of eczema, Am. J. Nurs. 64:3, 114.

Helfer, R. E., and Kempe, C. H. (eds.): The Battered Child, Chicago, Univ. Chicago Press, 1968.

Holter, F. R., and Burgeon, C. F.: Psychologic considerations of the skin in childhood, Ped. Clin. N. Amer. 8:719, 1961.

Johnson, B., and Morse, H.: Injured children and their parents, Children 15:147, 1968.

Leonard, M., Rhymes, J., and Solnit, A.: Failure to thrive in infants. A family problem, Am. J. Dis. Child. 111:600, 1966.

Rosenthal, M. J.: Psychosomatic study of infant eczema, Pediatrics 10:581, 1952.

Stone, H. M.: Psychological factors in infantile eczema, Am. J. Nurs. 53:449, 1953.

Sussman, S.: Skin manifestations of the battered child syndrome, J. Pediat. 72:99, 1968.

Svoboda, E. H.: Wilms's tumor and neuroblastoma: the child under treatment, Am. J. Nurs. 68:532, 1968.

Urbach, F., and Jacobsen, C.: Atopic dermatitis, Ped. Clin. N. Amer. 3:597, 1956.

Whitmore, W. F., Jr.: Wilms's tumor and neuroblastoma, Am. J. Nurs. 68:527, 1968.

UNIT 4

The Toddler (1 to 3 Years) and the Pre-school Child (3 to 6 Years)

Of the years between birth and adolescence no period is so unsettled and tumultuous as that which marks the conversion from infancy to early childhood. Physical growth is erratic, and appetite is often capricious. The toddler acquires locomotion (both horizontal and vertical) which permits his rash enthusiasm to lead him into hazardous situations. Although the total mortality rate for the age period falls to less than one-fifth of the rate for infants of 1 to 12 months, and to less than one-sixteenth of the rate for newborns, accidents become the leading cause of death, a position that is maintained during the rest of childhood. The disorders discussed in this unit are not limited to the toddler and preschool age but have been selected because of their frequency or special significance during this period of life.

Psychologically, the toddler discovers himself as a person independent from his mother. Hypnotized by the power of this new identity, his sense of self becomes reinforced as he vacillates between following his own whims and pleasing his mother. His mother bears the brunt of his incessant struggle to become a self-directing person and at the same time to hold onto some of the pleasures which eased his mind of worries and doubts in the past. Without patience and a good sense of humor she may find this to be an age to be endured rather than enjoyed. But from this very important period of psychosocial development the toddler will emerge with the rudiments of social behavior as his world expands from the intimacy of his family to embrace the local neighborhood, the nursery school and kindergarten.

Children in this age period fall into two groups:

1. The toddler, between the 1st and the 3rd birthdays.

2. The preschool child, between the 3rd and the 6th birthdays.

The term "toddler" is an apt one and is commonly used to designate the individual in transition from baby to child.

"Preschool child" is used to describe the individual in the second portion of this age span, largely for lack of a better term. Although many children of this age are in some type of school, the intent is to designate the child who has not yet entered the first grade.

16

Growth, Development and Care of the Toddler and the Preschool Child

PHYSICAL GROWTH

As the baby embarks on his second year of life the rate of growth slackens, and his growth curves bend accordingly. The most impressive changes in his appearance are the alterations in body proportions which follow the rapid growth of his legs relative to his trunk, and which advance him toward the body shape of the older child. The assumption of the erect posture emphasizes this new look and makes it increasingly possible for the adults around him to regard him as a child instead of a baby.

Height

Growth in height continues to be the steadiest of the changes taking place. During the toddler age it is difficult to measure because of poor cooperation; the preschool child begins to understand and enjoy being measured. Average heights advance from 30 to 46 inches (75-118 cm.) during this 5-year span. Less than one-third of the children will deviate from the heights which are average for the age by more than 1½ to 2 inches (3½-4½ cm.). The difference between the two sexes is very slight.

The slowing rate of growth can be appreciated from the following schedule of average performance:

During his first 3 months the infant grows 4 inches or about 20 per cent.

In 3 months of the 2nd and 3rd years he grows 1 inch, about 3 per cent.

In 3 months of the 5th and 6th years he grows 0.6 inch, about 1½ per cent.

The rapid growth of the legs is seen in a comparison of the infant whose legs comprise 30 per cent of his total length and the 6-year-old whose legs contribute 45 per cent of his height.

The height reached on the second birthday is a fairly good indication of the eventual size of a given child. Girls in general grow to a little less than twice the 2-year height; boys to a little bit more.

Weight

Mothers are often concerned that toddlers are not gaining weight during the second year. This is due to a sharp decline in the normal rate of weight gain. The 7 oz. per week which is expected of the newborn drops to about 7 oz. a month for the toddler. The average baby starts his second year weighing just over 20 lbs. and ends it weighing just under 30 lbs. During some portions of the year it may be true that a toddler fails to gain, for many pause momentarily, particularly during the winter months, and then spurt to catch up. Their weight curves reflect a step-like rather than a smooth advance. Illness or psychological factors may prolong such periods of standstill. However, after the third birthday the gains are usually consistent, and the weight curve parallels the standard curves.

Average weights move from about 22½ to 48 lbs. (10-22 Kg.) during the toddler and preschool years. More than two-thirds of the toddlers weigh within 3 lbs. (1.3 Kg.) of the average for their ages. The variation among preschool children may be wider. Four to 8 lbs. (2-3½ Kg.) represents a reasonable range on either side of the average. Boys begin to weigh a little more than girls.

General Body Proportions

The toddler appears top heavy when he first begins to walk. His trunk is long, and his legs are short. The diapers accentuate the low hang of his buttocks, from which emerge stumpy legs often still bowed by the residual effects of his intrauterine posture. His head rides on a chest which has caught up to and passed it in circumference. The abdomen at first is poorly

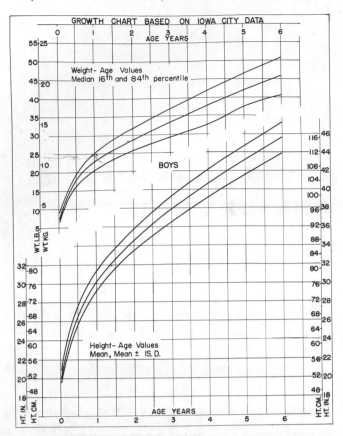

FIG. 16-1. Average height and weight of boys from 0 to 6 years of age.

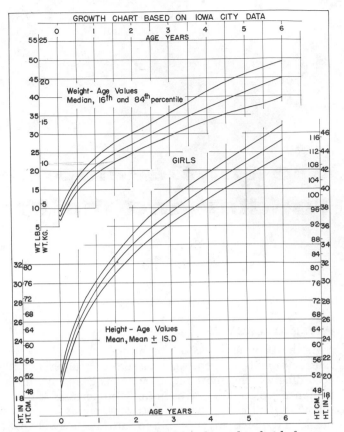

FIG. 16-2. Average height and weight of girls from 0 to 6 years of age.

guarded by muscle so that its contents bulge outward when the toddler sits or stands.

Growth during this period is faster in the legs than the trunk, and the infantile curves are straightened in the process. Because of a change in his fat-storing mechanism and an improvement in muscle tone, the toddler becomes less chubby as he replaces baby fat with solid muscle. His potbelly will gradually pull in so that by 4 to 5 years his abdomen will be flat, and the chest will be more prominent and better developed. The streamlining of his appearance gets an important boost when he is able to relinquish his diapers and wear less bulky underclothing.

The Head

The brain approaches its final size even at this early age; consequently the rapid growth of the head slows down suddenly. Whereas the head circumference increases by 4 to 5 inches (10-12 cm.) during the first year of life, it adds less than an inch during the second year and less than half an inch during the third year. The average circumference grows from 18½ to 20 inches (46.5-51 cm.) from the first to the sixth birthdays. Few children deviate by more than ½ inch from the average measurements. At the end of the sixth year the head has reached approximately 90 per cent of its final size.

Since further expansion of the skull is not needed, the suture lines begin to knit and the fontanel closes. Many small fontanels are closed before the age of 1 year; most of the large ones are replaced by bone at the age of 18 months. Delay in closure is a feature of disorders such as rickets, hypothyroidism and a few congenital abnormalities of bone.

The eruption of deciduous teeth which begins in the latter half of the first year proceeds to completion well before the third birthday. The usual order of eruption is the central and lateral incisors during the first year; the first molars which come in early during the second year; the cuspids which fill in between the incisors and the first molars during the latter half of the second year; and finally the second molars which appear during the first half of the third year. The final complement of 20 deciduous teeth remains unchanged until the permanent teeth begin to appear around the sixth birthday.

Other Changes

During the latter part of the second year the baby's skin changes from a delicate integument with high water content to a tougher more resistant epithelium. This is the age at which improvement in eczema is noted and the frequency of eruptions due to contact irritants declines.

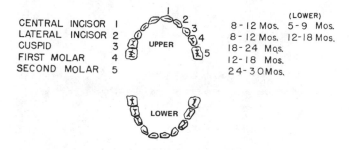

			(LOWER)	
CENTRAL INCISOR	1		8-12 Mos.	5-9 Mos.
LATERAL INCISOR	2	UPPER	8-12 Mos.	12-18 Mos.
CUSPID	3		18-24 Mos.	
FIRST MOLAR	4		12-18 Mos.	
SECOND MOLAR	5		24-30 Mos.	

Fig. 16-3. Time of eruption of deciduous teeth.

Maturation of the bones can be followed by roentgen examinations. Determination of the bone age in infancy is relatively crude because there are few significant centers of ossification which are normally anticipated. During the second and the third years, 25 to 30 new foci of ossification appear; in the preschool period an additional 15 or so can be expected. Girls generally have these evidences of maturity somewhat before their brothers.

The lymphatic tissue of the adenoids, tonsils and peripheral lymph nodes usually undergoes pronounced enlargement during this age period. In part this is due to stimulation by infections which the child is undergoing, and in part it appears to be a phenomenon of growth. By the end of the third year the adenoid tissue reaches its maximum size; subsequently it tends to decline in importance. The tonsils continue to grow until they reach their peak size at around 7 years of age and then start to diminish slowly.

The cellular constituents of the blood are approaching concentrations which are normal for the adult. However, the red blood cell counts remain below 4.5 million and the hemoglobin levels around 13 Gm. in most children of this age.

NUTRITION

Requirements

In amount and variety, the food required by the toddler for optimal nutrition differs little from that of the infant. The decline in his rate of growth is compensated by an increase in physical activity so that total caloric needs remain around 100 cals./Kg./day (45 cals./lb./day). Thus the average-sized toddler slowly increases his energy demands over the 2-year period from about 1,000 to 1,500 calories per day. The preschool child will need 1,400 to 1,800 calories per day. Within this the protein level should yield at least 3 Gm./Kg./day (about 30-50 Gm. for the daily total). The necessity for water diminishes perceptibly so that only 100 to 125 ml./Kg./day is necessary unless disease or hot weather is present. The total mineral and vitamin requirements do not change.

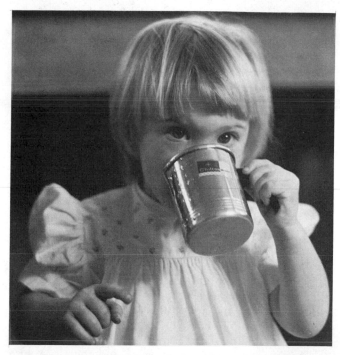

Fig. 16-4. With a growing sense of self and of autonomy, toddlers enjoy mastering the social amenities of mealtime rituals; nevertheless, their interest is often diverted toward other absorbing aspects of their environment. (Carol Baldwin)

Weaning to Deficient Diets

This is a critical period for toddlers reared in families living on deficient diets. Breast milk and many artificial formulas supply at least a basic minimum of nutriments throughout part of the first year. But when the child is weaned to a diet without animal milk or protein, he faces the risk of serious nutritional deficiency. Subsistence diets are composed almost exclusively of vegetable carbohydrates such as rice, potato, corn or yams. The protein content is low and the variety of amino acids is limited. Both B-complex and vitamin D are likely to be missing, and the intake of minerals such as calcium and iron is insufficient. A shift onto this type of diet may slow body growth almost to a standstill.

Psychological Factors

Even when economic factors yield an adequate supply of food, the toddler frequently decreases the quantity or variety of his food intake because of normal changes in emotional and intellectual development. Growing preoccupation with his own goals often brings the toddler into conflict with his mother's efforts to control his diet. He is likely to be faddish, demanding unlimited amounts of preferred food and rejecting unfamiliar foods. Some toddlers accept a well balanced diet, but many move more and more tenaciously toward a "white diet" which is composed

Talk to mother abt food abt weaning

of milk, sweets and starches and leaves them deficient in iron and vulnerable to anemia.

Because of field dependency (which will be discussed subsequently), the toddler is also fond of rituals at mealtime and often demands specific dishes, utensils and toys before he will accept food. With a growing sense of self and an urge toward independence, he will often reject help, selecting only preferred food. Unwillingness to become diverted for any length of time from an absorption in learning about his environment often complicates mealtime difficulties.

Mealtime strife can be avoided through anticipatory guidance. If the mother understands the child's innate impulses toward growth of self and independence she can encourage his explorations and support his learning and will be less anxious about his decreasing interest in food intake as his horizons become wider. Mothers should also be forewarned about declining appetite and accentuation of personal preferences so that their anxious overconcern does not precipitate a conflict of wills and accentuate the struggle over food. They should know that short periods of inadequate intake will usually be corrected when the toddler spontaneously changes his preferences and that it is wise to avoid forceful action to oppose the child's new assertiveness and independence.

Another important principle in dealing with capricious food acceptance is the conservation of appetite. Toddlers who are showing little desire for eggs, meat and vegetables should not be permitted to appease their appetites with carbohydrates or milk. These should not be proffered until the end of the meal. Sweets can profitably be dispensed with entirely. Milk should be limited to a maximum of a quart or less per day. Small portions of food are beneficial in that the toddler is not overwhelmed by feeding demands, but may request an additional portion. Vitamin supplements and sometimes iron preparations are helpful in ensuring adequate supplies of essentials.

Toddlers who reject all solid food and insist on milk from a bottle may be discouraged by progressively diluting the whole milk until hunger makes solid food more appealing. Occasionally it may be necessary to refuse demands for a bottle completely for a week or two until appetite for solid foods returns and interest in the bottle has decreased.

Beyond the third birthday, the strife and the rituals of mealtimes begin to abate unless the issue over food has become the habitual battleground for a conflict of wills between the mother and child. The child's appetite becomes more reasonable and the social aspects of eating take on new interest as the preschooler begins to enjoy the companionship of others at the table and becomes interested in imitating his parents' eating patterns. However, if mealtime is habitually unpleasant or unsociable, the example that the preschooler imitates will not further his attainment of cosmopolitan eating habits. When children of this

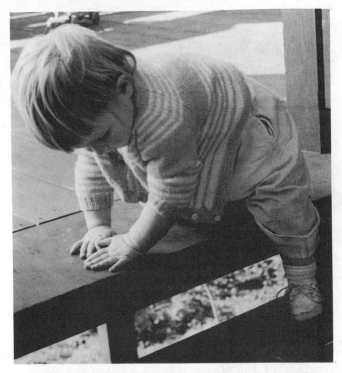

Fig. 16-5. Even though a toddler may not have achieved independent walking, stairs may pose no obstacle. (Carol Baldwin)

age period have meals at nursery or play school, it is not uncommon to hear that their eating habits at school are excellent even when the conflict over food continues at home.

NEUROMUSCULAR DEVELOPMENT

Continued interest in the factors which underlie development, including that of the neuromuscular system, is of significance in terms of the advisability of training technics to hasten motor skills. Complete answers are still not available as to the extent to which neuromuscular control and development are stimulated by inherent growth and maturational factors and the extent to which they are dependent on stimulation from the environment. Certainly there are enormous cultural differences in the beliefs regarding the effectiveness of training or stimulation in hastening neuromuscular control. It seems likely that some aspects of motor behavior are genetically determined, such as hand preferences which are related to cerebral dominance. Some sets of behaviors which occur in a sequential pattern, such as locomotion, seem to be dominated by neural growth and maturation, yet can be influenced by training. The conclusion now appears to be that the effects of experience and maturation are additive, and also that the effects of environmental stimulation will have different effects on very young children depending on their individual genetic endowment.

Keep milk till end of meal

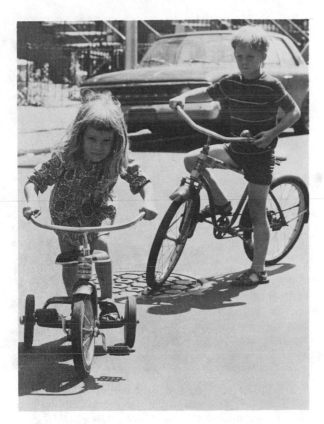

FIG. 16-6. Caught in the excitement of learning new motor skills, toddlers may need to be reminded of limitations to provide physical safety. (Carol Baldwin)

Locomotion

By the first birthday, a few babies have learned to walk unaided, but most acquire this skill during the first half of the second year. Infants who have not begun to walk alone by 21 months deserve special attention, for their lack of progress may signal their deprivation of environmental stimulation or may be an early sign of intellectual retardation due to other factors.

During the early stages, walking is normally accomplished on a broad base with feet that are often poorly positioned, toeing either in or out. The feet are commonly flat, and the infant has a tendency to turn his ankles inward. With practice and encouragement, balance is perfected so that he can take steps unaided, at first unsteadily and then with mounting assurance. The exact age at which toddlers acquire this skill varies in accordance with their fundamental disposition, the environmental stimulation and encouragement they have received from infancy and genetic factors affecting maturation of muscular skill. The trusting and enthusiastic child will attempt to master this skill as soon as he sees a prospect of success; a more cautious child may be able to walk quite well with minimal support before taking the plunge and

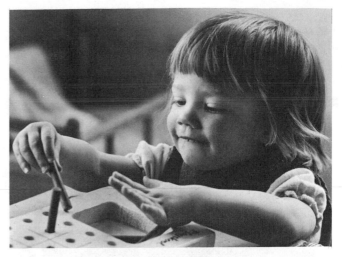

FIG. 16-7. With increasing age, eye-hand coordination improves. By age 3, most children are fairly accurate in placing objects where desired. (Carol Baldwin)

moving off from the security of a stationary object or his mother's hand. Most toddlers are running by 18 months of age and jumping by 2 years. During the third year the majority learn to balance on one foot and many will dance to music.

When the toddler first begins to walk, many mothers are concerned about the poor muscle tone of the legs and inefficient placement of the feet. They can be reassured that this is normal until children develop skill by practice and experience and the small muscles of the feet are better developed. This can be accelerated by allowing the child to go barefoot as much as possible and by fitting him with soft, pliable shoes when footgear is advisable. Too much corrected support denies him the opportunity to strengthen the muscles by exercise.

Some infants learn to crawl very efficiently and prefer to continue this mode of locomotion long into the second year. Climbing ability may also advance independently of walking. By about 15 months most are able to move up a flight of stairs and by 18 months to 2 years they are climbing onto chairs and other furniture, heading for ever more dangerous heights. Erect walking upstairs may be achieved before the age of 2; downstairs usually not before about 3.

By 12 to 18 months, the toddler has the muscular skill to satisfy his curiosity in exploring sinks, drawers and closets he could not reach before and by the age of 2 usually has the ability to open doors and run from his mother when approached. It is usually not until the latter part of the third year that he is able to manipulate a tricycle. By 4 years he can usually negotiate stairs without using the handrail, can walk backwards and hop on one foot. By 5 years of age, most children have learned to skip, to play in run-

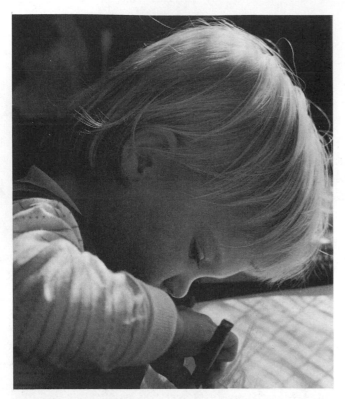

Fig. 16-8. Lacking the ability to move small muscles independently, the toddler uses his whole hand and arm to manipulate objects. (Carol Baldwin)

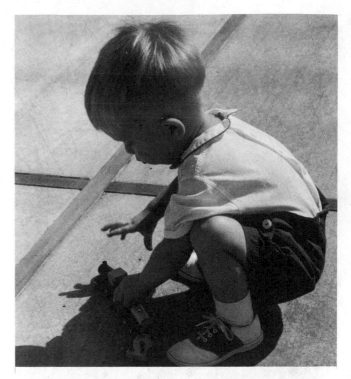

Fig. 16-9. Although at first the toddler engages in solitary play, toys enable him to initiate action and develop manual dexterity. (Carol Baldwin)

ning games, to jump rope, to jump off heights of several steps and perhaps are taking up roller skating.

Guidance. Freedom to explore, to satisfy curiosity about his expanding world and to develop skill in motor control during these early years promotes later self-confidence, creativity and intellectual curiosity, and prepares the child to compete favorably with others. If exploration and curiosity are not thwarted, but encouraged by providing opportunity for safe experience, progress in motor skill, social and intellectual capacity will be promoted. Children under 3 years of age need safeguards and adult watchfulness, however, in order to avoid accidents which not only constitute physical dangers, but may lead to a frustration of the drive to learn and to explore. Without limits, the toddler may also overextend himself to meet the continuous drive for mastery and to test his newly gained powers. Children over 3 years of age are usually more cautious regarding unfamiliar situations or equipment. Positive direction and encouragement will usually alleviate insecurity.

Abundant experience in exploration, in practice of motor skills, in following impulses to satisfy curiosity and in achieving a sense of mastery lay the foundation for all later physical, social and intellectual pursuits. Practice in learning muscle control is important to all children, and particularly boys, during the school years. The sense of freedom and encouragement to

seek answers through their own efforts will be important throughout life if young children are not inoculated by adult fears which frustrate their basic motivation to learn and achieve.

Manual Dexterity

Small muscle co-ordination also shows steady differentiation of motor responses similar to the development of large muscle control. As the child matures he progresses in ability to move muscles independently and becomes more able to make a single localized response. Movements also become more sharply articulated. The 10-month-old infant can usually probe with his index finger, place large objects one inside the other and throw them about. Skill with building begins with the use of two blocks and improves progressively until he can fashion towers of nine to ten blocks and begins to build bridges, houses, and the like by 3 years. At this age most children can also pour from a pitcher, string large beads, work simple puzzles and use paste. They can usually unbutton clothes, manipulate zippers successfully, put on shoes, wash their hands and brush their teeth after a fashion. By the age of 4, the child can generally cut out pictures and by 5, he can dress and undress himself and is in the process of learning to tie his shoes. Eye-hand co-ordination increases steadily until by 3 years of age most children are fairly accurate in hitting big pegs and within the next 2 years learn to utilize tools.

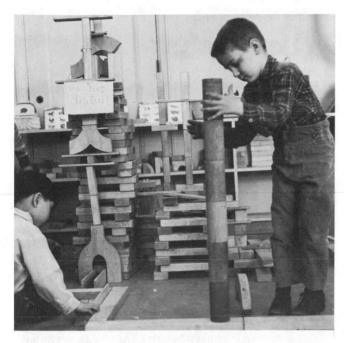

FIG. 16-10. Progress in the use of blocks develops rapidly between 1 and 6 years of age. Notice the challenge of the complexity in the structures which these children have erected. (Carol Baldwin)

This increasing co-ordination and articulation of small muscle movements is also seen in the manipulation of writing materials. Although the toddler can only make marks on paper, most 3-year-olds can imitate crosses and circles, and they glory in painting, using lines and masses of color. By the age of 4, children can usually copy a square and make a man with more than one part; by 5 the picture usually contains the main parts. Many children of this age

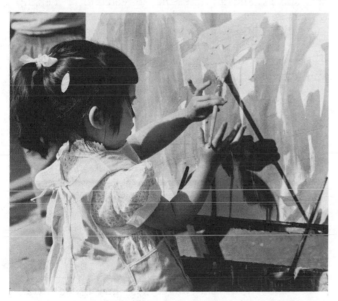

FIG. 16-11. Play also provides new avenues for expression of self and creativity. (Carol Baldwin)

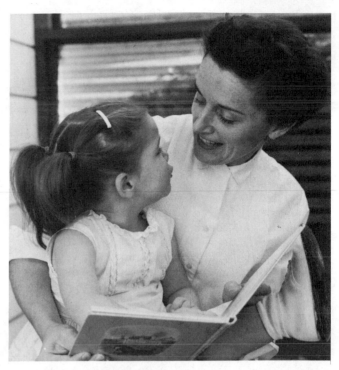

FIG. 16-12. Verbal communication with a child hastens language development and vocabulatory growth. (Carol Baldwin)

are also able to imitate triangles and show interest in copying letters.

The Purpose of Play. Play is the child's method of exploring his world, of testing new ideas and concepts, of venturing into the unknown, of testing reality and his own powers. Play permits the child to respond to challenge, to influence his environment, to initiate action and to observe the results. Through this medium, he acquires motor skills and manual dexterity, develops sensory and space perceptions and gains a beginning sense of mastery, confidence in his own powers and achievement and a positive self-image.

The toddler is intrigued by novelty and through play begins to learn problem solving. Although still unable to co-operate with peers, he uses play to translate his feelings, drives and fantasies into action and learns constructive ways to channel aggression and to handle frustration, fears and anxiety. As he progresses in age, play affords the opportunity to express imagination and creativity and to learn the delights and challenges of social relationships.

Supervision in the Use of Play Materials. Play equipment should be chosen with insight into the child's needs and with a view to providing motivation for learning and the expression of his emotions. Toys which help the child to develop concepts of size, color, shape, texture and relationships will aid in optimum intellectual progress. Objects which help the young child to build a concept of his own body, to distinguish people in his environment, to gain understanding of masculine and feminine roles, to come to terms with his feelings and to express aggressive feelings with acceptable actions foster maximum emotional development.

Low shelves or cupboard space with toys easily accessible facilitate self-directed activity. Property rights can also be learned through the experience of ownership and having his rights respected.

The toddler needs opportunity for free expression within the limits necessary to protect him, as well as other persons and his environment. Guidance should not be inhibitory to self directed activity; however, teaching in the use of equipment when the child indicates readiness, and limits in inappropriate use of equipment, are conducive to a sense of security and later social relationships. Adult interference in creative expression stifles further experimentation, self-confidence and the impulse to find solutions to the problems which prompted the selection of the particular activity.

Communication

Progress in language facility varies from one child to another as a result of individual characteristics, intensity of involvement in other phases of development or the demands for speech placed on the child. However, if speech fails to develop during the third year, evaluations should be done to determine the adequacy of hearing or intellectual capacity. Failure in speech development may also result from an inadequate relationship with the mother, in which he may suffer both from emotional deprivation and from lack of sufficient stimulation. In studying children who had been reared in orphanages without maternal care from birth to 4 years of age, Spitz* observed that 95 per cent of them had made no progress in learning to speak.

Preverbal Speech Development. From the time of birth, a child has the capacity to vocalize and to respond to sound. When the child's cries of discomfort bring his mother to his side, the rudiments of communication have been laid down. Most mothers soon distinguish the differential meaning of their children's vocalizations and this appropriate response becomes embedded in the child's experience.

Lewis† distinguishes three stages in the emergence of the discomfort cries and three in the emergence of the comfort sounds. At the outset, the discomfort sounds are vowel-like in quality. Later consonantal sounds begin to emerge and lastly, labial and dental consonants appear.

Through babbling or experimentation with sounds that are self-stimulating, self-reinforcing and pleasurable, the child acquires skill in vocalizing. He also evokes a response from his environment which is the

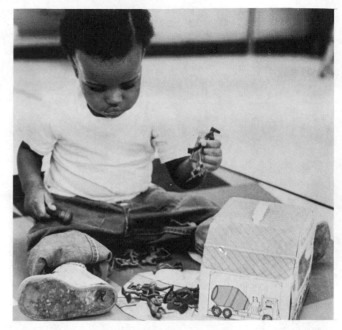

Fig. 16-13. Through endless play with toys the toddler learns how objects look and feel and eventually attaches names to them.

forerunner of verbal communication when mother and child are attuned to one another. Rudimentary imitation of sounds may be followed by a period in which imitation is in partial or complete abeyance, after which there is a vigorous rebirth of imitation.‡

When the child's imitation of sound approximates syllables or words, his parents' enthusiastic response creates a climate of approval which motivates him to repeat them and provides incentive to learning to communicate. He may watch his mothers' mouth as she speaks and imitate the movement of her lips, throat, gestures and facial expressions.

As the child learns to distinguish approving responses from those that manifest displeasure, he learns to associate meaning with what he hears and concomitantly to invest meaning into his own utterances.

The Development of Meaning. When the child evokes a response to his vocalization which corresponds to his intent, challenge and enthusiasm to understand and to speak is heightened. The first great landmark in understanding meaning of speech is evidenced by the appearance of the baby's specific action in response to the mother's specific words. This progress is highly complex and influenced greatly by the significance his mother holds for him and by the situation which evokes the affective response. A strong "no" from his mother arouses strong feelings, as does the "bye-bye" of parting.

The Growth of Language. The first pseudo-words,

---

* Spitz, Rene: Steps to maturity: what it means to grow up, *Child Study* 28:3, 1950-1951.
† Lewis, M. M.: Language, Thought and Personality in Infancy and Childhood, N.Y., Basic Books, Inc., 1963.

‡ Ibid., page 22.

or pattern of sounds with a consonant and one vowel, "ba," "za," etc., may have several meanings and refer to a number of objects. A "jargon" may then emerge, though in some children more than in others. At a particular point, a true word appears, and a large step is taken toward adult language! The first words are usually in response to an urgent need, whereas later words can be used to arouse feeling in another person. By 18 months of age, there is often quite reliable use of language with understanding of simple requests. The interaction between the child's growth of cognition on the one hand and linguistic development on the other, accelerates the growth of both processes simultaneously; each affecting the other. The reliable use of language also affects the process of perceiving the environment and aids in his growing ability in manipulating aspects of his expanding world.

The Development of Grammar. Within the second and third years, the toddler begins to learn to arrange words into meaningful assemblages. He learns that sequencing of words and the position of words in an assemblage marks something about the word's meaning.

In the beginning, the child is unable to discriminate parts of speech; but a rudimentary grammar appears as soon as words are joined together. This early grammar is not imitative of adult speech and the beginning sentences may sound odd to adults, e.g., "all gone sticky," or "more up."

Early speech and grammar are much reduced from grammatical adult speech; early speech seems almost telegraphic, and at the beginning is extremely egocentric. The young child does not communicate in the sense of waiting for answers; he does not take into account characteristics of his hearers, and early speech resembles a monologue. His speech is egocentric in that it relates to his own needs, desires and perceptions irrespective of those of the others in his environment.

Telegraphic speech reduces adult speech to nouns and words of action; the two-year-old, asked to repeat "I am tall," will state "My tall." It seems clear that there is a regularity in the reduction of adult speech. The young child cannot deal with six or seven sequential words and reduces the number into his own grammar. The result however, retains much of the meaning of the sentence, with the omissions of prepositions, tenses, and the like. The first sentences usually contain the subject, referent and action.

The young child may also have difficulty in dividing streams of speech which he hears into intelligible units. He must learn *segmentation,* or where one word ends and another begins. In the beginning he may hear them run together, such as "neckanears," and this is particularly evident if the heard material is too difficult for the child. Words such as "across the street," are originally organized in phrases, and one of the developmental tasks of this period is separation

of words for individual usage as building blocks for language.

Vocabulary Growth. By 2 years of age the average child has acquired a vocabulary of 100 or more words, and during the preschool years the comfortably adjusted child averages an increase of about 600 words a year. At 3 years of age, he is easily able to identify familiar objects in pictures and can retain and repeat about three numbers.

By 4 years speech has become a formidable weapon with which he boasts, exaggerates, threatens and distributes the family secrets about the neighborhood. He may acquire an imaginary playmate with whom he converses. He knows his age, can name one color and count to 4 or more. He will carry out commands more capably. By 5 years he is likely to be talking continually, and his understanding has progressed further so that he knows four colors, counts to 10, repeats fairly long sentences and describes pictures in detail. He is also showing some inquisitiveness about the meaning of words and is asking questions about the structure of the world around him.

Individual Differences in Language Development. Many factors are involved in the rate of acquisition of language, including the child's position in the family, his sex and his socioeconomic status. There are consistent sex differences, with girls more advanced than boys, although this difference usually disappears by middle childhood. Twins tend to be notably retarded in clear language development.

Children who develop in a crowded ghetto environment, or in institutional settings, are markedly retarded in acquisition of speech. This phenomenon tends to be related both to emotional and sensory deprivation in the institutionally raised child; whereas in the slum reared child, the retardation is related to lack of opportunity in learning well organized or "elaborated" language, in addition to probable sensory deprivation involving the entire cognitive structure. The closing off of intellectual curiosity and exploration, the limitations of opportunity in learning elaborated adult speech with the need for discriminating shades of meaning may be operative in both situations.

Understanding Limitations. During the period of language acquisition, limitations in understanding and in communicating verbally must be recognized. Directions must be given simply and accompanied by the act itself if they are to be fully understood. The young child often uses physical action in place of verbalization, and when emotionally aroused, he may be unable to express himself verbally and must resort to gestures in communicating his emotional state and needs. Lack of understanding of these limitations, or nonacceptance of cries of anger and fright increases the child's tension, feelings of helplessness and the problems with which he must cope.

When the young child is hospitalized, the nurse must be able to accept the ways he uses in expressing his feelings. The child not only needs this kind of understanding, but also requires help in controlling his body movements when this is necessary.

Support of Questions and Curiosity. Long before the child can speak, he demonstrates his curiosity by his quizzical facial expressions and investigative activity. Much of the toddler's behavior, which is often labeled "destructiveness," is actually a quest for knowledge. "What" questions usually come first in an effort to understand what he hears and sees: "What's zat?" "What is that man doing?" The three-year-old uses "when," "why," "where" and "how" questions: "Where's Mommy gone?" "When is shot time?" "Why can't I go home *now*?" "How are you going to fix that?"

Questions spring from a variety of needs and are usually asked after considerable pondering. They are a valuable source of information about the child's goals and worries and provide clues to the help he requires. The most obvious reason for questioning is to obtain information or to discover how things work or how they may be used. However, many more questions are posed in an effort to obtain relief from anxiety. Some questions are asked to find out the whereabouts of a beloved parent or to gain reassurance that he or she will return. Others reflect dread of a coming event or a wish to delay something that he is not quite ready to do or to have done for him.

A need for companionship is the purpose behind many other questions. Many adults use questions as a means of initiating a relationship with a child. Therefore, it is natural that children do likewise. The toddler cannot say, "I am lonely and miss my mother terribly. Please come and stay with me so I won't be frightened." But he can communicate his loneliness and need for support in questions like this: "What's your name?" "What are you doing?"

When questions are asked, the adult should pause, think and ask himself the following questions: "What is this child's problem?" "Is he afraid and if so of what?" "What else must I know to help him gain further understanding so that he can proceed with his play or get rid of his worry?" Too often the adult is too literal-minded and gives a quick answer without attempting to discover what really prompted the question or without waiting to see if his response resulted in greater relaxation for the child. There will be questions which are complicated or to which the answer is unknown. At such times it is best to acknowledge the difficulty or the impossibility of finding the answer. It will not result in loss of respect. The adult who responds to a child's question with, "I don't know, Skipper, but let's find out together," promotes an eager spirit of learning. Answering truthfully not only sustains the child's trust but also helps him to feel that he has the right to question further.

MENTAL DEVELOPMENT OF THE TODDLER

Although at the beginning of this period, the child

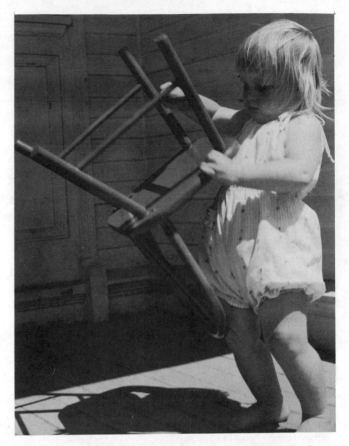

Fig. 16-14. Experimenting with objects and observing them from all angles facilitates concept formation and problem solving ability. (Carol Baldwin)

continues in the developmental phase which Piaget has termed the *sensory-motor* period, the changes and growth which take place in the child's ability to manipulate his world from the ages of 1 to 3 years are phenomenal. During these years, the development of language plays a tremendous role in the child's ability to conceptualize. It is during these years that active experimentation arises with elaboration of reality and the beginning of imitation and imagination. The child's ability to internalize images grows and he makes progress in the realms of causality, space and time.

New Constructions of Reality

During the first year of life, the infant perceived objects in his environment as extensions of himself and had great difficulty in distinguishing his inner from his outer world. However, by the middle of the second year, he is beginning to learn that objects have permanence; i.e., that they exist even though he cannot see them at the moment. Observation of the toddler demonstrates that he will search for an object that is hidden from his view. He is able to play "search games"; to follow a toy through several hiding places.

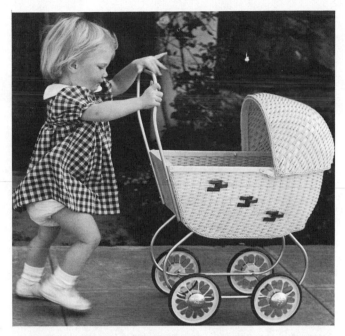

FIG. 16-15. The toddler's increasing ability to imitate behavior allows him to "play through" his experiences and to begin to understand adult roles. (Carol Baldwin)

The significance of this achievement lies in the fact that the object is now definitely seen as something apart from himself and subject to laws of space and time. It implies memory for relationships and the development of mental images. It also implies a dawning recognition of the fact that he is himself differentiated from his environment, thus allowing him to progress in his separation of himself from his mother and to begin establishing the concept of "I" and of autonomy.

Reality in Space, Time and Causality

With the acquisition of the concept of the permanence of objects, the toddler is simultaneously progressing in his sensitivity to differences in time, spatial arrangements and causality. Time becomes extended, both into the past and into the future as memory traces are laid down. Values of time are often identified with an immediate wish or with satisfaction for completed activity ("all done," etc.). Space begins to have meaning with the beginning primitive concepts of distance and allows the toddler to move toward objectivity; that is, that he also is an object moving through space.

Though the sense of time is still considerably circumscribed, the groundwork has been formed for the development of a sense of causality, in that there is a "beginning and an end," a "before and an after." The development of a mature and realistic sense of causality is a long and arduous developmental process which continues throughout childhood. Although the toddler is aware of cause and effect relationships, objective understanding of causal relationships is achieved as he moves further from the subjective or egocentric mode of thinking and increases his knowledge of the world about him. During this early stage of development, the young child still often confuses what he is feeling and thinking with objective reality. The "magical thinking" of the toddler is proverbial; he holds the belief that he can influence external objects or events through his own wishes and desires.

Role of Experimentation, Invention, Imitation and Imagination

With the child's growing ability to co-ordinate mental images, it becomes possible to experiment and invent; to anticipate possible outcomes. Where previously the toddler "discovered" ways of bringing toys and other objects within his field by groping, now he is able to experiment using various methods to attain his goals. This ability is assisted by the progression in development of motor co-ordination, which allows him to guide his movements in a sequence. He can search for new ways to solve problems, becomes excited with novelty and now has the ability to "invent" solutions to problems mentally rather than relying on blind trial and error. The enjoyment of pursuit of the novel can become all-absorbing.

With the growing ability to form mental images and with the acquisition of the concept of permanence of objects no longer in his visual field, imagination, make-believe and play become possible and pleasurable. Although in the beginning, play consists mostly of practice of motor activities not yet mastered and seems to have an aimless quality, yet there is a definite sense of intention and urgency. The toddler's imitative behavior is also deliberate and active and increasingly resembles the model. This imitation may be deferred; i.e., enacted when the model is no longer present, which allows for the beginning of the "work of play," wherein the child plays through complex events in his efforts to assimilate and understand them. With the organization of new skills, combinations appear and by the time the child is 3 years of age, he becomes able to neutralize his fear through play.

Role of Language in Mental Development

The *preconceptual* phase of development described by Piaget begins about the middle of the second year and lasts until the child is about 4 years of age. With the development of language, he becomes increasingly capable of mental symbols, or "symbolic functions." Conversely, when the child becomes capable of symbolic play, he also makes rapid strides in the acquisition of language. The first words mirror the *sensory-motor* stage, in that "use" is predominant: a chair is "to sit in," milk is "to drink." As imagery develops, the words increasingly become signs of actual objects and actions.

Within the second year, the toddler also becomes increasingly aware of the communication value of language. His incessant questions have been mentioned previously. Reasoning can also progress, though there remains gross distortion of reality. This reasoning can contain inference from the memory of previous events and thus also parallels developments in memory and in the sense of causality.

The rapid acquisition of language during this period influences the child's ability to organize and understand his environment and also profoundly affects his behavior. He is able to reconstruct past experiences and to anticipate future ones. Piaget* mentions three consequences of language development which are essential to further mental development:

(1) the possibility of verbal exchange with other persons which heralds the onset of the socialization of action; (2) the internalization of words, i.e., the appearance of thought itself, supported by internal language and a system of signs, (3) last and most important, the internalization of action as such which from now on, rather than being purely perceptual and motor as it has been heretofore, can represent itself intuitively by means of pictures and "mental experiments."

With the ability for thought, feelings and affect become more refined and the inner life can be communicated. Also, the child now has a new relationship with his parents and other meaningful adults who also can communicate more fully their thoughts and wishes, thus vastly enlarging the child's experience.

Global Organization of Thought

Toddlers and preschool children are proverbially ritualistic and sensitive to any change in their environment. The one-year-old may not recognize his parents in other clothes and the toddler may refuse his dinner if it is not served in the usual dish and in the usual place and manner.

Young children have great difficulty in distinguishing the essential from the nonessential. Experiences or events are known in terms of "qualities-of-the-whole" rather than in an articulated manner. The unaltered whole then is important in maintaining security and equilibrium since a situation seems to undergo a complete change, even if only minor alterations are made. Innovations are rejected because the child cannot yet grasp an experience or event as having numerous elements. Each element is as important as any other because all contribute to the situation totality. If any element is changed or left out, the entire experience is transformed from the one to which the child has become adjusted.

Such a view of "whole structures" contributes to the child's rigid traditionalism and makes him much more vulnerable to changes in his physical environment. When a toddler is hospitalized, he therefore not only loses the most meaningful person in his life, but the massive threat also includes the loss of the physical environment and the predictable sequence of events on which his security rests.

---

* Piaget, Jean: *Six Psychological Studies*, p. 17, N.Y., Random House, 1967.

PSYCHOSOCIAL DEVELOPMENT OF THE TODDLER

During this stage of development the child's major developmental task is the development of a sense of "I" or, as Erikson calls it, "a sense of autonomy." As previously discussed, this is based on the acquisition of the concept of the permanence of objects, of discrimination between his inner and outer worlds, and the idea of himself as a separate being with unique potentialities for gaining control over his body and his environment. Also implied is the need for direction which sustains the child's trust in himself and others and prevents the feelings of shame and doubt from becoming a part of his self-image.

Although this stage of development is generally said to encompass the period from 1 to 3 years, long before the end of the first year of life the child has already learned much through varieties of sensory stimulation. As memory traces are laid down, and through imitation and exploration, the baby develops

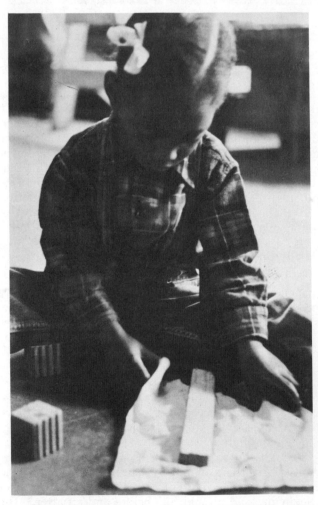

Fig. 16-16. Day after day this 3-year-old child wrapped and unwrapped a block in an attempt to gain intellectual control over her fear of separation. (Infant Welfare Society of Chicago)

new powers and his autonomy is expanded. During his first year, the baby began showing a wish for control; for instance, he wished to control his food at mealtime and was anything but passive when his mother placed him in a supine position for a change of clothing. There were times too, when he resisted cuddling and preferred solitary exploration. At such times, in many instances, the mother experiences the first pangs of "losing" her baby, and may be alarmed at the child's signs of wanting to govern himself. The mutuality of feeling which has existed between mother and child is threatened. However, no harm should befall either unless the mother holds on too tightly and does not allow her child the freedom he needs to develop his own way of asserting himself.

Strivings for Autonomy

A sense of trust encourages strivings for autonomy. When the baby's motor co-ordination and mental development become such that active exploration and experimentation become possible, his strivings to become a self-governing independent person become a predominant characteristic of his behavior. The infant who has developed trust in his environment during his first year has the impetus, motivation and courage to forge ahead, assert and test himself in the huge and exciting world he is discovering beyond and outside himself.

The toddler is a very egocentric, self-loving, uninhibited person who is deeply absorbed in his own importance and goals. He has discovered objects and himself, and since he cannot yet put himself in the place of another or understand the wishes and desires of others, he is very possessive. He says "mine" in words or gestures and holds toys away from any child who approaches him. If he wants the cookie the youngster beside him is munching contentedly, he snatches it and consumes it greedily since he is as yet mentally and emotionally unable to comprehend his contemporary's feelings.

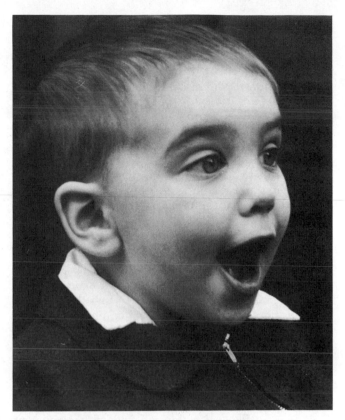

FIG. 16-18. The curious and the novel are of unending excitement to the toddler. (Carol Baldwin)

The toddler's interest in other children is exploratory and transient. He plays beside them (parallel play) but not *with* them, since true co-operation is not yet possible. His early speech during play is also egocentric and a little later may resemble a monologue, taking no consideration of his playmates' interests or answers. However, he curiously studies and explores them with the same consuming interest he displays for any novelty in his environment. At times he pushes, pokes, hits, bites and scratches without reference to the hurt he is inflicting since he does not himself feel pain. He is unable to comprehend the feelings and pain of another. He *enjoys* this activity without feelings of guilt, shame or pity since he still lacks controls within himself to check impulses that are striving for gratification. He has no inner standards (conscience) and his self-ideal is just being formed.

The toddler is consumed by his wishes. He demands without awareness that he cannot do or have everything he wants, nor does he realize that his impulsiveness can annoy others and endanger himself. In his quest for autonomy and mastery of his external world he experiments with abandon, ignoring his parents' cultural standards. He recognizes no limitations within himself, plunging ahead as if he were omnipotent, expecting no restrictions to stand in his way. When his wants are frustrated, he wails.

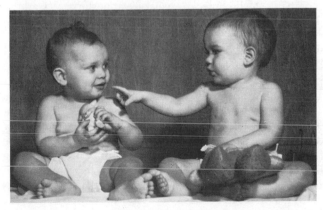

FIG. 16-17. Illustrating the toddler's mode of approaching children. Sometimes he tests cautiously, but more often his advances toward a new object are more aggressive. (Infant Welfare Society of Chicago)

Wishes are Frightening

Venturing into a bigger world on his own is exciting and challenging to the toddler, but it is also frightening and in many ways lonely. His insatiable wishes are new to him; being incapable of controlling them, he is uncertain of what they might lead him to do. Limits are reassuring and periodically he must go back to his mother as a safe base before exploring further. Even though he strives to do things by himself, there are times when he needs to be as clinging and dependent as a baby. Without his mother's understanding and readiness to comfort when the going gets rough, his adventurous spirit might fade before he finds himself.

Rituals and Security

Rituals are necessary and provide security. As mentioned in a previous section, toddlers experience the world in an unarticulated manner so that the unaltered whole is important to them in maintaining equilibrium. Minor alterations are unacceptable because they transform the entire experience.

The child also has a deep need for consistent routines since his inner world is so unpredictable and is rapidly changing. When daily routines provide sameness, he is able to predict them and therefore feels more in control of himself and his environment. Bedtime rituals are the most common, probably because the toddler is still engaged in managing separation from his mother. He is reluctant to relinquish her at bedtime because she has become all-powerful to him as a protector and he feels safest when she is nearby. Ritualistic behavior is at its peak at 2½ years. It is less pronounced at 4 years of age because of rapid strides in mental development which allow him to discriminate important elements in experience more readily and because his increased self-confidence makes adapting to changes in routine easier for him.

Bearable limits may need to be imposed on the toddler's self-devised rituals, if only for reasons of practicality. Understanding of the purpose which they hold for the child, however, and incorporation of rituals whenever possible into routines for care are supportive, both in the home and in the hospital. When the nurse realizes and respects the toddler's stage of intellectual development, she can find many ways of incorporating articles and routines from home which increase the child's security in dealing with a strange and frightening environment.

Co-operation vs. Self-Assertiveness

At first glance it appears as if the toddler has only three wishes: dominance, independence and acclaim. But there is a fourth wish—to please—and this leads to conflict. Evidence of this conflict appears when he is confronted with the restrictions and cultural standards that are necessary for an orderly society. His favorite word is "no" and he acts as if his independence

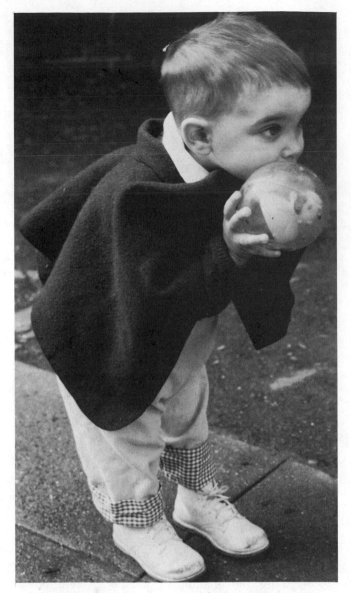

Fig. 16-19. The beginning of co-operative play initiates a lifetime of social relationships. (Carol Baldwin)

were contingent on his power to defy his elders. At the same time, however, he also needs and wants to please his mother; his security is dependent on her approval and the close emotional tie between them.

The toddler's "no" is an assertion of himself as an individual and of his new found powers of control over his environment. Resistance, nonetheless, may be frightening in that it has the potential for alienating him from the one person on whom he is most dependent. Even though resisting, he searches his mother's or nurse's face to determine her reactions. When threatened with disapproval he makes attempts to co-operate and thus to re-establish his security.

During convalescence Ted, age 16 months, had his meals in an armchair with a tray table over his lap. When he began to tip the tray, his nurse said, "Keep it still, Teddy."

In a flash, he repeated the act, watching the nurse out of the corner of his eye as he did so. Then, he clasped the tray to hold it still, lowered and raised his head and with coy flirtatiousness he said, "Hi," in an endearing tone of voice. His response to positive directives was not new; his mother had observed it often in the months preceding his admission to the hospital.

The toddler's wish to please his mother is a manifestation of intellectual and emotional growth. It demonstrates that he has made tremendous strides in separating himself from his environment and in recognizing his dependence on his mother. A background of satisfaction in his relationship with her has fostered the wish to give in return.

The child's wish to co-operate can be encouraged if statements are phrased with a bit of diplomacy. Questions such as "Do you want to take your nap now?" inevitably invite a flat "no." Such a question is also misleading, for it implies that the child is being given a choice. Not that the adult should invariably be dictative—it is good for the child if he is allowed to make decisions within his capabilities—but when specific action is desired, this must be clearly defined. "It's time to take your nap *now*. You can bring Teddy along and help me open your bed" gives the toddler direction in learning how to participate. An edict might be softened by a choice. "It's time to go to bed now. Do you want to bring Teddy or would you rather have your panda with you? I'll show you how to open your bed." (A child's adaptive capacities are strengthened when he is taught to do something for himself.) Some physical direction is usually necessary, too. Taking him by the hand is a subtle indication that all further resistance is futile, but it also provides the friendly warmth of a helping hand.

Dawdling

Dawdling is another characteristic of the toddler's behavior. Since he is in a transition period, not knowing fully how he should respond to his conflicting wishes, he has difficulty in making a choice. When his mother calls him, he does not know whether to come and please her or to stay and assert himself, so he tries to do both.

In such a situation the principle to follow is to help him to make the decision (taking advantage of his latent wish to co-operate) by firm but friendly—and immediate—action. He can be picked up with an affectionate hug, and forthwith taken where he is to go. Then quickly he should be helped to find pleasure in what is presently required of him. Once he learns that co-operation with his mother makes him feel more powerful and important, he will be able to make decisions more quickly and will cease to dawdle.

Temper Tantrums

It takes many reassuring experiences and much time for the child to learn to distinguish reality from fantasy. Early in this period the toddler imagines that his mother's love has been withdrawn each time she punishes him or disapproves of his behavior. He also hates with a vengeance when he is thwarted (he is still unable to delay gratification of his wants) and experiences the impulse to destroy the person who has opposed him.

Temper tantrums occur frequently with toddlers. His limited size and strength in comparison with adults, coupled with his many wants, makes for feelings of helplessness and hostility on occasion. These are easily aroused and vigorously expressed. However, once his destructive feelings are discharged, he quickly regains his composure and becomes loving again. (The word "hostility" refers to those feelings which have within them varying degrees of destructiveness and unfriendliness toward others.)

A toddler has difficulty in coping with severe frustration because he is as yet incapable of complex problem solving and is still verbally inept at expression of feeling. When experiencing intense emotion, he has difficulty in hearing his mother's words and she is too big and important to attack physically. He does not yet have the ability to control his emotions. Also, because of egocentrism (inability to see things from another's point of view) he believes his mother feels as destructive as he does. This is frightening since she is the person on whom he is dependent physically and emotionally. As a result of this complex of thoughts and feelings he expresses his conflicts in motor action by stamping and shrieking. Strong feelings cannot destroy if he gets them under his control, but first he must have help to conquer his fear of them. Then his mother can help him to find more fruitful and satisfying ways to expend his energy. However, a daily pattern of repeated outbursts should be cause for closer investigation. It may be that the child is under excessive pressure to adapt to too many restrictions at one time or is not being permitted to do those things he is capable of doing. Possibly, suitable play materials are not available, nor the space for tension-reducing exercise. It is also possible that he is not having sufficient outdoor activity, or is allowed to get overly tired and run down physically. Overdirection by an adult, such as commanding or intruding thoughtlessly on play without forewarning, can also lead to explosive resentment or stubborn balkiness.

It is during moments of anger that the toddler is most in need of his mother's support. This does not imply the satisfaction of every whim, for this would make him increasingly less tolerant of frustration and therefore more helpless. Calm acceptance of his need to express his helplessness and to master his fear of strong feelings is imperative. When the adult stands by to introduce an activity to restore his self-esteem when his fury abates, he will gradually learn that his fears are a product of his imagination and that he does not have to bear his scary feelings all alone.

Discipline

Discipline is guidance that helps the child to learn to understand and care for himself and to get along with others. Learning to get along with oneself and others is a difficult task, but one of the most important assets a child can acquire.

The first other people the child must learn to live with comfortably are his parents. In the first year of life this is comparatively simple, since his goals are less often in conflict with those of his mother. Now, while in the throes of finding himself and mastering a more complex external world, reconciling his own desires with those of his parents is often painful for everyone concerned.

Until the child establishes his own identity and achieves control from within, his mother (or her substitute) must act as his ego and conscience. She must teach him what is (1) appropriate in terms of his family's cultural standards, (2) safe from the standpoint of his physical or mental health, (3) suitable in relation to the comfort of others and the protection of his environment, and (4) within his power to accomplish.

The task of deciding on limits (controls) which are reasonable in terms of the child's current capacity to learn and at the same time serve to protect the rights of others is one of the knottiest problems that parents (and nurses, too) have to face. To know when to give a little and when to stand firm rests on understanding of the child and the particular problems he is dealing with at the moment; this calls for a great deal of self-examination on the part of the parent and an awareness of the values he deems important to transmit to his child.

This task is especially difficult for those parents who rebelled against the discipline that they had as children. To some parents the word "discipline" connotes punishment, intense frustration and withdrawal of love. Some of these parents strive to protect their children from the pain that they endured. Others cannot set limits, either because they are not aware of their tolerance for frustration, or because they fear their own aggression or that of their child. Others wait until they are provoked beyond endurance and then punish their children. This provides emotional release for them but serves only to frighten their offspring or to give them license to behave in the same way. Then there are those parents who have few resources within themselves to use in helping children to find constructive outlets for strong feelings because they have had meager help themselves. These parents need help to gain insight into the real meaning of discipline and its value for themselves as well as for their children.

Limits Lessen Worry and Fear. To establish permanent bonds with the world of reality and develop autonomy without residual feelings of shame and doubt the toddler must (1) have the steps toward maturation clearly defined for him; (2) know that his parents expect achievement; and (3) be taught practiced methods of expressing his impulses in socially approved ways. This help must include recognition of his efforts to co-operate and of his need for self-esteem. Shaming, threats and domination increase resistance or bring about unhealthy submission instead of mastery.

The child *wants* limits; he is frightened and worried without them. He feels loved when there is someone who cares enough to protect him from his own uncontrolled, primitive impulses. He wants to learn the ways of his world and remain secure in the affection of those adults on whom he is dependent and, eventually, of his playmates.

Limits are protective and provide security and freedom within bounds. When a child is certain that there is someone close by to protect him from destroying what he values the most, he can express himself freely. He does not have to worry lest he do something that will annoy others or injure his pride or his body.

Limits Gratify. Limits help the child to channel strong feelings into pleasure-giving activities. A child who is about to hurt another person or injure property can be removed from the situation or physically restricted temporarily. Then he should be redirected into an activity that will help him to learn as well as enable him to discharge his hostility. He can be given a hammering board, bean bags to throw or a puzzle to take apart and put back together again. A block-building project or washing doll clothes also can be beneficial.

Redirection communicates the adult's understanding of the child's feelings and also increases his independence. He feels less helpless and can venture farther away from his mother because he *feels* the controls that he has within himself.

Limits Help the Toddler to Find Himself and Grow. Through testing himself out against reasonable limits, the toddler learns what is safe and what is injurious for himself and his playmates. Eventually he accepts his limitations with more grace and is much less prone to tackle projects that are beyond his ability. He learns that heeding his mother's warnings often makes him more comfortable than when he has followed his own whims. He becomes more compliant to certain standards of his culture, and his conscience begins to form accordingly. He acquires many new skills which increase his powers to cope with the stress engendered by external restrictions.

Gradually, too, the child begins to grasp the idea that he both loves and hates persons who thwart him. Repeated experiences which reassure him that he is loved (even though his behavior may be deplorable on occasion) assists him in making peace with his ambivalent feelings and in seeing his parents in a more realistic light. As a result, his security with them becomes reaffirmed. At 3, the child is a more stable, comfortable person than he was at 2; he has become ready to broaden his horizons in the world outside his home.

Toilet Training

Acquiring Bowel Control. Training in the control of excretory functioning implies infinitely more than learning to use the toilet. The manner in which the child is taught control of body function influences the way he esteems himself and others, the manner in which he will assert himself, social relationships of giving and receiving, and his approach to new life situations. The physical, emotional and intellectual aspects of growth during this period of learning, as in others, are interdependent.

The fears, goals, mental functioning and conflicting wishes of the toddler also come into play throughout this experience. His behavior often reveals what he is unable to communicate verbally. If he receives understanding and time to adapt to the use of the toilet he will want to make sacrifices for his mother and will be able to gain control of his sphincter muscles without residual feelings of shame, self-doubt, hostility and/or fear.

A Shift of Interests

When weaning is over, the toddler's interest shifts to his anal area and to the products he excretes. He sees nothing shameful about urine and feces and is driven to explore them as a consequence of normal curiosity and the attempt to delineate the self from the not-self. He has not learned that they are wastes and inappropriate play materials or that the toilet is the socially approved place to deposit his excreta.

The impulse to explore and mess is natural and not shameful, but play with feces must be restricted, both because it is unsanitary and because of the emotion it arouses in others. The use of four safety pins to keep the toddler's diapers on snugly will prevent such play and protect him from disapproval.

The mother with insight into her youngster's need for gratification from smearing provides opportunities for play with sand, water, paste and eventually also with clay, mud and finger paint. This is known as *sublimation,* a psychological term which refers to the deflection of energy from primitive expression into pleasurable, creative and socially approved activity. (The mother is also helping her child to sublimate when she redirects aggression into constructive activity such as pounding or drawing.) Praise of the child's willingness to learn a new way to express his impulses is imperative in the development of the capacity to sublimate. It provides the satisfaction which makes giving up infantile pleasures worthwhile and provides incentive to further growth.

The outcome is different for the child whose mother condemns his impulse to smear and fails to help him find acceptable channels of expression. If his mother has made him feel that this impulse is something to be ashamed of, he will be forced to use energy in keeping it hidden from his consciousness (repressed). Rather than finding pleasure in the use of clay or paint, he will feel repelled and will express this in his behavior. The revulsion against messiness or untidiness may spread into other activities with the potential danger of overmeticulousness and unhappiness unless life is rigidly scheduled.

Readiness Essential for Active Participation and Mastery. After a period of unrestricted soiling, and from exploration which gives the toddler familiarity with his family's use of the toilet, he begins to demonstrate awareness of his need to defecate. This usually occurs when nervous system growth makes standing possible. The signals of awareness of a full rectum are individual. Some toddlers make grunting sounds or strain; others tug at their diapers, bring a diaper to their mothers or say some special word to communicate their readiness to learn. The mother's responsibility is to make known her expectations in a kind way and to expect functioning on the toilet only when he can co-operate. The toddler's reward comes from his mother's approbation and from his own pride in success. With this kind of help there is no deprivation that the child is unable to withstand. As a result his relationship with his mother becomes strengthened.

Acquiring Bladder Control. When physiologic functioning has progressed to the stage where a child's bladder can retain urine for a 2-hour period, he is usually ready to begin using the toilet or potty chair for urinating. Preceding this stage of development (15 to 18 months) the child will show awareness that he has already urinated. He will point to his wet panties or show the puddle he has made. This manifests intellectual growth and *merits commendation.* However, the fact that he notifies his mother that he is wet does not indicate that he has matured sufficiently to warn her *before* he urinates. This requires more growth and will come at a later date.

Training for bladder control also should be a gradual process. Again, the child's autonomy must be respected to prevent shame and self-doubt. When his bladder has held urine for a 2-hour period, the chances are that he will be able to co-operate. Then it is wise to put him on the toilet, let him know in simple words what is expected of him and maintain faith in his capacity to function as best he can. The child will respond to his mother's confidence in him and will welcome her approval. This recognition spurs him on to want to take the responsibility for his own toileting.

Gradually, during this period of development, the child will learn to desire cleanliness as his mother does. At times accidents are bound to occur, for they are a natural outcome of stress or absorption in play. The mother should not feel discouraged; to expect independence without occasional accidents before 3 years of age is to demand maturity which most children have not yet attained. Given a good relationship, it will come in time.

Acquiring Nighttime Control. After the child has attained daytime control, he becomes ready to succeed at night. Usually diapers are worn at night for some time after they are discarded in the daytime. When daytime control is achieved, nighttime use of diapers should be discontinued. Such a statement as the following indicates what is expected and gives the child the opportunity to take a further step toward maturity: "You don't need diapers at night anymore. Here are some new pajamas that you're ready for. Soon you won't need to urinate while you're asleep. You'll wake up when you need to use the potty. I'll leave it beside your bed and you can get up and use it all by yourself."

The child who has learned to use the toilet but is a bed-wetter at night may be taken up sometime between 10 P.M. and midnight and placed on the toilet, usually with some degree of success. This system may save wet beds, but the important lesson of unconscious control of the sphincter muscles of the bladder is not achieved. The child continues to urinate in his sleep. Moreover, it is difficult to waken a soundly sleeping child; if the attempt to do so creates antagonism or long periods of sleeplessness, it is wise to give up the routine. If there are neither physiologic abnormalities nor serious disturbances in the parent-child relationship, nighttime control eventually will take care of itself with the child's increased maturity and heightened awareness of the expectations of others. Usually this is achieved between 3½ and 4½ years of age.

Help Toward Independence. When a general pattern of care is followed, the child begins to help in his care. By the end of the first year, he begins to pull at the toe of his sock, to move his arms to get them into his clothing and to imitate the way his mother bathes him. In the second year he loves to help to put away his toys and, if hooks are within his reach, he will hang up his towel, toothbrush and clothes. He also appreciates arrangements which make it possible for him to do his own toileting.

When a child is ready to learn control of his bladder sphincters, he should be kept dry (so that he can become accustomed to dryness) and in training pants. The act of discarding diapers makes him feel grown-up, and training pants give him a way to help himself. A toilet chair is valued by the child because he can use it by himself without fear. When adult toilets are used, the noise of flushing must be anticipated for the child. When training is first begun, flushing away his productions distresses some toddlers. It is hard for them to comprehend why something their mothers have such interest in receiving in a specified way and they work so hard to give should be flushed away. From the child's frame of reference his productions are gifts, and he is usually delighted when they are received in the spirit in which they are given.

Regression. The child's current physical and emotional state influences his capacity for control. Illness produces regression because an ill child cannot concentrate on self-control. Intense feeling such as hostility and anxiety have a like effect. When a young child is separated from his mother, the source of his security, he regresses to babyish modes of behavior. The use of a bedpan and/or a urinal poses problems for many children unless their mothers have shown them how to use them. Sometimes children in the hospital are too frightened to make their needs known, or their appeals for assistance are not heard. When the child is admitted, the nurse should find out his way of signalling his need for toileting. She must be prepared to handle lapses with reassurance; if a child has gained self-control before entering the hospital, loss of control tends to heighten anxiety and lower self-esteem. Putting him back into diapers may be perceived as punishment or as belittlement; if it is absolutely necessary, it must be done in a way that preserves friendly relations with the child.

Regression may also occur if the young child is uncertain of his mother's love or is angry and unable to express it directly. This can happen when a new baby arrives in the family or when a favorite nurse appears to give more to another child than to himself. It can also happen when his mother's interest is diverted away from him to a new apartment or to herself during pregnancy.

Training During Hospitalization. If a child enters the hospital before he has acquired sphincter control, he will certainly not be ready for it during hospitalization unless a prolonged period of convalescence becomes necessary. (However, if a long hospital stay is required and the child is ready, such teaching should be instituted.) Ordinarily, unless the hospitalized child has his mother or one person who provides the daily periods of comfort which make it possible

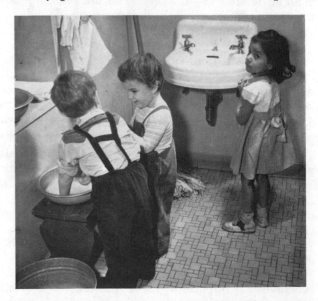

Fig. 16-20. Making self-care possible.

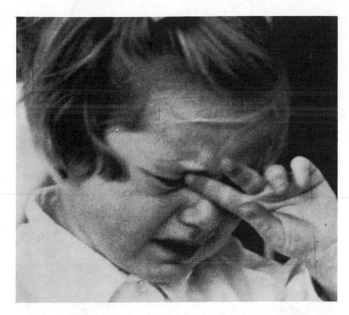

Fig. 16-21. Laura has lost her control. Her need for her mother is conscious and grief-laden. (Reproduced from the scientific film "A Two-Year-Old Goes to Hospital" by James Robertson)

for him to become attached to her, the advisability of toilet training is debatable, for he will have little incentive to make sacrifices. He may co-operate because he is afraid to do otherwise, but this is not the same thing as self-mastery.

The Child Who Retaliates by Soiling. A hospitalized child may soil to retaliate against the hostility which he feels is inflicted on him by his parents who placed him there. He may wet and soil his bed, urinate on the floor or call for the bedpan and then refuse to use it when it is received. (This habit may have resulted from a disturbed relationship with a parent.) The child may have had an accident during the acute phase of illness, or possibly at a time of loneliness. Instead of getting reassurance, he may have felt rejected or disappointed. Or he may have perceived that his soiling angered the nurse and gave him the attention that he needed. Through such experiences a child may become revengeful or may simply realize that he has acquired a weapon that he can use to punish or control the nurse.

Responding to the child's act with scolding, rejection or disgust intensifies the feelings which produced the asocial behavior. The only constructive approach is to seek out the underlying cause. The behavior is a symptom of emotional turmoil. Only as the child's emotional needs are discovered and met will he be able to find a nondefeating solution to his problem.

RESPONSES OF TODDLER TO LOSS OF MATERNAL CARE

The anxiety shown by young children on separation from their mothers has been the subject of widespread interest and investigation during the past 15 years.

Historically, awareness of psychological distress due to separation began with clinical studies reporting damage to institutionalized infants and to toddlers separated from their families during World War II. Subsequently, John Bowlby was enlisted by the World Health Organization to review the then current knowledge in the field. In a monograph published in 1952, he concluded that the mental health of the young child is dependent on experiencing a "warm, intimate and continuous relationship with his mother (or permanent mother-substitute) in which both find satisfaction and enjoyment."* Although focusing on the effects of long-term or permanent separation from the mother, he also reported that toddlers separated for shorter periods of time after a relationship with their mothers had been established, expressed distress resulting in somatic concomitants of anxiety, disturbances in activity, in severe regression, in behavioral deterioration and in withdrawal from reality with the potential for calamitous long-term aftereffects.

This report spurred research in the effects of maternal separation and led to the delineation of the many variables affecting the outcome of the experience, to the raising of questions relating to those children who escape severe reactions to separation and to the instigation of better controlled experimental studies of the separation phenomenon. Investigations were also launched as to the long-term or hidden effects of separation experiences, the results of multiple mothering in early childhood, the effects of psychological separations due to distortions or insufficiencies in the mother-child relationship and relating to conditions which influence the reversibility of the effects of separation.

In 1962, the World Health Organization reviewed the results of research in the intervening ten years and of the viewpoints and conclusions of various authorities in the field. From research reported in that monograph and from numerous studies completed in the past seven years, it seems clear that the young child's response to loss of mothering care is a complex process, influenced by multiple factors. These variables include: (1) the duration of the separation experience, (2) the number and effect of previous separation experiences, (3) the quality of the mother-child relationship prior to separation, (4) the quality of the preparation the child received for the experience, (5) the degree of concomitant stress or trauma; the timing of the separation experience in relation to developmental and environmental crises, (6) the events surrounding the actual separation or admission of the child to the hospital, (7) the meaning of the separation to the parents and their behavior and methods of dealing with this event, (8) the amount of contact with the parents during the separation, (9) the developmental level of the child; intellectual, phys-

* Bowlby, John: Maternal Care and Mental Health, World Health Organization, Geneva, 1952, p. 11.

ical and the level of ego strength; the child's capacity to relate to new adult figures, his ability to cope with anxiety through verbal communication or play, (10) inborn differences in responsiveness to the external environment or individual differences in vulnerability, (11) special environmental factors, such as the child's personal appeal, (12) the adequacy of the substitute mothering available to the child during the separation experience and the provision of supportive measures, (13) the manner in which the child is received by his parents following hospitalization and subsequent events.

Findings of studies agree that separation anxiety in the toddler becomes a crucial factor during hospitalization at the developmental point at which the child has made strides in differentiating himself from his environment and object relationships have been established. (This does not eliminate the possibility of grave damage due to depriving experiences during the first 7 months of life.) Several studies have concurred in suggesting that the critical period during which children are most susceptible to damage by hospitalization extends from 7 months to 7 years, with the most vulnerable period being 7 months to 3 years.

Although many questions remain unanswered, and much research is still needed to provide a sound base for nursing intervention, it seems clear that separation from the mother during this period should not be undertaken without serious reflection as to its necessity. When unavoidable, a single separation experience need not have lasting or irreversible consequences if the child is offered a major substitute maternal figure and if the separation does not lead to other deprivation experiences. However, *prolonged* deprivation of the young child of both maternal care and sensory stimulation *may* have grave and far reaching effects on intellectual, social and emotional development.

Clinical and experimental studies have determined that the effects of loss of mothering care can be mitigated through determined and planned efforts on the part of professional personnel during the separation of the young child from his parents, home and familiar surroundings. Branstetter found that when substitute mothering was provided for children aged 14 to 36 months and hospitalized for nonacute illness, the response of the children indicated substantially less anxiety than has been reported in studies where such care was not available. She suggests that much of the anxiety of the separated youngster may be due to need deprivation or to the lack of mothering care.*

Other factors which influence the child's reaction, such as feelings of helplessness, increased dependency, threats to body integrity, loss of self-esteem and autonomy, feelings of guilt and specific anxieties re-

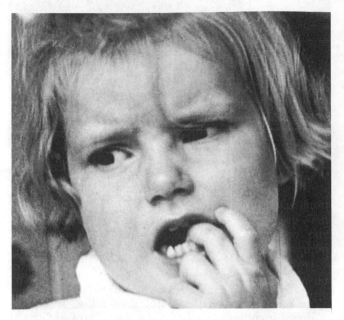

Fig. 16-22. Unfamiliar sights and sounds increase the young child's distress. Laura puts her finger in her mouth and scratches at her face to get relief from tension. (Reproduced from the scientific film "A Two-Year-Old Goes to Hospital" by James Robertson)

lated to developmental stages and conflicts (fear of mutilation, etc.) and specific deprivation due to hospital routines can also be reduced through the introduction of specific nursing measures.

Observation in a pediatric ward indicates that a toddler who has had a continuously rewarding relationship with his mother reacts violently when separated from her. Such toddlers indicate the feeling of tremendous loss and react with anger, fear, grief and revenge. On the other hand, children who have been denied such wholesome maternal relationships react more blandly to separation from their normal environment.

Robertson† observed children undergoing separation experiences between one and four years of age, in more or less depriving institutional settings. Three phases of responses to separation were observed in the process of defending themselves against loss and of "settling in" to the hospital environment. In describing the three phases—*protest, despair* and *denial*—Robertson pointed out that each phase merged into the next; none is sharply demarcated from the others. Thus, some children will be in a state of transition between two phases.

Heinicke and Westheimer‡ also found that young children react immediately to separation with protest in a desperate attempt to recapture the parents. Panic-like crying, longing and intense aggression were ex-

* Branstetter, Ellamae: The young child's response to hospitalization: separation anxiety or lack of mothering care? Am. J. Pub. Health 59:92, 1969.

† Robertson, James: Young Children in Hospitals, New York, Basic Books, Inc., 1958.
‡ Heinicke, C., and Westheimer, I.: Brief Separations, N. Y., Internat. Univ. Press, 1965.

pressed particularly in relation to the mother. These investigators felt that the loss of the parents was the crucial factor in the immediate response to separation of the children they observed.

After the initial response to separation, the children in this study directed psychic energy toward retrieving the lost relationship through defensively retreating to an earlier phase of development. Regression was seen in the children's ego functions with avoidance and withdrawal from adults in the new environment. A sense of despair also seemed to pervade the behavior of these children.

Resignation and cheerfulness appeared to mark the point at which the subjects adapted to separation through the denial of their need for their parents. Affect in relation to the parents was repressed along with increasing involvement with the environment.

The Phase of Protest. This initial phase may last for a few hours or may extend over several days depending on the child's energy and the quality of his hospital care. His longing for his mother and his grief are expressed through violent crying and intense aggression. Unless he is desperately ill, he will watch for his mother unceasingly except when he sleeps from sheer exhaustion. He uses all his energy and powers in attempts to recapture his mother, through extreme motor activity and through intense cries of "I want Mummy." On previous occasions she has always come when he needed her and he expects her to do so again.

The sense of being punished through abandonment by the parents is often expressed along with the fear of further punishment to come and the loss of self-esteem in a pervading feeling of "badness." Nurses and other adults may be consistently rejected, along with food and offers of physical comfort or bodily care. Physical aggression and hostility may be directed to all people and objects within reach.

For several additional reasons the toddler's need for his mother has now become more urgent than ever before. He is in a strange world without the objects and routines which have previously provided security and equilibrium. His need for love and stimulation have been denied to him and he sees and hears things which are frightening and threatening to his body integrity. He is terrified of complete desertion and in conflict regarding his anger at his mother whom he loves and for whom he is longing. Because of his egocentrism, he feels she is also angry with him and this increases his feelings of worthlessness and sense of insecurity. The child under 3 years of age lives in the here and now. The concept of time has not been fully attained so that when his mother is out of reach, she no longer exists for him.

He is also terrified by his own internal feelings of helplessness, and his newly gained sense of control and of autonomy is threatened. Simultaneously, he may also be experiencing unpleasant new body sensations which arise from disease. Like all people who are ill he longs for the old comforts that he knows his mother could provide and distrusts the strangers in this new environment. Finally, he may be seething with anger at admission procedures, which frightened him and made him uncomfortable and fearful of what may happen next.

The Phase of Despair. The second phase is one of increasing hopelessness characterized by subdued moans, a perpetually sad countenance and declining activity. Many toddlers try to comfort themselves by activities such as thumb-sucking, masturbation, head-banging, body-rocking, nose-picking, face-scratching or fingering their lips or a lock of hair. Others sit tightly clutching a toy or a blanket which serves as a link with home. The toddler's need and longing for his mother are still conscious. He may curl himself up in the fetal position or hide in a blanket, but he keeps constant vigil—not only for his mother but also to protect himself from danger.

During this phase the toddler makes few or no demands on his environment. He is anorexic, listless and withdrawn. The cessation of crying and overt protest does *not* mean that he has recovered from his loss. Careful study of his behavior proves otherwise. He is in a state of deep mourning and is suffering with an intensity which only one who has experienced it can imagine.

While in this phase, the child may no longer resist the nurse's approach as frantically as he did previously and may accept her ministrations without protest. At the same time, however, regression to an earlier stage of development may be seen in loss of sphincter control, in reduced verbal communication and in passivity.

The arrival of the toddler's mother during this phase precipitates a torrent of tears, and often signs of distrust and expressions of anger toward her. At points during the visit the child may reject his mother, acting as if he had to retaliate in kind for what she had done to him. He may turn his back on her or appeal to his nurse or attendant to take him out of her arms. But when he is returned to his mother he clings more anxiously than before. He does not understand why he is in the hospital or why his mother has failed him during his most urgent need. His piteous cries on her arrival and departure may make his mother dread to return and tempt her to stay away because she considers her visits detrimental to his welfare. The mother who has reacted with guilt to her child's illness often interprets his protests as rebukes. Taking flight from the ward may give the mother temporary relief from stress, but it neither relieves her guilt nor decreases her child's hostility toward her.

When liberal visiting hours were first introduced into pediatric units, many hospital personnel viewed them as detrimental to the adjustment of the children. Today, however, it is generally recognized that parental visiting is therapeutic to both children and parents. It allows suppressed feelings to come to the surface, helps to prove to the child that his mother

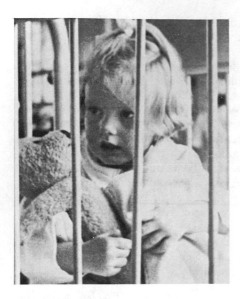

Fig. 16-23. Laura sits quietly clutching her teddy bear and "blanket baby" which her mother left with her when she left the hospital. She does not cry or demand attention. She is in the phase of despair. (Reproduced from the scientific film "A Two - Year - Old Goes to Hospital" by James Robertson)

is neither abandoning nor punishing him, and provides periods of essential comfort. Perhaps even more important is the fact that unrestricted visiting lessens the probability that the child will progress into the next stage of "hospitalism"—*denial*. Today sympathetic hospital personnel are helping parents to understand the reasons why children react as they do when they visit and offering them personal assistance in coping with their own distress. Support of this nature usually gives them strength to minister to their child and thus also relieves their own discomfort as well.

Some children who are in the hospital for short stays never enter the stage of despair but continue active protest until they are discharged. Others pass rapidly or slowly through this stage into one in which the mental suffering is eased temporarily by denial of the need for their mothers.

The Phase of Denial. The third phase is often erroneously interpreted as recovery. The child seems to have "settled in," to regain cheerfulness and to show more active interest in the ward. He no longer frequently calls for his mother, his appetite becomes improved and he makes overtures toward nurses and other adults.

This resignation, however, is an indication that he has defended himself against grief and pain through repressing the image of and all feelings for his mother. Continuous confrontation of the painful facts and of his hostility is no longer bearable and through the use of this psychological operation he becomes free to accept care from the nurses and attendants about him. Such a mechanism, however, requires much psychic energy.

Now, when visited by his mother, he may appear indifferent to her and behave as though he preferred her gifts to her presence. This lack of responsiveness is very painful for mothers who long to fulfill the maternal role. For the child however, it has become necessary to repress his intense longing and need in

order to keep his hostile and destructive feelings in check. Unless his mother is helped to see beneath this mask, their estrangement can only increase.

When hospitalization is prolonged, the child may fail to discover a person to whom he can attach himself for any length of time. If he finds someone he learns to trust and depend on and then loses her, the pain of the original loss is re-experienced. If this happens repeatedly (as it readily may in institutions) he will in time avoid involvement with and commitment to anyone because reactivation of the painful results of separation is too much to bear. He may deny all need for mothering and instead of investing his love and trust in others, he will confer it on himself and value material possessions more highly than any exchange of affection.

The Immediate Aftereffects. Children in this age period who have experienced short, painful periods of separation may show various behavioral changes when reunited with their families. They may show a lack of affect or resist physical closeness with their mothers because of the danger of losing control of aggressive and hostile impulses. On the other hand, they may regress to more infantile behavior, cling to their mothers and resist even a momentary separation from her in the fear that she may again disappear or continually test her responsiveness to their call. Intense need for affection and reassurance may be expressed in an acutely anxious manner. When the mother also feels anger at the child's "rejection" of her during hospitalization, re-establishment of the mutually rewarding relationship may be delayed. Conversely, mothers who have insight into their child's behavior and who can respond with extra babying and love allow the child gradually to express more directly his intense longing and anger and thus restore his trust and security. In order to prepare the mother adequately, the nurse should point out to her that such behavior is predictable.

If separation from the mother has been prolonged, the continuity of the mother-child relationship may be interrupted and a threat to its re-establishment posed when the child returns home. The child's response to reunion with his mother will depend on the experiences he has undergone, the defenses he has built to cope with his anxiety and the reception he receives. If subsequent events reinforce his loss of trust, self-esteem and independence, his potential for optimal psychosocial development may be threatened.

Emotional Support in Minimizing Anxiety

During the Phase of Protest. During this phase attention must be directed toward maintaining the child's emotional tie to his mother. His protest, crying and rejecting attitudes should be recognized as a healthy fright response to overwhelming anxiety. They are constructive and serve a useful purpose by decreasing tension and providing a measure of control over his environment and feelings of helplessness.

Through expression of aggression and hostility, the child has a greater capacity for responding favorably to his mother when she arrives.

Even when the therapeutic value of protest is understood, the child's behavior is difficult for the nurse to tolerate because it interferes with her ability to give both physical treatments and emotional comfort. It is frustrating to feel unable to satisfy a distressed child. Since the nurse is not familiar with his rituals for comfort, her care seems to add to his confusion rather than lessen it. The inexperienced nurse may readily conclude that her patient is rejecting her as a person and may feel angry and hurt. She may also fear that other children in the ward react in similar fashion and that her nursing colleagues draw the conclusion that she is ineffectual. The nurse may feel compelled to silence the child either through such lame and feeble reassurance as "Don't cry" or by trying to divert his attention from his main preoccupation. Neither will be effective. If the nurse looks back to her own childhood, she may remember that her parents did not condone free and uninhibited expression of distress and realize why she tends to suppress it in others.

If the nurse resists the temptation to withdraw and instead stays close by, the child feels accepted and not quite so helpless or deserted. Gradually, as he expresses himself, his tension is reduced and he becomes less hostile and more able to accept the ministrations of the nurse. With good nursing care he will feel protected and less frustrated by the lack of direct care from his mother; thus it will help to preserve the mother-child bond. On the other hand, if the nurse withdraws her support, his hostility will increase, as will his fear that his feelings are responsible for the separation. Then his hostility can easily become converted into self-hate and feelings of unworthiness. The following paragraphs describe the behavior of a child in the stage of protest. Two of the nurse's aims were: to help the child to regain her trust in and need for her mother and to sustain her will to protest.

Liza, age 14 months, had had a 5-day stay in another hospital during which her mother visited her for an hour daily. On Liza's return home, her mother, Mrs. Gee, observed that she was "nervous and jumped at every sound and acted as if she were afraid she was going to be left alone again." Mrs. Gee also reported that Liza had rarely been allowed to cry, had always been rocked to sleep, and was totally unaccustomed to strangers before her first hospitalization. She had repeatedly been entertained by adults and by her 2½-year-old sister rather than encouraged to develop her own resources to cope with frustration through self-directed play. The child was seriously ill and required intramuscular drug therapy and immobilization for intravenous fluid therapy (Salmonella organisms were found in her stool during her second hospitalization).

After a week at home, Liza was readmitted to a hospital with recurrence of severe diarrhea, vomiting, dehydration and a temperature of 39.5° C. Mrs. Gee slept on a cot in Liza's room during the first night of hospitalization. Then she decided to have her mother, Mrs. Jones, stay with Liza at night. This arrangement was continued until Liza's condition improved and she began to sleep through the night. Liza's parents visited for varying periods of time during the day and sometimes also in the evening when they brought Mrs. Jones to the hospital for the night.

When Liza was first observed on the morning after admission, she was alone and restrained on her back, a position she did not ordinarily use for sleeping. Her shrieks were piercing but not constant, for periodically she used her one loosely restrained arm to push a pacifier in and out of her mouth. Her skin and mucous membranes were pale and dry, she had deep circles under her eyes, and her hair fell over her puckered brow. Vomiting, which had occurred five times since admission, ceased soon after the fluid began to drip into a vein in her arm.

During the physician's examination Liza's protests grew louder. When the nurse moved closer to the crib to make it possible for the child to study her before receiving care, Liza focused her eyes on the nurse's masked face for a moment, seeming to look through her rather than at her. During the next 10 minutes, Liza occasionally turned toward the nurse again, but more often her eyes rested on the doorway. Her intermittent howl and sucking continued except during one short nap period. When the leg restraints were unpinned to permit some tensional outlet through kicking, she struggled persistently to roll over onto her abdomen.

A bath did not soothe Liza; instead, it increased the restlessness and made her wail more loudly. Petting did not comfort her either. She acted as if she would have rolled away from the nurse if her restraints had not prevented it. Wondering whether her presence was aggravating, the nurse moved to a spot where she could not be seen. The crying lessened. As the nurse moved back into view, Liza tossed her rattle away. The nurse returned it to her in order to communicate acceptance of the child's aggression and with the hope that she could use it again for a tensional outlet. She also spoke to Liza, not because she expected Liza to understand her words, but because the night nurse had reported that she showed the greatest degree of relaxation during periods when her mother talked to her. "Throw it again Liza. You miss your mommy and feel miserable. You'll feel better when your mommy comes back."

In an effort to assure Liza that comfort would be provided even during periods when she was angriest, the nurse applied firm pressure on her abdomen and against her back. The gesture helped Liza to relax. For the next half-hour she dozed fitfully, waking at every sound from the corridor, and then falling asleep. On awakening, her protests continued but grew fainter as the nurse changed her diaper and took her temperature. Because Liza seemed comforted by this care and from the sound of the nurse's voice, the nurse again tested Liza's response to fondling. This time Liza did not pull away, but her complaining and sucking continued until her mother reappeared. Occasionally Liza diverted herself by pulling tissues from a box or fingering a toy, but these activities were less satisfying than crying.

While fondling Liza, Mrs. Gee said, "Now you'll sleep because I'm here." She turned to the nurse and said, "She didn't have a *real* pain—only a pain in her heart." Then the nurse supported Mrs. Gee's awareness of Liza's need for her and took note of the way she comforted her baby. She remained close by, not only because she surmised that Mrs. Gee needed assistance in caring for her sick baby, but also to help Liza to see her as an extension of her mother rather than as a substitute. While Liza slept, Mrs. Gee talked about Liza's birth, the home routines of care, the child's illness and her feeling of guilt over having pressed Liza to take fluids which she could not tolerate.

During the few short intervals when the intravenous fluids were temporarily discontinued it was possible to accede to Liza's demands to be held. At these times the child alternated between relaxation on her mother's or the nurse's shoulder and pushing away from their bodies with angry howlings, indicating ambivalence of feeling. Several times when Mrs. Gee succeeded in helping Liza to relax in her arms she said, "I don't know if you know it, but this is a heavenly comfort for me." The nurse knew what she meant, for she, too, had often been distressed by Liza's punishing behavior. However, the nurse knew the value of using herself as a target for Liza's hostility.

A week later when oral fluids were begun, Liza's hostility was reflected in her response to nourishment. She wailed, spat and sometimes vomited. For a few days it seemed as if her destructive feelings would prevent her from taking nourishment. She could not sustain sucking on the nipple because her need to complain prevented it. Had she not opened her mouth occasionally to receive drops of Nutramigen, feeding would have been a completely discouraging process. During one of the feeding sessions Liza pulled aggressively at the threads of a frayed bed pad, and it was noticed that the child complained less frequently as she opened her mouth for food and showed some interest in it. From then on, an abdominal pad or a Kleenex which she could pull apart was placed within convenient reach. Her resistance at mealtimes lessened and finally vanished when her diet was increased and she was able to use her hands to feed herself bananas and cereal. At this time the diarrhea had ceased and she was beginning to make some progress in overcoming her fear of separation at nap time.

The task of helping Liza to overcome her fear of going to sleep on her bed was begun when intravenous therapy was discontinued. She was held and rocked a great deal then because she demanded it and because it helped her to regain trust. Efforts to keep her from awakening while being transferred from the nurse's shoulder to the bed were of no avail. She awakened and clung tenaciously, showing signs of panic. Not until Liza's behavior proved that she was becoming attached to her nurse did the latter attempt to hold her firmly in her accustomed sleeping position when she was tired. The first time the nurse used this method to help Liza grow through adaptation to frustration, she rebelled violently. Simultaneously, however, she clutched her cuddly doll and relaxed when she learned that the nurse trusted her capacity to withstand this amount of frustration.

The nurse stayed close by to prevent fear of separation when Liza first awakened. Soon Liza's fear of nap time vanished. She began to lay her head down when tired, put herself into her favorite sleeping position when placed on the bed, and after cuddling her doll for a while she was able to go off to sleep without being sung to or held. The nurse discovered that the act of raising the crib-side, which formerly awakened the child, now did not disturb her.

During the Phase of Despair. Despair sets in more quickly when the child has been taught to inhibit his feelings: that a display of anger is "bad" and punishable by physical means or withdrawal of love. Under such circumstances he must defend himself from his fear of the consequences of his hostility by withdrawing and becoming depressed.

The depressed toddler frequently expresses in his behavior his belief that both the "abandonment" which he is undergoing and treatment procedures are punishment for prior wrongdoing. He may be convinced that his illness and subsequent events are due to disobedience or defiance of his mother. The toddler has an immature concept of causality—of cause and effect—and often sees no relationship between his illness and efforts designed to assist recovery. Furthermore, he is in the stage of moral development when he believes that punishment is always justified; i.e., if he is punished, he believes he has done something to deserve such treatment. Such feelings underlie children's responses of "I be sorry, I be good" when nurses approach them to give injections or perform other painful procedures. When asked why they are in the hospital, some children will say, "I naughty," or "I bad."

The sense of worthlessness engendered by these feelings deepen depression and withdrawal from others. Such retreat is also heightened by his egocentrism. He is very bound to his own perceptions and believes that the intention of others is as hostile toward him as he himself feels. Unconsciously some children want punishment. If they feel anxious about some actual or imagined prior misdeed or their own anger, they will welcome painful treatment as punishment which relieves guilt.

Withdrawal from the environment may also be partially due to the young child's inability to shut out stimuli, or selectively to ignore massive sensory input as adults are capable of doing. The strange surroundings, the high level of unfamiliar noise, the sheer number of strangers who approach his bed may be overwhelming for the toddler and necessitate physical retreat beneath his covers. In addition, because he experiences his environment as a whole and none of the objects or routines surrounding him now are familiar, his insecurity is intense.

The goal of nursing care is to facilitate the overt communication of hostility, to encourage social interaction and to reassure the child that he is loved even though he may feel hatred toward those who want to help and comfort him.

The depressed child appears to be unresponsive to his environment and unwilling to develop any relationships with others. Underlying his passivity is the expectation of punishment which makes him suspicious of anyone who approaches him. Initially, the only sort of relationship such a child may be able to endure is to have a nurse sit passively beside him.

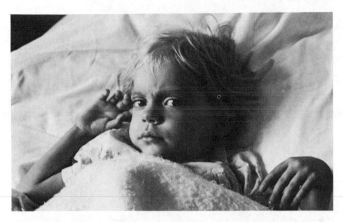

Fig. 16-24. The young child, separated from her mother, is suspicious of people until a meaningful relationship with her nurse is established. Note the lack of trust in her expression, which may be misinterpreted as rejection by the inexperienced nurse. (John Gorman)

This conveys to the child that the nurse cares for him personally despite his feelings of hostility and rejection.

At first the depressed child may reject the nurse completely and turn his back on her attempts to render physical care. By not retaliating or withdrawing herself, the nurse conveys to the child that she knows, understands and accepts his feelings of anger and fear, his right to withdraw, and his sense of helplessness and insecurity. She also communicates to him that despite his feelings she is available to him and ready to help as soon as he can accept it.

When the child responds to treatment as if it were punishment, the nurse should ask herself: "I wonder what Tim thinks he did that makes him scared." If the child cannot express his supposed misdeeds in words, something like the following communicates understanding: "Sometimes children think injections are given to punish them. They aren't given for that reason, Tim. They are given to make you well. When you're better you'll go home again."

The child's security can be strengthened through familiar objects and routines of his life at home. Often a particular dish may be important to the toddler's sense of the completeness of the mealtime experience or a well known blanket to the bedtime routine. Talking with the mother may provide much information which could be utilized in relieving the total strangeness of this new world for her child and alleviate her sense of guilt and helplessness. In addition, the loved and familiar object or routine provides a vital link to home and mother and thus maintains hope.

In raising the child's feeble self-esteem it is particularly important to watch for any indication of his renewed interest in a human relationship. Even a slight effort on his part to co-operate is sufficient. The nurse can take advantage of this to prevent him from feeling that he is a total failure as a person.

When a depressed child has continuity of under-standing care, he will eventually muster up courage to test the nurse's tolerance for aggression. At such times the nurse not only must show him that his aggressiveness is welcomed, but she also must remain close by to protect him from overly violent expressions of rage. If it boils up too rapidly, he may become afraid and retire again into his shell. By setting limits the nurse can prevent the child from destroying property and reassure him that he will be protected against himself on occasion. With such safeguards he can use play as an outlet for his hostility. The following illustrates the need for limits.

Tim was in acute despair, showing no interest in the toys beside him. During the early part of his mother's visit he lay silently with his back turned toward her. When the nurse called his mother out of the room, Tim grabbed two tinker-toy sticks and broke them into bits. Then he looked frightened, pulled the blanket up over his head and seemed far away in his own world when the nurse peeked under the covers in an effort to comfort him.

When Tim's mother left him, he lost control of himself. This frightened him and he had to withdraw once more. Tim eventually gained courage to play, but his initial attempts were cautious and without spontaneity. Only when Tim discovered that the nurse stopped him whenever his aggression began to get out of bounds was he able to play with abandon. On one occasion when Tim was about to hurl a block through the window the nurse said, "No, Tim, I'll not let you do that." The nurse rolled a laundry hamper to the bedside and said, "Throw them here just as hard as you want to. It won't hurt anything." When Tim used finger paint and was tempted to smear indiscriminately, the nurse restricted him, pointing out the area where it could be used without damage to property.

When the child is able to express his anger and discovers that the illness is no fault of his own, his feelings of despair subside and are replaced with hope. He has more energy to play actively; he begins to eat; he demands less attention after a period of clinging and possessiveness; and he begins to resist that which he formerly accepted passively. *This is progress; it indicates that he has taken steps to come to terms with his hostility.*

The following example illustrates another despairing child's behavior and how she was helped to overcome fear of her own aggression.

Ann, a Negro child, was 3 years old when she was brought from the South for repair of exstrophy of the bladder. She had never been away from home before and now found herself surrounded by a multitude of strange people and brand new experiences. Her malformed body was the object of many examinations and demonstrations. She had numerous treatments which were painful and restricting. After a 12-hour period of protest she complied submissively and showed no overt response to pain or restraints and no curiosity about the unknown.

The day following her operation Ann was silent and withdrawn. She never whimpered when the dressings were changed or needles inserted. She seemed oblivious to the nurse who was in constant attendance each morning. On the third day after the operation her doctor inserted a drain after probing the wound. Pain and anger were stronger than her controls. She shrieked: "No more. I hate you. Get out of here." Simultaneously she grabbed the physician's hand. Ann's face was contorted with terror.

Instead of being punished Ann received immediate understanding and praise. The nurse looked at Ann, smiled acceptingly, and said, "It hurts terribly when the doctor puts that thing in your tummy. I'm glad you told us how you felt." As she talked, the nurse stroked Ann's hand. Ann looked up at the nurse and nestled the hand into hers. It was the first time Ann had made any contact with her. (Previously the nurse had held her hand and stroked her head, but Ann's hand had remained limp. And her eyes never met the nurse's.)

Ann's nurse worked to demonstrate that her interest would not be withdrawn because of tempestuousness. A bond was established between them. From then on Ann dared to fight. She resisted treatment. Temper tantrums appeared. These expressions of feeling were encouraged because her nurse knew that bottled-up hostility would retard physical and emotional progress. Gradually Ann's despair lifted. She began to play and eat and became interested in all the activities of the ward.

Ann's mother, Mrs. Burr, was helped by a social worker to understand her daughter's aggressiveness. Since Ann's birth she had suffered from guilt over Ann's abnormality. Ann's behavior after admission increased this guilt to such a point that the mother stopped visiting. After receiving help Mrs. Burr returned to the ward, where she was encouraged to participate in her daughter's care. The nurse stayed close by to support Mrs. Burr when Ann's hostility was directed at her. At first this happened rarely, since Ann directed her hostility mainly at the nurse (because she felt safer in doing so). This provided an opportunity to demonstrate to Mrs. Burr that anger was not objectionable to the nurse, and thus Mrs. Burr was able to learn by example how to help her child to manage her aggressive feelings.

During the Phase of Denial. The prevention of this phase of "hospitalism" is far easier than the cure. Once the defense has been acquired, every means possible should be taken to re-establish the child's trust in people. Because he seems to have no preferences among those who care for him, the nurse may conclude that it is not important whether the child is served by one nurse or many. Yet, it is vitally important. Unless care is delegated to one nurse, the ways in which he can accept care may never be discovered and used to restore his trust in people, to encourage him to dare to make his wants known, to express his anger, and to face his longings for his mother. If the nurse can accept his initial rejection of her overtures of kindliness, fear of his own helplessness and anger will begin to diminish.

The paragraphs which follow describe the behavior of a boy who used denial to cope with stress.

Bill was 4 years old when he came into the hospital with leukemia. He sat in a chair hour after hour, his mind far away. A nurse, attempting to establish a relationship with him, told him she wanted to play with him. When she sat down beside him, he yelled, "Get out of here. I don't want you here. I want to be by myself." The nurse felt humiliated. (For a moment she doubted her adequacy in dealing with children and wanted to leave, but instead she reasoned: "Bill does not know me, so how could he dislike me? He does not know whether I am a good nurse or a poor one. If I go he'll never know I want to help him and I'll never discover whether my instructor's theories are valid or not. If I wait maybe I'll find a way to help him.") She tried again: "Bill, I want to stay with you and take care of you." Bill shouted at her again to go away. It was evident that the nurse's offer of help disquieted Bill. Why? For the next few moments the nurse pondered the question as she sat silently beside him.

During the remainder of the morning the nurse acceded to Bill's commands, but, at the same time, she made herself available to him. She placed him in the doorway where he could see her sitting at the desk and said, "Bill, I'm going to be at the desk. When you need something, call me. I'll hear you." But Bill never called her. He sat watching but did not seem to see what was going on about him. After lunch he condescended to let the nurse put him to bed. He was reluctant to go, though his pallor had increased from fatigue and a meager intake of food. When the nurse offered to read him a story, he shrieked again: "Get out of here! I don't want you in my room." Distressed by what she thought to be failure on her part, the nurse sought the instructor's help although all she really wanted at the moment was to have a change in assignment. Fortunately for her sake, and Bill's, too, the wish was not granted. Instead she was given an opportunity to express her helplessness and through this incident learned to understand Bill's behavior and something of how mothers feel when rejected by their children—a valuable experience for any nurse.

The next morning Bill's resistance to the nurse was equally pronounced, but now she knew how to discover the purpose that it was serving him. The nurse remarked, "I wonder why you don't want me to stay with you?" His response was revealing: "Do you know why? It's because you make me lonesome. That's why. Get out." The nurse said: "You want your mommy here. You need her so much and she can't be here because the hospital only lets mothers come after your resting time. That's the way all children feel." Bill's response, was filled with longing: "My mommy is the *goodest* mommy there is." Then his feelings broke through. He cried piteously, but at that moment he was able to accept comfort in the arms of the nurse. It was the beginning of a relationship which eventually led to acceptance of her care.

PSYCHOSOCIAL DEVELOPMENT OF THE PRESCHOOL CHILD (3 to 6 Years)

During this period of the child's life there is marked intellectual, social and emotional growth, in the course of which he seeks to consolidate a sense of autonomy and independence, to acquire initiative and to discover what kind of person he is to become. Since babyhood he has been learning to do the things that

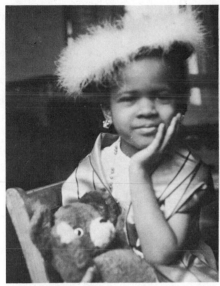 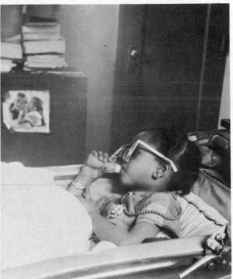

Fig. 16-25. (*Left*) This preschooler spent hours of her time in the nursery school dressed up in lady's clothing including high-heeled slippers. (*Right*) Sometimes in her hours of therapy with a psychiatric social worker she regressed and used a bottle to get some of the oral satisfactions that she had missed as a baby. However, she was not able to let herself regress until she had acquired greater maturity "as a lady" through identification with her woman therapist and through play in the nursery school. Even then regression was never massive. In those moments when she played at being a baby again she had bedecked herself with jewelry and held her purse against her body. Within the purse were treasured possessions—glasses, compact, lipstick and an odd assortment of jewelry. Her behavior showed the conflict between her wish to be a baby and her wish to be grown up. This conflict exists to some degree in all children, but usually the wish to grow up is much stronger than the wish to remain a child. (Infant Welfare Society of Chicago)

his parents do; their behavior, their mannerisms of speech and other characteristics. In psychological terms he has *identified* himself with both of them. When he has achieved separation from his mother, and a sense of himself as a person, his heightened love and admiration for his parents intensify his wish to be like them. Early in this period, however, signs of sexual identification begin to appear; that is, the boy concentrates on becoming like his father and the girl expends more energy in modeling herself in the image of her mother.

Hitherto, despite the father's influence, the mother, as the most consistent caretaker, was the most important person in the child's life—his protector and teacher. Now, in this period, the father's importance in shaping the personality of both the boy and the girl becomes magnified.

Increased mental growth contributes to extension of abilities and to character formation during this period. The elaboration of language improves communication between parents and child, gives the child better control of himself and of his impulses and deepens his concept of reality. As a baby and a toddler the child was dominated by striving for immediate satisfaction of his wants and impulses; in psychological terms he was governed by the *pleasure principle*. Now, however, with a background of satisfaction and with growth of his mental powers, he becomes less dependent on the immediate satisfaction of bodily needs.

He becomes increasingly able to postpone gratification because he knows that if he waits he will have greater pleasure in the future. He gains not only parental approval but also the satisfaction of knowing that he is behaving and feeling more like a grown-up. With such learning he has begun to function on what

is called the *reality principle;* in other words, the action that he takes toward the gratification of wishes is increasingly influenced by his awareness of objective conditions. During this stage the child's ego (the "I" of his personality) becomes strengthened. At the same time, mainly through parental influence, he develops a super-ego (conscience) which becomes an integral part of his personality structure. Thus he takes a long stride toward the achievement of responsibility.

Growth in locomotor power broadens the child's contact with a larger world of people, things and deeds. It stimulates his imagination, his curiosity and his drive to communicate verbally. The growth of his imagination is a new source of power and pleasure, but it has its dark side in that it can harbor fear to a more profound depth. Heightened curiosity increases his drive to learn more about himself, his world and his relationships with his parents, brothers and sisters (siblings) and playmates (peers). His strivings toward understanding and self-mastery draw heavily on his aggressive energy and include "the intrusion into other bodies by physical attack; the intrusion into others' ears and minds by aggressive talking; the intrusion into space by vigorous locomotion; the intrusion into the unknown by consuming curiosity."[*]

The preschooler's zest for living is probably more intense than the toddler's because his goals have expanded. He is self-activated; he has the capacity to love apart from himself; and he is secure enough to test his wings not only within his family circle but also in relationships with children and adults outside his home.

---

[*] Erikson, E. H.: Growth and crises of the "healthy" personality, reprint *from* Problems of Infancy and Childhood, p. 54, New York, Josiah Macy Jr. Foundation, 1950.

However, not all is smooth sailing during this period. Like all developmental periods it has its crisis or core problem which in this period can be summarized as initiative versus guilt. This problem centers around the child's changing relationship with his parents. There will be times when the preschooler basks in the glories of his successes, but there will also be moments when he is bitterly disappointed and enmeshed in worries concerning the integrity of his highly prized body and the new-found self contained within it. And there will also be periods in which he is deeply troubled by his changed and conflicting feelings toward his parents.

How the child handles this crisis will determine his feelings about himself as a boy or a girl and will influence the quality of his relationships with both sexes throughout his lifetime. To use and exploit his initiative without incurring a long-range guilt, the preschooler needs wise counseling from his parents and other adults. He must be taught some finer distinctions between fact and fancy. Thus he will be able to win certain important victories over himself and become a fit candidate for the demanding new world of school.

INTELLECTUAL DEVELOPMENT IN THE PRESCHOOL CHILD

With the increasing capacity to venture outside the home and with the heightened ability to communicate verbally, mental powers develop rapidly during the years between 3 and 6, for knowledge arises and becomes organized as the child interacts with his environment. The development of language also assists the child in overcoming the pull of his visual perceptions and thus to advance in the elaboration of reality.

Stages of Development. Throughout the age range of the toddler and the preschool period, the young child is in the *preoperational subperiod* as described by Piaget and at the beginning of the preschool period remains in the *preconceptual phase* (2-4 years). He is capable of distinguishing between the symbol or verbal label of an object and the actual object itself, an ability which forms the basis for logical thought. He devotes a great deal of time to imitation and symbolic play and as his memory span increases, he becomes able to plan future actions and to anticipate their possible consequences.

During this period, the child is still very rigid and is unable to see a situation from the viewpoint of another. He has great difficulty in disentangling an object from its background, a problem which has been termed *field dependency* and contributes to his need for sameness and routine. Time and additional experience are needed before he will be able to shut out unneeded stimuli and to discard unessential things from the total environment.

Until the age of about 4, the young child is also very bound to a single perception or one dimension of an object. Grouping of objects is usually carried out on the basis of one selected characteristic. The conspicuous, striking characteristics of objects automatically force them into one group. Thus blocks may be sorted by color or by form but never both. The child cannot take into account more than one characteristic at a time, a limitation which leads him to rejection of other important features and thus distorts reasoning. At this age, the young child is also unable to change his grasp of a situation to another one and thus is unable to change his image once it has been formed or to see an event from several points of view. His perception has become "set"; he conceptualizes on a single salient feature of his environment. Things are only what they appear to be. What a child of this age sees he takes on face value and accepts. Thus mothers and nurses must be aware that children of this age will make interpretations of situations which may be far different from their own.

From the age of 3 and often earlier, the questions a child asks become sprinkled with "why." "Why are you taking this road," "Why am I sick?" Children in this developmental stage wish to know both the cause and the purpose of all action, for to them nothing happens fortuitously or by chance. All events and objects must exist for human beings and have been created according to an established plan. The young child believes that there must be a reason for everything and therefore is troubled by the purpose of many events. His egocentricity is apparent in that all situations have a relationship to himself. Children in hospitals are thus perplexed and troubled by the many fearful occurrences which surround them.

From the age of 4 through 6 years, the child is in the stage of mental development which Piaget has termed the *intuitive phase*. He has progressed to the point where he uses numerous concepts although he is still unable to define them except through their usage; e.g., "a chair is to sit on." In this way, action and manipulation are still important to him in understanding his world. In order to comprehend an object, he must handle it, feel its texture and explore its surface. Nurses who have understanding of this developmental level of thinking in the child can help him to overcome fear of unfamiliar equipment, prepare him for what he will encounter in surgery, and other hospital departments to which he may be taken, by allowing him to handle and play with similar equipment.

The child's increased attention span, level of interest and ability to communicate and interact with his environment facilitate rapid acquisition of concepts and knowledge. As he meets contradictions or gaps in previous knowledge, he now has the capacity to cope with his problem, to experiment and to alter his previous mental constructs. He is still dominated by his sense perceptions in making judgments, nor does he feel it necessary to justify his reasoning, but he now has the new ability to see relationships and similarities and to compare objects or events. He also has the beginning ability to use numbers and to recognize quantities of things. He is increasingly capable of addressing himself to a specific task and to apply adapted intelligence to it.

At the end of this period, the rigidity of the toddler and the preschool child begins to lessen and he can be more flexible in his routine without disturbance to his equilibrium. With the growth of his mental abilities, affective life is also influenced, as he can now compare himself with others and thus begins to form a self-evaluation. With heightened interaction with others, he is also building a hierarchy of interpersonal values and acquiring the rudiments of moral knowledge and judgment.

Causal Relationships and Reasoning. The egocentrism of the young child, in which a lack of differentiation between himself and the outside world is seen, also influences the child's perception of cause and effect. The external world is linked with the ego and its needs and shares many of the characteristics which he senses within himself, i.e., awareness, intention, and the like. Reality becomes more objective as the child progresses in dissociating his responses from his environment.

Under the age of 4, children frequently establish a causal relationship between any two events that are contiguous in space or in time, contributing to magical thinking. Thus the color of an object may explain its floating, or the need for sleep may bring on darkness.

Egocentrism, or a centering within the self, may also be seen in the young child's conception of reality as a world that is organized in terms of human activity. For instance, the sun moves to provide warmth to people in other countries and dreams exist in order to punish children.

Young children may also hold man or God responsible for all objects or events and can thus interpret accident or illness as a deliberate design in retribution for their misdeeds. The child may also attribute life and consciousness to objects in his environment which make them capable of responding with the child's emotions. In this way, awe-provoking equipment may in itself harbor hostile intent.

For a long period, the concepts of necessity and chance remain alien to the child. The inevitability of death, the necessity for hospitalization are difficult for him to grasp. Conjunctions of motivation such as "because" and "since" are seldom employed by young children and therefore their inferences of happenings during illness may be grossly distorted from the adult's point of view.

PROGRESS IN EMOTIONAL DEVELOPMENT DURING PRESCHOOL PERIOD

With parental support, through relationships with children and adults and through successful coping and mastery of developmental and environmental problems, the child's ego grows and becomes strengthened. The interdependency in all spheres of development is again demonstrated in that with the increase of mental and physical powers, the ego is assisted in its function of testing reality. Intelligence and reason play a large part in the development and maturing of the capacities of the ego and the ego operates through the use of intellectual powers. Here also the role of experience is all important; it is through interaction with and exploration of the environment that the child learns to master reality.

Role of Identification

Although there are some differences of opinion related to the concept of identification, there is consensus that the preschool child is motivated to resemble the parent of the same sex, particularly if that parent is rewarding or perceived as powerful and salient. He may come to resemble not only what the parent is, but what the parent wishes the child to become. This process of identification is also strengthened if each parent approves of the other as a model for their children.

The process of identification is facilitated by the child's need for relief from anxiety, by his dependency and by his awareness that his parents expect compliance to cultural standards of behavior and sex role identity. It is also furthered by the acquisition of attributes or skills defining masculine and feminine behavior, by perceiving that others regard him as possessing a particular sex role, by experiencing of the model as nurturent and as being in command of desired goals, such as power or love from others. The child must also perceive objective signs of similarity between himself and his model. Gender role is also influenced through differential treatment of the boy or girl from birth, so that the child learns throughout childhood the behavior and mannerisms which are expected of sex role identity in a particular culture. For instance, dependency in girls is more rewarded in our culture than it is in boys. Finally physical factors, including sex hormones, may exert subtle effects on brain activity and behavior which influence the development of sex differences and sex identity.

Through identification, or the taking on of a "whole pattern," parental standards and ideals become internalized in the child's character so that he is no longer as dependent on his parents to regulate his behavior as he was formerly. Conscience formation, or development of the "super-ego," is the result of a constellation of factors including resolution of the primary identification with the mother, cognitive development and learning involving the acquisition of moral knowledge and judgment.

With the development of a conscience or "super-ego" the child is able to resist temptation without the physical presence of his parents. He begins to feel guilt for his misdeeds. The child under 5 years of age also feels guilty on occasion, but usually only *after* a rule has been broken or a forbidden desire reaches consciousness. Now the child feels guilt before an act is carried out which inhibits forbidden desires or

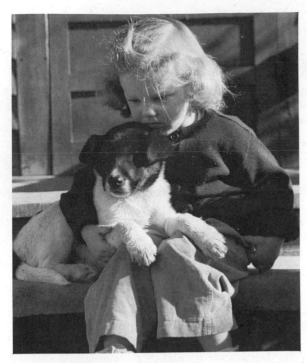

Fig. 16-26. The experience of caring for a pet often assists in the development of a sense of responsibility. (Carol Baldwin)

impulses or diverts the original wish to transgress into some action which will provide similar gratification without the penalty of self-reproach (sublimation). Parental warmth, use of love-oriented discipline technics and consistency of control facilitates the learning of moral expectations. Usually this process occurs without the child's being aware of it. At times when internal or external pressures are increased, the child may be alerted to danger by anxiety. In amounts that he can handle, anxiety serves a constructive purpose. It strengthens him to cope with increasingly more difficult crises of development. Only when anxiety is excessive and the child is given no help in coping with it does it become a deterrent to healthy personality development.

The internalization of moral standards involves three different components: the behavioral, emotional and judgmental aspects of moral action. The acquisition of internal control and the basic forces of moral character is accomplished chiefly during the first six years of life, whereas the ability to form sound moral judgments increases throughout childhood. The child's conscience becomes modified in later stages of development through meeting and adapting to the standards and conventions of his group, peers, teachers and eventually the wider community.

As the child begins to interact with others and acquires increasing cognitive capacity to define situations, his reasoning for moral action becomes more mature. By the time they enter school, most children know the basic moral rules and conventions of our society. Moral thought and judgment however, change and develop through a series of stages as social participation and intellectual ability increase. Moral role-taking involves the ability for empathy which is not yet possible for the preschool child because of his egocentrism.

During the preschool and early school years the child views rules as fixed and absolute and as passed down by his parents who are all-knowing and perfect. The young child tends to judge action as "bad" mainly in terms of its consequences. For instance, he may state that five cups broken while helping his mother is worse than one cup broken while stealing jam. He also views an act as totally right or totally wrong and believes that the adult's view is always the right one. During the preschool years, punishment is usually seen as deserved; i.e., if a child is punished, he must have done something to deserve it. (This characteristic of young children's thinking has been mentioned earlier in relation to the child's response to hospitalization as punishment for imagined misdeeds, influencing the sense of worthlessness.) Misfortune is also seen as occurring after misdeeds because it was willed by God or parents as retribution. As the child's experience increases, his moral judgment progresses toward more internal and subjective values and there is less concern for immediate external physical consequences.

Changes in Family Relationships

By 3 years of age, the child begins to assume behavior characteristic of sex role identity. The girl becomes aware of her appearance, dresses in her mother's clothes, studies herself in the mirror and is interested in choosing her own clothes and in helping out with household chores. A boy will show off, wear cowboy suits and carry guns or dress up in his father's hat and coat and imitate his behavior where previously his identification was predominantly with his mother.

During this period of development the child's interest turns to the parent of the opposite sex, giving rise to conflict, disappointment, anger and fear. Earlier the child was under stress when he discovered that he had to share his mother's love with his siblings. However, the conflicting feelings that he weathered then were of lesser intensity than are those that he must face between the ages of 3 and 6. Now the child may see his parent of the same sex as a rival because that person suddenly is a barrier to the child's desire to be the sole possessor of the parent of the opposite sex. He may become competitive, jealous and aggressive towards the thwarting parent and may have destructive wishes which are frightening. At the same time he loves that parent, on whom he is, of course, simultaneously dependent for help in learning his sexual role—hence the conflict.

This situation is especially frightening to small children because they are not equipped by experience to control such powerful emotions. Their thinking is also

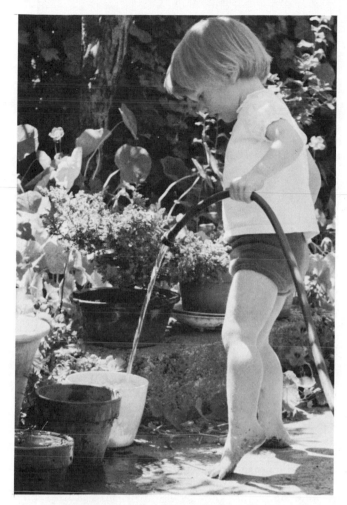

Fig. 16-27. Assisting mother in the care of growing things is an avenue of identification, and allows, as well, the enjoyment of play with water. (Carol Baldwin)

dominated by egocentrism and magical thinking. The preschooler still believes that his wishes may destroy, nor does he realize that they are different from deeds. He is frightened because he believes that his hostility may remove the person on whom he is dependent for protection and love, and because of subjective thinking also imagines that his parents feel equally destructive and retaliative. Until the boy has the experience he needs to prove that no injury can befall his genitals, he may clutch his penis periodically to reassure himself that he is safe. This behavior is often labeled "masturbation," but it is nothing more than a protective gesture.

Parental Support. Help from both parents in resolving the Oedipus Complex, as this crisis is often called, is necessary in furthering the child's preparation for successful marriage and parenthood. His parent of the same sex must be prepared to accept his intense love for the other and his hostility toward his person. For example, the mother should know that her daughter is not rejecting her completely and still loves her even when she says, "Mother, I hate you," or "I love Daddy more than you. Someday I'm going to marry him," or "I wish you'd go away and never come back. I don't love you any more." Acceptance of such feeling not only relieves the child of some emotional pressure and acknowledges understanding of the situation but it also helps to dispel fear of his parent's retaliation. Furthermore, and most important, it prevents the child from feeling guilt for *using his initiative* in meeting his goals.

Support from the parent of the opposite sex is just as important to the child. This parent also must help the child to submerge into the unconscious his impossible wish for exclusive love without causing him to feel ashamed of himself, inadequate or rejected. Of course, the child needs love and admiration from the parent of the opposite sex, but it must be the kind that protects him from sexual stimulation from which he can get no release.

It is not unusual for boys to want to sleep with their mothers and for girls to get into bed beside their fathers. Sometimes children try to separate their parents and crawl into bed between them. If this behavior is encouraged, the child will not be protected from overstimulation and will be deprived of help in learning that the parents have an intimate relationship which cannot be shared with him regardless of how much he is loved. When the child's parents are well adjusted to their sexual roles and to that of their mate, the child has the support that he needs. Unless the child's wish for exclusive love of his parent of the opposite sex is thwarted, he cannot take steps in developing ties of love to persons outside his family. Nor can he become more closely identified with his parent of the same sex, because hostility, guilt and fear of retaliation will be ever-present and will prevent full expansion of his relationship with him or her. This complex of problems leads to what is called *fixation* at this level of psychosocial development.

With support, the child's ego is strengthened as he succeeds in inhibiting his sexual and hostile feelings for his parents and makes a healthy adjustment to his sexual role and his place in the family. When this step in development is achieved, the child's love and hate become transmuted into friendliness toward both parents.

Anxiety created by frustration of the wish for exclusive love of the parent of the opposite sex and by envy and feelings of inadequacy are also often relieved by the defense of *denial*. In dramatic play, the child can pretend that he is "Mommy" or "Daddy" and do all the things that his ideal can do. In this way he becomes more capable of waiting for greater satisfaction which will be obtainable when he is an adult. Such play also is motivating to invest energy in preparing himself for his future sexual role.

Loss of a Parent. The child who loses a parent through circumstances such as illness, death or divorce needs careful guidance to prevent emotional disturbances from arising. This is especially true when a child loses his parent of the same sex because he may experience not only guilt but fear, since he may suspect that his hostility had something to do with his parent's death or disappearance. This vague sense of guilt may persist throughout his life.

When a child loses a person he loves, he should be allowed free expression of grief. Attempts to protect the child from this only increase his loneliness and indirectly tell him that overt expression of grief is unacceptable. When a child loses a parent, he needs repeated reassurance that the remaining parent will remain with him.

Sex Education

Sex education is not restricted to imparting the facts of reproduction and the sexual relationship; it is guidance that builds a foundation for marriage and parenthood. Specific knowledge must be imparted concerning the child's anatomy, the origin of babies and the process of birth. Such teaching is valuable because it helps the child to accept himself and his sexual role and protects his potentials for further learning. Josselyn* has observed that many learning problems have their origin in this period of psychosocial development. When sexual curiosity is repressed early because the child has learned that sex is a forbidden subject, the desire to learn about other aspects of living and of his world also may become submerged into the unconscious part of his mind. If this happens, full intellectual attainment may never be realized.

Sex education is influenced for good or ill by the quality of the child's interpersonal relationships. Before he has reached 3 years of age he has already had some of the most important lessons in sex education. Early care in an atmosphere of affection makes it possible for the baby to discover, love and respect himself; later it teaches him to receive and give love and to develop interest in assuming responsibility for himself and, eventually, for others.

Some adults have difficulty in believing that young children have sexual drives and wishes, but this has been proved by study of their play and of their interaction with parents, therapists and peers.

Curiosity. A child's tentative early questions concerning sex are nothing more than a reflection of that curiosity which embraces all things. Very often the directness of a child's questions about sex has a rather unnerving effect on his elders; but they should remember that to a youngster discussion of this subject is no more emotionally charged than that of the weather or any other natural phenomena. (Before long, however, the child does sense the peculiar emotional reaction which questions about sex always evoke in others, and thus the mystery becomes more profound and consequently more enticing—and, very often, frightening as well.)

A child's questions indicate that he has been pondering about the subject of his inquiry previously and is ready to learn, but he can assimilate only one idea at a time. He may even have to have an idea explained again and again before he can use facts to solve his problem of the moment. The adult should not conclude that he is obsessed with the subject. His quick transition from questions about sex to queries about other subjects proves that he has a myriad of accessory interests; it merely shows that he is trying to piece his observations together to gain some understanding of himself and life in a bisexual world. Because the experience of children is limited, the conclusions they draw are usually highly colored by imagination. Before an adult answers a question, it is wise to encourage the child to relate his own version of the subject. This can be done simply: "I'd like to hear the story you've told yourself about that. You tell me yours and then I'll tell you mine."

To hear the child out first is valuable. It reassures him that the adult is genuinely interested in everything that is of importance to him; it brings his fantasies with their emotional meaning to the surface where they can be dealt with constructively; it prevents his imagination from distorting the facts when they are given; and it encourages further questioning. A child who has repressed misconceptions because they were too frightening to think about has a difficult time gaining emotional understanding of truths at a later time. For example, a young woman who has been given factual knowledge of the birth process during her pregnancy and comprehends it intellectually may be unable to accept it emotionally because she has harbored childish feelings and fantasies which pictured birth as a gruesome process.

When the child's fantasies have been aired, the parent can correct them and then proceed to answer his question like any other—in the simplest and most truthful way possible. For instance, when a child asks, "How do babies get out?", a simple answer like the following one usually will satisfy his curiosity: "They come through a special opening in the mother's body."

Why Is My Body Different? When the child becomes aware of his body, he compares himself with others and develops an interest in the differences between boys and girls and men and women. When the little girl observes that a boy has something which she does not have, she may wonder if she once had a penis and, if so, what has happened to it. She may suspect that she has damaged herself by masturbating or has been punished for naughtiness. Some girls feel deprived and blame their mothers. Others reproach their mothers for having given more to their brothers than to them. In such instances they usually are not referring to material possessions; they are signalling their worry about their bodies.

---

* Josselyn, Irene M.: *Psychosexual Development of the Child*, p. 75, New York, The Family Service Association of America, 1948.

When the girl questions either verbally or by obvious investigations, she should be told simply that a boy is made differently and has a penis like his father, while she has just as much but her organs are inside her body, since she is feminine like her mother. Giving children the correct names of their organs increases their pride in their bodies and lays the foundation for later teaching.

A mother who enjoys her own femininity can give her daughter a feeling of pride in being a girl. Such a statement as the following, rendered at the appropriate moment, heightens self-esteem: "When you grow up, you'll have breasts and hair on your body just like your Mommy. When you're a grown woman you will have a husband as I do, and then you will have babies, too. You have a special place inside your body where babies grow. It is called a uterus."

During preschool years the girl wants to compete with her mother and "grow" a baby. Her wish for a penis is replaced by a wish for a child. She acts her wishes out in her play with dolls, real or toy animals, her younger siblings or playmates. They become "her babies," and in her play she imagines that she is a real mother; temporarily she feels grown up, powerful and victorious. In imagination, word and act she denies her childishness and overcomes her frustration at not being able to have a real baby immediately.

The boy is equally concerned when he first observes the body of a girl. He is perplexed because he wonders what has happened to her body and if the same thing might happen to him. He may imagine that she might have been punished for improper thoughts. This frightens him because he knows that he has been hostile and aggressive at times, too. He may directly question why the girl does not have a penis, or he may simply stare in wonder and fear. He may even clutch at his penis to reassure himself that he has not met with the same fate he imagines has befallen the other child. The boy should be told that he was born with a penis and will always have one because boys are made differently from girls. When the boy learns that girls and women are made differently because they "grow" babies, he should be told for the sake of his self-respect that men share in the process of creating a child. The boy also has a wish to "grow" babies during this stage but derives a substitute satisfaction in playing the role of father.

Before children can question they sometimes investigate and indulge in sex play to satisfy their curiosity. It is not uncommon to observe a little boy picking up a girl's clothing or suggesting that she undress. However, he is not being naughty or shameful; most likely he is merely trying to understand and free himself from worry. Nor should anyone take it amiss if a child peers under the skirt or looks down the front of his mother's or a nurse's dress. He is unsure of something and is searching for a solution to his problem.

When sex play is observed among children, it is unwise to inflict punishment or even to make much of a scene over it, for shame and anxiety connected with the genital region can upset psychosocial development with possible disturbance of sexual functioning in adult life. Of course, it is equally unwise to ignore it. Limits kindly imposed prevent children from becoming ashamed of and frightened by their natural sexual curiosity and impulses. They are a blessed relief to the child who is worried about his sexual fantasies and is uneasy about sexual play. They not only tell him that he can count on adults to define what is socially acceptable but also give him the courage to share his worries with an adult.

Where Did I Come From? As the child begins to relate himself to his parents as persons of opposite sex, he begins to wonder where he came from and how he grew. His curiosity is further stimulated by the changes occurring within him and in his relationship to his parents.

If the child's earliest questions were respected, he will turn to his parents in asking where he came from. "You grew inside Mother" is a simple and truthful answer. He will love hearing about himself when he was *in utero* and when he was a tiny baby unable to walk, talk or play. To relate stories concerning his parents' pleasure when he was born, first smiled, fed himself and talked will delight the child and increase his sense of belonging. Nothing will fascinate him more than accounts of his own care as a baby. In this period he continues to be greatly interested in himself, and if by any chance he is involved with problems relating to a new sibling, stories about himself will be doubly appreciated and reassuring as well.

How Are Babies Born? When the child asks, "Did it hurt when I was born?", the way in which this question is answered may have a far-ranging influence on the child's later attitude toward childbirth. This question often follows "How did I get out?" or it may not come until months or years have passed.

The mother who welcomed childbirth will convey this: "Yes, Mary, having a baby does hurt. It takes hard work to give birth to a baby, but you'll be able to do it. When the time comes for the baby to be born, the muscles of the mother's uterus begin to work. That hurts, but the mother wants to see her baby and she's glad to work to help it get born. When her uterus begins to do its work, the mother goes to the hospital. There the doctors and nurses help her to bring her baby into the world. If the mother needs it, the nurse will give her something to keep it from hurting at the time the baby is born. By the time the baby comes, the mother is tired, but she is also very happy. Then she can begin taking care of the baby outside her body."

How Does a Baby Begin? It will probably be a long time before the child begins to wonder what made the baby grow inside his mother. When he asks he can be told that it grew from a cell (ovum) which is as small as a speck, is alive, and is a part of the mother's body. Queries as to the father's role in reproduction usually come later. The child will probably be 5 to 8 years of age before he asks, "But how do babies start to grow?" And even later: "How does the father's seed get into the mother?" These are the most difficult of all questions for a parent to answer, for they are the most highly charged emotionally. The answers can be as simple as this: "When daddies and mothers love each other, they want to have a baby. It takes two of them. Daddies have special cells in their bodies just as mothers do. The daddy's cells or sperm must meet a seed in the mothers' body where the baby will grow. When the baby is ready to live outside his mother's body the baby is born." This is probably all the child will want to know during this age level.

Later when the child asks how the father's seed entered the mother's body, he probably will have surmised the answer already. All he will need then is a review of what he has already learned and help to clarify his understanding: "You know that boys and fathers have penises. You also know that girls and mothers have a uterus where the baby grows and an opening which leads from it to the outside of her body. The father uses his penis to place his cells in the opening of the mother's body. It is called the vagina. The father's cells can move. When the father's cell reaches the mother's cell, a baby begins to grow."

Self-Comforting Acts. As soon as the infant learns to use his hands, he finds different parts of his body and learns that there is pleasure in handling or rubbing them. He also finds that certain areas of his body are more pleasurable to touch then are others. In the beginning, stimulation of his mouth by breast or bottle led to satisfaction and to a release of tension. When growth is proceeding normally, interest is shifted from one area of the body to another as bodily functions are established. At the beginning of the second year the toddler finds pleasure in his excretory functioning and later, the preschooler's interest becomes directed to the genitals, where his erotic feelings become more specifically concentrated.

Masturbation, or rubbing of the genitals, is a normal activity in childhood and has as a purpose the discharge of tension, particularly the conflict of feelings toward his parents. A loving relationship with his parents is a precondition and gratification derived from handling his body is closely connected with his feelings toward his mother. In addition, its appearance indicates progress in the development of intelligence, of ego functions and in the differentiation of the self from the environment. Awakened sexual curiosity and increased fantasy life are contributing factors.

The act is not injurious in itself and can be used to discharge unpleasant bodily tensions connected with imperative body needs. However, the fantasies which accompany it may provoke guilt and worry (especially concern regarding genital injury), if the child is shamed or threatened with punishment or rejection, which may lead to impairment of sexual expression later in life.

Masturbation tends to occur less frequently when sexual stimulation is kept to a minimum, when the child's relationships with others are generally satisfactory and when a wide interest in the world about him has been encouraged. If the child's drive to care for himself and to grow less dependent on contact with his mother's body was utilized when it appeared, he will not be as likely to become overstimulated.

The child's approaches to gain intimate body contact from the parent of the opposite sex should be tactfully diverted to help him to gain control of his impulses. As the preschooler's intellectual development and sense of reality progress, the incidence of masturbation will also decline. If severe prohibitions or castration threats have not resulted in the giving up of masturbation completely and to the repression of all fantasies, emotional development will progress normally. On the other hand, the child's masturbatory activity should not be ignored completely. Provision of substitute gratification helps the child to achieve sublimation and conveys the feeling that his mother or nurse care enough about him to help him gain control of impulses that frighten him. He will not feel punished or ashamed if *they stay with him,* and he may also gain the courage to ask questions if he has fears relating to the safety of his body.

The following incident demonstrates the child's need for respect of his defenses.

Ted, age 5, had had continuity of nursing care by the same nurse for a week prior to the time this situation occurred. On this day his nurse suggested that he have a tub bath rather than sponging himself on his bed. The nurse took him to the bathroom in a wheel chair and helped him to remove his pajamas although he was capable of doing it himself. Beneath them were trunks, and he resisted having them removed for bathing. He scrambled into the tub with his genitals covered and clutched his pants when the nurse forcibly removed them from him. Then, instead of leaving him as he requested, she stayed in the bathtub cubicle and helped him with his bath. When she lifted him from the tub, he pressed his body tightly against hers, moved it up and down and resisted her efforts to put him on the chair for drying and dressing.

Ted's need for protection from uncontrolled impulses was not recognized; the nurse had not previously believed that children had sexual feelings. This experience increased her insight into the preschooler's instinctual development, and from then on she was able to support the defenses that children use to protect themselves from anxiety.

A child who masturbates excessively at home or in

the hospital is turning to himself for solace because he is not obtaining sufficient emotional satisfaction from others. Fear of bodily injury might be another reason why so much of his interest is devoted to his genitals.

Nurses can prepare parents to understand the developmental significance of masturbation. Although some parents may be unable to accept emotionally the theory of its origin, the nurse can point out the measures that will lessen the child's need to turn to himself for comfort.

Questions During Hospitalization. In the hospital nurses are often confronted with children's direct and indirect questions pertaining to sex differences, the origin of babies, birth and menstruation. Nurses must be prepared to help children to handle their curiosity. Sometimes the child's first experience in seeing the body of a child of the opposite sex occurs during his hospital stay. Because some parents prefer that their children be kept in ignorance, it is important that the nurse know the hospital policy in relation to giving information to children. There are parents who would be angry enough to sue a hospital if their children received information which they themselves have been unable to impart.

Whenever a nurse is confronted with this delicate problem, she should discuss the experience with the mother the next time she comes to the ward. The mother should be told the child's thoughts and questions and the nurse's answer. Such an incident can be a valuable learning experience for both the nurse and the mother. The former can observe the mother's reactions to her child's curiosity and to the help which was given. Often mothers are relieved because the child's questions have been answered, and they can seek further help from the nurse in order to be prepared to help their children later when more questions arise. Providing mothers with an opportunity to talk about their attitudes toward sex education often serves to help them to become more comfortable in talking with their children.

Development of Social Relationships

Nursery school and kindergarten experience can be of great value to those children who have the ego strength necessary to tolerate separation from their mothers for short periods of time and to turn to the teacher for help in learning to play and work with other children. In school the child can learn to become more independent and can express his feelings with greater freedom because his relationship to other adults is less emotionally charged than is his relationship with his mother. In a group the child's potentialities for socialization can unfold, and the teacher can help him to turn to playmates for an outlet of his affectionate feelings. When he succeeds in making friends with the children in the group, disappointment regarding family relationships becomes more tolerable.

Because anxiety on separation is still very much in evidence at this age, the child's adjustment to the nursery school is usually a gradual and conservative process. The child should be helped to feel that going to school is a progressive step rather than banishment for punitive reasons. Further apprehensions are allayed when he is assured that there will be an adult to take care of him, and when he is taken on a tour to see everything for himself. If the mother is able to stay with the child in the nursery school until he can go to the teacher for help and indicates readiness to remain without her, his adaptation to school will be facilitated.

Children have different methods of coping with the unfamiliar. Some children may plunge into a new situation and activity aggressively as if they had a need to explore and test themselves out in the new environment. Others are passive at first and need to survey the situation from a distance before entering into group activity. (Children's initial reactions to the ward or hospital playroom show similar wide variation.)

At first dramatic co-operative play involves "twosomes"; but there is an exclusiveness about it. "You can't play with us" is a frequently heard refrain. This exclusiveness—often a boy and a girl but not necessarily—may stem from the realization that they are unable to handle the problems which arise when more than two children play together (or it may well be their way of dealing with their feelings concerning exclusion from their parent's intimate relationship with each other). However, this period of isolation does not last long. Gradually children begin to welcome would-be joiners or else make known their availability to the larger group.

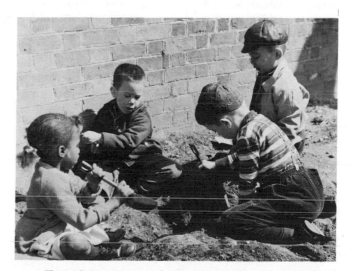

Fig. 16-28. During the preschool period, children develop the capacity for cooperating toward a common goal. Digging a hole offers many opportunities for creative expression and for working through fears. (Carol Baldwin)

Learning Co-operation with Others. Characteristics of generosity, consideration of others, and control of destructive impulses are not present from birth, but are acquired gradually through relationships with parents and other adults and through progress in intellectual development. Early in this period, the egocentricity of the child makes it extremely difficult for him to consider the viewpoint or feelings of other children. Although he is eager to make friends, the necessary development of empathy and capacity for co-operation takes time and help from meaningful adults.

Children learn to share their teacher and toys with others and to take turns through recognition of the expectation of their teacher and because they want and need her approval to feel secure. Learning to inhibit the impulse to strike out against offending playmates and to work together on projects is acquired by the same principle. However until the child's intellectual development progresses, consistent harmony should not be expected of the child.

Another reason why getting along with other children is difficult for many preschoolers is that their problems with their siblings have not been resolved. The child may have reacted to the birth of a sibling with jealousy and hostility because of the necessity to share the exclusive attention of his mother. Because the child knows that his mother expects him to adapt to the change in the family he must resolve his conflicts and *sibling rivalry* since his security depends on it. He really wants to be the most loved, and healthy response to this universal desire in children is to fight to keep their places in the sun. Regression, hostility and anxiety are natural and continue to be expressed either directly or indirectly until the child is reassured that he has not been displaced by the baby whom he perceives to be an intruder.

In nursery school (or in the pediatric ward) a preschooler's* relationships with his playmates will be governed to a great extent by his degree of success in dealing with the problem. Many will have made little or no progress. Some may have repressed their hostility and become submissive in order to maintain their security with their mothers. Others may have resorted to the defense called *displacement;* that is, instead of expressing their hostility to its object, they direct it toward their peers. This arrangement may serve to keep peace in the family, but the child's unpopularity with his playmates may cause him to be even more dependent on his mother.

The children who are not experiencing such conflicts nevertheless may be having their first experience in sharing an adult with others, and similar problems of rivalry and jealousy may arise.

When children become assured that they are loved although the teacher loves others, too, they relinquish their desire for an exclusive relationship with her and accept sharing her with their peers. At the same time, however, they demand that no other child receive more or be given privileges denied to them. If the teacher gives more to one child than another, it is deeply resented. If one child usurps the attention of the teacher, the other children in the group are quick to take steps to stop it.

Tale-bearing ("tattling") is common among preschoolers. A child may tattle to get even with a sibling or a playmate, but more often than not talebearing indicates that he feels neglected and believes that by tattling he will gain favor with the person in authority. The latter also should bear in mind that a child will report another's wrongful act because he has been sorely tempted to commit that very act himself. Since this is his way of appealing for help in restraining himself, the teacher should support the strength in his personality. The incident cited below shows a way in which this might be done.

Six children were lined up awaiting their turn to jump from an apparatus several feet from the ground. In the excitement which is invariably stirred up when preschool children are physically close to one another, Sally pushed Gina out of place in the line. As she did so Ned shouted, "Teacher, look! Sally is pushing." Immediately the teacher surmised that Ned wanted help to restrain himself from doing what Sally had done. She said, "Sally shouldn't do that." Ned's response provided evidence to support the validity of her hunch. He turned to Sally and said, "Hey Sally, Gina needs a place in the line." Ned not only derived strength to restrain himself, but, feeling understood, he also was able to identify himself with the teacher's values.

Some children handle their rivalry by competing excessively to be the best in the group. They seem to be driven to win a game, jump the farthest or build the tallest tower in the playroom. Although most adults are inclined to admire competitiveness in any form, very often this type of behavior is a sign of a child's inability to accept himself as he is. He may be striving futilely to outdo an older and more accomplished sibling of whom he is jealous, or he may be covering up a sense of inferiority from other causes. The teacher who makes it a point to demonstrate her continued approval—even though he does not always perform to perfection—may be able to help the child to relax a bit in his desperate effort to outdo his peers. Then he will have energy to relate to his peers and get the benefit of their approval. With closer relationships to them, his self-esteem and productivity can rise to greater heights.

When the ages of a group of children are widely divergent (as in a pediatric ward), rivalry within the group may be more pronounced. The youngest chil-

---

* Remnants of sibling rivalry will also be apparent in the behavior of many school-age youngsters and adolescents. Those who have had help in resolving this conflict constructively are fortunate indeed, for they are more adequately prepared to gain maximal benefits from school.

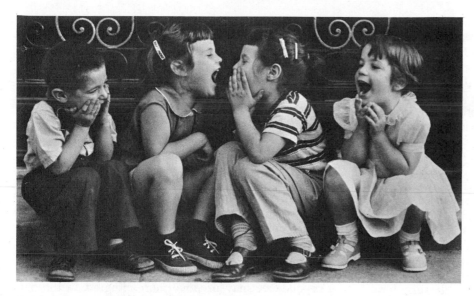

FIG. 16-29. Having the fun of sharing experiences with playmates decreases the child's dependence on his parents for emotional satisfactions. Notice the joyfulness and the spontaneity of these children in comparison to the young children seen in a hospital playroom. These children are healthy, but there are other reasons why they have energy to expend in developing themselves socially. They are in a known environment and within easy reach of their parents for help when they need it. (Photograph by Murray Zinn)

dren often want the privileges and the possessions they see the older ones receiving, but in most instances they are unready for them. It helps the younger child to be told that certain privileges come with increasing age, because this is another incentive for wanting to grow up. The oldest children in the group often resent the attention the youngest children require. Unless their need to be an important part of the group is recognized, they will see little value in their maturer status and revert to babyish ways of behaving to get what they would rather have in more mature ways.

Rivalry is lessened when each child is dealt with according to his individual requirements. To treat two children alike in that they are always given the same presents and the same amount and kind of attention is being rather too impartial because neither child's individuality is taken into account—and the children sense this. Instead of trying to discover the particular needs of each child, the nurse may plan to spend equal time with them all. If she prefers one child to another (and does not choose to admit this to herself), this arrangement may ease her conscience.

It is the quality of the interpersonal relationships, not the time devoted to them, which counts with the child. Children are more understanding than most adults would believe. If plans are shared with them, they know they will not be forgotten when the needs of others are being met. They are also reassured, for if they see that the needs of other children are being attended to, they can be more confident that theirs will be too. The following situation is presented to illustrate some of the ways in which the nurse can help children to learn to share an adult's attention with others.

On 4-year-old Suzie's 10th postoperative day after open-heart surgery, she became alerted to the cries of baby Jed in the adjoining room. When the nurse said that she would go and attend to him, Suzie became silent and looked angry.

When the nurse returned, Suzie looked more troubled. The nurse wondered whether her care of Jed had made Suzie jealous, or if the period of being alone had stirred up sorrow over separation from her mother. Or was Suzie worried about the dressing change she knew was going to be done that morning? Realizing that the sharing of troubles relieves a child's tension and gives the nurse knowledge to plan further action, the nurse said, "I wonder if you're worried about having your dressing changed today." Suzie answered angrily: "No! I want you to stay here if that baby doesn't yell anymore. He's not crying now." She had not only shared her worry but also had vented her anger, and she discovered that it did not lessen the nurse's affection for her.

"I won't go to Jed if he's quiet and not before you have a story. You can ring your bell if you want me. I won't be far away, and I'll come the minute I hear you ring." (The nurse wanted Suzie to know that she would be on the alert for her needs as well as for Jed's.)

"But I want you to *stay here.*" (Suzie's words and tone suggested that she could tolerate the nurse's absence only if she were sure the baby was distressed.)

The next time Jed cried, the nurse said, "Let's go see what's troubling Jed. I'll carry you to the door so you can see him. Then we'll both know what's bothering him." When they arrived within sight of Jed, the nurse asked "What do you suppose he needs?" Suzie said, "He's hungry." The nurse told Suzie that she would investigate to see whether or not that was his problem. Suzie accepted being placed on her bed, but first she made sure that the nurse would return as soon as Jed was satisfied.

In taking Suzie where she could see Jed, the nurse hoped that she would become interested in Jed and a participant in his care rather than a passive bystander. Being able to share in the care of a baby makes the child feel more powerful. As a result his ego is strengthened to cope with rivalry.

Dependency—Independence. Differences in amount of dependency in children who begin a nursery school experience can also be observed and in any individual child such behavior may vary considerably from one situation to another. A highly dependent child may cling to other familiar adults or strangers when separated from his mother. All children show less initiative when they feel insecure or anxious. The simple availability of a teacher or nurse will also increase dependency behavior in a child, particularly if that adult is busy or inattentive or when the normal relationship with his mother is being diluted for any reason. Thus preschoolers who are coping with the birth of a sibling may show less independence in nursery school or kindergarten.

The need for physical or emotional closeness is an incentive to learning. Experiments with children have demonstrated that they learn a task more quickly when they receive the approval of a nurturant adult. Children who have had a warm experience within their family and who are concerned about pleasing adults are more motivated to learn than are those who have no trust in adults or who are anxious about their dependency. This is not an unmixed blessing, however, for children who are very high in dependency are easily distracted from a task by their needs for approval and are more concerned with receiving the affection they wish for than with their successful completion of a task.

Dependency behavior may be more consistent in girls over situations and over time whereas it may be more fragmented in boys. This may well be due to the fact that dependency is more socially condoned in girls than it is in boys in our society.

The origins of excessive amounts of dependency are complex. Every child has strong incentives for the development of dependency. If strivings toward independency are delayed, however, the delay may be due to experiencing of reward for dependency responses in the home or through excessive amounts of anxiety. Children who are frequently made to feel insecure will be more dependent in new situations. Another factor is the degree to which they have been helped to find alternate ways of behavior, have been assisted in controlling their fear and helped to cope with separation.

When observed in a nursery school or hospital situation, children may demonstrate either active or passive dependency responses which are different and not usually found in the same child. The passive child may withdraw and wait to be directed, mainly because he has not been helped to progress toward independence or to find methods of coping with the unfamiliar. The other type of dependency is a constant, striving action in seeking physical and emotional closeness.

The abundance of warmth and closeness which a mother shows to her infant and toddler does not prolong his dependency on her. On the contrary, it gives him the trust and security he needs to develop autonomy and a sense of independence. Dependency bids during the preschool and school years are increased when the child is not certain of his parents' affection

for him or if discipline technics of withdrawal of love have been used consistently. Such methods of discipline create anxiety in the child regarding his affectional relationship with his mother. Thus parental rejection may be coupled with a high degree of preschool dependency, along with parental failure to help the child to find alternate methods of coping with his frustration. If independence is not supported or the child has been restricted in his early drives toward exploration, his sense of dependency on adults will be greater. Inconsistency of responses related to the child's dependency will also delay individual initiative. If parents have been highly nurturant to the child during infancy and toddlerhood, but become irritated with him for his dependency when he is a preschooler, dependency will be increased. Such a conflict in the child may result in a vicious circle: the behavior of the mother to detach herself and force independence may produce more clinging on the part of the child.

When the child enters nursery school or during hospitalization, he may need help in finding ways to cope with his frustration, to discover that his self-esteem is enhanced through independence of action and initiative and that he can receive affection and approval from a meaningful adult through successful completion of a task so that his relationships with other children can be facilitated. Increase in his self-evaluation will also be of assistance to him in coping with his conflicts at home, for as he learns new ways of behaving, the approval he receives from his mother may improve previous conflictual family relationships.

The Control of Aggression. In most societies there are prohibitions on the expression of aggression and conflicts in values about aggressive behavior. It is condoned in one sex more than in the other, in some situations more than in others and some modes of expression are more approved than are alternate methods. In almost all societies, aggressive and hostile behavior is inhibited within the family unit, for the continued existence of the family is dependent on keeping aggressive impulses under control.

The rules a child must learn in inhibiting his aggressive impulses are quite complex. Most children learn that expression of aggression toward their parents or other adults in authority endangers their security, whereas covert aggression toward children outside the home may be encouraged under certain circumstances. Boys must learn that aggression expressed overtly toward girls is discouraged whereas "holding their own" with other boys or defending themselves is often rewarded with approval.

During infancy, aggressiveness was expressed in physiological tension storms, while in the toddler, frustration often resulted in tantrum behavior or loss of behavioral controls. When a child reaches the preschool period, hostility may become more directed and intentional in character and physical expression of aggression may give greater place to verbal communication of anger.

The wide variation in the amount of aggressiveness expressed by children stems from numerous factors: (1) innate physical factors such as differences in inborn activity levels, differences in hormonal levels or body build, (2) difference in ego strength, in the ability to tolerate frustration, (3) the amount of help the child has received in controlling and redirecting his antisocial impulses into socially approved alternate methods of behavior, (4) environmental factors, such as the degree of conflict or harmony within family relationships, (5) the learning of prohibitions against aggressive behavior vs. reinforcement for aggressiveness. Learning that aggressiveness does "work" will reinforce such expression. In addition, severe physical punishment for aggressive behavior is related to later greater aggressiveness.

When young children are severely punished for aggression, displacement of aggressiveness to another object may also occur, or the defense of projection may be utilized so that the child senses himself as the target for the hostile impulses of others. Overt expression of aggressiveness may also become attenuated with vicarious enjoyment of aggressiveness in others or it may become directed to the self. If the child becomes acutely anxious about his own aggressive impulses, he may withdraw from situations which are threatening or employ strong countermeasures in condemning the aggressiveness of others. Severe punishment for the expression of aggressive impulses may also reduce later creativity, divergent thinking and the energy necessary for learning during the school years.

Although children should not become frightened of their normal feelings of anger, they must also have help in learning to control them and to redirect them into ways which are not hurtful to others. While learning to play together children meet many frustrating situations which provoke aggressive feelings. A child who suffers more frustration than he can bear may be benefited by removal from the group. However, prolonged separation is not desirable, since he needs other kinds of help to learn constructive ways to handle his aggression.

When children acquire increased facility in talking, they must be helped to solve their problems verbally rather than with temper outbursts or fighting. The following situation serves to illustrate steps which must be taken by the child before he can gain control of his anger.

For 10 minutes 4-year-old Sheila and Carol had had a hilariously happy time "jumping islands" as they called it. Large wooden blocks were scattered about the floor, and the children engaged themselves in gauging their jumps so that they would land on the nearest block. Then Ann decided that she would like to install a dumptruck on one of the islands. Sheila was infuriated. She kicked at the truck, increasing Ann's determination to have it where she wanted

it. With muscles taut, Sheila ran to the cupboard and pulled out a carton of records to play. Unfortunately, however, she was thwarted by her teacher who did not understand the purpose of her mission. Sheila clenched her fists, ground her teeth, raced to the table and used the hammer on the pounding board. "I'm mad," she cried as she hit the pegs. When another teacher observed the way she was dealing with her anger, she said, "Pounding helps when you're upset." Sheila's eyes met the teacher's and her facial muscles relaxed in a partial smile. Then she resumed her activity until she felt composed enough to rejoin her playmate.

A year later Sheila had taken another step in growing up. Instead of kicking and running away, she used words to express her feelings and initiated compromises which satisfied the playmate as well as herself. Note especially that Sheila had already taken the first and most important step in learning to control her anger before she was 4 years old; she had overcome her fear of it. She was able to say, "I'm mad," and vent her fury on the pounding board. She did not have to hide it from herself.

Overcoming Fears. As was mentioned earlier in this chapter, the preschooler is intensely afraid of pain and bodily injury. One cause of this in boys is a lingering fear of paternal retaliation. Also, after 3 years of age his body's value is heightened because it encloses the new-found self which he does not want to lose. Fraiberg says, "His wholeness as a personality, his psychic integrity, seems to be closely bound up with the completeness and integrity of the body."* Nurses have observed repeatedly that the preschooler is grossly threatened by intrusive medical and nursing procedures; that is, those which require entry into his body or cause it to be changed in any way. Examples are injections, withdrawal of any body fluids and surgery. Procedures involving the genital organs are especially terrifying. If an operation is required and the child has not learned the *real* reason for it, his fear of his father's retaliation may never be fully eradicated from the unconscious part of his mind.

Girls are also frightened by intrusive procedures, not only for the foregoing reasons but also because they, too, fear punishment for destructive wishes. Sometimes little girls think they have already lost a part of their bodies, in which case careful preparation is of the utmost importance for them as well as for boys. Without the continued support of both parents, preschoolers are likely to interpret treatment measures as hostile attacks.

Band-aids often work like magic after venepunctures and injections, but the purpose they serve for the child becomes understandable when the child's behavior after their application is observed. If children are permitted to put the Band-aid in place by themselves—or to remove the gauze protector if the wound

---

* Fraiberg, S.: *The Magic Years*, p. 130, New York, Charles Scribner's Sons, Inc., 1959.

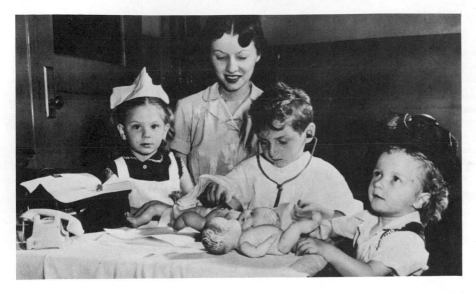

is out of their reach—their anxiety is reduced. The act of putting the Band-aid in place is one means by which they pull themselves together or gain control of their feelings about the situation.

Preschoolers are worried not only about their own injuries but also by the sight of injuries in others. Broken toys are also a source of concern. Having Scotch tape available for a repair job is often reassuring to children. The situation described below shows the way in which a nursery school teacher eased one child's worry about another's broken arm.

When Mrs. D. brought her oldest boy to school she had Dick, age 2½ years, with her. The day before he had had a cast put on a broken arm. When he entered the nursery school, Ellis, age 5, immediately noticed that a sleeve of Dick's coat had no arm inside it. He felt the sleeve, peeked inside it and pulled at the buttons to open his coat. His anxiety was reflected in his jerky movements and by the way in which he stammered out his words: "Where's his arm? Is it gone?" The teacher said, "He broke it but it's going to be well again."

Later when the children were having juice, the teacher explained that Dick had fallen and cracked the bone in his arm. She described how an x-ray picture is taken and a cast applied. "Will he be able to use it again?" asked Ellis in a trembling voice. "Yes, it will be just as it was before when the cast comes off." The children queried further, showing their wish to have her explain again and again. Ellis's worry was especially acute because his overt expression of hostility had alienated his mother from him. As a consequence he had not been able to make any progress in learning that his hostile wishes were different from deeds.

Play is an important means by which children overcome their fear of bodily injury. Adults can master painful and frightening feelings by talking about them. The young child cannot do this even if he has words at his command. To minimize anxiety relating to the safety of his body, his ego has repressed the source of his anxiety into the unconscious part of his mind. In studying the reactions of children to hospitalization, Prugh and his associates found that:

The fear verbalized most frequently was that of needles. In this regard an undoubted response to a reality factor involving pain was present. The impression was gained, however, that a great deal of the small child's fear of unknown procedures, of separation from the parents, of punishment, and of overwhelming attack was displaced much of the time onto such objectively less threatening but directly visible things as needles, tourniquets, etc. Fears of rectal temperature procedures or of throat sticks, for example, appear to have such a displaced meaning as well as the more specific meaning in terms of the erotogenic zone involved.[*]

When children are permitted to use toys in their own way, they can work through their problems in

[*] Prugh, Dane, *et al.*: A study of the emotional reactions of children and families to hospitalization and illness, Am. J. Orthopsychiat. 23:95, Jan., 1953.

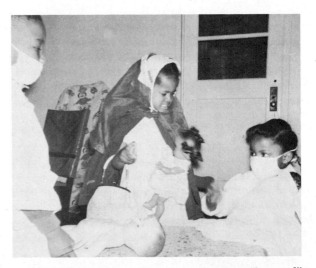

FIG. 16-31. These children engaged in "hospital" play. Notice the anger in the face of the girl who is about to inject her doll. The boy had just completed the act of "giving his patient a shot," and the masked girl clutched her doll close to her as she said, "I won't let cha give my baby one. She doesn't need it. She's all well already." (Infant Welfare Society of Chicago)

play. Erikson says, "to play it out is the most natural self-healing measure childhood affords."[*] Experiences which a child has had to endure passively are usually reproduced in their play of "doctor" or "nurse." The child thus identifies with the physician or nurse and actively relives upsetting experiences to gain control of the feelings that they aroused. In play he utilizes the ego defense which Freud[†] calls *identification with the aggressor.*

When hospitalized children are provided with appropriate play materials, most of them begin to gain control of their anxiety before they go home. With a nurse in attendance to supervise the play, a real syringe and needle, drainage tube, etc., can be used with benefit for the children, who are usually overjoyed and beg to play "hospital" repeatedly. (However, those who have been overwhelmed or traumatized usually repress the experience immediately and thus are unable to "play it out.") The situation described below tells of the way 4-year-old Ernest cured himself of his exaggerated fear of physical examination.

Ernest clutched his mother's skirt when they entered the door leading to the room where the Child Health Conference was held. He shrieked when he was weighed and had his chest examined but did not use his arms for fighting; instead he used his hands to protect his penis. A throat examination was not done because of his panic reaction when the doctor brought the tongue depressor to his mouth. Ernest's mother was embarrassed by his behavior, having no idea what was troubling him. She was greatly relieved when the nurse took time to explain the reason for his behavior and gave her blades to take home.

Three months later his mother brought him to the Conference again. As soon as he entered the door, he asked the nurse for more "sticks." During this visit he co-operated with weighing and a full examination. He showed pride in his willingness to have the tongue blade put into his mouth. His mother was elated with his progress: "Those sticks helped. He used them on himself and his twin sisters for days. His dad let him use his flashlight. Playing doctor has given him more fun than any other game he's ever played."

Factors Affecting the Child's Adjustment to Separation in the Latter Part of This Period

Before discussing medical and nursing care of the sick child, the factors which will have a bearing on the child's adjustment to experiences away from home during the latter part of this period will be presented.

Chronologic Age, Past Experiences and Ego Strength. *To adapt constructively to experiences away from home, the child must have sufficient ego strength and emotional freedom to transfer his dependence from his mother to others responsible for his care, to be able to participate in taking care of himself, to get along with children, to play and to express his feelings overtly.* As the child grows older, a satisfying

mother-child relationship eases the child's adjustment to separation rather than making it more painful as is true of the toddler.

After the age of 5, children are more able to tolerate separation from their families, have developed ego strength so that they no longer need their mothers as desperately to control their behavior, are more capable of interpreting events in terms of reality and have developed methods of coping with fear and frustration.

Those children who have had a school experience before entrance into kindergarten or first grade have become accustomed to the demands and expectations of its varied program of activities and to sharing their teacher with a group of children. If they were physically and psychologically prepared for the experience, they also have learned some rudimentary principles of human relations—enough so that with encouragement from the teacher they are able to make the compromises expected of them. They also have increased their attention span through discussion, music and play and story periods and acquired a greater degree of independence in their own care and thus become better prepared for the more rigorous demands of the primary school.

If entrance into primary school is the child's first experience with a teacher, he must know that she will expect him to do certain things at specified times, to take care of his own toilet needs and possessions and and to co-operate with his peers. It is the mother's responsibility to teach her child safety precautions to use in crossing streets and in protecting himself from strangers. If the mother expects her child to return home for play after school, he must be informed of this expectation.

Many parents will need help from a public health nurse in learning that their children need preparation for school. Appealing to the characteristic wish of mothers to have their children succeed at school often provides the motivating force for learning the importance of continued health supervision during this period—of adequate nutrition and of treatment for any existing physical or psychological defect which might impede their progress in school.

Cognitive Growth. When children have the variety of experiences and stimulation they need during the first few years of life, they develop a healthy curiosity and are eager to explore the wider world outside their home. They have also developed a sound basis for further intellectual achievement, differentiated themselves from their mothers, developed capacities for experimentation and problem solving and are ready to invest themselves in task performance.

During the end of the preschool period the child has made great progress in coming to terms with reality. His concepts of space, time and causality are further elaborated so that separation from home is no longer as threatening as it was a few short years ago. Memory span has also increased, along with the ability to sustain attention.

[*] Erikson, Eric: Childhood and Society, p. 222, New York, Norton, 1963.
[†] Freud, Anna: *Op. cit.*, p. 117.

Although much learning and intellectual growth lie in the years ahead, those children who have had the experiences they need to cause them to feel confidence in themselves and in their abilities will meet the challenge with enthusiasm.

Current Health Status. Optimal health is a support to the ego. If experiences away from home are necessary because of illness, the type of health problem the child is suffering with will have a direct bearing on his capacity for adjustment. The acutely ill or disturbed child is less able to handle new experiences constructively than, for example, the comparatively healthy child who enters the hospital for elective minor surgery. Even in these instances, however, preparation for hospitalization and surgical intervention is of the utmost importance in preventing personality distortions from occurring during this stage of development.

Preschool children who have been to a well-conducted nursery school have an advantage over the others if they must be hospitalized. For all children of this age group who are hospitalized for an appreciable length of time, provision should be made by the staff for an approximate equivalent of the nursery-school environment. Under these conditions hospitalization becomes tolerable.

SITUATIONS FOR FURTHER STUDY

1. How would you handle the problem if a mother displayed unusual concern because her 16-month-old boy had gained only 4 pounds since he was a year old?

2. What information would you need if a mother asked you for help in solving a "stubborn feeding problem" in her 18-month-old child?

3. What principles guide your behavior when you are with a child during a play period? Write a description of a toddler's play and your interaction with him. What purpose was his play serving? What problems did you encounter in this experience?

4. In what ways could a cleft palate interfere with a child's speech development?

5. John, 16 months of age, was a laborer's child. He had no toys to play with and whenever his mother took him shopping with her, she scolded him because he pulled the merchandise from the shelves while she looked over the stock. What results might this have on the child's learning at school? How could you help this mother to obtain play materials for John and how would you go about increasing this mother's insight into John's need for exploration?

6. What purpose do rituals serve in the life of the toddler? Interview a mother to discover the rituals her child devised for his care at home. Put them to use in your nursing care of him and describe his responses to you as you instituted them.

7. Discuss the ways in which your opinion relating to discipline for the toddler differs from the authors'. Cite the experiences on which you base your judgment.

8. During a period of care of a toddler, study his behavior to determine the decisions he is capable of making. How did he respond when you gave him choices and let him take the lead in showing you how he liked to have his care given?

9. Observe mothers with their toddlers in a tot-lot or on a playground. What were the different ways in which mothers handled their children when they were aggressive with each other? What variety of values did you note as you observed mothers supervising their children's play?

10. With what problems is the healthy toddler struggling? What behavior patterns might result from discipline which curtailed the toddler's efforts to find himself?

11. Read pages 57 to 65 in the book by Freud and Burlingham. Why were the children described so difficult to deal with? What did you gain from reading these descriptions of children's behavior which was helpful to you in the care of hospitalized toddlers?

12. Read pages 63 to 71 in Robertson's *Hospital and Children: A Parent's-Eye View* and comment on the values that the book might have for the public health nurse as she deals with mothers of young children who have been hospitalized.

13. Read the case of Alan on page 149 in Robertson's book. What were some of the reasons why Alan could not make a constructive adjustment to hospitalization? Do you think the mother's reactions to Alan's predicament were appropriate or inappropriate to the situation? How did the physician's response to the mother's anxiety as cited on page 151 affect her behavior? Why was her anxiety increased rather than assuaged by his behavior? What feelings might have motivated the nurse to pull down the shade between Alan and his mother? What other methods do nurses use to separate mothers and children? What might be the source of the urge to separate mother and child? After such an experience as Alan had, how do you imagine he might react when he becomes a parent and learns that his child must be hospitalized?

14. If you had been the nurse caring for 4-year-old Bill with leukemia, how would you have helped his mother to become more comfortable in visiting him? What might have prompted her infrequent visits to the ward? What responsibilities would you have toward Bill after he had begun to let himself depend on you for care?

15. What is the core problem with which the preschool child struggles? How does knowledge of psychosocial development during this period help you in the provision of care for the preschooler?

16. Read the story of Tommy's mother's activity in coping with her son's sexual curiosity (Fraiberg, page 212). What steps did she take in meeting the children's need to gain control of their impulses? Dis-

cuss her method in relation to your feelings relating to the way sex play should be handled.

17. Read the article by Joyce Robertson and comment on your reactions to the length of time it took her daughter to assimilate the experience of a tonsillectomy. Of what value was the hospital experience to her child? What effects did rooming-in have on the mother-child relationship? What benefits did you derive from reading this study?

18. After viewing the two films cited in the bibliography, contrast the adjustment that the two child patients made to hospitalization. Cite the behavior you observed which led you to conclude that each child's adjustment was constructive or nonconstructive. What signs of anxiety did you observe in Laura? In her mother? What changes did you see in Laura's relationship to her mother as the film progressed? Why do you suppose Laura was more responsive to her father than to her mother? What was the reason why it took Laura so long to respond to her mother when she arrived for visiting on the day after her operation? Why do you think Laura demanded that her crib side be raised? Had you been the nurse providing play periods for Laura, how would you have conducted them?

19. Read the monograph by Florence Erickson and write a report showing the way in which she conducted the study and the results that she obtained which provide insight into the way children feel about intrusive procedures. What recommendations did she make?

BIBLIOGRAPHY

Almy, M.: Young Children's Thinking, N. Y., Teachers College Press, Columbia, 1967.

Bettelheim, B.: Dialogues with Mothers, Glencoe, Ill., The Free Press, 1962.

Bowlby, J.: Maternal Care and Mental Health, Geneva, World Health Organization, 1952.

———: Separation Anxiety: A Critical Review of the Literature, N. Y., Child Welfare League of America, Inc., 1964.

Branstetter, E.: The young child's response to hospitalization: Separation anxiety or lack of mothering care? Am. J. Pub. Health 59:92, 1969.

Brown, R.: Language: The system and its acquisition, in Social Psychology, N. Y., The Free Press, Collier-Macmillan Limited, 1965.

Bruner, J., Oliver, R., and Greenfield, P.: Studies in Cognitive Growth, N. Y., 1966.

Caldwell, B.: What is the Optimal Learning Environment For the Young Child? in Chess, S. and Thomas, A. (eds.) Annual Progress in Child Psychiatry and Child Development, N. Y., Bruner/Mazel, 1968.

Child Welfare League of America, Inc.: Maternal Deprivation, N. Y., 1962.

Darmarin, F., and Cattell, R.: Personality Factors in Early Childhood and Their Relation to Intelligence, Monographs of the Society for Research in Child Development, Vol. 33, No. 6.

Doland, D., and Adelberg, K.: The learning of shared behavior, Child Development 38:695, 1967.

Erickson, F.: Play Interviews for Four-Year-Old Hospitalized Children, Monograph of the Society for Research in Child Development, Inc., Lafayette, Indiana, Child Development Publications, Purdue University, 1958.

Erikson, E. H.: Childhood and Society, N. Y., Norton, 1963.

Ervin-Tripp, S.: Language Development, in Hoffman, M., and Hoffman, L., (eds.) Review of Child Development Research, Vol. II, N. Y., Russell Sage Foundation, 1966.

Flavell, J.: The Developmental Psychology of Jean Piaget, D., Van Nostrand Co., Inc., Princeton, N. J., 1964.

Fox, F. N., and Campbell, D.: Young children in a new situation without their mothers, Child Development 39:123, 1968.

Freeberg, N., and Payne, D.: Parental Influence on Cognitive Development in Early Childhood: A Review, in Chess, S. and Thomas, A. (eds.) Annual Progress in Child Psychiatry and Child Development, N. Y., Burner/Mazel, 1968.

Freud, A.: The Ego and the Mechanisms of Defence, N. Y., Internat. Univ. Press, 1946.

———: The role of bodily illness in the mental life of children, Psychoanal. Stud. Child, 7:68, 1952.

Freud, A., and Burlingham, D. T.: Infants Without Families, N. Y., Internat. Univ. Press, 1944.

Glass, D. C. (Ed.): Environmental Influences, N. Y., The Rockefeller University Press and Russell Sage Foundation, 1968.

Goldberg, S., and Lewis, M.: Play behavior in the year-old infant: Early sex differences, Child Development 40:20, 1969.

Heinicke, C., and Westheimer, I.: Brief Separations, N. Y., Internat. Univ. Press, 1965.

Kagan, J.: Acquisition and Significance of Sex Typing and Sex Role Identity, in Hoffman, M. and Hoffman, L. (eds.) Review of Child Development Research, Vol. I, N. Y., Russell Sage Foundation, 1964.

Katan, A.: Some thoughts about the role of verbalization in early childhood Psychoanal. Stud. Child, 16:184, 1961.

Kidd, A., and Livoire, J. (Eds.): Perceptual Development in Children, N. Y., Internat. Univ. Press, 1966.

Kohlberg, L.: Development of Moral Character and Moral Ideology, in Hoffman, M., and Hoffman, L., (eds.) Review of Child Development Research, Vol. I, N. Y., Russell Sage Foundation, 1964.

———: Early education: A cognitive-developmental view, Child Development 39:1013, 1968.

Kuhn, D., Madsen, C., and Becker, W.: Effects of exposure to an aggressive model and 'frustration' on children's aggressive behavior, Child Development 38:695, 1967.

Lampl-de-Groot, J.: The Development of the Mind, N. Y., Internat. Univ. Press, 1965.

Laurendeau, M., and Pinard, A.: Causal Thinking in the Child, N. Y., Internat. Univ. Press, 1962.

Lewis, M. M.: Language, Thought and Personality in Infancy and Childhood, N. Y., Basic, 1963.

Maccoby, E.: The Development of Sex Differences, Stanford, Stanford Univ. Press, 1966.

Malmquist, C.: Conscience development, Psychoanal. Stud. Child, *23*:301, 1968.

Miles, M. S.: Body integrity fears in a toddler, Nurs. Clin. N. A., *4*:30, 1969.

Murphy, L.: The Widening World of Childhood, N. Y., Basic Books, 1962.

O'Connor, F.: My Oedipus Complex *in* Stories by Frank O'Connor, N. Y., Vantage, 1956.

Palmer, F.: Learning at two, Children *16*:55, 1969.

Piaget, J.: Six Psychological Studies, N. Y., Random House, 1967.

Prugh, D., *et al.:* A study of the emotional reactions of children and families to hospitalization and illness, Am. J. Orthopsychiat. *23*:70, 1953.

Read, K.: Nursery School: A Human Relationship Laboratory, ed. 3, Philadelphia, Saunders, 1960.

————: Young Children in Hospitals, N. Y., Basic, 1958.

————: Hospitals and Children: A Parent's-Eye View, N. Y., Internat. Univ. Press, 1963.

Robertson, J.: A mother's observations on the tonsillectomy of her four-year-old daughter, Psychoanal. Stud. Child, *11*:410, 1956.

Rutherford, E., and Mussen, P.: Generosity in nursery school boys, Child Development *39*:755, 1968.

Sears, R., Rau, L., and Alpert, R.: Identification and Child Rearing, Stanford, Stanford Univ. Press, 1965.

Seidl, F. W.: Pediatric nursing personnel and parent participation: A study in attitudes, Nursing Res. *18*:40, 1969.

Senn, M.: Early childhood education—for what goals?, Children *16*:8, 1969.

Siegel, I.: The Attainment of Concepts, *in* Hoffman, M., and Hoffman, L., (eds.) Review of Child Development Research, Vol. I, N. Y., Russell Sage Foundation, 1964.

Simon, W., and Gagnon, J.: Psychosexual development, Transaction *6*:9, 1969.

Vroegh, K.: Masculinity and feminity in the preschool years, Child Development *39*:1253, 1968.

Ward, W.: Reflection—impulsivity in kindergarten children, Child Development *39*:867, 1968.

Wexler, S. S.: The Story of Sandy, N. Y., Signet, 1958.

World Health Organization: Deprivation of Maternal Care, A Reassessment of its Effects, Geneva, 1962.

Yarrow, L. J.: Separation from Parents During Early Childhood, *in* Hoffman, M., and Hoffman, L.: (eds.) Review of Child Development Research, Vol. I, N. Y., Russell Sage Foundation, 1964.

Films

Robertson, J.: (1953) Film: *A Two-Year-Old Goes to Hospital:* 16 mm. sound, 45 min., English or French (abridged version, English only, 30 min.). Guide Book. Tavistock Child Development Research Unit (London); New York University Film Library; United Nations, Geneva, etc.

————: (1958) Film: *Going to Hospital With Mother.* 16 mm., sound, 40 min., English or French. Guide Book. Tavistock Child Development Research Unit (London); New York University Film Library; United Nations, Geneva, etc.

Books for Children

Coleman, L.: A Visit to the Hospital, New York, Wonder Books, Inc., 1958.

Ets, M. H.: The Story of a Baby, New York, Viking Press, 1939.

Gruenberg, S. M.: The Wonderful Story of How You Were Born, Garden City, New York, Hanover House, 1952.

Peller, L., and Mumford, S.: Our New Baby, New York, The Vanguard Press, 1943.

17

Prevention of Accidents and the Care of Injured and Poisoned Children

During the first year of life the infant was relatively safe in the hands of his guardians. Only a few general rules had to be observed to protect him from harm so long as he remained in his crib, high chair or playpen. If he was properly guarded against falls, the misuse of drugs and the mischievous experiments of slightly older children in the household, he was not likely to suffer injury. Accidental death forms only a small segment of the standard infant mortality rate, i.e., deaths during the first year of life. Thereafter the situation reverses rapidly. As the dangers of birth and congenital malformation begin to recede, accidents jump to the head of the list of causes of death and remain there throughout childhood.

With his ability to crawl, walk and climb the toddler is able to seek out trouble on his own. His normal curiosity leads him into a great variety of dangers, first within the house and later on the street or about the outdoor premises. He has little past experience or judgment with which to inhibit his explorations. Consequently, he must be continually watched until he is old enough to understand and abide by the prohibitions which are imposed for his safety. Boys are generally more aggressive and less tractable than girls and, accordingly, are more frequently the victims of accidents of every kind.

The great variety of dangers to which the toddler suddenly gains access (Table 14) makes the task of accident prevention a difficult one. His elders cannot foresee all the possible hazards. The best approach is to cultivate in parents an attitude of alertness toward the main types of danger and to encourage the neutralization of these dangers in ways which will still permit the toddler a maximal degree of freedom. He deserves an opportunity to explore his enlarging world and will be helped toward self-preservation if he learns from painful experience about some of its minor threats. Listed below are examples of the main types of accident to which he is prone. The order follows the approximate frequency with which each type is seen as a cause of death or serious injury. The discussion of accidents which follows is oriented toward safety in the home, but the same principles should govern the care of children who come temporarily under the nurse's responsibility when they are admitted to a hospital or a convalescent home.

The management of many of these forms of injury in childhood is traditionally within the province of the surgeon. Only a few of the varieties which require medical care will be considered here.

INCIDENCE OF ACCIDENTS

A National Health Survey in 1962 estimated that approximately 30 per cent of the children under the age of 5 years in the United States suffered some variety of accident or poisoning during each year.

Table 14. Common Mechanisms of Accidental Injury and Death in Early Childhood

1. Motor vehicles: Both as passengers and as pedestrians
2. Burns: From heating apparatus —stoves, heaters, humidifiers, radiators, irons
   From open fires—fireplaces, outdoor fires, matches, lighters
   From hot liquids—bathwater, cooking fluids, tea, coffee
   From electric circuits—defective wiring, unguarded outlets
   From strong acids and alkalis—lye, ammonia
3. Drowning: Bathtub, sink, wells, cisterns, swimming pool, ponds, ditches and large bodies of water
4. Falls: From furniture, stairs, porches, unguarded windows
5. Poisons: Drugs (aspirin, sedatives, tranquilizers, antihistamines, antihypertensives, ferrous sulfate, endocrine products)
   Insecticides and rodenticides
   Cleansing agents—kerosene, lye, ammonia, detergents, bleaches, dishwashing compounds
   Cosmetics, coldwave neutralizers, perfume
   Antiseptics
   Alcohol
   Cigarette butts
   Paints containing lead
6. Suffocation: Plastic bags, discarded refrigerators, carbon monoxide gas
7. Foreign bodies: Nuts (especially peanuts), dried beans, pins, (straight, safety and bobby), toys, coins, chewing gum, medals, nails, nuts, screws and bolts
8. Cuts and punctures: Knives, scissors, large needles, can openers, broken glass, power tools
9. Crush injuries from wringers

While the preponderance of these events were minor home accidents, the total amount of death and disability resulting during this single year was considerable: over 8,000 deaths; 40-50,000 survivors with permanent disability; over 200,000 hospitalized for this reason alone; unmeasurable quantities of psychic trauma to children and parents which impede normal growth and development of the child.

ACCIDENT PREVENTION

During infancy the parents or other caretakers are entirely responsible for the child's safety. But as he develops and gains independent action and a wider range of unsupervised activity, his safety depends increasingly upon habits of self-protection and prudence which have been inculcated by the explanation, discipline and example set by his parents. Physicians and nurses can exert their best influence by discussing potential hazards and methods of averting them with the parents of developing children, either through personal or group sessions or by the distribution of pamphlets and other literature calling attention to the hazards of the age (Table 15).

Table 15. Common Household and Outdoor Hazards for the Toddler

Hazard	Protection
Drugs, chemicals, sharp instruments	Keep in closets, cabinets or drawers which are locked, inaccessible, or tightly wedged with cardboard
Burns and scalds	Keep guards around stoves, heaters and fireplaces Keep matches well out of reach Keep stove utensils back from the edge Use no hanging table cloths or runners
Falls from unguarded stairs, porches	Use gates
windows	Use window guards or fastened screens
furniture	Make discipline consistent, and use gates
car doors	Use safety locks; discipline
Electricity	Use plastic plugs or tape over unused sockets Repair defective wiring Place fans, mixers and power equipment out of reach
Drowning	Never leave full tub unguarded Fence ponds and swimming pools Use consistent discipline at the beach
Traffic	Lock or hook outside doors Use consistent discipline on the street
Aspiration of foreign bodies	Keep small objects such as marbles, jacks, safety pins, buttons, nails out of reach in cupboards Make sure that toys have no parts that are easily removable, such as small wheels, eyes of dolls, etc.
Ingestion of lead	Repair defective walls and repaint peeling surfaces with lead-free paints

Many of the most serious accidents happen so rapidly that serious or even irreversible damage occurs before an adult can intervene. Prevention of these catastrophes is the most logical approach. The precipitous rise in our national rate of accidents and the multiplying hazards of modern life have stimulated a number of organizations to put on campaigns to educate the public toward better safety measures. The National Safety Council, the Children's Bureau, state and local health departments, insurance companies and many other public and private agencies are conducting such programs through the media of advertising, articles in popular magazines, pamphlets and talks on radio and television. Nurses and doctors can make an important contribution by relating these general principles to specific families and the actual risks which their members run. Well-baby and well-child conferences and contacts with the parents of sick children provide numerous opportunities to inquire about hazards and remind parents of the poisonous nature of drugs and household chemicals. The nurse who pays a home visit has a particularly valuable opportunity to make a safety check and offer specific suggestions. Table 15 lists a few of the more common sources of trouble.

A forward-looking safety program has the objective of gradually encouraging the child to learn how to exert his own controls. Restraint and discipline are necessary for the young toddler, but they should be carried out in such a way that he becomes neither resentful nor overcautious and fearful. With some of the trivial hazards he can be warned of the danger but permitted to discover by trial and error that what he proposes to do is unpleasant. If his mother thus becomes a reliable prophet, gradually he will learn to accept her cautions and be willing to divert his attention to the alternate amusement she suggests. Mothers should avoid constant nagging, since it rapidly loses force. They should also learn how to make constructive suggestions, substituting less dangerous toys or occupations for the ones which are forbidden. With potentially dangerous activities, discipline must be firm, prompt and consistent. Turning on the gas burners should not be treated as a cute performance which commands the sly approval of adults, for it may at a later time be responsible for a fire or carbon monoxide poisoning of the household. A similar attitude must be taken toward running into the street, dangerous climbing within the house and manipulation of hot water faucets and electrical equipment. However, the number of absolute prohibitions should be kept to a minimum so that the mother is not continually interfering with the toddler's need to gain knowledge about and mastery of his environment. It is also important that physical punishment be reserved for truly dangerous rather than merely annoying behavior.

As the toddler grows, he normally will have increasing faith in his mother's direction and will be able to dispense with some of the protections originally devised. Often he will not only begin to heed his own controls but may also keep the adults around him in line. However, when discipline has been nagging, spiteful, unjust or overanxious and inconsistent, the result may be anything but satisfactory. Some children respond to such discipline with timidity. They are afraid to try anything new, including perhaps even those enterprises that lead to success in school. Others abuse their newly acquired physical prowess in constant reckless experimentation to see how much they can get away with or to punish the person who has tried to inhibit their curiosity and drive toward mastery. As with other aspects of character formation, the toddler age is often most important in molding the attitudes toward safety which guide the child in later years.

The multiplicity of types of accident and poisoning makes it impossible to cover all the various situations which may arise. Only the more common and serious ones are here presented as examples.

BURNS

Pathophysiology

The degree of disturbance of general body function depends upon the extent and depth of the burn. *First degree* burns, such as sunburn, involve only the superficial layers of the skin and produce erythema, pain, mild blistering and peeling. But there are no significant constitutional changes, loss of fluid homeostasis or danger from local infection. *Second degree* burns imply deeper damage into the skin from prolonged contact with open flames, hot liquids or other objects. Death of tissue with loss of the cellular components, and more particularly, loss of the integrity of the vascular bed which serves the burned area account for some of the immediate disturbances of metabolism. Damage to blood vessel walls permits leakage of fluid through them into the surrounding tissues and the formation of local edema. There may be additional loss of protein and fluid from the surface of the burned area as necrosis progresses. If the burned area is extensive, i.e., exceeding 15 to 20 per cent of the total body skin surface, enough fluid may be lost from the intravascular compartment so that blood volume is reduced and the patient is threatened with hypovolemic shock. Renal blood flow is also reduced at a time when it is most needed to aid in the clearance of nitrogenous and potassium components of the cells killed by the burn. Later, the denuded skin becomes vulnerable to infection by bacteria from the environment because the normally thick epithelium is replaced with open granulation tissue. In *third degree* burns, the damage from more prolonged exposure to flame or to electric currents results in destruction of tissue completely through the skin layers and may

Table 16. Percentage of Total Body Surface Contributed by Different Regions at Several Ages

Area	Newborn	3 Years	6 Years	12 Years
Head and neck	18%	15%	12%	6%
Trunk	40	40	40	38
Arms	16	16	16	18
Legs	26	29	32	38

involve muscle, nerve, supporting structures and bone as well. Such deep burns exaggerate the metabolic effects for the amount of area involved. They also lead to later problems of restoration of missing skin and deeper structures if the patient survives. Since third degree burns coagulate the tissues and destroy the nerve supply, they can be recognized by their white color due to lack of blood and by their insensitivity to pinprick.

Extent

Since the metabolic consequences of a burn will depend mainly upon the amount of body surface involved, severity is usually measured in such terms. Table 16 offers a rough guide to the evaluation of surface area involved at different ages. It should be remembered that the percentages apply to involvement of the total length and circumference of the portions of anatomy and that the fraction of each percentage must be estimated from the individual burn. As a rule, second degree burns of less than 10 per cent of the surface can be managed with emergency local therapy. When 15 to 20 per cent or more is involved, hospitalization is probably desirable to observe and treat systemic effects. All third degree burns require closer observation and burns involving the face and neck or which threaten the airway must be regarded as emergencies.

Management of Minor Burns

The burned area should be covered with a clean, preferably sterile, cloth while the child is being taken for medical care. Cleansing and superficial debridement are usually performed and the area is then covered with nonadherent gauze and bandaged tightly. If no toxic symptoms occur, the bandage is usually left in place for 7 to 10 days. If fever or other suspicion of infection arises, it must be removed and the wound inspected, cultured and redressed and appropriate antibiotic therapy begun.

Severe Burns

Initial Management. Burns around the face or from inhalation of flame, smoke or noxious gases demand that the first concern be maintenance of an adequate airway. Since edema of burned skin and mucous membrane of the respiratory tract is likely to advance after the first few hours, whenever there is doubt about the adequacy of subsequent ventilation, endotracheal intubation or a tracheostomy should be performed.

Sterile precautions should be employed in the subsequent care of such tubes (p. 561) in order to avoid contamination of the lower respiratory tract.

Once the airway has been assured, the child should be weighed in order to provide a basis for later calculations. In anticipation of present or impending shock and the necessity for electrolyte therapy, an intravenous infusion must be placed and carefully maintained. The bladder is usually catheterized with an indwelling catheter to facilitate accurate determination of urine production. A nasogastric tube may also be placed to protect the child against aspiration of stomach contents. Tetanus prophylaxis with toxoid, and sedation to relieve anxiety and deaden pain should also be included in the early ministrations to the severely burned child.

Fluids and Electrolytes. An attempt must be made to anticipate the changes in intravascular fluid volume, the shift of electrolytes, the depression of renal function and the effects of severe stress. Initial measurements of hemoglobin, hematocrit, serum proteins and electrolytes and determination of urinary flow and specific gravity must be supplemented by repeated determinations and accurate knowledge of intake and output of fluids. Several general schemes are available for the initial programming of the administration of glucose, electrolyte solutions, plasma, dextran and whole blood. Any such scheme must be modified periodically according to the response of the patient. Consequently, the accurate monitoring and recording of the kind and amount of fluids administered and the output and loss of fluids as urine, vomitus and aspirate which is entrusted to the nursing staff may become a crucial factor in the survival of a badly burned child.

Therapy of the Skin. The major problem in managing the skin is to prevent or minimize bacterial infection until epithelial regeneration or grafting procedures have restored the protective surface. Systemic antibiotic therapy is useful but limited. Usually penicillin is administered to prevent invasion by beta-hemolytic streptococci. But the contaminants which too frequently appear are staphylococci, pseudomonas or proteus organisms which are indifferently susceptible even to the newer antibiotics. Consequently, a number of technics have been devised to discourage bacterial invasion. After initial cleansing and removal of dead tissue under sedation or anesthesia, one or more of the following technics may be employed.

OCCLUSIVE DRESSINGS. Occlusive dressings with antibiotic ointments (bacitracin, polymyxin, gentamicin) are very satisfactory for burns limited to the extremities where tight, circumferential dressings can be applied and left on for several days. Initial treatment by this technic is often successful in defeating secondary infection.

EXPOSURE. Exposure is necessary for burns about the face, perineum and trunk. An attempt is made to keep the child in as sterile an environment as possible by the use of sterile sheets and reverse isolation technic. Antibiotic ointments may be used in addition to prevent the infection of tissues beneath the crusts which will eventually form to render partial protection. Frequent changes of position of the child and adequate maintenance of body temperature complicate the nursing care.

WET DRESSINGS. Wet dressings of 0.5 per cent aqueous silver nitrate which are moistened frequently and completely changed twice a day decrease bacterial contamination and fluid loss from the burned area. They may, however, result in considerable losses of sodium, potassium and chloride from the burned area —losses which must be anticipated and corrected by adequate replacement through oral or intravenous administration. The use of Sulfamylon as a topical application with daily bathing is another technic used to protect against infection.

GRAFTING. Grafting of skin is necessary to bridge over third degree defects and is usually carried out when infection is under control, preferably during the first 2 to 3 weeks. Sometimes very early grafting is done as a temporary measure to protect against infection and excessive fluid loss.

Later Complications. In addition to the early hazards of shock, electrolyte disturbances and the ever present danger of systemic infection, there are a number of complications which must be of concern to the persons attending the child who is convalescing from a severe burn. Among them are malnutrition, duodenal ulcer, contractures from the scar tissue of the healing burn, hepatic failure, pneumonia, osteoporosis, renal calculi and urinary tract infection. Almost universal among these victims are major problems of psychologic and emotional rehabilitation after the trauma inflicted by the burn itself and by the necessity for painful treatments, immobilization, and acceptance of handicaps and disfigurement of the body and the body image. The problem of helping parents through the crisis may be as serious as that presented by the child.

Nursing Care. IMMEDIATE CARE OF THE SEVERELY BURNED CHILD. In severe burns, the first consideration must be given to the prevention of shock (or the treatment, if shock has already appeared) and of the toxic state that may ensue. In some instances, local treatment of the burn will be deferred until these dangers are over. Where it is necessary to carry out a debridement early, adequate anesthesia or sedation is essential not only for humanitarian reasons but to minimize pain which may otherwise aggravate shock.

In shock, insufficient cardiac output reduces the blood volume, which is further depressed by passage of plasma through the blood vessels and into the tissues. Such sluggish circulation does not meet the minimal metabolic requirements, so that normal function of vital organs may be impaired by anoxia and by slow interchange of nutrients and waste products

Fig. 17-1. Illustrating the care of a burned child on a Bradford frame. Waterproof material is used to protect from contamination the burned areas on the thighs. To collect urine specimens from an incontinent child, waterproof material should be used to construct the trough leading into the bed pan.

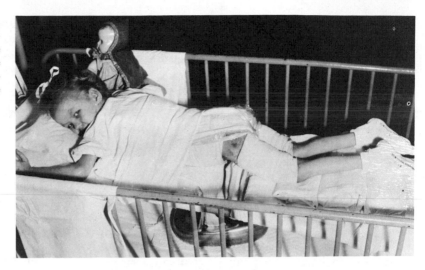

with the blood stream. The loss of plasma results in increased concentration of red blood cells. This affords a simple means of measuring the severity of the shock and the effectiveness of its treatment. Either the red blood-cell count or the hematocrit reading of the blood may be used as a rough guide.

The nurse must remember that shock after burns may be delayed because fluid loss is not as rapid as in the case of cutting wounds. Therefore she should be alert for symptoms of shock for some hours after admission, including decrease in systolic and diastolic blood pressure, drop in pulse pressure, pallor and clamminess of the skin. Children in shock may also complain of thirst and are extremely apprehensive. The nurse's activities immediately after admission of a burned child must be concentrated on close observation of these vital signs and the state of peripheral circulation in order that she may inform the physician of changes in the child's condition.

If shock is suspected, the lower extremities may be elevated to an angle of 45 degrees and the body aligned so that the thorax is slightly lower than the pelvis. The main element of treatment is to attempt to restore blood volume by intravenous injection of plasma expanders in amounts large enough to counteract the losses through the capillary walls. Oxygen may be required to combat anoxia and sedation to relieve pain. The room should be warm enough to maintain body temperature but application of external heat is not recommended since it may cause dilation of the peripheral vessels. If possible, the patient should be in a room where the heat and humidity can be controlled.

Once the blood volume has been supported adequately, additional parenteral fluids may be necessary to maintain an adequate fluid intake, promote urinary output and counteract acidosis.

The nurse must be alert to signs of respiratory distress, including restlessness, rapid respiration, cyanosis, coughing or crowing with inspiration. If the airway is endangered, oxygenation of the blood may be assisted by tracheal intubation, tracheotomy or by a mechanical respirator. The care of a child with a tracheostomy is discussed on page 561 of the Appendix.

On hospital admission of a burned child, emergency equipment, including tracheostomy and cut down tray, intravenous fluids, instruments and catheterization tray should be in readiness. In most hospitals, gowns and masks are required for anyone initially coming in contact with the child. After treatment of actual or impending shock, the nurse may assist in careful and gentle removal of the child's clothing and insertion of the catheter which is necessary for accurate measurement of urinary output. A nasogastric tube may also be necessary if there is nausea, abdominal distention or vomiting. Examination of the child and determination of the extent of the burn is done by the physician after emergency treatment has been given. If morphine is necessary, it is usually given intravenously because of poor subcutaneous absorption due to inadequate circulation. Sites for intramuscular injections for tetanus prophylaxis and for antibiotics may be limited if the burn is extensive, but any adequate muscle mass may be utilized.

The method chosen for treatment of the burned area will depend on the preferences of the physician. The goal in any case is the avoidance of infection and the promotion of healing. Prior to treatment of the burn, a bath with 3 per cent of hexachlorophene soap to remove gross debris or grease may be ordered, followed by a rinse with distilled water particularly if silver nitrate application is to be used. Gauze dressings, medication, stockinette or elastic rolls should be in readiness according to the method of treatment selected.

SUPPORTIVE CARE AND PHYSICAL HYGIENE. Subsequent nursing care varies according to the individual method of treatment selected. The plan of nursing care will also be influenced by the location and the extent of the burned areas and by the age and the needs of the particular child. The use of rigid isolation technics, masks and gowns varies according to the routines of the hospital and the type of treatment selected. Gown and mask technic and sterilized linen placed over the Bradford frame or the bed is an added measure to prevent cross-infection. In the nursing care of any burned child, frequent hand washing and the restriction of personnel with infections is mandatory.

A private room where heat and humidity can be controlled, or placement in a burn unit where oxygen, suction and hand washing facilities are available simplifies subsequent nursing care and reduces risk of infection. The use of a Bradford or Stryker frame or CircOlectric bed is highly desirable in extensive trunk and extremity burns (Fig. 17-1). Contractures can be prevented by maintaining good posture; urine specimens can be collected when the child is incontinent; and wound contamination from feces and urine can be lessened or prevented. If the head of the Bradford frame is hung higher than the foot, gravity will produce a downward flow of urine. By using two pieces of waterproof material, each 6 by 18 inches, to form a trough leading into a bedpan placed beneath the opening of the frame, urine can be collected more easily. One piece of the material should be placed under the buttocks and over the edge of the frame, while the other should be secured over the pubes and brought down over the perineum and into the bedpan. To determine kidney function, accurate measurement of urine must be recorded. The survival of the child may depend on meticulous determination of input and output with adequate fluid replacement. A chart for recording of intake and output should be in a prominent place near the patient's bed. The nurse is also responsible for monitoring the parenteral infusions, for frequent checks for leakage around the catheter site and to determine that the flow rate of the infusion is in precise relation to the patient's output.

Pressure areas, contractures and deformities can be prevented and the grafted area kept at rest by rigid adherence to a schedule for turning and repositioning. The patient should be turned from back to side at 2 to 3 hour intervals. Discomfort to the child can be reduced and touching of open wound areas avoided if several nurses assist the child in turning. When two beds with Bradford frames are available, the child can be lifted and turned directly onto a clean frame. The use of a Stryker frame also reduces turning discomfort. When the neck is burned anteriorly, a roll under the shoulders will hyperextend it and prevent disfiguring contractures. Sandbags or specially applied restraints may be indicated for immobilization. Constant supervision is essential to readjust appliances which prevent crippling complications that require traction or plastic surgery to correct. Measures to prevent foot drop are required. When the child is lying on his abdomen, a pillow placed beneath his thighs will keep his feet in good position.

Skin around the burned area can be kept free from irritating exudate and in good condition by frequent cleansing, massaging and application of petrolatum. When the lower extremities are burned, pressure on the heels can be prevented by supporting the thighs on small pillows to elevate the heels from the frame or the bed.

When the child is young and the burned area is irritating, arm restraints may be required to keep him from infecting the area with his hands. However, when dressings are utilized, snug coverings which keep the wound inaccessible can be applied. If the child is not too ill, suitable play materials will interest him and divert his attention from the skin irritation.

When the buttocks and the genitalia are burned, care to lessen dressing contamination and to promote healing is indicated. If enemas are necessary, waterproof materials must be used to prevent dressing contaminations. After bowel evacuation, the perineum should be cleansed with cotton balls and oil, and in some instances careful irrigation of the area with warm normal saline solution will help to cleanse the fecal material completely from the burned area. When the penis and the scrotum are burned, frequent cleansing and application of dressings reduce the incidence of infection. When the child is on his abdomen, a diaper sling under the frame opening will support the edematous organs and maintain the position of the dressing.

DRESSING CHANGES AND DEBRIDEMENT. Dressing changes are anxiety producing and emotionally exhausting for the child and also for the nurse. The necessity for them must be accepted by both and minute explanations given to the child before any treatment is attempted. Every opportunity to enlist the child's constructive assistance must be utilized and the individual child's needs to express his distress or for assistance in controlling himself during this painful procedure must be given every consideration.

When silver nitrate treatment is being utilized, dressings are kept continuously wet and changed twice daily. Thick gauze pads are applied to all burn areas and saturated with the silver nitrate solution. A catheter may be incorporated into the dressing to aid in later moistening which is done at 2 to 4 hour intervals. Application of petrolatum to healthy skin adjacent to the burn area contains the silver nitrate solution. With exposure to ultraviolet light, silver nitrate turns black and therefore results in housekeeping problems. Difficulties with staining can be reduced by protecting mattresses and pillows with plastic covers and by protecting floors with several coats of wax. Stainless steel utensils should be kept in the unit and stained linens washed with a solution of Wescodyne and soap.

If Gentamicin Sulfate ointment is the treatment of choice, dressings may be soaked off in a tub daily prior to reapplication of the dressing, held in place by

Kerlix gauze. In reapplication of both Gentamicin Sulfate or Sulfamylon ointment, gauze should not cover joint areas in long strips which immobilize the joint when dry.

When the eschar begins to separate from the underlying tissues, the nurse may be called on to assist in the debridement of loose crusts by the gentle use of dental forceps and scissors. Extreme care and patience are necessary to avoid bleeding and to cause as little pain as possible.

Physical therapy is often begun as soon as possible in order to assist in debridement, to maintain muscle tone and to prevent contractures. When silver nitrate application is the treatment method of choice, the patient is placed in a 50 gallon tub of temperature-controlled, balanced saline solution every 2 days for 20 minutes. Agitation of the water results in debridement of dead tissue. In any schedule of exercises, the nurse should consult with the physical therapist in order to continue recommended passive and active exercises at intervals throughout the day as the patient's condition permits.

NUTRITION. After the patient is able to tolerate clear liquids given orally, frequent feeding of foods high in calories, protein and iron is imperative to lessen the degree of hypoproteinemia and anemia. During the early stages of the illness, loss of nitrogen is great. It is lost when it passes from the surrounding areas into the burned tissue, when it is excreted from the body by way of the urinary tract and when exudate is formed. Frequently, poor appetite is encountered, and when protein intake is insufficient, hypoproteinemia develops rapidly. In encouraging appetite, the nurse should ascertain the patient's food preferences and accustomed mealtime habits. The timing for serving meals should be thoughtfully selected to avoid offering food when the patient is physically or emotionally exhausted—such as immediately following dressing changes. In some instances Amigen, a casein digest, is given orally. Through use of this material larger amounts of protein may be given than when unhydrolyzed protein alone is used. Often, vitamins B and C are given to accelerate healing and to stimulate appetite. Iron therapy is used when anemia begins to develop. Grafts do not grow well when the red blood-cell count and the hemoglobin are low.

Encouraging ingestion of fluids aids the body in eliminating toxins, maintains body-fluid requirements and prevents kidney damage when sulfonamide therapy is used to prevent or control infection. During the first few days, thirst from dehydration may be increased, and care must be taken not to give fluids too rapidly, for nausea and vomiting are produced easily. After this period, encouragement is usually necessary to keep the intake at desired levels. Accurate intake records allow for comparison with output, so that the onset of kidney impairment may be detected.

EMOTIONAL SUPPORT. Long periods of immobilization, isolation from family and playmates and overwhelming painful and frightening experiences involve mental attitudes that must be taken into account in the provision of nursing care. The accident itself is a harrowing experience. If it resulted from doing things that his parents had cautioned him not to do, the child may regard his pain as punishment for his misdeeds. If the burn resulted because he did not have his mother's protection when he needed it, he may have pronounced antagonism toward his parents. Such feelings may be expressed directly toward the parents, but much more commonly they are transferred to those people who care for him. Encouragement to express his aggression verbally or in play is highly important; if he represses it, his appetite may dwindle, his relationship with his parents will be further impaired, and his course in general will be affected.

Outwardly some children seem to accept painful experiences, but on closer observation one sees signs of anxiety. When a child reacts to pain with shrieks it is trying to the nurse in attendance, but this is one of the means by which the child's mental health can be protected, for it provides great release for his feelings. Keeping feelings buried is harmful. If a nurse whom the child likes accompanies him to the operating room or to the treatment room for dressings and remains to support him, dreaded experiences can be borne with greater fortitude.

Unless arms and hands are burned, play materials must be provided so the child can work through his feelings about the accident and his treatment. A folded sheet brought under the Bradford frame and pinned to the sides of the crib will form a hammock. This will provide support for his arms and space for toys. The use of the hammock will prevent position changes which result when a child retrieves his fallen playthings from beneath the frame.

The child will enjoy being read to and played with, and his need for companionship should be met. Placing his bed so that he may look out of the door or the window or into a ward of convalescent children will stimulate his individual activities and increase his desire to get well enough to join the group. In the convalescent period he will need the companionship of children and an environment that gives him increasing opportunity to prepare for life at home.

Through observation of the parent-child relationship, feelings of guilt—or lack of concern—will be detected in the parents. If the accident resulted from lack of protection during play or because the parents failed to teach the child about such hazards or to remove dangerous objects from his environment, profound parental remorse would be the expected response. If feelings of guilt are strong and if they adversely influence the parents' attitudes toward themselves or the child, the help of a social worker is indicated. If lack of concern is suspected, investigation into the circumstances leading to the accident should be made by the social worker before the child is discharged from the hospital. In these instances investigation into the stability of the family background might serve to prevent the return of the child to the same environment that played a part in precipitating the injury.

Assisting in a program of burn prevention is the responsibility of the hospital and the public health nurse. The mortality rate due to preventable accidents that produce burns is tremendously high. Little children are social beings. They enjoy the kitchen because they are with their mothers and because there is much there to interest them. For this reason kitchens must be made safe. Preschool children should be taught caution in the use of matches and in observing bonfires. Fires are fascinating to children, and admonition will not stifle their interest in them. Instead, positive direction should be given to teach children *how* to light a match and *when* they may do it and to teach them *how* to watch a fire safely. Adults must be taught to keep inflammable materials out of children's reach and to supervise all bonfires in their neighborhood. If these measures could be instituted, the incidence of burns would be reduced markedly.

TRAUMA

Injuries from falls, from motor vehicle accidents and from encounters with machinery produce a wide variety of anatomic lesions. As with burns, the first considerations are to maintain a patent airway and to watch for or deal with shock. The problems of identifying and evaluating the extent and mechanism of injuries within the skull, chest and abdomen are so diverse that the reader can be given only a synopsis of the management of some of the more common traumata. For detailed discussion, surgical, orthopedic and neurosurgical texts must be consulted.

Head Injuries

Concussion. Few children traverse the early years without suffering some variety of head injury. Most of these result only in bruising or laceration of the scalp. In a few there is evidence of temporary disturbance of cerebral functions which is referred to as concussion. In its mild form this may result in temporary dizziness, headache, vomiting or brief loss of consciousness. Sometimes there may be disturbances of vision or of motion of the eyes. Children usually recover rapidly from simple concussion and within a period of a day or two are restored to normal. The important point in management of concussion is to make sure during the early hours after the injury that no intracranial bleeding has resulted from the trauma.

The first 2 to 6 hours after injury is the critical period in which careful observation is required. During this time impending coma must be watched for.

The parent or the nurse should test the child's state of consciousness by arousing him periodically. In the hospital, accurate observation of pulse, respirations and blood pressure is desirable. Drastic change in these measurements or inability to arouse the child demands prompt investigation. If signs of bleeding are confirmed, neurosurgical exploration usually is indicated. Even though it be attended by a period of unconsciousness, only a very small fraction of children who suffer head injury will have bleeding, but this small fraction presents a dire emergency.

Skull Fracture. The management of skull fracture is primarily a neurosurgical problem. In many instances there is a linear crack in the skull which causes no displacement of the bones and is not associated with bleeding. Management in such instances is the same as for concussion. More serious disturbances result when the break in the bones occasions tearing of blood vessels or distortion of the brain by compression. Some form of operative relief usually is indicated in such instances. Recognition of depression of a skull fracture depends on roentgen examination or on the presence of localizing neurologic findings which indicate abnormal pressure on specific areas of the brain. With severe injuries the problem of managing shock and intracranial pressure is often of primary importance.

Chest Injuries

Crushing or perforating injury of the chest wall may lead to internal bleeding, which carries the risk not only of loss of blood from the circulation, but additionally may compress the lungs within the chest (hemothorax) and interfere with ventilation. Similarly, air under pressure may be introduced into the pleural space when a sucking wound of the chest wall is created, or a lung is punctured by a broken rib or external perforating object. In either event, drainage with negative pressure must be quickly established by the insertion of a thoracotomy tube with underwater seal. Injury to the heart by direct blow or by puncture of the pericardium may similarly lead to extravasation of blood into the pericardial sac and limitation of the filling of the heart due to tamponade. Aspiration or surgical relief must be carried out in this event.

Abdominal Injuries

Rupture of the capsule of the liver or spleen following blows to the abdomen must be recognized promptly to prevent sudden exsanguinating hemorrhage into the peritoneal cavity. Immediate surgical intervention and prompt transfusion are required. Rupture of a kidney may often be treated conservatively since the hemorrhage is contained within a tight space and may cease spontaneously before blood loss is great.

Injuries which perforate or indirectly tear hollow

organs such as the intestines, stomach and bladder must be dealt with by surgical exploration, for the extravasation of the contents of such viscera into the peritoneal cavity or surrounding tissues will be followed by serious infection or irritating inflammatory reactions.

Fractures

In general, children's bones tend to heal more rapidly than those of the adult and tend to correct deformities readily. Because of their greater pliability, long bone fractures are often of the "greenstick" variety without displacement of the full width of the bone. Such fractures are usually corrected by gentle manipulation and casting in corrected position. Long bone fractures with displacement of the fragments may require traction before the application of the cast in order to bring the ends of the bone into better apposition. Compound or multiple fractures will often require open operative reduction.

Flat bones such as the clavicle, ribs and pelvis are generally permitted to heal by simple immobilization. Fractures of vertebral bodies carry the important risk of compression of the spinal cord within the bony column. Head traction, laminectomy or other immobilizing procedures may be indicated for such injuries.

Nursing Care of Trauma

Many of the same principles apply to the nursing care of orthopedic trauma as were discussed previously under the care of burned children. If a fracture necessitates bed rest or traction, the maintenance of proper body alignment, frequent repositioning and skin care to prevent pressure ulcers are of prime importance. The use of massage and active and passive exercise to maintain normal range of joint motion and muscle tone, to improve circulation and to prevent deformities is an important nursing responsibility. In addition the nurse who is caring for a child in traction or a cast must have a knowledge of the musculoskeletal system, the principles behind various traction devices and an understanding of body mechanics.

Care of Children in Casts. The immediate responsibility of the nurse on the admission of a child with orthopedic trauma is to observe the vital signs to detect symptoms of shock. Changes in color, sensation or temperature of extremities distal to the injury should be carefully noted and brought to the attention of the physician. If debridement is necessary to remove debris from an open wound, rigid surgical technic should be employed.

If surgical reduction of the fracture has been necessary, postoperative procedures are followed until the patient is responding well. In either open or closed reduction, a cast is usually applied to maintain immobilization. Until the cast is completely dry, it must be handled carefully to prevent alterations which may result in pressure on a bony prominence or on the underlying tissues. Constant observation is imperative after cast application to detect changes in color of fingers or toes, pallor or blueness and coldness of the skin which may indicate circulatory impairment. Numbness, discomfort, complaints of tightness of the cast or edema and loss of motion should be reported immediately to the attending physician. Frequent turning of the patient reduces discomfort and allows the cast to dry evenly. Plastic covered pillows may be used to maintain proper positioning until the cast has completely dried.

Since plaster casts cannot be cleansed with water, waterproof materials must be used around the buttocks and perineal areas to keep the cast dry, clean and free from offensive odors. A pillow placed under the back during use of the bedpan will also help to prevent cast soiling. If the child is old enough, an overhead trapeze can be helpful in toileting and to prevent skin irritation of the elbows.

Meticulous care and observation of skin adjacent to the cast is of importance to prevent irritation and discomfort and to detect pressure areas. Careful cleansing with soap and water, massage and the application of a soothing ointment may prevent tissue breakdown.

Care of Children in Traction. When traction is used to immobilize a body part, to maintain correct position and to prevent contractures, the position in bed may necessarily be limited. Nevertheless, changes in position may be accomplished through the use of pillows and slight elevation of the head of the bed.

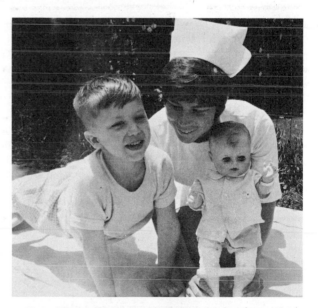

Fig. 17-2. Sensory stimulation and relationships of closeness and trust are essential for the immobilized child. The opportunity to be outdoors encouraged this boy to become physically active. Note the doll, also wearing a spica cast, through which the child was able to express concerns about his body image and treatment procedures.

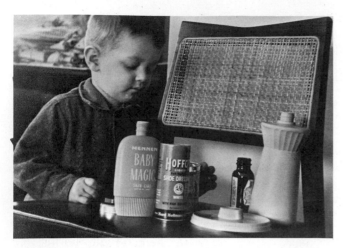

Fig. 17-3. Illustrating the toddler's temptation to explore even those things which his mother cautions him not to touch while she is cleaning high shelves.

The nurse should observe the patient frequently to detect pressure on the heels, irritation or redness of skin, swelling around pin insertions and to ascertain whether pulleys are working properly and weights are hanging freely.

Preventing Effects of Prolonged Immobility. Prolonged immobility may precipitate physiological stresses in addition to hazards to normal emotional and intellectual development. Because of orthostatic hypotension and because of increased heart load resulting from the recumbent position, cardiovascular function is affected. Secretions in the respiratory tract may become a problem because of less efficient clearing of the tract and because of a decrease in the rate and depth of lung expansion. Many children are anorexic after prolonged bed rest and problems of regular elimination are increased. Urinary dysfunction may increase the risk of urinary tract infections. With muscular atrophy and loss of muscle tone, efficiency and strength of muscle action is reduced. Changes in the normal texture of the skin result from circulatory impairment in addition to local pressure. Meticulous nursing care is required to prevent physiological difficulties from developing and prompt treatment is indicated when they do occur. Frequent changes of body position, massage, exercises and constant skin care are extremely important in preventing a large number of the above possible effects from prolonged immobility. Attention to deep breathing and coughing exercises, dietary modifications, environmental aids such as oscillating beds or pressure mattresses and emphasis on regular eliminatory habits are also very helpful in maintaining physiological equilibrium.

The hazards of lengthy hospitalization to healthy emotional development including separation from parents, loss of accustomed surroundings, subjection to frightening procedures and loss of previously accomplished control over body functions have been previously discussed. In addition, prolonged immobility may entail isolation (especially in the case of burned children) which reduces drastically the emotional stimulation and comfort available to the child. In both orthopedic trauma and trauma resulting from burns, former body image is altered radically and concern about future appearance and function may consume enormous amounts of emotional energy.

Because of an enforced recumbent position, sensory stimulation may be reduced radically so that the child is in a continually monotonous and homogeneous field. Such sensory deprivation is reinforced by isolation and by emotional withdrawal from the environment. Resulting habituation to the routine sights and sounds surrounding him and a turning inward of the self may be manifested by apathy, by lack of intellectual curiosity, by inability to concentrate and to learn, or by restlessness and disorientation. An important aspect of nursing responsibility is a constant alertness to detect the above symptoms and to provide for adequate sensory stimulation through provision of an organized play and reading program. Human companionship is extremely important in relieving both emotional and sensory deprivation. Other methods of altering sensory input include provision of radio and television, colorful decoration of the pediatric unit, changes in body position, kinesthetic stimulation through cuddling and skin massage or placement of the bed near a window. Providing for adequate stimulation to maintain mental functioning and to support adequate intellectual development under conditions of immobility entails a constant challenge to the ingenuity of the nurse. Such attention, however, must be an integral part of every nursing care plan.

POISONING

Poisoning ranks fourth among the causes of accidental death among young children (after motor vehicles, burns and drowning). It is estimated that well over a half-million poisoning incidents occur annually in the United States and that three-quarters of them involve children between their first and third birthdays. In 1963, 454 children died in this country from solid and liquid poisons.

The number of poisonous substances found in and around the modern home is growing steadily thanks to the skill of industrial and pharmaceutical chemists in synthesizing new drugs, cleaning and polishing agents, insecticides and materials for the extermination of rodents and weeds. The national Pure Food and Drug Administration requires such substances to be labeled as poisons, but it cannot control their careless use or the failure of parents to keep them away from children (Fig. 17-3). Because of the very great number of compounds and limitless trade names under which poisons are marketed, it is often difficult to discover exactly what has been ingested and the degree of its toxicity. Comprehensive handbooks and compendia are published, and many cities now have Poison Control Centers which make such information quickly available. Except for some of the more common substances, physicians and nurses need access to such additional sources of information to manage the poisoned child properly. This section will confine itself to a discussion of general principles and a few details about the more common kinds of poisoning.

Acute Poisoning

General Management. Some toddlers obtain poison without the knowledge or suspicion of their guardians so that the first sign of trouble is the appearance of symptoms of toxicity—drowsiness, coma, peculiar behavior, convulsions, excitement, nausea or diarrhea. The sudden appearance of bizarre illness in a toddler should always arouse the suspicion of poisoning. Detailed inquiry about the presence of potential poisons in the home may stimulate the parents to take an inventory and by a little detective work locate the probable offending substance.

When the ingestion of poison is observed or suspected by parents, quick action is of great importance, for the toxic substance may be recovered—at least in part—before significant absorption has taken place. Vomiting (except in the case of some substances, e.g. kerosene or lye) should be induced by inserting a finger or the handle of a spoon into the posterior pharynx. If this is unsuccessful, one or two cups of milk or water containing 1 tablespoon of mustard or 2 tablespoons of salt should be administered and the gagging repeated. If syrup of ipecac is on hand, doses of a half-teaspoonful every 5 minutes will eventually empty the stomach. Vomitus, unswallowed liquid or pills and the container should be kept as aids in the identification of the poison. These and the child should be taken promptly to a nearby physician or hospital. Thorough gastric lavage, identification of the kind and the amount of poison and appropriate treatment can then be instituted. If, at the time he is discovered, the child is unconscious or convulsing, attempts to induce vomiting should be omitted and he should be wrapped in a blanket and taken at once for more skilled medical care.

If the poisoning occurs at a distance more remote than a half-hour from medical assistance, vomiting should be induced several times in order to clear the stomach. Between episodes either milk or the universal antidote should be administered. The latter consists of 2 parts of powdered charcoal (burnt toast), 1 part of magnesium oxide (milk of magnesia) and 1 part of tannic acid (strong tea) given in a glass of warm water. Further directions should then be sought by telephone.

Once the child has been brought to a medical center, further treatment depends on the symptoms. Shock, convulsions and metabolic disturbances require prompt relief. Identification of the poison should be pursued through the manufacturer or the dispensing druggist, since specific antidotes are available in many instances. With some toxic substances exchange transfusion or the artificial kidney may prove to be lifesaving by reducing the circulating blood levels promptly.

Salicylate Intoxication. Aspirin heads the list of drugs which poison the toddler. It has become such a ubiquitous household remedy that many persons fail to recognize its danger to the young. Candylike preparations and poorly guarded containers add to the hazard of excessive ingestion. Even medicinal overdosage occurs with some frequency when parents or physicians overlook the cumulative effect of regular periodic dosage of the small child during an illness. (One gr./Kg./day is permissible if divided into 4 or 5 individual doses spaced through the day—if hydration is maintained.) In spite of reasonable precautions some infants and young children seem to have an individual susceptibility to aspirin which results in symptoms even from doses that are theoretically permissible.

The earliest symptom of aspirin intoxication is hyperpnea due to stimulation of the respiratory center by the salicylate ion. Acidosis follows within a few hours after ingestion, and heavy dosage may result in coma, convulsions or hyperpyrexia. Salicylates can be detected in the urine by appropriate chemical tests or by the use of Phenistix. An accurate indication of the amount ingested is obtained from measuring the salicylate level in the blood. Except in small infants, levels below 30 mg. per cent are usually nontoxic; those over 60 mg. per cent, dangerous; over 100 mg. per cent, fatal. Poisoning with methyl salicylate (oil of wintergreen) produces much more severe toxicity than do the medicinal forms of salicylate such as aspirin.

If the child is seen early after the ingestion of salicylates, gastric lavage should be done to recover as much of the substance as possible. If a half-hour or more has elapsed since ingestion, induced vomiting with syrup of ipecac is more likely to be effective. After 2 to 4 hours, such procedures are probably futile since the material will have been absorbed. Excretion of salicylate is through the kidney and takes place best in alkalinized urine. Intravenous administration of glucose, bicarbonate and potassium salts is given at a rate which is varied according to severity of the poisoning and the size of the child. Vitamin K_1 oxide may be administered to protect against bleeding, which may result from the dicumerol-like effect of the salicylates. In severe poisoning, more rapid excretion of salicylate may be required by peritoneal dialysis, the use of the artificial kidney, or by exchange transfusion.

Sedatives and Anticonvulsants. The barbiturates, sedatives and drugs used in the control of epileptic convulsions are commonly found in household medicine cabinets. Taken in overdosage by young children they produce depression of the central nervous system with drowsiness, coma or collapse. In addition to withdrawal of the drug from the stomach, attention must be directed to preservation of an airway, stimulation of respirations and maintenance of blood pressure and body temperature. Although stimulants are available, their use is generally considered to be unwise. If the essential cardiopulmonary functions can be maintained for 24 to 48 hours, recovery is likely.

Antihistamines, Tranquilizers and Ataractics. A large number of compounds are now sold for the purpose of combating allergic symptoms, seasickness, vomiting and emotional tension. Most of them produce drowsiness and mild circulatory collapse in children. A few result in stimulation of the nervous system. Treatment is similar to that used for oversedation.

Caustic Esophagitis. A number of strongly caustic substances such as lye, bleaches, Clinitest tablets, swimming pool neutralizers and less commonly, acids, when ingested will coagulate the tissues of the mouth, pharynx and esophagus. Initially they produce a painful burn which interferes with swallowing and may give rise to edema about the larynx threatening the airway. If the child recovers from the acute stage, later deep tissue destruction, particularly in the esophagus, may lead to stricture due to the contraction of scar tissue. Progressive difficulty with swallowing may ensue so that it becomes impossible to take food, liquids, or even to dispose of the normal salivary secretions.

Ingestion of corrosive or burning liquids of this sort requires long term observation. Neutralization of the fluids ingested is not useful for they create their destruction too rapidly. Gastric lavage is contraindicated because of the risk of perforation of the damaged esophagus. If inspection of the mouth reveals burns, careful esophagoscopy is indicated to discover whether or not the material has produced burns lower in the alimentary tract. If such are discovered, prednisone is generally given to reduce the inflammation and decrease scar formation. Repeated barium examinations of the esophagus must then be made over the subsequent 3 to 4 months to observe whether stricture is taking place and if so a program of esophageal dilatation is indicated. When damage has been extensive, a feeding gastrostomy may be required, with later esophageal dilatation from below. In the most severe instances, the patency of the esophagus cannot be regained and operative procedures to create a new esophagus in several stages must be undertaken—a difficult and tedious process.

Iron Salts. Excessive dosage with iron in the form of ferrous sulfate and similar compounds may produce serious poisoning. The iron is readily absorbed from all levels of the intestinal tract. Systemically it produces a severe acidosis and toxic effects upon the central nervous system. Locally, it creates a hemorrhagic gastroenteritis. Treatment consists of early lavage and the instillation into the stomach of bicarbonate or phosphate solutions to precipitate the iron salts and neutralize the sulfate. A new agent, desferoxamine, is of value in tying up the iron circulating within the blood stream by the process of chelation.

Kerosene Pneumonia. Toddlers occasionally · swallow kerosene, carelessly left around the home. Frequently, an extensive pneumonia ensues due to the irritant effect of kerosene which has been aspirated or is being excreted from the body by way of the lungs. (Vomiting should not be induced due to the danger of aspirating the kerosene.) Immediately after ingestion of kerosene the child may feel well except for nausea. Respiratory symptoms and fever appear during the first 48 hours and pursue a variable course, depending on the amount of kerosene taken. In mild cases there may be little or no pulmonary irritation and no fever. When large amounts are taken and retained, hyperpyrexia, dyspnea and convulsions may ensue. The roentgenogram of the chest usually demonstrates large areas of pulmonary consolidation extending out from the central portion of the lung fields. In the absence of hyperpyrexia and convulsions, the child usually recovers completely after a few days of dyspnea and cough. Diagnosis can be made from the characteristic odor of kerosene. Early treatment probably demands careful gastric lavage to recover as much of the kerosene as possible from the stomach. Treatment of the pneumonia, once it is present, is symptomatic with the addition of antibiotics since bacterial infection is a common sequel.

Lead Poisoning

In the adult, lead poisoning usually results in a chronic illness marked by abdominal colic and weakness due to peripheral neuritis and anemia. The infant or young child who suffers from lead intoxication is more likely to present a medical emergency because of the rapid appearance of cerebral edema with vomiting, headache, stupor, convulsions or coma. Early recognition of the disorder is highly important, for the longer the symptoms of encephalopathy persist the more certain it is that the child will suffer irreparable damage to the brain.

Etiology. The infant or the small child may ingest or inhale lead in a variety of ways. In the past, small infants have been poisoned by lead derived from lead nipple shields or from ointments containing lead which were used on the mothers' breasts. Teething powders, drinking water which passed through lead pipes and food contaminated by paint are other sources. The most common mechanism of lead poisoning is that of pica, or perverted appetite, which leads the small child to chew on any and all objects, including painted toys, furniture, household fixtures and plaster. In the course of time he consumes a significant amount of lead if these objects are coated with lead-containing paint. In the United States all children's toys and furniture must now be painted with lead-free paint by the manufacturers. However, this does not control the type of paint used by the amateur in his home. Lead also may be derived from inhaled gases such as burned storage battery casings or from the fumes of gasoline containing tetraethyl lead.

Lead that is taken into the body is deposited and stored in many tissues. In the bones it accumulates at the rapidly growing epiphyseal lines, where it is visible on roentgen examination. Its deposition in the brain leads to edema and signs of increased intracranial pressure. It is released slowly from the tissues when the blood level begins to fall and is excreted in the urine.

Symptoms. The symptoms of lead poisoning vary with the degree of cerebral irritation that is produced. Sometimes there will be warning signs of loss of appetite, periodic unexplained vomiting, irritability, changed disposition or ataxic gait. More frequently the encephalopathy appears abruptly with persistent major convulsions which are very difficult to control and may be followed by stupor or coma. A small fraction of children suffer from a more chronic form of the disease with anemia, weakness, colic and peripheral neuritis as the chief symptoms.

Diagnosis. The diagnosis is suspected from the history of lead exposure in combination with the appearance of symptoms as above. Several laboratory tests aid in its confirmation. An anemia is usually present which is associated with basophilic stippling of the red blood cells seen on the smear. Under ultraviolet light, fluorescence of red cells may be observed. There may be a mild degree of glycosuria. Coproporphyrins are regularly excreted in the urine where they react with ferric chloride reagent to give a simple diagnostic screening test. The spinal fluid ordinarily has an increased quantity of protein without much or any increase in the number of cells. It is under high pressure when encephalopathy is present. X-ray examination of the bones will demonstrate a band of increased density at the epiphyseal line. The width of this band gives some indication of the length of time that the lead ingestion has been in progress. Conclusive diagnosis can be reached by measuring the level of lead in the blood or the amount that is being excreted in the urine. Precautions are necessary in obtaining specimens in receptacles which are scrupulously freed of lead, for the amounts to be determined are minute, and contamination may result in a wrong interpretation.

Treatment and Nursing Care. The main problem in treatment is to get the lead out of the tissues, particularly out of the brain, and have it transported through the blood for excretion by the kidneys. To be effective this must be engineered in such a way that additional lead is not taken up by the brain during the process. This is accomplished by the use of chelating agents, which tie up the metal ions in the blood and tissues and prevent their entrance into cells, particularly of the nervous system. The complexes thus formed are then slowly excreted by the kidney. Before such treatment is attempted, residual particles of lead should be removed from the bowel. The most widely used chelating agent is edathamil calcium disodium (EDTA) which is given intramuscularly for a 5 to 7 day period every 4 hours. During active symptoms of encephalopathy, 2,3 dimercaptopropanol (BAL) is given as well to counteract the tendency of EDTA to initially increase cerebral edema. The urinary excretion of lead is measured during chelation therapy and, after a rest, the course is repeated until blood lead levels and the quantity excreted indicate that the child can safely be left to complete the process alone.

In addition to such attempts to immobilize lead in the blood stream, measures must be taken to terminate or prevent the convulsions that accompany encephalopathy. The usual sedatives such as phenobarbital are less effective than under ordinary circumstances and thus they must be used in large dosage. Paraldehyde is safer and is effective. Magnesium sulfate given intramuscularly in the same fashion as for hypertensive encephalopathy may aid in the control of cerebral edema. Surgical measures of decompression have been tried but are usually ineffective. Once the acute phase has passed, it is desirable to shield the child from acute infections that may reactivate his disease. Months are required to complete the process of deleading the tissues and thus removing the threat of recurrence.

The specific nursing care is that of a child with convulsions from any cause. Avoidance of unnecessary handling is desirable in order to give a minimal amount of stimulation to the central nervous system. In protracted coma it may be necessary to resort to gavage feedings and the skin care that is accorded to any unconscious patient.

Prognosis. In general the prognosis following lead poisoning is not very good. The mortality from acute encephalopathy even with early treatment is significantly high—around 25 per cent—and of those who survive, a high percentage will show evidence of neurologic disturbances, including mental retardation. How many of these victims were retarded children before the acute onset of encephalopathy is always hard to judge. The retarded child is more likely to be one who develops a perverted appetite for lead-coated objects, but pica certainly is not confined to the retarded group. Children who do not have acute encephalopathy, whose lead intoxication can be terminated early in its course, have a much more favorable prognosis for full recovery.

Prophylaxis. Because of the generally unsatisfactory results of treatment it is most important to try to prevent lead poisoning. The approach has been made through the passage of laws which forbid the use of lead paint on articles designed for use by children and through public education calling attention to the dangers of lead intoxication and indicating the common sources from which the child obtains lead. The nurse visiting a home can do much to discover and point out to the parents such potential dangers. In slum areas programs have been undertaken to screen the urine of all small children with ferric chloride reagent and measure blood lead levels of positive reactors. When significantly elevated levels are found, such children can then be admitted for prophylactic de-leading even if they present no symptoms. Unless their homes are improved, however, there is a strong likelihood that they will ingest more lead when they return home.

FOREIGN BODIES

The toddler loves to put things into his mouth and the other orifices of his body in order to see how they taste or whether they will fit. Most of such foreign bodies are relatively harmless, and serious illness results infrequently. To the mother they are a worrisome annoyance and to the toddler a source of discomfort before and during their removal. Occasionally when they occlude or damage an important body passageway they may be the source of real danger to the child.

Foreign Bodies in the Lower Respiratory Tract

Foreign bodies of small size and wide variety may be aspirated into the lower respiratory tract, especially by children. These may remain in the pharynx or pass into the bronchi. Seldom do they lodge in the trachea. In the larynx they are the cause of immediate and acute distress with violent coughing and with stridor due to obstruction to or spasm of the larynx. If the foreign body remains fixed in one place in the larynx, coughing subsides, but usually an inflammation occurs, the edema of which obstructs respiration, and operative relief becomes imperative.

When a foreign body passes into a bronchus, the effects vary with the size and nature of the foreign material. If the bronchus is completely occluded, the air in the lung beyond the obstruction is absorbed, and the lung collapses. If a large or primary bronchus is affected, the resultant pulmonary collapse may give rise to alarming symptoms, including cyanosis and dyspnea. A foreign body of any variety in a bronchus causes inflammation, but certain kinds, especially nuts, more easily induce inflammatory changes which are of a serious type. In a child who survives the immediate effects of a foreign body, the late result is likely to be a lung abscess or chronic pneumonia and bronchiectasis, unless the foreign body is removed early. The primary indication in treatment is removal of the offending material by laryngoscope or bronchoscope, as the need may be.

General Nursing Care. After the foreign body has been removed, the child should be placed in a ventilated "croup tent" or other source of moist air. The child should be observed closely for signs of respiratory difficulty. Trauma during laryngoscopic or bronchoscopic examination may produce edema of the larynx with accompanying respiratory embarrassment. Increased, labored respiratons, crowing, hoarseness, retraction of the soft parts of the chest on inspiration, cyanosis and restlessness are danger signals that should be reported immediately. If respiratory embarrassment occurs, tracheostomy may be necessary.

Foreign Bodies in the Intestinal Tract

Solid Objects. It is common for young children to place foreign bodies in the mouth. Small foreign bodies may be swallowed and cause no difficulty. Foreign bodies that reach the stomach usually are passed through the remainder of the tract without symptoms. If they are opaque, their progression should be observed with roentgenograms. Long bodies may be expected to cause some trouble in the sharp curves of the duodenum, and therefore should be removed through the esophagus with the help of an esophagoscope, or surgically through the abdominal wall. Large foreign bodies may become lodged in the pharynx or the esophagus.

A foreign body in the pharynx may cause gagging, choking and perhaps obstruction to respiration to an alarming degree. Except in definite emergency, attempts at removal with the fingers should not be made.

A foreign body in the esophagus may cause only moderate discomfort and difficulty in swallowing. Liquid foods may pass easily. Prompt removal is important, particularly in the case of sharp-edged objects, because of the probability of perforation and ulceration and extension of the inflammation to the mediastinum or the respiratory tract.

Bezoar. Most foreign bodies that reach the stomach pass on without trouble. Certain types of indigestible material, when swallowed in large amounts, tend to accumulate in masses so large that passage beyond the stomach becomes impossible. Any such mass is known as a bezoar. The most commonly encountered bezoar is composed of hair, which usually has been pulled from the head and swallowed over a long period. The hair becomes matted in a large ball or mass. The symptoms are vague, and health and nutrition suffer little. A tumor is felt, and a filling defect is shown by x-ray studies with barium. The only treatment is surgical removal, a relatively simple procedure.

Foreign Bodies in Other Sites

The Eye. Many foreign bodies which float into the eye are promptly removed by the pronounced tearing which follows. If pain, redness and discomfort continue, the toddler will require medical attention to ascertain whether the substance is embedded in the surface of the globe. Such examination requires at least a local anesthetic and frequently a general one, since the small child cannot be expected to cooperate with the search.

The Nose. Small objects which as peas, beans, buttons, bits of paper or crayon are sometimes inserted into the nose and lodge there. After a while they produce a chronic purulent discharge which may become blood tinged. Such a discharge, particularly if it is unilateral, should lead to further examination and removal of the object.

The Ear. Beads, beans, peas, crayons and pieces of paper may also get into the external auditory canal where they set up an irritating inflammatory reaction and may become further entrapped due to swelling of the canal wall. Their removal should be left to a physician.

The Genital Tract. In older children, objects may be inserted into the urethra of the male, resulting in pain on urination and a discharge from the urethra. Extraction of the foreign body requires the services of a urologist, since a urethroscope or cystoscope may be required. In the female, objects such as bobby pins or paper clips may be put into the vagina and become lodged so that they cannot be removed. A chronic discharge results. Extraction is usually easy if the examiner thinks of the possibility of a foreign body and makes appropriate rectal or roentgen examination of the tissues.

SITUATIONS FOR FURTHER STUDY

1. Study a child between the ages of 1 and 3 years after a tracheostomy to find answers to these questions: Could you detect his reactions to loss of his power to cry and talk? What reactions would you expect to see? Can you detect ways in which he tries to compensate for loss of communication? What did you do to encourage his use of substitute forms of communication? What other ways did you find to help him feel less threatened? What criteria did you use in evaluating your nursing activities? Do you think a child of this age would be comforted if he knew that you were aware of how frightened he was when he discovered that he could neither cry nor talk? Would telling him that he would be able to speak again be of benefit to a 1- to 3-year-old child? Test it out and report your findings in class.

2. How would you approach the subject of accident prevention with a mother of a 15-month-old child?

3. Read the study by Long and Cope to discover their findings relative to the frequency with which emotional disturbances occurred within the families of the burned children they studied. Of what significance were these findings to you as a nurse? What patterns of behavior did they observe in the subjects of their study? What insights did you gain which would be of help to you in understanding the behavior of a burned child?

4. How do you think you might react if on a home visit you observed that a mother became angry every time her 16-month-old son manipulated the TV controls, the light sockets or reached up to a table filled with dishes? How might you get a mother to talk about her feelings regarding her child's drive toward mastery of his environment?

5. How could you determine if a child's behavior was motivated by natural curiosity or by spite or revenge?

6. On arrival in a home a public health nurse discovered that 3-month-old Barry had been admitted to the hospital to have a foreign body removed from his throat. The nurse learned that it had been 2-year-old Bob who had put a small tin fish from his magnet game into his brother's mouth, thus necessitating an immediate operation. In the course of talking about the experience Mrs. J. said that Bob had had an unusually restless night. She took Bob in bed with her which angered Mr. J. so much that he told his wife to put Bob back into his own bed. Instead of doing this Mrs. J. took Bob into the living room and used the davenport for a bed. What feelings and thoughts might have prompted the behavior of Bob and each of his parents? How would you have handled the situation if you had been the nurse making this home visit? Do you think Mrs. J.'s actions were wise? Why?

BIBLIOGRAPHY

Artz, C.: The burn patient, Nursing Forum 4:87, 1965.

Assoc. for the Aid of Crippled Children: Behavioral Approaches to Accident Research, N. Y., 1961.

Barnes, C.: Support of a mother in the care of a child with esophageal lye burns, Nurs. Clin. N. Am. 4:53, 1969.

Chisolm, J.: The use of chelating agents in the treatment of acute and chronic lead intoxication in childhood, J. Pediat. 73:1, 1968.

Chisholm, J. J.: Accidents and poisoning, *in* Cooke, R. E. (ed.), The Biologic Basis of Pediatric Practice, p. 1, McGraw-Hill, N. Y., 1968.

Dalton, A.: Using a Stryker frame, Am. J. Nurs. 64:100, 1964.

Eaton, P., and Heller, F.: Therapeutic nursing care of orthopedic patients, Nurs. Clin. N. Am. 2:429, 1967.

Health Statistics from the U. S. National Health Survey, Ser. B, Nos. 16 and 37, U. S. Dept. HEW, Public Health Service, 1962.

Larsen, D., and Gaston, R.: Current trends in the care of burned patients, Am. J. Nurs. 67:319, 1967.

Long, R. T., and Cope, O.: Emotional problems of burned children, New Eng. J. Med. 264:1121, 1961.

Luschen, M.: Technique and temperament made the difference, Am. J. Nurs. 64:103, 1964.

MacMillan, B. G.: Management of Burns in Children, *in* Shirkey, H. C. (ed.), Pediatric Therapy, ed. 3, St. Louis, Mosby, 1968

Maxwell, P., Linss, M., McDonnough, P., and Kinder, J.: Routines on the burn ward, Am. J. Nurs. 66:522, 1966.

Miles, M.: Body integrity fears in a toddler, Nurs. Clin. N. Am. *4*:39, 1969.

Noble, E.: Play and the Sick Child, London, Faber and Faber, 1967.

Olson, E.: The hazards of immobility, Am. J. Nurs. 67:781, 1967.

Petrillo, M.: Preventing hospital trauma in pediatric patients, Am. J. Nurs. *68*:1468, 1968.

Price, W., and Wood, M.: Operating room care of burned patients treated with silver nitrate, Am. J. Nurs. *68*:1705, 1968.

Rubin, M.: Balm for burned children, Am. J. Nurs. *66*:297, 1966.

Sherman, R. T.: Burn fluid management, Nursing Forum *4*:93, 1965.

Simeone, F. A.: The nature of shock, Am. J. Nurs. *66*:1287, 1966.

Sister Mary Claudia: TLC and Sulfamylon for burned children, Am. J. Nurs. *69*:755, 1969.

Skellenger, W. S.: Treatment of poisoning in children, Am. J. Nurs. *65*:108, 1965.

Stoll, C.: Responses of three girls to burn injuries and hospitalization, Nurs. Clinics of N. Am. *4*:77, 1969.

Strathie, N., and Swanson, C.: Problems in one patient's care, Am. J. Nurs. *66*:524, 1966.

Suchman, E., and Scherzer, A.: Current Research in Childhood Accidents, N. Y. Assoc. for the Aid of Crippled Children, 1960.

Wood, M., Kenny, H. A., and Price, W. R.: Silver nitrate treatment of burns, Am. J. Nurs. *66*:518, 1966.

18

Nursing Care of Children With Viral Infections

Viruses, which cause a number of our common infectious diseases, are submicroscopic particles with certain common properties. In some measure these properties explain the characteristics of viral infections. The general remarks about viruses which follow are not strictly applicable to each of the viral infections subsequently described, but they may give the reader a theoretic framework which will aid in the understanding of the symptomatology, prevention and treatment.

Unlike the bacteria, viruses cannot survive for long unless they are in intimate relation with living cells. Some viruses are quite precise in their requirements and must parasitize not only a certain type of tissue cell but even require also a certain species of animal. Virus particles are regarded as incomplete forms of life which must borrow enzyme systems from living cells in order to carry out their metabolic processes and to reproduce. Once furnished with an appropriate environment, many of them will increase at an extraordinarily rapid rate and overwhelm the tissues which they infect. Recent laboratory technics have made it possible to support virus life outside the animal body by supplying the proper living cells in tissue culture media.

In general, viruses enter the body and then remain clinically dormant through an incubation period which is at least a week in length and sometimes much longer. During this period they presumably are migrating toward the cells which they seek to invade. Symptoms of disease do not appear until virus multiplication is well advanced and the favored cells are being attacked. Thus, by the time a clinical diagnosis can be made, the virus already has gained a foothold in the tissues.

Treatment of most viral infections is relatively ineffectual in controlling the growth of virus particles which already have entered cells. In this sheltered location it is impossible for specific antibodies or antibiotics to affect them. (There are a few exceptions to this statement.) Under natural circumstances the disease is brought to a conclusion when the body begins to produce a specific antibody against the infecting virus. This antibody probably does not enter the cells but it limits infection to those cells which already have been attacked and disposes of virus which is circulating among or being released from them. In some instances artificially given antibody or antibiotic may speed this process, but in general they have little advantage over natural controlling mechanisms. Clinical recovery is frequently abrupt and probably corresponds to the point at which antibody has gained the upper hand over the infecting virus. For most of the diseases discussed the quantity of antibody production is sufficiently great to result in a long period of protection from reinfection: often the protection lasts for the rest of the person's life.

Prevention of viral diseases may be achieved in two ways: (1) by artificially stimulating the body to produce antibody through the administration of a vaccine and (2) by administration of antibodies which have been formed previously by another person who has had the infection. The first method (*active immunization*) is used before the person encounters the disease in question and is the best method of providing a long-standing protection. Unfortunately, it is not available for many viral diseases. The second method of *passive immunization* may be used during the incubation period when known exposure has occurred but before the virus has been able to get an irreversible foothold in the tissues. A general view of the prevalence of the viral diseases in the United States is given in Table 17, together with the methods available for their control.

ACUTE RESPIRATORY INFECTIONS

Infections of the upper respiratory passageways are by far the most common diseases among children. Clinical classification is hampered by the lack of pre-

Table 17. Control and Prevalence of Viral Infection*

Disease	Active (Lasting) Immunization	Passive (Temporary) Immunization	Incidence in U.S., 1966	
			Cases	Deaths
Smallpox	Vaccination (Jenner, 1798)	Hyperimmune gamma globulin	0	0
Vaccinia	(Jenner, 1798)	Hyperimmune gamma globulin	Millions	10
Rabies	Rabbit-brain vaccine (Pasteur, 1885) Duck-embryo vaccine	Hyperimmune horse serum	2	2
Poliomyelitis	Salk vaccine, 1955; live oral vaccine, 1960	Gamma globulin	113	9
Influenza	Tissue culture vaccines, 1944		†	2,830
Measles	Enders vaccine, 1960	Gamma globulin	204,136	261
Rubella	Vaccine, 1967	Gamma globulin	46,975	12
Other respiratory viruses			Legion	Rare
Mumps	Tissue culture vaccine	Hyperimmune gamma globulin	128,295	43
Infectious hepatitis		Gamma globulin	34,356	757
Viral encephalitis	Tissue culture vaccines used mainly for animals		2,121	579
Varicella			136,149	137

* Figures from Annual Supplement to the Morbidity and Mortality Weekly Report, U.S.P.H.S., HEW, 1967 and from Vital Statistics of the U.S., 1966.
† Reporting of these diseases not required in all states; figures incomplete.

cise knowledge about etiology and by the confusing overlap of the symptoms produced by different infections and by their complications. A number of terms such as "coryza," "acute rhinitis," "nasopharyngitis," "viral infection" and "undifferentiated respiratory disease," have been applied to illnesses of this sort. The respiratory infections with clear-cut clinical pictures and accepted etiology (influenza, measles and streptococcal pharyngitis, etc.) are considered separately.

It is desirable for the nurse to have some idea of current theories concerning the manner in which these infections arise and spread, and of the factors that determine the amount of damage they do. Newer methods for studying these infections make it probable that these ideas will soon be modified through the accumulation of more precise knowledge about etiology and epidemiology.

Epidemiology

The agents that produce upper respiratory infections are passed around from one individual to another mainly through the air. From the nose and throat of an infected person they are discharged into the surrounding atmosphere where they remain suspended for a time on minute drops of water vapor or particles of dust. During the act of breathing the nose and throat of the child are continually sampling this atmosphere several times a minute. When it is contaminated by infectious agents, they lodge on the mucous membranes of the nose or throat during inspiration and, if they find a favorable climate there, proceed to multiply rapidly and produce disease in the new host. The newly infected child then serves as a fresh point of dissemination to the air about him.

Since the infectious agents die off more rapidly in outdoor air when exposed to unfavorable temperatures and the action of ultraviolet light from the sun, the chain of transmission becomes more difficult during the summer months when children spend much of their time out of doors and when windows are open and houses are well ventilated. At the fall opening of school, children are congregated into enclosed rooms containing warm air. Introduction of an infectious agent into one member of such a group is readily followed by its dissemination to others. Consequently, it is the usual experience to find that after a period of grace, respiratory infections begin to make the school rounds during the late fall and continue to do so until spring. Exclusion of infected children from the school group has only a partial effect in breaking up the chain of spread, for each victim serves as an unwitting dispenser of germs for a day or two before obvious symptoms of his disease are present. Isolation is thus imposed a bit too late to provide complete protection for the group.

Age is an important factor in epidemiology. From long experience it seems clear that the older the child is the better he is able to resist infection. He appears to develop immunity from repeated experience with the infecting agents. This accounts for the high incidence of disease among children in kindergarten or nursery school and for the much lower incidence among the teen-agers. In a general way it seems as though most children must spend one or two bad winters before they begin to combat infections successfully. Individual exceptions are noteworthy, for each class has a few children who never seem to be affected by the illnesses of the group, and a few others who acquire immunity at such a slow rate that they continue to have trouble at short intervals for several years.

Etiology

Certain bacteria can be cultivated regularly from the noses and throats of healthy children. Staphylococci, micrococcus catarrhalis, probably alpha-hemolytic streptococci and some varieties of pneumococcus fall within this group. This "normal flora" of the respiratory passages presumably is held in check by the natural body defenses. Other bacteria, notably the beta-hemolytic streptococcus, certain varieties of pneumococcus and the influenza bacillus are associated more regularly with respiratory disease and are considered to be at least potential pathogens. Perhaps at times upper respiratory infections are initiated entirely through a loss of resistance to those bacteria comprising the normal flora. But a more generally accepted mechanism is that a viral agent invades first, establishes an infection which lasts only 2 or 3 days, but in so doing breaks down the local resistance to bacteria so that they are able to infect tissues which normally resist their activity. The later symptoms of upper respiratory infections and of many of the complications are blamed on such a secondary bacterial invasion of the tissues.

The popular lay idea that wet feet, fatigue and exposure to cold can initiate respiratory infections probably has some basis. Reflex changes in the nasal mucous membrane are known to occur when the body is suddenly chilled. It is likely that temporary loss of local tissue resistance follows and permits the invasion of bacteria or viruses which are already present in the passageways.

A number of viral agents that are capable of producing the symptoms of early respiratory disease in monkeys and human volunteers have been isolated. The new tissue culture technics have revealed a confusing situation in which the same agent may sometimes be found associated with a simple cold, at other times with a more severe influenza-like illness or pneumonia, and sometimes can be recovered from persons with no illness at all. Under usual circumstances the necessary viral studies are not undertaken and the common cold is managed without precise knowledge of its etiology. The names of some of the agents involved are the adenoviruses, influenza and parainfluenza, Coxsackie viruses, respiratory syncytial virus, rhinoviruses, rheovirus and Eaton agent (mycoplasma). The clinical picture of a few of the more distinctive illnesses are described below.

The Common Cold (Coryza, Acute Rhinitis, Undifferentiated Respiratory Disease)

Symptoms. The symptoms of acute upper respiratory infection are too well known to require elaborate description. The common cold begins with sneezing, clear nasal discharge and general malaise, but little or no fever. Conjunctivitis may be present, due to the invasion of the mucosa of the eye. Headache usually is due to the distention of the paranasal sinuses with fluid. Cough may be due to the irritation of the larynx by posterior nasal discharges or to primary infection of the laryngeal tissues. Upper respiratory infections may also begin with fever, headache, cough or sore throat. The clinical picture of the disease is not necessarily reproduced exactly in the succeeding victims to whom it is passed.

After the early catarrhal stage of the infection, bacterial invasion is apparent in the purulent character of the discharge from nose and sinuses and in the compli-

cation of otitis media which may follow retrograde extension from the pharynx up the eustachian tube.

Prognosis and Prevention. The strictly viral phase of upper respiratory infection is often a brief affliction with good prognosis. However, the bacterial complications may protract the symptoms and lead to annoying complications such as sinusitis, bronchitis and otitis media. In small infants or children with debilitating disease or with poor general resistance, bacterial invasion initiated by an apparently mild upper respiratory infection may progress to serious or even fatal disease such as pneumonia, bacteremia or meningitis. In this latter group it is essential to protect them by isolation from known infections and in certain instances by prophylactic administration of antibiotics when exposure cannot be foreseen. Prevention of respiratory infections in the school population is a difficult problem only partially solved by exclusion of infected children. In general it is probably best to permit the child to attend school as regularly as possible in order to acquire immunity through exposure, since no effective vaccination is yet available. Delicate children or those whose upper respiratory infections precipitate bronchitis or asthma may require protection with small doses of antibiotics taken regularly during the winter months. The problem of tonsillectomy and adenoidectomy is discussed in a later section.

Treatment and Nursing Care. In uncomplicated coryza the most important measure is to keep the nose clear in order that the child may breathe comfortably. Free breathing can be accomplished in the early stage by dropping into the nose a very small amount of a solution of ephedrine (0.5 to 1.0%) or Neo-Synephrine Hydrochloride (0.25%), which decreases the swelling of the mucous membrane and permits drainage. When dropping solutions into the nose for the purpose of treatment, the child should lie down and the head should be allowed to drop backward until it is below the level of the shoulders. After 3 or 4 days, when the discharge has become purulent, suction may be used for the removal of the secretions.

Solutions containing oil should not be used in the nose, since they are known to pass unchecked through the larynx and into the trachea. Their accumulation in the lung may be responsible for lipid pneumonia.

When the nasal secretion is profuse and irritating, the nostrils and the upper lip should be protected with cold cream or petrolatum. If symptoms are acute, and if the child is irritable and uninterested in his food, no attempt should be made to encourage him to take the accustomed amounts. When fever is present children often reduce their own diet, a procedure that tends to prevent gastrointestinal disturbances. Water should be encouraged. Increasing the humidity of the room helps to keep secretions fluid and relieves cough.

Rest in bed is necessary as long as fever persists and should be continued for 48 hours longer. When the child's temperature becomes normal, he will feel much better. Unless interesting play materials are provided for him, bed rest will be difficult to maintain in the home. In order to prevent the spread of infection into the eustachian tube, children should be taught a safe method of clearing their nasal passages. They never should be directed to "blow hard." Instead, they should be taught to keep their mouths open while they ease the secretion from both nostrils at the same time.

Sedative or antipyretic drugs are often used to decrease discomfort and restlessness. The drugs used include aspirin, codeine and the barbiturates. Although sulfonamides and antibiotics are widely used in the treatment of colds, they should be reserved for use in complications or to terminate a protracted infection. However, in debilitated children the immediate administration of antibiotics is rational as a prophylactic measure.

Influenza

Influenza is a specific respiratory viral infection caused by a group of closely related viral agents. The symptomatology is well known—chills, fever, muscular aches, headache and sore throat. A similar train of symptoms may be observed with other acute respiratory infections, particularly adenovirus infections, and differentiation is possible only by special laboratory examination or by suspicion during the course of an epidemic. In general, children are not so seriously affected as adults, and for this reason, prophylactic immunization with influenza vaccine has found little favor except for children with chronic cardiac or respiratory disease. Treatment consists of bed rest, aspirin for relief of symptoms and protection against superimposed bacterial infections.

Herpes Simplex Infections

The herpes simplex virus is commonly seen as the cause of fever blisters in the adult or the older child. It is an almost universal infection of man, lying dormant within the tissues of the mouth during health and producing its characteristic lesions only when the body is placed under stress. In young children the virus is picked up from adult associates. A few children suffer an uncomfortable illness at the time of this initial infection when they have no protective immunity. This disorder, herpetic stomatits, is marked by diffuse redness, swelling and ulceration of the gums and the mucous membranes of the mouth and the pharynx. It may be accompanied by fever and localized enlargement of the lymph nodes. Eating becomes uncomfortable, and occasionally the child suffers from restricted fluid intake. Milk is tolerated better than any other food or liquid. The disease lasts for 1 to 2 weeks when spontaneous healing begins. Local treatment is not very satisfactory. Administration of broad-spectrum antibiotics is thought by some to speed the healing process. Once having had this initial infection the child may in later life have fever blisters or a few ulcerations in the mouth at times when his immune response is low.

Herpangina

This form of mouth infection is caused by infection with Group A Coxsackie viruses. It is marked by the sudden onset of fever and sore throat. Small vesicles are found on the palate and in the pharynx, but there is no diffuse inflammation of the mouth and the gums. The disease is self-limited, subsiding in 1 to 4 days. Treatment is symptomatic for the relief of fever, and occasionally convulsions.

Croup

Viruses of the parainfluenza group are now recognized as a chief cause of croup. The clinical management is discussed in Chapter 14.

Viral Bronchitis and Bronchiolitis

Adenoviruses and the respiratory syncytial virus may produce bronchitis in infants or small children. The clinical features are discussed in Chapter 14.

Primary Atypical Pneumonia

This is a type of pneumonia, caused by a virus-like agent (mycoplasma), which produces symptoms of cough, fever and general malaise. Its course is likely to be protracted to 2 or 3 weeks in length, but the child is seldom alarmingly ill, and the prognosis is universally good. Diagnosis is suspected by exclusion of bacterial pneumonia and by the discovery of various types of pulmonary consolidation in the roentgenogram of the chest, often in the absence of physical signs in the chest. The mycoplasma (or Eaton agent) can be cultivated from secretions by special laboratory technics. A rise in specific antibody in the patient's blood may also be used to confirm the diagnosis. The treatment is entirely symptomatic. Tetracycline is effective in shortening the course of the illness. There are no complications of this type of pneumonia.

THE ACUTE EXANTHEMS

Measles (Rubeola, Morbilli)

Measles is a disease having symptoms of respiratory infection and a characteristic enanthem and exanthem (Plate 1).

Etiology. Measles is caused by a virus which, during the active stage of the disease, is present in the nose, mouth, throat and eyes and in the discharges from them. Measles is one of the most highly communicable diseases. It is communicable from the beginning of the respiratory symptoms and before the appearance of the rash. The period of greatest communicability is at the height of the respiratory symptoms, and it diminishes as these symptoms subside. Measles occurs chiefly in the late winter and the early spring. Infants under 6 months of age usually do not acquire measles even though thoroughly exposed to it, because their mothers transmit protective antibody to them via the placenta. After this age, the susceptibility at all ages is great. One attack usually protects permanently against a second attack. Second attacks occur occasionally, but in most instances of reported recurrence one of the two illnesses probably was due to some disease other than measles. Relatively few adults acquire measles because of the protection afforded the majority by a previous attack in childhood.

Symptoms. Symptoms of measles begin to appear after an incubation period of from 10 to 11 days. Approximately 14 days elapse between exposure and development of the rash. The invasion is gradual, with fever and coryza. During this early stage, it is difficult to distinguish measles from an ordinary cold. The enanthem appears on the 2nd or 3rd day, and the exanthem on the 3rd, 4th or 5th day. The original respiratory symptoms continue and extend. Lacrimation and photophobia are associated with the conjunctivitis. The discharge from the eyes becomes purulent. Sneezing is frequent at the onset, and complaint is made of soreness of the throat. The infection may extend to the ears and cause otitis media. It always extends to the larynx, trachea and bronchi, and frequent cough, sometimes modified to a "brassy" sound by the laryngitis, is a distressing symptom. The white count is normal or low throughout the course of measles except when pyogenic complications occur.

The fever reaches its height within a few days of the onset and remains high until the rash is fully developed over the body. In a few instances, a transitory decrease in fever occurs just before the appearance of the eruption. In the absence of complications, the fever either ceases by crisis or decreases rapidly by lysis with full development of the rash. The constitutional symptoms usually correspond in severity and duration to the course of the temperature. Irritability, malaise, drowsiness and often chilly sensations are present. Headache is common, and delirium may occur. As with other infections, the child may be affected mildly, moderately or severely. The illness may be so severe that the child dies before the rash appears, or the rash may be hemorrhagic. Such severe varieties of measles are uncommon, and death seldom occurs as a direct result of measles but only as a result of complications.

ENANTHEM. The most characteristic feature of the enanthem is bluish-white spots, pinpoint size, surrounded by a red areola on the mucous membrane of the mouth. These spots are known as Koplik's spots and are important in the early diagnosis of measles before the rash appears on the skin. Koplik's spots disappear quickly, sometimes by the time the rash has appeared.

EXANTHEM. The exanthem or rash appears first somewhere on the head and spreads gradually over the body. From 3 to 4 days are required for it to reach its greatest extent, and then it persists for from 1 to 6 days longer. The rash consists of small dark-red papules which increase in size and coalesce into groups. Between these groups of papules the skin appears to be normal. The contrast between the blotchy, raised areas of redness and the normal skin surrounding them produces the appearance characteristic of the rash of measles. The character of the rash is thus very different from that of scarlet fever, in which the appearance from a distance is that of diffuse redness with no normal skin in the same area as the rash. Unlike scarlet fever, the rash of measles always involves the face in the same manner as other parts of the body. After the rash has faded, there remains in the same blotchy areas a pigmentation of the skin which persists for several days.

The superficial layer of skin begins to desquamate during the second week in very fine flakes, the desquamated skin never being of the size or the thickness found after scarlet fever. This process lasts from 5 to 10 days. In rare instances when the illness and rash are unusually severe, petechial hemorrhages occur in the areas of eruption, causing what has been termed "black measles."

Complications. Bronchopneumonia is the most important of the common complications of measles. Otitis media, though frequent, is not so serious. The stomatitis which is a part of measles in the early stage usually causes no difficulty and requires no special attention, but it prepares the way for the more serious ulcerative variety which sometimes occurs as a complication. Nephritis is infrequent. Encephalitis, although not common, occurs approximately once in a thousand cases. It is a cause of death in a few instances. Complete recovery may be expected in more than half the cases; residual defects of varying severity persist in the remainder. Measles is reputed to be an activator of pre-existing tuberculous infection. In severe measles, as in any other severe infection, the intoxication may be great enough to affect the myocardium and cause dilatation of the heart and a rapid feeble pulse. If the circulation fails for this reason during the eruptive stage, the rash fades or even disappears. The popular fear of the "rash going in" has no foundation except as this event may be dependent on circulatory failure. Keeping the rash well out by the use of heavy clothing or a hot room is more of a disadvantage than otherwise.

Isolation. The isolation period of measles should be for the duration of the catarrhal symptoms. This period is from 1 to 2 weeks after the beginning of symptoms and from 2 to 3 days after the temperature becomes normal. In most instances, 5 days after the appearance of the rash is a sufficient isolation period.

Prognosis. The prognosis in measles is dependent in part on the age and also on the previous condition of the child. The younger the child is and the poorer the physical condition, the more likely is the disease to result seriously. In the general population, the mortality rate is seldom more than 1 per cent, and it is usually less. In a hospital where children already are ill, especially in a ward for infants, the mortality rate may be expected to be several times that in the general population.

Prevention. The widespread use of the tissue culture vaccine developed by Enders in 1960 and subsequent modifications has led to a dramatic decline in the incidence of the disease in the United States. The original vaccine administered to infants or older children beyond the age of 1 year is frequently followed by 1 or more days of fever and rash about a week after inoculation. However, the important complications of bacterial otitis and pneumonia and viral encephalitis are abolished. A more attenuated strain developed by Schwartz has yielded a lower incidence of febrile complications. The use of killed vaccine has been disappointing in its ability to maintain protection. Peculiar sensitivity reactions have been observed when live virus vaccine is subsequently given to such subjects.

Unvaccinated, susceptible children who have been exposed to measles may be temporarily protected by the administration of commercial gamma globulin during the first 5 days after exposure. A dose of 0.25 ml/ Kg. of body weight will generally prevent the disease; 0.05 ml/Kg. may be used to permit a mild case of measles to develop with the hope that permanent immunity will be established. Active immunization should be delayed at least 2 or 3 months after the administration of gamma globulin.

Diagnosis. Typical measles offers little difficulty in diagnosis. The rash may be simulated by that of German measles, in which respiratory symptoms are mild or lacking, and Koplik's spots never are present. Some drug eruptions may resemble measles for a short time. These rashes may be distinguished from measles by the history of drug ingestion and by the absence of respiratory symptoms.

Treatment and Nursing Care. The child should be kept in bed as long as fever persists and as much longer as cough and physical signs of lung infection are present. No special diet is indicated, except that in any acute febrile illness the diet during the acute stage should be light and easily digestible, consisting chiefly of liquids. Because of photophobia, the eyes should be protected from light until it is no longer unpleasant. For this purpose, some means other than darkening the room is preferable. The child's bed may be placed in such a position that he does not have to look directly into the light of a window. Wearing dark glasses or placing a screen behind the bed will shield the child's eyes from bright light. Unusually high fever is controlled by hydrotherapy. Cough is controlled by sedatives when severe enough to disturb sleep and rest. Often moist air is used in the management of laryngitis or bronchitis. Any itching associated with the eruption may be controlled as suggested for scarlet fever.

All of the complications of measles except encephalomyelitis are the result of bacterial invasion of mucous membrane surfaces which have been debilitated by the infection with measles virus. Antibiotic therapy controls these complications. In some instances antibiotics are given during the febrile period of measles in order to forestall bacterial invasion.

Rubella (German Measles)

Rubella is a contagious disease characterized chiefly by a skin eruption and mildness of constitutional and associated symptoms. It is a relatively unimportant disease because of the slight and fleeting incapacity produced. Its chief importance is from the standpoint of diagnosis because of its resemblance to measles or scarlet fever and also because of its serious effects upon the fetus when transmitted through the placental circulation (Chapter 10).

Etiology. Rubella is caused by a virus which is present during the early stage in the upper respiratory tract. The incubation period varies from 7 to 22 days. The disease does not commonly occur in the first 6 months of life. The immunity produced by the disease is permanent, and recurrences are rare.

Symptoms. Symptoms of invasion are often absent. When present, they consist of slight fever and malaise and mild catarrh. The fever rarely lasts more than 2 days, usually less. The catarrhal symptoms consist of coughing and sneezing. Congestion of the mucous membranes of the nose and eyes is present. Even though no complaint may be made of sore throat, there is to be seen almost constantly a diffuse redness of the pharynx and often slight swelling of the tonsils. In many cases, there is an enanthem on the soft palate, consisting of red spots pinhead in size. Koplik's spots never are found. Slight general glandular enlargement occurs. Enlargement of the posterior cervical and occipital glands is of some diagnostic importance. The white blood count is normal or low.

RASH. Soon after the onset of the symptoms of invasion, or in their absence, the eruption appears on the face and in the course of from a few hours to a day spreads over the body. The first thing calling attention to the disease may be the finding of a rash covering the body. Sometimes the rash has faded from the face and neck by the time the extremities are involved. The total duration of the rash is not more than 2 to 4 days, often less. The eruption consists of erythematous spots, slightly papular, which vary in size from that of a pinpoint to several millimeters, and they are usually discrete. In some areas these spots may become confluent and assume the blotchy appearance of measles. The eruption varies considerably, even in different cases in the same epidemic. It may resemble closely the rash of measles in one case and of scarlet fever in another. A faint desquamation similar to that found in measles sometimes follows the eruption.

Complications. On rare occasions encephalitis, arthritis or thrombocytopenic purpura occurs as a complication of rubella. The only other complications of importance are certain congenital malformations of the fetus when the mother develops the disease. If rubella affects the mother during the first 3 months of pregnancy, the fetus may develop congenital malformations. Later in the pregnancy rubella has no effect on the fetus.

Isolation. Isolation is not considered necessary except in institutions if the diagnosis is certain. By the time the diagnosis is made, the remaining infective period is brief. The child probably is not a source of infection after the rash has faded.

Prognosis. The prognosis in rubella is good except in those few instances in which encephalitis occurs as a complication. In many instances, recovery from encephalitis is complete.

Prevention, Diagnosis and Treatment. Sometimes prevention is attempted when a susceptible woman is exposed during the first trimester of pregnancy. Gamma globulin is used, but its efficacy is not well established.

A tissue culture vaccine has now been developed which, in early trials, appears capable of providing active immunity against rubella.

Diagnosis is relatively easy in an epidemic but difficult in sporadic cases. The disease can be simulated by various toxic and drug eruptions and by very mild scarlet fever. It lacks Koplik's spots and the more severe catarrhal symptoms of measles.

Treatment other than brief isolation is not required.

Exanthem Subitum (Roseola Infantum)

(See Chapter 14.)

Chickenpox (Varicella)

Chickenpox is a highly communicable viral disease in which the chief feature is a generalized vesicular eruption (Plate 1).

Etiology. The virus of chickenpox is present in the nose and throat, in the vesicles of the eruption and probably in the crusts resulting from the drying of the vesicles. The disease is rare in the first 3 months of life but occurs at the first exposure after this age. It is one of the most highly communicable diseases.

Symptoms. The incubation period is from 14 to 16 days. Prodromal symptoms usually are absent or are limited to a slight fever of which no complaint is made. Rarely, high fever may be present and even convulsions. Commonly, the first thing noted is the rash, which appears first on the face or trunk and a little later on the extremities. New lesions continue to appear over the entire body for a period of from 3 to 4 days. Each lesion appears first as a macule, which quickly develops into a vesicle, or first a papule and then a vesicle. The vesicle rapidly increases in size to 3 or 4 mm. in diameter within 24 hours of the first appearance of the macule. The characteristic mature chickenpox lesion is a vesicle with a red areola and filled with clear fluid. The vesicle then dries gradually, first becoming depressed at the center, and later becoming a flat crust. The crust falls off in from 1 to 3 weeks.

After the eruption has been present for a day or two, all stages of it may be seen on the skin in the same area. In the same general area may be seen macules, papules, immature and mature vesicles and crusts of dried lesions. The presence of many stages of eruption at the same time is due in part to the development of the lesions in successive crops and in part to beginning retrogression of a large number of lesions before maturity, perhaps because of developing immunity.

The lesions of chickenpox also appear on the mucous membrane of the mouth and the vagina. In these areas no vesicles are seen, but the appearance is as if a vesicle had been present and the top rubbed off, that is, a gray-white spot surrounded by a ring of redness.

Complications. Complications are infrequent. Scratched or traumatized lesions offer a portal of entry for pyogenic bacteria, with resultant local suppuration and sometimes the development of cellulitis. The virus of the disease sometimes causes encephalitis, but complete recovery is the rule. Unlike measles, the small infant obtains little temporary immunity from his mother. At this age the disease tends to be more severe.

Children who have not previously had varicella and who are receiving steroids in high dosage for the treatment of leukemia, malignancies or collagen disease, are high risks since they may suffer from overwhelming disease if exposed. Reduction of steroid dosage to maintenance levels and administration of very large doses of gamma globulin soon after known exposure may provide some degree of protection.

Isolation. An isolation period of from 10 to 14 days is generally considered sufficient, but in institutions that care for children it is preferable that isolation be continued until all crusts are off.

Prevention. When chickenpox occurs among children in their own homes, preventive measures other than isolation are not carried out because of the mildness of constitutional symptoms and the rarity of serious complications. On the other hand, the disease becomes important when it occurs in a children's hospital, where it may cause postponement of the treatment for which the child was admitted, for example, a surgical operation. Other reasons why an epidemic cannot be allowed to continue in a hospital are obvious.

Diagnosis and Treatment. The disease most likely to be confused with chickenpox is smallpox. Usually, smallpox is a serious disease with great prostration, but it may be mild and resemble chickenpox. Smallpox has only one crop of lesions in any one skin area, and all are in the same stage of maturity at any one time. Smallpox affects more prominently the exposed parts, the extremities and the face, while chickenpox affects chiefly the trunk, with scattered lesions on the face and the extremities. The vesicular lesions of chickenpox are superficial in the skin, and the early lesions contain obviously clear fluid. Smallpox lesions are more deeply seated in the skin, and the early vesicular lesions have a pearly appearance, never that of containing obviously clear fluid.

Herpes Zoster (Shingles)

This disorder, commonly known as shingles, consists of a group of itching or painful blisters that are confined to the distribution of one of the sensory nerves emanating from the posterior root ganglia of the spinal cord. It is recognized by its sharp limitation to one side of the body within a skin area corresponding to a dermatome. It is now thought that herpes zoster is caused by the same virus as chickenpox and that it often represents a reactivation of chickenpox in a person who had his first attack previously. The disease is not very common in children.

Smallpox (Variola, Alastrim)

Smallpox is a highly contagious communicable disease which has been virtually eliminated from the United States, Canada and Europe by universal vaccination of populations and immigrants. It is considered here only briefly because the nurse is unlikely to encounter it unless she serves in Asia or Africa where dangerous foci of the infection still smoulder.

Etiology. The virus which causes smallpox is very similar to that which is used for vaccination. In the infected individual it invades widely—the skin, mucous membranes and blood stream. Exposed persons who have not been vaccinated are universally susceptible at any age. It is spread by contact with the scabs or the contents of the lesions and by air-borne passage of virus from the respiratory passages of an infected subject. The period of contagion lasts until the last scabs have disappeared—at least a month from the onset. Infected material which is passed along on intermediate articles may also be a source of spread.

Symptoms. The incubation period is 10 to 12 days after exposure. The onset is abrupt with headache, backache and fever of 103° to 104° F. The eruption appears on the 3rd day after onset, usually on the forehead or wrists. In contrast to chickenpox it emerges as one crop and is heaviest on the extremities, face and scalp. The individual lesions are hard, umbilicated vesicles with necrotic centers which become pustular and often secondarily infected. They are deep-seated and leave permanent scars when they heal.

Complications include corneal ulceration and scar-

ring, respiratory tract obstruction, furunculosis, septicemia, pneumonia and encephalitis.

Prognosis. The outcome depends on the virulence of the strain of virus involved. In alastrim, which is a mild variety of smallpox, the mortality is around 1 per cent. In other epidemics among unprotected persons, rates of 25 to 50 per cent or even higher have been observed.

Treatment. This must be carried out in a hospital with facilities for rigid isolation in order to limit the spread of the disease. Antibiotics to prevent secondary infection of the lesions and general supportive measures comprise the basis of therapy.

Prevention. This is accomplished by universal vaccination of population groups which are free of smallpox. The technic, devised by Jenner, is the oldest prophylactic measure known. If a case appears in a community, revaccination should be undertaken at once. Persons vaccinated after exposure are not necessarily protected. A group of drugs known chemically as thiosemicarbazones have been shown to be effective in preventing smallpox if used soon after exposure. They are not useful after the eruption has appeared.

Vaccinia

Vaccinia is a local skin lesion produced by the inoculation of cowpox virus for the purpose of protecting against smallpox. Cowpox is a pustular disease affecting cattle and is communicable to man. It is a less virulent and less serious disease for both cattle and man than is smallpox for man. A man who has had cowpox is thereafter immune to smallpox. This view was current among the country folk of England during the life of Edward Jenner (18th century). Jenner was the first to take advantage of this knowledge by making the experiment of inoculating a human being with cowpox (1796). Since then, cowpox vaccination has become customary in many countries and compulsory in some.

Cowpox acquired naturally is a generalized disease, as is smallpox. Inoculation into the skin produces only a local lesion, but it gives immunity to both cowpox and smallpox. The virus of cowpox is contained in the pustules of this disease. Early in the history of vaccination, inoculations were made from the pustule of one human to the skin of another. Complications were not uncommon. Sometimes pyogenic and other bacteria were carried along with the virus. Inoculation is no longer made from the human. In commercial production the virus is obtained from calves under most carefully controlled conditions. The safeguards are such that complications of the variety mentioned are all but impossible. Some of the available vaccine is produced by growing the virus in the chorio-allantoic membrane of the chick embryo with still further elimination of the hazard of bacterial contamination.

Vaccination. Vaccination or the inoculation with cowpox virus may be carried out as follows: The skin of the site chosen for inoculation is washed first with soap and water and then with ether or acetone. After drying, the skin is scratched or punctured through a drop of the prepared vaccine. The object is to infect the skin with the virus and with the virus alone. If the scratch procedure is used, two or three short parallel scratches are made with a needle, not deep enough to draw blood. If the multiple puncture method is used, the skin is punctured lightly several times with the needle. Usually the needle is held almost parallel with the skin surface in order to control the depth of puncture. After the inoculation, the vaccine remaining is wiped off. No dressing is applied.

Site. The inoculation site usually chosen is the left arm at the insertion of the deltoid muscle. In girls and women, the lateral surface of the calf of the leg is sometimes chosen, or the inoculation may be made on the thigh. (In these areas the risk of secondary infection is greater.)

Course of the Lesion. After the lapse of 2 or 3 days, the inoculation site should appear normal except for slight evidence of the original trauma. On the 4th or the 5th day, a papule appears (Plate 2). This increases rapidly in size and becomes vesicular. The vesicle is pearly gray and surrounded by an area of redness. The vesicle is a pustule or quickly becomes pustular. It increases in size and reaches its maximal extent by the 9th or 10th day. At this time, there may be some swelling of the axillary glands and constitutional symptoms consisting of fever, malaise and irritability. After the 10th day, the pustule begins to dry and the neighboring inflammation to disappear. The constitutional symptoms subside rapidly. The crust which forms as a result of the drying of the pustule gradually loosens and falls off, usually late in the third week, leaving a scar which later becomes white and depressed and is characteristically pitted.

Management of the Lesion. Many prefer no dressing at any stage of the lesion. Some suggest that gauze be pinned inside the sleeve over the pustule. A very good procedure is to place a plain gauze dressing over the pustule and hold it in place by adhesive tape in such a manner that constriction of the swollen arm by the tape is not possible. The object of the dressing is to prevent secondary infection in case the pustule should be broken accidentally. If the pustule should rupture, the dressing will adhere to it. Then if it is desired to change the dressing, the outlying portions of the gauze are cut away, leaving the small circle of gauze stuck to the lesion. Then a new dressing is applied over the old one. A "vaccination shield" should not be used.

Complications. Complications in vaccinia are uncommon. The most common are those arising from secondary infection of the pustule, such as erysipelas and sepsis. Sometimes a child will rub the freshly vaccinated spot with a finger, then with the same finger rub the skin elsewhere and produce a second lesion.

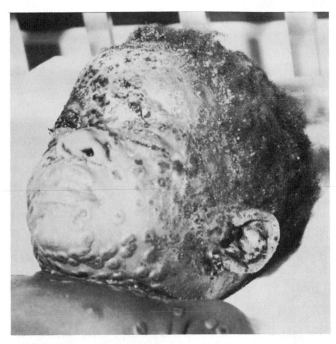

Fig. 18-1. Child with generalized vaccinia superimposed upon chronic eczema. The vaccinia was contracted from a sibling with a normal taking vaccination. After a long and stormy course this child recovered.

Generalized vaccinia or cowpox is a rare complication but is potentially serious (Fig. 18-1). Infants with exuding eczema are particularly susceptible. They should be neither vaccinated nor exposed to others who have been vaccinated recently. Children with permanent imperfections of immune response such as the Swiss type of agammaglobulinemia, and those with temporarily suppressed immunity due to treatment with radiation and immunosuppressive drugs must be defended against exposure to vaccinia virus for they may develop generalized or progressive vaccinia. Postvaccinal encephalitis is a serious but rare complication. The mortality rate may be as high as 25 to 30 per cent. The survivors usually escape without brain damage.

Treatment. Usually the constitutional symptoms are not severe enough to require treatment. For severe symptoms, remaining in bed is sufficient. The treatment of any pyogenic complication is that which is applicable irrespective of vaccinia.

Treatment of generalized vaccinia includes measures to reduce fever, to prevent secondary infection of the extensive skin lesions, to maintain hydration and nutrition and to support the infant or child through an illness which may be as severe as an extensive burn. Specific immune gammaglobulin is available through the American Red Cross which is usually effective in preventing the disease in those exposed unwittingly to vaccinia, and is somewhat effective in reducing the severity of the infection once it has appeared. Thiosemicarbazones may be of additional assistance in those rare individuals who have progressive vaccinia, a complication in which the original lesion fails to heal and advances locally even to destruction of an extremity and ultimate death.

Vaccination Failure. Vaccination may fail to "take" because of faulty performance of the procedure. When properly done, two reasons exist for failure. It will be unsuccessful if the person is immune because of previous vaccination or smallpox. In these circumstances, an immune reaction will appear. This reaction consists of the development of a small area of induration and redness within a day or two of vaccination. More often, vaccination is unsuccessful because the virus used is no longer living. The virus as dispensed commercially will remain living for many months if kept cold and away from sunlight. Continued exposure in a warm room will soon make it useless.

Revaccination. Although a single vaccination may protect for life, immunity for so long a period cannot be relied on. Vaccination in infancy and revaccinations every 3 to 5 years are to be recommended. When the first vaccination is performed in early infancy, the reaction is much less severe than at later periods of life. After successful vaccination all subsequent vaccinations tend to have milder reactions.

ENTEROVIRUS INFECTIONS

In the course of the extensive studies on the agents that produce poliomyelitis, two other groups of viruses have been encountered which have somewhat similar properties. These are the Coxsackie viruses and the ECHO viruses. All these agents are small viruses which can be found from time to time in the stools of children and adults. They are more prevalent in warm climates and during the summer months. Most of the individuals who harbor them are not affected by their presence, either because of specific immunity or because the agents remain confined to the interior of the intestinal canal. Some persons, children more commonly than adults, suffer disease because their lack of immunity permits the viruses to invade other parts of the body, particularly the blood and the central nervous system.

Poliomyelitis (Infantile Paralysis)

Etiology. Poliomyelitis is caused by a small virus which, when it gains access to the central nervous system, produces dysfunction or death of nerve cells, particularly those in the anterior horn of the spinal cord and the corresponding regions of the brain, i.e., the cells that supply motor nerves. Three general types of poliomyelitis virus have been separated by immunologic methods. These are designated Type I (Brunhilde), Type II (Lansing) and Type III (Leon). In nature, the viruses infect man alone; experimentally, the disease can be produced readily in monkeys and, under special circumstances, in a few other animals. The work of Enders, Weller and Robbins, which won a

Nobel prize, accelerated the study of poliomyelitis by providing a simple means of cultivating these and other viruses in tissue culture media and of rapidly testing for antibody against them.

Method of Invasion. The manner in which the virus enters the body and gains access to the cells of the spinal cord or the brain has been under study for a great many years but is not understood thoroughly. Entrance into the body is probably through the mouth, the pharynx and the intestinal tract, perhaps occasionally through the nose.

There is reason to believe that asymptomatic infection with the poliomyelitis virus is a common, almost a universal, event among children. During past epidemic periods virus was found in the stools of children living in association with poliomyelitis victims, children who themselves showed mild or no evidence of disease. It is judged that fewer than 1 out of 10 children who excrete virus in the stools will have evidence of clinical disease. Furthermore, examination of the blood of adults shows that a high percentage have antibodies against poliomyelitis, even though they never have had the disease. The belief is growing that most children acquire viral infection early in life, but that only a few permit the virus to migrate from their intestinal tracts to their nervous systems. The reasons why some fail to keep it localized have yet to be discovered. Vaccination against poliomyelitis provides the child with a better defense against the transmission of virus from intestine to nervous system.

Types of Disease. Infection with the virus of poliomyelitis can result in a great variety of clinical manifestations:

THE CARRIER STATE. This merely signifies that the child has poliomyelitis virus in his stools but no evidence of the disease. The condition goes unrecognized except when special epidemiologic studies are in progress. No treatment is required.

The symptoms may include brief fever, headache, sore threat, mild diarrhea, abdominal pain, nausea and vomiting. Signs of involvement of the nervous system are lacking, and the spinal fluid is normal. Since the symptoms subside rapidly, no treatment is necessary.

NONPARALYTIC POLIOMYELITIS. This is similar to the foregoing, except that symptoms may be prolonged over several days' time, and in addition there is clinical evidence of meningeal irritation. The latter is manifested by pain in the neck or the back with limitation of flexion of the spine. There may be increased sensitivity of skin or muscles and peculiar sensations such as tingling or transient weakness of muscles. The spinal fluid shows an increase in the number of lymphocytes and a slight increase in protein content. Treatment consists of bed rest and observation until the fever and other symptoms disappear and it is clear that no paralysis will occur.

SPINAL FORM OF PARALYTIC POLIOMYELITIS. *Symptoms.* In what might be called the average or typical case, the onset is sudden, with fever, headache and prostration, sometimes vomiting and, rarely, convulsions. The fever, the headache and the prostration continue. Irritability, general or local hyperesthesia and neck and back rigidity develop. The child may be mentally clear or drowsy. In severe infections, coma may occur.

After the symptoms described have persisted for a variable period, often from 2 to 3 days, paralysis and other phenomena appear. Such true paralysis as occurs is flaccid in type, and the muscle fibers affected cannot function and therefore cannot exhibit spasm. Either the maximal amount of paralysis appears at once or it increases in degree and extent for a period of 3 or 4 days. In the order of their frequency, paralysis occurs in the following parts of the body: one or both legs, one or both arms, combined arms and legs, legs and trunk. The legs are involved in the majority of cases; other parts, to a much lesser extent.

The constitutional symptoms characteristic of the early stages of poliomyelitis seldom last more than 6 or 7 days. Sometimes the hyperesthesia and the irritability last longer. After the paralysis has developed fully, it remains stationary from 1 to several weeks. Although no change occurs in the paralysis during this time, those muscles or portions of muscles which already are paralyzed undergo more or less atrophy. After this short stationary period, improvement in power of the paralyzed parts takes place. Some show complete recovery in a few weeks; others will be completely well in 3 months. The most rapid improvement occurs in the first 6 months. After this time, nearly half of the children will have recovered completely, while the remainder will show permanent paralysis of varying extent. If the permanent paralysis extensively involves a limb, its further growth, in both size and length, is stunted, the skin is cold and mottled from poor blood supply, and unless proper care is given, contractures occur and result in deformity.

Treatment and Nursing Care. In the absence of useful specific therapy, the treatment is symptomatic and supportive. The diet should be suitable to the severity of the illness and fluid intake should be maintained but not forced. Usually a soft diet is appropriate except when bulbar involvement causes difficulty in swallowing.

The maintenance of good body alignment on a firm flat mattress and frequent repositioning is important in prevention of deformities. If the legs are affected, the heels and toes should be allowed to extend over the end of the mattress or a foot board should be used.

The pain of muscle spasm is relieved in the first few days by hot applications (Kenny treatment). When spasm and pain have been relieved, passive motion is used to maintain muscle nutrition and joint sense. Active motion done by a physiotherapist is permitted and encouraged (under water when desired) when such activity does not increase spasm and tenderness, pain or fatigue.

Muscle training and re-education prevent contractures from muscle shortening and should continue for as long as evidence exists of return of muscle function. Braces and splints may be prescribed for support when the child is ready to attempt locomotion. The final step in treatment may require operative procedures to improve the efficiency of permanently paralyzed extremities.

BULBAR POLIOMYELITIS. *Symptoms.* When the inflammatory reaction of poliomyelitis attacks the higher portions of the central nervous system, especially the bulb, or medulla oblongata, nervous control of vital functions is threatened, and the prognosis for survival is reduced. In favorable instances the muscles of the eye, the face, the jaws or the palate alone may be affected. Recovery is complete in most cases, and no serious effects are suffered from the temporary disability. But when the lower cranial nerves and the upper portions of the spinal cord are involved there may be serious disturbance of swallowing, of respiration or of the central control of circulation. Paralysis of swallowing not only prevents the intake of food but also interferes with the disposition of the normal accumulations of mucus and saliva in the pharynx. Aspiration into the trachea may result in pneumonia or atelectasis. When certain areas of the brain stem are involved there may be serious disturbance of the general circulation with progressive cyanosis and a weak, feeble pulse. Disturbances of respiration may be due either to involvement of the respiratory center which governs the automatic effort to breathe or to paralysis of the muscles of respiration such as the diaphragm, the intercostal muscles and the pectoral muscles. Most of the fatalities in poliomyelitis are caused by disturbances of the circulation or the respiration.

Treatment and Nursing Care. The management of bulbar poliomyelitis is frequently difficult and demands the best medical judgment and skillful, attentive nursing. Gentle suctioning of the pharynx and postural drainage may protect the airway. Because of inability to swallow, feeding is accomplished by gavage or by a nasal tube left in place and by additional parenteral fluids. A tracheostomy may be necessary to maintain a clear airway.

Patients who require care in a respirator because of failing respiratory muscles present a complicated problem which is handled best by a staff of doctors and nurses who are specially trained for this purpose. Some of the difficulties which must be met are those of maintaining an airway, preventing aspiration, providing mechanical aids in exchanging air, maintaining nutrition and morale, prevention of intercurrent respiratory and urinary tract infections and, eventually, rehabilitation of a patient who sometimes is extensively paralyzed and fearful of being weaned from the respirator.

Diagnosis. The diagnosis of poliomyelitis after

paralysis has occurred presents no difficulty. Diagnosis in the preparalytic stage with any degree of certainty is obviously not so easy. The preparalytic symptoms which have been enumerated, together with the results of an examination of the cerebrospinal fluid, will give strong presumptive evidence of a correct diagnosis. The cerebrospinal fluid in poliomyelitis, whether preparalytic or abortive, always shows moderate but definite abnormality. The cells are increased, often up to 100, seldom to 500 for each cubic millimeter, and rarely sufficiently to cause the fluid to be definitely cloudy. The proteins of the fluid are increased, and the colloidal tests (Lange, etc.) are positive.

Poliomyelitis may be confused with other infections of the central nervous system such as Coxsackie virus disease, mumps encephalitis, infectious polyneuritis or the viral encephalitides. Spinal fluid examination usually permits a ready distinction between poliomyelitis and acute meningitis.

Isolation Precautions. To limit the spread of virus from a hospitalized child with known infection, the same sort of precautions as those taken with typhoid fever are required, namely, aseptic technic and careful disposal of stools. The period during which this must be continued is determined arbitrarily and usually is set at about 2 weeks after the onset of symptoms. The child who is cared for at home already has contaminated his environment with virus by the time his disease is discovered, so that enforcement of such isolation measures is probably useless.

Prevention. Active immunization is now available in two forms: (1) Salk vaccine which is an inactivated preparation of the three main strains of poliomyelitis virus, and (2) live-virus vaccine which consists of preparations of avirulent virus of the main types which can be taken by mouth. Since 1955 the practice of routine immunization of infants and children with first Salk, and then the more convenient and possibly more effective Sabin vaccines has produced a miraculous and sustained drop in the incidence of the disease. The practical elimination of poliomyelitis is mirrored in the fact that in 1952 there were over 35,000 cases of paralytic polio in the U.S., whereas the figure has dropped progressively so that in 1965, only 43 such cases were reported.

Infectious Polyneuritis (Guillain-Barré Syndrome)

Although the viral etiology of this disorder has long been suspected, it has not been proved. Infectious polyneuritis is considered here because it is frequently confused with poliomyelitis at the onset. It is a disorder characterized by generalized, often extensive weakness and pain in various muscle groups. It is ordinarily a self-limited disease which progresses for a period of 2 to 4 weeks and then abates. During this interval there may be considerable atrophy of the involved muscles. The chief importance of this disorder is its confusion with poliomyelitis. Distinction between the two diseases is made from the presence of sensory changes in infectious polyneuritis and from the appearance of the spinal fluid, which usually contains a marked increase in protein but little or no increase in cells. Nursing care of polyneuritis is similar to that for poliomyelitis.

Coxsackie Virus Infection

Coxsackie viruses (pronounced cook'-sock-ee) are a family of viruses closely related to the polio viruses and sometimes found in association with them. They primarily inhabit the intestinal tract where they produce infrequent disease. Occasionally they spread to other portions of the body where a variety of clinical disorders can result. Their serious effect upon newborn infants has been discussed in Chapter 10. Less commonly they may produce myocarditis in older children. Aseptic meningitis comparable to nonparalytic poliomyelitis, pleurodynia and upper respiratory infection are also the result of infection with these agents. There is no specific treatment or prevention available. Nursing care is symptomatic.

ECHO Virus Infection

This group of viruses was isolated before they were known to produce disease in man. The name is derived from the initials of "enteric cytopathogenic human orphan" viruses and signifies that they are found in the intestinal tract, produce changes in tissue culture cells and were formerly orphans, i.e., had no relation to human disease. Subsequently they have been found associated with aseptic meningitis and other epidemic febrile diseases usually appearing in the summer months. Infection is self-limited and requires no treatment. Recovery is almost always complete. Some of the summer epidemics of ECHO virus infection are accompanied by morbilliform and other types of rashes.

Mumps (Epidemic Parotitis)

Mumps is an acute contagious disease affecting chiefly the salivary glands, especially the parotid glands. It causes swelling of these glands, local discomfort and usually moderate constitutional symptoms.

Etiology. Mumps is a virus disease. It occurs infrequently under 2 years of age and is not common in adults. The period of greatest incidence is between 4 and 15 years. Closer contact is required for the transmission of mumps than for most of the contagious diseases, and only a small proportion of those exposed acquire the disease. One attack usually protects the individual from subsequent attacks. The incubation period varies. It is usually between 2 and 3 weeks, with an average of 18 days.

Symptoms. In most instances there are no prodromal symptoms. When present, they consist of slight fever, malaise, headache and anorexia. These are of short duration before the swelling of the parotid gland begins, associated with local, dull, aching pain. Sometimes both parotids are involved simultaneously; sometimes the disease remains limited to one; but more often one parotid gland is involved first, and after an interval of several days the disease in the other parotid becomes manifest.

The parotid becomes swollen, tender and painful. Much individual variation exists in the number and the severity of local and general symptoms. In the majority, the disease is mild, and most of the discomfort is local. It is difficult to confine such children to bed. Some children have high fever and are prostrated. Opening the mouth may be impossible because of swelling and pain. The swelling begins to subside within 2 or 3 days, and at the same time the constitutional symptoms subside rapidly. By the 8th to the 10th day the swelling and all signs of the disease usually have disappeared.

Frequently, the submaxillary and the sublingual salivary glands are involved coincidentally with the parotid glands. Occasionally, the submaxillary or the sublingual glands alone are affected.

Complications. Although complications occur frequently in some epidemics among adults, they are uncommon in childhood. The most common complication among males past puberty is orchitis. This occurs usually 1 week (sometimes up to 2 weeks) after the onset of mumps, and the local and the general symptoms are severe. The testis becomes greatly swollen and subsequent atrophy occurs in about half the cases. A similar inflammation may occur in the ovaries, the uterus and the breasts or the external genitalia of the female. Pancreatitis is occasionally suspected when mumps is accompanied by abdominal pain.

Meningo-encephalitis of mild degree is the most common complication in the younger child. Increase in the pressure and the cellular content of the spinal fluid may be suspected when headache, vomiting or delirium is marked. Relief of symptoms often follows a lumbar puncture. Recovery is complete in all instances.

Deafness also rarely occurs as a complication, but when it does it is usually unilateral and permanent.

Isolation. Isolation of those with mumps should be continued for 2 or 3 days after the swelling has disappeared. Thus, most children can be released by the end of 2 weeks. Any complication prolongs the course of the disease approximately 1 week.

Diagnosis. A common error in diagnosis is confusion of cervical lymphadenitis with mumps. The lobe of the ear is at the center of parotid swelling, while the swelling of lymphadenitis is slightly lower in the neck. An aid in diagnosis is redness and swelling of the outlet of the parotid duct in the mouth. The blood leukocytes are normal in number or decreased in uncomplicated mumps and increased in acute lymphadenitis.

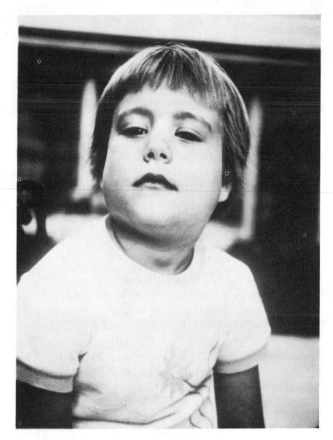

Fig. 18-2. Mumps.

Laboratory assistance in confirming the suspicion of mumps is now available in that specific antibodies can be found in the blood. A skin test with inactivated virus is useful in distinguishing between susceptible and immune persons. An inflammatory response at the site of injection of the killed virus indicates immunity.

Prevention. Vaccines for active immunization have not been widely accepted because the disease is usually mild in children and the duration of vaccine induced immunity is short.

Treatment and Nursing Care. Treatment and nursing care are symptomatic. Often no treatment is required. For local pain, the application of heat usually gives relief. It may be necessary to restrict the diet to articles of food which do not require chewing. Acid foods tend to increase the pain. It is common belief that rest in bed helps to prevent complications. Observation of soldiers in World War I showed that this was not the case, particularly as regards orchitis. Complications usually require treatment in bed.

MISCELLANEOUS VIRAL INFECTIONS

Infectious Hepatitis (Catarrhal Jaundice)

Infectious hepatitis is the most common cause of jaundice after the period of infancy. It is caused by a virus whose effects in human volunteers have been studied. The virus itself has eluded isolation in animals and tissue cultures, preventing the development of specific diagnostic tests and vaccines.

The virus passes from one individual to another by the oral route through the ingestion of food or other substances which have been contaminated by infected feces. It circulates in the bloodstream for a time and can be transferred to another individual by transfusion or by the use of needles contaminated with blood. A closely related virus (serum hepatitis) passes only by way of the blood and produces a similar disease.

Symptoms. There is reason to think that the disease occurs in such a mild form that it is overlooked in a great many children. When symptoms are present they appear within 2 to 6 weeks following natural exposure to infectious hepatitis virus but not until 2 to 4 months after injection of blood which is contaminated with the serum hepatitis agent. The outstanding symptom, and in mild cases the only symptom, is jaundice. With increasing severity of the disease there may be nausea, abdominal pain, loss of appetite and vomiting. Occasionally a fulminating form is seen in which death occurs within 2 weeks. Severe protracted cases may result in important degrees of liver damage with cirrhosis.

The diagnosis in children is easily made from the presence of jaundice due to direct-reacting bilirubin in the blood. There are very few other causes of obstructive jaundice in the child. Confirmation is obtained by serial studies of liver function.

Prognosis. In children the prognosis is almost always good—a contrast to the adult who runs a more serious risk of permanent liver damage.

Treatment and Prevention. No specific treatment is known. Rest in bed until the jaundice has begun to subside is desirable. The diet should be low in fat and high in carbohydrate and vitamins. Isolation precautions must be observed to protect other patients from the virus being discharged in the stools for at least a week after the onset of jaundice. Exposed susceptible individuals can be given a measure of protection by the injection of gamma globulin in a dose of 0.02 ml. per Kg. of body weight.

Viral Encephalitis

Epidemiology. Since 1930 a number of specific viruses (arborviruses) have been shown to cause epidemics of encephalitis in the United States and other parts of the world. Viruses isolated from specific geographic areas can be separated from one another in the laboratory, although the diseases they produce are clinically very similar. Each has acquired the name of the general area and circumstances under which it was first discovered—St. Louis, western (U. S.) equine, eastern (U. S.) equine, Japanese B, Russian spring-summer, Venezuelan. The term "equine" indicates that this form of encephalitis exists primarily in horses rather than in man. Now it is known that each of these forms is transmitted from animal to man by a particular variety of mosquito or mite. In some instances the epidemics are restricted to certain times of the year (usually summer) because of the life cycle of the insect required for the spread of the infection.

Symptoms. The onset of the disease is generally abrupt, with fever, vomiting, stiff neck, convulsions, delirium and coma present in varying degree. In some instances there may be a preceding period of illness that simulates influenza. In many respects the symptoms imitate meningitis, and the distinction must be made from examination of the spinal fluid, which contains relatively few cells, usually lymphocytes instead of polymorphonuclear leukocytes, and is sterile on bacterial culture. The fatality rate and the incidence of enduring neurologic disturbances is higher among infants than in older children or adults. Exact figures depend on the variety of agent responsible for the encephalitis.

Diagnosis. Usually this is made from the clinical picture and the examination of the spinal fluid. At a later stage in the illness, specific virus antibodies appear in the blood which can be used for laboratory confirmation of the type of illness.

Treatment. No specific treatment is known. General good nursing care, control of convulsions and support of nutrition are indicated until the disease subsides spontaneously.

Rabies

Rabies is a uniformly fatal disease resulting from a specific viral infection of the nervous system, usually acquired through the bite of an animal afflicted with the disease. Presumably, all warm-blooded animals are susceptible, although in settled communities the dog is the animal most commonly affected. Skunks, bats, wolves and foxes are the wild animals which most often harbor virus.

The virus of rabies is present in the saliva of rabid dogs and is introduced into the body by means of a bite. The virus travels along nerves, eventually reaching the central nervous system by this route. The time of travel represents all or most of the incubation period, which is widely variable, depending on the quantity of virus introduced, the virulence of the virus, the nerve supply and the distance of the point bitten from the central nervous system. Rabies from bites about the head has a short incubation period. The incubation period is rarely shorter than 2 weeks and may be as long as 6 or 7 months. The average time is from 1 to 2 months. If the virus is introduced in small quantity in an area poorly supplied by nerves, the disease may never develop. Bites through thick clothing are not very dangerous because of the small quantity of virus inoculated. Only from 15 to 20 percent of those bitten by rabid animals develop the disease.

Symptoms. Regardless of the length of the incubation period the symptoms are equally severe when they occur. The onset and the course are rapid. An outstanding feature is hypersensitiveness and increased reaction to external stimuli. Excitement, convulsions and spasm of the muscles of deglutition characterize the final stages of illness, which terminates fatally in 3 to 4 days.

Treatment. Once symptoms appear, treatment is completely futile. Heavy sedation to make the child's final days as comfortable as possible is all that can be done.

Prevention. Because of the long incubation period between the bite and the appearance of symptoms, there may be time in which to build up an active immunity before invasion of the central nervous system takes place. Bites on the distal portions of the extremities offer a more favorable chance than those which are closer to the brain and cord, i.e. on the face and neck. Because the materials to be used in producing the immunity are not innocuous in themselves, a carefully planned series of steps is usually followed in which decisions depend upon knowledge of the health of the biting animal. Therefore it is highly desirable to capture and observe the attacker if at all possible. If the biting animal shows no symptoms of rabies in 5 days, preventive measures can be omitted or discontinued.

Local care of the wound should include thorough washing with green soap and debridement if indicated. Zephiran or 50 per cent alcohol can be used to flush out the wound and destroy any unabsorbed virus. For severe wounds, local injection of antirabies serum may be made.

Passive temporary protection may be given with antirabies serum prepared in animals. The subject must be tested for sensitivity to the serum before it is used. Serum alone is not sufficient if exposure to virus has occurred and active immunization with rabies vaccine must be started at once. Vaccines prepared from animal brain tissue which has been infected and then inactivated are the most potent antigenically, but carry a significant risk of producing encephalopathy if the recipient is sensitive to the tissue included in the vaccine. A newer vaccine prepared in fertile duck eggs is less likely to produce untoward reactions, but its antigenic potency may be less. Injections of either vaccine are made subcutaneously daily for 14 to 21 days depending upon the severity of the wounds and their proximity to the brain and cord. If neurologic manifestations appear, the vaccine must be discontinued.

Table 18. WHO Recommendations for Management of Rabies

Exposure	Status of Biting Animal		Treatment
	At Exposure	After Observation	
No lesions / Indirect Contact / Licks of un-abraded skin	Rabid		None
Licks on mucosa or abraded skin	Healthy	Clinical or lab. evidence of rabies	Start vaccine at first sign of rabies
Mild exposure	Suggestive rabid behavior	Healthy	Start vaccine at once; stop if animal is well on 5th day
	Rabid, escaped, killed, unknown		Start vaccine at once
	Wild animal bites		Give serum followed by vaccine
Severe exposure	Same as for mild exposure but invariably give serum at once		

Adapted from WHO Expert Committee on Rabies, Fifth Report, WHO Technical Report Series, #321, Geneva, 1966, p. 34.

The World Health Organization has issued a set of recommendations to guide the use of antiserum and vaccine. It is presented in abbreviated form in Table 18.

SITUATIONS FOR FURTHER STUDY

1. How do symptoms of German measles differ from those of rubeola? Do infants under 6 months of age acquire measles? What is the period of greatest communicability in measles? In what age period is the mortality rate of measles the highest?

2. Compare the lesions of chickenpox and smallpox. How do they differ? What is the difference in the distribution of the lesions?

3. What specific protective measures against communicable disease can be given during the period of infancy?

4. If you were a public-health nurse and visited a family with a 9-month-old baby and a toddler who had had no immunizations, how would you go about motivating the mother to use the facilities that were available to her?

5. What is entailed in the convalescent care of a child with poliomyelitis? What problems would be need help in facing during the convalescent period?

6. A child has been bitten by a neighborhood dog. The mother asks you for advice. What suggestions would you make?

7. What should parents teach their children about dogs?

BIBLIOGRAPHY

Agar, Ernest A.: Current concepts in immunization, Am. J. Nurs. *66*:2004, 1966.

Calafiore, D.: Eradication of measles in the United States, Am. J. Nurs. *67*:1871, 1967.

Creighton, H., and Armington, Sister Catherine: The bite of a stray dog, Am. J. Nurs. *64*:121, 1964.

Freidman, R.: Interferons and virus infections, Am. J. Nurs. *68*:542, 1968.

Geis, D., and Lambertz, S.: Acute respiratory infections in young children, Am. J. Nurs. *68*:294, 1968.

Gregg, Michael B.: Communicable disease trends in the United States, Am. J. Nurs. *68*:88, 1968.

Kempe, C. H.: Smallpox and Vaccinia, *in* Cooke, R. E. (ed.), The Biologic Basis of Pediatric Practice, N. Y., McGraw-Hill, 1968.

Krugman, S.: Rubella—new light on an old disease, Am. J. Nurs. *65*:126, 1965.

Parrott, R. H., and Chanock, R. M.: Respiratory Viruses, *in* Cooke, R. E. (ed.), The Biologic Basis of Pediatric Practice, N. Y., McGraw-Hill, p. 657, 1968.

Plotkin, S.: The future of vaccines against viral diseases, Pediat. Clin. N. Am. *15*:447, 1968.

19

Nursing Care of Children With Bacterial Infections

Many different bacteria are capable of producing infection in children. In this text it will be possible to consider only the more common invaders which produce characteristic symptoms. Some of these have already been discussed in the units concerned with the newborn and the infant.

In comparison with diseases caused by viruses, the bacterial infections tend to have incubation periods which are a matter of a few days rather than a week or more. Their courses are not as brief and self-limited. Many will linger or recur unless controlled by effective treatment. Fortunately, almost all of them can now be modified by antibiotics—substances that are completely ineffectual against viruses. For this reason it is desirable to arrive at a rapid and accurate diagnosis so that the proper form of antibiotic treatment can be started early in the disease. With viral infections, exact early diagnosis seldom speeds recovery, for no specific measures are available. Bacteriologic technics are sufficiently quick so that with a few exceptions the infecting germ can be identified in a day or two, and its antibiotic sensitivity worked out in another 24 to 48 hours. Recovery of viral agents or proof of their transit through the child more frequently takes a week or even longer.

Even before the antibiotics were discovered, methods were devised to bring the three dangerous childhood diseases under control—diphtheria, pertussis and tetanus. Active immunization is practiced routinely against these, and on particular indication against a few others (Table 19). Against the most prevalent bacterial infection of children — streptococcal — no prophylactic vaccine has yet been developed. However, for most bacterial infections a wide range of antibiotics are now available which, if properly used, can be expected to shorten the course and improve the prognosis.

STREPTOCOCCAL INFECTIONS

General Considerations

The streptococci are a large and ubiquitous family of bacteria which have in common the properties of round shape, positive staining by Gram's method and a tendency to form chains during the process of reproduction. They are of great importance in human disease, particularly in pediatric infections. Unlike the typhoid bacillus, there is not one single variety of streptococcus but rather a large family, the members of which have widely differing abilities to create disease. Some are natural inhabitants of the body; others are harbingers of important disease. A general understanding of the classification is desirable in order to interpret bacteriologic reports.

To differentiate among the streptococci it is first necessary to discover what type of hemolysis the growing colony produces on a blood agar plate. Streptococci that are productive of *alpha* or *gamma* type of hemolysis are common inhabitants of the upper respiratory and gastrointestinal tracts, and their presence does not indicate disease in these locations. On the other hand, if found in blood or urine cultures, they assume pathogenic importance. The streptococci that

Table 19. Control of Bacterial Infections

Disease	Active Immunization (Lasting)	Passive Immunization (Temporary)
Diphtheria	Toxoid (Park, 1922; Ramon, 1923)	Antitoxin
Pertussis	Vaccine (Leslie and Gardner, 1931)	Hyperimmune serum
Tetanus	Toxoid	Antitoxin
Typhoid	Vaccine	
Tuberculosis	B.C.G.	

are of major importance in pediatric disease produce a type of hemolysis known as *beta* hemolysis. The more nearly exact term "beta-hemolytic streptococcus" often is shortened to "hemolytic streptococcus" in everyday usage. Actually, about a dozen groups of beta-hemolytic streptococci can be identified by immunologic methods. Only those in Group A are important in human disease. However, few laboratories actually test the grouping of the streptococci; instead they assume that a beta-hemolytic streptococcus isolated from a person with an illness is probably a member of Group A. Occasionally, this assumption is wrong, and the streptococcus that is isolated turns out to be a harmless member of one of the other groups (B to N).

Group A·beta-hemolytic streptococci can be subdivided further into some 40-odd types by a different immunologic procedure. Determination of these types has utility in the investigation of certain aspects of epidemiology but is not practiced commonly in clinical medicine. Group A streptococci produce a number of substances which exude from the bacterial cells and have a bearing on the type of disease which results. Among these substances are erythrogenic toxin (or Dick toxin), streptolysin O and streptolysin S, streptokinase (or fibrinolysin) and hyaluronidase. As a result of streptococcal infection the body may produce antibodies against these substances which are known respectively as streptococcal antitoxin, antistreptolysin, antistreptokinase and antihyaluronidase.

Types of Streptococcal Disease. The most common site of infection with Group A beta-hemolytic streptococci is the upper respiratory tract. Many infections such as pharyngitis, tonsillitis, cervical adenitis and otitis media are initiated by these organisms. (The same sort of infection by a strain that produces a large amount of erythrogenic toxin and happens to infect a person who has no antitoxin immunity will result in scarlet fever.) These upper respiratory infections constitute the common form of beta-hemolytic streptococcus infection in childhood.

In another group of disorders, the hemolytic streptococcus infection is not a primary one but is favored by previous illness such as measles, pertussis or diphtheria. Secondary streptococcal infection of this sort is particularly troublesome after the viral infections.

The skin may be invaded by hemolytic streptococci in three characteristic ways: erysipelas, impetigo and cellulitis. *Erysipelas* has almost disappeared. *Impetigo* was discussed in Chapter 14. *Cellulitis* usually results from the invasion of a break in the skin by beta-hemolytic streptococci. It is a diffuse erythema and edema of the skin which surrounds the local wound. It may be accompanied by lymphangitis and local adenitis.

The Group A beta-hemolytic streptococci have an additional role in human disease. Glomerular nephritis, rheumatic fever and perhaps some other systemic diseases are preceded regularly by hemolytic streptococcus infections. The resultant disease is not due to direct streptococcal invasion of the organs affected but is rather a secondary phenomenon associated with the development of antibodies during recovery from the local streptococcal disease.

Hemolytic streptococci also may be responsible for pneumonia, septicemia, osteomyelitis, pyogenic arthritis and meningitis. Fortunately, these are rare varieties of infection.

Epidemiology. Streptococcal disease is endemic in most areas of the United States. It tends to be more prevalent during winter and early spring, probably owing to the collection of children indoors during the school year and during inclement weather. It is most prevalent in those in the first or second year of schooling and presumably in the process of having their first contact with such organisms. In families where there are several children the school-age children may introduce the infection into the family and transmit it to preschool siblings or even infants. In the latter the disease is likely to be more severe and persistent. Younger children who suffer from repeated infections over many months sometimes are said to have "streptococcosis" analogous to the first infection with tubercle bacilli.

In addition to infected school contacts, children may acquire the infection from carrier adults who are well or suffer only minor symptoms in spite of the fact that they harbor virulent streptococci in their noses and throats. Search for and treatment of such carriers is often essential before the recurring infections of the child can be terminated.

The density of streptococcal infection varies in a given community from one winter to the next. Usually, the incidence of scarlet fever, nephritis and rheumatic fever parallels the amount of general streptococcal infection in any given year.

Diagnosis. Precise diagnosis by culture of the nose, throat or purulent discharges should be made so that rational management of the patient can be carried out. If Group A beta-hemolytic streptococci are recovered, the child must be regarded as contagious until therapy is well under way. Furthermore, it is important to continue appropriate therapy well beyond the period of symptomatic cure as noted below. Confirmation of remote streptococcal infection which has passed the infective stage may be made by use of the antistreptolysin O titer of the blood—an antibody which appears in the wake of streptococcal disease and remains present for weeks after the organisms have disappeared from surface infections.

Treatment. Penicillin is universally effective against Group A beta-hemolytic streptococci. No strain has been found to be resistant to it! Treatment should be planned so that even with minor infections, an effective level of penicillin is maintained for a period of 10 days. Failure to do so may lead to suppression rather than elimination of the organisms so that the child has a return of symptoms and contagiousness after temporary improvement. For the ordinary streptococcal infection, 600,000 or 1,200,000 units of benzathine penicillin G given intramuscularly and repeated in 5 days is usually sufficient. When infection is severe, treatment may be started with the more rapidly acting procaine penicillin and followed by benzathine penicillin after severe toxicity has been brought under control. Oral penicillin is effective if regularly taken in a dosage of 250,000 units 4 times a day. It is less reliable for home treatment since children and parents may tire of, or forget the medication once the acute stage of the illness has passed.

For patients who are sensitive to penicillin, full dosage with erythromycin by mouth may be substituted for the 10 day period.

Prophylaxis. Rheumatic subjects and others with chronic illness who require special protection against new streptococcal infections receive an adequate defense in most instances if they are given continuously either benzathine penicillin intramuscularly once a month, or penicillin 250,000 units orally twice a day, or sulfadiazine 0.5 Gm. orally twice a day.

Scarlet Fever (Scarlatina)

Etiology. Scarlet fever is an upper respiratory infection with Group A beta-hemolytic streptococci accompanied by a generalized erythematous skin eruption and toxic manifestations due to the effects of erythrogenic toxin on a susceptible person. In occasional circumstances the initial streptococcal infection is in a wound or a burn rather than in the upper respiratory tract.

The disease occurs rarely in the first year. The incidence is at its height in the 5 to 8 year age group, after which it decreases. The disease occurs chiefly in the fall and winter months, only rarely in summer.

The incubation period varies from 1 to 7 days; most frequently it is from 2 to 4 days. The period of greatest communicability is during the height of the febrile period, the first 3 to 5 days. The causative streptococcus is abundant in the throat and in all discharges from this site. Streptococci gradually decrease in number and may be expected to have disappeared within 5 weeks of the onset if no antibiotics are given.

Symptoms. The onset of scarlet fever is sudden, with sore throat, vomiting, prostration and fever. The onset is so sudden that the mother often can state an exact time. The appearance of the throat is that of acute tonsillitis. Within from 24 to 36 hours both an enanthem and an exanthem appear, and the fever reaches its height. This period is marked by restlessness, great thirst and often delirium. Also, the pulse rate is high and out of proportion to the temperature. After reaching the maximum, the temperature remains elevated continuously for several days, then gradually declines, reaching normal in from 10 to 14 days after the onset in the untreated child.

Enanthem. The enanthem consists of closely packed, minute, dark-red macules on the palate and the fauces, which later spread to the cheeks and the gums. The macules may fuse to a diffuse redness. The tongue in the beginning is coated, then first the edge and finally the entire tongue becomes clean. As the tongue clears, a swelling of its papillae is apparent. Very early in the disease, usually after the 3rd or the 4th day, the tongue assumes the appearance known as "strawberry tongue," due to the general redness and the swollen papillae extending above the surface. Although strawberry tongue occurs in most cases of scarlet fever, it occurs also in other disease and is not characteristic of any disease.

Exanthem. The exanthem, or rash starts about the neck and the upper trunk; it spreads over the body and it attains its maximum in from 12 to 24 hours. It lasts from 3 to 7 days and gradually disappears. It is followed by desquamation, which begins about the 8th day or later. From a distance the rash looks like a diffuse red blush but on closer inspection is seen to consist of small points of redness, closely grouped. The appearance on the face is that of a diffuse blush, with the exception of a narrow area about the mouth, which by contrast appears to be white. When the rash is fully developed, the entire surface of the body is red except for the small area of pallor about the mouth. When the disease is mild, the skin, especially of the extremities, may be involved incompletely by the eruption.

Complications. The most common complications are otitis media, cervical adenitis and nephritis. Less common are arthritis, carditis and pneumonia. The otitis and the adenitis are extensions of the process in the throat. Although nephritis may appear earlier or later, it starts most commonly in the 3rd week. Carditis and pneumonia may be expected to occur only when the illness is severe.

Isolation. The isolation period should be based on the persistence of streptococci in the throat or the continuation of suppurative discharges.

Prognosis. In general, scarlet fever as it occurs at the present time is less severe than that of former years, and few deaths result directly from the toxic effects of the disease. Children nearly always recover from the nephritis of scarlet fever. The infectious complications tend to be more serious than the toxic effects.

Diagnosis. Eruptions similar to the rash of scarlet fever may be produced by certain drugs. In such instances, sore throat and other characteristic symptoms are likely to be absent. Sometimes erythematous eruptions from other causes are distinguished from the rash of mild scarlet fever with some difficulty. In such instances, the Schultz-Charlton test is of value.

Schultz-Charlton Reaction. The injection of immune serum into the skin in an area of scarlet-fever eruption, if made early in the course of the eruption, will cause a blanching of the rash in the area surrounding the site of injection. No other rash responds in this manner.

Prevention. Children known to be exposed to scarlet fever or other hemolytic streptococcus infections can be protected in many instances by prophylactic administration of a small dose of sulfadiazine, penicillin or other antibiotic given early during the incubation period.

Treatment and Nursing Care. In most instances the treatment is the same as that for any hemolytic streptococcus respiratory infection.

PNEUMOCOCCAL INFECTIONS

Pneumococci are most characteristically associated with pneumonic infections. However, otitis media, pharyngitis and occasionally cervical adenitis may be caused by these organisms. Treatment is effectively carried out with a wide variety of antibiotics. Penicillin is almost always quite adequate.

INFLUENZA BACILLUS INFECTIONS

The influenza bacillus, *H. influenzae*, produces its most serious infection as a purulent meningitis in infants and small children (Chap. 14). It may also be responsible for otitis media or pneumonia. The older the child, the more likely this agent is to be an unimportant inhabitant of the respiratory passages. One exception to this is described below. Treatment with penicillin is not effective. Treatment with ampicillin, sulfonamides or chloramphenicol is more effective.

Acute Epiglottitis

A variety of croup which is a surgical emergency is acute epiglottitis, a condition usually caused by *H. influenzae* and characterized by inflammation and edema of the tissues above the larynx. Its danger lies in the fact that the loosely swollen tissue may be drawn into the larynx at the beginning of an inspiration, occluding the airway completely and leading to sudden death. In contrast to ordinary croup, the symptoms include snoring or flapping sounds during *expiration* in addition to the inspiratory stridor. When epiglottitis is suspected clinically, it should be immediately confirmed by laryngoscopy and an emergency tracheostomy performed.

DIPHTHERIA

In regions where routine immunization against diphtheria has been established as a program for all children, the disease has been eliminated. But even in the U. S. where widespread immunization is practiced, it continues to erupt in localities in which the coverage is incomplete. In 1965 there were 165 cases reported. Periodically epidemics occur in the larger cities following migration of infected children from rural areas.

Etiology and Pathophysiology

The disease is caused by the diphtheria bacillus, *Corynebacterium diphtheriae*, which grows on mucous membrane surfaces, usually of the nose and pharynx, rarely in the vagina or upon open wounds of the skin. The bacterium exerts its main effect through the production of a soluble toxin which locally destroys the underlying tissue, producing a coagulum which is visible as the characteristic membrane. The same toxin may be transported by the blood stream of an unimmunized individual to produce damage in distant tissues such as the heart, where myocarditis may result, or the peripheral nervous system, where neuritis occurs. The local membrane is hazardous only insofar as it obstructs important channels such as the larynx. Of much greater concern are the widespread effects of the soluble toxin which may be lethal.

Symptoms

Faucial Diphtheria. Diphtheria of the tonsils and the tonsillar region is known as faucial diphtheria and is the variety most frequently observed. It has an incubation period of from 1 to 4 days. In the average or typical case the symptoms consist chiefly of fever, sore throat, malaise, headache and often general aches and pains. An early throat redness is followed quickly by an exudate which coalesces, becomes thicker and resembles a membrane. The membrane at first is grayish white but later becomes a dirty gray (Plate 3). The breath has an unpleasant, rather characteristic odor. When the membrane is removed forcibly, a bleeding surface remains. When no treatment is given, the membrane spreads in all directions. It may involve the posterior pharynx, the uvula and the soft palate. The cervical lymph glands are moderately to greatly enlarged, with proportionate visible swelling of the neck. Prostration increases as the disease progresses. Death results in a high proportion of those who are untreated.

Nasal Diphtheria. When the lesions of diphtheria are limited to the nose, little and often no constitutional disturbance results. Internal examination of the nose reveals areas of membrane. Nasal discharge is present, sometimes thickly purulent, but more often thin and tinged with blood. The discharge excoriates the upper lip. The disease may extend to the pharynx and the fauces. Nasal diphtheria tends to remain chronic over a period of weeks.

Laryngeal Diphtheria. Diphtheria may occur primarily in the larynx and remain limited to it. More commonly, laryngeal diphtheria occurs in association with and probably as an extension from faucial diphtheria. Usually, the obstruction is caused by inflammatory edema and by membrane and sometimes by an additional factor of spasm of laryngeal muscles excited by the infection. A croupy cough is present, and the voice is lost because of involvement of the vocal cords. Otherwise, the symptoms are chiefly those of respiratory difficulty. The breathing is noisy or stridulous on both inspiration and expiration. The accessory muscles of respiration are brought into use by voluntary effort. Retraction of the tissues of the neck above the clavicle, of the intercostal spaces and often of the abdomen at the chest margin occurs during inspiration. Cyanosis is present, the degree depending on the amount of obstruction. Death from asphyxia is frequent.

Isolation

Isolation is maintained until several consecutive cultures of the nose and throat fail to grow the diphtheria bacillus.

Prognosis

In general, the mortality rate is between 5 and 10 per cent. It is higher with laryngeal diphtheria and lower when the infection is limited to the nose. For those who live, complete recovery is to be expected.

Prevention

In the event of known exposure of a nonimmune child, temporary protection can be given by antitoxin, which usually is injected intramuscularly for this purpose. A satisfactory prophylactic dose is 10,000 units. A previously immunized child should be given a booster dose of toxoid.

Active immunization produces long-lasting immunity. Alum-precipitated toxoid is most commonly used and usually is combined with tetanus toxoid and pertussis vaccine. Although a single injection of this material may give satisfactory immunity, it is preferable to give 3 injections a month apart. The time required to produce satisfactory immunity varies from 2 weeks to 6 months. The majority are immune within 2 months. It is desirable to verify the existence of immunity subsequently by means of the Schick test. If the test is positive, the child should have more immunizing injections. Some physicians give booster injections every 3 years arbitrarily without Schick testing.

Diagnosis

The diagnosis of diphtheria is made by means of the clinical features which have been described and by the finding of the diphtheria bacillus in material from the site of the local lesion.

Treatment

The administration of diphtheria antitoxin is of primary importance. It alone can neutralize the effects of free toxin which has not yet become attached to cells. It probably has no effect on toxin which already is combined with cells. A single dosage with antitoxin is to be preferred to repeated small doses, and the common practice is to give 40,000 units intramuscularly. In children who exhibit symptoms of severe toxicity, an additional 40,000 units may be given intravenously. In either circumstance it is imperative to test the child first for sensitivity to horse serum. Unlike toxoid, antitoxin is prepared in horses and is capable of producing a severe or even fatal reaction in a child who is sensitive to it. Testing is done by conjunctival or intracutaneous inoculation of a small amount of the diluted material. An immediate inflammatory reaction appears if the individual is sensitive.

Several antibiotics are effective against diphtheria bacilli. The neutralization of the antitoxin should be followed by full dosage with penicillin or one of the broad-spectrum antibiotics such as erythromycin or tetracyline.

In addition to administration of antitoxin and antibiotics, certain other treatment measures are important. The child should be kept in bed until afebrile in all cases—for at least 2 weeks in cases of moderate severity and for at least 3 weeks in cases of greater severity.

Cleansing gargles or similar appropriate measures add to the comfort of the child. The diet should be modified according to the amount of soreness of the throat and the degree of prostration. If myocarditis should develop, absolute rest in bed is the chief therapeutic measure of importance. Confinement to bed should be maintained until the child has recovered entirely and for several weeks thereafter. The necessary inactivity should be aided by full doses of morphine or other sedative at short intervals. Digitalization is usually employed to augment the activity of the cardiac muscle.

Laryngeal Stenosis. If laryngeal stenosis is present, the breathing of warm moist air (croup tent or steam room) and the administration of such drugs as antipyrine and ipecac will relieve whatever part of the stenosis is caused by spasm of the larynx but will have no effect on stenosis due to edema and membrane. Almost without exception hospitals now resort to tracheotomy when relief of laryngeal obstruction is indicated. The nursing care is discussed in the Appendix. Tracheostomy tubes are left in place until the membrane formation has been controlled by specific treatment—usually only a matter of a few days.

Diphtheria Carriers

Individuals who are found to harbor diphtheria bacilli in their throats without being ill themselves are known as carriers. They are a potential menace to the community and should be isolated until freed of their organisms. Penicillin in full dosage for from 1 to 2 weeks is usually effective. If it fails, one of the broad-spectrum antibiotics should be used. If this too fails, removal of tonsils and adenoids or thorough drainage of infected sinuses may be required.

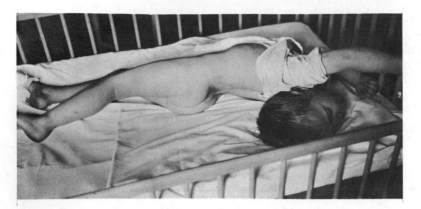

FIG. 19-1. Opisthotonos of tetanus.

TETANUS

Pathophysiology

Tetanus (lockjaw) is characterized by tonic muscular spasm, either local or generalized, a manifestation of toxic effects on the nervous system produced by the exotoxin of the tetanus bacillus. Unlike diphtheria, it is not contagious or transmissible by contact. It resembles diphtheria in that symptoms are due to a soluble exotoxin which disseminates from the infecting bacilli.

The tetanus bacillus (*Clostridium tetani*) commonly is found in the soil and in the fecal discharges of man and animals. It is anaerobic. Puncture wounds, crushing injuries and burns are particularly apt to provide favorable soil for the tetanus bacillus. In the newborn infection enters via the umbilicus. Its growth produces no identifiable local tissue damage and therefore no characteristic lesion, but it is accompanied by the production of an exotoxin. The toxin has a special affinity for nervous tissue and finds its way to the central nervous system along the various motor nerves.

Incubation periods vary from 3 days to 1 month or more, falling between 7 and 14 days in a high proportion of cases. It has been stated as a rule, not strictly true, that the prognosis is bad in the newborn and when the incubation period is less than 9 days and relatively good when the incubation period is longer.

Symptoms

Sometimes the earliest symptom is twitching of the muscles in the neighborhood of the wound. Usually, however, the first symptoms are associated with the shortest motor nerves of the body, namely, those of the head. Thus a stiffness of the muscles controlling the jaw, a condition known as trismus, is the outstanding first or early symptom. The jaw is held tightly closed and it cannot be opened. Involvement of the muscles of the throat and the tongue causes difficulties in swallowing and in speech. Soon the muscles in the distribution of the spinal nerves are affected, and all the voluntary musculature of the body assumes a tonic state. Superimposed on the continued tonicity are

paroxysms of increased muscular spasm. These paroxysms are termed convulsions, though they differ considerably from the cerebral type of convulsion. Consciousness is not lost or impaired, unless through asphyxia from spastic fixation of the thorax. The convulsions are precipitated by relatively small external stimuli, such as noises, bright lights or jarring of the bed. When all the muscles of the body are in strong contraction, the position of the body is determined by the strongest muscle groups. The characteristic position is one of opisthotonos, often extreme, with the head drawn back and the back arched (Fig. 19-1). Such strong muscular contractions are very painful, and are felt particularly in the back and head. During severe paroxysms, the thorax is held immovable, so that the respiratory movements are feeble or absent. This results in cyanosis and anoxia and in many instances in death by asphyxia.

In the children who survive, the symptoms remain unchanged for a period of from 5 to 10 days or more, and then gradually subside, their complete disappearance requiring from 2 to 3 weeks or longer. The temperature may be normal throughout the course of the disease or it may rise to 104° F. or higher. In those who die, terminal pyrexia is common. Death may occur from exhaustion or from aspiration pneumonia. The most common cause of death is asphyxia from fixation of the respiratory muscles. Bad prognostic signs are a short incubation period, early complete trismus, rapid general development of spasms and high fever. Without treatment by antitoxin the average mortality from tetanus was as high as 80 to 90 per cent. With antitoxin and modern methods it has been reduced to 20 to 50 per cent.

Prevention

Passive Immunization. Tetanus may be prevented by parenteral administration of human antitetanus immunoglobulin or antitoxin soon after the injury which permitted the introduction of the tetanus bacilli. The antitoxin is similar to that used in diphtheria and is prepared in the same manner in horses. Testing for sensitivity to horse serum is essential before it is used. The usual prophylactic dose is 3,000 units. The human immunoglobulin requires no test for sensitivity. Dosage is 250 to 500 units. If the wound is large or grossly contaminated, it is sometimes desirable to repeat the dose within a week or 10 days. Decision as to which wounds require antitoxin administration and which do not is sometimes difficult. In cases of doubt the antitoxin should be given. Burns, compound fractures, wounds from explosives and any wound in which soil contamination is likely, require tetanus prophylaxsis.

Active Immunization. Immunity produced by injection of tetanus toxoid (alone or in combination with diphtheria toxoid) produces a long-lasting immunity which may be more or less permanent. At least 2 doses of toxoid are required, spaced from 1 to 3 months apart. The basic immunity thus established may be reactivated within 4 to 6 days if a booster injection is given. Thus, in children known to have basic immunity, fluid toxoid rather than antitoxin is given as prophylaxis. No test for horse serum sensitivity is necessary when toxoid is used.

Treatment

Surgical Treatment. Any foreign body should be removed, any cellulitis or inflammation treated appropriately. The existence of tetanus does not call for radical or emergency operative measures, for the reason that antitoxin will neutralize any toxin that is present or that will be formed in the wound. In most instances, the wound will be healed and require no attention by the time tetanus develops.

Antitoxin Treatment. Enough antitoxin to neutralize all the free toxin within the body and any which is being newly formed in the wound should be given at once. Tests for serum sensitivity are imperative before the dose is administered. For a child, 50,000 units intramuscularly and an equal amount intravenously suffices.

Intramuscular human immunoglobulin can be used instead of antitoxin in dosage of 10,000-20,000 units.

Antibiotics. Pencillin and/or oxytetracycline in full dosage should be given for 10 days to be sure that all tetanus bacilli and spores are killed in the local wound.

Control of Spasm. Every effort must be made to minimize the occurrence of muscular spasms and convulsions, which may exhaust or asphyxiate the child. Well planned, considerate and continuous nursing care is probably the most important factor in the child's survival. Sedatives (phenobarbital, avertin, chloral hydrate), tranquilizers (chlorpromazine, diazepam) and muscle relaxants (mephenesin, methocarbamol) may be used in various combinations. Feeding by nasogastric tube will decrease the disturbance to the patient and permit administration of a high caloric diet which is necessary to support the strenuous muscular activity. Airway maintenance must be carefully attended by suction, or when indicated, by tracheostomy, perhaps supplemented with positive pressure intermittent assistance.

Nursing Care

The life of the child depends in large measure on meticulous nursing and medical attention. A nurse should be with the child constantly, for unless continuously watched, the child who suddenly develops a convulsion may die before his plight is discovered. Sedatives may also be required in sufficient quantity to render the child unconscious, in some instances the state of unconsciousness may be maintained from 1 to 2 weeks. In such a circumstance, food must be given by gavage and parenteral fluid administration is often necessary. Bowel and bladder function must be watched and accumulated mucus must be aspirated from the throat. The pneumonia that may occur under these circumstances is extremely severe and may cause death. Frequent respiratory stimulation with a breathing mixture of carbon dioxide and oxygen is desirable. A respirator is used only with inadvertent overdose of sedative.

When the child is conscious, the nurse is also faced with grave responsibilities. In addition to maintaining a clear airway through frequent suctioning of the throat or of the tracheostomy tube, she must be constantly alert for muscle spasms or convulsions and monitor the required parenteral infusions. An important responsibility of the nurse is to reduce external stimulation, which often results in involuntary spasms. A calm, low tone of voice and an unhurried manner can be extremely beneficial in supporting relaxation. In no nursing circumstance is it more important to give the child clear explanations before attempting any nursing or treatment procedure. Because of the sense of helplessness produced by loss of control over his body, the child is usually extremely fearful and therefore the emotional support which the nurse can give is of vital importance.

PERTUSSIS (WHOOPING COUGH)

See Chapter 14.

STAPHYLOCOCCAL INFECTIONS

The group of organisms known as staphylococci are very common saprophytic (presumably harmless) bacteria which are found on the skin and in the dust of homes, schools and hospitals. Under usual circumstances these agents are not important incitors of disease, for the bodily defenses prevent them from invading. When resistance is low, they may initiate infection of the skin (furunculosis or impetigo; see Chap. 14) or may extend beneath the skin to form abscesses, or may even gain access to the blood stream and produce a bacteremia with distant foci of infection such as osteomyelitis, meningitis or pneumonia. The circumstances which permit their invasion by reason of lowered bodily resistance are those of chronic debility from other disease or certain age factors, notably prematurity, the newborn period (Chap. 10) and, to a lesser extent, adolescence. Occasional sporadic generalized staphylococcal infections are encountered in individuals without obvious reason for such reduced resistance. Treatment is based on isolation of the organisms, determination of antibiotic sensitivity and heavy dosage with the appropriate antibiotic. Pneumonia, osteomyelitis and meningitis may require special mechanical procedures to aid in the drainage of localized collections of pus.

It has become apparent that the staphylococci capable of invading the body have a great facility for acquiring resistance to the antibiotics in general use. Thus, although penicillin was originally a potent weapon against most staphylococci, today in hospital environments only one-quarter or less of the organisms isolated may be found to be susceptible to it.

Such resistance depends upon their ability to produce an enzyme—penicillinase—which destroys the penicillin being used for treatment. New modifications of penicillin (oxacillin, methicillin, nafcillin) are now available which are not destroyed by penicillinase if the strain isolated from the given patient proves to be resistant to ordinary penicillin. The penicillinase producing strains of staphylococci are most likely to be found around hospitals and particularly among convalescent surgical patients. Strains of staphylococci acquired outside in the general community are more likely to be sensitive to penicillin. Resistant staphylococci may be transported from the surgical or other units of a hospital to newborn nurseries where they have sometimes been responsible for epidemics of infection which are difficult to control.

OSTEOMYELITIS

Acute osteomyelitis is an infection of cancellous bone most often, but not exclusively, due to staphylococci. Exceptions are in small infants whose infections are more likely to be due to organisms of the intestinal canal; in children with sickle cell anemia in which salmonella organisms are usually responsible; and in a minority of older children who suffer from streptococcal or other pyogenic infection of bone. Bone tuberculosis is another form of osteomyelitis, but one which pursues a more chronic course.

For a fuller discussion of the pathophysiology, symptoms and treatment of acute osteomyelitis, see Chapter 29.

TYPHOID FEVER

Typhoid fever is an acute infectious disease most typically characterized by fever, prostration, stupor, enlarged spleen and inflammation of the intestine.

Etiology

The causative bacterium is the bacillus typhosus, *Salmonella typhosa*. The portal of entry is the alimentary tract. In areas where water supplies are supervised and sewage disposal is adequate, typhoid fever is uncommon. In such areas, the infection is acquired chiefly from persons who have the disease or are carriers of the typhoid bacillus. Typhoid fever has its greatest incidence in late childhood and early adulthood (15 to 25 years). It is uncommon in infancy and early childhood.

Pathophysiology

The infection is implanted first in the intestinal tract, and the greatest anatomic damage occurs at this site, but the organisms also reach the mesenteric lymph glands and the blood stream and are distributed throughout the body. The organisms are found in the blood during the first week of the disease but usually not subsequently. It is the lymphoid tissue (Peyer's patches) of the intestine that is affected most severely. The patches of lymphoid tissue become swollen and then ulcerated. The ulcerations may cause hemorrhage within the intestine, or an ulcer may extend entirely through the bowel wall into the peritoneal cavity and cause peritonitis. The inflammation of the intestinal mucosa, other than in the lymphoid tissue, is only moderate, but it is sufficient in most instances to cause diarrhea. In a few cases, constipation is present.

The disease is spread from man to man through the transmission of organisms in infected stools or urine. Animals do not play a role in transmission. Either a person ill with the disease or an asymptomatic carrier, or a contaminated water or milk supply is the usual source of infection.

Symptoms

The incubation period is variable and because of the insidious onset it is difficult to determine. In general, it may be stated as being from 1 to 2 weeks.

The symptoms vary greatly with the age of the child. The younger the child is, the less severe is the disease. As children approach the age of puberty, the disease occurs with a severity approaching that observed in the adult.

The prodromal symptoms may be malaise, anorexia, headache and thirst. In a few cases in childhood, the disease develops abruptly without prodromal symptoms. In the more severe case, the fever is high and usually remittent. It reaches its peak within the first week. Prostration is severe. The mental state is affected sometimes by delirium, sometimes by stupor. It is the stupor that gives rise to the term "typhoid state."

Abdominal distention is the rule, often requiring special treatment measures. The pulse rate is low, out of proportion to the fever. The white cells of the blood are not increased and frequently are decreased. The spleen becomes palpable during the first week of the disease and remains enlarged throughout the illness. Late in the first week an eruption (rose spots) appears on the abdomen in a large proportion of cases. The rash disappears within a few days. When the disease is severe, degenerative changes may occur in the liver, heart and kidneys. Albuminuria may be present.

In the young child, the disease is less severe. The onset is often indefinite and ill-defined, and the disease is of shorter duration, often only from 2 to 3 weeks.

In infants, typhoid fever may manifest itself chiefly by vomiting and diarrhea and resemble in every way, except duration and response to dietary therapy, a gastrointestinal disturbance due to improper food or to parenteral infection.

Complications

Intestinal hemorrhage and perforation are the usual complications and are the cause of most of the deaths in childhood.

Isolation

Isolation should be continued until several successive stool cultures fail to grow the typhoid bacillus.

Prognosis

The mortality in children is less than half that in adults because of the relative mildness of the disease and the infrequency of complications.

Prevention

Typhoid vaccine is as useful for children as for adults. It is to be recommended especially if the family is sojourning in places where the food and water supply may be subject to poor sanitation. The vaccine is used in the same manner as for adults in one half the adult dose for a child; one quarter for an infant. Children have less reaction to the vaccine than do adults. Seldom does it cause inconvenience. Protective immunity may be expected to last for from 2 to 3 years.

Treatment and Nursing Care

To the symptomatic treatment of typhoid fever there have been added effective antibiotics—chloramphenicol, ampicillin and tetracycline. The child should be kept in bed regardless of the mildness of the illness or how well he feels. The diet should be complete with high energy value but with little rough residue. Foods should be finely divided and of a character which will not aggravate existing diarrhea. Milk, eggs and puréed fruits and vegetables should be prominent in the diet. Sugar may be used to increase energy value. Hydrotherapy for nervous symptoms and fever is not indicated as often as in adults.

When diarrhea is present, specific nursing care is indicated (see Diarrhea). Dehydration is especially likely to occur in infants. Moderate anemia is common with severe typhoid fever. Sometimes trans-fusions are desirable to promote quick recovery. When a child is confined to bed for a long period, especially if he is in a state of stupor, special nursing care is required to keep the skin free from pressure areas and to keep the mouth clean. Nursing measures to prevent distention are required.

When the disease is severe, the nurse should be alert for symptoms that indicate intestinal hemorrhage or perforation. Restlessness, rise in rate and change in quality of the pulse, abdominal pain and distention are symptoms of perforation that require immediate attention.

Chloramphenicol is highly effective in shortening the course of typhoid fever. Administration in high dosage (50 to 100 mg./Kg. of body weight per day) usually will produce reduction of fever and sterilization of the blood stream in from 24 to 48 hours. Treatment is continued for at least 3 weeks in order to assure the eradication of organisms from all recesses of the intestinal tract. Ampicillin in dosage of 50 mgm./Kg./day is also effective.

In instituting aseptic technic the nurse must bear in mind that the alimentary tract is the portal of entry and the chief exit of the typhoid bacillus. The stools contain an abundance of the organisms. For a short period early in the disease, the organisms are present also in the urine in many instances.

SALMONELLA INFECTIONS

The Salmonella group of organisms is a very large family with characteristics similar to the typhoid bacillus. Unlike the latter, infection generally is spread to man from contact with the products of infected animals. The resultant disease is in some instances quite similar to, although usually milder than, typhoid fever, requiring the same sort of diagnostic measures, isolation precautions and treatment. Occasionally, these organisms produce acute food poisoning. In small infants there may be insidious infection with unexplained fever and mild diarrhea. As long as the infection remains confined to the intestinal tract it tends to be mild, albeit often protracted. If a heavy infection of the blood stream occurs, there may be more serious consequences, such as osteomyelitis or meningitis, which are more difficult to eradicate. Antibiotic therapy is not required except during symptomatic illness of this sort.

TUBERCULOSIS

Tuberculosis is an ancient scourge which man has learned to control under optimal conditions of public health but which still disseminates widely and dangerously among people who live under crowded and unhygienic conditions. It is a chronic disease which comes and goes so subtly that it escapes recognition in a high percentage of its victims. Only through constant search and vigilance can all of its infectious victims be identified and proper methods of control be invoked so as to interrupt its spread. Since children are particularly vulnerable to its serious forms, it is highly important for persons concerned with their care to understand the stealthy habits and elusive behavior of tuberculosis.

Etiology

The tubercle bacillus (*Mycobacterium tuberculosis*) differs from most other bacteria in important respects. It fails to grow on the usual artificial media of the laboratory and multiplies so slowly on the media specifically designed for it, that a result is not obtained for 2 or more weeks after the original inoculation. However, a waxy coat which surrounds the bacillus is able to take up and hold the stain of certain dyes even when subjected to treatment with acid. Thus, tubercle bacilli are said to be "acid-fast" and can be differentially identified in smears made from sputum, pus, urine or spinal fluid. The bacillus also produces a characteristic type of cellular reaction in the tissues which it invades, so that in biopsy material, even if the organisms are not found, their presence may be suspected from the type of cellular response seen under the microscope. Another special property of the organisms is their ability to hibernate. Outside the body they can remain alive in spite of drying and can exist for weeks in dust or an article of clothing and furniture or the pavement or floor. Within the body, too, they may escape the body defenses by taking up sequestered positions deep in the tissues where they remain inactive for years but are able to revive and produce new disease if the circumstances around them become favorable. Much of the sneaky behavior of tuberculosis is due to this ability of the organisms to

remain dormant but alive over long periods of time.

Once admitted to the body the tubercle bacillus produces an allergic response to its protein component, tuberculin. Our most important diagnostic test in children, the tuberculin test, depends on the recognition of this allergic state which may be incited by a small number of tubercle bacilli. The relation of allergy to immunity in tuberculosis has long been debated. Probably mild degrees of allergy assist the immune response to localize organisms and destroy them within the tissues. The more intense variety of allergic response can produce necrosis and sloughing of tissue which may actually encourage the dissemination of organisms rather than confining them.

The main source of tubercle bacilli is an infected human. Transmission to a new individual depends on the numbers of bacilli being produced in the body excretions (mainly the sputum) and on the frequency and intimacy of the exposure. Casual contact is not nearly so likely to effect a transfer of organisms as close living in which there is repeated exposure to coughing, kissing, the joint use of eating utensils and the environmental dust. The result within the exposed child will depend in part on the numbers of bacilli received but will also be influenced by his age, nutrition, general state of health and the administration of certain drugs such as steroids or immunosuppressive agents.

The cow used to be a significant source of infections for young children. A bovine strain of organisms was recognized and found in association with intestinal and cervical node infection. In the United States this type of tuberculosis is rarely seen thanks to the care-

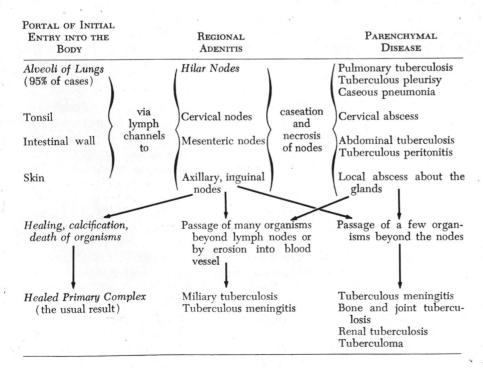

FIG. 19-2. Routes of tuberculous infection—the pathways followed by tubercle bacilli after their entry into the body *en route* to the production of various clinical forms of tuberculosis.

ful controls exerted over dairy herds to prevent contamination of milk.

Pathogenesis

The tubercle bacillus cannot enter the body through unbroken skin. However, it can pass across the more delicate protecting membranes of the upper respiratory passages, intestinal tract and pulmonary aveoli. Under special circumstances it is carried beneath the skin by wounds or is rubbed into pre-existing abrasions. In more than 90 per cent of the instances of tuberculous infection, the evidence points to the lungs as the portal of entry, indicating that the organisms have been inhaled on dust or particles of moisture suspended in the air. In Figure 19-2 the routes which such organisms may travel once they have gained access to the tissues of the body are presented in schematic form.

From the portal of entry the organisms most commonly invade the local lymphatic structures and pass to the regional lymph nodes where they multiply and produce more obvious physical evidence of infection. It is a general rule that little disease remains at the site of entry and that the maximal disturbance is seen in the lymph nodes which drain this point. In the common types of infection, this aspect of the disease passes unnoticed, since the enlarging glands are out of sight in the chest or abdomen. Only when the portal of entry is through the tonsils or the skin, is attention attracted to the resulting adenitis. From this point, a great many of the infections heal spontaneously as the organisms are contained within the lymph nodes and are either killed or immobilized for long periods of time. A healed primary complex results, and the child acquires only a positive tuberculin reaction and perhaps some spots of calcification in the lymph nodes visible on a roentgenogram.

Unfortunately this happy outcome does not always result. If disease in the regional lymph nodes is extensive, the tubercle bacilli, aided by the allergic response of the tissues, may destroy the lymph nodes and replace them with the caseous material which is characteristic of tuberculous infection. If the capsule of the gland remains intact, it creates damage only by virtue of its enlargement and the pressure it exerts on neighboring structures (the trachea or the bronchi in the case of the hilar lymph nodes). But the capsule of the gland may burst and discharge its contents into the surrounding tissues. In the lung this is usually a bronchus, with resultant dissemination of organisms through the lungs and the production of a caseous pneumonia. Elsewhere an abscess forms which attaches itself to surrounding skin or other structures and may eventually create a fistula through which its contents are discharged.

With or without destruction of the lymph nodes by caseation, the tubercle bacilli can filter on into the blood stream and be disseminated to distant parts of the body. If large numbers are thus spread, miliary tuberculosis results. If only a few organisms seep through, they create localized tuberculous infections in places such as the brain, liver, spleen, bones or kidneys.

In the case of primary invasion of the lungs, a large dose of inhaled organisms may also set up a focus of parenchymal disease at the portal of entry into the alveoli.

Diagnosis

To be recognized, tuberculosis must be suspected and actively sought. When clinical disease is present in the child an associated positive tuberculin reaction is important presumptive evidence, but it is not proof. The latter must be sought through the identification of tubercle bacilli in body fluids such as sputum, aspirates of gastric contents, pus from abscesses, the urine and pleural, ascitic or spinal fluid. Recognition of tubercle bacilli may be made from direct smears if the density of organisms is great. More often, bacteriologic confirmation must await the results of cultures or animal inoculations. Another important means of diagnosis is the microscopic appearance of tissue removed at biopsy or during the evacuation of an abscess.

The younger the child is the more significant is the tuberculin test, for it denotes fairly recent invasion of his body. In older children and adults, a positive tuberculin reaction may mean only that the individual has a healed primary complex with residual allergy. When no clinical disease is apparent, the search for tuberculous infection is conducted among children with the tuberculin test; among adults by means of chest roentgenograms.

The *tuberculin* test is a test for the presence of allergy to the protein of the tubercle bacillus. With a few exceptions a negative reaction to a properly performed test excludes the possibility of tuberculous infection. Several methods are available for the performance of this valuable skin test.

The Vollmer patch test uses squares of tuberculin-impregnated ointment attached to the skin by adhesive tape and left in place for 48 hours being read 48 hours after removal. It has value as a screening test for large numbers of children or in routine testing when infection is not seriously suspected. Although convenient, the patch test is subject to both false positive and false negative results. It must be checked with an intradermal test before final conclusions about tuberculin allergy are drawn.

The intradermal Mantoux test uses a measured quantity (0.1 mg.) of old tuberculin (O.T.) diluted in 0.1 ml. of saline and injected into the skin. The site of injection is examined after 48 hours; 10 mm. or more of induration at that time indicates a positive response (Plate 2). Negative responses should be checked with a repeat test using 1.0 mg. of old tuberculin.

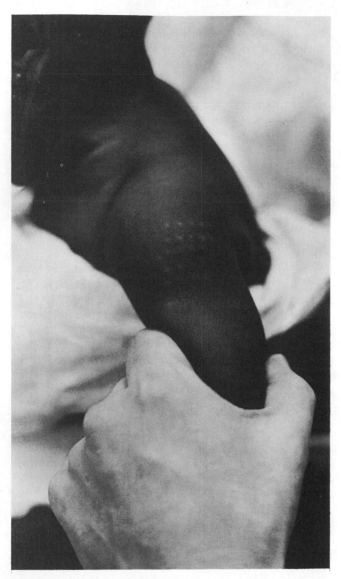

FIG. 19-3. Grid scar from BCG vaccination.

Similar to the Mantoux test is a chemically purified fraction of tuberculin which can be used with less chance of nonspecific reactions. This material is known as purified protein derivative (P.P.D.) and is provided in first, second and intermediate strengths. If the child fails to respond to the second strength of this material, tuberculin allergy is lacking.

The "tine" test inserts tuberculin into four small puncture holes in the skin. It is a simple screening test approximately equivalent to intermediate strength P.P.D. but less reliable. Any induration reaction should be checked by re-testing with P.P.D.

Tuberculosis may be confused with histoplasmosis or coccidioidomycosis (Chap. 20), two fungus infections that produce similar lesions in the lung and also tend to heal with the deposition of calcium. In geographic regions where these diseases are prevalent, distinction can be made by the use of histoplasmin and coccidioidin skin tests which are comparable to the tuberculin test.

Incidence

Even before modern drugs for the treatment of tuberculosis were developed, the incidence of the disease was declining in the United States. Whether this was due to better public health measures, better nutrition or increasing resistance of the population is not clear. Since chemotherapy has been available, the fall in the incidence of tuberculous disease has been accentuated.

The incidence of tuberculosis is increased within communities and families in which the standards of hygiene, housing and education are poor. Crowding increases the ease of passage of the disease from one person to another, as does the lack of attention to disposal of sputum, hand washing and general cleanliness. Economic need and poor education usually mean less access to medical care or less understanding of the aims of treatment and prevention. Thus in the United States, tuberculosis is found mainly among urban slum dwellers, particularly among Negroes, Puerto Ricans, Mexicans and Chinese.

Prevention

The most important part of prevention lies in keeping the child from making contact with infectious individuals. This can be done directly for the newborn infant by making sure that neither his parents nor other members of his family are suffering from tuberculosis. Most maternity services require at least a a chest roengenogram of the mother during the course of her pregnancy. This protection does not cover the other members of the family and hence by itself is imperfect assurance. Indirect protection of the child is gained through community measures of tuberculosis case-finding which seek out active cases in the community and attempt to bring them under proper care. Mass tuberculin testing of school children and routine periodic testing of children in clinics and physician's offices aid in the discovery of positive reactors and through them of their infectious contacts. Adult surveys are also conducted by industry, health departments and other interested organizations that offer free chest roentgenograms to all.

Active Immunization

By propagating bovine tubercle bacilli though successive transplants on artificial media for many years, Calmette produced a strain (*Bacillus Calmette-Guérin* or BCG) of low virulence with which he claimed to be able to produce immunity of perhaps several years' duration. He advocated its use especially for infants of tuberculous parentage. The vaccine was given in 3 doses by mouth on alternate days in the first 10 days after birth. Currently in the United States this vaccine is administered by multiple puncture, scarification of the skin or intracutaneously (Fig. 19-3). If a positive skin tuberculin reaction does not develop or if the skin reaction later becomes negative, vaccination is repeated. The procedure is used extensively in Scandinavian countries and elsewhere, not only for infants but also for older persons who have negative reactions to tuberculin tests. It has had only limited and experimental use in this country, where there has been a steadily declining tuberculosis rate despite the absence of an immunization program. Although the vaccine is believed to be relatively safe, its value as an immunizing agent remains controversial. It should not be regarded as a substitute for approved hygienic measures or public-health practices. Its use should be restricted to selected groups of those nonreactors most likely to be exposed to tuberculosis.

Clinical Forms of Childhood Tuberculosis

Description of tuberculosis in the child is difficult because of the great variation in severity and character of the disease which results from the entrance of organisms into the body. A few of the general problems encountered are described. Modern improvements in prevention, case-finding and treatment are rapidly changing the spectrum of disease encountered. The antituberculous drugs (isoniazid and streptomycin) have brought a revolution in the prognosis, so that recovery is now expected in a high percentage of patients.

Pulmonary Tuberculosis. More than 90 per cent of infections affect the lungs. In general the pathologic changes produced are accompanied by less clinical evidence of disease than would be expected from the extent of invasion seen in a chest roentgenogram. Hence, it is very important to pursue the study of children with positive tuberculin reactions at least as far as obtaining a chest roentgenogram, for even in the absence of symptoms or signs of illness, there may be extensive pulmonary involvement. Within the lungs tuberculosis can behave in such varied ways that each case must be considered independently. The separation into clinical types of disease which is given below is an artificial and incomplete representaton.

Tuberculin Allergy Without Manifest Disease. In many children a positive tuberculin test will be found which is not associated with evidence of illness or changes in the chest roentgenogram. The management of such children must begin with an attempt to discover the source from which the positive test was obtained so that continued exposure to an infectious adult can be terminated. *Unlike other infectious diseases, the immunity obtained from a first infection with tubercle bacilli does not yield adequate protection against additional exposure.* The second consideration is the infectiousness of the patient for others. Experience over many years has shown that children without roentgenographically demonstrable lesions in the lungs are usually not infectious. However, where

doubt exists or there is reason for particular caution, a search for organisms in the sputum should be made. This is done by recovering the stomach contents by gastric lavage on each of 3 consecutive days in the morning before breakfast. The material is digested, concentrated and examined by smear and culture or animal inoculation. A positive result should, of course, serve as a warning that the child is potentially infectious to others.

Whether a child with no evidence of disease other than a positive tuberculin test should receive specific drug treatment is a much debated point. Logically the best time to attack the organisms is during the early stages of invasion when they are fewest in number and before they have a chance to find refuge in fibrotic or calcified lymph nodes where drugs will not reach them readily. For this reason most physicians now believe that any child under 3 to 4 years of age with a positive tuberculin reaction should receive isoniazid therapy. The oral dosage is 10 to 20 mg./ Kg./day and is usually continued for about a year. Toxic reactions are very infrequent in children. Many also believe that older children whose tuberculin tests have presumably converted recently should also be treated. If calcification is seen in the hilar lymph nodes, the probability is that the infection is 2 or 3 years old, and the desirability of drug therapy diminishes.

Children without symptoms or signs of disease do not require bed rest or restriction of activity. They should be protected against measles and should receive steroid therapy only after careful consideration of the risk of aggravating the tuberculous infection.

Hilar (Mediastinal) Lymphadenitis. Some degree of enlargement of the hilar lymph nodes is an almost inevitable feature of pulmonary infections which can be seen in the chest roentgenogram. The amount of associated infiltration of the lungs and the presence of signs of active infection such as fever and increase in the sedimentation rate are quite variable. If the latter are absent and there is little or no parenchymal lung involvement, management is the same as that for asymptomatic infections. When fever or increase in the sedimentation rate of the red blood cells is present, restriction of physical activity is required in addition to isoniazid therapy.

Enlarged hilar nodes may create mischief by compression of the adjacent trachea or bronchi. Brassy cough has been attributed to compression irritation of the trachea. More serious is the partial or complete occlusion of branches of the bronchial tree which may produce emphysema of a lobe or atelectasis, depending on the extent of the luminal occlusion. Bronchoscopic examination is usually required to clarify the mechanical situation and rule out the possibility that a foreign body is present within the lumen of the tube. Specific treatment can be expected to relieve the obstruction gradually, since the size of the nodes diminishes as the infection within them is brought under control.

ENDOBRONCHIAL TUBERCULOSIS. Enlarged nymph nodes which adhere to a bronchus may erode through its wall and produce a chronic granulomatous fistula through which the infected contents of the node are discharged into the bronchus, producing tuberculous pneumonia. This form of pulmonary disease is often stubbornly resistant because the drug therapy fails to clean out the infection present within the core of the node. Even though the pulmonary portion of the disease responds to drug therapy, there is repeated reinfection from the discharging node. Maximal therapeutic efforts are required. In addition to isoniazid, streptomycin and para-aminosalicylic acid (PAS) are given in order to prevent the tubercle bacilli from becoming resistant to the single drug.

CASEOUS PNEUMONIA. When the eroding bronchial node described above discharges a large amount of its infected contents into the bronchial tree, a widespread pneumonia may develop in the distal segment of the lung. The child with this form of the disease is usually quite ill with fever, malaise and loss of weight. Recovery depends on prompt and intensive drug therapy.

PROGRESSIVE PRIMARY DISEASE. When the initial dose of organisms is large, the child may have a pronounced infiltration in the lungs around the portal of entry. This may or may not be accompanied by fever and other signs of systemic illness. Usually such foci progress for a time without treatment but respond promptly to proper use of the antituberculous drugs. However, the regression of the chest lesions as seen by x-ray is considerably slower than the disappearance expected with pneumococcal infections of similar appearance.

TUBERCULOUS PLEURISY. In some instances there is a collection of fluid or fibrinous exudate in the pleural cavity over the surface of involved lung. This seldom is present in amounts sufficient to interfere with respiration or produce chest pain. It is usually an incidental discovery from the roentgen examination of the chest. Fluid removed by thoracentesis is clear and serous in character in contrast to that seen with pyogenic empyema. It usually contains tubercle bacilli. No particular additional treatment is required.

CAVITATIONAL TUBERCULOSIS. Even in small children, pulmonary tuberculosis may sometimes advance to the point where lung destruction is so marked that cavities can be seen in the chest roentgenogram. The treatment required is usually more prolonged and the prognosis somewhat less favorable.

MILIARY TUBERCULOSIS. When tubercle bacilli are discharged in quantity into a blood vessel, there is a rapid seeding of the body tissues (including the lungs) with small foci of infection. The child becomes acutely and seriously ill with sudden fever and prostration.

The spleen is usually enlarged, and the lungs commonly present the findings of bronchiolitis. The chest roentgenogram shows a uniform diffuse seeding of the lungs with tiny foci of infiltration, often described as a "snowflake" infiltration. Untreated, this form of the disease is uniformly fatal. It is often accompanied by tuberculous meningitis. Treatment with all three types of drugs is required at first, with persistent administration of isoniazid for a year to 18 months after the acute stage of the illness has passed.

Extrapulmonary Tuberculosis. CERVICAL GLAND INFECTION. This form of tuberculosis is not usually accompanied by symptoms other than the progressive enlargement of the cervical lymph nodes on one or both sides of the neck. Unlike pyogenic adenitis there is usually no history of preceding fever or acute sore throat. The nodes tend to be firm and discrete at first but gradually become attached to the under surface of the skin and soften in the center where a characteristic area of thin, shiny skin overlies the collection of necrotic material beneath. If left alone, the skin eventually ulcerates at this point, and a draining fistula appears which heals only after weeks or months of drainage. The discharge from such a fistula contains tubercle bacilli so that the child is potentially infectious to those about him. Usually the chest roentgenogram shows trivial or no involvement of the lungs.

Treatment of tuberculous cervical adenitis in the early stages before the nodes have become matted and attached to the skin is by surgical excision combined with streptomycin and isoniazid administration to ensure healing and the eradication of disease in the tonsils or other nodes which have not been extirpated. If rupture of the nodes has taken place, drug therapy should be given first in the hope of encouraging the fistula to close after which excision may be performed. Frequently, there is a combined infection with pyogenic organisms so that antibiotics in addition to the antituberculous drugs may be indicated.

AXILLARY AND INGUINAL ADENITIS. The appearance of the glands and their treatment is similar to that of cervical node tuberculosis. If the portal of entry is a distal abrasion of the skin, a chronic ulcer may be present which heals only when adequate treatment by drugs is instituted.

ABDOMINAL TUBERCULOSIS. The primary form of abdominal tuberculosis which follows the ingestion of milk contaminated with bovine organisms is rare in the United States. Mild infections pass unrecognized except when calcified mesenteric lymph nodes are found in the roentgenogram of the abdomen. Heavy infections may produce ulceration of the intestines with chronic diarrhea and tenesmus. Extension into the peritoneal cavity may lead to either an ascitic accumulation or a dry adhesive peritonitis. Similar types of abdominal involvement may occur from the constant swallowing of heavily infected sputum during the course of pulmonary tuberculosis. The treatment of both types is the same as that for active pulmonary tuberculosis.

TUBERCULOUS MENINGITIS. This type of tuberculous infection is discussed in Chapter 14.

BONE AND JOINT TUBERCULOSIS. Tubercle bacilli transported by the blood stream may lodge in bones and there set up tuberculous disease. In the long bones, the site of the lesion may be in the shaft, but usually it is near an epiphysis, where the line of least resistance for extension is toward the neighboring joint. It is in this manner that tuberculosis of the joints most frequently originates. The weight-bearing joints are affected most commonly, possibly because resistance is lowered by trauma. Joint tuberculosis is characterized clinically chiefly by pain, muscle spasm, limitation of motion and early muscle and bone atrophy. The prognosis as to life is good, especially in childhood. The outlook for function depends somewhat on the adequacy and the promptness of treatment. In some instances good function results, but in most a stiff joint may be expected.

The spine is a common site for bone tuberculosis, and the thoracic spine is the part most frequently affected. The disease always arises in the anterior portion of the vertebra and erodes the vertebral body. The erosion soon permits a kyphos, which is the characteristic deformity. Muscle spasm and referred pain are constant when the spine is not at rest in a good position.

Tuberculous abscesses are common in bone and joint tuberculosis. These usually progress slowly and may burrow for considerable distances before coming to the surface. Often they are referred to as "cold abscesses" because of the lack of heat characteristic of the usual pyogenic abscess. With good treatment of the bone and joint tuberculosis, the abscesses often are resorbed without having been drained. The treatment for bone and joint tuberculosis consists of the general care suitable for a child with any type of tuberculosis and, in addition, mechanical or surgical measures which immobilize the parts in proper positions.

RENAL TUBERCULOSIS. The kidneys are infrequently involved by tuberculosis in children except during miliary dissemination of the organisms. In older children, however, chronic pyuria, hematuria or hydronephrosis is occasionally found due to a tuberculous lesion in the kidney. Treatment with isoniazid and streptomycin is indicated with careful urologic evaluation of the function and the degree of infection of each kidney separately.

General Nursing Care of Tuberculosis

Children whose disease is mild enough to permit full activity require little symptomatic nursing care. Those whose disease requires lengthy hospitalization and bed rest will require the care accorded to any child with a chronic illness. Maintenance of morale is highly important for the older child who may become discouraged with the slow progression of his cure. Sensory stimulation technics previously discussed are vital to prevent lethargy, to support contact with the environment and to aid in intellectual development. In most cases, school work can be continued and if isolation is not ordered, occupational therapy and constructive play with other children should be provided. The infant or the toddler requires consistency in personnel in order to develop an adequate relationship to substitute for the mother's care which often must be denied him.

Administration of isoniazid is not difficult, and its toxic reactions are infrequent in children. Occasionally, stimulation of the central nervous system may result in excitement or convulsions. Administration of pyridoxine usually controls this effect of the drug.

Streptomycin must be given intramuscularly to be effective. Only in serious forms of tuberculosis is it continued for long periods. It may damage the vestibular nerve producing dizziness and unsteady gait. Other toxic manifestations include rashes and depression of the bone marrow.

Para-aminosalicylic acid is given in such large dosage that the mere volume sometimes creates a problem in dosage of small children. The nurse may find her powers of persuasion taxed by the recurring necessity to get numerous pills or large volumes of liquid into a small child. The only toxic symptoms are those of gastric irritation and vomiting.

Nurses also have an important responsibility in casefinding, in arranging for initial diagnostic procedures, in assisting parents to cope with the impact of the illness on family life and in helping them to make the necessary treatment arrangements. Consistent and frequent visiting is usually required by the nurse in the community to assist parents and relatives of children with tuberculosis to understand the necessity for prolonged treatment and for exclusion of infectious adults from contact with small children. She must also help parents to examine and accept their feelings related to the origin of the illness in their child, for unless this is done, the unresolved sense of guilt may interfere in the proper management of treatment through the failure to accept arrangements necessary for the child's protection. Frequent consultation between the nurse caring for the child in the hospital and the nurse supporting the parents in the community is vital to a comprehensive and continuous nursing care plan for both child and family.

BACTERIAL MENINGITIS

Meningitis due to bacterial infection with meningococci, pneumococci, influenza bacilli and the tubercle bacillus is discussed in Chapter 14.

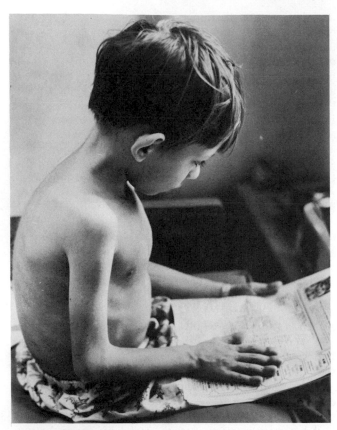

Fig. 19-4. The chronic lung disease of cystic fibrosis of the pancreas produces increased depth of the chest due to the persistently overinflated lungs from the entrapment of air within the alveoli by sticky bronchial secretions. Note also the clubbing of the fingers.

PNEUMONITIS DURING CYSTIC FIBROSIS OF THE PANCREAS (CFP)

No single bacterial agent is responsible for the infection of the lungs which so frequently complicates the course of cystic fibrosis of the pancreas and ultimately determines the life span of its victims. The management of such children is a constant struggle against changing bacterial flora with shifting resistance to antibiotics and slowly progressive interference with pulmonary function.

Pathophysiology

The genetic mechanisms and disturbances of respiratory physiology have been discussed in Chapter 13. In essence, the genetic defect is expressed as an abnormality in the character of mucus secreted by the bronchial glands. Unusually thick and sticky secretions interfere with the normal movement of secretions and entrapped particles which have been inhaled, from the lower reaches of the tracheobronchial tree up toward the pharynx where they can be swallowed or expectorated. Thus accumulation of

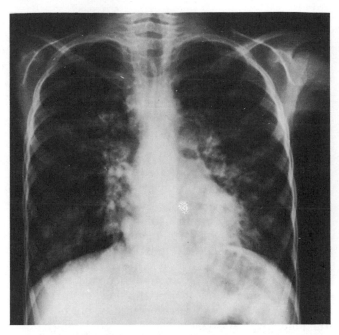

Fig. 19-5. Chest x-ray of the boy in the preceding illustration showing the increase in total intrathoracic volume, the upper and lateral areas of overinflated lung, and the concentration of densities due to collapse or pneumonia in regions around each of the hila.

thick secretions with entrapped bacteria fosters obstruction of small radicles of the tree, pooling of infected secretions and chronic or intermittent infection of the lungs. Air-trapping behind partially obstructed bronchioles leads to distal emphysema. Complete obstruction of bronchial radicles produces areas of actelectasis beyond. Behind such obstructions the further complications of diffuse emphysema, pneumothorax, lung abscess, bronchiectasis and pulmonary fibrosis may eventually produce serious and ultimately fatal reduction in pulmonary function.

Symptoms

In the early stages there may be no symptoms at all, and the presence of pulmonary changes is discovered only by chest x-ray which shows an increase in the bronchovascular markings of the lungs. Ultimately, cough becomes a chronic symptom as the child attempts to bring up the thick mucus accumulations. With more advanced disease, the chest assumes the overdistended appearance of persistent emphysema, and an increase in respiratory rate and decrease in pulmonary function with limitation of activity are noted. In the advanced stages of the disease there may be cyanosis, clubbing of the fingers and cardiac failure due to interference with the circulation of blood through the pulmonary circuit.

Periodically, acute pneumonia may be superim-

PLATE 1

PLATE 2

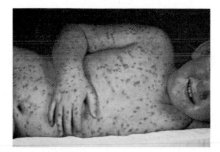

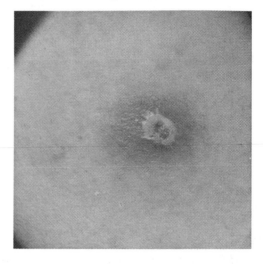

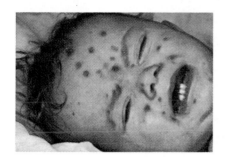

A taking vaccination with scar of previous vaccination next to it, demonstrating that immunity is not necessarily permanent. (From Franklin H. Top, M.D., *Communicable Diseases*, St. Louis, Mosby, 1955, and *Therapeutic Notes*, Parke, Davis and Company)

(Top) The rash of measles.
(Bottom) The rash of chickenpox.

PLATE 3

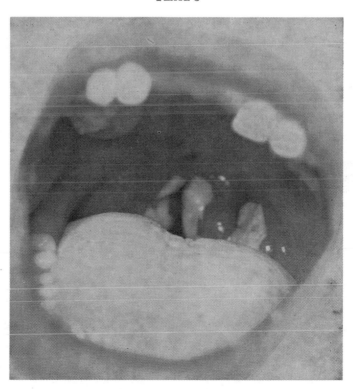

Diphtheritic throat showing membrane on the tonsils.
(From Franklin H. Top, M.D., *Communicable Diseases*, St. Louis, Mosby, 1955, and *Therapeutic Notes*, Parke, Davis and Company)

PLATE 4

ORIGIN AND DEVELOPMENT OF BLOOD CELLS

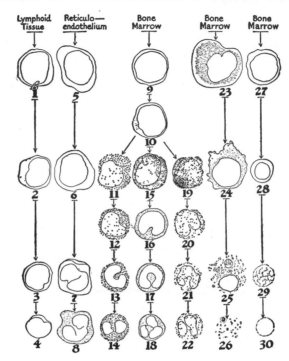

1. Lymphoblast
2. Large lymphocyte
3. Intermediate lymphocyte
4. Small lymphocyte
5. Monoblast
6. Large monocyte with azure granules
7. Monocyte with a few granules
8. Mature monocyte with azure granules
9. Myeloblast
10. Premyelocyte
11. Eosinophilic myelocyte
12. Juvenile eosinophil
13. Band eosinophil
14. Segmented eosinophil
15. Neutrophilic myelocyte
16. Juvenile neutrophil
17. Band neutrophil
18. Segmented neutrophil
19. Basophilic myelocyte
20. Juvenile basophil
21. Band basophil
22. Segmented basophil
23. Megakaryocyte (bone marrow)
24. Later megakaryocyte (bone marrow)
25. Megakaryocyte (peripheral blood)
26. Thrombocytes (platelets)
27. Megaloblast
28. Normoblast
29. Reticulocyte
30. Normocyte (erythrocyte)

PLATE 4

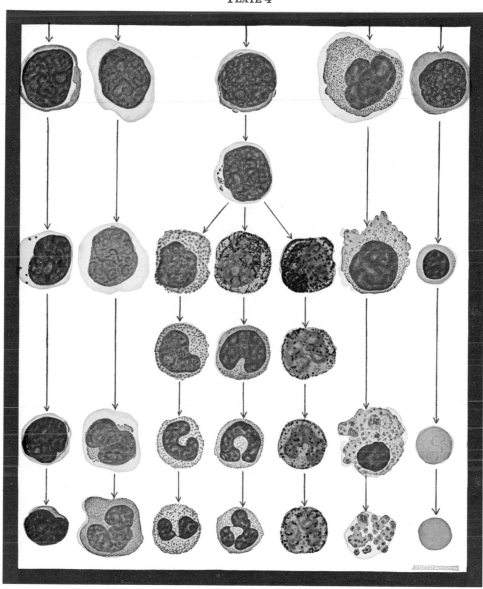

Blood cells.
(Kracke, Roy: Diseases of the Blood and
Atlas of Hematology, Philadelphia, Lippincott)

PLATE 5

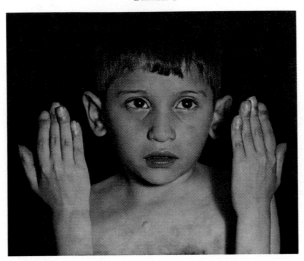

Cyanosis and clubbed fingers in a boy with
tetralogy of Fallot.

posed upon the more slowly advancing symptoms of declining respiratory competence.

Treatment

The two main objectives of treatment are to prevent or suppress infection through appropriate use of antibiotics, and to improve pulmonary aeration by relieving the mechanical factors which block the air passages. General attention to nutrition, rest and emotional support are obviously important adjuncts. The late complications of disease may require special measures.

Antibiotics. Only a few fortunate children with CFP will escape persistent or intermittent infection of their respiratory passages. Once the diagnosis has been made, a decision is required about whether or not to attempt prophylactic protection against bacterial invasion. Some physicians avoid such measures on the grounds that antibiotics given before infection occurs only encourage the more rapid appearance of resistant strains of bacteria. Others believe that once evidence of pulmonary infection has appeared, the child is a victim of persistent low grade bacterial invasion at the very least. These latter keep the child on daily dosage with sulfonamides or tetracyclines even when symptomatically well. Some select three or more antibiotics, which they use in arbitrary rotation to decrease the likelihood of the appearance of resistant strains. During acute superimposed infection it becomes very important to identify the invading bacteria by culture and to determine the antibiotic susceptibility to guide selection of antibiotics. Full dosage by parenteral or oral administration is indicated. Since these children often acquire organisms in their respiratory flora which are resistant to all the antibiotics that may be safely given systemically, others such as neomycin and polymyxin may be added to aerosols and given by inhalation.

Initially, staphylococci are the most common invaders. After repeated or continuous use of antibiotics, the predominating organisms in the secretions may change to the gram-negative coliform organisms, pseudomonas, klebsiella or others.

Relief of Obstruction. Some liquefaction of secretions can be obtained by adding moisture to the air which the child breathes. The ordinary devices for humidification may have some effect, but if a significant change is required, *mist therapy* must be employed. Only very small particles of water vapor will find their way into the deeper recesses of the lungs where the significant obstruction is taking place. Consequently, the inspired air must be prepared with a nebulizer which adds water vapor in very finely divided droplets. The fog which results must then be confined to some type of tent in which the child is kept. Such arrangements are most often used just during the night when the child is sleeping. With

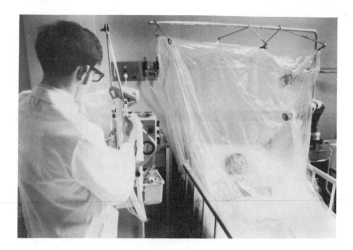

Fig. 19-6. Mist tent in use. The fogging within the tent should be heavy enough to partially obscure the patient.

more serious obstructive respiratory difficulties, the tent may be used continuously.

Expectorants such as iodides, glycerol guaiacolate and desoxyephedrine are frequently given orally to promote liquefaction of secretions. Mucomyst (acetylcysteine) and proteolytic agents such as streptokinase, streptodornase and pancreatic dornase are administered in the form of aerosol sprays several times a day. Care must be taken that sudden solubilization of the secretions does not result in such a sudden outpouring of fluid that the child drowns because he is unable to clear it by his coughing efforts.

Bronchodilators which relax the constricting musculature of the bronchial tree are also employed. They may be given by mouth in the form of Tedral, Quadrinal or similar preparations; or as aerosols of isoproterenol or phenylephrine well diluted and sprayed into the child's respiratory passages as he inhales.

Physiotherapy is employed when accumulation of secretions is significant or when obstruction of the larger branches of the bronchial tree is apparent. Periodic postural drainage by inversion of the child with cupped hands percussion over blocked areas of the lungs is often effective in improving ventilation of the lungs. Skilled operators can teach parents and nursing personnel how to carry out these procedures. Breathing exercises may also be taught to the older child to foster fuller expansion and aeration of the lungs.

The management of complications such as atelectasis, pneumothorax, heart failure and lung abscess is similar to that described under those headings elsewhere in the text.

Nursing Care

Nursing care of the child with cystic fibrosis who is hospitalized because of pneumonitis is focused on supporting respiration through measures aimed at

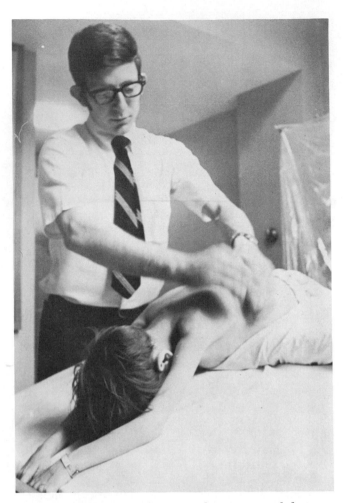

FIG. 19-7. Physical therapy during postural drainage. By percussing with cupped hands over collapsed areas of lung, the operator tries to dislodge mucus plugs in the child who has previously received bronchodilating and mucolytic medications.

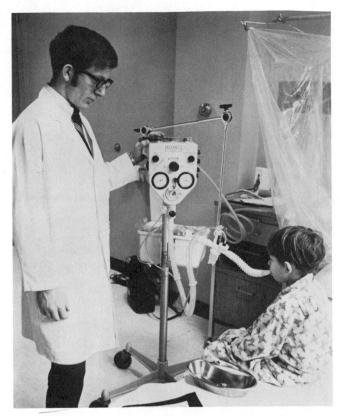

FIG. 19-8. Intermittent positive pressure breathing. The child must cooperate by holding his mouth closed around the mouth-piece while the machine administers a pulse of medicated air under pressure.

thinning secretions and through assisting the patient in clearing the mucus from the respiratory tree. Liquefaction or thinning of secretions is accomplished through aerosol therapy usually produced by nebulizers powered by compressed air. While the child is receiving mist therapy within a tent, frequent observation is indicated to check that the equipment is working properly, that the density of the mist is adequate and that the temperature within the tent is maintained at between 75 and 80° F. If the child becomes fatigued during the procedures, short rest periods should be permitted. Enclosure in a tent may be frightening to the small child. The presence of his nurse, or of his favorite toys within the tent may help to relieve his loneliness. Medications used in the treatment often clog the equipment; therefore the latter should be thoroughly washed and rinsed after each treatment.

Although in most larger hospitals physiotherapists

usually supervise the postural drainage and the clapping and vibrating used to clear the bronchial tree, nurses are often called upon to assist in the treatment, to carry it out when the therapist is not available or to supervise treatment in the home. When accumulation of secretions is considerable, postural drainage and treatment are usually necessary three times daily. The procedures must be carefully explained to the child and his cooperation enlisted before any treatment is begun. The child may be placed in a leaning position over the side of the bed or in a jackknife position over an elevated joint of the bed. The position will vary to give greatest access to the most affected lobe of the lung. Clapping over the affected lobe is carried out with the cupped hand gently for 1 to 2 minutes at a time for a total length of approximately 30 minutes. Such clapping aids in dislodging mucus plugs which obstruct the flow of secretions. Following each period of clapping, the child is encouraged to cough and raise the mucus freed by gravity and the treatment.

The nurse in cooperation with the physiotherapist should assist parents in learning these technics and in feeling secure in their execution. Parents may also need support in encouraging regular periods of deep diaphragmatic breathing and in vigorous exercise according to their child's tolerance level. Many parents of children with cystic fibrosis feel overburdened with the necessity of daily and prolonged treatment, with this constant reminder of their child's illness and with their responsibility in maintaining their child's health. They often feel insecure and inadequate in their performance of the exercises and uncertain as to how much they should protect their child from contact with others or the extent to which they should enforce limitations on his play and exercise. An important responsibility of the nurse, both in the hospital and in the community, is to offer understanding, encouragement and support to parents in their efforts toward continuing measures to improve pulmonary ventilation when the child returns home.

During hospitalization, it is also an important responsibility of the nurse to assist the child in accepting his medications and to assure that the time he receives them is appropriate. Pancreatic enzymes must be given with meals. Cotazyme may be crushed and mixed with soft foods if the child is too young to take the capsule easily.

The maintenance of adequate nutrition is of vital importance and may prove challenging since many children are anorexic with pulmonary infection. Others may have a voracious appetite symptomatic of their disease. A high protein, low fat diet can be made more attractive through inclusion of the child's food preferences whenever possible, through frequent between-meal snacks, through careful substitition for foods not allowed on the diet and through avoidance of excessive persuasion to eat when the child has little appetite. Eating with others at an attractive table may stimulate appetite and encourage constructive relationships.

Meticulous attention must be given to cleanliness and to personal hygiene of children with cystic fibrosis. Frequent bathing and shampooing of the hair are necessary to remove sticky residue caused by the aerosol therapy. Special consideration must be given to mouth care because of frequent expectoration of mucus. Bedpans and soiled diapers should be removed immediately to avoid unpleasant odors.

Measures aimed at supporting the child's emotional and intellectual development have been previously discussed and must be emphasized as an integral part of the nursing care plan. Prolonged hospitalization may entail specific measures to alleviate sensory deprivation, to counteract depression and lethargy and to provide for discharge of tension and anxiety. Parental reactions to a diagnosis of probable fatal illness in their child have been discussed in Chapter 2. Continuous support for both child and parents is imperative in order to assist them in coping with fear and anxiety. The collaborative efforts of the social worker, nurse, physician, clergyman, physiotherapist and others is indicated to aid the family through all stages of this chronic stressful circumstance.

SITUATIONS FOR FURTHER STUDY

1. How can diphtheria be prevented?

2. How can tetanus be prevented? If you were notified that a 2-year-old child with tetanus was coming to the ward, what precautions for his care would you make? What equipment should be in readiness for his medical and nursing care? What symptoms would lead you to believe that the child was near the point when he needed more rectal Avertin?

3. What are the common complications of scarlet fever? How can they be prevented?

4. How do symptoms of typhoid fever differ in infancy and in childhood? How does nursing care differ in infancy and childhood?

5. To confirm a diagnosis of tuberculosis, sputum examination is often desired. How would a sputum specimen be obtained from a 2-year-old child? What equipment would be necessary? How would you help a child to face the experience? How would you help him to dissipate the feelings that the procedure aroused after it was completed?

6. Read Plank's report and discuss the role she suggests for the nurse in a program she reported on. Discuss her findings concerning children's reactions to ward personnel on return clinic visits. Of what value was Plank's interpretation of the children's behavior to you in fulfilling your role as a nurse?

7. If a tuberculin patch test was done and the child's mother asked you to explain the reason for it, what would you tell her about it?

BIBLIOGRAPHY

Bruton, M. R.: When tetanus struck, Am. J. Nurs. 65:107, 1965.

Burgess, L.: Morale boosting in cystic fibrosis, Am. J. Nurs. 69:322, 1969.

Cohen, N., and Baker, G. D.: Jean's story—a child with cystic fibrosis, Nurs. Outlook 11:721, 1963.

Carnevali, D., and Little, D.: Tuberculosis patients and nurse specialists, Nurs. Outlook, 13:78, 1965.

Dubo, S.: Psychiatric study of children with pulmonary tuberculosis, Am. J. Orthopsychiat. 20:520, 1950.

Hlohinec, E.: Hospital care for the tuberculous child, Am. J. Nurs. 68:1913, 1968.

Johnson, M., and Fassett, B.: Bronchopulmonary hygiene in cystic fibrosis, Am. J. Nurs. 69:320, 1969.

Krugman, S., and Ward, R.: Infectious Diseases of Children, ed. 7, St. Louis, Mosby, 1968.

Kurihara, M.: Postural drainage, clapping and vibrating, Am.J. Nurs. 65:76, 1965.

Milio, N.: Family-centered care for cystic fibrosis, Nurs. Outlook 11:718, 1963.

Musklin, I., and Burns, A. J.: Tracking down tuberculosis, Am. J. Nurs. 65:91, 1965.

Plank, E. N., *et al.*: A general hospital child care program to counteract hospitalism, Am. J. Orthopsychiat. 29: 94, 1959.

Rosenburg, M., and Gottleib, R.: Current approach to tuberculosis in childhood, Pediat. Clin. N. Am. *15*:513, 1968.

Schwab, L., Callison, C. B., and Frank, M. P., Cystic fibrosis I. Medical care and treatment, Am. J. Nurs. *63*:62, 1963.

————: Cystic fibrosis II. Nursing care, Am. J. Nurs. *63*:67, 1963.

Schwachman, H., and Khaw, K., Cystic Fibrosis, *in* Shirkey, H. C. (Ed.): Pediatric Therapy, St. Louis, Mosby, 1968.

Shapiro, C.: Typhoid fever, trained nurse and hosp. rev. *118*:120, 1948.

Steigman, A. J., and Epting, M. H.: Diphtheria in children, Am. J. Nurs. *57*:467, 1957.

Report of the Committee on the Control of Infectious Diseases, Evanston, Ill., American Academy of Pediatrics, 1969.

20

Nursing Care of Children With Infection and Infestation by Other Forms of Life

In the temperate zones of the world, the bulk of childhood infections are produced by viruses and bacteria. But a variety of other forms of life are also able to create illness by invasion of the tissues or by residence on the skin or in the intestinal tract. The list includes rickettsia, fungi, spirochetes, protozoa, mites and worms. Most of these disorders are common to the warm climates and properly belong within the province of tropical medicine. Brief descriptions are given here for the purpose of orienting the student toward those ailments which may be encountered in the United States.

RICKETTSIAL INFECTIONS

The infectious agents called rickettsia are larger than viruses and barely visible through the ordinary microscope. They are agents which primarily infect ticks, mites, fleas and lice but may be transmitted to man in some instances. Like the viruses they are incapable of surviving unless in close association with living cells. The rickettsial diseases of man are not transmissible from man to man but require the mediation of one of the small parasites mentioned above. The diseases that rickettsia produce have some common characteristics— fever, headache, skin eruption, leukopenia, self-limited course and favorable response to chlortetracycline (Aureomycin), oxytetracycline (Terramycin) and chloramphenicol.

Rocky Mountain Spotted Fever (Tick Typhus)

This is the most severe rickettsial infection seen in the United States. As the name suggests, it is found in the Rocky Mountain area (and, to a lesser extent, along the eastern seaboard) and is transmitted to man by infected ticks. The onset is abrupt with high fever and severe headache followed by a measles-like rash which generally is more marked on the extremities than on the trunk. The prognosis of the untreated disease is rather serious, but rapid response to tetracy-

clines or chloramphenicol is to be anticipated. A vaccine is available for active immunization.

Murine Typhus

Murine typhus is transmitted to man by fleas and mites which live on rats. It is seen in the southern part of the United States. The symptomatology is similar to tick fever but less severe. It responds to the same treatment.

Rickettsialpox

This is a new disease which thus far has been observed almost exclusively in New York City. A mouse mite is responsible for its transmission to children. A local lesion develops at the site of the infecting bite and before the appearance of the rash which is distributed over the entire body except palms and soles. The disease is self-limited and improves under tetracycline or chloramphenicol treatment.

Q Fever

This is a rickettsial infection which simulates protracted influenza. It is derived from infected cattle which excrete organisms in their feces. Transmission to man takes place through inhalation of contaminated dust. It too responds to chlortetracycline.

FUNGOUS INFECTIONS

The common varieties of fungous infection in man are superficial invasions of the skin (epidermophytosis) or of the oral cavity (monilia). A few varieties of fungus are capable of producing systemic disease. Both coccidioidomycosis and histoplasmosis are similar to tuberculosis in their clinical manifestations.

Coccidioidomycosis (San Joaquin Valley Fever)

This disease is confined to the southwestern portion of the United States where the climate is hot and arid. The fungus spores are disseminated with the dust

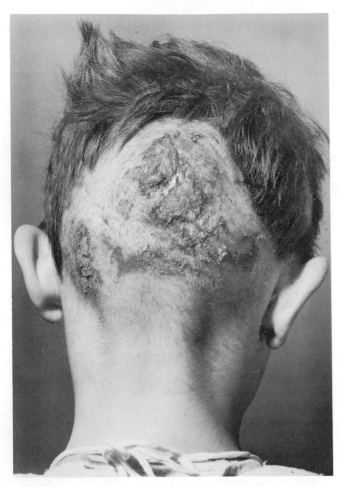

FIG. 20-1. Ringworm of the scalp (tinea capitis or tinea tonsurans).

and gain entrance into the body either through the respiratory tract or through cuts and abrasions of the skin. The initial invasion may be accompanied by an influenza-like illness or it may be unrecognized. Roentgen examination of the chest reveals enlargement of hilar lymph nodes, soft patches of infiltration in the lung fields and occasionally cavities. Allergy to the fungus may be demonstrated by a skin test similar to the tuberculin test. Erythema nodosum is present in some instances during the onset of allergy. Widespread dissemination of the fungus takes place in a small fraction of infected persons. Manifestations similar to those of disseminated tuberculosis, including meningitis, may occur. No specific therapy is available. Ordinarily, the disease is self-limited, but the uncommon generalized form carries a significant mortality. Sulfonamides are moderately effective in suppressing proliferation of the fungus. In severe infections amphotericin B is used, but it is a highly toxic drug which should be reserved for desperately ill patients.

Differentiation from tuberculosis may be difficult on clinical grounds but usually can be achieved through skin test reactions and immunologic procedures.

Histoplasmosis

Histoplasmosis is the result of infection with a fungus that occurs widely in the Mississippi Valley and to a lesser extent in areas along the eastern seaboard of the United States. It, too, is confused frequently with tuberculosis but generally is discovered accidentally through roentgen examination of the chest. The early lesions simulate primary tuberculous infection, and the healed lesions calcify. Differentiation is made through the use of skin tests which demonstrate allergy to the protein of the fungus and through complement fixation reactions of the blood. In severe cases the fungi may be seen in the bone marrow.

In most instances the disease is asymptomatic and presents purely academic interest. In a few children the infection may be heavy and produce severe pulmonary disease with cavitation or a generalized bloodstream involvement which is progressive and attended by a high mortality. As with coccidioidomycosis, no treatment is required for the benign form. Sulfonamides offer some protection against the disseminated form. Amphotericin B is somewhat effective once dissemination has occurred.

Tinea (Ringworm)

Superficial fungous infections of the skin commonly are called ringworm and technically are known as tinea. The varieties of tinea are designated by the part of the body or the shape of the resulting lesion. Thus, ringworm of the scalp is *tinea tonsurans* or *capitis;* of the body, *tinea circinata;* of the nails, *tinea unguium* or *onychomycosis;* of the feet, *tinea pedis* or *dermatophytosis* or *athlete's foot.* A number of fungi, some of which are obtained from young domestic animals, may be involved. Since fungi fluoresce under ultraviolet light, the Woods lamp can be used to aid in diagnosis and gauge the adequacy of treatment. Accurate identification of the fungus requires special laboratory facilities but is sometimes essential to direct adequate treatment.

Ringworm of the Scalp. This infection may have its start at the site of a single hair, but the lesion increases in extent up to an inch or two in diameter. The patches are roughly circular. The base of the hair is invaded by the spores of the fungus. The hair becomes brittle and breaks off close to the skin, leaving the area apparently bald. The skin of the area is scaly and shows no other evidence of inflammation except that secondary infection may occur with the formation of pustules in the hair follicles. Mycelia of the fungus are found in the scales. (Fig. 20-1)

The treatment of ringworm of the scalp has been

greatly improved by the development of an antifungal antibiotic, griseofulvin. It is given by mouth, preferably with a fatty meal which improves its absorption. The dosage is 10 mg./Kg./day for ordinary severity; greater for stubborn infections. The head is usually shaved and fungicidal ointments are used locally. The adequacy of treatment may be followed by examination with the Woods lamp.

Ringworm of the Body. This differs unimportantly from ringworm of the scalp, except that hair is not affected so obviously. The lesion occurs also on the face. In any location the lesion extends by enlargement at the edges: the newer part is pinkish and slightly elevated; the older part at the center is paler or pigmented and moderately scaly. Thus the lesion may be suggestive of a ring. Itching may be present, but little inflammation is apparent except where the origin was animal, and then there may be much inflammation. The responsible fungus is found in the scales. A customary treatment consists of the application of Whitfield's Ointment, which relieves the itching promptly. Griseofulvin is usually curative.

Ringworm of the Feet. This infection is located most often between the toes. The moisture of these regions prevents the usual scale formation; instead, the macerated superficial epithelium tends to desquamate, leaving a raw surface with fissures and often with vesicles. The itching is likely to be intense. Like all ringworm, the disease is contagious. It is acquired in gymnasiums, at swimming pools and other similar places where people go barefoot. For the purpose of avoiding this infection, it is desirable to wear some kind of foot covering when walking where others walk barefoot. Also, it is important to keep infected persons away from places where people are likely to walk with bare feet.

Treatment for the ordinary type, such as occurs between the toes or on the soles of the feet, consists of application of an ointment such as Desenex. Other and often more vigorous methods of treatment are advocated by various physicians. The more vigorous methods are much more likely to cause treatment dematitis. In addition to treatment of the skin, the foot coverings previously worn should be sterilized or discarded. Thin, ventilated shoes help to avoid the sweating that aggravates the condition. Oral griseofulvin may be used in stubborn cases but must be continued for several weeks.

Other Fungous Infections

In rare instances children may be infected with other types of fungus such as those that produce actinomycosis, blastomycosis and sporotrichosis. The characteristics of these infections are not distinctive in children, and their rarity makes them unsuitable for discussion in a brief text. For specific information reference should be made to the standard treatises on internal medicine.

Moniliasis, or thrush, is considered in Chapter 7.

SPIROCHETAL INFECTIONS

Spirochetes are a special type of bacteria which are long, slender, coiled and highly motile. The most prevalent disease producer is the *Treponema pallidum* which causes *syphilis*. This disease is considered in Chapter 10.

In one variety of ulcerative stomatitis (*Vincent's infection*) a spirillum is present which is thought to be partly responsible for the symptoms. It also responds to adequate treatment with penicillin.

Rats may transmit spirochetal disease to children in two ways. *Rat-bite fever,* as the name implies, is due to the bite of an infected rat. It is uncommon and responds well to penicillin. *Leptospirosis* is usually transmitted by indirect contact with infected rats which excrete spirochetes in the urine. Children consuming water or food which has been contaminated by rat urine in wells, sewage or ponds may suffer an illness marked by fever, meningeal symptoms and a rash resembling measles. Penicillin and the tetracyclines are effective in treatment. Prognosis is good unless renal failure intervenes. Prevention of the disease depends on rat control.

PROTOZOAL INFECTIONS

Malaria

Malaria is the most important of the protozoal diseases. It is of little concern in the United States where control of the mosquito which transmits the disease from one person to another has been achieved. However, many areas of the world are still plagued by this disease. In addition to mosquito control, protection or suppression of symptoms may be obtained by regular prophylaxis with quinine or one of the newer antimalarials such as chloroquine and primaquine.

Toxoplasmosis

Toxoplasmosis is a protozoan disease which is seen mainly during the newborn period. It is discussed in Chapter 10.

Amebiasis

The pathogenic amoeba, *Entamoeba histolytica*, thrives in the intestinal tract of man and is discharged with the stool. An infected person may pass the infective cysts on to others by routes which involve contamination of food or water supplies. Thus, amebiasis appears where standards of hygiene are low. The infective cysts are rapidly destroyed by drying, heat and heavy chlorination of water.

The disease is more common in adults and older children than it is in the toddler or the infant. It produces varying symptoms. Many infected persons are asymptomatic. Others have diarrhea of varying degrees of severity because the amoebae create an inflammation within the wall of the intestine. The diarrhea is often bloody and sometimes severe. Liver abscess is an occasional complication but is rarely seen in children.

Prevention of the disease is mediated under favorable circumstances by proper personal hygiene and disposal of stools. Fecal contamination of the water supply must be forestalled. In areas where amebiasis is prevalent, raw fruits and vegetables should be avoided unless they are carefully washed or freshly peeled.

Diagnosis is achieved by the recognition of cysts in the recently passed stool. The cysts lose their typical microscopic appearance unless examined at once or refrigerated until the specimen can be handled. Treatment of the disease during the acute stage is begun with a tetracycline antibiotic which usually relieves diarrhea and tenesmus within a few days. Sterilization of the intestine must be pursued until carefully examined stool specimens are free of cysts. Drugs used for longer term therapy include Diodoquin, Milibis, chloroquine and carbarsone. Investigation of family contacts is necessary to discover and treat carriers.

PARASITIC INFESTATIONS OF THE SKIN

Pediculosis

Three varieties of lice are found inhabiting the hair or the clothing of children.

The most common form is *pediculosis capitis,* in which the lice dwell in the hair of the scalp and lay their eggs or nits on the shafts of the hairs. The lice themselves are often difficult to see, but the nits are small, fixed, ovoid, white bodies which can be seen with the naked eye. Scalp lice cause itching which eventually may lead to infection of the scalp by pyogenic bacteria at sites of trauma from constant scratching.

Body lice (*pediculosis corporis*) actually live in the clothes but irritate by their excursions onto the skin surfaces for the purpose of biting and feeding.

Pubic or crab lice (*pediculosis pubis*) dwell in the pubic hair of older people but may invade the eyelashes or eyebrows of young children. The nits are seen easily; the lice themselves are found less commonly.

Modern treatment of louse infestation is relatively simple and quite effective. Clothes can be laundered or dusted with 10 per cent DDT in talc, which kills both lice and nits. Various preparations for use in the hair are available. Topocide contains DDT and benzylbenzoate as its main constituents; Kwell and Eurax contain other types of synthetic pesticide. Usually, 2 applications about 12 hours apart are sufficient to eradicate the lice and the nits.

Scabies

Scabies is a contagious skin disease caused by *Acarus scabiei* (*Sarcoptes scabiei*) or itch mite. The human disease is caused exclusively by the female acarus, which burrows into the skin for the purpose of depositing eggs. The parts of the body involved are chiefly those in which the skin is thin and moist. In the older person, one may expect to find the lesions most abundant between the fingers, on the underside of the wrists, in the axillae and about the genitalia. In the infant, they may be almost anywhere. The most characteristic lesion in infants is the infected burrow on the palm, present as a small pustule with the black wavy line of the burrow on the surface. The primary lesions are the burrows produced by the travels of the acarus. These usually are less than ⅛ inch in length. With a hand lens they are seen as dark or black lines, the color being produced by fecal deposits of the parasite. Typical burrows may be difficult to find because of secondary inflammation. Scabies causes severe itching. The reaction of the parasite, together with infection produced by scratching, causes inflammatory changes which may take the form of papules, vesicles or pustules.

The treatment of scabies is similar to that for pediculosis as noted above. Occasionally, the modern agents are not available, and the old-fashioned sulfur ointment (5%) may be used. It is important to discover all of the infested members in a family so that they may be treated simultaneously in order to kill all the mites within the household and prevent return of the disturbance.

Ticks

Ticks (and mites) are small arthropods which have biting and sucking parts and attach themselves to man or animals for the purpose of sucking the blood. After satiating themselves they let go and drop off. In the process of feeding they may transmit viral or rickettsial infection to a child or may cause paralysis or fever by the injection of toxic substances. These latter events depend on the presence of poisons or infections within the biting tick. In the United States, most ticks are harmless, and the bite is inconsequential except for the local discomfort. Some of the diseases which may be transmitted by ticks or mites are Rocky Mountain spotted fever, St. Louis encephalitis, typhus fever and rickettsialpox. The uncommon circumstance of tick paralysis clears up when the tick is discovered and removed.

SPIDERS

The black widow and the brown spider found within the boundaries of the U.S. are capable of inflicting toxic bites. The amount of venom injected is ordinarily small and a painful local lesion results without the systemic manifestations of headache, vomiting, muscle cramps, rigidity and a paralysis which may follow the injection of larger doses of venom. These latter symptoms can be relieved by the intravenous administration of calcium gluconate. Antivenin is available for the treatment of serious poisoning.

SNAKES

Several poisonous snakes are found in the U.S.: rattlesnakes, moccasins and coral snakes. A multivalent antivenin is commercially available and should be used, if obtainable, in preference to the traditional methods of incision and sucking of the bite, freezing, or other procedures which devitalize the local tissues and increase the risk of local tissue destruction. Information about antivenin and how to obtain it is best sought from a local zoo, forest ranger or public health station.

INTESTINAL PARASITIC WORMS

Intestinal worms have been blamed erroneously for a wide variety of symptoms such as nose-picking, restless sleep, grinding the teeth while asleep, circles under the eyes, and convulsions. Most of these symptoms are related to emotional disturbances in the child and have nothing to do with intestinal parasites. Children who do harbor worms usually have no symptoms. An accurate estimate of the frequency of worm infestations is possible only by intensive and repeated study of stools and anal swabs. Such studies usually demonstrate a remarkably high prevalence of pinworm and roundworm infestations not only in the southern climates but also in the northern cities of the United States.

Pinworm (Threadworm, Seatworm, Enterobiasis, Oxyuriasis)

This is by far the most common variety of intestinal parasite. The worms are small white threads from ⅛ to ½ inch in length which are seen most commonly about the anus after the child has been asleep for an hour or two. Sometimes they are found on the surface of a stool. Infestation occurs when eggs are swallowed. The eggs hatch within the intestinal tract, and the gravid female worms inhabit the cecum until ready to lay their eggs. Then they crawl out of the anus, usually after the child has gone to sleep. They either lay their eggs shortly after emerging or are broken open and scatter the eggs about the child's perineum and into his clothing. The eggs survive for several days and are the source from which the same or another individual in the environment may acquire a new infestation. The period between ingestion of the egg and appearance of the gravid female at the anus is about 6 to 8 weeks.

Symptoms. Symptoms of pinworm infestation may be entirely lacking, and the condition may be discovered only by finding the worms. When infestation is heavy there may be itching about the anus or about the vagina in the female. The scratching that results traps new eggs under the finger nails and affords an easy means of their transfer back to the mouth.

Diagnosis. Diagnosis usually is made by finding and recognizing the worms as they emerge from the anus. The eggs may be found by swabbing the anal region with Scotch tape and examining it under a microscope. Since the females do not lay eggs within the intestinal tract, eggs are not found in the stools.

Treatment. Treatment attempts both to intoxicate the worms so that they will leave the intestine before completing their maturation, and to eliminate the eggs deposited in the environment before they can cause another infestation. Gentian violet in enteric-coated tablets is the standard vermifuge for pinworms. It may cause nausea and mild abdominal pain and must be used over a 10-day course to be effective. Piperazine citrate (Antepar) in a single morning dose of 0.25 to 2.0 Gm. depending upon body size and repeated for 7 days, and pyrvinium pamoate (Povan) in a single dose of 5 mg./Kg. are more modern and equally effective treatments. After a rest of 2 weeks the treatment should be repeated to be sure of expelling any worms on a different cycle. Underclothing, night clothing and bed linen should be boiled at least twice a week in order to destroy eggs deposited therein. Careful cleansing of the perineum, the hands and the nails should be carried out several times a day. Application of a soothing ointment, such as ammoniated mercury or blue ointment, may allay the itching and reduce the viability of the eggs that have been deposited. All individuals in the family who have any suspicion of being infested must be treated simultaneously if success is to be attained.

Roundworm (*Ascaris lumbricoides*)

The adult roundworm is a large (6 to 15 in.) white or pink parasite about the diameter of a lead pencil. It lives for periods up to 6 months in the intestinal tract, during which time the females lay enormous numbers of eggs that are discharged in the patient's stools. The eggs require from 2 to 4 weeks and a moist, shaded environment to develop into an infective stage. The infestation is passed from one individual to another only in regions where flush toilets are absent and defecation is performed in outhouses or on the open ground.

An egg that has developed to the stage of infectivity and is ingested follows a somewhat complicated development within the child. It is transformed first into a larval stage within the intestine. The larva is able to migrate through the intestinal walls; it gains access to the portal venous system and the general circulation and then reaches the lungs, where it breaks out of the blood stream into the alveoli. From the lungs the larvae are coughed up and swallowed to complete their growth into adult worms in the intestinal tract. The full development requires from 4 to 6 weeks.

Symptoms. Roundworms produce no symptoms except when present in unusual number so as to block the intestinal tract, or through unusual migrations as into the bile tract.

Treatment. Antepar given in heavy dosage on 2 consecutive days is highly effective in removing roundworms from the gut. The dosage varies from 1.0 to 3.5 Gm. according to the size of the subject.

Hookworm (*Uncinaria americana*)

The hookworm is a small (¼ to ½ in.) worm that lives in the upper intestinal tract where it is attached firmly by a mouth with teethlike parts through which it derives nourishment by sucking blood from the intestinal wall. The females lay large numbers of eggs which are passed in the patient's stools. The eggs require warm sandy soil for their development into larvae within about 2 weeks. Larvae may be ingested, or, more commonly, they penetrate through the skin of a child who is going barefoot. They enter the blood stream and circulate to the lungs where they enter the alveoli, are coughed up and swallowed and complete their development in the upper intestinal tract. Hookworm disease is limited to the southeastern portion of the United States and depends for its spread on outdoor toilets and barefootedness.

Symptoms. The symptoms of hookworm disease depend on the number of worms present in the individual. When the number is large, the loss of blood to the worms may be sufficient to cause anemia. Chronic infestations also produce anorexia, malnutrition and chronic fatigue. A sensitized child may develop itching at the site of entrance of larvae into the skin of his feet.

Diagnosis. Diagnosis is made by finding the ova in the stools.

Treatment. Tetrachloroethylene is given in the morning following a light liquid meal the preceding evening. The dosage is 0.1 mg./Kg. of weight. Fat containing foods are withheld for another 12 hours after medication. Occasionally transfusion for anemia is indicated. Usually attention to the general diet is indicated.

Beef Tapeworm (*Taenia saginata*)

The beef tapeworm requires an intermediate host, the cow, for its passage from one individual to another. It is acquired by eating infested beef which has not been cooked sufficiently to kill the larvae present within it. A larva so ingested develops in the upper intestinal tract into an adult worm with a tenacious head which attaches itself to the intestinal wall. It grows by progressive segmentation until it reaches considerable length—10 to 12 feet or more. Segments of the worm may break off and be noticed in the stool, or the end of the worm may protrude from the anus. There are no symptoms.

Treatment. Treatment attempts to intoxicate the worm so that it will release its hold on the intestinal wall and pass out of the tract. Atabrine, 15 mg./Kg., is divided into 2 doses and given an hour apart. The treatment is preceded by one day of liquid diet and a cleansing enema and followed by a saline purgative. It is important to save all segments of the worm which are passed, for the head must be identified in order to be sure that treatment is complete. If some of the worm is broken off and the head is left behind, it will continue to grow.

Trichina (*Trichinella spiralis*)

This is a fairly common infestation obtained from the ingestion of uncooked pork in which the encysted larvae of the worm reside. Digestion in the stomach of the patient frees the larva from its thick capsule and permits it to develop in 3 to 5 days in the intestine into the adult form. Adults then burrow into the intestinal wall and release larvae which enter the blood stream and take up residence in the skeletal muscles. Infestation by a few trichinae may pass entirely unnoticed, but heavy infestation may produce severe or even fatal disease.

Symptoms. Symptoms of a heavy infestation may begin within a few days of the ingestion of the contaminated pork. The activity of the developing worms in the intestinal mucosa may produce diarrhea and fever. Marked constitutional symptoms of fever, pains in the muscles, swelling of the eyes and myocarditis may accompany the invasion of larvae into skeletal and heart muscle during the first 3 to 6 weeks. There is no effective treatment.

LARVA MIGRANS

Creeping Eruption

Infestation with the larvae of the cat or dog hookworm (*Ancylostoma braziliense*) produces an uncomfortable itching of the feet as the larvae burrow about in subcutaneous tunnels. The tunnels are visible to the naked eye. The disease can be terminated by freezing the larvae *in situ* with ethyl chloride.

Visceral Larva Migrans

Eggs from cats or dogs infected with the worms *Toxocara cati* or *canis* if swallowed by small children may produce their larval forms within the intestinal tract and thence migrate to the child's liver where they produce a granulomatous chronic disease. Eosinophilia, fever and enlarged liver result. In very heavy infestations there may be distant granulomata in the lungs, brain or eye. No treatment is available. The disease slowly subsides after many months.

BIBLIOGRAPHY

Barrett-Connor, E., Connor, J. D., and Beck, J. W.: Common parasitic infections of the intestinal tract, Pediat. Clin. N. Am. *14*:235, 1967.

Brown, H. W.: Parasitic Diseases *in* Shirkey, H. C. (ed.), Pediatric Therapy, St. Louis, Mosby, 1968.

Noojin, R. O.: Pediatric Dermatology *in* Shirkey, H. C. (ed.), Pediatric Therapy, St. Louis, Mosby, 1968.

Rivers, T. M., and Horsfall, F. L., Jr. (eds.): Viral and Rickettsial Infections of Man, ed. 3, Philadelphia, Lippincott, 1959.

Tobias, N.: Essentials of Dermatology, ed. 6, Philadelphia, Lippincott, 1963.

Wexler, L.: Gamma benezine hexachloride in treatment of pediculosis and scabies, Am. J. Nurs. *69*:565, 1969.

21

Nursing Care of Children With Hematologic Disorders

PHYSIOLOGIC CONSIDERATIONS

Blood consists of a fluid portion known as plasma and of formed components or cells. The plasma comprises slightly more than 50 per cent of the volume of the blood. Among the many functions of the plasma are the carrying of food materials to all parts of the body and the carrying away of waste products for excretion.

The plasma contains the elements necessary for blood clotting. A blood clot is formed by conversion of fibrinogen of the plasma to fibrin, which forms the coagulum. Fibrin is formed under the stimulus of thrombin. Thrombin is formed from the prothrombin of the blood through the action of thromboplastin derived from damaged blood platelets and from injured tissues. The calcium of the blood also is necessary for clot formation. That part of the plasma which remains after the fibrin is separated is serum.

The formed components of the blood consist of red cells (erythrocytes), white cells (leukocytes) and platelets (thrombocytes) (Plate 4).

In fetal life and earliest infancy the red cells are formed in the liver, the spleen, the bone marrow and other lymphatic structures; after birth they are formed in the bone marrow alone. The mature red cell has no nucleus, but a nucleus is present in an early stage of its formation. In fetal life, nucleated red cells are common in the blood, and some may be found in the early days after birth, particularly in prematurely born babies.

After the earliest period of life, the finding of nucleated red cells means an abnormally rapid formation of red cells to supply a demand, as in the case of some of the anemias of infancy. A lesser degree of immaturity of red cells is shown by persistence in the cell of material known as reticulum, which is identified easily in a specially stained preparation of blood. Normally, red cells are being destroyed constantly and being replaced by new ones. The average period of red cell

survival in the blood stream is 120 days. As evidence of normal speed of generation and replacement, approximately 1 per cent of the red cells of the blood are reticulated (reticulocytes). An increase above this proportion indicates rapid cell generation. Conversely, a paucity of reticulocytes connotes abnormally slow formation of red blood cells. Thus in the anemias, a knowledge of the proportion of reticulocytes is important for diagnosis and prognosis.

The chief function of the red cells is to carry hemoglobin, and the chief purpose of hemoglobin is to take oxygen to the tissues and remove carbon dioxide for excretion by way of the lungs. Hemoglobin is formed by the reticuloendothelial cells of the bone marrow. In the normal disappearance of red cells from the blood, the cells are removed by the reticuloendothelial tissues, especially those of the spleen. The hemoglobin of the cells is broken down. The iron of the hemoglobin is split off and is largely reused. The pigment is changed to bile pigment and is excreted (p. 147).

The rate of red cell production in the bone marrow appears to be related to the production of a hormone-like substance by the kidney. This substance, erythropoietin, is present in the blood stream in large amounts when anemia or anoxemia is present; absent when red cell levels and oxygenation are normal. The exception to this rule is in anemia secondary to kidney disease wherein the production of erythropoietin is defective.

The white cells of the blood consist of granular leukocytes or granulocytes, lymphocytes and monocytes (large mononuclear leukocytes). The mature lymphocytes and monocytes have no important subdivisions. Granular or polymorphonuclear leukocytes are of 3 varieties: neutrophils, eosinophils and basophils. The granular leukocytes are formed in the bone marrow; the lymphocytes develop in the spleen, the lymph nodes and thymus; and the large mononuclear leukocytes have their origin in the reticuloendothelial

Table 20. Normal Blood Values at Different Ages

	Birth	12 Wks.	6 Mos.	2 Yrs.	12 Yrs.
Red cells (millions/cu. mm.)	4.5-5.5	3.5-4.5	4.0-4.5	4.3-4.7	4.5-5.0
Hemoglobin (gm./100 cc.)	15.5-18.5	10-12	11-13	12-13.5	13.5-15
White cells (average/cu. mm.)	20,000	12,000	12,000	10,000	8,000
Platelets (average/cu. mm.)	350,000	300,000	300,000	300,000	300,000

lining of the blood sinuses of the spleen, the bone marrow, the liver and the lymph nodes (Plate 4).

In the course of development of granulocytes, the type of cell immediately preceding the mature cells is known as a "myelocyte." Myelocytes differ from mature cells in their appearance and staining characteristics when a stained preparation is examined microscopically. The presence of myelocytes in the blood indicates an unusually rapid formation of granulocytes. An abundance of myelocytes characterizes the disease myelocytic leukemia.

The mature lymphocyte is small in comparison with the larger and more deeply staining immature form. The immature forms are found abundantly in lymphatic leukemia.

Plasma cells are infrequent but important units of the lymph nodes and bone marrow which are also found in the circulating blood at times. Their special significance is due to the fact that they form the gamma globulin of the plasma. This is the blood fraction which contains the antibodies.

The white blood cells seem to have no physiologic function in health other than to serve as a part of the defense mechanism of the body against infections. They are actively motile and penetrate tissues, especially at the site of infection. An increase in the number of neutrophils in the blood is often evidence that an infection is present and is stimulating the increase. After these leukocytes have migrated to the site of infection, they ingest and destroy many, though not all, varieties of bacteria. The so-called "pyogenic infections" stimulate an increase in the polymorphonuclear leukocytes. Other types of infection cause an increase in the lymphocytes of the blood. The eosinophils are increased especially in parasitic infestations.

The blood platelets or thrombocytes are formed in the bone marrow. The chief function of the platelets concerns blood coagulation. Platelets adhere to injured surfaces. In a wound, they quickly become damaged. Damaging of platelets releases thromboplastin, which initiates clot formation. When platelets are decreased greatly in the blood, spontaneous bleeding or purpura results. While platelets are important in the prevention of spontaneous bleeding, they are of less importance than the injured tissues in stopping hemorrhage from a wound. Injured tissues are a more important source of thromboplastin in these circumstances. Another important function of platelets is associated with their tendency to agglutinate. Thrombi in blood vessels sometimes consist mainly of agglutinated platelets. Agglutination of platelets in the terminal vessels of a wound assists in stopping bleeding.

The expected quantities in numbers of each of these formed elements in the blood at different ages are listed in Table 20. A great deal more variation from the average is permissible in children than in adults, particularly so in small infants.

ANEMIA

Pathophysiology

Anemia literally means without blood. Sometimes the term is used in this sense in relation to organs of the body, such as anemia of the brain, a condition in which the supply of blood to the brain is greatly reduced. More commonly the word "anemia" is used to designate a condition in which the concentration of red blood cells or of hemoglobin or of both in the circulating blood is reduced below normal. Usually, in childhood anemia the level of hemoglobin is the more important figure to consider.

Normally, red cells and hemoglobin are formed at the same rate at which they are destroyed. Anemia occurs whenever formation is decreased or destruction is increased. In the growing child the rate of formation also must keep pace with the demands of a body which is increasing in size. Except for the circumstance in which blood is lost from the body by hemorrhage, these two mechanisms are the sole fundamental causes of anemia. However, in many conditions there is a combination of the two mechanisms (or even of three mechanisms if we include blood loss) taking place, and a strict classification of anemias on this basis is not made easily. In Table 21, the principal mechanisms of anemia are outlined with examples of specific

Table 21. Principal Mechanisms Producing Anemia in Childhood

Blood loss (hemorrhage)
  Acute (trauma, operation, purpura, hemophilia)
  Chronic (ulcerative colitis)
Inadequate rate of blood formation (hypoplasia)
  Poor hemoglobin synthesis (prematurity, iron deficiency)
  Delayed red cell maturation (megaloblastic anemia, scurvy)
  Combination of above factors
  Infection (chronic respiratory, nephritis, rheumatic fever)
  Drugs (tridione, folic acid antagonists, nitrogen mustard)
  Poisons (lead, benzol)
  Bone marrow invasion (leukemia, tumors)
Other idiopathic anemia, hypersplenism, radiation injury)
Increased blood destruction (hemolysis)
  Antibody reactions (erythroblastosis, transfusion reaction)
  Hereditary trait (congenital hemolytic jaundice, sickle-cell anemia, Mediterranean anemia)
  Drugs (sulfanilamide, acetanilid, primaquine)
  Poisons (naphthalene, fava bean)
  Infections (malaria, septicemia)
  Other (acquired hemolytic anemia, glucose-6-phosphate dehydrogenase deficiency, Lederer's anemia)

disorders in which these mechanisms operate as the main cause of the resulting anemia.

Symptoms

The symptoms of anemia are similar regardless of the cause. Lassitude, listlessness and fatigability are the early manifestations. As the severity increases, pallor, weakness, tachycardia and palpitation may occur. It is surprising how well a child with chronic anemia can get along. Compensations for the low level of hemoglobin often permit fairly normal activity when the concentration is reduced to a third of the normal value. However, persistence of such levels results in mental sluggishness, irritability and cardiac enlargement. Fatal anemia is a consequence of the inability of the heart to perform its normal work.

General Treatment and Nursing Care

The management of anemia will depend on the severity and on the presumptive cause in the individual case. Transfusion is the obvious and most widely applicable method of correction. It is imperative and often lifesaving when acute blood loss or severe chronic anemia has progressed to the point of interfering with cardiac function. It also may be useful in supplying missing blood elements other than red blood cells and hemoglobin (coagulation factors in hemophilia and platelets in purpura, for instance). Even in anemia of lesser severity it often provides the child with a sense of well-being and permits better appetite and a more active resistance. In some forms of anemia it is the only possible method of ameliorating the failure of an inactive bone marrow. The nursing management of transfusion is considered in Chapter 4, and in the Appendix.

Anemia which is due to insufficient intake of iron or to loss of the body stores of iron through hemorrhage requires an increase in the iron intake. This supplies the missing elements necessary to build new hemoglobin and also stimulates the activity of the bone marrow. Iron may be given by mouth in a number of ways. Ferrous sulfate, ferric ammonium citrate and ferrous glycinate are some of the compounds in common use. In infants particularly, it is desirable to start with a small dose and work up to the desired level gradually because it sometimes irritates the gastrointestinal tract, and vomiting and diarrhea may result. When adequate dosage is achieved the stools usually assume a dark-green or black pigmentation. In occasional circumstances iron is given intramuscularly. Sometimes copper and cobalt salts are added to the iron medication in the hope of augmenting its erythropoietic powers.

Vitamin B complex factors such as folic acid, vitamin B_{12} and liver or liver extracts are essential adjuvants in treating some of the anemias associated with a megaloblastic bone marrow. In scurvy the correction of the deficiency by treatment with vitamin C rapidly helps the associated anemia.

Splenectomy is usually curative in congenital hemolytic jaundice and sometimes is used to advantage in Mediterranean anemia and other forms associated with tremendous enlargement of the spleen.

The nursing care of the child with anemia should be directed toward the maintenance of good general hygiene in order to build up resistance to intercurrent infection. Of these measures, one which the nurse will find especially demanding of her ingenuity is helping the child to adhere to his diet (foods high in vitamins, calories and iron). Anorexia is common and, although many such children are too weak to feed themselves the entire meal, they may resent being dependent on someone else to do this for them. The nurse's unobtrusive assistance with a second spoon can prevent injury to pride by making the child feel that he is in control of the situation.

Children with anemia tire easily. They should be allowed activities within their capacity in order to support efforts toward independence, to counteract boredom and to sustain intellectual functioning and interest in the environment. On the other hand, the nurse must be alert to signs of beginning fatigue—irritability or hyperactivity—and divert the child's interest to a more sedentary project such as a puzzle or modelling clay.

Transfusions can be made much more bearable if the purpose of the treatment is made clear to the child. Interest may be stimulated by showing him a blood smear under the microscope and explaining that the blood he receives gives him the power to do things that other children are capable of doing. It is not uncommon to see a child with anemia face transfusions courageously once he finds that they make him feel better and stronger. Giving approval when the child is able to cooperate also enhances his self-esteem and his willingness to endure such treatments. The stress of repeated blood counts can be reduced if the technician recognizes the child's need to control certain aspects of the procedure, such as cleansing the area of puncture, and gives him opportunity to investigate and handle the apparatus.

In some instances of anemia, the child's condition may become acute. Constant nursing care is then required to monitor the vital signs and to report any changes in the child's condition. Blood pressure readings should be taken frequently and precautions taken to protect the child in the event of a convulsion. If edema is present, daily weighing should be done along with accurate measurement and recording of the intake and output. Meticulous care of the skin is also indicated to prevent tissue breakdown.

Should the child go into cardiac failure, the administration of oxygen is usually required. Constant observation of the rate and depth of breathing is necessary along with frequent checks to assure proper functioning of the equipment.

If the course of the illness is chronic and frequent hospitalizations are required, subsequent admissions are facilitated if the child feels secure in the knowledge that his individual needs and interests are known by the nursing staff. When a child is greeted by nurses whom he knows, his concern about separation from his parents may be reduced. A favorite toy may be in readiness and in some instances it may be feasible to allow the child to select his own bed location. Encouraging him to make his own preparations for the hospital trip may bring satisfactions that compensate in part for the uncomfortable aspects of the experience.

The nurse can also be very helpful to the parents of a child with chronic anemia by assisting them to understand the origin, nature and treatment of the illness. She can assist them in planning ways to protect him from respiratory infections without placing stringent restrictions on his activities. In cooperation with a nutritionist, she can also help the mother to plan a diet for the child which is adequate for his particular needs and consistent with the resources of the family. Supporting parents through anticipatory guidance and by conveying understanding of their concerns and frustrations related to this chronic illness, the nurse is also helping the child by reducing the amount of transferred parental anxiety.

Anemia Due to Blood Loss

When there is sudden loss of blood from the body as from a severe epistaxis, a freely bleeding wound or a gastrointestinal hemorrhage, the disturbance in body physiology is not related to the loss of blood cells alone; in addition there is a loss of the plasma portion of the blood with reduction in the circulating blood volume. Thus, in addition to the effects of anemia, the child also may be suffering from shock. Treatment consists of transfusion and, of course, appropriate measures to terminate the hemorrhage.

The common causes of excessive blood loss vary with the age of the child. In the newborn the common causes are an improperly tied umbilical cord, birth injury from a difficult delivery and free bleeding from the gastrointestinal tract. In the infant, bleeding from the bowel is most common. In the older child it is more commonly the result of a traumatic accident or a defect in the clotting mechanism of the blood, such as hemophilia or purpura.

When blood loss occurs at a slower rate, as from chronic ulcerative colitis or bleeding from an intestinal polyp, the reduction in blood volume does not take place, and the symptoms are due chiefly to the resulting anemia. Treatment is directed at the underlying cause and may include transfusion as a temporarily supportive measure.

Nutritional Anemias

Hypochromic or Iron-Deficiency Anemia. See Chapter 12.

Megaloblastic Anemia. During fetal life the bone marrow contains very large cells (megaloblasts) which are the precursors of the fetal red blood cells. Normally, these large cells disappear from the bone marrow during the last weeks of intrauterine life and are replaced by a smaller type of cell (erythroblast) which is the precursor of the adult type of red blood cell. Under certain clinical conditions megaloblasts may persist in the bone marrow after birth or may return to it. Their presence in the bone marrow can be detected only by marrow aspiration, but it may be suspected when the circulating blood contains red cells which are larger than normal (macrocytes) or when anemia is accompanied by a sharp decrease in the number of red blood cells in the circulating blood in addition to the reduction of hemoglobin. In hypochromic anemia, each red blood cell carries an abnormally small quantity of hemoglobin, but the number of cells is close to normal. In megaloblastic anemia the number of cells is decreased, but each cell may carry a normal quantity of hemoglobin (normochromic) or even an increased quantity (hyperchromic), due to its large size.

A variety of clinical circumstances may precede the development of megaloblastic anemia. These have in common a disturbing effect on the normal metabolism of folic acid, folinic acid (citrovorum factor), pyridoxine, vitamin B_{12} or vitamin C. These disturbances in turn interfere with the synthesis of nucleoproteins which are necessary for the maturation of the red blood cells. The clinical conditions which may result in megaloblastic anemia are not very common. Among them are scurvy, dietary deficiency of folic acid, pernicious anemia, celiac disease and certain varieties of liver disease. Treatment depends on the exact nature of the metabolic disturbance, but in most instances correction can be achieved by giving liver extract, vitamin B_{12}, folic acid or vitamin C.

Anemia of Infection

With repeated acute infections or with chronic infection of long standing, some degree of anemia usually is found. Increased red cell destruction is sometimes a factor, but the more severe effect of infections is on the blood-forming tissues. The formation of hemoglobin is retarded in most instances, with a secondary effect of decreased formation of red cells. In other instances, in addition the blood generative cells are affected adversely, a condition known as hypoplasia when the decreased formation is partial and as aplasia when it is complete. Hypoplasia may outlast the infection. In many instances, the hypoplasia does not affect the generation of white cells; rather, a leukocytosis occurs. A few infections cause deficient generation of both white cells and platelets. If aplasia of granular leukocytes (agranulocytosis) occurs, the condition becomes serious, and death is likely to result. In the case of most of the infections, the anemia is neither severe nor serious.

Hypoplastic Types of Anemia

Under this heading are included those forms of anemia in which the *main* abnormality is the inability of the bone marrow to manufacture new red blood cells and hemoglobin at a rate which will support a normal concentration of these substances in the circulating blood.

Diagnosis of hypoplastic or aplastic anemias is made from the decrease in circulating red cells and particularly an absence of reticulocytes which cannot be corrected with the usual bone marrow stimulants. Bone marrow aspiration or biopsy also shows a marked reduction in the red cell precursors.

Anemia of Prematurity. See Chapter 9.

Drugs and Poisons. A number of substances which are used in treatment of childhood diseases or are ingested accidentally by children may interfere with the formation of red cells and hemoglobin by the bone marrow. Tridione, Chloromycetin, sulfonamides, the folic acid antagonists used in the treatment of leukemia and nitrogen mustards are examples of therapeutic agents which must be monitored by periodic blood examinations. To this list the effects of radiation from roentgen therapy or from the use of radioactive compounds in the treatment of neoplastic diseases must be added. Lead and benzene derivatives are the most common types of poison that may depress bone marrow activity.

Bone Marrow Invasion. In leukemia and in some of the tumors of childhood which have widespread metastases (neuroblastoma of the adrenal, for instance) there may be so much replacement of normal marrow tissue that an insufficient quantity remains available to form new blood cells. This type of anemia also is called myelophthisic anemia.

Miscellaneous Causes. Congenital and idiopathic types of hypoplastic and aplastic anemia are known to occur. In the congenital variety the failure to form sufficient red cells is present at birth. In the idiopathic variety the deficiency appears later in life for unknown reasons. The term "hypoplastic anemia" implies that the rate of formation of red cells is slowed; "aplastic anemia" implies that the formation of red cells has stopped altogether. Usually there is an associated defect in the formation of the other elements of the blood, such as the platelets and the white blood cells. Stimulation of the sluggish bone marrow is sometimes possible through the administration of ACTH or cortisone in conjunction with androgenic hormones such as testosterone. Where this fails, repeated transfusions must be given in the hope that a spontaneous remission will occur.

Certain disorders associated with splenic enlargement may be accompanied by anemia. Both the excessive destruction of red cells by the spleen and a depressant effect on the bone marrow by unknown substances produced in the spleen have been blamed. In some instances removal of the spleen causes improvement in the anemia. In other instances the splenic anemia is part of a more widespread disorder which cannot be treated in this fashion.

HEMOLYTIC TYPES OF ANEMIA

In the hemolytic varieties of anemia the predominating mechanism is too rapid destruction of the red blood cells. The speed at which excessive destruction takes place determines the nature of the symptoms. Very rapid destruction takes place in the types of hemolytic anemia which are mediated by antibody reactions. These include erythroblastosis fetalis and transfusion reactions. Under these circumstances a large quantity of pigment resulting from the breakdown of hemoglobin from destroyed red cells is presented suddenly to the liver for excretion. Since the liver is unable to clear the blood of this pigment, jaundice develops. The process is acute, often serious and usually limited to a brief time. In congenital hemolytic jaundice a slower degree of hemolysis takes place continuously, with superimposed "crises" during which the rate of hemolysis is accelerated temporarily. A similar but less marked phenomenon may occur with sickle-cell anemia, but in Mediterranean anemia the hemolysis tends to be slow and steady. Jaundice in these latter disorders is ordinarily difficult to detect except during a crisis. However, increased levels of bilirubin are present in the circulating blood. In all varieties of hemolytic anemia the bone marrow responds to the demands for a more rapid production of red cells. It hypertrophies and occupies a larger than normal share of the inner structure of the bones. Microscopic examination of a sample of bone marrow obtained by aspiration reveals evidence of great acceleration of red blood cell formation. Reticulocytes and in some cases nucleated red blood cells appear in the circulating blood in increased numbers.

Transfusion Reaction. When mismatched blood is transfused there is rapid agglutination of red blood cells, due to admixture with agglutinins of the same type as the agglutinogens of the transfused cells. Once agglutinated, the red cell masses are destroyed rapidly, and their hemoglobin is released. Jaundice results. No aggravation of the pre-existing anemia takes place, since only the transfused cells are being destroyed.

Erythroblastosis Fetalis. This disorder, also known as acute hemolytic anemia of the newborn, is discussed in Chapter 10.

Congenital Hemolytic Jaundice. This disease occurs only in the white race. The outstanding clinical features are mild jaundice and enlarged spleen. Anemia may be only moderate. In the typical case, the red cells show increased fragility when suspended in salt solution of decreasing concentration in a series of test tubes. Hemolysis normally begins when the concentration has been decreased to 0.42 per cent and is complete with a decrease to 0.32 per cent. In congenital hemolytic jaundice, hemolysis may begin before the salt concentration has been reduced to 0.50 per cent and is complete at concentrations higher than that required for normal blood. The increased fragility in the test tube does not explain the increased fragility in the body, because similar osmotic conditions do not exist. In some instances in which the disease cannot be otherwise distinguished from congenital hemolytic jaundice, the fragility in the test tube is unaltered from the normal. Other evidence that the red cells of this disease are abnormal is shown when a preparation of fresh blood is examined under a microscope. Many of the red cells are more or less spherical in shape (spherocytes) instead of being the usual biconcave disks.

The disease makes its appearance at any time after birth and persists indefinitely. Often the health apparently is unaffected. In other instances, severe anemia may develop. An acute hemolytic crisis may occur abruptly with fever and chill and may last for several days or weeks. Recovery is usual.

The treatment consists of splenectomy. Removal of the spleen always causes improvement and often apparent cure. Increased phagocytic activity for red cells has been demonstrated in the spleen. Immediately after splenectomy, a major increase in red cells and hemoglobin equivalent to an autotransfusion occurs. However, the red blood cells retain their abnormal shape and increased fragility to laboratory tests.

The classic variety of congenital hemolytic jaundice depends on a hereditarily transmitted abnormality of the red blood cells. Transmission is through the passage of a dominant gene. Other members of the child's family, including at least one parent, will show the same abnormality in fragility. The extent to which the abnormality bothers an individual is variable, since some have no symptoms while others may have recurring severe hemolytic crises. In the classic form of the disease, splenectomy is curative. When hereditary transmission is not apparent or other features are missing, the disorder may not be improved by splenectomy.

Other Types of Hemolytic Anemia. Drugs, poisons and infection may produce an accelerated rate of red blood cell destruction which eventually leads to anemia. Sulfanilamide, acetanilid, naphthalene and fava beans are examples of substances whose ingestion may lead to hemolytic anemia. During the course of malaria the parasites disrupt the red blood cells and produce hemolysis which eventually leads to anemia. In various types of septicemia, notably that caused by the hemolytic streptococcus, acute hemolysis may occur. Lederer's anemia is a severe acute form of hemolytic anemia seen among children. Its mechanism is not entirely understood, but it frequently appears to be the result of an acute infection. Ordinarily, it does not recur.

Genetically transmitted defects in red blood cell enzymes (glucose-6-phosphate dehydrogenase, pyruvic kinase) may also be responsible for hemolytic anemia under certain conditions of stimulation.

Hemoglobinopathies

Several varieties of hemolytic anemia are associated with the presence of abnormal types of hemoglobin in the red blood cells. Changes in the morphology of the red cells usually afford the clue to the presence of unusual hemoglobin which can then be confirmed by electrophoresis. Normal adult hemoglobin is designated as A; that present in fetal life and for a while after birth is called F; letters and names are attached to more than 50 other varieties which are occasionally encountered. Genetic transmission of the type of hemoglobin is well established with recessive autosomal transmission. In unusual instances a child may have a combination of two hemoglobinopathies such as sickle-cell thalassemia (S and A_2) or sickle-cell C disease (S and C). The severity of the symptoms varies with the type of hemoglobin involved. Only the two most common and severe varieties are described here.

Sickle Cell Anemia. Sickle cell anemia occurs almost exclusively in the Negro race. The red blood cells tend to assume a crescentic or sickle shape, due to the presence of an abnormal hemoglobin which is designated as hemoglobin S. The tendency of the cells to sickle can be demonstrated by the following test: A drop of blood on a slide is mixed with a drop of normal saline, covered with a thin cover-slip which is rimmed with petrolatum and allowed to stand 24 hours at room temperature. The number of cells which sickle depends on the proportion of hemoglobin S as compared with normal hemoglobin in each cell. When the dominant sickling trait is inherited from one parent alone (heterozygous state) it does not cause an anemia. But when it is inherited from both parents (homozygous state), an anemia develops as a result of the rapid breakdown of red cells carrying a large proportion of hemoglobin S, and the child shows all of the signs of a chronic hemolytic anemia, i.e., enlargement of the spleen, jaundice and widening of the marrow spaces of the bones visible by x-ray. The active disease may start during the first year but seldom before 3 to 4 months of age. Its onset may be gradual or by the sudden appearance of a crisis with fever. Treatment is symptomatic and directed at reversing the agglutination of sickled cells within the small blood vessels. This latter is accomplished to a degree by the administration of oxygen and by expanding the blood volume through hydration with fluids low in electrolyte content. Transfusions are avoided whenever possible, for they add to the iron content of the body and

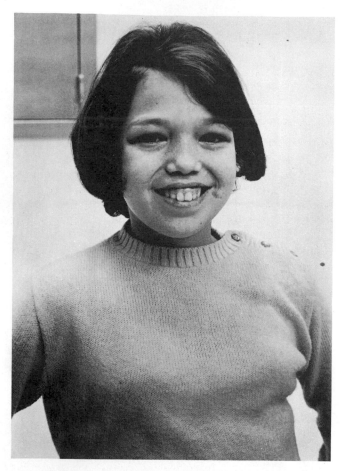

FIG. 21-1. Older girl with thalassemia, showing mildly mongoloid features.

in time may lead to abnormal deposition of iron in the tissues of the body (hemosiderosis).

Mediterranean Anemia (Cooley's Anemia, Erythroblastic Anemia, Thalassemia). This hemolytic anemia is both hereditary and racial. It occurs in families whose national extraction can be traced to the races inhabiting the Mediterranean Sea, predominantly Greek, Italian and Sicilian. It is congenital and familial. Although congenital, the signs of the disease are rarely present in the newborn period but develop within the first few months of life. The anemia progresses slowly and is severe; it is characterized by marked distortion of the shape and the size of the red blood cells and the presence of large numbers of nucleated red cells (erythroblasts and normoblasts) in the peripheral blood. Most of the hemoglobin in the red cells is A, but abnormal amounts of F or A_2 are usually present. Like sickle-cell disorder, the condition may occur as a mild, heterozygous trait (thalassemia minor) or as the homozygous, full-blown disease (thalassemia major).

The characteristic feature of the disease is the extreme activity of the blood-forming organs, which produce large numbers of immature and defective red cells which are destroyed rapidly. The distinctive clinical signs—enlargement of the spleen and the liver and thinning of the long bones of the skull and the face—result from the combination of excessive blood formation and destruction. The physical appearance of severely affected children is similar; physical growth is stunted, the pallor is muddy, the faces are broad with high malar prominences and shallow orbits, the abdomen is enlarged, the posture is poor, and the musculature is flabby. Roentgenograms of the bones reveal progressive evidence of dilatation of the medullary cavity and atrophy of cortical and cancellous bones. The anemia eventually becomes severe and causes death. No satisfactory treatment is known. Transfusions are necessary to support life but cannot correct the anemia adequately or indefinitely.

LEUKEMIA

Prior to 1948 leukemia in childhood was a rapidly progressive, invariably fatal disease with a course of 3 to 6 months from the time of its discovery. Today it is still a lethal disease but the advent of therapeutic agents permits many of its victims to enjoy prolonged remissions so that the average life span has increased from a few months to over 2 years. Much of the management can now be carried out at home with periodic hospitalization during exacerbations or complications. Types of leukemia are designated by the predominating variety of white cell in the peripheral blood and by the chronicity of the untreated process. In children the most common types are (1) acute undifferentiated or stem cell, (2) acute myeloblastic and (3) acute monoblastic leukemia. Subacute and chronic forms of lymphatic or myelogenous leukemia are quite rare in children.

Pathophysiology

In all three types of acute leukemia, immature white blood cells or blast forms are produced in large numbers in the blood-forming tissues throughout the body, while the production of normal cells is reduced progressively. The immaturity of the leukemic blasts may limit their identification by any of the specialized hematologic technics, and it is often impossible to distinguish among the different types of cells involved in the acute forms of the disease. However, certain characteristics are common to all of the blast cells typical of leukemia: (1) they multiply rapidly; (2) they fail to develop into the mature cells of the strain which they represent; and (3) therefore they are unable to function as mature white blood cells. The factors which stimulate production of these cells and limit their maturity are unknown, but at present it is felt that leukemia has many of the features of a neoplasm. The immaturity of the blasts and their infiltration into tissues outside the centers of blood formation support this concept of the disease.

Although it is true that an overproduction of a

single cell type always occurs in leukemia, the number of leukemic cells which circulate in the blood is not always high. When the white blood count is high, the blasts are present in high percentage, and the blood picture is said to be "leukemic." When the count is low, with a low percentage of blasts, it is spoken of as "aleukemic." In the latter case it may be necessary to confirm the diagnosis by a study of a sample of the bone marrow, which is obtained by aspiration of fluid marrow.

Anemia develops rapidly in the early course of leukemia in children. It is a hypoplastic type of anemia in which the hemoglobin and red cell count are reduced proportionately, and a low reticulocyte count reflects the failure of red cell formation.

Platelet production is impaired, and the level of platelets in the blood is reduced severely. The hemorrhagic manifestation of the disease is due largely to the lack of platelets and the consequent oozing of blood from the smaller blood vessels.

The lymph nodes throughout the body enlarge, and the liver and spleen may grow to great size unless the development of the leukemic tissue can be controlled. The bony skeleton may be involved as a result of widening of the medullary spaces and infiltration of the periosteum with leukemic cells.

Children whose course has been prolonged by therapy may suffer an infiltration of the meninges by the abnormal cells, producing increased intracranial pressure and its attendant symptoms.

The peak of the age incidence of leukemia occurs in children between 3 and 8 years. This curve is similar to that of the acute communicable diseases. However, to date, no relationship has been demonstrated between leukemia and infections. The disease may occur at any age; several cases are recorded of congenital leukemia recognizable at birth. It occurs throughout childhood, adolescence and young adult life. The acute leukemias are rare in people over 30.

Symptoms

In general, the symptoms of the acute leukemias are the same regardless of the cell type involved. The onset may be gradual or rapid. Common first symptoms which date the onset of the disease are low-grade fever, pallor, tendency to bruise, enlargement of the lymph nodes, pain in the legs or the joints and lassitude. When pain in the bones occurs early, the condition may be confused with rheumatic fever. The early symptoms must be differentiated from many of the acute infectious diseases which involve the peripheral lymph nodes and the spleen. As the disease progresses, fever of a relapsing type, hemorrhagic manifestations, increasing pallor and enlargement of the liver and spleen develop. The symptoms vary greatly in individual cases, as might be expected in a disease which affects not only the blood-forming organs primarily, but all of the tissues of the body, either by infiltration

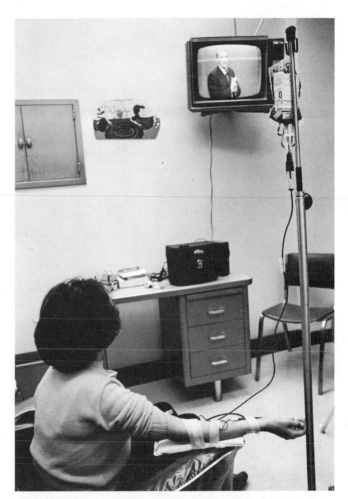

Fig. 21-2. Transfusions can be given in comfort in the out-patient clinic.

or indirectly by the changes in the blood which is brought to them. In the natural course of the disease, the complications which develop from a lack of normal white blood cells are usually fatal; ulcerations of the mouth and the pharynx form as a result of bacterial invasions of the buccal mucous membrane, and hemorrhages from these sites are common. The low level of blood platelets causes purpuric and petechial hemorrhages in the skin and elsewhere throughout the body. Intracranial and visceral hemorrhages are not uncommon. Anemia is progressive, and although it can be supported with transfusions temporarily, the child becomes weaker, and death results either from the disease itself or from an intercurrent infection.

Diagnosis

Leukemia often is suspected from the combination of weakness, pallor, hemorrhagic manifestations and enlargement of lymph nodes, spleen or liver. If immature cells are present in the peripheral blood, the diagnosis is made easily from the differential blood smear. When there is doubt, microscopic examination

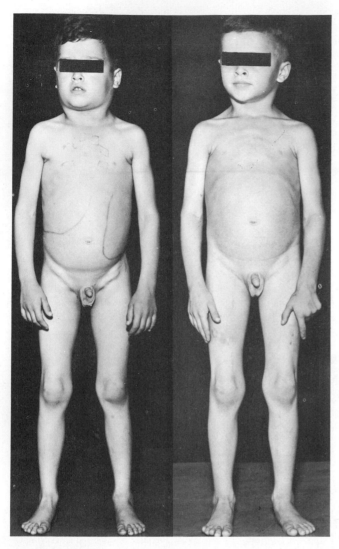

FIG. 21-3. (*Left*) A child with leukemia before treatment with ACTH. Note enlargement of cervical and inguinal lymph nodes and the penciled outline of liver and spleen. (*Right*) Same child after treatment with ACTH, showing decrease in size of lymph nodes of neck and groin.

of bone marrow is usually conclusive. In some instances the suspicion of leukemia may arise through histologic study of a lymph node biopsy.

Sometimes leukemia is confused with other disorders which produce an increase in the number of circulating white blood cells or an alteration of their appearance. Pertussis, severe infections, infectious mononucleosis and occasionally the iron-deficiency anemia of infancy may cause temporary confusion until study of the bone marrow eliminates the possibility of leukemia.

Treatment

The general measures in the management of leukemia include correction of severe degrees of anemia by transfusion, control of hemorrhagic phenomena by the administration of blood, platelets or platelet-rich plasma, and control of the infections to which the child may be more than usually susceptible, by the appropriate use of antibiotics. Highly important is the maintenance of an optimistic environment around the child and the granting of permission for him to assume as normal a life as possible in spite of the known seriousness of his prognosis.

Suppression of the leukemic process itself is usually possible through the administration of one or more of the following general classes of drugs: (1) steroids (ACTH, cortisone, prednisone, etc.) which act through their ability to lyse lymphocytic cells; (2) purine antimetabolites (6-mercaptopurine, thioguanine) which interfere with cell reproduction by blocking the incorporation of purine into nucleic acids; (3) folic acid antagonists (aminopterin, methotrexate) which interfere with the production of DNA and RNA necessary for cell reproduction, and (4) agents which destroy cells (Cytoxan, vincristine). Since these drugs are also toxic for normal cells as well as the leukemic tissues, their use must be carefully supervised by someone familiar with their toxic effects. Not all children will respond to a given drug; nor will such a response be continued indefinitely even when successful. The usual procedure is to start treatment with one of the steroids or antimetabolites and follow the child's peripheral blood count carefully. Improvement may occur within a few days or may be delayed as long as 6 weeks. Amelioration of symptoms (Fig. 21-3) and improvement in peripheral blood count does not necessarily indicate a full remission. This latter success can only be confirmed by examination of the bone marrow. Relapses may occur at any period after the complete remission has been achieved. Consequently, although apparently well, the child must have repeated bone marrow examinations about once a month to be sure that a relapse has not begun. If it has, a change in his therapy to another agent is indicated even before he shows symptoms. Programs of therapy are constantly being modified as new drugs are found to be effective and as careful study reveals which ones are most successful in producing remissions.

Toxic manifestations of treatment vary somewhat with the drug in use. The effects of the steroids are the same as when these agents are used for treatment of other diseases. Nausea, vomiting, loss of appetite and ulceration of the mouth or the intestinal tract are common complications of treatment with the antimetabolites and cytotoxic agents. Severe bleeding from the intestinal tract may require transfusion and cessation of the drug in use. Sometimes depression of the bone marrow with severe reduction in circulating cells and platelets dictates termination of therapy.

Both the disease and the therapy tend to lower resistance to infection. Protection against bacterial infection and suppression of established infections may be attempted by administration of the appropriate antibiotic. Unfortunately, resistant organisms often play a role in children who have received prolonged or repeated therapy. Viral infections may be particularly serious for leukemic children under treatment. They should be protected from exposure to varicella and measles. When such exposure is known to have occurred inadvertently, full dosage with gamma globulin is indicated. Live virus vaccines against measles and smallpox should not be administered although oral poliomyelitis vaccine is permissible.

When intracranial invasion by the leukemic process occurs, it can usually be ameliorated with a course of intrathecal methotrexate.

Nursing Care

The physical nursing care of a child with leukemia is as concerned with the toxic side effects of the chemotherapy as with the effects and complications of the disease itself. The nursing care required during prolonged use of steroids has been described in Chapter 4. In addition, other chemical agents used in conjunction with steroid therapy may produce side effects requiring specific protective measures in addition to those which relieve discomfort.

Since the mucous membrane is particularly sensitive to the drugs used in treatment of leukemia, lesions may occur in the oral cavity and the rectum. Gastrointestinal distress, including nausea, vomiting and diarrhea may precipitate dehydration requiring the administration of parenteral fluids and attention to the electrolyte balance. Because of thrombocytopenia, bleeding may occur in the conjunctival membranes and those of the buccal mucosa.

As a result of bleeding and ulceration of the lips and mouth, maintenance of adequate fluid intake and nutrition may be difficult. A bland ointment applied to the lips may relieve discomfort and prevent the adherence of tissues. Liquids should be offered frequently but must be bland to avoid discomfort to exposed tissues. If anorexia and gastrointestinal complications are severe, accurate intake and output records should be kept. Careful attention should also be given to oral hygiene with gentle brushing of the teeth with a soft brush and frequent rinsing of the oral cavity with a warm saline solution.

Constant alertness is required to detect new evidences of bleeding, including skin manifestations such as petechiae and ecchymotic lesions. Gentle handling during care of the body is extremely important to prevent bruising and necessary injections should be given with great care. All previously discussed measures to enlist the child's cooperation should be used to avoid hematomas at the injection site. Pressure applied to the area after the injection has been given may also help to prevent continued bleeding.

Because of the disease process itself and as a result of chemotherapy, children with leukemia are extremely sensitive to infection. Care should be taken to assure that personnel coming in contact with the child are free from infectious processes. The child can also be protected by careful body hygiene and prompt treatment of breaks in the skin. Any sign of infection, including temperature elevation, chilling, reddening of the skin or furuncles should be promptly reported.

When vincristine is used in chemotherapy, side effects to nerve tissue may produce foot drop and constipation. The use of a foot board, careful body positioning and measures to relieve stool retention are necessary.

The necessity for frequent transfusions of whole blood, platelets or platelet-rich plasma is a challenge to the ingenuity of the nurse in making the constantly recurring, distressing procedure as tolerable as possible for the child. Prior warning that the procedure is to be done allows the child to mobilize his available coping strategies. Allowing the child some measure of control reduces feelings of helplessness, and approval for his efforts toward control of his body will enhance his cooperation. Permission for expression of feelings is essential along with calm acceptance and understanding of the child's distress.

Since the possibility of central nervous system involvement is always present, constant observation of the child is important to detect any changes in behavior or physical condition. Persistent nausea and vomiting, headache, lethargy or irritability should be promptly reported. More specific manifestations such as dizziness or ataxia may herald a sudden convulsion.

The administration of intrathecal methotrexate 3 to 5 times at intervals of several days is usually ordered to treat meningeal complications. When this is done, fluids must be forced or given parenterally to prevent toxicity. A padded tongue blade should be kept at the child's bedside in the event of convulsions and constant observation is necessary to detect early toxic symptoms including stomatitis, fever, headache, pallor or gastrointestinal distress.

Diagnostic procedures, such as bone marrow aspiration and lumbar puncture, are frequently necessary throughout the treatment of leukemia. The prior preparation of the child and continued support throughout the event are necessary not only to reduce his distress but to ensure successful completion of the procedure.

Because the child with leukemia usually requires many periods of hospitalization with uncomfortable diagnostic procedures and treatment, it is especially important that his parents be in attendance as much as possible. This will be of benefit to them, too, because the opportunity to help care for their child will provide additional strength to face the inevitable outcome. It is imperative that the attending nurse have the complete confidence of the parents. Often the nurse who is sought by the mother is the one who has made an effort to learn which care measures the child enjoys and is accustomed to. With such a person in charge, the mother is assured that her child will not be deprived of his special sources of comfort in her absence.

In the terminal stage of leukemia, the child is miserably uncomfortable, irritable and often demanding as his need for physical relief and emotional comfort increases. His gums may be sore and bleeding (Fig. 21-4); his extremities are painful. He may be dyspneic and the mucous membrane of his rectum is usually inflamed and necrotic. He is often nauseated, yet thirsty. He is easily fatigued and annoyed by changes in routine and by being cared for by a succession of nurses who are unfamiliar with his particular preferences.

During this terminal stage of the child's illness, the nurse can give comfort by keeping his mouth and nose clean and his lips and tongue moistened; by administering sedatives regularly, by bathing his feverish skin and turning him when she sees that he is becoming fatigued. Remaining with him and his parents to lend her strength to them during the period of acute crisis is vitally important.

As discussed in Chapter 2, the child's fear may be acute because of the contagion of the anxiety of others along with his awareness of the changes taking place in his body. He is anxious when alone and may make a great effort to control those who care for him in an attempt to draw them to himself. This behavior should be understood and accepted; his demands met as far as possible, since such understanding care helps in allaying his fear and loneliness and lessens his feeling of helplessness.

Parental reactions to the loss of a child have been discussed in Chapter 2. The amount of denial necessary for parents is related to the length of time since the diagnosis was made, their inner resources and the environmental support they have received. Some parents may need to continue to deny the possibility of the child's death into the terminal stage hoping for remission or possible cure. For such parents the actual death of the child will be overwhelming despite their prior intellectual knowledge of the prognosis.

If the child's parents are unable to endure being with their dying child, the staff's support must be sustained. At such times the child must have the security of knowing that he has not been abandoned. Although he may lapse into unconsciousness from intracranial hemorrhage or from chemical changes in his body, the parents must have the comfort which comes from knowing that constant vigilance is being maintained.

The nurse who ministers to the dying child must be able to accept the parent's individual expression of grief as well as devoting her best efforts to the comfort of the child in his final hours. Such a responsibility demands a personal philosophy which will permit her to be empathic toward all concerned and yet leave her effectiveness unimpaired. It takes time, experience and thought to evolve such an attitude toward death. It is necessary however, since leaving the parents alone during such a crisis conveys that the nurse is uninterested or deliberately avoiding them. This is particularly true if the parents have expressed their emotions overtly. Formal condolences are unnecessary. What parents usually wish is sympathetic understanding of their need to relive experiences that they have enjoyed with their child, to express their grief and sometimes also their resentment against the fate which has befallen them, and to share with valued friends the meaning which the loss has to them personally.

MALIGNANT LYMPHOMA (HODGKIN'S DISEASE, LYMPHOSARCOMA, RETICULUM-CELL SARCOMA)

The several types of malignant lymphoma are closely related neoplastic disorders affecting the lymph glands and the related lymphatic tissue. Differentiation among the three types is made by the histologic appearance of the tissue in the enlarged lymph nodes which are characteristic of the disease. All of the types are progressive but at a variable rate. In Hodgkin's disease the progression may be very slow; in reticulum-cell sarcoma, very rapid.

The cause is unknown. In some respects, the lesion appears to be neoplastic in much the same manner as does lymphoid leukemia, except that a different type of cell is involved in the hyperplasia. The disease runs a much slower course than leukemia of childhood.

In the beginning, only a few glands are affected. Often these are in the neck, where the increase in size becomes obvious. Later, other groups of glands are involved. The spleen usually is enlarged. Lymphoid tissue of the bone marrow increases and gradually replaces blood-forming tissue.

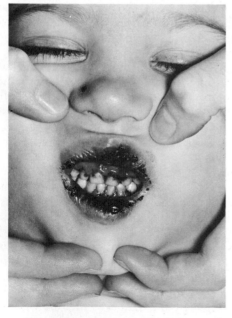

FIG. 21-4. The mouth lesions of leukemia.

Symptoms

At first symptoms are meager or absent. As the various groups of glands enlarge, pressure symptoms are likely to appear. Glands in the mediastinum may press on the trachea and the bronchi, causing respiratory embarrassment. Other groups may press on blood vessels, causing edema or ascites. Many types of pressure symptoms are possible. After the disease has progressed sufficiently, constitutional symptoms appear. Fever of remittent and intermittent type is present. Anemia of hypoplastic type gradually increases. Weight loss occurs. Death occurs eventually when the disease is discovered too late for effective therapy, from general weakness, or because of disturbance of some vital function from gland pressure.

Diagnosis

Diagnosis is made with certainty only by histologic examination of a lymph gland and the finding of cells characteristic of the disease.

Treatment

In a few fortunate instances the process may be discovered early when it is limited to a few lymph nodes which can be completely removed surgically. More often, by the time the diagnosis is made, widespread changes are apparent. Roentgen therapy is effective in reducing the size of the nodes, but there is a limit to the amount which can be given safely to any one area or to the body as a whole. Usually, such treatment is given to nodes which are causing pressure symptoms by impinging on adjacent vital structures. The nitrogen mustard compounds, antileukemic agents and triethylene melamine are also effective in reducing the size of lymph nodes by destroying the more rapidly growing cells. The frequency and the dosage of administration must be regulated carefully, since these compounds also have a depressing effect on the bone marrow in general.

DISORDERS OF BLOOD COAGULATION

Pathophysiology

Serious consequences follow when sizable amounts of blood are lost from the intravascular space. Equally serious difficulties may follow if the blood coagulates within the channels of the vascular tree. The very complex biochemical mechanism which permits the circulating blood to remain fluid under conditions of health and to coagulate rapidly following injury to the branches of the vascular bed is now known in some detail. Numerous factors are involved some of which are simple chemical entities, others complex materials which have not yet been identified and which bear the names of their discoverers; others are enzymes and protein components of the tissues. The full ramifications of the clotting process cannot be presented here. An abbreviated outline is presented in Figure 21-5

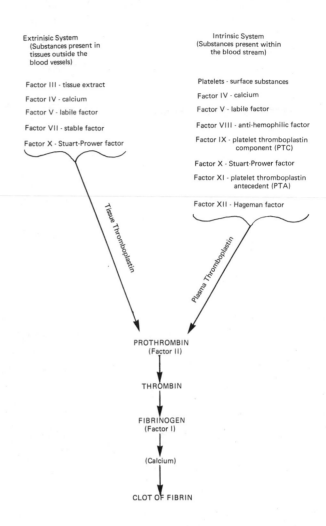

FIG. 21-5. Outline of Blood Coagulation.

in order to offer a general scheme of the manner in which clotting proceeds and to enumerate the substances involved. Factors which are designated by Roman numerals do not necessarily participate in any sequential way in the clotting mechanism. Their order is in part due to the sequence in which they were discovered and added to the earlier theories of blood coagulation.

In addition to the substances named in the figure, there may be antagonists or inhibitors of some of the substances present in the blood stream during pathologic states. Only a few of the clinical conditions of defective clotting will be described here. Rarer defects and those conditions in which the blood becomes hypercoagulable cannot be included in this elementary discussion.

Purpura

Purpura is a term used to denote conditions of spontaneous hemorrhage from small blood vessels. Its effects are most obvious in the skin where small capillary rupture produces petechiae; more extensive cutaneous bleeding causes ecchymoses. Purpura is generally due either to a deficiency of platelets in the circulating blood or to a disorder of the smallest radicles of the vascular system, the capillaries.

Idiopathic Thrombocytopenic Purpura (ITP). This, the most common variety of purpura, has a wide variation in the severity of its symptoms. In the milder forms there are few constitutional symptoms and the hemorrhagic lesions are limited to the skin. With more severe types of the disease there may be fever, involvement of and hemorrhage from the mucous membranes, epistaxis or hematuria. A fortunately rare but serious complication which tends to occur early in the course of the illness is intracranial hemorrhage. Spontaneous disappearance of symptoms occurs in a high percentage of children after a few weeks without serious hemorrhage. A small fraction will continue to have purpura for several months or even enter a chronic form of the disease.

DIAGNOSIS. The platelet count on the peripheral blood is markedly reduced, usually below 30,000 per cu. mm. Since the platelets of the peripheral blood play an important role in several phases of the clotting mechanism—release of thromboplastin, plugging of vessel defects by forming agglutinated masses, facilitation of enzyme reactions—the bleeding time after skin puncture is prolonged. In addition the clot which forms in a test tube fails to retract properly and there is a decrease in the consumption of prothrombin during its formation. Application of a tourniquet to the arm generates petechiae distally. The clotting time of blood in the test tube, however, is usually normal. Platelets are derived from the megakaryocytes in the bone marrow, but contrary to expectation, these cells are found in normal numbers in the marrow of patients with ITP. The defect in circulating platelets is ascribed to a combination of excessive utilization and inhibition of production by the megakaryocytes. An "auto-immune" mechanism is postulated.

TREATMENT. Untreated ITP usually runs a self-limited course with spontaneous recovery. Because of the hazard of intracranial bleeding, however, treatment with corticosteroids at least during the early weeks of the disease is commonly practiced. The steroids will produce at least a temporary increase in the platelet count and in some children will terminate the disease within a few days. This result cannot be expected in all subjects and in a few the long-term use of steroids may actually interfere with ultimate cure. Transfusions and platelet infusions may be used when there has been an unusual loss of blood or when the child is suffering from serious constitutional symptoms. Splenectomy is used successfully if the disease enters a chronic stage; usually, however, a spontaneous remission is awaited for 6 months to a year before this somewhat hazardous operation is undertaken.

Congenital Purpura. Mothers who have or have had ITP may bear infants suffering from the same disease. Usually the disorder is mild and the platelet count rises within a short time after birth. Treatment is the same as for ITP. Transplacental passage of an antiplatelet antibody from mother to baby has been demonstrated in some cases.

Aldrich's Syndrome. The association of thrombocytopenic purpura, eczema and unusual susceptibility to infection has been noted in certain families in which the disorder is transmitted as a sex-linked recessive trait. Treatment is symptomatic and relatively ineffective since most of the subjects die within the first few years of life.

Purpura Due to Bone Marrow Suppression. In contrast to the types of purpura described above, defects in the number of circulating platelets may also occur because of interference with bone marrow function by drugs, by invasion with tumor or leukemia, by destruction from irradiation or owing to the effects of severe infections such as meningococcemia, fetal rubella and septicemia. Management of this type of purpura depends upon the correction of the primary disease.

Allergic Purpura (Henoch-Schönlein Purpura). This variety of purpura is not really a disorder of coagulation but rather an allergic reaction of small blood vessels throughout the body. Blood counts and platelet counts are usually normal. The skin lesions tend to be located on the lower portion of the body. There may be swelling and tenderness of joints and more frequently abdominal pain. In the older child, a type of nephritis is seen in nearly half of the victims. Treatment with corticosteroids is of some value but usually not necessary unless renal involvement is present.

The Hemophilias

Hemophilia A. The classical type of hemophilia is due to an inherited defect of Factor VIII or antihemophilic factor. The defect is transmitted as a sex-linked recessive trait which is seen only in the male. It is now known that variations in the severity of the disorder occur and that the degree of deficiency of Factor VIII tends to remain constant within a given family. Severe symptoms are usually associated with levels which are less than 2 per cent of the normal.

SYMPTOMS. In contrast to purpura, the hemorrhagic manifestations tend to be deep rather than cutaneous. Rupture of blood vessels from minor, even normal trauma, may result in extensive hemorrhage beneath the skin, into muscle, behind the peritoneal lining of the abdominal cavity or into joint spaces. Cutting or puncturing injuries and surgical operations are particularly hazardous because loss of blood may be severe before it can be staunched by appropriate treatment. Uncommonly, bleeding may take place into the central nervous system or the urinary tract.

Pain is usually localized to the swollen area into which hemorrhage is taking place and distending the tissues. It is particularly severe when the bleeding is into a joint capsule. Weakness, pallor and tachycardia may follow even when actual escape of blood from the body is not taking place. Often the loss of blood out of vascular spaces and into the tissues is much larger than can be judged from external appearances. Consequently the fall in hemoglobin must be carefully watched.

Repeated bleeding into the same joint or muscle group may lead to atrophy and ankylosis. However, the ability of affected joints to recover their function after severe hemarthrosis is often remarkable.

DIAGNOSIS. The peripheral blood elements including the platelets are normal in hemophilia. The platelets, however, although present in normal numbers, fail to produce thromboplastin at the normal rate when damaged. This defect can be measured by special tests. In contrast to purpura, the bleeding time in hemophilia when tested from a small skin incision is not prolonged, whereas the clotting time in the test tube is greatly prolonged. Methods are available now for the specific determination of levels of circulating Factor VIII which is less than 25 per cent of the normal level in untreated hemophilias.

TREATMENT. Replacement therapy with Factor VIII in order to stem the bleeding is imperative and can be carried out in a number of ways. Transfusion with freshly drawn whole blood or plasma will supply Factor VIII and at the same time combat shock and anemia if blood loss has been severe. Preparations of frozen plasma and plasma concentrates are also available which can be used very effectively in the early stages of bleeding when blood loss has not been severe. These preparations are sometimes given to prevent or abort early bleeding episodes and in preparation for operations.

Management of hemarthrosis is always conservative. The general measures which stop the bleeding usually relieve pain rapidly even while the joint is still much swollen. Rest and splinting against excessive motion or weight bearing is desirable at first, but once the bleeding has been surely controlled, passive motion and early resumption of the use of the joint is desirable to prevent ankylosis and muscle atrophy. Aspiration of a hemarthrosis to remove blood is a hazardous procedure.

Hemophilia B. This variation of classical hemophilia is due to an inherited defect of Factor IX (PTC) and is also known as Christmas disease. It is less common than hemophilia A but the symptoms and management are much the same. Because Factor IX is more stable at ordinary temperatures of refrigeration, blood or plasma which has been so stored can be used for periods up to 3 weeks.

Hemophilia C. This is a milder form of hemophilia due to a deficiency of Factor XI (PTA) which is transmitted genetically as an autosomal rather than a sex-linked recessive trait and can therefore occur in both males and females. Symptoms and management are similar to the other types.

NURSING CARE IN HEMOPHILIA. Although most bleeding episodes in hemophilia are internal and spontaneous, constant vigilance is required by the nurse to prevent external trauma while the child is hospitalized. The sides of a baby's crib must be padded and only toys which cannot cause even a minor wound should be provided. Toddlers and older children who are not bedfast must be continuously supervised to protect them from potentially dangerous encounters in an unfamiliar environment. However, the temptation to keep the child confined unnecessarily to his crib or bed to avoid the responsibility of constant surveillance should be resisted. Nurses caring for children with hemophilia should be knowledgeable regarding measures which can be taken to control bleeding without a physician's order should accidental trauma occur. They must also be constantly alert to detect new bleeding sites or the symptoms of impending shock.

Children who are hospitalized because of bleeding into the joints require skillful and gentle handling. Careful consideration for the least painful method of changing the child's position conveys the concern of the nurse for his comfort, increases his security and lessens his anxiety. When the child is able to direct the nurse in moving him it lessens his pain and also his sense of helplessness. Both patience and skill are necessary when procedures are required. Injections must be given slowly and pressure applied subsequently to prevent continued bleeding.

Children with hemophilia usually have many hospital and clinic experiences and frequent periods of extended bed rest for blood transfusions or other treatments. They are in great pain when bleeding into the joints and may suffer from severe joint deformities. They are often fearful and anxious, not only because of past and present experiences, but because the possibility of death is ever present. Because of the chronicity and nature of the illness their dependency needs may be very high and they may therefore require a nurse who has a large supply of patience and is continuously attentive.

Living with hemophilia is a constant, exhausting strain not only for the child but for the total family. Because of the genetic factor, the mother may carry a load of guilt. Such children also demand constant care and sacrifice. As a result of guilt and conscious or unconsciously felt hostility related to the sacrifices which the family must make and the father's resentment of a son who is unable to compete athletically, the child may be overprotected or suffer from various degrees of rejection. Goldy and Katz found that parental supervision of hemophilic children fell into three classes: (1) overprotective, (2) realistic or permissive and (3) indifferent. Although hemophilic children usually expect their mothers to carefully limit their activities, fathers who deny physical activity may be resented by boys as a denial of their masculinity. When both parents are overprotective, the boy's urge toward independence and maleness may be throttled.

Goldy and Katz also found that the amount of dependency displayed by hemophilic children and their self-concept as different from other children are related to the degree of isolation and alienation felt, the restriction from usual boyhood activities experienced and the amount of time spent with their mothers. Avoidance of body contact injuries is difficult for the boy of school age since physical activity is valued in this developmental period and because his physical appearance is normal. Many children learn early to conceal their illness in order to gain peer acceptance and to avoid the fear displayed by others when in contact with them.

The degree of family stress has also been found to influence the number and amount of spontaneous internal bleeding episodes. The child's ability to handle such stress is directly influenced by the parent's response to the illness and their attitudes to the child.

Garlinghouse and Sharp concluded from their study of 18 hemophilic children that when stress was low, a high self-concept was associated with fewer bleeding episodes and a low self-concept was associated with more bleeding episodes. However, when stress was high, bleeding tended to be high regardless of other variables.

The importance of assisting parents to deal with hemophilia is vital, therefore, to help them in handling their anxiety constructively and in promoting optimum physical, mental and emotional development for the child. The fine line between necessary caution and support of independence is extremely difficult to maintain. During the toddler stage, prevention of falls and potentially dangerous exploration without keeping the child in constant fear or making him feel inadequate is a constant problem. The aggressive energy of the toddler and headlong curiosity tend to overrule any sense of caution. If overprotected however, in later years a child may submit completely and in so doing deny himself new experiences or over-react to restriction and deliberately court disaster.

Parents of children with hemophilia are constantly plagued with questions and with conflicts between a desire to support normal peer relationships and independence and fear lest the child be hurt and they be criticized as neglectful. These parents also need a nurse who is understanding of their problems, sympathetic and who can assist them in preventing harmful overprotection through helping the child to learn his own limitations.

Other Types of Coagulation Defect

Prothrombin deficiency (Factor II) is seen as a more or less normal phenomenon in the newborn infant. When very marked it may produce *hemorrhagic disease of the newborn* which is considered in Chapter 10. In later life a tendency to bleed may be seen with severe or chronic liver disease because of inability to fabricate prothrombin. Anticoagulant therapy has the same effect but is very infrequently used in children.

Congenital afibrinogenemia is a rare disorder due to inability to produce Factor I. Blood from such individuals will not coagulate in the test tube. The newborn may suffer a severe hemorrhagic disorder at birth, or in later life trauma will result in serious loss of blood. Surprisingly, these individuals may have no bleeding manifestations except under stress.

SITUATIONS FOR FURTHER STUDY

1. Review fetal hematopoiesis. How does hematopoiesis of a normal 2-month-old infant differ from that of a baby with anemia?

2. If you encountered a 7-month-old baby in a well-child conference who had a hemoglobin level of 8.0 Gm. and a red blood cell count of 4.0 million, how would you approach the problem with his mother? What information would you need and how would you attempt to motivate her to institute the measures that you deemed advisable to correct his iron deficiency?

3. While making a home visit, Mrs. Jany told the public-health nurse that she was going to take Jim, her 4-year-old son, into the hospital on the coming Monday because her neighborhood doctor had told her that he had a "serious blood disease." Mrs. Jany had 2 other children, one 6 months old, the other 6 years of age. Currently, Mr. Jany, an auditor, was unemployed and was greatly distressed about "Jim's weakness." Mrs. Jany's neighbor had a daughter who died of leukemia and in talking with the nurse she expressed the fear that Jim might have this trouble, too. If you were the public health nurse and had gathered this information during the early part of your visit, what would you do? If you had the opportunity to make another home call before Jim's admission to the hospital, what would be the purpose of your visit?

4. What personal problems did you encounter in caring for a child during the terminal stages of his illness? How did you cope with them?

5. How do you imagine a mother might feel when she discovers that her child is a hemophiliac? Spend time with a mother of a hemophiliac to observe her reactions to her problems and to discover ways in which you could be helpful to her.

6. How might hemophilia magnify the natural problems which beset the preschool boy? In what different ways might the mother's overprotectiveness threaten the preschool boy's resolution of the Oedipal conflict?

BIBLIOGRAPHY

Agle, D. P.: Psychiatric Complications of Hemophilia, *in* Hemophilias: International Symposium (1963), Brinkhouse, K. M. (ed.), Chapel Hill, N. C., U. of N. Carolina Press, p. 350, 1964.

Armiger, Sister Bernadette: Reprise and dialogue, Nurs. Outlook *16*:26, 1968.

Brodish, M. S.: The nurse's role in the care of children with acute leukemia, Am. J. Nurs. *58*:1572, 1958.

Cobb, Beatrix: Psychological impact of long illness and death of a child on the family circle, J. Pediat. *49*:746, 1956.

Conley, C. L.: The anemias, Am. J. Nurs. *52*:957, 1952.

Cooke, R. E. (Ed.): The Biologic Basis of Pediatric Practice, Section 5—The Hematopoeitic and Reticuloendothelial Systems, N. Y., McGraw-Hill, p. 421, 1968.

Finland, M.: Serious infections in splenectomized children, Pediatrics *27*:689, 1961.

Fleming, J. W.: The child with sickle cell disease, Am. J. Nurs. *65*:88, 1965.

Folck, M. M., and Nie, P. J.: Nursing students learn to face death, Nurs. Outlook *7*:510, 1959.

Garlinghouse, J., and Sharp, L. J.: The hemophilic child's self-concept and family stress in relation to bleeding episodes, Nurs. Res. *17*:32, 1968.

Goldy, F. B., and Katz, A. H.: Social adaptation in hemophilia, Children *10*:189, 1963.

Gutowski, F.: Nursing the leukemic child with central nervous system involvement, Am. J. Nurs. *63*:87, 1963.

Hartman, J. R., and Bolduc, R. A.: Hemophilia, Am. J. Nurs. *56*:169, 1956.

Lindemann, E.: Symptomatology and management of acute grief, Am. J. Psychiat. *101*:141, 1944.

Lunceford, J. L.: Leukemia—disease process, chemotherapeutic approach and nursing care, Nurs. Clin. N. A. *2*:635, 1967.

Lyman, M. S., and Burchenal, J. H.: Acute leukemia, Am. J. Nurs. *63*:82, 1963.

Mead, Margaret: The right to die, Nurs. Outlook *16*:20, 1968.

Norris, C. M.: The nurse and the dying patient, Am. J. Nurs. *55*:1214, 1955.

Richmond, J. B.: Psychological management of children with malignant disease, A.M.A., Amer. J. Dis. Child. *89*:42, 1955.

Shepard, M.: This I believe . . . about questioning the right to die, Nurs. Outlook *16*:22, 1968.

Smith, C. H.: Anemias of infancy and childhood, Am. J. Nurs. *48*:617, 1948.

White, D. W.: Living with hemophilia, Nurs. Outlook *12*:36, 1964.

Wilson, H. E., and Price, G.: Leukemia, Am. J. Nurs. *56*:601, 1956.

Wintrobe, M. M.: Clinical Hematology, ed. 5, Philadelphia, Lea & Febiger, 1961.

Wolff, I. S.: Should the patient know the truth? Am. J. Nurs. *55*:546, 1955.

22

Nursing Care of Children With Congenital Malformations of the Heart and the Great Vessels

Thirty years ago it was necessary to assume a fatalistic attitude toward the child with a congenital malformation of the heart. Once the basis of his trouble was determined, the only available therapy was the regulation of his activity within the limits of tolerance of his abnormal circulation. Today these children face a totally different prospect. Based on the detailed studies of the anatomy and the embryology of the heart made by Abbott and by Taussig, and the bold surgical innovations of Gross, Blalock and others a complex technology has arisen which now permits accurate *ante mortem* diagnosis of even the complex aberrations and the successful correction of many of them. The nurse cannot hope to understand the intricacies of this technology without an extensive knowledge of cardiac anatomy, embryology and physiology, but she must have an understanding of the general principles in order to render intelligent care to her patients.

The placement of this discussion in the unit concerned with the toddler and the preschool child is an artificial convenience. These disorders may be of crucial significance in the newborn period or may gain recognition and therapeutic importance at any age up to and including the seventh decade of life. The same principles apply at any age.

NORMAL ANATOMY

The circulating blood has two great circuits: one of these is the pulmonary; the other, the systemic circulation. The heart is divided into two parts, known as the right and the left hearts. Each acts independently of the other, although they act synchronously. The right heart receives blood which is returning from the body tissues and pumps it into the capillaries of the lungs for aeration. The blood returns from the lungs to the left heart, which then propels it to the various parts of the body (Fig. 22-1).

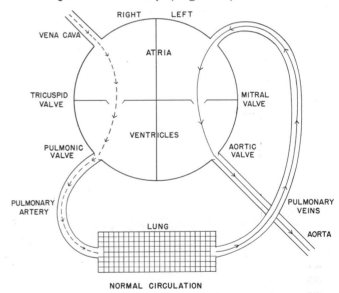

NORMAL CIRCULATION

FIG. 22-1. Diagram of the normal circulation of blood. Unoxygenated, or venous, blood is indicated by the dotted line from its entrance into the heart through the vena cava, thence into the right atrium, through the tricuspid valve into the right ventricle, out the pulmonic valve into the pulmonary artery and thence into the lungs, where it becomes oxygenated. The solid line indicates the course of the oxygenated blood through the pulmonary veins, the left atrium, the mitral valve, the left ventricle, the aortic valve and the aorta. The last distributes oxygenated blood to all the body tissues, where it loses oxygen in the capillary circulation, is collected by the veins and returned to the heart by way of the vena cava for recirculation. (Adapted from Cassels, D. E., and Morse, M.: Blood volume in congenital heart disease, J. Pediat. *31*:485)

Fig. 22-2. The fetal blood circulation. Arrows indicate the direction of blood flow. The solid lines between the arrows indicate that the blood is fully oxygenated; dotted lines denote partially oxygenated blood. See text for detailed description of the circulation.

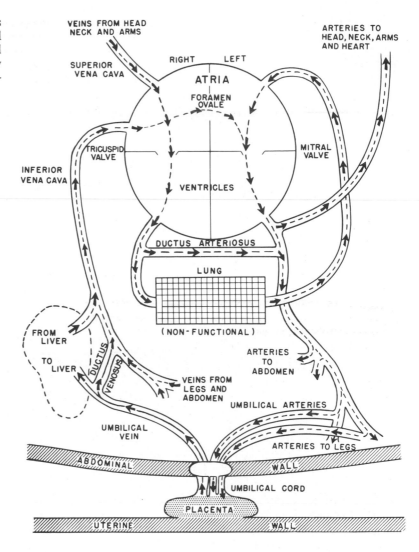

In the normal child, blood returning from the body by way of the great veins (venae cavae) and filling the right side of the heart and the branches of the pulmonary artery is venous or unoxygenated blood (dotted line in the diagrams). Its relatively low oxygen content gives it a dark purple color. Once the blood has passed through the lung capillaries and is fully oxygenated, it is bright red. Oxygenated blood (solid lines in the diagrams) normally is found in the pulmonary veins, the left side of the heart and all the branches of the aorta and the arterial system. It gives the skin its pink color.

EMBRYOLOGY AND PATHOGENESIS

The Period of Organ Development

As early as the second week of embryonic life the heart appears in its rudimentary form. At first it is a simple tube which receives blood at one end and pumps it out at the other. Within the short space of 6 weeks this tube undergoes a series of complicated changes, folding on itself, forming septa and valves within its lumen, and modifying its connections with the main blood vessels that serve the lungs and other parts of the body. By the 8th to the 10th week of fetal life these changes are completed, and the heart has acquired the form which it will retain until birth.

The period during which most congenital malformations are determined is this initial transformation from a simple tube to the complex heart. It is easy to appreciate how any error in the sequence of developmental rotations and invaginations or in the speed of growth of septa and closure of orifices could upset the final structural result. Thus it is believed that this first 2 or 3 months of the gestation is the time during which adverse influences may wreak their greatest damage on cardiac formation. What such influences are is still conjectural. It is assumed that heredity and maternal nutritional deficiencies or disease play some role. Thus far the only factor which has been definitely incriminated is the occurrence of rubella in the mother during the first trimester of pregnancy. However, this accounts for only a small percentage of the cases of cardiac malformation.

The Fetal Circulation

From the end of the second fetal month until birth the heart grows in size, but its basic structure and connections remain the same. Since the oxygenation of blood must take place at the placenta rather than the lungs, the route of its circulation differs from that which will be followed after birth.

As described above, the normal postnatal circulation makes a sharp separation between the unoxygenated blood of the venous system and the oxygenated blood of the systemic arteries. However, the fetus gets along with mixed venous and arterial blood, but the arrangement is such that the most important organs receive blood of the highest oxygen content. The major pathways are shown in the expanded scheme of Figure 22-2.

The only stream of completely oxygenated blood is that which is carried in the umbilical vein running from the placenta to the liver. This organ, which is busy making protein and other important products necessary to growth, thus has first priority on the oxygen supply. Some of this oxygenated stream goes through the liver cells and thence into the vena cava; some bypasses the liver cells through a fetal channel (the ductus venosus) and enters the vena cava still fully oxygenated but is immediately mixed with venous blood from the lower portion of the body. The combined stream of blood then passes into the right atrium where it is directed at once through another fetal channel (the foramen ovale) into the left atrium and ventricle and sent to the vessels serving the heart, the brain and the thyroid. Thus, these important organs are next in line to the liver in the receipt of oxygen. The venous blood from these organs returns to the superior vena cava and again enters the right atrium, but on this round it passes into the right ventricle and through the pulmonary artery toward the lungs. Since the latter are not yet functioning, they require very little blood. The main portion of the stream is diverted through the third fetal channel (the ductus arteriosus) into the aorta and thence to the lower portion of the body including the umbilical arteries which return some of the blood to the placenta where it is oxygenated again.

Changes in the Circulation at Birth

With the clamping and cutting of the umbilical cord, the umbilical arteries, the umbilical vein and the ductus venosus immediately lose their functions, and their channels are rapidly obliterated by thrombosis and fibrosis. The lungs expand with the first respirations, and a marked increase in the volume of blood sent through the pulmonary circulation results. At the same time, rapidly increasing pressure in the left atrium effectively closes the valve-like curtain which

hangs over the foramen ovale and stops the flow of blood between the right and the left atria. The ductus arteriosus also contracts and diminishes flow through its lumen which eventually closes. With these changes the two circulations—the systemic and the pulmonary—become separated because of the closure of all the fetal shunts. Henceforth all blood must traverse these circuits alternately.

Cardiac anomalies may result from the failure of these fetal channels to close at birth. Continued patency of the ductus arteriosus is seen either as an isolated abnormality or as a part of one of the more complicated syndromes. A foramen ovale which fails to close may act like an anomaly—atrial septal defect (ASD). No functional difficulties result from persistence of the ductus venosus.

INCIDENCE

Because of the many varieties of malformation and the variability in their clinical manifestations it is difficult to fix an exact incidence. Less than 1 per cent of newborn infants will have anomalies which are sufficiently severe to produce clinical symptoms that require attention.

GENERAL PROGNOSIS

The prognosis for a child with a cardiac malformation ranges from a life expectancy of a few minutes or hours to a normal span of life unhampered by any functional disability. The outlook depends on the extent to which the body metabolism is impaired. The earlier in life that clinical evidence of malformation appears, the more serious is the prognosis unless surgical correction is employed. Infants who begin to show cyanosis, poor weight gain, failure to grow or signs of heart failure during the first year have a very poor outlook. Those in whom the diagnosis rests on the physical findings of murmurs which are not associated with dyspnea, cyanosis or poor growth, have a favorable future—usually for many years and often for a full adult life. The decision to subject an asymptomatic child to diagnostic procedures or to surgical correction can be made only by a physician who is versed in the numerous varieties of malformation and their potential hazards. The main diagnostic technics used in congenital heart defects are discussed below.

DIAGNOSTIC PROCEDURES

Several special methods of examination are now in use which yield information about the anatomic and the physiologic state of the heart—information which in cases of congenital malformations is often essential to an exact diagnosis and to the decision to attempt surgical amelioration. These procedures are highly technical ones; only the general type of information sought can be discussed here.

Three main classes of congenital heart disease (CHD) are distinguished on the basis of the abnormal communications (shunts) which exist between the general circulation and the pulmonary circulation. In *acyanotic CHD* no shunts exist and the two circulations are normally independent of each other. Cyanosis occurs only when the internal derangement of the system throws such a strain upon the heart that myocardial failure results. In *cyanotic CHD* there is an abnormal opening between the two circulations with pressure relationships which permit unoxygenated blood to flow into the general circulation, diluting the oxygen concentration because red blood cells which have not passed through the lungs are mingling with those which have. In *potentially cyanotic CHD* an abnormal connection exists, but the pressure relations are such that blood flows in the other direction; i.e., from the oxygenated side to the unoxygenated side, or from the general circulation back into the pulmonary circulation. No cyanosis is present in this situation unless some change in pressure relationships occurs which reverses the flow of blood through the shunt. Thus the diagnostic procedures to be described are attempting to answer such questions as: Is there a shunt? If so, where is it? What effect does it have upon the pressures within the various chambers of the heart? How does it alter the delivery of oxygen to the peripheral tissues?

Physical Examination

Valuable clues are obtained from general examination of the patient. The presence of a murmur on auscultation of the chest is a common indication of CHD but not necessarily a conclusive one since many babies and children have benign or "functional" murmurs heard with an essentially normal cardiovascular system. Other suspicious findings are cyanosis, dyspnea, pallor and tachycardia. Severe degrees of physiologic interference may be reflected in the infant's failure to thrive or the older child's failure to grow, or in indications of heart failure such as enlargement of the liver and puffiness of the eyes.

When cyanotic CHD is suspected, blood studies may help to support the suspicion and to evaluate its severity. The red blood cell count and hematocrit reading rises above normal levels and the arterial saturation with oxygen falls from the normal of 95 to 100 per cent to ranges below 85 per cent.

Phonocardiography

Considerable skill and experience are required to analyze the murmurs heard with a stethoscope over the chest of a small infant or even an older child. A phonocardiogram provides a permanent visual record of the sounds which permits analysis and interpretation at the examiner's leisure. It is particulary valuable in infants with rapid heart rates where precise timing of the sequence and duration of cardiac sounds and murmurs is important. The advantages in

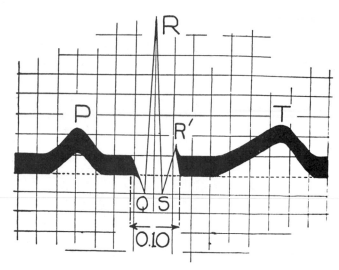

Fig. 22-3. Components of an electrocardiogram complex. Electrical neutrality is represented by the dotted baseline. The P-wave corresponds to atrial contraction. The P-R interval measures the length of time it takes the impulse to travel from the sino-atrial to the atrio-ventricular node. The Q-, R-, S- and R'-waves correspond to ventricular contraction. The T-wave is a phenomenon of recovery of electrical balance within the heart muscle.

helping unskilled listeners to improve their clinical acumen are also obvious.

Electrocardiography

The electrocardiogram (EKG) measures changes in the electric potentials of the heart muscle. Analysis of tracings taken with the three standard leads and the unipolar limb and chest leads discloses the contractile state of the underlying heart muscle and permits the recognition of relative hypertrophy of the atria or ventricles. These determinations help to decide which portion of the heart is being called upon for unusual effort either against an obstruction or in order to move an unusually large volume of blood. The EKG and more particularly the vectorcardiogram shows also the progression of the contractile impulse through the heart muscle. The vectorcardiogram gives a three dimensional view of this progression. EKG tracings in children must be interpreted with an understanding of the way in which normal tracings differ from those of the adult. For details of the technology of EKG interpretation the reader is referred to the text by Ziegler.

Radiologic Procedures

Plain Chest Films. To the experienced radiologist, plain chest films contribute significant diagnostic information with respect to the overall size of the heart, its position and the state of the ventricles and atria. In addition, the condition of the pulmonary vascular bed—normal, engorged, or collapsed—can be esti-

Table 22. Normal Cardiovascular Pressures in Children Beyond the Newborn Period

LOCATION	Pressure in mm./Hg.	
	Systolic	Diastolic
Right atrium		2-5
Right ventricle	15-30	2-5
Pulmonary artery	15-30	8-15
Left atrium		5-8
Left ventricle	80-130	5-10
Peripheral artery	80-130	40-90

mated. Lateral and oblique views of the chest may be required to outline the particular segments of the cardiac silhouette under study. Sometimes a swallow of barium will reveal the displacement of the esophagus by an enlarged left ventricle or by abnormal vessels comprising a vascular ring. Fluoroscopy may also be used to supplement the films and permit visualization of the motion of the structures being viewed.

Cardiac Catheterization and Angiography. Although several of the more common varieties of CHD can be diagnosed accurately by the methods detailed above, the special technic of cardiac catheterization with or without angiography is required for an understanding of the more complex abnormalities and for an exact determination of the physiologic abnormalities present prior to surgical correction.

With the usual technic a catheter is inserted into an arm vein of the sedated infant or child and advanced under fluoroscopic control into the superior vena cava, the right atrium, the right ventricle, and the pulmonary artery. In each of these locations it is possible to measure the pressures encountered and to take blood samples to determine the oxygen content of the blood. When abnormalities are present, the catheter may either fail to pass through the normal channels as in atresia of the tricuspid or pulmonary valves, or it may pass into abnormal openings such as a defect in the atrial or ventricular septum or a patent ductus arteriosus. Measurements of pressures and oxygen concentrations at the various sites and comparison to the normal values (Table 22) provide information from which the direction and volume of abnormal blood flow can be calculated.

With special apparatus such as the image intensifier, which permits longer fluoroscopic exposure without the hazard of excessive radiation, it is possible to inject radiopaque dye through the catheter and take moving pictures of its passage through the heart, providing a graphic view of the chambers and their vascular connections.

Catheterization of the left side of the heart in the absence of shunts such as ventricular, atrial or ductus arteriosus channels through which the catheter can be passed, is more difficult and must be done either through the aorta or by penetrating the atrial septum within the heart or by direct entrance into the left ventricle through the chest wall.

There is some risk associated with the use of any of the above technics. Since the risk is higher in the small child, such specialized studies are usually delayed until after 4 or 5 years of age if there is no urgent need for the information they provide. However, in cyanotic heart disease or when there is cardiac failure or failure to thrive from CHD, accurate diagnosis becomes imperative so that the child may profit from appropriate surgical correction. Before attempting catheterization, the infant or child should be brought to as optimum condition as possible by medical management of cardiac failure or electrolyte imbalance.

ACYANOTIC CONGENITAL HEART DISEASE

A few types of malformation of the cardiovascular system are incapable of producing cyanosis by the admixture of venous blood in the arterial circulation because there is no abnormal communication between pulmonary and systemic circulations. When symptoms develop, they are due to abnormalities in the course or the caliber of the vessels which leave the heart.

Coarctation of the Aorta

Coarctation is a narrowing of the aorta in a short segment just beyond the point of emergence of the left subclavian artery. The severity of symptoms depends on the degree of constriction. When the narrowing is slight, the defect goes unrecognized until late childhood or adulthood when elevation of blood pressure in the arms and low pressure in the legs provides the clue to its presence. Somewhat greater degrees of constriction may interfere with growth during childhood or may produce symptoms of fatigue and weakness in the legs. Severe degrees of constriction result in cardiac failure and enlargement which demands treatment during early infancy.

The diagnosis is usually suspected from the blood pressure changes mentioned above. It can be confirmed by aortography which will delineate the site and the extent of the narrowing. Surgical repair by excision of the constricted area is now possible. Direct anastomosis can usually be made although grafts of aorta sometimes must be inserted to complete the channel. Operation in middle or early childhood is preferred. If the symptoms are severe during infancy and treatment of cardiac failure is not sufficient to tide the child over, repair is undertaken as an emergency measure, although the technic is more difficult in the small baby.

Aortic Stenosis

Obstruction to the flow of blood out of the left ventricle may result from congenital malformation of the valves, the aortic ring or the tissue below the valves (subaortic stenosis). If the degree of constriction is mild, no symptoms result, and the diagnosis is made through the finding of a systolic murmur in the aortic area on routine physical examination. Treatment is not necessary for the asymptomatic individual.

More severe degrees of constriction produce symptoms of fatigue and fainting spells. The pulse pressure is usually low; i.e., there is only a small difference between the systolic and the diastolic blood pressures. Angiocardiography shows a delay in the exit of dye from the left ventricle. Catheterization of the left heart may permit better visualization of the constriction and measurement of the pressure difference on the two sides of the valve. Surgical relief is obtained by division of stenotic valves or dilatation of the constricting ring. These procedures are done best under the direct vision afforded by the open-heart technic.

Stenosis of the Pulmonic Valve

Like aortic stenosis, obstruction to the outflow of blood from the right ventricle may occur due to abnormality of the valves or the ring of the pulmonic valve. As an isolated finding it may have no implications for the child except the presence of a loud murmur over the valve. The more severe degrees produce symptoms of dyspnea on exertion which may require surgical correction similar to that employed for aortic stenosis.

Vascular Rings

During its early development the aorta has several arches, only one of which persists into late fetal life. Occasionally two arches remain which, in conjunction with the ductus arteriosus, may form a constricting ring around the trachea and the esophagus, thus interfering with swallowing or breathing. The diagnosis can be made by roentgen study of the upper esophagus and the trachea with contrast media. Surgical treatment consists of dividing one of the components of the constricting ring.

Myocardial Abnormalities

Particularly in small infants, cardiac failure without abnormal shunts may present a serious threat to the child's survival. *Endocardial fibroelastosis* is probably the end result of an intrauterine infection in which sclerotic changes in the inner wall of the heart muscle prevent proper relaxation and contraction of the ventricular chambers. As the child grows the symptoms become more severe and death in early infancy is the usual result. *Glycogen storage* disease of the heart may also be responsible for enlargement, poor contractile power and repeated cardiac failure. An *anomalous origin of the left coronary artery*, when it comes off the pulmonary artery instead of the aorta, results in unoxygenated blood being supplied to part

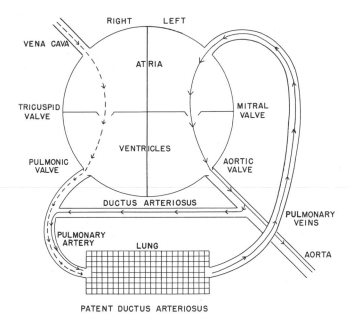

Fig. 22-4. Diagram of the circulation in patent ductus arteriosus. This is similar to that in Figure 22-1 except that oxygenated blood in the aorta can leak back through the open ductus into the pulmonary artery, thus adding to the volume of blood circulating through the lungs. Cyanosis does not develop, because the pressure relations are such that the blood in the ductus flows from the oxygenated side to the unoxygenated side, except under unusual circumstances. (Adapted from Cassels, D. E., and Morse, M.: Blood volume in congenital heart disease, J. Pediat. *31:*485)

of the heart muscle with symptoms of early cardiac failure. It can be distinguished from the above by characteristic EKG changes and is correctable by early surgery.

POTENTIALLY CYANOTIC CONGENITAL HEART DISEASE

In the potentially cyanotic group of malformations an abnormal communication exists between the pulmonary and the systemic circulations, but the pressure relations are such that the blood flows through this shunt from the arterial side to the venous side so that no cyanosis results. Under unusual stress, such as superimposed disease or myocardial failure, it is possible for the flow in the shunt to reverse its direction and produce cyanosis by admixing venous blood with arterial. When reversal of flow occurs, it is usually a terminal phenomenon; consequently, this group of disorders also is called the late cyanotic type of congenital heart disease.

The entities presented here are only examples of a larger number of possible defects which may occur singly or in combination. Larger texts must be consulted for more detailed discussion.

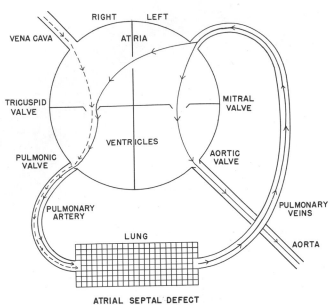

FIG. 22-5. Diagram of the circulation in atrial septal defect. This is similar to that of Figure 22-1, except that oxygenated blood returning to the left atrium can flow through the defect in the atrial septum into the right atrium, thus decreasing the volume of blood sent to the left ventricle and increasing the volume in the right side of the heart. No cyanosis develops unless the distention of the right side of the heart becomes excessive and reversal of the flow through the atrial defect takes place. (Adapted from Cassels, D. E., and Morse, M.: Blood volume in congenital heart disease, J. Pediat. *31:*485)

Patent Ductus Arteriosus

The ductus arteriosus is a fetal connection between the pulmonary artery and the aorta. Ordinarily, this channel spontaneously constricts, closes its lumen and atrophies shortly after birth. In some infants this change fails to take place, and the fetal communication between the pulmonary and the systemic circulations persists. Symptoms result when the opening is large, because there is leakage of blood from the aorta back into the pulmonary circulation (Fig. 22-4). No cyanosis results, but the volume of blood which the heart must pump in order to meet the requirements of the peripheral tissues is increased. A small channel has no effect on growth or physical activity, for the heart can hypertrophy enough to meet the slightly increased burden. When the volume of blood flowing through the ductus is large, both physical activity and growth may be hampered.

Diagnosis. The diagnosis is suspected from the presence of a typical machinery-like murmur over the pulmonary artery. It is confirmed by the presence of a low diastolic blood pressure and by various roentgen maneuvers which demonstrate enlargement of the pulmonary artery and increased blood flow to the lungs

or by actual visualization of the ductus itself after injection of opaque dye during cardiac catheterization.

Surgical Treatment. Surgical treatment consists of ligation and division of the abnormal channel. Usually it is performed after the age of 2 or 3 years. Even if symptoms are lacking, the ductus usually is closed, because its continued patency carries a risk of subacute bacterial endocarditis. In skilled hands the operative mortality is very low, and relief of symptoms can be confidently expected.

After the permanent ligature or division of the ductus is made, blood pressure reading discloses a rise in diastolic pressure. Blood pressure remains high for 4 to 5 days postoperatively and then stabilizes at a new level.

Atrial Septal Defects

Openings in the septum between the right and the left atria may occur from any of three embryologic faults: (1) persistence of an opening in the foramen ovale, which rarely produces any physiologic abnormality; (2) a high (ostium secundum) defect, or (3) a low (ostium primum) defect. The functional effect on the circulation is similar in the latter two defects. Oxygenated blood flows from the left to the right atrium through the defect and then is recirculated through the lungs (Fig. 22-5). A disproportion between the amount of blood circulating in the pulmonary and the systemic circulations ensues, producing enlargement of the right heart and distention of the pulmonary vessels. It has been postulated that the relatively meager flow to the rest of the body may lead to the slender, delicate habitus and poor tolerance for exercise which sometimes is observed. Susceptibility to pneumonia and rheumatic fever is increased. The diagnosis may be suspected from the presence of a murmur in the area of the pulmonary artery, with enlargement of the heart and roentgen evidence of congestion of the pulmonary circulation. It may be confirmed by insertion of a catheter into the right atrium and through the defect into the left atrium (cardiac catheterization). Surgical repair is possible both by closed and by open-heart technics. Since life expectancy is good for many of these children, the benefits of surgical correction must be balanced against the operative risk in each situation.

Ventricular Septal Defects

Two general types of defects in the septum between the ventricles are recognized: (1) small defects in the lower or muscular portion of the septum, which have a good prognosis, and (2) large defects in the upper or membranous portion of the septum, which usually cause significant symptoms.

The low septal defects (maladie de Roger) are characterized by loud systolic heart murmurs not accompanied by symptoms or evidence of cardiac enlargement or electrocardiographic strain. The life expectancy is normal, and no treatment is indicated. Recently it has been determined that some of these defects close spontaneously during childhood. Of course, it is highly important to recognize such defects so that the child will not be restricted merely because he has a heart murmur.

With larger defects high in the septum the situation is quite different. Blood under high pressure from the left ventricle flows into the right ventricle and increases its work load by augmenting the volume of blood in the pulmonary circulation. The heart enlarges, and there is evidence of right ventricular strain. Growth may be impaired, and the infant may suffer from dyspnea, feeding difficulties and repeated respiratory infections. Diagnosis is made from the loud systolic murmur heard over the defect together with cardiac enlargement and engorgement of the pulmonary circulation. Cardiac catheterization is usually performed in order to confirm the diagnosis and to study the pressures in the several chambers which are accessible. Operative repair is possible using open-heart surgical technics. Atrial and ventricular septal defects may be repaired by direct closure or by suturing a patch of specially prepared plastic sponge material into the opening. The plastic material acts as a framework for final healing by the heart's own tissue. Immediately after the patch is sutured in place, fibrous tissue begins to invade the hundreds of tiny openings contained within it. Thus, reopening of the defect or rejection of the plastic patch becomes impossible. The result will depend on the amount of resistance which has developed in the pulmonary vascular bed. If the latter is high, the child will not do well, with or without surgical correction.

CYANOTIC CONGENITAL HEART DISEASE

In cyanotic congenital heart disease there is a communication between the pulmonary and the systemic circulations in which the blood is flowing continually from the venous to the arterial side. The blood delivered to the periphery of the body by the aorta never is fully saturated with oxygen, and the tissues take on a bluish hue instead of the normal pink. Cyanosis may be apparent at birth and persist or it may be inapparent at birth but develop during the first year of life. In either event it tends to become more marked during the early years of life. In part this is due to an increase in the number of red cells per unit volume of blood (polycythemia), which represents an attempt of the body to improve the oxygen-carrying power of the blood. When polycythemia is marked, the peripheral capillaries of the skin and the mucous membranes become distended with purple blood, the fingers and the toes may take on a clubbed shape (Plate 5), body growth is delicate and retarded, the capacity for exercise is reduced, and the

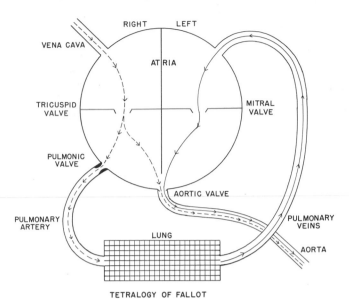

FIG. 22-6. Diagram of the circulation in the tetralogy of Fallot. Venous blood entering the right ventricle is diverted from the pulmonary artery because of the narrowed orifice at the pulmonic valve. Some of it escapes through the defect in the interventricular septum into the left ventricle and almost immediately into the abnormally placed aorta. Partly because of anatomic relations and partly because of hypertrophy of the right ventricle, the venous blood is able to flow into the aorta. A decrease in the volume of blood sent to the lungs and a continual contamination of the stream of oxygenated blood from the left ventricle result. Cyanosis is present, and an increased volume of blood is present in the greater circulation. (Adapted from Cassels, D. E., and Morse, M.: Blood volume in congenital heart disease, J. Pediat. *31*:485)

child runs the hazard of complications due to spontaneous clotting of the thickened blood within his vessels. In very cyanotic children, periodic hematocrit determinations should be made. If the reading approaches 70 per cent the child is in danger of spontaneous thrombosis, which, if it occurs in a cerebral vessel, can be very serious. Infections tend to elevate the hematocrit reading owing to attendant dehydration so that a child with cyanotic heart disease must have careful attention to his fluid intake during febrile illnesses and perhaps should receive antibiotic treatment early to abort as many of these incidents as possible.

Paradoxically, children with cyanotic heart disease may suffer from functional anemia. Because of the abnormal blood flow they need a certain optimal, high concentration of hemoglobin and often will be benefited by transfusion or iron therapy when their blood counts are in the average range for normal children—a range which is too low for their particular requirements.

Tetralogy of Fallot

The most common variety of cyanotic heart disease which permits survival consists of a combination of abnormalities. Blood leaving the right ventricle toward the lungs encounters an abnormally narrow opening into the pulmonary artery (Fig. 22-6). In the same vicinity there is an opening in the interventricular septum which provides a ready diversion of blood into the left side of the heart and particularly into the aorta. Cyanosis arises because of the contamination of the aortic contents by venous blood. The direction of flow through the shunt is determined in part by the position of the aortic opening and in part by the fact that the right ventricle has hypertrophied because of its excessive task and thus is able to overbalance the pressure of the left ventricle. Poor oxygenation of the tissues is furthered also by the fact that the rate of blood flow through the lungs is decreased. Diagnosis is made from the combination of findings from several types of examination of the heart. Roentgen examination demonstrates enlargement of the chambers of the right side, decrease in size of the pulmonary artery and decrease in blood flow through the lungs. The electrocardiogram shows right ventricular hypertrophy. Catheterization demonstrates high pressure in the right ventricle which falls off rapidly in the pulmonary artery. The catheter tip also may demonstrate the ventricular septal defect.

Medical Management. Medical management consists of preventing intercurrent infections and dehydration and alleviating attacks of paroxysmal dyspnea which tend to occur during the first 2 years of life. These attacks are characterized by air hunger, deep cyanosis and loss of consciousness with or without convulsions. The child's discomfort can be relieved by placing him in a knee-chest position to increase cardiac efficiency and by increasing oxygen saturation of the blood.

The child with tetralogy of Fallot usually limits his own activity because of fatigue and dyspnea. His play is usually interspersed with rest periods during which he squats to relieve the dyspnea. In spite of the fact that such children have a chronic circulatory disturbance to the brain with some degree of relative anoxia, many of them are of average or above-average intelligence. Fainting spells and occasional convulsions also may occur in children over 2 years of age when the degree of anoxia is increased temporarily.

Surgical Treatment. The optimal age for operation is between 2 and 15 years. The original "blue-baby operation" done by Blalock and Taussig was designed to ameliorate the abnormality. In this operation a branch of the aorta is anastomosed to the pulmonary artery. In older children the subclavian artery is used. In the Potts operation the side of the pulmonary artery is anastomosed directly to the side of the aorta. Both of these shunting operations increase the pulmonary blood flow by creating an artificial patent ductus arteriosus. Neither operation corrects the original defects, but they do add a compensating one which increases blood flow through the lungs and thereby reduces cyanosis and dyspnea and improves the child's tolerance for activity. Improvement also may be achieved by an operation which widens the pulmonary valve opening.

With the newer technics of open-heart surgery which utilize extracorporeal circulation it is now possible to make a complete correction of the defects. The operation is a formidable one which requires a large group of technical specialists. When possible it is deferred until the child is at least 6 or 8 years old.

Other Forms of Cyanotic Heart Disease

Tricuspid Atresia. In this serious malformation there is no opening between the right atrium and the right ventricle. Blood returning from the body via the venae cavae can leave the right atrium only through a persisting defect in the interatrial septum and thence into the left atrium and the left ventricle. Unless there is an additional defect in the ventricular septum or a patent ductus arteriosus, there is no way for blood to circulate through the lungs. Even if one of these channels is open, the efficiency of oxygenation is poor. Consequently, these infants are cyanotic early in life and do so poorly that many of them die within a year unless surgical correction is accomplished. The diagnosis is suspected from the electrocardiogram which shows that the left ventricle is assuming an unusual work load. It can be confirmed by cardiac catheterization. The same types of shunting operations as those employed for the tetralogy will give improvement, although the results are less dramatic.

Transposition of the Great Vessels. This anomaly results when the aorta emerges from the right ventricle and the pulmonary artery from the left ventricle. Unless there are connecting defects in atrial or ventricular septa, two separate circulations result which have no interchange and, since oxygenated blood cannot get into the general circulation, extrauterine life is impossible. If there is some crossover between the two circuits, the infant may live for a while, but the prognosis is very poor and operative relief is possible only through a very complicated procedure which carries a very high mortality. Diagnosis is made by angiocardiography.

Truncus Arteriosus. In this malformation the aorta and the pulmonary artery are fused into a single tube, which takes its origin from a defective interventricular septum in such a way that it can receive blood from both the right and the left ventricles simultaneously. The severity of cyanosis, dyspnea and growth failure in an individual child depends on conditions which regulate blood flow through the lungs. If pulmonary blood flow is plentiful, the symptoms will be mild, but more commonly the child does poorly. Diagnosis is suspected from the presence of a loud murmur over the point of origin of the truncus. It can be confirmed by angiocardiography. Treatment is symptomatic, since no form of surgical relief has yet been devised. Protection against infections and management of heart failure are the main objectives of medical management.

Anomalous Drainage of Pulmonary Veins. The pulmonary veins which normally carry the oxygenated blood back from the lungs to the left atrium sometimes empty elsewhere into the venous system, thus depriving the systemic circulation of the oxygenated blood that they contain. If all of the pulmonary veins drain into the right side of the circulation, life is not possible without a defect in the interatrial septum which permits some oxygenated blood to get back to the left atrium and ventricle. Under these circumstances there will be cyanosis, fatigue and congestive heart failure. Partial anomalous return, i.e., when some of the veins connect with the left atrium and others do not, is accompanied by milder symptoms. Diagnosis is made by the discovery of abnormally high levels of oxygen in the blood of the right atrium during cardiac catheterization. When the symptoms are severe, open-heart surgery must be performed to correct the venous connections and close the interatrial septal defect. In some instances of partial anomalous drainage the child may get along reasonably well without operation.

PRINCIPLES OF MEDICAL MANAGEMENT

Children with congenital malformations of the heart should be permitted to lead lives which are as nearly normal as their individual disabilities will permit. If they are able to engage in full activity and participate in sports without discomfort they should be permitted to do so in spite of the presence of murmurs which indicate a structural abnormality. There are a few exceptions to this generalization, and for this reason it is desirable that all such children be seen by a physician skilled in the interpretation of cardiac murmurs in order to decide whether more extensive diagnostic study is imperative for the child's safety. Those who demonstrate poor growth, fatigue, dyspneic spells, cyanosis or fainting attacks obviously should have the benefit of thorough study and evaluation of the benefit that they might derive from surgical correction.

The complications of spontaneous thrombosis and paradoxic anemia have been mentioned in the discussion of cyanotic heart disease. These children and others with noncyanotic heart disease also may suffer from cardiac decompensation or, rarely, from subacute bacterial endocarditis.

Cardiac Decompensation

A damaged heart or one subjected to excessive strain is said to be compensated when it has hypertrophied and adjusted its performance sufficiently to overcome its handicap completely. If it fails to maintain an adequate circulation, it is decompensated.

Etiology. The heart may fail for a variety of reasons: oxygen supply to the myocardium may be insufficient because of its low concentration in the coronary vessels; peripheral resistance may be increased by vascular constriction during hypertension, or by increase in the volume or the viscosity of the blood which a ventricle is expected to move; excessive demands may be placed on a ventricle which has to pump blood through an abnormally small orifice; or disease may weaken the inherent power of the cardiac muscle as in rheumatic fever and other forms of myocarditis.

Symptoms. When the circulation is inadequate, blood accumulates in the venous system. In the lungs, the congestion of the vessels causes symptoms resembling bronchitis. Small amounts of blood may appear in the sputum. Congestion of the systemic venous system causes digestive disturbances, enlargement of the liver and accumulation of fluid in the tissue spaces (edema) and in the serous cavities (ascites). Nausea and vomiting may be the first outstanding symptoms of decompensation. The congestion of the liver may lead to dysfunction sufficient to cause jaundice. Only rarely does the ascites become great enough to embarrass respiration or heart action.

An adequate gas exchange between the blood and the tissues is impossible in the presence of circulatory failure. Cyanosis and dyspnea result. Cyanosis is noted best in the lips and the fingertips; dyspnea may be so severe as to require the child to maintain a sitting posture.

Treatment. The treatment of decompensation consists of reducing to a minimum the amount of work required of the heart, administering cardiac stimulants to help the heart to meet the circulatory needs and, finally, when compensation has been attained, providing favorable conditions for the heart to recover as much reserve as possible. The child should be in bed, absolutely at rest. If dyspnea is present elevation of the shoulders is usually desired. Not only rest but also an abundance of sleep is necessary. Sedative drugs usually are strongly indicated, and no hesitancy need be shown in the use of morphine. In fact, morphine is a very important drug in this condition. The early administration of oxygen is valuable. In cases of most severe decompensation, removal of blood from the circulation may be desirable unless anemia is present. However, removal of blood is seldom necessary when the other measures mentioned are carried out appropriately.

DIGITALIS. This drug serves to slow the heart rate by prolonging diastole, thus allowing more cardiac rest and at the same time permitting better ventricular filling. Digitalis increases cardiac tone. It increases the extent of ventricular contraction and relieves or prevents dilatation beyond the physiologic limit, making possible maximal cardiac output.

To be therapeutically useful, digitalis must be given in sufficient quantity to saturate the cardiac muscle and produce the desired physiologic effects. However, the margin between therapeutic and toxic quantities is narrow, and toxic manifestations may do more harm than good to the decompensated child. Usually a total digitalizing dose is computed according to the child's age and size, and a schedule of doses is planned which will reach this amount in 24 to 48 hours. If the appropriate effect is achieved the child is then placed on a daily maintenance dose of ⅒ to ⅕ of the total digitalizing dose. Two preparations are commonly used for such gradual digitalization: (1) digoxin, which reaches its optimum peak within the body in about 4 hours and is fully excreted in 48 to 72 hours, and (2) digitoxin, which peaks in 4 to 8 hours and is excreted more slowly, taking 10 to 14 days to disappear from the body. For extreme emergencies only, lanatoside C (Cedilanid) may be given intravenously with an expected effect within 15 minutes. It is rapidly excreted so that another preparation must be used after 24 to 36 hours. *It is of the utmost importance to decompensated children that accurate records of time and dose be maintained during digitalis administration.* Table 23 lists the preparations in general use with suggested dosage schedules and times of peak action and excretion.

A digitalizing effect is determined by improvement in dyspnea, tachycardia, liver enlargement and venous pressure or by alterations in the electrocardiogram. Overdosage may be heralded by irregularity of the heart action, excessive slowing due to heart block, nausea, vomiting and visual disturbances. When toxic symptoms are present it is, of course, important to withhold additional digitalis until the basis for the symptoms has been clearly determined. Particular care must be exercised in regulating the dosage for children who have or may have received digitalis previously.

OXYGEN. For the child in cardiac decompensation, oxygen is generally indicated to improve the oxygenation of his blood and relieve dyspnea.

DIURETICS. The increased blood and interstitial fluid volume which accompanies congestive failure throws an additional burden upon an already overworked myocardium. Hence measures to reduce the fluid volume are usually indicated through limitation of the intake of fluids and sodium and through the promotion of diuresis. In children the xanthine diuretics (theophylline, theobromine) the mercurial diuretics (Mercuhydrin, Thiomerin) and enzyme inhibitors (Diamox, Diuril) are used under various circumstances. Measurements of fluid intake and excretion are helpful in evaluating the effectiveness of these measures.

After all signs of decompensation have disappeared, the child should be kept at rest until some cardiac reserve has been attained. Then activity should be permitted gradually. If the pulse rate becomes much accelerated or remains increased after exercise, the exercise has been too severe or too prolonged. It may be that the child never will have the normal degree of cardiac reserve and that his activities always must be somewhat restricted. Any noteworthy recurrence of decompensation is an indication for renewed convalescent care for weeks or months and calls for prolonged restriction of activity. Nursing care of children with heart disease is discussed in Chapter 27.

Subacute Bacterial Endocarditis

Children with malformations of the cardiovascular system (and those who have heart valves damaged by rheumatic fever) are vulnerable to infection of the lining of their abnormal channels by bacteria which occasionally circulate in the blood stream. The most common offender is the alpha-hemolytic streptococcus which is normally found in the upper respiratory passages. If it succeeds in setting up residence on an abnormal valve or a portion of the vascular system where stagnant eddies are present, a chronic granulomatous infection results which produces anemia, fever and embolic phenomena in various parts of the body including the spleen, the liver, the kidneys and the lungs. Fortunately this complication is rare in children and when diagnosed can usually be treated successfully by intensive and prolonged therapy with penicillin or other appropriate antibiotic.

PRINCIPLES AND COMPLICATIONS OF SURGICAL MANAGEMENT

In advance the surgeon plans whether he can make the necessary correction without interrupting the action of the heart and directing the blood through an artificial heart-lung machine. If he can, the operative procedure will be comparable to a thoracotomy performed for any type of thoracic surgery, and post-

Table 23. Digitalis Preparations

General Type	Digoxin	Digitoxin	Lanatosides
Trade Names	Lanoxin	Crystodigin Purodigin	Cedilanid D
Peak Activity	4 hrs.	4-8 hrs.	15 minutes
Excreted after	48-72 hrs.	10-14 days	24-36 hrs.
Digitalizing Dose Newborn & premature	0.03-0.05 mg./Kg.	0.022 mg./Kg.	0.022 mg./Kg.
	(0.6-0.75 mg./M.²)	(0.3-0.35 mg./M.²)	0.3-0.35 mg./M.²)*
Older child	0.04-0.08 mg./Kg.	0.03-0.45 mg./Kg.	0.025 mg./Kg.
	(1.5 mg./M.²)	(0.75 mg./M.²)	(0.75 mg./M.²)
Route	Oral, I.M., I.V.	Oral, I.M., I.V.	I.M., I.V.
Maintenance	⅒-⅕ above	⅒ above	

* mg./M²—the dosage calculated for body surface area.

FIG. 22-7. Circuit of helix-reservoir machine conducts blood from two catheters inserted in venae cavae to bottom of mixing chamber. Bubbles of oxygen rising through the chamber are removed in the debubbler. Thence the blood flows into the helix reservoir and is pumped back into the femoral artery of the patient. The machine also can be used to stop the heartbeat by chilling the heart. This is done by passing part of the blood through a cooling coil and returning it directly to the coronary artery. Blood flowing from the coronary circulation into the chambers of the heart is aspirated and returned to the heart-lung machine for oxygenation. (Lillehei, C. W., and Engel, Leonard: Open-heart surgery, Scient. Amer. *202*:80)

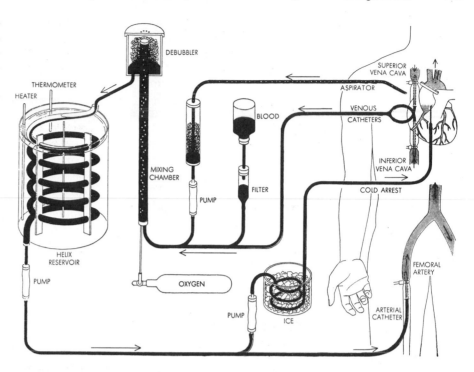

operative nursing care will be the same. If he cannot avoid by-passing cardiopulmonary circulation, then an extensive team effort becomes necessary, and the operative hazard to the child increases.

By-passing the cardiopulmonary circulation requires the use of the heart-lung machine which was perfected in 1955 (Fig. 22-7). The machine makes it possible for the surgeon to open the heart, remove the blood within it and repair the septal defects and/or the valves under direct vision and without the hurry which was necessary prior to its development. The machine withdraws carbon dioxide-laden venous blood by gravity through two catheters securely fastened into the venae cavae and sends it into a tube that admits oxygen through holes which are big enough to form large bubbles. The flow of oxygen into this tube causes the blood to rise up into the debubbler chamber where the exchange of carbon dioxide and oxygen takes place. Excess gas and clots are removed from the blood within the debubbler chamber to prevent emboli from getting into the child's blood stream. From the debubbler chamber the oxygenated blood passes into a reservoir, where it is warmed to body temperature before it is pumped into the child's arterial system through a catheter which is inserted into the femoral or the subclavian artery. In young children with small arteries, both femoral arteries must be used to prevent oxygen deprivation. The machine is regulated so that it pumps the amount of blood that the heart would pump if it were doing its usual work. Thus the machine supplies the entire systemic circulatory system with oxygenated blood and returns carbon dioxide-laden blood back to the heart via the venae cavae. There it is picked up by

the catheters in the venae cavae and redelivered by gravity to the machine for reoxygenation.

Before the machine is used it must be primed* with 2 to 4 pints of fresh, venous heparinized blood from compatible donors. Heparin, an anticoagulant, is also given intravenously to the child to prevent clotting in the system.

Without a heart-lung machine, any interruption in the functioning of the heart and the lungs for even a brief interval would result in irreversible damage to the oxygen-sensitive tissues of the brain and the kidneys. For difficult and extensive repairs which require a motionless and bloodless heart, heart beating must be stopped by cold arrest. This is accomplished by circulating small amounts of cooled blood through the coronary arteries of the heart while the remainder of the child's body is kept at a normal temperature. When the cooled blood reaches the chambers of the heart, it is aspirated and returned to the heart-lung machine for reoxygenation. Cooling the heart to 65° F. reduces its need for oxygen to such a degree that its requirements can be met satisfactorily with small amounts of circulating blood.

Such bold procedures as those described above require expert surgeons and anesthetists, a trained team to monitor the operation of the heart-lung machine

---

* It is estimated that approximately 30 per cent of the child's blood is donor's blood when the operation is completed. It has been suggested that an allergic response to the donor cells may be the cause of the temperature elevation which occurs 48 to 52 hours postoperatively. Brick red urine may also be produced as donor cells are hemolyzed. Parents are often concerned when they learn that large quantities of donor blood are required. They need to know that priming the pump is required and that all donor cells remaining in the child's body after operation will be destroyed and replaced with cells of his own.

and continuous electrocardiographic and perhaps electroencephalographic recordings of the child's condition. After the defects in the heart are repaired, the normal blood channels must be restored and the spontaneous contractions of the heart reactivated by supplying warm blood and/or by administering calcium chloride. The effects of heparin also must be counteracted with such drugs as protamine sulphate or polybrene. Whatever blood is lost is replaced by transfusion before extra-corporeal circulation is discontinued.

Ventricular fibrillation, a disorganization of the heartbeat which renders the cardiac muscles useless as a pump, may occur from cooling as the heart recovers from arrest. However, it is not so prolonged or so dangerous as the fibrillation that occurs when the heart muscle is deprived of oxygen during "drug" arrest. Usually, recovery from "cold" arrest occurs quickly and spontaneously.

In addition to closing the wounds of the chest and those made to expose the femoral artery, chest tubes must be inserted to drain fluid and air from the pleural cavity. If retained, these would prevent complete expansion of the lungs and serve as a culture medium predisposing the child to empyema.

The use of a transistorized battery-powered electric pacemaker has been another means by which mortality from open-heart surgery has been reduced. Normally the heart maintains its proper rhythm from imperceptible electrical impulses which are conveyed through a band of muscle and nerve tissues called the "bundle of His" after the German research worker who identified it. Sometimes the needle used to suture the plastic patch into the cardiac defect strikes the neuromuscular fibers which carry the heart impulse from the heart's natural built-in pacemaker to the ventricles. When this happens, the impulse cannot reach the ventricles, and the atria and the ventricles cannot synchronize their beats and heart block results. The artificial device (the pacemaker) stimulates and regulates ventricular contractions through a wire implanted directly into the heart muscle. The wire is removed from the muscle of the ventricle when healing has restored the heart's capacity to maintain a normal beat.

Under some circumstances the technic of hypothermia is used. The body temperature is gradually reduced to 86° F. by cooling the anesthetized or sedated child in a tub of water or by wrapping his body in a rubber blanket through which a refrigerant is circulated. Such muscle relaxants as curare or succinylcholine are given to prevent shivering which aids in the maintenance of body heat. Hypothermia decreases the metabolism of the body, particularly the brain, and renders the latter organ less susceptible to damage if the oxygen supply is reduced during the course of the operation. During periods of hypothermia there is a decline in the performance of the circulatory system. The pulse rate drops from the effects of cold on the

heart's built-in pacemaker, and the volume of blood in the circulation lessens as the plasma becomes isolated in the peripheral capillary beds. With this technic, the surgeon can shut off the already reduced flow of blood through the heart for 8 to 12 minutes and repair the defects in a bloodless heart by direct vision. Then the child is *gradually* warmed to a normal temperature again. Hypothermia, or "cold sleep" as it is often called, has been used since 1952 for closed-heart operations and for some open-heart surgical procedures in which repair can be made quickly before the brain and the kidneys become endangered from oxygen deprivation.

Although there are numerous chances for fatal errors in the complex procedures cited above, well trained teams are able to hold the operative mortality to a surprisingly low figure. However, vigilance to guard against complications must be constant to prevent serious complications and death during the postoperative period. The chest cavity which is drained of air and fluid with water-sealed chest drainage apparatus must be kept functioning at an optimal level for the reasons cited previously. Concealed hemorrhage into the chest may occur from imperfect anastomosis of vessels or from the effects of the anticoagulant used during the operation. If fluid administration has not been sufficient, operative dehydration may foster cerebral vessel thrombosis in children with polycythemia. Thrombi in other arteries can also occur. Because the heart-lung machine is less efficient than the lungs in removing carbon dioxide from the blood, some degree of acidosis is to be expected in the early postoperative period. Low serum sodium and, more importantly, low serum potassium levels are also characteristic findings in children who have been sustained on extracorporeal circulation during the operation. The potassium level must be closely watched and replacement therapy instituted when it falls to dangerously low levels.

Administration of intravenous fluids and blood is determined by periodic measurements of the chemical constituents of the blood, by careful appraisal of the urinary output in relation to intake and by measuring the quantity of blood and fluid lost via chest drainage. To protect the child from electrolyte imbalance and from too rapid increase in blood volume which would create cardiac overload, meticulous care in following orders concerning the *kind* of fluid to be administered intravenously and the *rate* at which it should be given is *absolutely* essential. Cardiac arrest from ventricular fibrillation can occur at any time even with the use of the artificial pacemaker. Vomiting can cause aspiration and undue stress on the heart. For this reason Wangensteen gastric suction may be employed for the first 24 postoperative hours. The usual postoperative dangers of atelectasis and failure to clear bronchial secretions also may complicate recovery and make a tracheostomy necessary.

NURSING CARE

Preparation of the Child for Cardiac Surgery

The child with a congenital cardiac defect should receive a full explanation of the nature of his infirmity at the earliest age at which he is able to understand. If the parents suppress the truth out of shame or guilt, the child not only will remain in a state of prolonged confusion and uncertainty but also will be poorly prepared for medical treatment. Ideally, this information should be imparted early enough so that the child will be able to explain the situation to his playmates. His brothers and sisters also must be told so that they will not resent his receiving special attention or feel ashamed of his differences.

The child should be able to grasp the essential facts of his cardiac defect at about the time that he begins to understand the facts of gestation and birth.

At this time the child may question the reason for repeated and lengthy physical examinations and diagnostic procedures. He may also become puzzled by differences between his physical functioning and that of his playmates and by his mother's greater protectiveness. When he is able to ask specific questions, information can be given slowly until the child has gained greater understanding of his condition and of his need for medical care.

Admission of the child to the hospital will be difficult for the parents as well as for the child. Preschool children will respond with anxiety to separation and painful procedures and in addition will reflect the stress of their parents. Parents however (as well as school-age children and adolescents) have acute awareness of the life-threatening implications of open-heart surgery. Although parents often find it difficult to comprehend the complexities involved in the repair of a malformed heart, they have usually been informed about its risks. Often this decision has involved months and perhaps years of worry, many moments of painful indecision and agonizing fears lest their decision lead to the death of their child. It is understandable, therefore, why parents are unnerved, frightened, fatigued and in need of a person with whom they can share their burdens and from whom they can obtain information which will clarify their understanding of the treatment and nursing care plans.

The concerns and fears of parents show wide variation depending on their personality make-up and their dealings with professional persons since the defect was first discovered. Some parents have had a great deal of helpful guidance and feel assured that they have made a wise decision to permit the operation. Others have had meager help and continue to harbor feelings of guilt about the defect. Some are badly confused as to why an operation is necessary, particularly in instances in which their children appear to be healthy and show no obvious symptoms.

Some degree of irritability, retardation in emotional and mental development and insecurity can be expected in the child with a congenital heart defect. The constant concern of his parents, transmitted to the child through verbal and nonverbal cues, results in insecurity in the child regarding his own safety. Because most parents naturally do everything possible to lessen the distress of a cyanotic child, he has had fewer opportunities for developing a tolerance for frustration. On the other hand, he has been subjected to repeated stress situations which healthy children are not called upon to withstand.

Parental overprotection prior to surgery may be extreme because such measures reduce anxiety and guilt in the parents. Many children with heart defects respond with emotional problems and a lack of control and independence. Other children may rebel against such severe restrictiveness and refuse to accept the role of the sick child which their mothers have bestowed upon them. Most children come to value the secondary rewards of the sick role although it intensifies sibling rivalry problems. Lack of self confidence may be apparent (or carefully covered) because their opportunities for accomplishment have been limited and because their lack of physical stamina may result in feelings of inferiority. Rewards in school may be lacking, because of frequent absences, emotional insecurity, lower energy levels and because of a lag in intellectual as well as motor development. Such defeat may result in depression and feelings of alienation and isolation.

The child admitted to the hospital for cardiac surgery usually has had previous hospital experience. Knowledge of the circumstances and results of these experiences will help the nurse to understand the child's present behavior and to help him in mastering current fears and stresses. The child who has had a constructive experience during the time of diagnostic studies will be infinitely better prepared for cardiac surgery than the child who has been traumatized by them.

Before preparing a child for any type of operation, answers to the following questions must be obtained: (1) What new experiences will the child meet before and after operation? (2) What evidence do I have that suggests that he is ready to depend on me to help him to face it? (3) How can I prepare him so that his trust in his parents and me can be sustained? (4) How much information can he assimilate at one time?

Preparing the child for surgery may include a tour of the pediatric ward (if he is unfamiliar with it) and a preparatory trip to the operating room, where he can become familiarized with the garb of the personnel and the room where the anesthetic will be given. If a trip of this nature cannot be planned, the child must know how he will be taken to the operating room and what he will see there. He must also learn about the preoperative injection and the particular anesthetic he will receive through graphic though simple explanations on his level of understanding.

The child is benefited by learning what is going to be done* after he has gone to sleep, what he will see and feel postoperatively and the purpose of treatments which will be done. He will also need to know where the stitches and the chest drainage tubes will be and the importance of repositioning, coughing and deep breathing exercises. It is imperative that he be prepared for the pain these procedures will precipitate; otherwise the child may hamper his progress by immobilizing himself. Practice in deep breathing, coughing and turning will teach him how to work *with* the nurse postoperatively. At this time, the nurse can demonstrate how she will hold her hands firmly against his chest wall to support it while he coughs. He can also be told that he will probably feel like giving the nurse suggestions about turning and feeding him, and that these will be welcomed. The nurse also can tell him that he will probably be irritated with her when she disturbs his rest to check vital signs and to turn him, thus conferring upon him the freedom to express himself when the operation is over.

The purpose of the chest and the urinary drainage tubes, the pacemaker, the oxygen tent, intravenous therapy, tracheal aspirations and intramuscular injections must also be explained so that the child is not caught unawares. Learning that tracheal aspirations are uncomfortable but are done to make him breathe easier will increase his tolerance for the most distressing of all postoperative measures. He should not be left with any doubt that nurses will be with him every minute to keep him as comfortable as possible.

Of course, such preparatory information will be given over a period of time. Some details can be given the child at home. Other parts, especially those relating to postoperative care, should probably be postponed until the child and the parents have acquired confidence in the persons who will provide care. However, many school-age children and adolescents may seek knowledge about postoperative care from their physician or clinic nurse before they come into the hospital for operation. School-age children and adolescents are benefited by the use of diagrams and other visual aids. A doll with drainage tubes attached to it and with the area of incision marked out helps the preschooler to visualize the changes that he will see in his body after operation. Typical questions are concerned with how long the tubes will stay in and how they are removed, when he will be able to get

up and when he can eat and how stitches are removed. But in the nurse author's experience, one of the questions asked most frequently by children over 6 years of age revealed their need for reassurance that she would be available to them at the time of anesthesia and in the postoperative period. Two of the group the nurse author studied stated that they would not go to the operating room unless she was with them. For this reason she always made a point of reemphasizing the details of her nursing role on the evening before the operation (incidentally, this was as important to the parents as it was to the children).

The child can be expected to regress to a considerable extent during this experience, and the nurse should convince him that a temporary return to infantile behavior is entirely acceptable. This is accomplished best by demonstrating tacit approval of regression during the time the child is adjusting to hospitalization. Regression is a natural human response to stress, and for a child to resist it simply imposes an additional burden on him. And, as will be explained later on, the state of regression can in itself be beneficial. An example of the kind of regressive behavior which may be observed is 4-year-old Suzie's interest in using a feeding bottle during play before her operation. Sucking on the bottle not only relieved her distress associated with separation and with preparation for her operation, but it might also have been her way of testing the nurse's response (and her own, for that matter) to babyish behavior. If a child shows resistance to regression before his operation, every effort should be made to help him to maintain his self-esteem in the face of it.

The more closely the nurse observes a child's individual mode of coping with stress before operation, the better prepared she will be to provide help in the postoperative period. The following incidents illustrate the value of such observations.

Entrance of the medical staff into 4-year-old Suzie's room invariably caused her to withdraw into pensive contemplation while she fingered her lips. When her hand was free for this self-comforting activity, she was able to maintain control during frightening procedures. The defensive value of this gesture became apparent one day when the physician removed her fingers from her lips as he examined her heart. With her defense gone, she was unable to control herself. She shrieked loudly and kicked until the physician permitted her to resume her accustomed activity. Postoperatively, the nurse made sure that one arm was free so Suzie could comfort herself when she needed it.

Sara, age 9, became acutely distressed whenever venepuncture was necessary. The large syringes frightened her, and on the physician's arrival she tried to hide under the bed. With persuasion, Sara positioned herself on the bed, but she could not hold herself still or adapt to the restraint the nurse tried to use. When Sara saw the needle she was horrified. Then, in a demanding way which showed the intensity of her fear, she said, "Count! Don't stop! Keep on counting 'til he's gone." The results of counting were dra-

---

* Unless a very young child will see that a part of his body has been removed, it is better if the words "removed" or "take out" are avoided in preliminary explanation. Preparation for tonsillectomy is an exception because almost universally children hear parents and children talking about the time they had these organs "taken out." The following type of explanation is appropriate: "Tim, your tonsils are the cause of your sore throats and the doctor is going to take them out. You don't need them as you do the other parts of your body."

matic. For some reason which never became fully understood, the counting minimized Sara's fear to such a degree that she could participate by immobilizing her arm.

On the evening after operation, the initial administration of positive pressure increased Sara's tension to a considerable extent. The nurse remembered the effects of counting and tested out this measure to see if it would be as effective in relieving symptoms of stress as it had been preoperatively. The results were more dramatic than previously. Sara relaxed when counting accompanied the administration of positive pressure, and also when other uncomfortable measures were carried out.

To assure the parents that they can depend on the nurse's support during the operation and immediately following it is another important nursing item. Such help can reduce the parents' anxiety at the time the child is taken to the operating room and during the agonizing period when they are waiting for news of the outcome. It is during the period of waiting that parents tend to ask the most questions. They want to know what they will see after the operation and how they can be of material help to their children. The parents can be told that chest drainage and a rise in temperature postoperatively are to be expected, and that turning, deep breathing and coughing, etc., cause pain, but that the child's cries help him to inflate his lungs and promote drainage from the pleural cavity. (By crying he gives himself positive pressure.) The parents can learn why the nurse will be preoccupied with such activities as the frequent checking of vital signs, monitoring of intravenous apparatus and observing the many other physical responses to surgical intervention. Unless the parents are informed of these routines, they are likely to interpret the nurse's busy concern as a sign that the child's condition has worsened. If both parents and the child know that these activities are *protective measures* they are not only reassured when they see them performed, but they also will refrain from interrupting the nurse during the time when she is busiest.

Care During the Immediate Postoperative Period

When the operation is over, the child is weighed and transported to the recovery room where he is placed in a previously flushed, humidified oxygen tent or croupette. Then the drainage tubes are connected to a water-sealed suction drainage system, and a Foley catheter is placed in the bladder and connected to tubing which carries the urine into a bottle for careful measurement. While the patient is in the recovery room constant electrocardiograph and blood pressure recordings are made and observed constantly by a member of the medical staff. In most instances some type of cardiac monitoring is now being used.

This period is one of special threat for the child both physically and psychologically. In health, the outer covering of the body serves as a protective barrier against painful and frightening stimuli from the outer world. Upon responding after the effects of the anesthesia and sedatives have worn off, the child not only has strange body sensations and a changed body to cope with, but he is also confronted with a frightening new world. Even though he may have seen the recovery room before, he has had no opportunity to discover what really happens there. From the adult's point of view his immediate environment is protective, but to him it is full of peril. He cannot use motility as a defense against danger as he did before his operation because movement is painful and his critical state prevents it. Furthermore, he is trapped under an oxygen tent and his body is festooned with tubes and other apparatus. Nor can he get into the arms of his mother as he was accustomed to doing when he was a little child and frightened. The result of such circumstances is intolerable helplessness and anxiety. Being incapable of dealing actively with such an overwhelming accumulation of threats, massive regression and withdrawal result.

In the immediate postoperative period this state is beneficial because it gives the child the temporary retreat and protection needed for self-preservation. It allows the body to recoup its forces for physical adaptation to the changes within it. It also protects the child from feeling the full effects of surgical trauma, and from dealing with a frightening environment, until body integrity and security have been restored.

During the period of massive regression, most children become oblivious to what is going on around them and being done to them after their first intense reaction to their plight on regaining consciousness. Occasionally during the first postoperative evening they may manifest varying degrees of awareness of familiar persons and express their need for security by such appeals as "Stay with me," or by calling for their mother, but most of the time they make no overt response to care. They may resist being moved or try to fight against the positive-pressure mask or being suctioned, but resistance is feeble and lessens appreciably when they are forewarned of what is going to take place. Encouraging the child's retreat from the outer world by cutting down the glare of bright lights, eliminating needless noise and disturbing him as little as possible as the physically supportive measures listed below are carried out are other important means by which his trust can be regained.

1. Have the following equipment at bedside:
Oxygen tent and humidifier
Water-sealed suction apparatus
2 clear plastic Levin tubes
2 nasal oxygen catheters
1 tube Amphojel
Endotracheal tray
Tracheostomy set
Thoracentesis set
Intravenous solutions, sets and standards (2)
Positive-pressure machine

4 pointed glass connectors
2 small straight glass connectors
2 large straight glass connectors
Sterile instruments: 2 curved Halstead clamps; 2 Kelly clamps; knife handles No. 3, No. 4; knife blades No. 10, No. 20
1 jar Zephiran sponges
Emergency drugs, needles, syringes
Syringes: 10 cc. (3); 20 cc. (1); 5 cc. (6)
Needles: 5 No. 24; 3 No. 18; 6 No. 26; 6 No. 20
2 Jones snaps
2 mosquito clamps for use with intravenous apparatus
   Armboard, arm splints
   Sterile gloves (3), size 7½-8
Adhesive tape, bandage, tongue blades, ankle and wrist restraints, safety pins, 4x4 inch gauze (2 pkgs.), Band-Aids, mouth wipes.

2. Study the chart to learn the operative procedures which were carried out, the amount of blood, intravenous fluids and medications given during the operation, and the orders prescribed for the child's nursing care.

3. Check the intravenous apparatus frequently to make sure that fluid is flowing into the veins at the designated rate. This is especially important after the child's position has been changed because speed of flow can be rapidly increased as his extremities are moved. This is important in order to avoid overloading the circulatory system. On the hour the amount and the kind of fluid absorbed during the previous hour must be recorded. Observations must also be made to determine whether or not fluid is infiltrating into the tissues and to prevent kinking or compression of the intravenous tubing. Whenever fluid is added to the intravenous system, the time, the amount and the kind of fluid absorbed and begun must be recorded. An 8-hour and a 24-hour total of all fluid intake and output must be made.

4. Take vital signs hourly and more frequently if a change in condition warrants it. Notify the physician if the child's systolic blood pressure rises or falls more than 15 points and whenever there is marked change in the functioning of the heart or the lungs or in the child's temperature.

(a) Note the rate and the depth of respiration and whether or not chest expansion is equal on both sides.

(b) Observe the quality, the rate, the rhythm and the volume of the pulse. Compare the difference between the radial and the pedal pulse rates. Take the apical rate if there is a change in the rate, the rhythm or the quality of the radial pulse rate. When the Blalock-Taussig operation is performed, the radial pulse will be absent on the operative side.

(c) Notify the physician immediately if irregularity in pulse rate occurs simultaneously with a drop in blood pressure, because these symptoms forewarn of impending cardiac arrest.

(d) Observe for signs of neck vein distention which indicates overburdening of the circulatory system.

(e) Note the blood pressure as well as variations in it. (Use a cuff which covers ⅔ of the distance between the shoulder and the elbow.)

(f) Report immediately signs of hemorrhage (drop in blood pressure, rise in pulse and respiration rates, and extreme thirst).

(g) A subnormal temperature is expected in the immediate postoperative period. Unless there are orders to the contrary, the child's temperature should be allowed to return to normal without the application of external heat. After the temperature has returned to normal, adjust the amount of covering over the child to his body requirements. Give aspirin suppositories, alcohol sponges or use an ice-water mattress or hypothermic blanket as ordered by the doctor to reduce an elevated temperature which increases the metabolic rate and the speed of flow of blood through the body.

5. Examine the chest drainage apparatus to make sure that: (1) the tubing is long enough to allow for movement of the child; (2) there are no kinks in or pressure on the tubing at any time; (3) fluid in the tubing is fluctuating with respiration; (4) there is no bubbling or gross increase in the amount of drainage; (5) all tubing is securely taped to the glass connectors to prevent leakage; and (6) the drainage bottle and the bottle of water are securely fastened to the floor with adhesive tape or confined in a holder which prevents them from *being raised from below the lowest level of the child's chest.* Record the amount of drainage from the pleural cavity hourly and report immediately any bright blood. To ensure accurate readings a strip of adhesive tape can be placed vertically on the bottle for marking the hourly level of drainage. All blood lost from the chest cavity is usually replaced by transfusion. Keep 2 Jones clamps snapped to tape on the head of the bed for use in clamping the chest catheters near the child's body if any of the tubing should become disconnected or a drainage bottle breaks. Milk the chest tubes in the direction of the drainage bottles to clear the tubing of clots and pockets of serum if ordered.

6. Record hourly the amount of urine excreted through the Foley catheter. Note changes in color and notify the physician if no urine is excreted during a 2-hour period. Placement of a calibrated burette into the bladder drainage tubing lessens the burden of hourly measurement. Each hour the amount of urine can be ascertained before the spigot of the burette is turned to let the urine pass into a 24-hour urine bottle beneath the bed.

7. Support the child's chest firmly with both hands and encourage him to take deep breaths and to cough

every 2 hours. Coughing raises mucus, prevents mucous plugs from forming, increases intrapleural pressure and promotes drainage of air and lung expansion. A respirator may be used for intermittent positive pressure breathing. All signs of willingness to cooperate must be praised and patience exercised when the child is unresponsive to suggestions or too exhausted to participate. At these times, the physician must be informed so that he can ascertain the degree to which mucus is collecting in the respiratory tract.

8. Change the child's position hourly. After the first 24 hours, encourage the child to participate in turning to prevent fear of moving and self-imposed immobilization. Some increase in chest drainage can be expected after turning and coughing and also after removal of one of the chest tubes. Support the child's back and arms with pillows and keep his legs extended as much as possible to prevent contractures.

9. Keep the temperature in the oxygen tent between 66° and 70° F. except when there is a marked change in body temperature. At such times the temperature within the tent must be adjusted to meet the child's requirements. Keep the tent well tucked in around the mattress to prevent the escape of oxygen. Flow of oxygen into the tent is usually ordered at 8 to 10 liters per minute.

10. Keep steam vapor flowing into the tent constantly to make breathing easier and to prevent drying of mucus in the respiratory tract which can result in the necessity of tracheostomy.

11. Remove mucus from the respiratory tract. Lubricate the catheter with Amphojel or water, insert it through the nostril until it reaches the approximate level of the tracheal opening and manipulate the thumb for suctioning and for withdrawal of the catheter. Because the airway is occluded during suctioning and causes the feeling of suffocation, the catheter must be withdrawn quickly and a period of rest allowed before it is reinserted. Some physicians order suctioning at specific intervals. Others prefer that it is done only when rapid, noisy breathing indicates that there is an accumulation of mucus in the respiratory tract.

12. Give positive pressure as ordered to increase expansion of the lungs. Note change in color and depth of respiration during its administration.

13. Observe the color of the child's skin, nailbeds and earlobes and determine whether or not the skin is warm, dry, cold and clammy, or perspiring. A jaundiced hue to the skin can be expected from hemolysis of donor cells.

14. Observe the extremities during the first 2 postoperative days to detect blanching, cyanosis or coldness which may indicate the presence of thrombi in the arteries.

15. Examine the wounds to detect blood loss from them or around the insertion of the intravenous needles and to note any beginning signs of infection.

16. Observe for early signs of nausea. When these appear, turn the child on his side immediately. Record the amount and description of the vomitus.

17. Observe for abdominal distention and record the time when flatus is first expelled.

18. Report immediately such neurologic symptoms as: twitching or paralysis of the extremities, unusual irritability or restlessness, headache, dizziness, blurring of vision or irrational behavior.

19. Check vital signs and carry out all comforting measures to reduce anxiety before sedatives are given.

20. Begin exercising the child's arms and leg muscles on the second postoperative day to prevent thrombus formation and contractures. Telling the child that exercise will become less uncomfortable with each movement will make him less inclined to resist when it is first begun.

21. Take pulse and respiration rates before and after new activities such as a test period out of oxygen, dangling and placement in a wheel chair are carried out.

22. Prepare the following equipment for chest tube removal: stitch removal set, one set of Jones clamps, sterile petrolatum gauze, gauze squares, straight glass connector, nonwaterproof adhesive tape.

23. Prepare the following equipment for removal of the pacemaker wire from the heart muscle: stitch removal set, one No. 25 and one No. 26 needle, 2-cc. syringe, procaine 1 per cent, gauze squares, swabs, Merthiolate and adhesive tape.

24. Check vital signs hourly for 8 hours after the chest tube and the pacemaker wire are removed.

Care During the Period of Infantile Dependence

The period of massive regression is followed by one in which there is a gradual return to full awareness of a changed body and the world surrounding it. During infancy the child signaled his need for relief of bodily tension by crying. Physical contact with his mother's body and food relieved his discomfort. Therefore, it is natural that he resort to old patterns of behavior when he longs for cuddling again. It can be expected that he will call for food and physical comforts—the unconscious symbols of love—to express his need for relief of discomfort. (Children must do something to relieve their tension. After major surgery they do not have the energy to read or play and if their bodies are painful, moving about in bed is frightening. Lying inert puts undue strain on their bodies.) The type of nursing care which communicates "you will not be abandoned"* is necessary to help the child to regain trust in his own capacity to

---

* This is most difficult to achieve unless the nurse is assisted by a mother who is prepared to provide comforting physical contact, or by a second nurse in whom the child has confidence. Many of the procedures which are necessary to protect the child physically take a great deal of the nurse's time, preventing her from concentrating on meeting the child's need for physical and emotional closeness to a person.

deal with threats. Understanding the origin of the child's demanding attitude in his attempt to cope with frustration of his wish for cuddling supports him in acquiring the courage to face the treatment regimen. Without this support from his parents and nurses, mistrust, mounting anxiety and retreat from the world may be prolonged and depleting.

Care During the Period of Struggle to Regain Autonomy

As recovery takes place, the demands made on the child's fortitude do not lessen; rather, they increase. He not only has to undergo the repetition of uncomfortable known procedures, but he also is confronted with new ones, such as removal of drainage tubes, intravenous needles, stitches and the wire which was implanted into his myocardium. When intravenous fluid, nutrient and antibiotic administration is discontinued he has to have additional intramuscular injections of antibiotics. He is also expected to take more fluids by mouth. Under such circumstances feelings of rebellion, helplessness and despair are bound to arise.

How the child reacts to this situation depends on various considerations discussed earlier in this book. The natural healthy response is to fight for control of it. Such a child is not afraid to ask questions or express himself. He may devise rituals, as in his past quest for autonomy. He may become dictatorial in order to restore his self-esteem and assert his right of independence. (This is especially true of the adolescent.) In addition he will work hard to gain self-mastery in play when he has energy for it.

Physical debilitation not only prevents the child from actively upholding his self-esteem but also weakens his defenses against anxiety. This state of affairs frightens the child and increases his helplessness. The result may be that he lapses into a state of resignation, and it is vitally important that the nurse help to prevent this. The most effective means for doing this is to make use of the child's own powers to gain control of the situation—to encourage him to assert himself. In so doing the nurse in effect tells him that she values his efforts and respects him as someone with a mind of his own. It also supports his efforts to re-establish his identity and to regain the autonomy he lost when the anesthetic was begun. With this accomplished, the child usually regains his physical strength quickly and begins to focus on adjusting himself to his wounds. Very soon after this he also will have energy available for reconquering the negative counterparts of the other core problems he had faced prior to his operation.

Care During Convalescence

This is a transitional period marking the child's progress from a state of acute illness and helplessness to physical recovery and further assimilation of the experiences he has endured. In this period, activity is usually unrestricted, but, even then, waiting to go home poses problems for the child. The child who has regained his physical strength, trust and autonomy and re-established his identity earlier, anticipates new experiences. He signals his readiness to do more for himself and to share his nurse with other children and to play with them.

Many mothers have difficulty in relinquishing the pleasure that they derived from overprotectiveness. Time must be allowed for them to prove to themselves that their children have become capable of increased activity, of learning to care for themselves and of tolerating increasingly larger doses of frustration. With reassurance by a trusted person and help in seeing their child's freedom from signs of overexertion during periods of self-directed play, most mothers conquer their fears and find substitute statisfactions for those that they enjoyed when their children were more dependent on them. However, if there is no progress in this direction, referral to a social worker is usually indicated.

SITUATIONS FOR FURTHER STUDY

1. Read the articles by Barton and Bear cited in the bibliography and discuss the ways in which Kathy was prepared for an open-heart operation. What preparation would you need to succeed in helping a child to face his operation?

2. What reasons might a mother have for not visiting her child during the period when he is being prepared for open-heart surgery and on the first few postoperative days?

3. What help could a mother be to her child in the days following open-heart surgery? How would you prepare her to give this help?

4. What help do you think parents would need when they visit their child initially after he has had open-heart surgery? What preparation would you need to give this help?

5. When caring for a child during the first 8 postoperative hours after an open-heart operation, what physical and behavioral signs would indicate the child's need for the physician immediately?

6. In what ways does knowing how the heart-lung machine functions help you in providing care for a child with repair of an interventricular septal defect?

7. What would be your goals of nursing care of a 5-year-old boy after repair of an interventricular septal defect during the period he was becoming aware of the treatment regimen and the changes which had been made in his body?

8. What might be the consequences if a 4-year-old girl sensed that her nurse could not accept self-assertion and expression of feeling about the care she was receiving after her heart defect was repaired? Became anxious whenever she was aggressive with her dolls?

BIBLIOGRAPHY

Adams, J. G., Jr.: Hyperbaric oxygen therapy, Am. J. Nurs. *64*:76, 1964.

Adriani, J.: Anaesthesia for infants and children, Am. J. Nurs. *64*:107, 1964.

Bailey, T. F.: Puppets teach young patients, Nurs. Outlook *15*:36, 1967.

Barnes, C.: Working with parents of children undergoing heart surgery, Nurs. Clin. N. Am. *4*:11, 1969.

Barton, P. H.: Play as a tool in nursing, Nurs. Outlook *10*:162, 1962.

Bear, E. M.: Operation—"open heart," Nurs. Outlook *10*:158, 1962.

Belling, D.: Complications after open heart surgery, Nurs. Clin. N. Am. *4*:123, 1969.

Betson, C., Valoon, P., and Soika, C.: Cardiac surgery in neonates: a chance for life, Am. J. Nurs. *69*:69, 1969.

Creighton, H., and Richard, Sister Gabriella: When you are scared, Am. J. Nurs. *63*:61, 1963.

Dumas, R., and Leonard, R.: The effect of nursing on the incidence of post-operative vomiting, Nurs. Res. *12*:12, 1963.

George, J. H.: Electronic monitoring of vital signs, Am. J. Nurs. *65*:68, 1965.

Gillon, J.: Continuity in nursing care of cardiac infants, Nurs. Clin. N. Am. *4*:19, 1969.

Gross, R. E.: Surgery of Infancy and Childhood, Philadelphia, Saunders, 1958.

Hammes, H. J.: Reflections on "intensive" care, Am. J. Nurs. *68*:339, 1968.

Hickey, M. C.: Hypothermia, Am. J. Nurs. *65*:116, 1965.

Honamey, R.: Teaching patients breathing and coughing techniques, Nurs. Outlook *13*:58, 1965.

James, E. E.: The nursing care of the open heart patient, Nurs. Clin. N. Am. *2*:543, 1967.

Lillehei, C. W., and Engel, Leonard: Open heart surgery, Sci. Am. *202*:75, 1960.

McBride, M. A.: Nursing approach, pain and relief: an exploratory experiment, Nurs. Res. *16*:337, 1967.

Merrow, D., and Johnson, B. S.: Perceptions of the mother's role with her hospitalized child, Nurs. Res. *17*:155, 1968.

Minckley, B. B.: A study of noise and its relationship to patient discomfort in the recovery room, Nurs. Res. *17*:247, 1968.

Nadas, A. S.: Pediatric Cardiology, Philadelphia, Saunders, 1963.

Oestreich, P.: Children's reactions to cardiac catheterization: play interviews and interpretation, Nurs. Clinics of N. Am. *4*:3, 1969.

Peay, R.: The emotional problems of children facing heart surgery, Children *7*:223, 1960.

Pitorak, E. F.: Open-ended care for the open heart patient, Am. J. Nurs. *67*:1452, 1967.

Potts, W. J.: The Surgeon and the Child, Philadelphia, Saunders, 1959.

Rasof, B., Linde, L. M., and Dunn, O. J.: Intellectual development in children with congenital heart disease, Child Development, *38*:1043, 1967.

Rawlings, M. S.: Heart disease today, Am. J. Nurs. *66*:303, 1966.

Roe, N. M.: Caring for patients following open heart surgery, Am. J. Nurs. *63*:77, 1963.

Roy, Sister Mary Callista: Role cues and mothers of hospitalized children, Nurs. Res. *16*:178, 1967.

Stanley-Brown, E. G.: Pediatric Surgery for Nurses, Philadelphia, Saunders, 1961.

Watson, H. T.: The role of the school nurse in support of children with certain cardiovascular disorders, Nurs. Clin. N. Am. *1*:31, 1966.

Ziegler, R. F.: Electrocardiographic Studies in Normal Children and Infants, Springfield, Ill., Thomas, 1951.

Congenital Heart Abnormalities (Nursing Ed. Series, Pamphlet No. 7), Columbus, Ohio, Ross Laboratories, 1961.

If Your Child Has a Congenital Heart Defect (pamphlet), American Heart Association, 44 E. 23rd St., New York 10, New York.

23

Nursing Care of Children With Metabolic Disorders

MALABSORPTION SYNDROMES

In 1889 Gee described a clinical condition which he called celiac disease. The combination of chronic or recurrent fatty diarrhea, poor growth, distention of the abdomen, malnutrition and vitamin deficiencies is now recognized as the hallmark of a number of conditions in which there is difficulty with absorption of foods from the intestinal tract. The most common of these, cystic fibrosis of the pancreas, has been considered in Chapter 13. The other member of the group which is encountered with some frequency is gluten-induced enteropathy which is also called the celiac syndrome and which is described below. Brief statements about the less common forms of malabsorption are also given. A more detailed discussion of these disorders must be sought in the references given in the bibliography.

Gluten-induced Enteropathy (Celiac Disease)

Pathophysiology. The tendency for this disorder to occur in more than one individual in a family suggests that the basic mechanism is inherited. Following certain triggering incidents, susceptible individuals lose their ability to absorb carbohydrate and fat from the intestinal tract at the normal rate. The triggering incidents may be parenteral infection, dietary deficiency or psychologic disturbances. Thereafter, continued ingestion of wheat or rye which contains the offending protein, gluten, is followed by retention of carbohydrates and fats in the intestinal lumen. This in turn leads to abdominal distention; to chronic diarrhea with bulky, greasy stools which float; to progressive malnutrition due to failure to utilize ingested calories; and, in longstanding cases, to deficiency of absorption of vitamin D, producing rickets or tetany. Crises associated with electrolyte imbalance, rapid dehydration and severe acidosis may also occur.

Improved recognition and early treatment of this disorder has led to a marked decline in its incidence in severe form in areas where pediatric care is good. The disorder tends to be self-limited, so that even a poorly treated child who survives will eventually outgrow the disorder and those under proper therapy can expect to have a gradual relaxation of dietary restrictions.

Symptoms. The disease seldom begins before about 6 months of age and is most common during the toddler age period. It is of slow onset, and marked by poor weight gain, abdominal distention, loss of fat depots, particularly in the area of the buttocks, by irritability, anemia, and chronic or recurrent diarrhea. The stools are watery during episodes of acute diarrhea; bulky, fatty and float on the surface in the toilet bowl during intervening periods.

Diagnosis. After other possibilities have been ruled out—particularly cystic fibrosis and infectional diarrhea—the finding from laboratory studies of a marked increase in the fat content of the stools and a decrease in the ability to absorb sugars as demonstrated by abnormal glucose or xylose tolerance tests, adds nonspecific suspicion to the nature of the disorder. The only positive proof is obtained by eliminating wheat and rye protein from the diet and producing a remission of symptoms. Foods which have had these proteins added must also be eliminated.

Treatment. In addition to the dietary measures noted above, the vitamin requirements must be met by the addition of water-miscible vitamins A and D in at least double the usual protective quantity. A high caloric intake should also be offered in skimmed milk, banana, and protein foods other than wheat and rye. Such a diet will usually be necessary for a period of 6 months to a year before tolerance for other foods is regained.

During episodes of acute diarrhea, dehydration and acidosis must be combated in the same fashion as for acute diarrhea from other causes. Attention to the emotional climate around the child is likewise of great importance.

Nursing Care of the Child with Celiac Disease. The child with celiac disease is malnourished, anemic and his appetite may be capricious. Feeding experiences should be thoughtfully managed with understanding of the child's feelings pertaining to food deprivation. Foods should be given slowly in small amounts and with no attempt to force him to take what he does not want. As the dietary regimen is instituted, marked change in digestion and desire for food will be noted. The kinds and the amounts of food eaten and the child's behavior during feeding should be recorded. After the initial period when new foods are added to the diet, the stools, the degree of abdominal distention and the child's disposition should be noted to determine the tolerance to each one. Stools must be described accurately, for they are a guide in prescribing the diet. Should symptoms of indigestion be

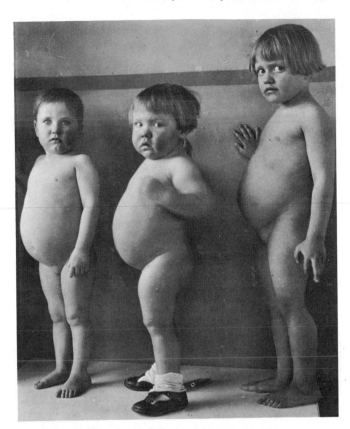

Fig. 23-2. Three children with celiac disease who are making good growth progress under treatment.

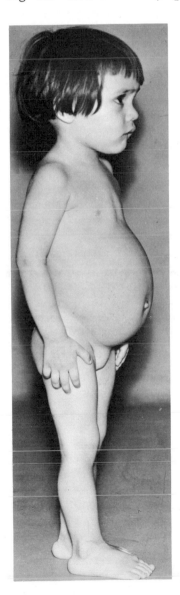

Fig. 23-1. Celiac disease showing protuberant abdomen.

increased, the new food should be eliminated temporarily from the diet. Although appetite may increase markedly, new foods should be limited in quantity, because hastily introduced foods increase bulk and do little to improve the child's nutritional state unless his digestive capacity has improved.

When the child is hungry and is deprived of food, he will react angrily. Some children develop anorexia and vomiting. The child with celiac disease needs freedom to complain because this will minimize withdrawal symptoms. Babies express their fury by crying or incessant whining. The older child puts his anger into words if he knows that his nurse can accept them.

Because of anemia and lowered physical resistance, the child with celiac disease must be protected from infections. His temperature is often subnormal and his extremities are cold; hence, he must be dressed appropriately. Since he perspires freely and tends to lie in one position, he is prone to develop respiratory infections which increase his indigestion. Careful personal hygiene and frequent changes in positioning are therefore important in nursing care.

For diagnostic purposes the proportion of ingested fat excreted in the stools is determined while the child is receiving a diet with an amount of fat customary for a normal child. Such a study may be made for a period of 24 hours or longer. During the period chosen, the amounts and the kinds of foods eaten are recorded accurately. The beginning of the stool collection period is marked by passage in the stool of carmine given previously by mouth. The dye is tasteless and can be given in a portion of the milk; the time of ingestion of the carmine must be recorded. Beginning with the first appearance of the dye, all stools are saved until the carmine appears again after ingestion of a second capsule given exactly 24 hours, or other longer time period chosen, after ingestion of the first. The stools should be placed in a covered container in a laboratory refrigerator. The normal child excretes approximately 10 per cent of the ingested fat that is in the diet, while the child with celiac disease may excrete as much as from 50 to 70 per cent or even more.

In celiac disease, irritability usually accompanies symptoms of indigestion. The older child may be withdrawn, depressed and unable to play actively. Former pleasures, such as thumb-sucking and dependence on certain objects or toys may be frequently noted. The nurse who is patient and understanding of mood changes and regressive behavior can add materially to emotional satisfactions. Gradually, as he begins to gain weight and his physical condition improves, he will evidence interest in his surroundings and a desire for increased stimulation. His dependence on infantile satisfactions will decrease as he finds satisfactions in play and in his relationship with others.

Since the period of medical supervision is a long one, the mother must understand the child's dietary regimen, his need for general hygienic measures to prevent infection and the necessity for follow-up medical examinations. Before the child leaves the hospital, the nurse can emphasize these points in her contacts with the mother, and initiate contact with the community health nurse. With good supervision and care, most of these children can recover completely.

The nurse can include several practical suggestions for making the child's life more pleasant. For example, he may be deeply resentful of being deprived of foods which others about him are enjoying. Cookies can be made of dried fruit or egg whites and artificial sweetening. Ice cream and cakes can be made of gelatin. Diabetic candies, while not as tasty as those made with sugar, nevertheless can do much for the child's morale.

It would be wise for the nurse to sound the mother out to determine whether there may be special problems from her standpoint. If there has been a history of difficult feeding experiences since the child's birth, having the child follow the new dietary regimen will not be easy. Also, if the mother has believed herself to be somehow responsible for the child's condition, she may have tried to compensate through overprotection.

Other Forms of Malabsorption Syndrome

Postsurgical Malabsorption. If it becomes necessary to resect a portion of the small intestine because of disease, or to make a bypassing operation, the amount of absorptive surface left may be insufficient for the child's nutritional needs and a celiac-like disorder requiring permanent dietary management may ensue.

Obstruction of Intestinal Lymphatics. When intestinal parasites such as *giardia lamblia* or invasive disease such as Hodgkin's disease or abdominal tuberculosis interfere with the flow of lymph from the intestinal wall, malabsorption may result and the child may present the symptoms of the celiac syndrome.

Idiopathic Steatorrhea. The passage of fatty stools with other manifestations of the celiac syndrome is sometimes unresponsive to removal of gluten from the diet and is presumably due to some other, as yet undetermined cause.

Disaccharidase Deficiency. In recent years, inherited defects in the intestinal enzymes which split the double sugars such as lactose, sucrose, fructose and maltose have been found to be an explanation for chronic diarrhea with failure to thrive. Normally, the disaccharides are split by enzymes present within cells of the intestinal mucosa and the resulting monosaccharides are then readily absorbed. Interference with this process results in an accumulation of the double sugars within the intestine which leads to fermentation by bacteria and irritation of the intestine. These disorders are more characteristic of infants during the first year of life. They respond to diets lacking in those sugars which cannot be metabolized.

DISTURBANCES OF RENAL FUNCTION

In some respects, nephritis of children differs much from that of adults. The child's kidneys have a power of regeneration after injury far greater than do those of the adult. The commonest type of nephritis in childhood (acute glomerular) is the least common among adults and is the most benign of all the varieties. Nephritis of the older person is likely to be complicated by degenerative changes, whereas such changes are not common in childhood. Pure nephrosis that is fully reparable seems to occur only in children. Nephrosis of adults is usually a part of chronic nephritis which ultimately leads to irreparable and fatal kidney damage. Those classifications dealing with adults largely or exclusively are likely to contain statements concerning nephritis which are wholly true for adults but do not apply to children.

Acute Glomerular Nephritis (Acute Hemorrhagic Nephritis)

Acute glomerulonephritis is characterized by changes in the glomerular capillaries which permit the passage of blood cells and protein into the glomerular filtrate.

The finding of blood in the urine is a constant feature of the disease. Associated changes in other parts of the body are commonly but not necessarily present. These include edema, hypertension, azotemia and the secondary phenomena which may result from them.

Pathophysiology. This variety of nephritis is also called postinfection nephritis because it is invariably preceded by an infection with beta-hemolytic streptococci of Group A. It is now recognized that a few of the more than 40 different types of such streptococci are much more likely to produce nephritic complications than are other members of the group. (Types 4, 12, 25 and 45 are mainly responsible.) The site of infection is not in the kidney but rather in the upper respiratory tract, most frequently in the tonsils and adjacent lymph nodes. Scarlet fever, which is also a streptococcal sore throat in essence, may be the initiating disease. Less commonly, nephritis follows streptococcal infections of the skin—impetigo, burns, eczema or scabies.

Presumably, the strains of streptococci responsible for nephritis contain antigens similar to those of basement membrane of the renal glomeruli. The body then makes antibody not only against the invading streptococci, but also against the glomerular tissues. The resultant inflammatory reaction in the kidney is a response to antigen-antibody combination. The blood vessels of the body generally may also be involved with a loss of capillary integrity and spasm of arterioles secondary to the changes taking place in the kidney.

Symptoms. Nephritis may occur at any age but is most common in the toddler and preschool or early school-age group. When the onset of the preceding streptococcal infection can be dated, a latent period of 1 to 3 weeks ensues before the appearance of symptoms of nephritis. Undoubtedly, many children have such mild nephritis that their disease goes completely unrecognized. Usually, the initial symptoms are puffiness of the face or grossly bloody urine, or headache and vomiting. These symptoms may occur alone or in combination. Occasionally, the disease is announced by dyspnea due to impending heart failure. Oliguria is frequent but transient; anuria occurs rarely. Later in the disease, chronic fatigue, anemia and malnutrition may constitute the chief symptoms.

In the majority of affected children the symptoms rapidly reach their maximum intensity and trail off within a week or two, leaving the child symptomatically well but with evidence of the continuing disease apparent in various laboratory tests. Azotemia is seldom responsible for symptoms unless its severity is sufficient to produce uremia. The chief mechanism responsible for the symptomatology is the consequence of a general vascular disturbance which leads to edema and spasm of arterioles. Combined with hypertension, these processes lead to varying degrees of cerebral edema and myocardial insufficiency. Occasionally in children serious or even fatal complications ensue—hypertensive encephalopathy with convulsions or coma, or congestive heart failure.

Diagnosis. Usually, the history and the symptoms alone strongly suggest the diagnosis. Examination of the urine should disclose red blood cells, albumin and casts. If the casts contain red blood cells, there is no doubt about the diagnosis. Hypertension and azotemia may or may not be present. Renal biopsy is seldom necessary to confirm the diagnosis.

Prognosis. Recovery from acute glomerulonephritis is to be expected in nearly all children. Even among those in whom the disease is severe enough to require hospitalization, more than 85 per cent recover completely. Mild illnesses last as little as 2 to 3 weeks; in the more obstinate cases evidence of continuing renal disease may last from 1 to 2 years before recovery takes place. In exceptional instances the disease is progressive and takes on the characteristics of chronic nephritis. A small number of children succumb to the early effects of hypertensive encephalopathy or heart failure.

Treatment. INFECTION. Although antibiotic therapy is of no avail in the treatment of the nephritis itself, complete eradication of the beta-hemolytic streptococcus infection which preceded should be assured through the use of penicillin.

BED REST. During the acute stage and for as long as hypertension persists or appreciable amounts of blood appear in the urine, the child should be kept at bed rest. If the disease is prolonged and enters a subacute stage in which there are minimal findings in the urine, the child may be allowed complete activity but should be protected from further infection and from chilling, which seems to reactivate the nephritic process.

DIET. Contrary to previous belief, the diet need not be restricted in respect to protein but should contain a full complement of all nutrients as soon as the appetite returns. In the presence of edema, salt intake usually is restricted. Except during evidence of cardiac failure no fluid restrictions need be imposed.

CARDIAC FAILURE. The management of cardiac failure is essentially the same as described in Chapter 22. Morphine, oxygen and digitalis may be required. Diuretics are contraindicated in the presence of nephritis.

HYPERTENSION. The control of hypertension is a very important aspect of treatment. Magnesium sulfate may be given for this purpose by mouth, intramuscularly or intravenously, depending on the severity of the cerebral symptoms. Prevention of convulsions is highly desirable, so that oral administration of a 50 per cent solution in doses of 1 or 2 ounces usually is given as soon as appreciable elevation of the blood pressure is detected. The drug has surprisingly little cathartic action during the course of nephritis. The rectal route may be substituted for the oral if vomiting is present or if the child refuses to take the medication. At higher levels of blood pressure, magnesium sulfate is given intramuscularly in a 50 per cent solution at a dosage of about 0.2 ml. per Kg. of body weight. If symptoms are severe or other forms of administration have been ineffective, the drug may be given slowly intravenously in a 2 per cent solution at a dosage of 10 ml. per Kg. Overdosage with magnesium sulfate may produce respiratory depression, which can be counteracted by intravenous administration of a soluble calcium solution which should be readily available whenever intramuscular or intravenous treatment is being employed.

A combination of hydralazine (Apresoline) by intramuscular injection of 0.1 mg./Kg. and reserpine

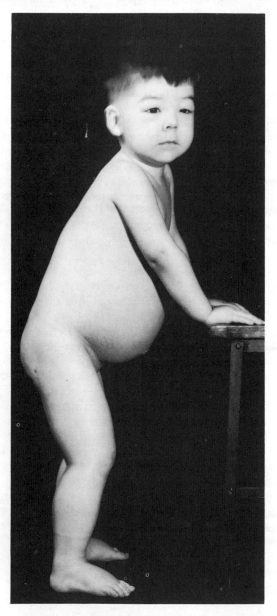

Fig. 23-3. The nephrotic syndrome showing generalized edema and the pendulous abdomen full of fluid.

0.07 mg./Kg. will often relieve hypertension and is preferred by some to the use of magnesium sulfate. The dose may be repeated after 12 hours or may be continued by mouth if thought necessary.

The use of steroids in acute nephritis has been found to be generally ineffective and sometimes harmful.

Nursing Care. During the acute stage, when rest in bed is required, play activities should be provided in order to keep the child occupied and in contact with his environment. The blood pressure should be observed at intervals throughout the day and night and any elevation reported immediately. Should this occur, increased observation is indicated to detect cerebral changes and cribsides or a crib bed should be provided for his protection. Equipment to give magnesium sulfate intravenously and intramuscularly should be in readiness in the child's room.

When complete activity is permitted, the child should be dressed warmly enough to prevent chilling and protected from contact with other children or adults with infections. Appetite can be stimulated through special attention to the preparation and serving of meals and to the child's individual food preferences.

The Nephrotic Syndrome
(Nephrosis, Lipid Nephrosis)

The nephrotic syndrome is a clinical condition characterized by generalized edema, often with anasarca, by proteinuria of marked degree, by lowering of the plasma proteins primarily in the albumin fraction, and by an elevation of the blood lipids including cholesterol.

Etiology. The most common or classical form of nephrosis in childhood arises without relation to any known causative agent and is called *idiopathic nephrosis,* signifying that its etiology remains obscure. Experimental and clinical observations have accumulated a number of bits of evidence which suggest that it is an abnormal immune response to chemical substances, tissue antigens, or both. However, no completely satisfactory theory to explain its genesis has yet been devised.

Less frequently in children, the nephrotic syndrome may occur in association with certain diseases—amyloidosis, disseminated lupus erythematosus, diabetes, syphilis, renal vein thrombosis, chronic glomerulonephritis. It may also follow the toxic effects of mercury, Tridione, penicillamine or a bee sting. The relation of these forms of nephrosis to the more common idiopathic variety is still obscure.

Pathophysiology. Kidney biopsy during the initial stages of nephrosis shows minimal changes in the glomeruli and tubules under ordinary light microscopy. However, in the greater details which can be observed with the electron microscope, a characteristic lesion of the foot processes of the glomerular epithelium is regularly observed. The extent of the enlargement and smudging of these processes correlates fairly well with the extent to which the patient is losing protein in the urine. As proteinuria progresses, the plasma proteins decrease and the blood loses some of its ability to hold fluid within the vascular compartments by osmotic pressure. At the same time the passage of water into the interstitial spaces and the peritoneal cavity is increased by overproduction of aldosterone, an adrenal hormone which increases the retention of sodium within the body.

Symptoms. Edema. The disease usually appears insidiously without any antecedent infection, beginning as the slow, asymptomatic accumulation of edema, which is noticed first about the eyes. As the swelling advances, it may involve the legs, the arms and the back to varying degrees (Fig. 23-3). Accumulation of fluid in the peritoneal cavity and the scrotum is frequent. Shifting of the edematous areas is common, depending to some extent on the position of the child during sleep or during waking activity. With moderate stretching of the skin over the subcutaneous fluid, there is pronounced pallor which is out of proportion to the degree of anemia; with severe degrees of edema, striae may appear from overstretching— striae which simulate those seen on the abdomen of the pregnant woman.

Malnutrition. Excessive fluid accumulations impede activity and appetite and may embarrass respirations by limiting the excursion of the diaphragm. As the disease continues, inapparent malnutrition takes place, which is revealed clearly only when diuresis and loss of subcutaneous edema occur.

Anemia. Anemia of moderate degree usually appears during the course of the illness.

Resistance. Poor resistance to infection is characteristic. Before modern chemotherapy, death occurred in a considerable proportion of children with nephrosis because of the ravages of septicemia, peritonitis and meningitis. Formerly, streptococci and pneumococci were usually responsible for these severe infections; more recently, there has been an increasing prevalence of other organisms.

Nephrotic Crisis. A nephrotic crisis simulates peritonitis by producing abdominal pain, fever and sometimes an erysipeloid skin eruption. These events may occur without demonstrable infection. They usually subside within a few days and may be followed by a spontaneous diuresis.

When the course of nephrosis is complicated by one of the contagious diseases such as measles or chickenpox, spontaneous diuresis and loss of edema may result. Although the remission is ordinarily temporary, occasionally it is permanent.

Laboratory Findings. Urine. In the urine the constant findings are those of heavy albuminuria with casts and white blood cells. Red cells may appear transiently, in small amounts persistently, or in larger numbers when the disease is changing its characteristics toward those of chronic nephritis. The urea clearance test of kidney function is commonly normal, sometimes supernormal. Lipid granules are almost always present in the urine and aid in diagnosis of the disease.

Blood. The changes in the blood involve the proteins and the lipids. There is a reduction in total protein level from the usual 6 to 8 Gm. per cent to less than 4 Gm. per cent. Most of this reduction is in the albumin fraction, which may be reduced to less than 1 Gm. per cent. Gamma-globulin is also reduced. The levels of blood lipids, including cholesterol, are usually at least double the normal values and frequently produce a cloudy appearance of the blood plasma when it separates. During active stages of disease the sedimentation rate is greatly increased.

Course and Prognosis. The course of nephrosis invariably is prolonged unless death occurs from an early complication. Few children endure a course that is less than 18 months. During this period there may be fluctuations in the severity of symptoms, even to the extent of complete remission. With modern protection against infection and suppression of proteinuria by steroid therapy, as many as 75 to 80 per cent of children with the idiopathic form of the disease can eventually expect a favorable outcome.

Treatment. At best, the management of nephrosis is a long-term problem which must be continued for years. Parents must be aware that immediate success in reversing the symptoms does not mean that the disease is permanently gone. Optimism is justified but the necessity for attention to detail and for prolonged supervision must be stressed. While some children who are protected from infection and given symptomatic relief from excessive accumulations of fluid can be expected to have a spontaneous remission of the disease in 1 to 2 years, steroid therapy will increase the percentage of eventual cures and will shorten the period of invalidism.

Steroids are usually given in heavy dosage to produce a diuresis once the diagnosis has been made. Prednisone or its equivalent in dosage of 30 to 80 mg. per day depending upon the age of the child is given orally in 4 evenly spaced doses. Diuresis is usually produced within 10 to 14 days but steroid treatment is continued until the sedimentation rate returns to normal, protein disappears from the urine, and the serum albumin level rises. When this point is reached, usually in 3 to 4 weeks, the steroid dosage is tapered rapidly and replaced by intermittent therapy, either every other day or three days in the week. Either hospital or home testing of urine for protein is continued in order to identify a relapse, for if this occurs full steroid dosage must be resumed. After the child has been free of proteinuria for several months, progressive slow reduction in dosage may be attempted.

Antibiotics are generally given to protect the child against bacterial infection since his already low resistance is further depleted by the administration of steroids. Although most of the bacterial agents to which he is susceptible are sensitive to penicillin, a broad spectrum antibiotic such as a tetracycline, sulfonamides, or ampicillin is preferable in order to cover the possibility of infection with gram-negative bacilli. Once the active stage of the disease has been brought under control by steroids or by spontaneous remission, the necessity for prophylactic antibiotics is less urgent.

Antihypertensives may be required if the blood pressure rises during the early treatment with large doses of steroids. The same therapy as for acute hemorrhagic nephritis may be used.

Potassium is usually given during the time of diuresis in order to protect the child from hypokalemia.

Diuretics have generally been found to be ineffectual in nephrosis and are now used mainly as a last resort when proper steroid therapy fails. In unrelieved anasarca it may be necessary to remove fluid from the peritoneal cavity by paracentesis if the discomfort is too great or respirations are compromised.

During the edematous stage of the disease the child's appetite is generally poor and the *diet* cannot be well regulated. With remission of his disease and return of appetite it is desirable to offer a high protein, high caloric diet to permit restoration of lost plasma and tissue proteins as rapidly as possible. The restriction of salt in the diet is not generally necessary and only serves to decrease its palatability.

Exercise need not be restricted. The child should actually be encouraged to do whatever he can unless he is in a period of hypertension. Both within the hospital and at home, permission to do as much as he is able is often an important morale booster.

When the usual therapeutic measures fail to produce a remission of the disease within a reasonable time, other measures may be tried such as the use of intravenous salt-poor albumin to increase the oncotic pressure of the plasma; or immunosuppressive drugs such as nitrogen mustard, chlorambucil, or some of the agents used in the treatment of leukemia.

Nursing Care. The supportive care of a child with nephrosis is highly important. During the stage when edema is present, the appetite is poor and malnutrition and anemia may be hidden. Frequently the child's appetite is stimulated by serving small quantities of special-diet foods initially, by attractive tray arrangements and by permitting the child additional amounts at his discretion. Catering thus to a capricious appetite the child may be encouraged to eat food that is necessary for his maintenance and final recovery.

During periods of marked edema, close observation of the child's entire body is necessary and areas of transient edema should be carefully noted. Meticulous care of the skin and frequent changes in body position are important to prevent tissue breakdown. When the external male genitalia are extremely edematous, special local care becomes necessary. The genitalia should be bathed several times daily and dusted with a soothing powder. The scrotum should be supported by a cotton pad held in place by a T-binder lightly applied. Cotton to separate the skin surfaces will prevent intertrigo. When the child is lying on his side, pressure on the edematous organs can be eliminated by placing a pillow between his knees. When edema of the eyelids is marked, circulation of lacrimal secretion over the eyes is impaired. Warm saline irrigations can be used to keep the eyes free from exudate. By maintaining head elevation during parts of the day, eyelid edema can be minimized.

The child should be weighed 2 or 3 times weekly to note changes in the degree of edema. Accurate records should be kept of intake and output.

As a result of the disease process, the restriction of usual activities and because of the administration of steroids, the child with nephrosis may be irritable or appear demanding. The mood swings accompanying medication may be bewildering and challenging to the nurse's ingenuity. A balanced, planned program of rest, quiet activities and recreation designed to stimulate normal mental and emotional growth is an important part of the nursing care plan. Other comfort measures and efforts designed to maintain the child's tie to his parents and home have been discussed previously and are particularly important to the child with long-term illness.

Every effort must be made to avoid respiratory infections. The child with nephrosis must be protected from other children and adults with any infectious process.

When ascites is present to a marked degree, *abdominal paracentesis* is required to relieve the pressure symptoms. If the child knows that the discomfort of the procedure will be less than the discomfort from the collection of fluid in his abdominal cavity, he usually will cooperate and assist by maintaining quiet during the procedure.

Puncturing the bladder during the paracentesis should be avoided by having the child void just prior to the treatment.

Sterile equipment required for an abdominal paracentesis consists of hypodermic syringe, hypodermic and aspiration needles, procaine (Novocain), scalpel, cannula, trocar, rubber tubing, needleholder, suture needles, sutures, forceps, gloves, towels, graduated receptacle, cotton balls, gauze squares and an abdominal dressing.

Unsterile equipment consists of a preparation tray, test tubes, a pail for the collection of fluid, a scultetus or abdominal binder and safety pins.

Two nurses are required to assist in this procedure. One nurse prepares the area, collects samples of ascitic fluid for culture and checks the child's pulse, respirations and color during the procedure. The second nurse is responsible for maintaining the child's position close to the edge of the examining table. When the child's cooperation has been secured through careful preparation, no restraint is necessary. Satisfactory position usually can be maintained if the nurse stands behind the child, supports his back with her body and clasps his hands which are held at his side.

After the doctor has anesthetized the area with procaine and has made a small incision through the skin, he inserts the cannula and the trocar until fluid begins to flow from the peritoneal cavity. Then he attaches the rubber tubing to the cannula, regulates the flow to prevent sudden withdrawal of fluid and directs the flow into the graduated receptacle. Sudden and too rapid withdrawal of fluid reduces intra-abdominal pressure, causes the blood to distend the deep abdominal veins and reduces the normal supply of blood in the heart. If too much fluid is withdrawn, symptoms of shock develop. When sufficient fluid has been withdrawn to reduce pressure symptoms, the cannula is removed, sutures are taken, and the area is cleansed with alcohol and covered with a dressing. After a scultetus or an abdominal binder has been applied snugly, the child is returned to his bed. After the treatment, the amount of drainage from the wound and the child's condition should be observed and charted.

For most and sometimes all of the long period of illness, these children have no prostration or discomfort. When the degree of edema lessens and the child is permitted to be out of bed, activities in a playroom will be enjoyed and will contribute toward making his hospital stay constructive.

Before the child is discharged from the hospital, parental guidance will be necessary to ensure adequate continued care. The mother should be given complete information concerning the child's diet, the measures necessary to prevent upper respiratory infections and the need for continued medical supervision.

Chronic Nephritis

Chronic nephritis (chronic glomerular nephritis) is a terminal illness which is the result of progressive destruction of nephrons, leading to severe loss of renal function. Although the clinical manifestations are fairly uniform, the avenues by which individual children enter are diverse.

Etiology. There is no uniformity of opinion about the etiology of chronic nephritis, and it is probable that the term encompasses the end result of several different disease entities. Some children are discovered to have well-advanced chronic nephritis without having suffered any recognizable renal disease previously. Others first pass through a period of nephrosis which gradually changes over to chronic nephritis. A few suffer from chronic or recurrent bacterial infection of the kidney. Rarely does the child pass directly from a classic episode of acute glomerular nephritis into the progressive form of the disease.

Lupus erythematosus and anaphylactoid purpura are sometimes recognized as etiologic antecedents of chronic nephritis.

Symptoms. When there has been no recognized renal disease previously, the symptoms are insidious and the onset is gradual. Fatigue, anemia, headache and mild degrees of edema of the face or the feet are the most common early symptoms. Often the disease is discovered accidentally during a routine urine examination or during a physical examination which reveals the presence of mild hypertension. In the early stages symptoms are frequently mild or intermittent, and the child is able to pursue normal activities.

The terminal symptoms are those of uremia or hypertension. Activity may be hampered by severe headache, nausea, fatigue or acidosis. In the final days of his illness the child usually passes into coma due to hypertension or uremia.

Diagnosis. The diagnosis of chronic nephritis depends on the interpretation of laboratory tests. The earliest abnormalities are found in the urine, where albumin and casts are regularly present, together with varying degrees of hematuria. The urea-clearance, phenolsulfonphthalein and urine-concentration tests indicate marked loss of renal function. In the later stages of the disease, blood-chemical determinations show retention of nitrogen products (uremia), acidosis and the accumulation of phosphates and creatinine above their usual levels. The blood pressure, particularly the diastolic pressure, usually is elevated.

Renal biopsy should always be done to assure the diagnosis when chronic nephritis is suspected. The child deserves the benefit of every diagnostic aid before his prognosis and treatment are determined.

Course and Prognosis. Recovery from fully developed chronic nephritis is not to be expected. The course may last only a few weeks after discovery of the disease or may permit survival over a period of many years. In very unusual instances children have been known to reach a point of permanent stabilization of the disease.

Treatment. No treatment is known which will stem the progress of chronic nephritis toward a fatal termination. When the diagnosis has been established with certainty, the most charitable attitude is to permit the child to follow normal activities within the limits of his physical comfort. This regimen allows him the maximum enjoyment of his remaining months or years and supports his morale.

General hygienic measures are important. The diet should be designed to maintain optimal nutrition. Salt restriction should be imposed if there is edema. Prevention and prompt treatment of all infectious illnesses should be provided. During the periods of hypertensive or uremic symptoms, hospitalization usually is required to provide comfort through such measures as sedation, transfusion, relief of heart failure and correction of acidosis.

Peritoneal dialysis is of temporary benefit and not

very useful for children with irreversible nephritis. The technic of dialysis with the artificial kidney may be used with the older child but has some practical limitations when indefinite usage is contemplated. Renal transplantation is gradually being perfected to a point where it may ultimately offer prolongation of of useful life to some victims of chronic progressive renal disease.

Nursing Care. If peritoneal dialysis is employed in renal failure, it is the responsibility of the nurse to assemble the equipment, to prepare the child and his parents for the procedure, to remain with the child during the dialysis, to observe for complications and to comfort the child after the treatment has been completed. Several commercial dialysis sets are now available including peritoneal catheters and connecting sets. In addition, the nurse should have available at the bedside: the peritoneal dialysis solution and a standard, a paracentesis tray, antiseptic solution, sterile gloves, 2-inch adhesive tape and a dialysis record form.

The procedure must be carefully explained to the child *prior* to beginning the treatment. He will be less frightened and better able to cooperate if he has had the opportunity to handle similar unsterilized equipment, to discuss his concerns and fears regarding the treatment and to communicate to the nurse the methods she can use to best support him. Small children who will be unable to cooperate in holding still will need to be restrained to avoid contaminating the sterile field.

Before the treatment is started, the child should empty his bladder and his weight should be recorded. The physician may ask that the abdomen be shaved and surgically scrubbed.

During the dialysis, it is the responsibility of the nurse to support the patient, to observe the vital signs, to be alert for signs of nausea or vomiting or difficulty in respiration, and to make notes on the dialysis sheet. It is essential that meticulous aseptic technic be maintained throughout the procedure. The tubing must be kept patent through periodic checks for kinking of the catheter or obstructions. Irrigations or changing of the catheter should be done by the physician.

Careful records of intake and output must be maintained throughout the period of hospitalization. Daily weights should also be recorded and blood pressure readings taken several times daily. The nurse must be constantly alert for signs of peritoneal infection, including rise in temperature and localized discomfort and report such signs to the attending physician immediately.

Children in renal failure need a nurse who is knowledgeable and whom they have learned to trust. It can be expected that such children will have fears for their ultimate safety intensified by the visible evidence of physical dependence on complicated apparatus. The fears and concerns of children with

chronic illness and a poor prognosis are discussed in Chapter 2. Children with chronic nephritis and their parents need the constant understanding help and support of all members of the health team.

SITUATIONS FOR FURTHER STUDY

1. How does nephritis in children differ from that in adults? Can nephritis in children be prevented? What are the complications of this disease?

2. Observe a toddler with nephrosis who has had several hospital admissions. Describe his behavior in relation to you, his mother, father and roommates. How do you think he feels about himself, the hospital and his treatment regimen? On what observations do you draw your conclusions? What is the pattern of his play? Has he the inner strengths that you would expect in a child of his age? In the article cited in the bibliography, Korsch and Barnett make the statement that the body image a child is forming of himself can become adversely affected by nephrosis. In what ways could nursing care affect the way the child feels about himself? In what ways can a prolonged illness like nephrosis affect family relationships? Describe your care of this child, giving details which show your observation of the child's concern with his body and the way in which you helped him to deal with it.

3. Study a young child with celiac disease. What personality characteristics did he show during the first week after admission? What symptoms caused the mother to seek medical attention? How did she feel about her child's symptoms? What part of his care distressed her the most? Make a record of the changes in behavior you observed during the course of treatment in the hospital. Did you detect any feelings of deprivation in the child during meal times? If so, how did he express them and how did you deal with them? In what way have you attempted to help his mother to adapt herself to his changing needs?

4. Read Korsch's results of meetings held with parents of children with nephrosis and give your opinion of their value.

BIBLIOGRAPHY

Bois, M., Barfield, N., Taylor, E. E., and Ross, C.: Nursing care of patients having kidney transplants, Am. J. Nurs. *68*:1238, 1968.

Brand, L., and Komorita, N. I.: Adapting to long-term hemodialysis, Am. J. Nurs. *66*:1778, 1966.

Calcagno, P. L., and Rubin, M. I.: Physiologic considerations concerning corticosteroid therapy and complications in the nephrotic syndrome, J. Pediat. *58*:686, 1961.

Fellows, B.: Hemodialysis at home, Am. J. Nurs. *66*:1775, 1966.

Korsch, B., and Barnett, H. L.: The physician, the family and the child with nephrosis, J. Pediat. *58*:707, 1961.

———: Fraad, L., and Barnett, H.: Pediatric discussions with parent groups, J. Pediat. *44*:703, 1954.

O'Neill, M.: Peritoneal dialysis, Nurs. Clin. N. Am. *1*:309, 1966.

Prugh, D. G.: A preliminary report on the role of emotional factors in idiopathic celiac disease, Psychosom. Med. *13*:220, 1951.

Riley, C. M.: Nephrosis, *in* Shirkey, H. C. (ed.), Pediatric Therapy, ed. 3, St. Louis, Mosby, 1968.

Shebelski, D. I.: Nursing patients who have renal homotransplants, Am. J. Nurs. *66*:2425, 1966.

Steele, S.: The preschooler with nephrosis, Nurs. Outlook *12*:50, 1964.

Struempler, R.: A clinical specialist works with a mother in the care of a chronically ill child, Nurs. Clin. N. Am. *4*:111, 1969.

Watkins, F. L., and Downing, S.: The patient who has peritoneal dialysis, Am. J. Nurs. *66*:1572, 1966.

24

Nursing Care of Preschool Children Requiring Surgical Treatment

Although in this chapter no attempt will be made to include all conditions requiring surgical correction, those described herein were selected as being typical of or peculiar to the age group under discussion. As the student has noted from her study of Chapter 16, the experience of a surgical operation is a particularly critical one in the life of the toddler and the preschooler.

CRANIOSTENOSIS

In order to allow for postnatal growth of the brain, the infant's skull is composed of bones separated by suture lines which do not normally fuse intimately until early adult life. If the brain fails to grow at the expected rate because of congenital abnormality, the skull does not expand at the expected rate and the sutures may close early (microcephaly). In some children the potential for brain growth is normal but, due to unknown causes, one or more of the suture lines may close prematurely and prevent growth in a direction perpendicular to it. If all the sutures close prematurely the situation is critical since the attempt of a normal brain to expand within a closed box will lead to increased intracranial pressure and may damage important structures such as the optic nerves. Early recognition and the provision of artificial suture lines by removal of strips of bone parallel to the closed sutures is essential to preserve sight and intellect. When the sagittal suture alone is prematurely closed, the head becomes narrow and elongated in the fronto-occipital dimension, but no increase in intracranial pressure occurs and the child develops normally except for the abnormal appearance of the skull. Surgical relief is seldom indicated for other than cosmetic reasons. When only the coronal sutures are prematurely fused the head becomes wide and short in the anteroposterior dimension. This type of defect is more likely to be associated with other abnormalities and to interfere with the normal development of the orbits so that corrective procedures may be necessary to protect vision.

EPISTAXIS (NASAL HEMORRHAGE)

Epistaxis may occur as a symptom of heart disease, typhoid fever, whooping cough and diseases of the blood, such as purpura and leukemia. It may be due also to inflammation within the nose. Frequently recurring nasal hemorrhage in the absence of systemic disease is usually due to an ulceration of the anterior part of the septum. Very commonly, hemorrhage results from injury: an external blow, as from a fall, or internal trauma—picking the nose or inserting an object into it.

In the common variety of nasal hemorrhage, the bleeding is from the anterior and inferior portion of the nasal septum. Such a hemorrhage is controlled easily. If the child remains quiet, the hemorrhage may stop spontaneously in a few minutes. Pressure on the bleeding point by pinching the nose is accomplished easily and usually is effective. In case the hemorrhage persists, it always can be stopped by packing into the anterior part of the nose a small piece of cotton or strip of cloth, either dry or moistened with thromboplastin or a vasoconstrictor such as epinephrine or ephedrine. In case of the more severe and less common type of hemorrhage from some other part of the nose, posterior packing may be necessary.

CLEFT PALATE

Nursing Care

Surgery for closure of the anterior hard palate is usually done when the child is 6 to 12 months of age, whereas second stage soft palate closure may be done from 12 to 24 months after birth. The child should be free from any infectious process, and his hemoglobin level should be adequate before he is admitted to the hospital. During hospitalization, nursing care will be of utmost importance to the entire habilitative program. Ideally, the child should enter the hospital several days prior to operation in order to be familiarized with the treatment which he will require afterwards. He should have an opportunity to develop trust in the nurse, who must anticipate his needs when he is unable to speak. In this period the nurse can also assist his mother in preparing him psychologically for surgery and postoperative care. The introduction of arm restraints and mouth irrigations prior to surgery allows the child time to become familiar with the equipment and reduces later fear and resistance.

During the preoperative period, isolation technics may be recommended to protect the child from respiratory infection. On the day before operation, frequent feedings of sweetened fluids should be encouraged as a shock protective measure.

In the immediate postoperative period, the child should be placed on his abdomen to prevent aspiration of mucus or blood and suction apparatus should be available at the bedside. Constant nursing attendance is necessary to monitor the vital signs, to observe for signs of shock or hemorrhage and to prevent injury to the child's mouth. Elbow restraints should be applied as soon as the child regains consciousness. Basswood splints which have been padded with sheet wadding and extending from the axilla to the wrist will prevent damage to the operative site while allowing some freedom of motion.

A tray with sterile saline solution, a sterile rubber ear bulb and an emesis basin should be at the bedside for postoperative mouth irrigation. This is done most effectively with the child in a sitting position with his head tilted downward. Slight pressure should be used to produce a gentle stream directed over the suture line. During the first 6 hours after surgery, the suture line should be moistened frequently with saline solution to give the child comfort and to promote healing.

When the child's nausea and vomiting have ceased, fluids can be given by cup or from the side of a spoon; they are never given by straw, nipple or syringe. For the first 3 days, clear liquids with additional carbohydrates are given at 2-hour intervals. After this period, milk, eggnogs and creamed soups can supplement the diet. Sips of water should be given after feedings to cleanse the mouth. Most children will accept their food and irrigations more readily if their arms are unrestrained and if they are allowed to hold the glass for drinking and the basin for the irrigation. A fluid diet is continued until all sutures are removed. The child should be weighed periodically to assure that his nutrition is being adequately maintained.

After the initial postoperative period, adjustment to a liquid diet is difficult for the child because of his increased appetite. Substitute satisfactions are essential to prevent feelings of deprivation. If his mother cannot stay with him, play and a satisfying relationship with his nurse are necessary to minimize the dis-

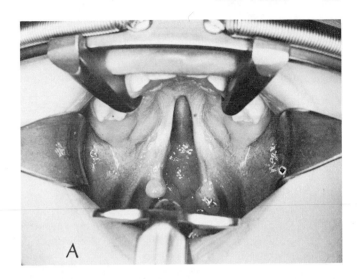

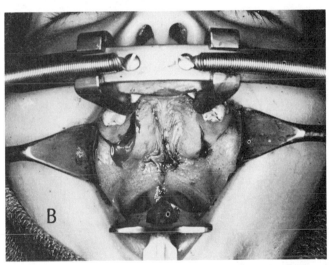

FIG. 24-1. Cleft palate (A) before and (B) after operative repair. (From Dr. H. Zarem)

comfort that he feels from the operative manipulation on his mouth, from restraint and from the limited diet that he is served.

Children with a cleft of the palate are handicapped in both emotional and intellectual development in addition to the physical defect. In the preschool period, they become aware that they have difficulty in making themselves understood. During the early school years, they may be avoided and ridiculed by their peers, particularly if their speech defect is pronounced. They may have fewer opportunities to express themselves and are thus hampered in receiving satisfactions from academic pursuits. As a result these children may withdraw from both emotional relationships and intellectual stimulation; they may develop an inferior self-concept and grow overly dependent on their mothers.

When these children are admitted to the hospital for operation, they will need additional help to feel comfortable in the ward. Opportunities for social relationships should be provided as soon as the child's physical condition permits. They need opportunities for creative expression from which they can gain recognition and satisfaction. If a social worker is available on the hospital staff, the parents might welcome an opportunity to discuss with her their problems in rearing a handicapped child.

Frequently the child who has had his cleft palate repaired is discharged from the hospital before all sutures are removed. In these instances, the mother will need instructions concerning his dietary requirements, his need for elbow restraint and the importance of restricting his impulse to put objects into his mouth. In the home greater difficulty will be encountered in restricting the child to the prescribed fluid diet, since food will be more accessible and the temptation greater.

When speech clinic facilities are available, arrangements for the child's referral should be made. If the cleft palate is repaired before speech patterns are set, much can be accomplished with skillful guidance and training. Parents may have to be convinced of the value of speech therapy for the sake of the child's future welfare.

CYSTS OF THE NECK

There are two common types of malformation about the neck which, although anatomically present at birth are either unnoticed in the small infant or left alone until the child grows larger and the operative procedure becomes technically easier. If surgical treatment is indicated, it is most commonly undertaken during the period of early childhood.

Thyroglossal Duct Cyst

In embryologic life the thyroid gland develops as an outpouching from the primitive intestinal tract, taking origin from the base of the tongue. Ordinarily the primitive connection between the thyroid and the tongue atrophies and disappears. In a few children, a remnant of this channel persists and secretes small amounts of fluid, forming a cystic mass on the anterior surface of the trachea close to the midline (Fig. 24-2).

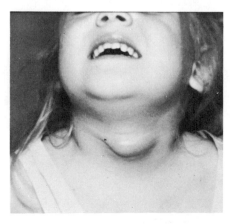

Fig. 24-2. Thyroglossal duct cyst. (From Dr. H. P. Jenkins)

No symptoms are present unless the cyst becomes infected, in which case it may rupture and produce a chronically draining sinus with irritation of the surrounding skin.

Treatment requires complete surgical removal not only of the obvious cyst, but also of the slender tract which connects it with the base of the tongue. Incomplete removal of this tract results in recurrence.

Branchial Cleft Remnants

Early in fetal life the region of the pharynx is pierced by a series of slits comparable to the gills in fishes. Normally these tracts close and leave no vestige. Occasionally an epithelium-lined communication persists either as a branchial cleft sinus or as a cyst. A sinus appears as a pinpoint opening on the side of the neck and drains a small amount of fluid. A branchial cleft cyst forms a lump beneath the skin, similar to a thyroglossal duct cyst but off to one side. Such cysts may appear for the first time in the wake of a respiratory infection and be mistaken for cervical lymphadenitis.

Treatment of either variety of branchial cleft remnant is by thorough surgical excision.

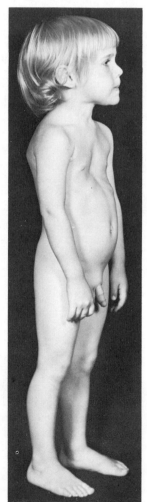

Fig. 24-3. Moderately severe pectus excavatum. (From Dr. M. Ravitch)

FUNNEL CHEST (PECTUS EXCAVATUM)

Recession of the lower end of the sternum occurs quite frequently in mild degree as a minor congenital abnormality of the chest wall which requires no treatment. In some children the deformity is quite marked, displaces the heart to the left and in later years may be associated with a stooped, hunched posture and create a cosmetic defect which is psychologically disturbing to the child. In the latter instances, an extensive remodeling of the chest wall may be undertaken to free the sternum from its posterior attachments and permit more normal expansion of the thoracic cavity. In competent hands the operative risk is low in spite of the extent of the procedure. It is usually deferred until at least 3 years of age when the supporting structures such as ribs and costal cartilages are assuming enough rigidity to keep the sternum in its new position.

INTESTINAL POLYPS

Benign polypoid growths occur within the intestinal mucosa of children and lead to passage of blood in the stool. Most frequently the source is a solitary polyp in the rectum. Sometimes such a polyp on a long pedicle extrudes from the anus, but usually they must be sought by proctoscopic examination and be removed through this instrument. Less commonly, polyps occur higher up in the large bowel and cause painless bleeding. They may be demonstrable by contrast barium enema, employing both air and barium to make them visible on the roentgen film. Rarely, a child has multiple polyps throughout the whole colon. This is a serious disorder which can interfere with growth and eventually may lead to malignant degeneration of the masses. Total colectomy is usually required in extensive polyposis to forestall malignant degeneration.

SUBLUXATION OF THE HEAD OF THE RADIUS

A common arm injury occurs in toddlers who are pulled by an adult with forcible internal rotation of one arm which dislocates the radial head from its ligamentous attachments. An immediate snap is heard; pain in the elbow is felt momentarily, and the child then keeps the arm slightly flexed and is unable to supinate the hand. X-rays fail to disclose any broken bones. Reduction and restoration to normal function is accomplished by forcible supination of the forearm while exerting pressure upon the displaced head of the radius. If properly done, the radial head pops back into position and the child is at once able to use the arm normally.

TUBERCULOUS SPONDYLITIS (POTT'S DISEASE)

Tubercle bacilli which gain access to the blood stream, either during primary infection or by miliary spread, may lodge in the bones where they produce smoldering foci of osteomyelitis. The most common such localization takes place in the vertebral bodies. After a period of back pain and the assumption of guarded postures, roentgen examination reveals destruction of a vertebral body with loss of the normal space between it and an adjacent vertebral body. Pressure upon the nerves emerging from this portion of the spine, due to the formation of a local cold abscess (psoas abscess) or to kinking of the spinal cord within the bony canal, may produce neurologic disturbances of the legs such as paraplegia. As early diagnosis and treatment of tuberculosis in general is advanced, Pott's disease decreases in frequency. Treatment is the same as for general tuberculosis when the disturbance is recognized early. If destruction of the bony structures is advanced or neurologic signs are present, immobilization on a Bradford frame may be necessary until some healing is achieved. If severe kyphosis results from the destruction of vertebral bodies, spinal fusion may be necessary.

POSITIONAL ABNORMALITIES OF LEGS AND FEET

As the infant passes into the toddler stage, the aberrations of the position of his legs and feet, which were ascribed in Chapter 7 to the effects of intra-uterine pressure, become more apparent when he adopts the erect position and tries to use his legs for locomotion. Knock-knees, bowlegs, pigeon-toes and externally rotated flat feet are very commonly observed by parents during this period of early walking. Most of these irregularities correct themselves gradually as muscle power improves, the bones undergo further growth and the child and his skeleton gradually accommodate to a more efficient manner of bearing and moving his weight. Ordinarily, no special shoes or braces are required and the child is best left alone. When deformity is unusually marked, the use of a Denis Browne splint at night may hasten the correction of tibial torsion and rotation of the feet. In extreme instances, osteotomies may be required to permit the development of more normal postures. In these latter instances it is important to be sure that no generalized disease of bone such as chondrodystrophy or resistant rickets is present.

CONDITIONS REQUIRING EYE SURGERY

A limited number of afflictions of the eyes during childhood require treatment by surgical means. Since no particular age period predominates in eye surgery, these conditions have been assembled here for convenience. Nursing care is of considerable importance both preoperatively and postoperatively in lessening the natural anxiety which a child feels about the threat to his most precious sensory organ. Because the technics are similar for all types of operation, discussion of the principles of nursing care is postponed to the end of the section.

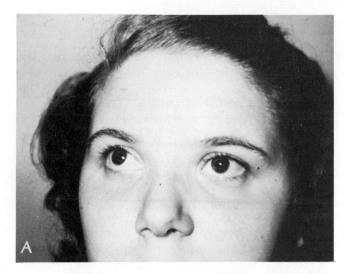

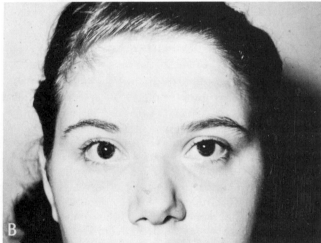

Fig. 24-4. A, Divergent strabismus prior to operative correction. B, Postoperative result following operation on the extra-ocular muscles. (Courtesy of Dr. Albert M. Potts)

Small children in particular must often be anesthetized for minor procedures such as adequate funduscopic examination, refraction, removal of foreign bodies or the incision of chalazions. These are usually outpatient procedures which do not necessitate admission of the child to the hospital.

Cataracts

A cataract is an opacification of the lens of the eye which has several possible causes. Some result from intrauterine influences during the course of fetal development—rubella is the outstanding example. Others appear during the course of metabolic diseases such as galactosemia, diabetes and parathyroid disorders. Some follow trauma to the eye or severe infections.

Cataracts are recognized by funduscopic examination of the eye which reveals areas of opacity in one or both lenses. The symptoms are dimness of vision

and nystagmus. Treatment depends on the position and the extent of the cataract. Small opacities are usually left alone, since they do not interfere with vision. Larger ones are removed by an operation in which the capsule of the lens is opened and the contents are washed out or permitted to resorb gradually under the influence of the aqueous humor. The result is an eye that admits light but can no longer focus without the aid of strong glasses.

Glaucoma

This disorder is due to an overproduction of aqueous fluid within the eye which tends to enlarge it, makes it tense and painful and gradually decreases vision. It may be on a congenital basis or associated with other disease or injury of the eye. The condition is suspected in infancy by the appearance of the cornea, which looks too large (buphthalmos or ox-eye). Operative procedures attempt to provide better drainage of the aqueous humor so that the internal tension will be reduced. Goniopuncture and iridectomy are two of the technics used. Medical management with miotics and diamox are seldom adequate to control the fluid accumulation in children.

Retinoblastoma

This is a fortunately rare malignant tumor of the retina seen exclusively in infants and young children. It may be discovered by ophthalmoscopic examination or by observation of an abnormal color of the light reflected from within the eye—loss of the normal red reflex. Early treatment may save the child's life if the condition is discovered early enough. The eye and the adjacent optic nerve must be removed. This sometimes is followed by radiation or drug therapy. Unfortunately, many retinoblastomas are bilateral and metastasize before they are discovered.

Strabismus (Squint)

Strabismus is a condition in which the eyes cannot be used at the same time for looking at an object. A person with strabismus is commonly said to be cross-eyed. Normally, the lines of vision (visual axes) of the eyes are parallel when the object is at a distance of 20 feet or more. When looking at a nearer object, the visual axes converge to meet the object. In strabismus the visual axis of only one eye goes to the object.

Many varieties of strabismus exist. Strabismus from prenatal causes may become apparent at any time from birth to the sixth year. Development of strabismus after this time usually is caused by disease. Sometimes the muscles that move the eye outward or those that move the eye inward are overactive or underactive, and the resulting condition may be referred to as paralytic strabismus. When strabismus is caused by underaction of the muscles of one eye, the affected eye does not have as full ocular movements as the fellow eye. In non-paralytic strabismus the affected eye moves with the eye used for vision, but always with a visual axis not corresponding to that of the seeing eye, a condition known as concomitant strabismus. Concomitant strabismus may be either monocular or alternating. In monocular strabismus, one eye is used constantly for vision and the other eye is turned either inward (convergent strabismus) or outward (divergent strabismus). In alternating strabismus, either eye is used for vision, and the other eye becomes the affected eye. (Fig. 24-4)

Concomitant strabismas usually is due to error of refraction. When the eyes change fixation from a distant to a near object, the pupils contract, the lenses change power for an exact focus, and the eyes converge. The error of refraction may be such that the focus (accommodation) is not accurate at the same time that both eyes are able to fix accurately on the object. The child must choose between accurate fixation with poor vision and accurate accommodation with double vision. The choice resulting in strabismus may be made at any time in early infancy.

When both eyes cannot be brought to bear on an object, double vision (diplopia) results, and the images in the eyes differ. The person with strabismus quickly learns to disregard the image in the affected eye. As a result, vision in the affected eye may be reduced markedly. Usually the false image of the affected eye is suppressed by the time the child comes under care.

Because of danger to vision, as well as for cosmetic effect, treatment for strabismus should be undertaken as soon as the condition is observed. Usually, the earlier the treatment is undertaken, the better are the results, and, conversely, the later the treatments, the slower the progress and the less satisfactory the final status. The objectives of treatment are to improve the vision of the poorly functioning eye, to produce or restore single vision when both eyes are focusing together and to correct the deformity.

In early infancy the better eye should be occluded by a patch or a cover until the baby is old enough to wear glasses, which may be at the age of from 12 to 14 months. With use of the poorer eye the vision should improve, and often it can be brought to normal. Correction of the refractive error helps to restore single vision and is fully effective in many instances. For some children, correction of the deformity by operation may be necessary, but operation is not indicated until maximum improvement by glasses and training has been attained, usually not before 3 or 4 years of age. Correction of the deformity early, particularly before the child goes to school, is important for psychological reasons. Otherwise, the child is taunted and is likely to develop behavioral changes which thwart his potentials for personality growth. If operation has been necessary, further treatment must be given to help the eyes function together.

Spurious Strabismus. During the early months of life, infants are not expected to maintain parallel vision at all times. Brief periods of convergent or divergent strabismus usually have little significance. Frequently, too, parents and relatives may be misled by an optical illusion which causes them to believe that the young infant with a broad nose and epicanthal fold is suffering from convergent strabismus, when actually he is using parallel vision. The explanation lies in the fact that during lateral gaze, the eye that is turning toward the nose appears to go too far inward because the epicanthal fold obscures more of the white sclera than the observer thinks that it should. The superficial conclusion of strabismus is drawn easily. A simple test will permit a distinction between real and spurious strabismus. If a bright point of light is directed into the infant's eyes, the reflections from the two corneas should be seen in the same relative position with respect to the center of the pupil in each eye. If the eyes are not parallel there will be an obvious difference between them.

Injuries

Injuries of or about the eye are potentially serious threats to vision and should aways be seen promptly by an ophthalmologist. Many superficial cuts and bruises will heal without difficulty, and foreign bodies will be dislodged without causing any damage. However, if a wound or a foreign body penetrates the globe or if infection of the internal structure of the eye takes place, there is danger of *sympathetic ophthalmia*. This condition is a plastic inflammation of the opposite eye which may appear 2 to 8 weeks later, threatening to destroy vision in the remaining good eye. Thus, at the time of eye injuries a competent, thorough examination must be made to be sure of their extent. Although modern treatment with steroids and antibiotics has greatly improved the prognosis, mature clinical judgment is needed to decide whether the injured eye should be removed to forestall sympathetic ophthalmia in its mate.

Nursing Care of Children Undergoing Eye Surgery

There are differences of opinion as to the amount of restraint that is necessary after cataracts have been extracted from a child's eyes. Some surgeons believe that restriction results in more tension within the eyes as the child fights against it. They suture adequately and eliminate the need for body restraint, recommending only the use of elbow restraints to prevent the child from removing the dressings and rubbing his eyes. Others recommend the use of jacket and elbow restraints to prevent tampering with the dressings, and insist on keeping the baby flat on his back. Often sandbags are used on either side of the head to immobilize it completely. The infant must be fed in this position until the surgeon allows him to be moved into a sitting position for feeding. Fluids should be given cautiously until tolerance for large quantities is assured. Every measure to prevent vomiting must be taken because it increases intraocular pressure and poses the threat of aspiration, especially when the baby is restrained on his back.

Care should be taken to prevent startling the infant when he is approached. Talking pleasantly to him before the cribside is lowered lessens the danger of frightening him and prepares him for being handled. The immobilized infant will miss the comfort of being held for feedings and of play with his parents. Stroking the infant's head, talking to him in gentle soothing tones and carrying out all measures that ensure comfort and prevent loneliness will lessen his need for sedatives, which will be required if he is restless and tearful.

Opinion also varies as to the need for eye dressings after strabismus has been corrected. Some surgeons feel that psychic trauma can be prevented by eliminating the fear that is attendant on awakening from anesthesia with eyes blinded by dressings. In instances in which the surgeon uses eye dressings, the child must be prepared for them preoperatively and also for elbow restraints, which will be necessary to remind him that his eyes must remain covered until healing takes place. His parents and nurse must also anticipate the fears that he may experience after operation (awakening in the dark, permanent loss of vision) and give him assurance that they will be within call when he needs them.

The child with eye dressings enjoys the privilege of knowing what foods are on his tray and of controlling the order in which they are fed to him. He also appreciates the feeling of independence that comes from removal of his restraints so that he can feed himself with his fingers.

In most instances prolonged visiting periods are necessary for the child who has had an operation on his eyes. Most children are acutely anxious when their eyes are covered, not only because of pain and temporary blindness but also because their eyes have been one of their greatest sources of protection. In a strange world filled with sounds which can become easily distorted into signals of danger, constant contact with trustworthy persons is essential to prevent insecurity

which may extend beyond the time when successful correction of the deformity has been achieved.

When exercises are recommended postoperatively, the nurse must assist the mother in understanding the reasons for them. If the child is attending school at the time of operation, it is advisable to notify the school nurse so that she can ensure continuation of the orthoptic training.

SITUATIONS FOR FURTHER STUDY

1. How would you prepare a child with a cleft palate for the fact that soreness of his mouth would make it difficult for him to talk with you after his operation?

2. What preoperative observations would be necessary to prepare you to give a child emotional comfort in the period after a cleft-palate repair has been done?

3. Investigate community facilities available for speech training of children with cleft palates. Visit a speech clinic to observe methods of speech training and to learn ways in which a nurse can help parents to continue speech training at home.

4. Observe a child whose mother could not be with him after correction of strabismus and observe his responses as he comes out of anesthesia and faces the discomfort of painful eyes and partial or complete loss of vision. Describe the methods that you used to relieve the discomfort you observed and the results you achieved.

BIBLIOGRAPHY

Atkinson, H.: Care of the child with cleft lip and palate, Am. J. Nurs. 67:1889, 1967.

Buckley, J. J.: Pitfalls in anaesthesia for emergency pediatric surgery, Postgrad. Med. 29:575, 1961.

Lis, E. F., *et al.:* Cleft lip and cleft palate, Pediat. Clin. N. Am. 3:995, 1956.

McDermott, M.: The child with cleft lip and palate on the pediatric ward, Am. J. Nurs. 65:122, 1965.

Millard, D. R., Kuszaj, J., and Wirch, B.: Nursing care of the patient with cleft lip and palate, Nurs. Clin. N. Am. 2:483, 1967.

Ripley, I. L.: The child with cleft lip and palate, through his years of growth, Am. J. Nurs. 65:124, 1965.

Ophthalmologic Staff of the Hospital for Sick Children, The Eye in Childhood, Chicago, Year Book, 1967.

UNIT 5

The School Child (6 to 13 Years)

For children in general the elementary school years are challenging, predictable and healthy. Physical growth is slow but steady until the final surge, which appears toward the end of the period to herald the beginning of puberty. Muscle and fat are added more rapidly than height so that bodies become sturdier. The baby teeth are replaced by permanent structures. Many of the illnesses which have already been considered are still seen during the school years, but disease and psychological handicaps now begin to resemble those found among adults. The low rate of illness encourages laxity in periodic health examinations and in stimulation of previously given immunizations, but school health authorities recognize how necessary these are to maintain optimal physical condition.

The sexes begin to separate from each other more noticeably, both in their physical appearance and in their social intercourse. It is a period of marked psychosocial growth with progressive addition of new skills and controls which make children more comfortable with themselves and in their community.

25

Growth, Development and Care of the Child During the School Years (6 to 13 Years)

PHYSICAL GROWTH

Typically the child enters his elementary school years with a body type and rate of growth to which he steadfastly adheres until the changes of puberty begin. It is important for parents and teachers to accept the fact that in general, short children remain short, thin ones thin, and tall ones tall. The characteristic body type of the child usually emerges out of his period of erratic growth as a toddler, becomes apparent during the preschool years and then is confirmed during the school years. There are some exceptions. Very few healthy children change their relative height positions in the class. A large percentage change in respect to weight. However, it is amazing how many who return for annual measurements turn up each year in exactly the same position with respect to the average curves.

Height

Inspection of the height curves shows that on the average boys grow from about 45 inches (114 cm.) to about 60 inches (153 cm.) over the 7-year period—a little better than 2 inches (5 cm.) a year. The variations on either side of the average measurement for a given age do not generally exceed 2½ inches (6½ cm.). The curves for girls are not greatly dissimilar, but careful inspection will show that although the average girl begins her school years a trifle shorter than the corresponding average boy, she is significantly taller than he by the age of 12 years. This is due to the fact that pubertal changes with their attendant spurt in growth appear about 2 years earlier in girls than they do in boys. Consequently, more girls than boys in the later years of elementary school suddenly will receive a forward push in growth. However, the advantage which the female sex gains at this

time is a temporary one because puberty eventually causes a fusion of the epiphyses at the growing ends of bones and brings further extension in height to an end. Those who enjoy an early puberty run ahead temporarily but also reach their final height sooner. The social implications of these height discrepancies are well known to anyone concerned with school dances.

Weight

The average weights for boys move from about 45 lbs. (20.5 Kg.) to about 90 lbs. (41 Kg.) during the 7-year period, reflecting an annual gain of 6-7 lbs. (3 Kg.). Variations from the average weight for age are usually less than 5 lbs. in the early years but may be as great as 15 lbs. in the older members of the group. The differences between the sexes behave much as those described for height, and for the same reason.

Other Physical Changes

The Head. Although there is only a slight further increase in the size of the skull, differential growth of the features takes place which emphasizes the individual facial characteristics. In particular, the jaw grows longer and more prominent, providing the child with more chin and a place into which his new and larger teeth will be able to erupt. Not visible except on roentgenograms are changes taking place in the paranasal sinuses, which enlarge rapidly during the period of the school years. The lymphoid tissue also hypertrophies to maximum size, so that on inspection the average school child displays a set of tonsils which are relatively large.

Dentition. At or just before the age of 6 years the first permanent molar teeth erupt, appearing behind the deciduous second molars. As the other permanent teeth come in, they usually push out the corresponding deciduous teeth ahead of them. Occasionally the permanent incisor teeth will come through behind the still present deciduous incisors, arousing concern lest they do not take up their proper position in the jaw. It is surprising how much rearrangement will take place after the deciduous incisors have been shed. The order of eruption of the permanent teeth is shown. Most children have all their permanent teeth except the 2nd and 3rd molars by the age of 12 years.

Skeletal Maturation. By the early school years the skeleton has produced most of its centers of ossification. Estimations of bone maturity depend to a large extent on the size and shape of characteristic centers as seen on roentgenograms. The distance between these centers and the adjacent bones narrows progressively and, in the following period of puberty, fusion will be visible between epiphyses and shafts of many

of the long bones—a phenomenon which announces the cessation of growth in the particular bone.

The growth in bones often proceeds faster than the increase in strength of muscles and ligaments, particularly in children who are growing rapidly. Consequently, loose-jointed, gangling and sway-backed postures are not uncommon. Spurts of growth may also be accompanied by muscle aches, particularly at night. These "growing pains" are a real phenomenon for many children when their muscles are trying to catch up with the new skeletal size.

Neuromuscular Skills. By the time he is ready to enter school the child has acquired all of the basic mechanisms which he will use in later life. However, he will spend these years in perfecting his muscular skills and in acquiring and developing intellectual concepts. Progress in these respects becomes a more individual matter as age increases, so that the athletic, the bright and the personable children become iden-

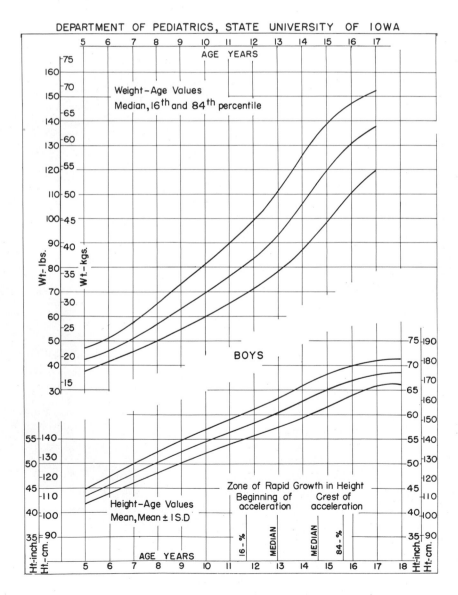

FIG. 25-1. Average measurements of boys from 5 to 18 years of age.

FIG. 25-2. Average measurements of girls from 5 to 18 years of age.

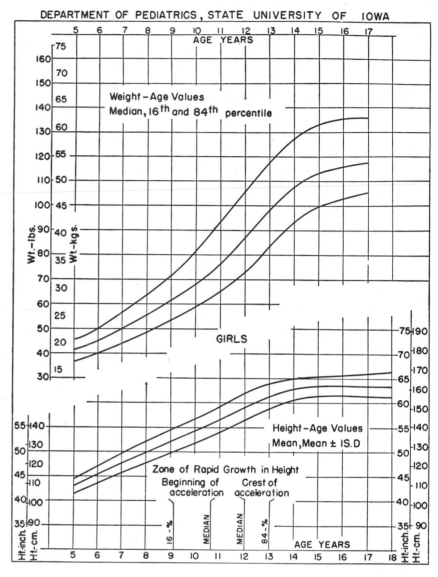

CENTRAL INCISOR
LATERAL INCISOR
CUSPID
FIRST BICUSPID
SECOND BICUSPID
FIRST MOLAR
SECOND MOLAR
THIRD MOLAR

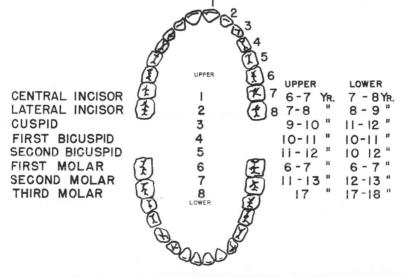

		UPPER	LOWER
CENTRAL INCISOR	1	6-7 YR.	7 - 8 YR.
LATERAL INCISOR	2	7-8 "	8 - 9 "
CUSPID	3	9-10 "	11 - 12 "
FIRST BICUSPID	4	10-11 "	10 - 11 "
SECOND BICUSPID	5	11-12 "	10 12 "
FIRST MOLAR	6	6-7 "	6 - 7 "
SECOND MOLAR	7	11-13 "	12 -13 "
THIRD MOLAR	8	17 "	17-18 "

FIG. 25-3. Time of eruption of permanent teeth.

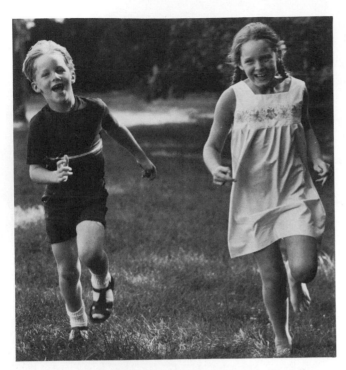

Fig. 25-4. The school aged child has boundless energy and demonstrates the sheer exuberance of running and large muscle activity. (Carol Baldwin)

tified in any group and contrast with the clumsy, the dull and the asocial. Some general statements can be made about the characteristics of the several age levels, but the analysis and evaluation of the progress of an individual child become an increasingly more complex task as the neuromuscular, intellectual, social and emotional facets of his behavior become intertwined.

Six-year-olds reflect the tension of transition to elementary school life in endless energy and constant bodily activity with a tendency to overdo. Boys and girls play together in rough and tumble fashion like bear cubs. Inhibitions are weak, and self-centered strivings create frequent crises and frictions due to showing-off and bossy attempts to dominate. Hand co-ordination is enough to permit banging with a hammer and printing large letters. Athletic endeavors are rudimentary—bouncing and throwing a ball, jumping and running games, elementary stunting on a bar.

At 7 there is a more cautious approach to activity and less vehemence in demands and opinions. The child is easier to deal with. Muscular skills show improvement. Boys can catch as well as throw a ball and may begin to try a baseball bat. Most will want to learn to ride a bicycle if they have not done so already. Fine hand movements are improved. Pencils are preferred to crayons, and printing has become smaller and easier to do.

At 8 there is greater smoothness in muscular movements. Boys prefer baseball, soccer and hiking, and

girls concentrate on jumping rope and playing hopscotch. Cursive writing skills are developing and replacing the printed letter.

By 9 the child is working intently on the perfection of skills already acquired. The disparity between the abilities of different individuals within the group becomes more noticeable.

The latter half of this age period is marked by increasing physical strength and endurance among the boys. For many the perfection of individual skills begins to approach an adult level of proficiency.

NUTRITION

Requirements

The amount of food required per unit of weight continues to fall gradually. The young school child needs about 80 calories/Kg./day (or 35 calories/lb.); by 12 years this has slumped to 70 calories/Kg./day or 30 calories/lb. Thus the range of total calories runs from about 1,600 to 2,800 calories/day. More important than weight is the energy expenditure of the individual child. Girls tend to be more quiet and sedentary, and, consequently, their caloric needs are somewhat more modest. A simple scheme for computing approximate energy requirements in this age period is to allow 1,000 calories plus 100 for each year of age. Thus, a 6-year-old will need about 1,600; an 8-year-old 1,800; and a 12-year-old 2,200.

Within the total calories protein is required at about 2 to 2.5 Gm./Kg. or about 1 Gm./lb. Thus, the daily protein intakes will range from about 50 to 80 Gm. Vitamin and mineral requirements remain about the same.

Those older school children who are approaching puberty often will have a rapid increase in food requirements. At this time of life it is desirable also to make sure that calcium and vitamin D intakes are adequate to support the rapid enlargement of the bones. About 1.5 to 2.0 Gm. of calcium per day and at least 400 units of vitamin D are desirable.

Water is needed at the rate of 75 ml./Kg./day, yielding a total between 1,500 and 3,000 ml. depending on the size of the child.

Diet and Mealtimes

The wisdom of evaluating the daily diet of a school child to ensure its adequacy cannot be questioned. Likes and dislikes for food are frequently a product of the eating experiences of the toddler and the preschool period. Acceptance of an adequate diet by the child is seldom attained through his mother's insistence that particular foods are "good for him." The child who has been badgered too much will continue to thwart his mother's efforts to determine what he eats. Family attitudes toward foods and eating are mimicked readily once the child becomes a regular member of the group at mealtimes. Father's refusal of vegetables

FIG. 25-5. By the age of 6 carpentry begins to take on new interest. (Photographer Edgar Bernstein)

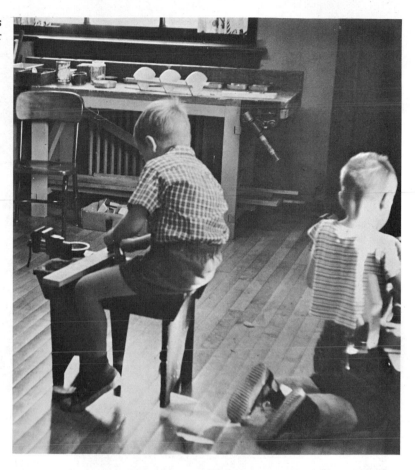

or mother's concentration on starches and sweets does not pass unnoticed.

Other factors begin to have an influence on the diet. School children often are too busy with other affairs to take the time to eat. Play and television easily take priority unless a firm understanding is reached and mealtime is made enjoyable. A period of rest from the excitement of these diversions is often desirable so that the meal may be consumed in a relaxed state of mind.

Some school children tend to express their individuality through food preferences. Hamburgers and hot dogs may be the only forms of meat accepted willingly. Dishes which they have never tasted are consistently rejected. If the total intake is sufficient in basic content, it is generally wise for the mother to yield to these fads rather than nag, persuade or discipline. A change of heart is more likely to occur spontaneously or under the influence of schoolmates or other outsiders than under the mother's persuasion.

In homes where mothers work or sleep late in the morning, breakfast may be inadequate because the school child is left to fend for himself. The piece of cake and glass of milk (or cup of coffee) which usually results is not a sufficient bulwark against midmorning hunger. A small fraction of otherwise normal children seem to be physiologically unable to eat much breakfast. Most of them make up this deficiency at other meals. However, an inadequate breakfast is a common cause of headache and lassitude during the late morning.

Lunches are arranged in different ways according to the school arrangements. Many schools now serve an adequate midday meal. Others require the child to bring his lunch or to return home for it. Mid-afternoon snacks are a common practice with school children, and no adverse effects follow if the food taken at this time does not interfere with a proper intake at dinner. However, in working families the interval between after-school snacks and the evening meal is often very brief, and poor appetites result.

PSYCHOSOCIAL AND COGNITIVE DEVELOPMENT

Formation of Personality During Early Years

At birth the infant's personality was undifferentiated and his impulses were directed toward the attainment of immediate gratification. As he grew physically, intellectually and emotionally, he achieved neuromuscular control, separation of himself from his environment, acquired a sense of trust and learned to communicate verbally with his family. Subsequent steps in develop-

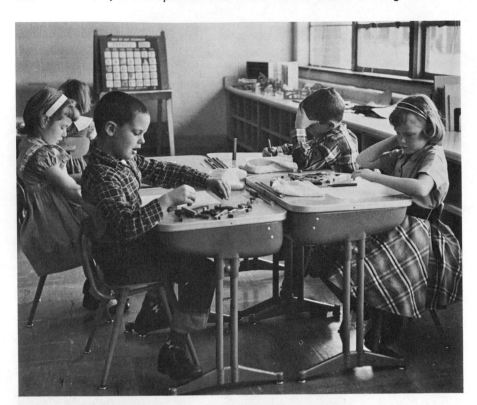

FIG. 25-6. Notice the intentness with which these children are working on their problems, being able to divert their attention away from the children beside them. (Photographer Edgar Bernstein)

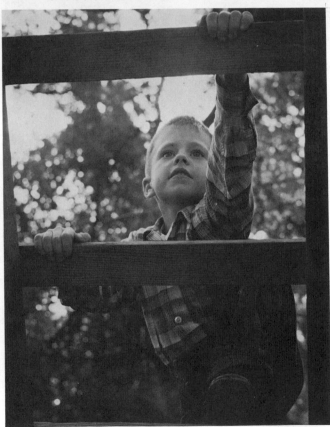

FIG. 25-7. Our society expects boys to achieve athletically. Fear may be denied with an air of independence which may be misleading. (Carol Baldwin)

ment included elaboration of reality, an urge toward exploration and experimentation, the acquisition of autonomy and some power over his impulses and environment. The struggle that he had in relationship to his parents, in defining his sex role and in learning independence, resulted in identification with his parent of the same sex, in fearlessness in the use of his initiative and in the formation of a structured personality consisting of three parts, defined in psychoanalytical terminology as: (1) the id, or instinctual drives, (2) the ego, or executive force and (3) the super-ego or conscience and ego-ideal. Adaptation to new core problems will affect the relationship which each part of the personality has to the other parts, but it cannot produce a new structure because its basic form has already been established.

Mastery of earlier crises in psychosocial and intellectual development prepares the 6-year-old child to begin tackling his next core problem—industry vs. inferiority. The first grader is eager to learn about his world, to affirm his sexual identity, to become master of himself and all he surveys, and to find his place in a group of peers. Support in acquiring a sense of industry is derived from encouragement of his efforts to develop his special interests, to meet the demands of his teacher and peer group and to move toward reliance on his friends for intimate companionship. With this help, inferiority can be conquered, and in its wake there can arise a sense of adequacy with genuine enjoyment of work, co-operation and competition.

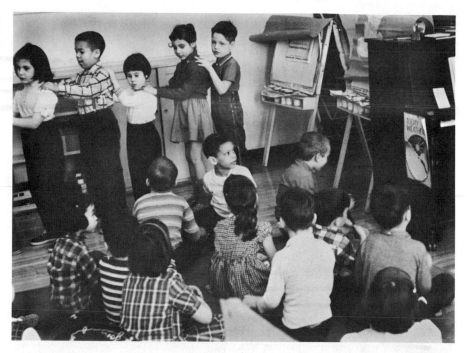

Fig. 25-8. Sitting still while others do what they want to do requires control and a desire to stand well with the teacher and the child's classmates. (Photographer Edgar Bernstein)

Importance of This Period

The importance of this period of middle childhood, or "latency" as it is often called, rests on the fact that the child's ego is now relieved from concentration on strong basic drives. Although many children continue to be concerned periodically with sexual curiosity and impulses, most have succeeded in repressing the intensity of interest in the parent of the opposite sex which was necessary for nonconflictual relationships with both parents. This period of respite makes it possible for the child to direct his energy into learning and intellectual growth, into development of new social relationships, into the formation of socially important defenses against his basic impulses, and into modification of his super-ego or conscience to meet the demands of the world beyond his home.

However, not all school-age children have this advantage. When sexual feelings are aroused in the child through experiences which may not have been meant as consciously seductive, he has no appropriate way to discharge tension. Such stimulation also prevents the child from directing his energy toward progress in intellectual and social development. Protection from overstimulation through human contact, movies, books and television programs is necessary so that the child's ego may become strengthened to meet the demands of puberty. At puberty his sexual drive is biologically re-aroused and his aggression is increased markedly.

Factors Affecting School Adjustment

Past Experiences. When a child enters first grade, many new demands are made on him. He is expected to learn how to deal with a new authority figure, a large group, new routines and restrictions on his activity. In kindergarten his teacher helped him to play with others, to use equipment and to develop manual and motor skills. Now, emphasis is placed on learning to listen, recite, read and write and to fit into all group activities.

For some children the transition from home to school is accomplished rapidly. Others may be temporarily insecure in a less intimate environment and feel as if they were losing their identity. Some may regress from overextending themselves. An affectionate send-off from his mother, a similar reception on his return home and willingness to listen to his account of the day's activities make the child feel that his efforts to meet the demands of school were worthwhile. Support in adapting to school also comes from the mother's readiness to respect her child's need to proceed slowly and from her confidence in his ability to separate himself from her. Sound physical health and emotional freedom to learn are also necessary for success in school. Middle childhood is the time for the development of mental skills. Unless the tools for learning are acquired in this period, the child will not be able to perform the more difficult tasks required of him during adolescence.

Learning is a complicated process which requires the capacity to give as well as to receive. It also requires the use of aggressive energy. The child must be able to listen, to look and to use his initiative in the search for knowledge. He must be able to make connections between what he has learned in the past and knowledge presented to him now. He must also be able to conceptualize, draw conclusions from the facts at hand and put ideas together in a way that has meaning for him. These are not new experiences for the first grader. He has been gathering data and learning from them since birth unless his natural, aggressive, investigative pursuits were thwarted early in life and resulted in a block or inhibition in learning.

Blocks in learning do not suddenly appear in school; they are directly related to the past. The incidence of failure in school is high, eight to ten times more frequent in boys than in girls, and is as commonly due to emotional problems as to mental retardation. School failure may involve one area, such as reading, but often there is general inability to learn. Investigators estimate the incidence of reading failures in normally intelligent school children to be from 8 to 10 per cent.

The causes of learning difficulties are multiple and are difficult to uncover and correct. School failures may result from conflict stemming from problems in interpersonal relationships and cannot be overcome unless their underlying causes are eliminated. Tutoring often increases the intensity of the conflict, especially if the child's parent tries to assume this role.

Sometimes failure in learning represents a regressive tendency in the child; he does not dare to grow up for reasons that are hidden from conscious awareness. He may unconsciously equate success in school with winning his parent of the opposite sex. In such instances, he must fail his school work in order to protect himself from anxiety. Another child may not feel secure in his parents' affection and so cannot relate himself to his teacher and a new social group. Despair is at the roots of some children's failure. There is no one who cares whether they succeed or not and, as a result, they do not get the recognition that they need to become emotionally free to work. Sometimes what the child gives to his parents is never enough. No matter how hard he tries, his parents always want more. Criticism and needling bring old suppressed feelings of inadequacy to the surface before he has had time to master them. Then his anxiety is increased, and anger makes it impossible for him to give something of himself to please his parents.

Intellectual Readiness for Formal Education. Children who have received the optimum levels of stimulation in the first years of life, encouragement and support of normal curiosity and drives for exploration, and recognition of success in mental endeavors are eager to continue development of their intellectual skills through formal education. Learning to read is exciting for those children who have become skilled in communication and language ability through encouragement to speak, extensive verbal interaction with their parents, acquaintance with books, listening to stories read to them, and systematic expansion of sentence structure.

Many children, however, have not had such opportunities during their preschool years. Children who live in culturally deprived environments often do not have the variety of sensory stimulation and experiences necessary for optimum intellectual growth or the acquisition of basic concepts. It has been demonstrated that environmental deprivation stunts the development of intelligence during the preschool period and contributes to the progressive decline of I.Q. scores during the school years unless remedial steps are taken. Effects may also include poor perceptual discrimination skills, inability to use adults as sources of information, and paucity of information. When exposure to language is limited in the home, auditory discrimination tends to be poor; there is a deficiency of abstract vocabulary, language-related knowledge, and understanding of the environment. The child's entire orientation to language is concrete, immediate and particularized, contributing to delay in reading readiness.

It is now known that the first four years of life are crucial in building the foundation for achievement of full intellectual potential. In addition, children who have lived in conditions of deprivation may also have failed to develop the sense of adequacy necessary to accept the challenge entailed in education, the motivation to succeed in intellectual endeavors or the responsiveness to adult guidance in the learning process.

Such children benefit from compensatory preschool education which enriches their experience in the areas previously cited. In addition, as they enter formal education, special attention should be given to developing listening, memory and attention skills, to furnishing models for language development and to gearing the educational process to the child's mode of thinking through providing more concrete, empirical props and opportunities for direct physical manipulation. Although future rates of growth are limited by previously attained levels, an optimal learning environment during the school years may arrest and in part reverse the existing degree of environmentally produced retardation in the acquisition of mental skills.

School Environment. The teacher is the most powerful influence in the child's school environment. She affects his attitudes toward school and proves to him that the world of adult authority is trustworthy. She sees that his environment is safe, stimulating and satisfying. She teaches him about his society and supports him in getting the knowledge and skills which he needs to get along in it.

The teacher's relationship with the children must be of the quality which supports them in making full use of the school environment. To accomplish this, she must understand the goals toward which they are striving and handle her feelings in such a way that *all* the children are benefited. Furthermore, she must know how to adapt her expectations to individual abilities and to help each child to enjoy being a member of a group.

Most children entering first grade are eager to identify themselves with their teacher's goals but also feel as if they must compete with other children for her attention. This situation arouses jealousy and heightens the child's admiration for his teacher. It also helps him to learn that the school environment is different from the intimate family life of his home.

Accepting the limited share of the teacher's attention is no problem for the emotionally healthy child unless there is obvious inequality shown, though most children secretly yearn for more of the teacher's personal interest. However, along with this wish is the need to escape from family Oedipal entanglements and to master tasks which make him more competent in the management of his own affairs. The school-age child manifests these strivings by separating himself from and becoming cool to adults; he is relieved from anxiety when he discovers that his teacher respects his need to emotionally distance himself from her.

The teacher who communicates that she is a *teacher* and not a *mother* supports the child's need for a respite from instinctual urges. In other words, the teacher who concentrates her energy on achieving group solidarity and productiveness strengthens the children's motivation to settle down to the job of learning. Holding up expectations which are appropriate to the individual child's ability is another way to free him from preoccupation with his impulses. The healthy child *wants* his teacher and parents to make demands on him, for, without challenge, he cannot conquer the negative counterpart of his core problem.

Hospital Environment. The school-age child in the hospital also will communicate his need to distance himself from his nurse and to direct his energy into work when he recuperates from acute illness. However, children with long-term illnesses may have problems as they attempt to involve themselves in their work. Deprivation of normal sensory stimulation may dull their ability to concentrate on intellectual tasks. Children who are bedridden for long periods or who are allowed only limited ambulatory privileges often become preoccupied with their bodies and have more trouble than do healthy children in keeping their sexual impulses under control. Manifestations of this difficulty can be observed when the children are being prepared for the night. They seek an outlet for pent-up aggression and goad each other into using the nurse to gain outlet for their affectionate feelings. It is not unusual to observe school-age boys demanding kisses from their nurse. Girls may act similarly when physicians make their night rounds. After a frustrating day in bed with little opportunity for emotional outlet and a long evening of stimulation from television programs, it is little wonder that the children have trouble in settling themselves down for rest.

Children need concrete help in dealing with such feelings rather than rebuff which conveys rejection of them personally. If the unit is small, the nurse might suggest that the children tell stories or play records

which encourage relaxation. If it is obvious that the children are too stimulated to sleep, the nurse might turn on the lights again for a game of cards with them or allow a pillow fight to be terminated. Sometimes initiation of a discussion of the problems which they have had during the day gives them relief from tension and helps them to feel understood. Nursing intervention of this kind communicates the fact that the nurse is not a mother but a person who is there to help the group to make the most of their experience in the hospital.

The nurse also can reinforce the value that the teacher places on the child's participation in the school program. Children worry about keeping up with their classmates in their own school. When the child's lessons are related to the world outside the hospital, he will be motivated to resume life there as before. Helping the child to keep his mind occupied with interesting activities releases energy to restore his body to health.

The child who resists going to the hospital classroom needs support in meeting his responsibilities. Discovering the reasons for his lack of interest in school and then working with the teacher to find ways to help him to enjoy the group experience usually proves beneficial. Encouragement of each sign of interest in the resumption of responsibility for his own learning (an ego strength) supports him in overcoming his regressive tendencies.

Hospitalized children are benefited when nurses and teachers work together to provide a stimulating environment for them. Unless teachers are kept informed of the children's medical progress through active participation on the health team, they may miss the point at which children become ready for more challenging work experiences.

Intellectual Development During Middle Childhood

It is during the elementary school years that intense intellectual and conceptual growth occurs and that reasoning becomes logical through the acquisition of mental constructs involving relationships which permit the co-ordination of differing points of view. Until the child is approximately 7, his thinking has been dominated by a lack of objectivity or completeness of separation between himself and his environment. Perception of the world was subjective, centered within the self; thus reality for the child held distortions, and true co-operation with others was not yet possible.

It has been previously observed that children go through certain successive stages in mental development as they do in emotional development, although the specific age at which a certain stage is reached may vary from individual to individual. Piaget stresses the age of 7 as a decisive turning point in mental development, for at this time new forms of organization appear which mark the beginning of logical thought.

During the years from 7 to 12, the child is in the phase of mental development which Piaget has termed the subperiod of *concrete operations.* The term "operation" refers to a mental action involving thought to reach a conclusion. Classifying objects into a hierarchy of classes, arranging items in a continuum and the reversibility involved in doing arithmetic are examples of mental operations.

During the preschool period, the child acquired the concept of the permanence and "constancy" of objects, i.e., that objects continue despite his absence and remain invariant through differing perceptual impressions due to changes in distance, perspective, brightness, and the like. During the school age period the child acquires the concept that certain properties of objects such as quantity of matter, weight and volume are also invariant although transformed in different ways. This awareness is termed *conservation*—the ability to be aware of the constancy of properties of objects in the face of transmutations. The development of this concept is vital and prerequisite to the subsequent development of logical thought.

As mentioned in previous chapters, the preschool child was dominated by his sense perceptions of his environment so that reality was only what it appeared to be. His thinking was subjective and tied to a perceptual domination from the environment. This can be demonstrated by showing a young child two balls of clay of the same size and weight. One of the balls is then flattened, shaped into a sausage, or cut into bits. Before the age of 7, the child believes that the quantity of the matter, the weight or the volume has been altered through the transformation. During the years between 7 and 12, the child will recognize the invariability or constancy of matter, weight and volume in that order.

The importance of the acquisition of the concept of conservation lies in the fact that it reveals: (1) the child's release from the domination of what he perceives through his senses or the illusion of the moment; he is no longer fooled by appearances and can differentiate appearance from reality, (2) the ability to utilize the deductive process and (3) the ability to see and use relationships. With the recognition of relationships, the child becomes capable of reasoning and of logical thought; he is able to form attitude and value systems, interpersonal perceptions and a concept of self. The child's ability to see relationships is also critical to increasing ability to deal symbolically with words, classes and numbers and to think in categorical terms in a more objective manner.

The difference in mental organization between the preschool and the school age child is that the older child has a cognitive *system* by which he organizes his world and through which he can construct the present in terms of the past. His mental structures are in equilibrium, he is capable of reflection, and new knowledge can now be assimilated into this flexible and plastic, yet enduring cognitive bedrock.

Concepts of Time, Space and Causality. The mastery of concepts of time becomes possible when the child has the ability to recognize relationships, can place events into successive order and can comprehend duration of intervals separating events. Time begins to exist for the child as a constant flow at approximately age 7 to 8 years. The comprehension of speed becomes possible with the co-ordination of distance and time relationships.

The construction of the concept of space also becomes elaborated during this period. At about the age of 7, children begin to manipulate objects actively and systematically and gradually acquire the capacity to differentiate cognitively between squares, triangles and circles. At this time they can also indicate comprehension of dimensions and somewhat later achieve complete relativity of perspectives.

Increasing liberation from egocentric thinking, wherein the world shares the characteristics of the self, is also seen in the child's elaboration of causality. Through progressive differentiation of the self from the external world, he becomes gradually more conscious of objective reasons for the occurrence of events and of physical causality. However, until the age of 12 (and sometimes later) individual children will, on occasion, continue to see life and energy in surrounding objects. Ascribing life to inanimate objects will dissolve first, while the tendency to ascribe energy to moving objects similar to human muscular energy may remain for some time.

Table 24. Simple Tests of Mental Proficiency

Age	Numerical Skill	Other Concepts
6	Counts forward to 30 Repeats 4 digits	Tells right from left Tells A.M. from P.M. Draws a man with head, neck, hands and clothing Defines objects in terms of how they are used
7	Counts by 2's and 5's Repeats 5 digits forward; 3 backward Can tell time	Copies a diamond Recognizes parts left out of a drawing
8	Makes change from a quarter Counts backward from 20	Knows days of the week Has an idea about distant places Can give similarity and difference between simple objects
9	Can do simple multiplication and division	Knows correct date Can arrange weights in order of heaviness
10	Uses fractions Knows numbers over 100 Repeats 6 digits forward	
11		Defines abstract terms such as honesty, fair play, deceit Can give the moral of fables

Beginning of Co-operation. As the child reaches middle childhood and becomes increasingly able to differentiate aspects of himself from his environment, he becomes capable of true co-operation because he no longer confuses his point of view with that of others. He can now see himself in the place of another and in relationship to his environment, appreciate various opinions, and value and respect both his personal autonomy and the viewpoint of others. This development allows for true friendship, for collaboration in group work, for real discussion and exchange of ideas, for the capacity to share in a common goal and for acceptance of individual responsibility in reaching that goal.

This new ability for co-operation can be seen in the emergence of games with rules at about the age of 7 years. A collective game is possible since they can agree on rules, adhere to them, control each other and compete on mutually accepted grounds. "Succeeding" takes on new meaning in terms of measuring the self against an accepted external standard.

A new sense of respect for himself and for others is also seen in the emergence of a stronger system of personal values and a moral code. Honesty in playing takes on importance, along with a sense of justice and fair play, camaraderie, sharing, empathy and an organization of the will.

Implications for Nursing Care. Children of school age need opportunities to manipulate objects, to handle and become familiar with equipment with which they will come in contact during hospitalization. Since their thought processes are situation-directed, they need experiences that will assist them in coping with unfamiliar places and routines. Tours of hospital wards, of playrooms, intensive care units and the like are beneficial in supporting their methods of coping when they have less energy due to illness or surgery.

Children of this age also benefit from discussions in which they can learn about their illness, its origin and the proposed plan of treatment. With a more mature concept of causality, they have the capacity for understanding that neither the illness itself nor treatment efforts are imposed on them because of their own misdeeds. With the ability for logical thinking and deduction and with a more mature grasp of reality and recognition of relationships, they are better able to understand the relationship between their illness and its symptoms and the treatment to be instituted. Co-operation in adherence to prescribed therapeutic measures is possible, for children of this age are able to think before acting. From experiences with medical and nursing personnel they can learn to identify themselves with professional goals and values.

School age children can express their feelings in words and this ability eases the adjustment to painful events. Children, particularly boys, want to be courageous. If they are allowed to grumble and project blame onto others until they mobilize their defenses, they will be able to face feared situations with the bravery that is necessary to their maintenance of a positive self-concept.

With a greater grasp of time sequences, they are able to maintain emotional contact with their homes and families during the intervals during which their parents cannot remain with them. Separation is also less painful for them since they are moving away from complete dependence on their parents. They are also better able to project into the future, to comprehend the duration of time required for medical treatment and to accept physical limitations that have a projected termination.

Since children of school age have developed a greater ability for attention and concentration, they can benefit from activities designed to maintain their interest in the environment. Literature, school work, puzzles, games, drawing, and other such activities can be utilized to relieve the monotony of life on the pediatric ward. Competitive games with rules, played with nurses or other children, are also welcomed as opportunities for the child to support self-concept, to release aggressive feelings and to reach out to the environment. Games can also be used as a tool to promote communication between nurses and school age children. The mechanics of the game give the child something easy to talk about; he gets a chance to size up the nurse, and in many instances he becomes confident enough to discuss his hobbies with her. When the nurse makes it fun for him to talk about his own interests, he begins to see her as a person who can help him to become adjusted to the hospital and will talk about his experiences there when rapport has been established. If the nurse makes herself available to him when he is under stress and expresses resentment, he can get relief from sharing his burdens with her.

Children who are hospitalized for long periods need experiences that help them learn about the world outside the hospital. A child who spends his sixth year on a Bradford frame or in a ward for children with rheumatic fever will not know what school life is like even though the hospital teacher shows him pictures and describes the school activities. He cannot develop realistic concepts about life in the community unless he has firsthand experiences with it. However, various parts of the hospital, such as the kitchen, telephone systems, storerooms and animal and chemical laboratories can be used to satisfy the child's quest for knowledge about the hospital, his body and the way in which disease is affecting it. Without concrete facts, learning to differentiate reality from fantasy is retarded. Co-operation in learning to protect his own health can be obtained when knowledge of the disease and the rationale of treatment is shared with him.

The personnel in some hospitals take chronically ill

and handicapped children on excursions to baseball games, circuses, beaches and restaurants to give them concrete experience, to keep their interest in learning alive and to prevent boredom, listlessness or unruly behavior. They also have cook-outs and invite celebrities in to entertain them or teach them something about the skill or the art in which they are proficient. Educational movies are also used. Such stimulation speeds children's progress toward adjustment to their handicaps.

Intelligence, Productive Thinking and Creativity. Differences in intellectual performance have been obvious from the beginning of history. Until fairly recently it was thought that cognitive processes developed through maturation and that potential or capacity was entirely inherited. It was also felt that intellectual performance was fairly homogenous and that an intelligence test measured all that was of significance in intellectual capacity. It is now known, however, that intellectual talent is multidimensional, composed of a cluster of special abilities, and that it can be modified through environmental variables and is affected by personality correlates. Types of thinking processes now generally differentiated are cognitive memory, convergent thinking or the analysis and integration of data, divergent thinking or the ability to produce new and original ideas, and evaluative thinking.

Intelligence is a potential or capacity to interact adaptively with the environment, the ability to work with symbols and to solve new problems based on past experience. However, capacity or naked ability in itself cannot be measured without the underpinnings of culture and previous experience. Standard intelligence tests measure performance relative to age as based on previous experience and language skills. As such they are quite predictive of success in the educational system which builds on such early experience.

The reliability of intelligence testing with very young children is limited and scores are only slightly correlated with later scores obtained in late childhood and adulthood. This is due to the fact that in the first years of life tests measure sensory-motor capacities, whereas at later ages there is a much higher contribution of symbolic processes in intellectual performance. Young children also have a short attention span, have difficulty in shutting out distractions, and are affected to a greater degree by the rapport established with the administrator of the test and by momentary emotional and physical states of well-being. Scores obtained through intelligence tests tend toward stabilization at age 6 and are reasonably predictive of adult performance at age 10. The constancy or fluctuation of test scores obtained throughout childhood, however, may often be erratic and influenced by environmental and personality variables. Children with ascending test scores are characterized by be-

havior indicating greater independence and competitiveness, moderate aggressiveness, willingness to strive for a distant reward, curiosity, self-initiating behavior and a drive for mastery and achievement. Those whose scores tend to decline progressively are characterized by a sense of parental rejection or lack of love, dependence and passivity.

Parent-child resemblance in intelligence also tends to increase with age. A relationship begins to develop in the second or third year of life and increases throughout childhood, until an average correlation of .50 is reached. This relationship points to the genetic component of intellectual performance, but the size of the correlation indicates that a great deal of the variance is due to environmental influences.

In recent years it has been found that intelligence tests do not necessarily predict greater creative abilities or the capacity for divergent thinking. Divergent thinking and creativity have been defined as the ability to generate new information out of known information, to produce new and original ideas and the capacity for breaking away from the conventional. Qualities of the individual which are prerequisite to a free flow of ideational possibilities include a lack of rigidity and tolerance for ambiguity, a strong sense of personal autonomy and the ability to experiment with concepts.

The cognitive processes involved in creative expression seem to have a close link with emotional development and personality structure. Creative awareness tends to occur in an atmosphere of permissiveness and openness to experience without undue concern for personal success or failure as evaluated by others. This implies a sense of inner trust and personal autonomy, and relative comfort with impulsiveness. There must be a tolerance for non-logical thinking stemming from primitive processes. Severe repression of earlier modes of thinking and feeling cuts off the individual's ideational supply, his ability to explore combinations of ideas which seem illogical and makes large portions of his own experience unavailable to him. Tolerance for temporary regression to more childlike modes of thinking allows the individual greater freedom to consider the unique in an attitude of playful contemplation. Thus the psychoanalytic concept of "regression in the service of the ego" has application to this aspect of cognitive process.

Other personality variables correlated with high creative ability are: a sense of self-confidence in striking out from the known and expected, a positive self-image and lack of undue concern for the evaluation of others or of feelings of inferiority, a tolerance for risk taking, a sense of independence and the motivation to persevere.

The creative child usually has a home background of satisfying relationships and parents who support individuality and divergence, aesthetic sensitivity and progress toward independence, and refrain from coerciveness toward conformity or frequent evaluative comments of the child's productions which engender fear of error.

Emotional and Social Growth During the Early School-age Period (6 to 10 Years)

Development in Personality Structure. The school-age child does not need to endow his parents with omnipotence because he has gained increased control of himself and of his environment. He begins to see his parents in a more realistic light, dares to argue with them, and learns that there are other persons worthy of emulation.

Early in this period the child's defenses are weak and break easily when demands are excessive or when he is faced with more frustration than he can bear. Malfunction of his body depletes him of energy and disrupts his sense of identity. When ill, he again becomes vulnerable to separation anxiety and irrational fears and is likely to regress markedly for a time. However, if he was emotionally healthy before the illness, he will quickly remobilize his defenses during convalescence because his newly internalized conscience and ego-ideal prevent him from enjoying babyish behavior as he did in the past.

During the period of middle childhood, the child's conscience is undergoing modification through influences both within his home and in the wider community. In addition, growth in cognitive ability releases him from the limitations of his former intense egocentricity and allows for the development of empathy and for growth in moral judgment. It becomes possible for the child to understand feelings of others in opposition to his own. The learning of cultural rules and of sanctioned social behavior also operates to smooth the transition of the child into the wider community. Modification of the conscience through interaction with peers and adults continues throughout childhood with an emphasis on the "morality of co-operation" and mutual respect.

The super-ego is also influenced by growth of the ego. As the ego becomes strengthened, it becomes increasingly able to deal with primitive impulses and the outside world and thus modifies the super-ego. The super-ego is greatly influenced by the cognitive factors of the ego; as the ego and reality-testing ability of the child become stronger, moral judgments become more rational.

Under the super-ego is subsumed both the conscience aspects and the ego-ideal. The ego-ideal is an expression of what "one wishes to be," whereas the conscience is the agent of self-criticism in terms of what "ought to be." The roots of the child's ego-ideal are in past experiences with his parents. The ideals of his parents for themselves and for the child become his ideals and throughout his lifetime he will strive to attain the goals that he acquired early in life. Experiences outside the home will modify them, but

his aspirations will always be colored by the image that he formed of himself when he was a young child. As he begins to see his parents more realistically, he fears them less. However, now when he fails to meet the demands of his conscience, he suffers from guilt and self-criticism. If he does not live up to his image of himself, he suffers from shame and is burdened with unconscious fear of abandonment.

Self-esteem, the self-image or self-concept is a result of the child's determination as to how well he lives up to his ego-ideal and represents an expectancy in regard to his present and future behavior. It is also greatly influenced by the way his peers and meaningful adults evaluate him. Judgments about himself are made by the child in relation to the manner in which he meets and copes with problems in his environment and developmental tasks. A sense of self-esteem has been achieved when the child confidently predicts success in meeting new or important experiences.

The foundation for a positive self-concept is built through a satisfying mutuality between mother and child in infancy and early childhood wherein the child internalizes the sense of being loved and trusted. With such a background of experience, the child of school age can look upon himself as competent and trustworthy. If, however, the child has not been so fortunate, he may enter the school years with a self-judgment of incompetence and untrustworthiness.

There is usually some discrepancy between the ego-ideal or "ideal self" and the "real self" or what the child considers himself to be. If the discrepancy is not too great, the self-concept will be integrated and in equilibrium and he will not need to resort to defensive maneuvers to protect the ego. On the other hand, if the child's self-concept varies markedly from the judgment and evaluation of others, there may be impairment in his ability to test reality.

Through the school years self-esteem is influenced through experiences of success and failure, through the opinion and reactions of significant others, the degree of comfort in ethnic and racial belongingness and the vicissitudes of developmental and environmental crises.

The restrictions of the super-ego are often as severe as external parental control (and sometimes more so); the guilt and shame felt as a result of infringements against the dictates of the conscience are as painful and frightening as parental disapproval or temporary withdrawal of love. It is fear of being punished by guilt or by loss of self-esteem and the increasingly higher standards of his elders which motivate the child to direct more of his energy into learning. It also stimulates him to strengthen the defense of *reaction formation*. Instead of overtly expressing an impulse, he reacts against it, represses it and replaces it with the opposite characteristic. For example, in place of the exhibitionism he demonstrated at age 4, he becomes modest in toileting, bathing and dressing. He dislikes being exposed and, when hospitalized, is uncomfortable when the nurse fails to pull the curtains around his bed when he is bathed or toileted. Cleanliness replaces messiness. He does not need to be reminded to wash his hands before meals; fear of punishment by his conscience motivates him to wash if he has previously learned that clean hands are important to his mother. At times he will be sloppy as he rebels against parental standards, but there will also be times when tidiness becomes the rule of the day. Co-operation and willingness to share replace greediness, and sympathy for close friends becomes more characteristic than cruelty. These characteristics are also influenced by the growth in his cognitive processes.

School-age children use a variety of other defenses to cope with anxiety, dependence and feelings of inadequacy. Denial of fear is usually expressed by an air of independence which can be misleading. It is important for the nurse to know that school-age children often "whistle in the dark" and display the greatest amount of bravado when they are feeling the most helpless. Such behavior conveys to the nurse that she is of no importance to the child; however, if she remains with him, she will discover that her presence strengthens the child's ego and makes it possible for him to protect himself from loss of self-esteem. The capacity to identify himself with important adults and peers becomes strengthened; he uses this defense to protect himself from fear of ridicule. Dressing like his friends or having long hair is not whimsical; it meets a need to be like his friends. Flight into active dramatic play provides a temporary escape from worrisome problems and gratification which is acceptable to his conscience; it gives him renewed energy to tackle his problems at a later time.

School-age children also defend themselves from anxiety with the use of compulsive rituals or "magic incantations." They step over cracks in the sidewalk chanting to themselves as they go: "Step on a crack, and you'll break your mother's back; step in a hole, and you'll break your mother's sugar bowl." They hold their breath as they ride by a cemetery, clutch at their clothing as a hearse rides by and mumble magic words when they get trapped in uneasy situations. Asking a child why he does these things does not produce much response. They feel safer when they do these things, but cannot say why. Magic rituals, which are a part of children's folklore, neutralize anxiety related to aggression. They may also express their new awareness of death and fear lest something dreadful might happen to them or to their loved ones.

Magic rituals comfort children and are normal unless they become so obsessive that they prevent them from functioning efficiently without them. The following anecdote illustrates the way in which a nurse used her understanding of children's magic to alleviate anxiety.

A father brought his two sons and a daughter to a child health conference for their first physical examinations since infancy. After the examinations were over, they huddled close to him as he talked with the nurse. They stood stiffly, not speaking or fingering any of the articles on the desk. Ted, the 3-year-old looked especially frightened. When the nurse took him on her lap to comfort him, she noticed that two fingers on each hand were crossed. When the nurse asked him why he had crossed his fingers his body stiffened more. "You must think something awful is going to happen here. Parents bring their children here to make sure that they are healthy. I'll bet your big sister told you to do that while you're here." Both children nodded. Then the nurse noticed that his sister's fingers were crossed, too.

The situation below illustrates some of the defenses used by a 7-year-old boy on the day after admission for repair of an interventricular septal defect. Although the boy's behavior betrayed the stress he was enduring, his defenses remained intact during the preoperative period.

When Bob was in the hospital for diagnostic studies, he had learned the purpose of oxygen tents, drainage tubes, etc. While conferring with Bob's mother at the time of his second admission, the nurse learned that she had shared with Bob some of the preparation for operation which she received from the physician. She also learned that Bob was an aggressive boy who coped actively with anxiety. During the week before admission, Bob became more active than usual. He cut off locks of his hair and after his mother reprimanded him, he sheared hair from his dog. He had also been obsessed with a new interest in the refrigerator. He stopped his play repeatedly, opened the refrigerator door, peeked inside, slammed the door shut and then resumed his former activity. In all probability, this compulsive act was useful to Bob in mastering his fear of having his chest opened and closed. Evidence to support this conjecture is based on the fact that interest in the scissors and the refrigerator was acquired immediately after he learned that a bed would be available for him in a week.

The next morning after Bob had dressed himself, he hurled linen into the hamper, clutched his soiled pajamas against his body and said, "They're mine" and then jammed them into the drawer of his table. His need for his mother was soon expressed: "Me and that other nurse are betting on something. We're betting my mother will be here when she said she would." He held his robe up to his face and blinked away tears. An aid brought him an x-ray gown and said, "Now you know where you are going."

While awaiting his turn for an x-ray, Bob sat pensively swinging his legs, picking his fingers or twirling his sash. Not once did he look at the nurse who had been introduced to him as a person who wanted to visit with him. He co-operated with the technician as he struggled to control his tears. The nurse observed carefully to find ways in which she might be useful to him. An opportunity came when visitors pushed their way into a crowded elevator. The nurse encircled Bob's body with her arms to prevent him from toppling over. Immediately, he looked directly into her eyes for the first time. (On the day of operation, Bob's father reported that Bob had told him about the experience on the elevator. In chatting with his father about the nurse, he always referred to her as his "bodyguard.")

Upon return to his room, Bob changed into his own pajamas and wanted to go to the solarium to watch TV. Enroute there, he ripped a "Nothing by Mouth" sign from the foot of an empty bed and bellowed angrily: "When I had my heart test, the doctor took tape from my arm just like that. Wow. That hurt bad!" The nurse recognized the reality of his feelings and surmised that he was dreading a similar event. They walked to the solarium with Bob striding far ahead of the nurse. Upon arrival there, Bob continued to ignore the nurse as he watched TV and the door alternately. Then he said, "Guess I'll go get my Army set." He accepted the nurse's offer to accompany him and told her how glad he was that he would not have to be moved to another room after his operation: "I just hate it when the nurse moves my bed."

Bob gathered up his trucks and guns, refused to have help in transporting them and dashed back to the solarium with a self-sufficient air. However, his periodic shift of interest from shooting suction cup bullets to watching the doorway for his mother betrayed the fact that his independence was more assumed than genuine. When Bob's mother arrived on schedule, he did not run to her immediately: he said "Hi" without enthusiasm. Ten minutes elapsed before he left his play to go to her, and then he asked her for a dime so that he could call his father.

The above kind of behavior is characteristic of the school-age boy unless he is markedly regressed from illness. He wants his mother near by but at arm's length to protect him from Oedipal conflict. He also wants freedom to play with his friends. Bob's mother recognized his needs and in no way tried to divert his attention from his playmate. Even in the face of threat, Bob was able to maintain emotional distance from her.

The arrival of an older boy in the solarium supported Bob in maintaining his defenses. No words passed between the boys until Ronnie helped Bob by retrieving a bullet from a spot on the wall which was out of his reach. Then Bob said, "You can play with me. I'll show you how to use this gun. We can aim at any old thing but not at people. We'd be dead ducks if we did." Bob's apathy vanished, and he laughed loudly when Ronnie missed his target. Occasionally he smiled at the nurse when he succeeded in hitting the mark. For another hour Bob assumed the role of a bomber pilot, worked off considerable aggression, and seemed to forget how needful he was of his mother earlier in the day.

Influences of Parental Child Rearing Practices. The technics that parents use in socializing their children during the preschool years have lasting effects, as indicated by the fact that the behavior of children in middle childhood is very predictive of personality characteristics in adolescence and maturity.

The children of mothers who are quite restrictive during their preschool years often later indicate greater submissiveness, dependency and shyness, show less mastery and dominance, but are more courteous, obedient, neat and generous. Such children are often conforming and indicate less curiosity and self-initi-

ated activity. Parents, however, who encourage independence and self reliance in their children in the years 3 to 6 promote the need for mastery during school age. If severe restrictiveness continues into middle childhood, the child may begin to show hostility and aggression toward his parents and, as adults, boys frequently demonstrate both dependency and aggression toward their mothers (hostile dependency). When such restrictiveness also includes elements of parental hostility, children may later turn their aggressive impulses inward into aggression against the self. Under the same conditions, girls in adulthood may indicate less hostility toward their mothers, but greater passive and dependent behavior.

The children of mothers who are highly protective during middle childhood often respond passively to frustration and are fearful of physical harm. Boys are less interested in typical masculine pursuits. On the other hand, such boys seem to strive harder toward academic excellence and show more need to achieve in school work.

The amount of aggression demonstrated by boys in middle childhood is related both to high parental permissiveness for aggression and to severe physical punishment for such behavior. In the first instance, the child fails to develop inner controls against his aggressive impulses. In contrast, parental punitiveness instigates anger in the child and resistance to authority and also constitutes a model for such behavior. Children in this age period who indicate internalized standards and guilt in response to transgressions, and who accept responsibility for their behavior, generally have parents who are warm and use psychological technics of discipline, such as withdrawal of love, use of praise, reasoning and isolation. Resistance to temptation has also been found to be related to love-oriented types of discipline rather than to external control.

Knowledge of parental attitudes toward discipline and the methods they practice in assisting their child to meet the demands of society is helpful to nurses in understanding the behavior of children when hospitalized and in providing optimum support throughout the experience. Nursing intervention related to encouragement for verbalization of hostility, setting of limits and provision for acceptable methods for discharge of tension and aggression, encouragement toward specific avenues for achievement and increasing self-esteem must be individualized in relation to the child's present personality characteristics and needs as based on his past experiences within his home.

Interaction with Peers. In this period the child becomes keenly interested in becoming a member of a group and there is an urgent need for friends to share experiences. He senses that he can become less dependent on his family only through group association, and he wants to shift from the contentment he ex-

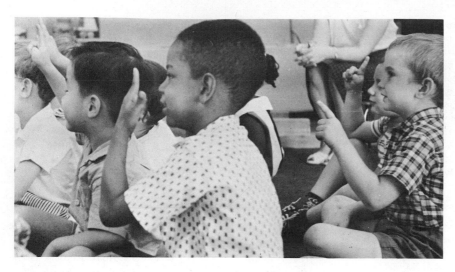

Fig. 25-9. Notice the way in which these children are giving; they are actively participating with their teacher. It is also evident how much they want to share their ideas with others. (Photographer Edgar Bernstein)

perienced within the small and personalized community into a larger environment of persons significantly like him and where the threat to control of his aggressive and sexual impulses is substantially less.

To become a valued member of a group, the child must be able to forego some of his own desires and to contribute for the benefit of others. Intellectually, he has achieved the ability to cooperate with others, to feel empathy and to understand and respect the viewpoint and opinions of his playmates. He now wishes to exchange ideas with his friends and to talk endlessly, comparing opinions and experiences. He can respect their rights, seeks their approval and wishes both to co-operate and compromise and to compete. In the beginning, a special friend must be rather similar in many ways to himself and they must have much in common, although some differences lend interest to the relationship.

As children progress through middle childhood, rules become increasingly important to them. When they have tested their powers in competition with others and mastered a game with one set of rules, they devise new ones to make the game more difficult to win. Such experiences help children to develop skills, and master feelings of inferiority, and teach them that rules benefit all players and can be changed through co-operative effort.

Children's interest in legislation is also expressed in their love of clubs. They compete for election to offices, vote on passwords, secrets and meeting places and formulate rules to control themselves and others. Such activity gives children the thrill of governing themselves and prepares them for membership in teenage and adult organizations.

After the age of 8, children begin to associate themselves with a group of their own sex to reinforce their sexual identity and to practice the role which they will assume in later life. Fighting within the group is common, but it rarely lasts long and when it is over, the bond between them is strengthened. Boys fight physically while girls tend to express their hostility with sarcasm and derision.

Teacher Influence on Socialization. The nature of the interaction between the personality characteristics of the child and the teacher's behavior and instructional style has a pronounced effect on the progress of the child's learning and in his sense of self-esteem. During the first few grades, teachers who are warm and nurturant are more effective with children who are less independent and self-reliant, while children who are characterized by curiosity and by self-initiating behavior are motivated to learn through enlisting their interest in the subject matter. The warmth which the teacher conveys is also important in protecting the self-esteem of children who are below the average in intellectual ability. When the teacher of such children genuinely likes them as individuals, their self-concept and achievement are considerably higher, whereas there may be no relationship between a bright child's achievement and the teacher's personal regard for him.

Experiences with success and failure influence the child's level of aspiration. If the rewards set by the teacher are entirely related to academic achievement, the child who has lesser ability experiences continual failure. Teachers who broaden the basis for evaluating students, allow freedom to students in setting individual goals, and are alert to reducing the prominence of relative standing in the class as based solely on academic achievement, will assist children in evaluating themselves realistically and protect their positive self-concept.

The degree of compulsiveness or conception about exactness and order and the amount of anxiety which a child feels when perceiving a threat to self-esteem also interacts with the prevailing climate of the classroom in influencing his level of achievement. Children who are generally conforming and somewhat compulsive are helped by a high degree of structure in teacher presentations. Continuance of structuring

Fig. 25-10. Notice the way in which these children are receiving from the teacher—with their mouths as much as the rest of their bodies. Their delight in listening to the teacher is also apparent, although one boy seems to be more interested in the girl at a distance from him than in what the teacher is saying. (Photographer Edgar Bernstein)

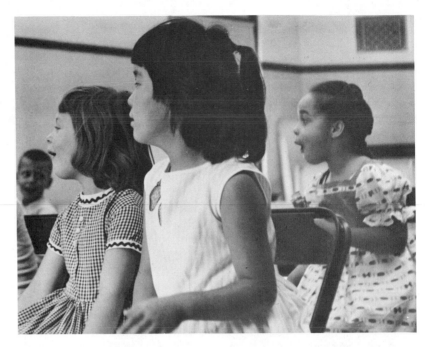

throughout the period of elementary education, however, may perpetuate a sense of dependence on authority. The performance of highly anxious children also deteriorates in an unstructured or permissive classroom since they risk failure due to lack of clearly perceived directives. When previous behavior patterns become ineffective in dealing with the environment, the resulting loss of self-esteem induces further anxiety and maladaptive behavior. On the other hand, children who are secure, confident of their ability and who can cope constructively with novel situations progress rapidly in a permissive atmosphere and are more productive in divergent thinking and creativity.

Continued Importance of Play. School-age children need space to run, jump and work off hostility and tension. In school the child must keep his energy channelled into learning and productivity, but when the bell rings he bolts from the door, seeking freedom for other pursuits. Physical activity is necessary to exercise large muscles, and skills in this area are valued by school-age children because they give them status in the group and assurance of their competency. Girls spend more time in crafts, doll and house play than in sports, but boys desire physical prowess. They are generally more aggressive than are girls and recognize that society expects them to achieve athletically.

Aggressive play involving symbolic conquering of an enemy is common in this period and is accompanied by shrieks of delight. Vicarious mastery over others is also sometimes obtained from reading comic books or watching Westerns and competitive sports on television, but is not a substitute for active creative play. Dramatic play may often be utilized to master anxiety.

Bob, the 7-year-old boy mentioned in the previous anecdote, had many reasons to be angry but was struggling to control himself. In play with Ronnie he separated his soldiers into two groups: one group was the "good" Americans; the other, the "bad" Russians. Bob shot down some Russians, ambushed others beneath his truck and surrounded them with the "good" soldiers. The Russians never

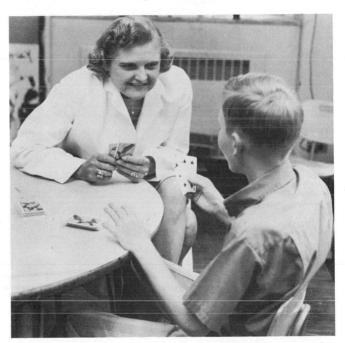

Fig. 25-11. The hospitalized school-age child has a need to win competitive games as a reaffirmation of a positive self-concept and as an outlet for aggressive feelings. Note that the nurse reinforces his self-concept by her obvious pleasure in the boy as an individual. (Bill Bargagliotti)

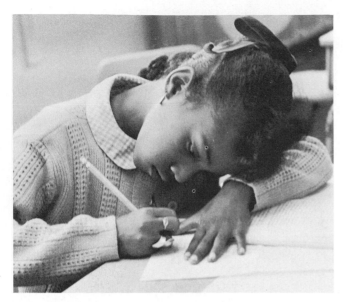

Fig. 25-12. The child in middle childhood is engrossed in the development of mental skills. The ability to concentrate has become highly developed. (Carol Baldwin)

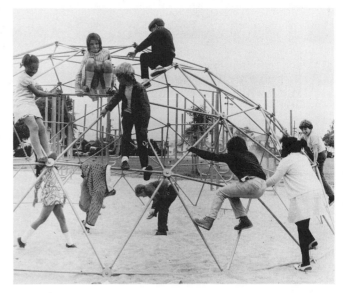

Fig. 25-13. During this period, children are keenly interested in group activities and physical skill is valued. (Carol Baldwin)

won a battle; there were too few of them to overpower the Americans.

Bob's aggression frightened him; anxiety aroused by conflict between his conscience and id warned him that he must get his "bad" feelings under control. Bob also had "good" feelings toward others and undoubtedly hoped that they were strong enough to conquer those which were a threat to him. When the enemy was overpowered, Bob laughed and talked more freely because his play made him feel that he was in control of himself, and therefore powerful.

Convalescent children are equally dependent on active play for comfort. During the day reasonable aggressive behavior is often markedly restricted by the limits imposed by hospital routines to facilitate the work of physicians and nurses. As a consequence of this the children often explode from accumulated frustration when the authority figures leave the ward. It is the evening nurse who has the problem of helping children to deal with their tension. Pillow fights, wrestling matches and arguments are staged because the children cannot control themselves any longer.

Prevention is the most therapeutic method of handling the above problem. Aggression may be discharged in play and discussions in the daytime, and outdoor activity is especially valuable. Creative activities provide outlets. Children enjoy such crafts as soap carving, jewelry making, carpentry, weaving and pottery. They also like to paint such objects as airplanes, boats and cars. Making murals, playing games of all kinds and staging plays in which they can wear costumes absorb their interest, too.

Children in the hospital vary greatly in their capacity to do creative work. Some will create spontaneously if they are given raw materials because they have talent and have already learned that they get relief from tension when they use it. But because of chronic illness or discouragement other children have few ideas of their own. They are preoccupied with themselves and have little surplus energy to develop latent talents. Selecting projects which they are capable of finishing quickly prevents further loss of self-esteem. Samples of finished products stimulate interest. When the nurse demonstrates confidence in the child's ability and is ready to help him when he shows signs of discouragement, he will generally exert himself to please her. Then when he succeeds in completing a project, pride in himself and relief from tension gives him energy to think up ideas for another one.

Like all school-age children, hospitalized children enjoy collecting things which have symbolic meaning to them. One 10-year-old girl in the authors' acquaintance collected her stitches, intravenous tubing, needles, medicine vials and paper cups to make a "medical museum." Children like to catalogue and organize their possessions. They are not always consistent in keeping them in order, but progress in this direction indicates that they are beginning to perceive benefits in regulating their lives more systematically. Children's interest in hobbies thrives with encouragement but vanishes quickly when adults interfere in their development. Most hobbies are of a transient nature. They meet a temporary need and then are replaced with another.

Books and story periods absorb most children's interest because they teach and give them relief from their worries. Comics may be read because friends

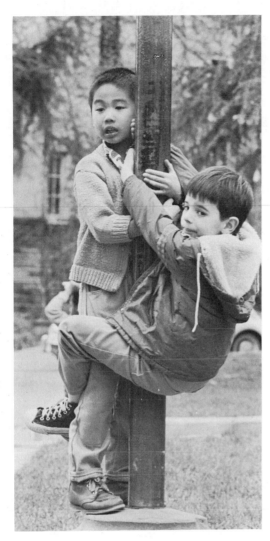

FIG. 25-14. Children who have the opportunity to learn, appreciate and value friends with varying cultural heritages can develop a basis for sound social relationships in adulthood. (Carol Baldwin)

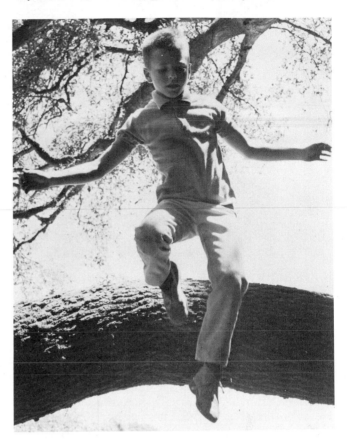

FIG. 25-15. Climbing and jumping not only reinforce feelings of self-esteem, but also facilitate discharge of feelings of frustration, aggression and tension. (Carol Baldwin)

expect them to know about Superman, or they may satisfy the child's longing for adventure. Contrary to adult opinion, not all comics are "trashy"; some do an excellent job of dramatizing real events. Favorite comics are those which portray the "good" person triumphing over the "bad." However, substitutes which provide varied kinds of pleasure must be provided or children will continue to spend much of their leisure time on comic books and television.

Individual Guidance. The previous sections have illustrated the complexity of the child's problems and cited some of the causes of maladaptive behavior during this stage of development. Impulses which were formerly expressed freely now must be restrained. This requires ego strength and the ability to handle considerable tension. Children who have been allowed to dissipate their anger in words and in active play

do not find it necessary to act out their aggression in the classroom or to keep it under such rigid control that no energy is left for learning.

Children with problems in relationship to their parents, teachers and playmates may reflect their distress by psychosomatic illness or by such symptoms as tics, obesity, enuresis, stealing, nose boring, truancy or malnutrition. Unruly and withdrawn behavior is also symptomatic of emotional turmoil.

The unruly, aggressive child never goes unnoticed in the classroom or the ward. He may be cruel, destructive, inattentive, domineering and/or unable to participate in group activity. He annoys the teacher and the children as well. He cannot understand that the pleasure he gets from his impulsive behavior is minimal compared to that which he would receive from learning and from constructive relationships with others. He is frustrated, troubled and bewildered but does not know how to change his patterns of behavior, and he could not do it alone even if he were told how he might do it. He needs understanding and help in learning how to get satisfactions which win approval.

The quiet, withdrawn child also needs study and

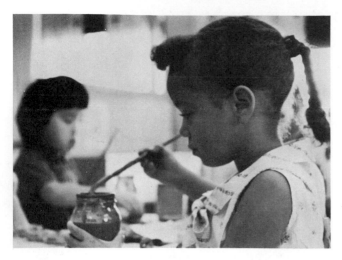

FIG. 25-16. Notice how carefully this 8-year-old uses her brush and compare it with the way in which a preschooler paints. This girl wants to make the most of her tools—just manipulating a brush does not satisfy her. (Photographer Edgar Bernstein)

special help. He may not be noticed by adults because he rarely complains and presents no disciplinary problems. But he, too, is lonely, confused and afraid. He has little initiative, becomes easily discouraged and rarely questions or contributes to group discussions. He cannot let himself become involved in relationships because he is afraid of his aggression and must dissipate his energy in keeping it under control. He may slip into a world of fantasy because reality has been too painful to bear.

The school-age child who is not progressing in his relationship with other children needs help. He will be handicapped in preadolescence if he has not become a part of a group. Children who never become part of the group are often referred to as "isolates." Most of these lonely children need a warm relationship with an adult before they become secure enough to participate in group activity. A few may respond favorably to a group leader who discovers their special talents and helps the group to appreciate the contribution which they can make to it. This gives them more security and assists them in freeing themselves from dependence on adults.

Observation in the School. Today many schools have counseling programs which are available to children who are having adjustment problems in school. Physical examination and psychological studies are made as a basis for care and guidance. Individual counseling is provided, and there are consultation services with professional workers in other fields as well. The school nurse is an important part of these school health services. Through study of the home situation she often is able to contribute knowledge of the causative factors in school maladjustment. She helps the mother to study her problems with her child

and to find ways in which she can lessen pressure on him at home. Not infrequently the trouble lies in the fact that the mother is harassed by extraneous family problems which make it impossible for her to be giving to her child. With help in resolving these problems, she can become more receptive to knowledge concerning the value of correcting physical defects and of implementing whatever suggestions the counselor makes. If psychotherapy has been recommended, the mother may turn to the nurse for help in understanding its purpose.

The mother may not understand why her child cannot confide in her but needs treatment designed to give him relief from his worries so that he can achieve in school. The nurse can expand the mother's insight into her child's needs to become less dependent on her. She can also stimulate the mother's interest in psychotherapy by assuring her that the therapist will help her to discover ways in which she can become more helpful to her child. Thus her fear lest the therapist might alienate her child's affection from her can be minimized. Referral for psychiatric treatment threatens most mothers. Therefore, it is wise to learn what referral means to the mother before helping her to understand the purpose of psychotherapy.

Observation in the Ward. When children are hospitalized for psychosomatic illnesses and emotional disturbances, recording of their behavior is valuable for all members of the team trying to help them to solve their problems in healthier ways. Therapists like to know their patients' choices of play materials and the way in which they use them. They also appreciate learning how they respond to their parents' visits, to authority, treatments, school activities and to the children and adults in the ward. A description of the social interaction which precedes or occurs concurrently with exacerbation of symptoms of body dysfunction is also useful. The therapist in turn can help the nurse to identify the child's particular needs for nursing care.

The child with a physical disease or handicap needs to be observed similarly. Some children need to be assured of the nurse's continued interest in them as they become convalescent and begin to socialize with their age-mates. If they can count on their relationship with her even though they loosen their dependent tie to her, they are better able to progress toward their previous level of independence.

Emotional and Social Growth During Preadolescence (10 to 13 Years)

Preadolescence is the 2- to 3-year period preceding the onset of physical maturity. The beginning of the period varies in children depending on their inborn timetable for sexual maturation. Much of the behavior described below continues to be manifest during adolescence. Unsolved problems from the past which reappear during preadolescence do not suddenly

FIG. 25-17. This girl is getting ready to make a mural. The boy is involved in screen painting. Both of them are more interested in expressing themselves and using paint than in each other. (Photographer Edgar Bernstein)

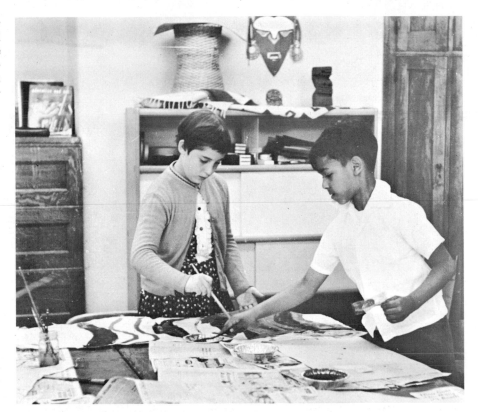

vanish at puberty; they continue to trouble the adolescent until he finds satisfying solutions to them.

Although this period is unsettling for the preadolescent because of new and unfamiliar sensations from his body and beginning changes in his emotional response to others, there is as yet no significant alteration in the strength of his sexual drive. During pre-puberty the child is struggling with several potent forces: (1) an increase in physical activity and energy made available from successful solution to some of his earlier problems and through hormonal and other physiological changes, (2) active anticipation of puberty with ambivalence and conflicting feelings regarding sex, (3) revival of the struggle between desires for dependency on the mother and a wish for independence, (4) an increase in the urge to master his environment through attainment of knowledge and skill, and (5) stirrings of interest in the opposite sex with resultant increase of effort toward becoming more closely related to members of his own sex. Toward the end of this period, physical growth is stimulated through hormonal action and interest becomes focused on bodily changes, resulting in increased anxiety.

Concern Regarding Body Changes. Because of the relative freedom from sexual stirrings early in this period, the child can learn biological facts comfortably. Later, however, he becomes quite conflicted about sex, receives information with mixed interest and apprehension, and may rebuff parental efforts toward preparation for the biological and emotional changes of puberty. At this time, sex information which is offered at home or in the school may be incompletely assimilated or rapidly forgotten. Children also become aware of the ambivalence and conflict within our society regarding sex. On the one hand, they learn cultural prohibitions and condemnations of sexual activity, while absorbing the emphasis on sexuality in all channels of mass media. They may also recognize parental discomfort in discussing sexual matters and thus turn to their peers for information. Unfortunately, this often leads to misconceptions and misinformation and prevents them from fully understanding the way in which their bodies will function when they become physically mature. Within their peer group, curiosity may be intense, with examination of their own bodies and those of their friends, secret conversations and exchange of information gleaned from magazines, novels or television.

When a child has learned throughout childhood that his parents answer his questions without evasion or obvious discomfort, he will be more likely to approach them when he feels a need for knowledge at this time. Girls can understand simple descriptions of the menstrual cycle or explanations of the female generative tract which will reassure them that their bodies are responding normally if their menstruation begins at a different time from that of their friends.

As the girl approaches adolescence she will need to have her own supplies and to know the approximate length of a period. She should also know that menstrual irregularity is characteristic during the early

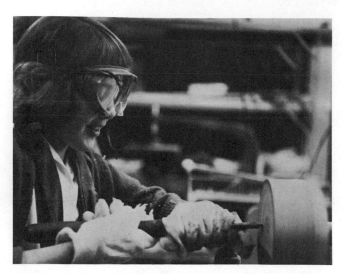

FIG. 25-18. This 9-year-old girl is in the process of learning a new skill. Notice the way in which her face expresses the pleasure she is having as she begins to make a wooden bowl. She is not afraid to use her initiative in learning something new. (Photographer Edgar Bernstein)

period of adolescence. If she accepts menstruation as a natural feminine function, transition into adolescence will be smoother.

Preadolescents must also learn that seminal emissions mark the beginning of the boy's progress toward maturity. Involuntary discharges of semen which occur during sleep are as natural for boys as menstruation is for girls. Unless boys understand this natural phenomenon, they may be frightened and think that it is caused by masturbation or disease or a sign of weakness. Seminal emissions require acceptance as do the boy's changing voice, growth of a beard and spurt in physical growth. Boys may worry needlessly about their rate of maturation unless they are reminded that normally there are wide variations in the time when adolescence begins.

As the child learns more biologic and social facts he will become motivated to bring more questions and ideas to his parents for discussion. When his parents have accepted his curiosity before adolescence, he will seek further help from them when sexual feelings become re-awakened. Then much of his concern will be centered on learning to deal with his impulses when he is in the company of the opposite sex.

Behavior Changes. The most common characteristic of the preadolescent is his boundless energy. He plays with increasing vigor to ease his tensions and anxieties related to approaching puberty and the reconfrontation of old and unresolved problems. In school he is restless and has difficulty in sitting still, and in his free time he immerses himself in competitive sports, club activities or hobbies in a seeming fear of passivity. Impulses toward aggression become

stronger in play and in fantasy. There may also be a marked increase in appetite to support the beginnings of rapid growth and to lessen anxiety.

Girls are more active too, and some express their increased energy and aggression in "tomboy" activities, horseback riding, and the like in a seeming denial of their femininity, whereas others accept this role more quickly and with more equanimity. Some children may cling to their activities of former years in what appears to be an attempt to postpone the changes and problems of adolescence.

Preoccupation with fantasies of the future may lessen the preadolescent's ability to concentrate in school and lead to an insensitivity to adult directives; yet, conversely, boys become closer in their relationships with their fathers and perceive men as friends and allies. Their relationships with their mothers are more conflictive, in that they simultaneously wish to be dependent, yet fear surrender and desire independence. This struggle may also be reflected in their abhorrence of feminine sentimentality and in their conviction of the unfairness of all female teachers.

Many changes in behavior occur during preadolescence because the balance between the id and the ego which sustained equilibrium during middle childhood is becoming loosened and upset. The child's conscience also cannot keep his impulses under control as well as previously. Unsolved problems from the earliest periods of development reappear. He becomes less interested in his appearance. Greediness, cruelty and exhibitionism may be striking. He again finds comfort in eating and his approach to food is like that of the young child. Table manners deteriorate and so does punctuality for meals. His interest in chores dwindles appreciably, and each new one that is added arouses antagonism and argument.

Negativism and assertion of independence may be even more marked now than when the child first discovered himself as an individual. His resistive behavior expresses his need for time to learn to do things independently. The behavior changes of preadolescence are disconcerting and threatening to parents unless they understand the purpose that they serve in preparing the child for adolescence.

From an adult standpoint, increased activity, the revival of old problems and a change in the strength of the conscience are disadvantageous. But for the child, temporary disorganization of his personality is necessary because the changes of adolescence cannot take place without prior loosening of the personality pattern and the destruction of previous modes of behavior.

Purpose of the Gang. Children begin to separate themselves from their parents during the early school-age period, but the detachment which occurs during preadolescence is more complete. Preadolescence is the *early* psychological weaning period, with final emancipation from parents at the end of adolescence.

Children expect their parents to respect their need for privacy as they respected their demand for it previously. The situation below shows how preadolescents manipulate their environment so that they can gain their independence.

Jackie, Madeleine, Caroline and Rose met each other in the hospital and became close friends. They asked for permission to room together and then called the unit "the girls' dormitory." On discovering that they had little privacy, they found an isolated area used to store equipment and set up a clubhouse. Using furniture from the playroom, they set up a kitchen, bedroom and clubroom. They spent hours each day taking care of their sick dolls, keeping house and going to meetings.

These preadolescents took steps to ensure their privacy. They put a screen in front of the door with a sign on it which read: "No Admittance Here. Please Keep Out." Their wishes were respected. When they wanted adult help or company, it was available to them, but when they wanted the joy of independence, it also was granted to them.

In cliques like the one above, preadolescents reveal their curiosity to each other and deny the worth of the opposite sex. In groups of either boys or girls there is speculation regarding the nature of sexual activity built in part upon realistic information they have received, but also upon fantasies, distortions and rumors which have come to them from many sources. Although girls are already indicating their interest in the opposite sex in subtle ways, boys respond to these overtures with avoidance or in an aggressive and teasing manner while continually reaffirming their strongly negative view of girls to adults and to each other. The interest of preadolescents in the opposite sex is expressed in negative terms because they are as yet unsure of their own positive identity and appeal and because they lack social finesse.

Preadolescents are absorbed in charting the beginning signs of sexual maturity and compare themselves with each other. The boy's fear of bodily injury and his envy of the childbearing ability of females may be evident in such activities as the raising of animals or fish, the observation of birth and the protection of the resulting offspring. The girl's envy of the masculine body also comes to the surface again and is reflected in aggressive and boyish behavior.

Groups which are made up of pairs of friends and held together by leaders serve many purposes for the preadolescent. Relationships with special friends are different from those of younger children. The preadolescent develops keen sensitivity to the needs of his "best" friend and helps him to achieve status in the group. This movement toward closeness to a person of his own sex provides the friends with mutual satisfactions and the security of knowing that they are important to one another. It gives each child an opportunity to get a new look at himself through the eyes of a friend who cherishes his friendship. It also gives him the security of knowing that he is not as

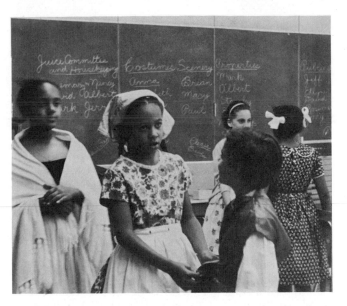

Fig. 25-19. Putting on plays not only provides avenues for self-expression, but it requires organization activity as well. Notice the blackboard to see some of the ways in which these 10- and 11-year-old children organize their work. (Photographer Edgar Bernstein)

different from other children as he had imagined himself to be. Together they can face their common problems in growing up. As the pairs of best friends unite to form a group and move toward the formulation and realization of a common goal such as organization of a hockey team, for example, skill in getting along with members of their own sex is attained. Until the youngster becomes secure in his relationship with members of the opposite sex during adolescence, he will continue to rely on his gang for support in solving his problems.

However, association with the gang is not without conflict for the preadolescent. The codes of the gang are stricter than the rules made by younger children and are often quite different from parental standards. Shifting from adherence to parental standards to those of the group arouses guilt and fear of punishment. Conflict arises from opposing goals. The child wants to please his parents, but he also must obtain the recognition of his peers if he is to succeed in emancipating himself during adolescence. When parents understand his dilemma and continue to support him with their approval, he acquires the courage to experiment with new ways of dealing with his problems.

Value of Hero Worship. The preadolescent needs an adult friend of the same sex to idealize and from whom he can get support during the period he is loosening his ties to his parents. The girl selects an older girl or young woman, endows her with protectiveness and warmth, "worships" and emulates her. With this source of gratification of her dependent needs, she can dilute her hostility toward her mother by criticizing her appearance, for example, or by suggesting better ways to run her house and manage the younger children. She may also take over some of her mother's responsibility, but somehow she always seems to irritate her when she does so.

Boys go through a similar phase of development, but, since they have learned that their society frowns on strong masculine attachments, their friendships with older people are usually less intense than those seen in girls. Boys more often master their fear of dependence by obtaining jobs outside the home. Since this solution does not generally have parental sanction for girls, they must form closer attachments to friends to emancipate themselves.

Parental stability in the face of the youngster's scorn prevents the preadolescent from becoming overwhelmed by fear of his obnoxious impulsivity. The preadolescent does not hate the parents he deprecates; he is merely trying to prove to himself that he does not need them as much as he did before.

During hospitalization the preadolescent girl may perceive her nurse as a mother figure. She may become critical of her though her attacks probably are not intended as a personal affront. Or, the nurse may become the girl's ideal. In such instances the nurse can meet the needs which are expressed in this behavior by showing interest in her as a person through such gestures as teaching her how to arrange her hair, for example, or by helping her to become successful in her relationships with the girls in the ward.

Guidance of the Preadolescent. Maintaining warm adult-child relationships throughout this period of disequilibrium supports the preadolescent in dealing successfully with the frightening changes which are occurring within him. Democratic guidance protects his self-esteem and strengthens his adaptive capacity. Overt demonstrations of love are distasteful because they remind him of his childhood. Love is welcomed in the form of tolerance of his irritating behavior, freedom to associate with his pals and interest in those personal affairs which he is willing to share with adults. The preadolescent rebels when he is disciplined like a younger child. He loathes hearing how amiable he was before and being compared to his siblings in a derogatory manner. *However, he does want limits set on his behavior to support his wish to adapt to reality.* He recognizes the fairness of punishment if it is appropriate to his age, fits the offensive act from his point of view and he knows *why* it is being imposed.

The healthy preadolescent knows when he has infringed on the rights of others and expects to pay a penalty when his behavior gets out of bounds. If he destroys something, he should pay for replacement from his allowance or through work assignments by his parents. He should return articles which do not belong to him. Suggestions to rectify situations which he knows are wrong will not provoke resentment. Instead they support his healthy inclination to take responsibility for his own actions.

The youngster who loses control of himself repeatedly and does not respond favorably to understanding guidance and reasonably imposed limits needs help before sexual maturity is reached. Guidance is indicated which helps him to gain inner controls and rewards his efforts to become more socialized. In most instances this help must be given by a psychiatrist. Immaturity and a need for psychiatric help are also being manifested by the preadolescent who never dares to rebel, to assert his independence and to become closely associated with a group.

To grow emotionally, the preadolescent must have freedom to use his increased energy in furthering the expansion of his ego. The more success he has in directing his energy into constructive pursuits which provide recognition and prove his worth, the less aggressive he will be in his relationship with others. He will also be better prepared to meet the demands of adolescence.

By preadolescence, the youngster has learned to size up people quite accurately. When he learns to make constructive use of this ability to appraise the strengths and the weaknesses of people, it will enhance his interpersonal relationships considerably. The preadolescent has not acquired this ability. Instead, he uses it for his own selfish purposes. Preadolescents know what behavior irritates their parents the most and then use this knowledge when they feel helpless and do not know any other way to handle it. Bedridden preadolescents are apt to do the same thing. While nurses are concentrating their attention on the provision of care, children take stock of their personality characteristics. When a preadolescent's image of himself as an independent person is threatened, he is apt to do those things which he knows will provoke the nurse the most. A response which focuses the preadolescent's attention on his strengths is appropriate in these situations because it furthers his acceptance of temporary dependence on others for the care which he would ordinarily take pride in giving to himself.

SITUATIONS FOR FURTHER STUDY

1. How does guidance during earlier periods of personality development affect the child's adjustment and growth during this period?

2. From what does the 6-year-old's sense of inadequacy stem? What motivates him toward acquiring a sense of industry?

3. In what ways might emotional support for the 6- to 10-year-old child differ from that provided for the 4-year-old child?

4. In what ways can the nurse help the convalescent school-age child (6 to 10 years) to regain his former level of functioning after an acute illness?

5. What made it possible for Bob to maintain his defenses during his earliest days in the hospital? What elements were a part of the nurse's role in this period? What purpose did cutting hair serve Bob? What do you think prompted Bob to ask his mother for a dime to call his father?

6. When a child acts directly opposite to the way he feels, what defense is he using? Of what value is it to a nurse to recognize a child's defenses against frightening feelings?

7. What personality strengths would facilitate the school-age child's adaptation to the hospital milieu?

8. Observe first-grade children in a public school. Describe what you saw and felt as you observed the situation. What behavior did you observe which made you believe that the children were reacting to the pressure of the demands of the teacher? During what situation did they feel the most comfortable? What behavior manifested this change in feeling?

9. What personality characteristics in a 7-year-old child would lead you to believe that he was well-adjusted? Poorly adjusted and in need of special study?

10. Observe school-age children on a playground. Describe the behavior and the activity of the group. How did the children's behavior differ from that which you observed on a playground of preschool children?

11. What legislative activity have you observed in small units of school-age children in the hospital? What rules did they make for their own comfort?

12. Describe the behavior of a 6- to 10-year-old child in a stress situation. Cite the problem as you think the child views it and discuss the ways in which he attempts to cope with it and you intervene to give him support.

13. What physical and behavioral changes appear in the preadolescent period of personality development? What produces the behavioral changes? How might you interpret the meaning of these changes to a pre-adolescent's parents?

14. What are the preadolescent's goals?

15. Observe fourth and sixth grade children in a public school and compare the behavior of the two groups. What differences in behavior did you observe? How did their teacher's guidance differ? How did the teacher of the sixth grade children use their initiative in planning their program of study? What did you learn from this observational experience which will increase your skill in working with preadolescents in a hospital ward.

16. Describe the behavior of a 10- to 13-year-old youngster in a stress situation. Cite the child's problem as you think he perceived it. What strengths did he have to cope with it? How did you intervene to support him?

17. Read the article by H. Creighton and Sister Gabriella Richard cited in the bibliography and be prepared to discuss the following points in class: (a) What attitudes did the nurse reveal in her behavior which made it possible for Christopher to share his fears with her? (b) What strengths and needs did Christopher's behavior reveal? (c) How did the nurse support his strengths?

BIBLIOGRAPHY

Becker, W.: Consequences of Different Kinds of Parental Discipline, *in* Hoffman, M., and Hoffman, L. (eds.), Review of Child Development Research, N. Y., Vol. I, Russell Sage Foundation, 1964.

Beflin, I. N.: Working with children who won't go to school, Children *12*:109, 1965.

Bettelheim, B.: The decision to fail, The School Review *69*: 377, 1961.

———: To nurse and to nurture, Nurs. Forum *1*:60, 1962.

Blos, Peter: The initial stage of male adolescence, Psycho-anal. Stud. Child *20*:145, 1965.

Bresner, J., Olver, R., and Greenfield, P.: Studies in Cognitive Growth, N. Y., J. Wiley and Sons, 1966.

Breznitz, S., and Kugelmass, S.: Intentionality in moral judgment-developmental stages, Child Development *38*: 469, 1967.

Brodie, R., and Winterbottom, M.: Failure in elementary school boys as a function of traumata, secrecy and de-rogation, Child Development *38*:701, 1967.

Bronfenbrenner, U.: The psychological costs of quality and equality in education, Child Development *38*:909, 1967.

Brooks, B.: Aggression, Am. J. Nurs. *67*:2519, 1967.

Bruce, S.: What mothers of 6-10 year olds want to know, Nurs. Outlook *12*:40, 1964.

Campbell, J.: Peer Relations in Childhood, *in* Hoffman, M., and Hoffman, L. (eds.), Review of Child Development Research, Vol. I, N. Y., Russell Sage Foundation, 1964.

Committee on Adolescence, Group for the Advancement of Psychiatry: Preadolescence *in* Normal Adolescence: Its Dynamics and Impact, N. Y., Charles Scribner's Sons, 1968.

Creighton, H., and Richard, Sister Gabriella: When you are scared, Am. J. Nurs. *63*:61, 1963.

Cromwell, G.: The child in the school, Nurs. Outlook *13*:27, 1965.

Deutsch, H.: Prepuberty *in* Psychology of Women, Vol. 1, N. Y., Grune, 1944.

Erickson, F. H.: When 6-12 year olds are ill, Nurs. Outlook *13*:48, 1965.

———: Helping the sick child maintain behavioral control, Nurs. Clin. N. Am. *12*:695, 1967.

Feshbach, N., and Roe, K.: Empathy in six- and seven-year-olds, Child Development *39*:133, 1968.

Fredlund, D.: The route to effective school nursing, Nurs. Outlook *15*:24, 1967.

Freud, A.: Orientation of the Process of Defense According to the Source of Anxiety and Dangers *in* The Ego and the Mechanisms of Defense, p. 58, N. Y., Internat. Univ. Press, 1946.

———: The Latency Period *in* Psychoanalysis for Teachers and Parents, N. Y., Emerson Books, 1947.

Gallagher, J.: Productive Thinking *in* Hoffman, M., and Hoffman, L. (eds.), Review of Child Development Research, Vol. 1, Russell Sage Foundation, N. Y., 1964.

Garari, J.: Formation of the Concept of "Self" and the Development of Sex Identification *in* Kidd, A., and Rivoire, J. (eds.), Perceptual Development in Children, N. Y., Internat. Univ. Press, 1966.

Gardner, R., and Moriority, A.: Personality Development at Preadolescence, Seattle, Univ. Washington Press, 1968.

Glidewell, J., Kantor, M., Smith, L., and Stringer, L.: Socialization and Social Structure in the Classroom, *in* Hoffman, M., and Hoffman, L. (eds.), Review of Child Development Research, Vol. II, N. Y., Russell Sage Foundation, 1966.

Godden, R.: An Episode of Sparrows, N. Y., Viking Press, 1955.

Hartup, W., and Coates, B.: Imitation of a peer as a function of reinforcement from the peer group and rewardingness of the model, Child Development 38:1003, 1967.

————: Glazer, J., and Charlesworth, R.: Peer reinforcement and sociometric status, Child Development 38: 1017, 1967.

Heath, H.: Three eight year olds, Child Development 38: 747, 1967.

Herbert, E., Gelfand, D., and Hartman, D.: Imitation and self esteem as determinants of self-critical behavior, Child Develop. 40:421, 1969.

Humphreys, A. L.: Heaven in My Hand, Richmond, Va., John Knox Press, 1950.

Hundleby, J., and Cattell, R.: Personality Structure in Middle Childhood and the Prediction of School Achievement and Adjustment, Monographs of the Society for Research in Child Development, Vol. II, No. 5, 1968.

Josselyn, I.: The Happy Child, N. Y., Random, 1955.

Kagan, J., and Moss, H.: Birth to Maturity, N. Y., J. Wiley and Sons, 1962.

Kuhn, D., Madsen, C., and Becker, W.: Effects of exposure to an aggressive model and frustration on children's aggressive behavior, Child Development 38:723, 1967.

Lee, H.: To Kill a Mockingbird, Philadelphia, Lippincott, 1960.

Lewis, G.: Interpersonal relations and school achievement, Children 2:235, 1964.

Malmquist, C.: Conscience development, Psychoanal. Stud. Child 23:301, 1968.

Medaris, E.: Incorporating health concepts in school nursing, Nurs. Outlook 15:60, 1967.

Nass, M.: The superego and moral development in the theories of Freud and Piaget, Psychoanal. Stud. Child 21:51, 1966.

Parks, G.: The Learning Tree, Greenwich, Conn., Fawcett Publishing Co., Inc., 1963.

Patterson, G., Littman, R., and Bricker, W.: Assertive Behavior in Children: A Step Toward a Theory of Aggression, Monographs of the Society for Research in Child Development, Vol. 32, No. 5, 1967.

Patton, F. G.: Good Morning, Miss Dove (Pocket Book edition), Dodd Mead, 1954.

Piaget, J.: Six Psychological Studies, N. Y., Random House, 1967.

Proshansky, H.: The Development of Intergroup Attitudes, *in* Hoffman, M., and Hoffman, L. (eds.), Review of Child Development Research, Vol. II, N. Y., Russell Sage Foundation, 1966.

Redl, F.: Pre-adolescents: What makes them tick, Child Study 21:44, 1943, 1944.

Rooke, M.: What does the teacher expect of a school nurse? Nurs. Outlook 13:33, 1965.

Rubin, R.: Body image and self esteem, Nurs. Outlook 16: 20, 1968.

Schroeder, C.: Mental health facilities in the school, Nurs. Outlook 13:30, 1965.

Sears, P., and Sherman, V.: In Pursuit of Self Esteem, Belmont, Calif., Wadsworth Publishing Co., 1964.

Shore, M., Geiser, R., and Wolman, H.: Constructive uses of a hospital experience, Children 12:3, 1965.

Siegel, I., and Hooper, F.: Logical Thinking in Children, N. Y., Holt, Rinehart and Winston, 1968.

Stobo, E. C., Shoobs, D., McKevitt, R., and Matsunaga, G.: The Nurse in the Elementary School: Promotion of Mental Health, N. Y., Teacher's College Press, 1968.

Stuart, H. C., and Prugh, D. G.: The Healthy Child, Cambridge, Harvard, 1960.

U. S. Dept. of Health, Education & Welfare, Children's Bureau: Health of Children of School Age Supt. of Doc., U. S. Govt. Printing Office, Washington, D. C., 1964.

Walker, R.: Some Temperament Traits in Children as Viewed by Their Peers, Their Teachers and Themselves, Monographs of the Society for Research in Child Development, Vol. 32, No. 6, 1967.

Wallach, M., and Kogan, N.: Models of Thinking in Young Children: A Study of the Creativity-Intelligence Distinction, N. Y., Holt, Rinehart and Winston, 1965.

Ward, W.: Creativity in young children, Child Development 39:737, 1968.

Wayne, D.: The lonely school child, Am. J. Nurs. 68:774, 1968.

Yando, R., and Kagan, J.: The effect of teacher tempo on the child, Child Development 39:27, 1968.

Your Child from 6-12 (pamphlet), Washington, Federal Security Administration, Children's Bureau.

26

Nursing Care of Children With Disorders of the Endocrine Glands

GENERAL DISCUSSION

Knowledge about the endocrine glands, the hormones they produce, their functions, interactions and abnormalities has increased rapidly within recent years. New concepts are being added as biochemical research clarifies the role which these organs play in normal and abnormal growth and in disease.

The endocrine glands consist of the thyroid, the parathyroids, the adrenals, the pituitary, the islands of Langerhans of the pancreas, and the gonads (ovaries or testes). The pineal and the thymus glands have sometimes been included in the list, but the function of the pineal gland remains uncertain and the thymus is now recognized as being a basic organ of the immune response of the body.

The endocrine glands secrete hormones which are absorbed into the blood. The hormones are "chemical messengers" which have their effect on other organs of the body. Hormones of several glands may act together and enhance the effects of the others; or they may act antagonistically, maintaining a balance of activity.

The pituitary hormones activate or inhibit secretion in so many other endocrine glands that the pituitary often is called the master gland. The pituitary gland (or the hypophysis) has two parts: an anterior and a posterior lobe, each with separate functions. When injected, posterior lobe preparations cause increased blood pressure, increased intestinal tonicity and peristalsis, increased respiratory rate and powerful contraction of the uterus; they also have an antidiuretic effect in diabetes insipidus. The most important hormones of the anterior lobe are those that promote growth and those that increase the function of the generative, the adrenal and the thyroid glands. Many other effects have been recorded.

Several of the hormones of the anterior lobe of the pituitary have been isolated in relatively pure form.

Of these, the adrenocorticotropic hormone (ACTH) which stimulates the cortex of the adrenal glands is the most widely used in treatment of children. Growth hormone, gonadotropic hormones which stimulate the generative organs, and thyrotropic hormone which increases the activity of the thyroid gland, are also available for limited therapeutic and diagnostic use.

The effect of hormones in some instances depends on the ability of the receptor organ to respond. For example, if the epiphyses have not yet fused and the bones still have capacity for growth in length, abnormally increased secretion of the growth-promoting hormone of the anterior lobe of the pituitary gland results in exaggerated symmetric growth of the body (gigantism). After fusion of the epiphyses, the increased secretion results in acromegaly, a condition of distorted growth in which various parts of the body increase in size without increase in body length.

Carbohydrate metabolism is controlled by the pancreas and the pituitary, the adrenal and the thyroid glands. The main hormone of the pancreas, insulin, regulates the storage of glucose as glycogen. The pancreas also produces glucagon, a substance which increases blood sugar levels by changing liver glycogen back to glucose. One of the pituitary hormones is antagonistic to insulin. Hyperpituitarism produces hyperglycemia and glycosuria. Hypopituitarism has the opposite effect. Epinephrine causes increase in blood sugar by calling out the glycogen stores from the liver and has other effects on sugar metabolism. The thyroid hormone causes increased combustion of sugar.

The thyrotropic hormone of the anterior pituitary stimulates the thyroid to increased activity. In excess, it may produce hyperthyroidism; a deficiency may result in hypothyroidism.

Growth and maturation of the body are dependent upon proper functioning of the pituitary, the thyroid, the adrenal and the gonads. The pituitary is concerned directly with growth and also indirectly through stimulation of the gonads and the thyroid. The general maintenance of growth of body organs, especially of epiphysial and periosteal bone growth, is the chief function of the growth-promoting hormone of the pituitary. The thyroid also directly affects growth because of its effect on metabolism.

The parathyroid glands control the level of blood calcium, using bone as the reservoir of calcium. Hypoparathyroidism produces tetany from low blood calcium. In addition to producing high blood levels and a high rate of excretion of calcium, hyperparathyroidism causes disappearance of bone mineral, with resulting osteoporosis.

The outer portion of the adrenal glands (the cortex) is the site of production of a number of hormones which are chemical derivatives of cholesterol and re-

ferred to as steroids or corticosteroids. Their production is largely under the control of the pituitary gland through the mediation of ACTH. This group includes aldosterone which regulates salt metabolism; the glucocorticoids, such as cortisol, which affect carbohydrate metabolism; the androgens, estrogens and progestins which are concerned with protein metabolism and with sexual development and function.

The inner portion of the adrenal glands is embryologically closely related to the tissues of the sympathetic nervous system. This medullary portion of the gland produces epinephrine and norepinephrine, both of which maintain blood pressure. Epinephrine has additional influences upon carbohydrate metabolism which are useful during sudden stress.

Under the stimulation of gonadotropins during and following puberty, the gonads produce their corresponding hormones—estrogens from the ovaries and androgens from the testes—which in turn govern the appearance of secondary sex characteristics and influence the skeletal growth and maturation.

NORMAL SEXUAL DEVELOPMENT

The physical changes characteristic of puberty (see also Chapter 30) are dependent on the presence of gonadal sex hormones that are formed as a result of stimulation of the gonads by the gonadotropic hormones of the pituitary gland. The amount of secretion of gonadotropic hormones by the pituitary is negligible in early childhood but increases in late childhood to give the impetus to puberty development. These pituitary hormones maintain gonadal activity for many years.

The sex characteristics, particularly the secondary characteristics, are determined by the type of hormone formed in the greatest quantity and by the relative proportions of the two types of sex hormones. The sex hormones, both male and female, are similar chemically. Each person elaborates both types of hormones. Androgens give the body the male configuration and cause the normal hypertrophy of the male sex organs. Estrogens give the body the female configuration and cause normal hypertrophy of the female sex organs. Both types of gonadal hormones stimulate fusion of the epiphyses through repression of the pituitary growth hormone, bringing growth in length to a stop. The process of epiphysial fusion is slow, so that growth proceeds for a considerable time after puberty. The gonadal hormones have a powerful influence on attitudes and general health.

The endocrine sex mechanisms in boys are relatively simple in comparison with the complicated cyclic changes which take place with menstruation in girls. The gonadotropic hormones of the pituitary not only stimulate the production of estrogen by the ovary but also stimulate the maturation of ova. As soon as the ovum begins to ripen, the follicle in which it is developing secretes further amounts of estrogen. This in-

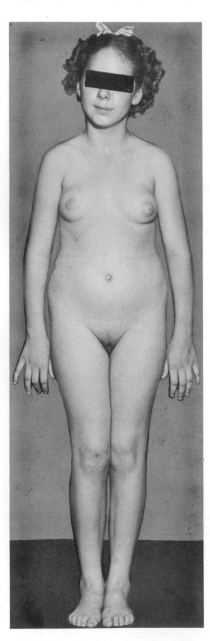

FIG. 26-1. Constitutional sexual precocity in a girl of 7 years.

creased amount of estrogen causes increased growth of the inner lining of the uterus (endometrium) and increase in its vascularity. After the ovum has matured fully and has been extruded, the follicle site becomes filled with cells to form the corpus luteum. This is formed under the stimulus of a luteinizing hormone from the pituitary. The corpus luteum produces the hormone, progesterone. The effect of this hormone on the uterus is to cause still further increase in the thickness and the vascularity in the endometrium. The endometrial changes are in preparation for reception of the fertilized ovum. When the ovum is not fertilized it is not implanted in the uterus, and the corpus luteum immediately atrophies, and progesterone disappears. With the sudden decrease of progesterone, the outer portions of the hypertrophied endometrium slough off, producing menstrual flow.

SEXUAL PRECOCITY

Constitutional or Idiopathic Precocity

Sexual development is regarded as precocious when secondary sex characteristics appear before the age of 8 in girls (Fig. 26-1) and before the age of 10 in boys. Such an acceleration is about 4 times as common among girls as it is among boys. The most common variety of sexual precocity is called constitutional or idiopathic precocity, signifying that there are no obvious associated abnormalities which might be presumed to set off the maturing effects of the pituitary gland prematurely. In some instances there appears to be a hereditary predisposition within the child's family. The effects of this variety of sexual precocity may be upsetting to the family and to the child because of his or her abnormally mature appearance. No serious consequences result otherwise, and the child's agemates eventually catch up in development. The ultimate height of such boys and girls tends to be below the average, for, although a marked growth spurt usually occurs when sexual development first appears, the process also leads to early epiphyseal closure in the long bones of the skeleton, which in turn limits the duration of growth to an abnormally brief period.

Intracranial Lesions

Intracranial lesions such as a preceding encephalitis or an unrecognized brain tumor may stimulate the precocious appearance of puberty. Usually there are other evidences of neurologic disturbance when this is the exciting cause.

Adrenogenital Syndrome in Boys

Either hypertrophy or tumor of the adrenal cortex may lead to excessive production of androgens which in turn stimulate premature development of male sexual characteristics but without proportional enlargement of the testes. Benign hypertrophy occurs most frequently and is due to perverted activity of the adrenals which are unable to synthesize the normal corticosteroids. Treatment with cortisone results in rapid decrease in the production of androgen, cessation of further virilization and a fall in the level of 17-hydroxy-ketosteroids in the child's urine. If the underlying defect is due to a tumor, this therapeutic result will not be obtained, and other diagnostic procedures are in order.

Tumors of the Gonads

Rarely, tumors of the gonads may be responsible for precocious pubertal development. Interstitial-cell tumors of the testis usually can be recognized by palpation, since they produce enlargement of one testis. Granulosa-cell tumors of the ovary are likewise discoverable by palpation. In such circumstances the tumor must be removed.

THYROID DISORDERS

Goiter

The thyroid gland which lies on the anterior surface of the neck has the responsibility of manufacturing thyroid hormone which is an essential regulator of the body metabolism and of growth. Iodine in small amounts is needed in the process. Ordinarily, the gland is seen or felt with difficulty. Under certain conditions it may enlarge and become visible. The resulting tumor is called a goiter. The presence of enlargement does not indicate what the nature of the underlying abnormality is. This must be worked out by additional investigations, particularly of thyroid function.

Simple Goiter. This term implies a physiologic enlargement of the thyroid which occurs particularly in girls at the time of puberty when the gland is called on to produce an increased amount of hormone. It requires no treatment. It may also occur with pregnancy.

Endemic Goiter. Enlargement of the gland occurs in geographic regions where the soil is lacking in iodine and the local vegetables thus fail to provide adequate amounts for the fabrication of hormone. The enlargement is a response to the attempt to make hormone with insufficient materials. It can be stopped or corrected by administration of iodine. In the United States it has become very rare, since it is prevented automatically by the addition of iodine to most commercial table salt.

Goitrous Cretinism. Cretinism may be due to an inability of the gland to manufacture hormone in spite of an adequate intake of iodine. This variety of hypothyroidism requires the same treatment as that described for cretinism due to congenital absence of the gland (see Chap. 13).

Toxic Goiter. This is enlargement of the gland associated with an abnormally large production of hormone. It is discussed below under Hyperthyroidism.

ACQUIRED HYPOTHYROIDISM

Occasionally, hypothyroidism of lesser degree than that of cretinism is encountered in childhood. All degrees of hypothyroidism exist, from the obvious to that detected only with special tests. When the condition is of at least moderate degree, both physical and mental growth is slowed (Fig. 26-2). The basal metabolic rate is decreased. The "bone age" is less than the chronologic age. Puberty is delayed. The child tends to be lethargic. The skin is cool and dry and of a poor color. The cholesterol content of the blood is increased, and the phosphatase content is decreased. The creatine output in the urine is below normal.

The treatment of these children consists of giving an appropriate dose of thyroid. The amount should be that which corrects the symptoms and less than that which produces nervousness or other evidence of hyperthyroidism. The child with hypothyroidism has good tolerance to thyroid medication. When thyroid is given in case of an erroneous diagnosis of hypothyroidism, as often happens in obesity, the tolerance is poor, and nervousness develops quickly.

HYPERTHYROIDISM (TOXIC OR EXOPHTHALMIC GOITER)

Hyperthyroidism as it occurs in childhood is more frequent in girls than in boys and has its onset most

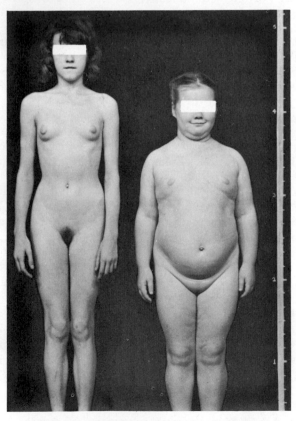

Fig. 26-2. Normal 12-year-old girl (*left*) contrasted with 13-year-old girl with hypothyroidism.

often near the time of puberty (Fig. 26-3). The cause of increased thyroid secretion is not known. Toxic goiter has been observed with pituitary tumor and has been relieved by treatment of the tumor. In most instances, however, hyperthyroidism is associated with a circulating long-acting thyroid stimulator (LATS) which does not derive from the pituitary but rather from lymphoid cells in the body. A second abnormal substance (exophthalmos-producing factor or EPS) does apparently originate in the pituitary and produces the prominent eyes seen in some victims of the disease.

The onset usually is gradual. All the symptoms that develop are attributable to excess thyroid secretion. These include nervousness, increased pulse rate, increased blood pressure, muscle weakness, easy fatigue, increased metabolic rate and sweating. Fine tremor of the extended fingers and the tongue is present. Despite increased appetite and food intake, many have weight loss because of increased metabolic rate. The rate of growth is increased, and the bone age ultimately advances above the chronologic age. The thyroid gland increases in size (goiter), and the eyeballs may become prominent (exophthalmos). The urinary excretion is increased, and blood cholesterol is decreased from the normal. In the more severe intoxications, vomiting, diarrhea, cardiac palpitation and dyspnea are likely to be present.

Aids in diagnosis include tests for the protein-bound iodine (PBI) and butanol-extractable iodine (BEI) content of the blood, the T3 uptake of red blood cells and the basal metabolic rate, all of which are elevated but may need careful interpretation to exclude extraneous influences.

The course of the disease varies, but the illness does not become dangerously severe so often in children as in adults. In some instances it may become progres-

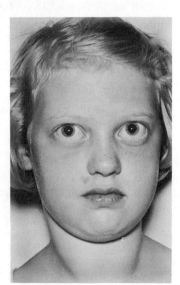

Fig. 26-3. Exophthalmos and goiter in a girl with hyperthyroidism.

sively and rapidly worse from the onset and cause death if no relief is given. More often, it progresses slowly with remissions. The so-called thyroid crisis is not common in children. A crisis represents a sudden large outpouring of thyroid secretion, resulting in prostration, high fever, vomiting, diarrhea and greatly increased nervous and mental symptoms.

Treatment. Since the introduction of drugs such as propylthiouracil, methylthiouracil and Tapazole which suppress the formation of thyroid hormone, the treatment of hyperthyroidism in children has shifted from a surgical to a medical approach. Appropriate dosage with one of these drugs can be expected to produce gradual reduction of the metabolic rate and disappearance of the symptoms, including the enlargement of the gland. Prominence of the eyes may not reverse, but it usually does not advance after treatment is started. Addition of thyroid extract to the regimen aids in the decrease in size of the gland. The antithyroid drugs must be monitored for evidence of toxic reaction in the form of rashes or serious depression of the white blood cell count. In the absence of these complications, hyperthyroidism usually can be brought under sufficient control to allow the child to pursue a normal life. The duration of treatment must be individualized. In many instances the drug has to be continued for several years before the disease burns itself out.

If toxic reactions to the drug cannot be avoided, or if the parents or child fail to cooperate with medical management, surgical removal of part or all of the thyroid must be undertaken. If all of the thyroid is removed, the child will require permanent substitution therapy with thyroid preparations.

Carcinoma of the Thyroid

Occasionally, neoplastic change in the thyroid gland is found in girls. Usually there is nodular enlargement of the gland or enlargement of the adjacent cervical lymph nodes to which the tumor has metastasized. The condition is a very slowly progressive one and can often be controlled by removal of the tumor if it is recognized in an early stage. There is strong suspicion that the use of x-ray therapy to the neck and the chest in early infancy may play a role in initiating neoplastic changes in the gland.

PARATHYROID DISORDERS

Primary disorders of the parathyroid glands, which regulate calcium and phosphorus metabolism, are quite rare in children. A familial type of hypoparathyroidism is seen occasionally which gives symptoms of chronic tetany comparable with the acute form observed in rickets. Treatment, consisting of large doses of vitamin D, is difficult to regulate appropriately.

PITUITARY DISORDERS

Pituitary Dwarfism

Children who remain unusually small but well-proportioned are suspected of suffering from a deficiency of the growth hormone of the pituitary gland. Actually, there are two varieties of symmetric dwarfism which are very difficult to distinguish from one another during childhood. In one type there is actually a lack of pituitary function, but the proof of this fact is not clinically apparent until the child passes through adolescence without maturing sexually. The other type of dwarfism is hereditary or constitutional in type, and the child matures sexually at the expected time. Laboratory tests are now available to detect the presence of growth hormone in the blood. A limited supply of hormone is also available for treatment.

Diabetes Insipidus

Diabetes insipidus is a condition in which the water excretion by the kidneys is abnormally large, with the result that the intake also must be large in compensation. The kidneys are normal but do not function normally because of lack of the controlling posterior pituitary hormone. This lack causes a lowered threshold for water. Because of the large quantity of water excreted, the urine has a very low specific gravity (1.002).

Diabetes insipidus may be caused by various conditions that disturb pituitary function. Thus, it may occur in cases of brain tumor located in or near the pituitary gland, particularly in the neighboring hypothalamic region. It may occur as a result of encephalitis or other inflammation of the hypothalamic region. In some instances it has resulted from traumatic injury to the brain. In many instances no lesion can be demonstrated, and the disease is on an idiopathic basis.

The symptoms of the idiopathic disease may consist only of drinking and excreting large amounts of water. The nutrition may suffer because the drinking of so much water is likely to interfere with the taking of sufficient food.

The treatment consists of regular daily administration of posterior pituitary hormone and of attention to the underlying brain lesion, when such exists. Such conditions as brain tumor are more dangerous to life than diabetes insipidus. Certain of the brain lesions are not amenable to treatment.

When the disease is idiopathic, administration of posterior pituitary hormone is the only treatment needed. Pitressin tannate in oil is the preparation usually employed. Dosage must be regulated by trial for the individual child, but usually amounts of 1 or 2 ml. per day will bring the volume of urine excretion to normal levels. A pitressin-resistant form of diabetes insipidus is encountered in which the kidney fails to respond to the hormone.

DISORDERS OF THE ADRENAL GLANDS

Adrenal Cortical Insufficiency

Insufficient production of corticosteroids may be due to congenital hypoplasia or to hemorrhage into the glands at birth; it may occur during severe infections; it may occur in a more chronic form (Addison's disease) when the glands are destroyed by tuberculosis or autoimmune disease; it may occur as a consequence of insufficient production of ACTH by the pituitary; or it may appear as a consequence of the too rapid withdrawal of steroids which have been given in treatment of some other disease. Except for the latter, defective production of corticosteroids is uncommon in children. Symptoms include weakness, vomiting, circulatory collapse, hypotension and coma. Laboratory studies show low blood values for sodium, chloride and corticosteroids and high levels of potassium. The blood volume is decreased. Dehydration and acidosis may occur rapidly if appropriate treatment is not instituted.

The life-threatening aspects of cortical adrenal insufficiency are in large measure due to the failure to produce aldosterone, the substance which controls the loss of sodium in the urine. When sodium is not retained adequately, water too is lost and the blood volume shrinks, blood pressure cannot be maintained and a wide variety of bodily functions suffer in consequence. In addition there is an attempt to compensate for the loss of sodium by retention of potassium which in high concentration may compromise normal cardiac action. Insufficient production of cortisone may result in hypoglycemia and long-term disturbances of carbohydrate and protein metabolism which compromise growth and lead to general weakness and poor resistance to infection.

Treatment must include not only adequate replacement of cortisone, but attention to hydration and most importantly to substitution therapy which permits adequate retention of sodium and water. Aldosterone itself is not available for therapeutic use, but desoxycorticosterone (DOCA) can be given intramuscularly during the acute stage of the illness and one of the fluorinated hydrocortisone compounds (Florinef, F-cortef) may be used orally for long-term administration. The relative potency of some of the commercially available steroid preparations with respect to their ability to substitute for cortisol and their effect on salt retention is displayed in Table 25.

Adrenal Cortical Hyperfunction

Nowadays the effects of overproduction of corticosteroids are most commonly observed as the consequence of long-term treatment with cortisone or ACTH. They include obesity, especially rounding of the face and the development of a buffalo hump, hypertension and virilism with acne and increased growth of body hair. The same changes may occur spontaneously as Cushing's syndrome which is rare in

Table 25. Equivalent Potencies of Common Steroids

Trade Names (Partial List)	Chemical Name	Glycocorticoid Effect Compared to Cortisone	Sodium Retaining Effect Compared to DOCA
Percorten	Desoxycorticosterone acetate (DOCA)	0	1
Not available	Aldosterone	(1/3)	(10 ×)
Cortone Cortivite Cortigen, etc.	Cortisone acetate	1	1/20
Hydrocortone	Cortisol, hydrocortisone salts	1.2 ×	1/20
Delta-cortef Deltasone Hydeltra Deltra Meticortelone Meticorten Paracort Sterane	Prednisone and prednisolone	5 ×	1/50
Medrol	Methylprednisolone	6 ×	0
Aristocort Kenacort	Triamcinolone	6 ×	0
Haldrone	Paramethasone	12 ×	0
Florinef F-cortef	Fludrocortisone	19 ×	10 ×
Decadron Deronil Gammacorten Hexadrol	Dexamethasone	30 ×	0
Celestone	Betamethasone	40 ×	0

children. Also rare are adrenal cortical tumors which may produce either virilization or feminization. The adrenogenital syndrome has been discussed briefly in Chapter 11. In this instance the inability of the infant or child to make cortisol in normal amounts due to a congenital enzymatic defect in the adrenal glands, results in an absence of control of the output of ACTH from the pituitary and, in consequence, excessive stimulation of the adrenals results in an overproduction of those hormones, mainly androgens, which they *are* capable of manufacturing. When therapeutic cortisone is given it depresses the production of ACTH from the pituitary and this in turn decreases the production of virilizing substances by the adrenals.

Pheochromocytoma

Hyperfunction of the adrenal medulla with overproduction of epinephrine and norepinephrine is occasionally seen in children due to the presence of a tumor of chromaffin tissue. Such tumors (pheochromocytomas) may be in the adrenal gland or in the sympathetic nervous tissue along the lumbar or thoracic spine. The primary symptom is hypertension associated with headache, flushing or excessive sweating. Diagnosis can be made by demonstrating abnormal amounts of catecholamines in the urine or by showing

urine, but two of them are acids
lization. Thus base is removed
rise to acidosis, which if allowed
o coma and death.

ar in the urine is important but
ice, since a few children have a
or sugar (renal glycosuria) with
oolism and blood sugar. The re-
of glycosuria, together with in-
blood, may be considered as con-
vishes to confirm or to exclude
tes definitely, a glucose-tolerance

Test. The test is useful only for
the determination of the amount
permitted a child with diabetes. Dex-
akfast after a night of fast. Dex-
ven in solution by mouth in the
for each Kg. of body weight, or
rd dose is given regardless of
ld the urine are examined before
als after the dextrose has been
l child will not excrete sugar or
ir values in these circumstances,
liabetes will. Normally, the blood
at all times, the amount varying
for each 100 ml., depending on
s. At slightly above this higher
n the urine of the normal person.
vith diabetes has a renal threshold
ind fails to spill sugar even with

gement

o distinct methods of treating the
The traditional (strict diet or
implies that the child must be
meticulously if he is to have the
g life and freedom from the late
disease. This method makes use
ed diets, permits no departures
exact substitution of equivalent
ie insulin dosage so closely that
in the urine at any time. Advo-
nt (free diet, glycosuric) method
ich exact regulation is necessary
glucose in the urine is not harm-
el that the child should be given

dence being a state of coma due to the development of
severe acidosis.

Acidosis. When carbohydrate is not available for
energy production, fat is mobilized for energy in
amounts greater than can be burned completely. When
the fat is oxidized incompletely, ketone bodies (acetone, diacetic acid and oxybutyric acid) accumulate.
These substances are only slightly toxic and are ex-

freedom to follow a diet of his own choosing, provided
that he avoids excesses and that his insulin need be
regulated only with a view to keeping him from excreting ketone bodies. Those who advocate this method
doubt that late complications are more frequent with
this regimen. They also believe that the child is much
better off without the regimentation implicit in the
aglycosuric system. Although the general principles of

management are the same in each system, there is a considerable difference in the exactness of physiologic correction sought. Each system will be described, since the approaches are not the same. First, however, the nurse should have knowledge of the types of insulin and their different uses.

Varieties of Insulin

Three general types of insulin are available—regular, long-acting, and intermediate—each of which has its place in the management of the diabetic child. None can be used orally.

Regular Insulin. Regular or unmodified insulin begins to exert its effect upon carbohydrate metabolism within ½ to 1 hour after injection, reaches its peak activity in about 3 hours and has lost its effect in 6 to 8 hours. It is used to bring the child into initial regulation because its relatively short period of action decreases the risk of overshooting and sending the child into prolonged hypoglycemia. While it is possible to manage a child indefinitely on regular insulin alone, 2 to 4 injections per day will be required. Once stabilized, most children are carried on the insulins with more protracted effect so that the number of injections per day may be minimized. Regular insulin is also valuable as a supplement to other regimens during acute illness or other conditions when the requirements are temporarily increased.

Long-Acting Insulin. When insulin is combined with zinc and protamine, a complex is formed which acts as a depot in the tissues from which insulin is slowly released. Such preparations—protamine zinc insulin (PZI), extended insulin zinc suspension (ultralente insulin)—do not release enough insulin to start having an effect on carbohydrate metabolism until 5 to 8 hours after injection, reach their peak of activity in 12 to 24 hours, and may still be having a hypoglycemic effect as long as 36 hours after injection. Thus, they are not as immediately effective during an acute need for insulin, but they maintain a more constant release of insulin which makes multiple daily injections unnecessary. They carry the hazard, however, that by a gradual accumulating effect extending beyond one day, the child, if overdosed, may suffer a prolonged hypoglycemic reaction.

Intermediate-Acting Insulin. To utilize the advantages of each type of insulin, combinations of regular insulin and long-acting insulin given once in the morning can be worked out for the individual child. The regular insulin thus provides for his needs immediately after breakfast, while the long-acting insulin with its delayed effect keeps him under control for the rest of the day and night. These preparations may be given in either separate syringes or mixed in a single syringe. The same advantages are now available in several commercially prepared mixtures with intermediate action—globin, lente, and isophane (NPH) insulins—

whose effective action begins within ½ to 1 hour, peaks at 8 to 18 hours, and has dissipated within 24 to 28 hours.

Strict Diet Management

A precise balance between food intake and insulin dosage is desired so that the blood sugar levels stay within narrow limits and no sugar is spilled in the urine. To do this the diet must be carefully weighed or measured, its exact components taken at the same time each day, and insulin doses arranged so as to keep the child aglycosuric. Adjustments in the diet for growth, changes in activity or illness are carefully planned.

Food Requirements. Once his disease has been brought under control with insulin, the child with diabetes has the same food requirements as a normal child of the same age. From the known nutritional requirements a diet with optimal calories, proteins, vitamins and minerals can be constructed from tables which give the composition of various foods. For the sake of variety it is possible to provide exchanges of equivalent amounts of food, but the daily caloric intake must remain constant and must be consistently divided between the three meals. Although water can be taken *ad libitum*, no foods other than those in the planned diet are permitted. It is expected that meals will be taken at the same time each day, and that the whole meal will be consumed.

Insulin. All children with diabetes require insulin. Unlike some adults whose mild disease permits adequate regulation by dietary measures alone, or with the aid of the orally administered sulfonylurea compounds (Orinase, Diabinese), childhood diabetes cannot usually be kept under control without injectable insulin. Even when the food intake is rigidly controlled, insulin requirements vary from child to child and in the same child from one time to another because the disease itself varies in severity. Thus, a child with severe diabetes may require 4 insulin injections per day given 30 minutes before each meal and once at bedtime, while a child whose disease is milder may be closely controlled on 3 or even 2 doses per day. With some children the disease becomes quite stable after the initial period of regulation, so that the same diet and insulin can be used day after day without glycosuria. In others it will be necessary to make frequent adjustments in order to achieve this objective.

The initial doses of insulin frequently are based on the amount of excess sugar in the blood, and the subsequent doses on the amount of sugar lost in the urine. For this reason, it is desirable to collect the urine in 4 separate portions: (1) from breakfast to dinner, (2) from dinner to supper, (3) from supper to bedtime or the time of the night dose of insulin and (4) from previous collection until breakfast. By means of this division the adequacy of each dose of insulin is indicated. When diabetes is brought under control in this manner, it is customary to find that the child recovers some of his lost sugar tolerance, and as a consequence the insulin dosage must be lowered. Usually, a stability in the insulin dosage is attained in the course of from 3 to 6 weeks, and the daily dosage becomes relatively constant. Certain uncontrollable factors, such as the amount of exercise and the occurrence of infection, may cause moderate variation from day to day. For this reason, constant checking and alertness are necessary. The insulin requirements will change also as the child's food intake increases with growth. Blood-sugar determinations are made at intervals, as it is possible for the blood sugar to be maintained at a level above normal without sugar appearing in the urine.

Free Diet Management

With this management, excretion of sugar in the urine is permitted, and the precise controls over diet and insulin are relaxed. This does not mean that supervision is abolished. Until the child and his parents learn the general principles of diabetic physiology and the vagaries of the individual child's disease, frequent consultations about diet, insulin adjustment and general hygiene are needed. Regular examination of the urine for the presence of sugar and acetone is required also.

The mother and the child are instructed in the requisites of a good diet. Although an exact intake is not prescribed, regularity and consistency are urged in order that insulin adjustment may be regulated easily. Periodically, the child's food intake is analyzed by the physician or the dietitian in order to be sure that he is meeting his requirements for calories, proteins, minerals and vitamins. If he is lacking in any dietary respect, acceptable modifications of the diet are suggested. Excessive carbohydrate intake and between-meal feedings are discouraged but not forbidden.

Since exact control of glycosuria is not a goal, the administration of insulin usually is reduced to a single injection of globin or NPH insulin once a day or a combination of protamine and regular insulin given simultaneously in 1 or 2 syringes. The urine is tested 3 or 4 times a day for both sugar and acetone. If there is intermittent glycosuria without acetone in the urine, the regulation is considered as being adequate. If glycosuria is continual but without acetone, periodic quantitative estimation of the amount of sugar being excreted per day is desirable. If more than 30 Gm. is being lost in the average 24-hour period, the glycosuria is considered excessive, and insulin is increased in an attempt to decrease the spillage. Acetone in the urine is a sign of danger. When it appears, physician's examination is necessary to adjust the diet or the insulin dosage and to search for symptoms of an infection. If the urine is consistently free of sugar, insulin is usually reduced to avoid insulin reactions.

The proponents of the free diet management of diabetes recognize the danger that parents and children may become lax and casual in the regulation of the disease. However, they believe that in the long run most families can achieve a satisfactory regulation and avoid the emotional rebellion which the stricter regimen often induces.

Medical and Nursing Management of Special Problems

Initial Effect of Treatment. When a child first comes under care, the insulin requirement is always higher than it becomes subsequently. With the return of blood sugar to normal levels the child's ability to produce insulin increases. In fact, for a time after the initial adjustment some children are able to get along without any insulin at all for a few months. This return of the ability to produce insulin is particularly important in the strictly managed child who may be pushed into chronic insulin reactions if appropriate reductions in dosage are not made. The phenomenon is temporary, and after a period of 4 to 12 months the insulin requirements begin to rise slowly.

Insulin Shock. In addition to the alterations of the disease cited above, overdosage with insulin may result from errors in measurement, from unusual exercise, from vomiting or from failure to take the expected amount of food. A variety of symptoms may be observed: nervousness, irritability, stubbornness, silliness, drowsiness or lassitude, unusual hunger, pallor, flushing, dilated pupils and sweating. If insulin shock becomes more profound, the child slips into unconsciousness and may suffer localized muscle jerkings or generalized convulsions.

Mild insulin shock can usually be managed effectively by getting the child to take a lump of sugar or an ounce or two of orange juice or milk. If no relief is obtained within 15 minutes, additional food should be given. For severe insulin shock, prompt infusion with glucose is desirable to forestall damage to the brain which can result if the reaction persists.

The distinction between insulin shock and diabetic coma is not always easy to make on clinical grounds. Laboratory tests reveal low blood sugar and an absence of sugar in the urine in shock; high blood sugar, glycosuria and ketonuria in coma. No significant harm is done by treating for shock when the distinction cannot be made quickly, but *a child already in insulin shock must not be given more insulin.*

Exercise. Exercise has a striking effect in reducing the insulin requirement. Increase in muscular activity requires compensation either by increasing the food intake or by decreasing the dosage of insulin. Failure to make this compensation is the most frequent cause of insulin shock. When the increase in activity is temporary, a relatively constant dosage of insulin is maintained and additional food is given at mealtime. A boy in active camp life requires less insulin than he does when he returns to the sedentary life of school in the fall.

Emotional Disturbances. The effect of emotional

disturbance may be as severe as that of infection and may require increased insulin. The insulin dosage is much easier to regulate for the emotionally stable child.

Acute Infections. The child's ability to use sugar properly is lessened. As soon as signs of any infection appear, insulin is increased to prevent glycosuria. If glycosuria occurs, insulin is increased again, and, if symptoms of shock develop, the dose is decreased. The diet should consist of easily digested soft or liquid foods. With severe infections, fat should be reduced or eliminated. The regular regimen is re-established when the infection subsides.

Surgical Operations. Children with diabetes withstand operations well if proper care is given them. Details of management vary with the circumstances of operation. Insulin is given before and during the postoperative period. Regular insulin usually is employed because of its short period of activity. If food cannot be tolerated, calories are supplied by intravenous infusion of glucose. Many children are restored to their usual regimen on the day after operation.

Acidosis. The mechanism by which acidosis develops already has been described. As long as the ketone bodies are formed in only moderate amounts and the body is able to excrete them without excessive drain on its supplies of base, acidosis does not develop. The condition then is known as ketosis. This is not a desirable or a healthy state of affairs, but the immediate danger is slight. With increased formation of ketone bodies the base of the body is depleted, and acidosis develops. As it becomes severe enough to become clinically manifest, the following symptoms and signs may be noted: the respiration becomes deep, rapid and without pause (air-hunger breathing) and remains thus until the child is *in extremis,* when it may become slow and shallow; the cheeks are flushed, the skin and the mouth are dry; nausea and vomiting are frequently present; thirst usually is extreme; the pulse is rapid and thready; the temperature may be either normal or elevated; the white cells of the blood may be increased markedly; severe abdominal pain may be present.

As the acidosis increases in severity, the child becomes stuporous and then comatose. Death is the usual sequel to untreated diabetic coma. These various signs and symptoms usually do not appear suddenly but increase in severity rather insidiously during several days as a result of some infection or dietary mismanagement. If the urine is tested daily, as it should be, sugar and increasing amounts of acetone will be found, giving warning and making it possible to prevent or to relieve the acidosis promptly.

If the urine contains much acetone and sugar but symptoms of acidosis have not developed, the child should be confined to bed, kept comfortably warm and given abundant fluids. The diet should consist of liquids; most of the fat-containing foods should be ex-

cluded. The dextrose equivalence of the previously prescribed diet or of a diet slightly lower in energy value should be maintained. The insulin dosage should be increased sufficiently to make the urine sugar-free. Usually this also will cause the disappearance of acetone. The amount of insulin needed cannot be foretold. When the sugar excretion has lessened demonstrably, the extra insulin administration should be discontinued and the child put on the regimen described for the treatment of diabetes.

If symptoms of acidosis are present, the treatment is similar to that just described but it must be more vigorous. The sugar content of the fluids ingested should be recorded, and every 2 to 4 hours the child should receive one unit of insulin for each gram of sugar ingested in the preceding period. If the child is vomiting excessively, 5 per cent dextrose in normal salt solution, to which insulin has been added (one unit for each gram of sugar), may be ordered. In addition, extra insulin will be prescribed to metabolize the excess of sugar already present in the body.

When acidosis is extreme, the treatment is extended to include intravenous sodium bicarbonate or sodium lactate to counteract the acidosis. As recovery takes place potassium solutions are added in order to replace the large amounts lost in the urine during the acute stage of acidosis. When the child is able to take oral fluids, liquids such as tea, fruit juice and milk will provide potassium. After the acidosis has disappeared, as evidenced by the disappearance of acetone from the urine, the former dietary and insulin regimen is re-established. However, it is usually preceded by a low-fat, liquid diet for 2 or 3 days.

Other Aspects of Nursing Care

The child with untreated symptoms of diabetes, acidosis or insulin shock is unstable physically and frightened by it. As a consequence he responds with changes in behavior which alert his parents to danger who in turn communicate their anxiety to him. Emotional disturbance and anxiety may produce a high level of spilled sugar. Therefore, it is important to explain the purpose of each test and treatment to him and to his parents with the utmost poise. If the child is too young or too ill to understand, responsiveness to his needs for physical support will increase his security and influence the development of wholesome attitudes toward his disease as he grows older.

Learning to distinguish between changes in behavior which result from an emotional upset and those which are caused by acidosis, insulin shock or infection is an important protective measure. When any of these complications are suspected, careful observation at the bedside of the child is indicated. When no signs of improvement can be detected in 10 minutes, the physician should be notified so that treatment which has been cited in the above section can be instituted before sugar metabolism has been markedly affected.

There are many ways in which the nurse can support the child in dealing constructively with problems relating to his responses to his disease and its treatment. Alleviation of worry about his physical status, his prognosis and the reasons why he needs insulin and a special diet lessens the incidence of altered carbohydrate metabolism and of behavior disturbances. Some children interpret the treatment of diabetes as punishment. Unless unrealistic concepts concerning the cause of the disease and the need for insulin are discovered and corrected, they will derive little therapeutic benefit from instruction.

There are several precautions to take when administering insulin. Careful sterile technic must be used in handling the equipment as is the case when giving any injection. The syringe should be dry before the insulin is drawn up. Care should be taken to make sure that the measuring scale of the syringe matches the unitage on the bottle of insulin. Injections should be rotated to prevent atrophy of subcutaneous fat or a lipomalike swelling which occurs when insulin is given repeatedly in one area. These conditions interfere with insulin absorption and can be avoided by methodical rotation of injection sites, using the tissues of the outer thighs, the arms, the abdomen and the buttocks. Careful recording of the injection site will be helpful in maintaining rotation.

Injections should be given into the deeper layers of the subcutaneous tissue in order to prevent local skin reactions and to promote absorption. The skin over the selected site should be stretched, cleansed with an alcohol sponge and the needle inserted at a 90 degree angle. A 25 gauge, ½-inch needle is usually employed, unless the child is quite obese. If, on the other hand, there is a small amount of subcutaneous fatty tissue, a skin fold should be formed prior to injection. Following insertion of the needle, slight traction should be exerted on the plunger of the syringe. If traces of blood are drawn into the barrel, the needle should be extracted a few millimeters before the insulin is injected. Following injection, firm pressure exerted with the alcohol sponge will prevent bleeding and massage of the area will aid absorption of the medication.

When the child is encouraged to express his feelings about the injections, the nurse will discover the meaning which they have to him and the point at which he becomes ready to learn to prepare and to give them. The nurse will also be instrumental in helping him to accept himself as a person with a particular kind of disease. Mastery of his fear of injections and of being different from other children is obtained when he is given opportunities to gain control of the situation through play, active participation in supplying himself with insulin and through the reception of knowledge about his disease. At first the child may only want to cleanse the injection site or keep the nurse posted on the areas previously used for injection.

A few children younger than 8 years of age are

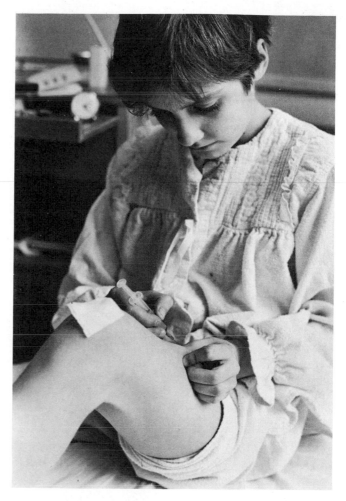

Fig. 26-4. The well adjusted diabetic child soon learns to administer her own insulin.

capable of injecting insulin prepared by the nurse. Generally, however, fine finger and eye control are not sufficiently developed until the age of 8 to 10 years when most children can be taught to measure the prescribed dose in the syringe and learn to inject it in a safe and capable manner.

Grouping children with diabetes on the ward can be helpful to the child in lessening the sense of being different from other children. It can also aid in teaching self-care in diet and in the administration of insulin. Those children who have mastered initial reaction to the reality of chronic illness in a healthy manner can benefit the ones who have not attained this therapeutic goal.

Getting specimens of urine to the laboratory at the time when they are ordered protects the child's rights to a predictable schedule of care. Sufficient bottles plainly and correctly labeled must be on hand for fractional specimens. Children need to be informed in advance of the time specimens are required and of the importance of getting them to the physician at specific times. Eventually, the child will show readiness to learn how to collect his specimen, test it and report results to medical personnel or to his parent when he is at home.

Collection of specimens becomes an irksome task for the older child or for the adult who assumes the responsibility for the preschool child. Awareness of the toddler's struggle to gain autonomy during the time he is being toilet trained will guide the nurse in preventing specimen collection from thwarting his attainment of it (see Chap. 16). During the preschool period and thereafter resistance to cooperating with the mother in collecting specimens often becomes manifest in boys as a defense against their fear of their instinctual urges. In such instances, respect for the boy's wish for privacy and assurance of the father's or intern's help usually solves the problem.

A restricted diet is prescribed, and in the hospital it is prepared by the dietitian, but it is the nurse who shoulders the responsibility for helping the child become well adjusted to a diet which is different from that served to other children. Segregating the child from other children may protect him from temptation in the hospital, but it does not help him to deal with a problem that he will be faced with at home. In addition, segregation increases his worry lest he is different from other children. When he has his meals at a table with others, questions arise which give the nurse an opportunity to help the group to learn about the particular dietary needs of children with diabetes.

Food likes and dislikes are as characteristic of the child with diabetes as they are of nonhandicapped children. Forcing and urging a child to eat disliked food creates problems which are more difficult to treat than is the diabetes. Better results are obtained when the child participates with the dietitian in planning his meals.

Resistance to the impulse to eat forbidden foods is acquired slowly and depends on the strength of the child's ego and the degree of hunger he is dealing with at the time he has access to it. When the blood sugar is low, the child is usually famished and may easily yield to pressure from his instinctual drives. The preschool child's conscience is not strong enough to check his drives. The nurse and eventually the mother will have to protect him from overindulgence until he accepts their standards as his own. When the mother-child relationship is sustained at a constructive level during the period of adjustment to his particular needs for care, inner controls against temptation can be expected during the early school-age period. But even then he will need support when he is threatened with overwhelming hunger.

Preadolescence is a particularly trying time for the child with diabetes. Demands for oral gratification are increased at the same time as his conscience is undergoing change from association with peers. It is also the time when his need to be like others is intensified.

All children are frightened by their impulses during preadolescence, but for the informed child with diabetes, the threat is greater. He knows that dietary indiscretion can affect his body, but even then he cannot always resist temptation. Support at these times is derived from knowledge that his wish for forbidden food is understood and that he will be given help in finding new ways to deal with his problem so that tension and relief from worry about his health can be eliminated. Tom's behavior, the subject of the next illustration, demonstrates the conflict that arises when a preadolescent cannot resist the temptation to take forbidden food. Had Tom been punished, relief of guilt or arousal of hostility and a wish to revenge might easily have resulted in more indiscretion (or, if he had been a child who had never dared to face his hostility directly and instead turned it against himself, symptoms of a metabolic complication might have appeared). Furthermore, punishment would have given Tom no help in dealing with his problem more constructively in the future.

Eleven-year-old Tom received insulin b.i.d. and was on a restricted diet. Tom's nurse learned that he had taken a piece of cake from the food cart and went to talk to him. She found him pacing the floor looking remorseful and frightened. It was some time before Tom could talk about the subject of his concern. Then he said, "I took some cake from the cart. I couldn't help it. Something inside of me kept saying: 'Tom, go take the cake. You'll like it!' The minute I ate it, something inside of me said, 'Tom, you shouldn't have done it!' " (Tom was not fabricating; he was putting his conflict into words. His impulses were stronger than his conscience, but the moment that the cake was eaten, his conscience punished him with guilt to prevent further indiscretion. Tom knew that he had done wrong; his guilt was sufficient punishment.) The nurse understood his longing for sweets and showed her trust in him: "Tom, it's hard to resist taking food when you want it so much. I think we could find a way to make it easier for you. All boys have this problem sometimes, especially when they are growing up. Tell me when you need help and I'll call the doctor and you can talk with him. If he knew how hungry you get, I'm sure he would ask the dietitian to help the two of you plan a diet which would satisfy you."

Parental attitudes toward the child and his disease should be studied before the child is discharged, for adjustment to treatment may be complicated by environmental problems. In most instances parents need repeated reassurance that the prognosis is favorable when adequate care is given. Concrete help is necessary before parents can assume responsibility for the calculation of diets, the giving of insulin and the detection and emergency treatment of early symptoms of acidosis or insulin shock. Self-assurance is gained through the reception of knowledge and practice in the care of the child before he goes home.

The administration of insulin is the most difficult part of the child's care for most parents. Supervision of the mother in giving insulin is more effective if it is preceded by conferences which give her an opportunity to talk about her feelings. Mothers who have guilt and ambivalent feelings toward their children often perceive the administration of insulin as the infliction of punishment and protect themselves with resistance to learning. Considerable help is necessary before they become able to accept emotionally the fact that the injection of insulin is an act of giving to the child what he cannot supply by himself.

The adolescent may have problems which are quite different from those of the younger child. When he reaches puberty without self-esteem and knowledge of his disease, he has a more difficult time than the healthy adolescent in resolving his conflict between dependence and independence. Diabetic coma occurs more frequently between the ages of 10 and 15 than at any other time. The physiologic changes of puberty produce metabolic complications in some instances, but they do not account for all of them. Problems in maintaining self-control continue during early adolescence. There is also a powerful urge for recognition, to be like others and to rebel against authority. The adolescent must depreciate parental attitudes and judgment to solve his core problem. If he reaches puberty with a weak ego, he may use his disease as a focus for his anxiety and take over the management of his treatment regimen before he is prepared to do so. Routines bore the adolescent, and he may discard them to prove that he is more knowledgeable than and independent of his parents. He often indulges in dietary indiscretions because he is hungry and wants to hide his affliction from his friends. One excess in his diet produces no immediate catastrophe, but a cumulative effect may occur without his realizing it. When this happens, his adequacy becomes threatened, and he is forced to assert himself again to maintain the image that he has of himself as an independent person.

In order to survive, the child with diabetes must learn to take responsibility for his own health. This character trait is rooted in self-respect, acceptance of and knowledge about his limitations. When he has gained these strengths through encouragement of his readiness for self-direction, he can become a member of the health team long before adolescence. Then through more active participation on the team during adolescence, he can gain status and freedom from fear of his dependence on others.

Mothers who have been gratified by their handicapped children's dependence on them need help before they can permit them to move toward closer relationships with others. The example* which follows illustrates one way in which resentment and anxiety

------

* Material pertaining to Gus was prepared by Mrs. Betty Butler, Department of Social Service, The Children's Memorial Hospital, Chicago.

caused by such a situation can be expressed. It also illustrates the way in which a social worker can help a mother to gain insight into her use of her child's handicap to solve her own problems. The importance of the father's participation in making plans for the child's care at home is also demonstrated.

Gus was a 13-year-old boy who had been under medical care for 3 years. His general adjustment had been satisfactory before. Then his behavior changed. His parents became alarmed when they were notified that their son was failing in school. Gus's physician asked the social worker's help in discovering the cause of his problem at school when he learned that his blood sugar level was fluctuating to a serious degree. In early interviews with Gus's mother, the social worker learned that the parents were having marital difficulties and that Gus was becoming increasingly more rebellious about his diabetic regimen. He refused to eat his breakfast and to let his mother test his urine. He had also "skipped school" and refused to reveal his whereabouts when he was late to meals. In spite of the mother's concern and her pleas for "any solution," she resisted the suggestion that her husband come to the hospital for an interview. It was not until Gus was hospitalized for insulin regulation that he and his father were seen by the worker. Once Gus's father began to talk about his role in the family, it became clear that the marital difficulty was the family's major problem. Gus's mother wanted to keep him as her "little boy." She used his small stature and his disease to control him. Gus vacillated between wanting this attention and proving that he was as adequate as other boys. He refused to talk with either of his parents for several days at a time and remained aloof from the children in the ward. Gus's nurse reported that he dreaded discharge. Gus had also complained to her that his mother had looked at his urine "just like you would check on a baby."

After several conferences with the family, the social worker concluded that Gus's father was capable of changing his role in the home. Gus's mother complained that her husband left all decisions up to her. However, in the same interview she admitted that she had "hidden problems" from him, including the fact that Gus had been out of diabetic control for several days before admission.

Before Gus's discharge, the team discussed the situation together and made plans for care at home. Gus wanted to take the responsibility of testing his urine with his father's supervision. At first Gus's mother responded as if she felt that the team couldn't trust her. She needed further help before she became aware of Gus's need for a change in routine. Gradually she became aware that she had been using Gus as a threat against her husband. Both parents eventually recognized their need to discuss their marital problem with a family agency, and a referral was made.

SITUATIONS FOR FURTHER STUDY

1. If diabetes were discovered while a 5-year-old boy was hospitalized for the treatment of furunculosis and you had the responsibility for giving his first dose of insulin, what goals would you have and how would you go about achieving them? What criteria would you establish to evaluate the results of your work?

2. If a 4-year-old boy with diabetes took a cookie from another child's tray, what would you do? If this happened when he was at the table with a group of children, how would your nursing intervention differ from that used in the foregoing situation?

3. Study a preadolescent boy with diabetes. At what age did the disease develop and how did his mother respond to the diagnosis and treatment? What meaning does diabetes have to the child and how did you discover it? Describe the child's behavior at the time insulin was due and during the period it is given. How did observation of his behavior at this time guide you in formulating plans for this aspect of his care? Describe the child's reactions to your plan when you implemented it. Did he offer suggestions as to how the plan might be modified to meet his needs more adequately? Were your goals achieved when you used his suggestions? If they weren't achieved, how did you cope with your frustration? Describe this child's relationship with you, and with peers, parents and physicians. What did you learn from observation of his interaction with others which guided you in designing your plan of nursing care? How did you use knowledge of growth and development in providing care? From your study of the child, what do you perceive his problems to be and on what behavior did you base your conclusions? What help do you anticipate that his parents will need before he is discharged?

4. Describe another method that might have been used to help Tom to solve his problem of temptation to take forbidden food. State the reasons why you believe the method that you propose might result in greater growth in adjustment for the child.

BIBLIOGRAPHY

Bruch, H., and Hewelett, E.: Psychologic aspects of medical management of diabetes in childhood, Psychosom. Med. 9:205, 1947.

Coates, F., and Fabry, K.: An insulin injection technique for preventing skin reactions, Am. J. Nurs. 65:127, 1965.

DiGeorge, A.: The Endocrine System, *in* Nelson, W. E., McKay, R. J., Vaughan, V. C. (eds.), Textbook of Pediatrics, 1173-1237, Philadelphia, Saunders, 1969.

Etzwiler, D., and Sines, L.: Juvenile diabetes, J.A.M.A. *181*:304, 1962.

Fischer, A. E.: The emotional factors in the treatment of diabetic children, Proc. Am. Diabetes Ass. 7:217, 1947.

———: Factors responsible for emotional disturbances in diabetic children, Nerv. Child. 7:78, 1948.

———: and Horstmann, D. L.: Handbook for Diabetic Children, ed. 3, New York, Grune, 1960.

Geis, D.: Nursing at Camp Needlepoint, Nurs. Outlook *15*:47, 1967.

Joos, T. H., and Johnston, J. A.: A long term evaluation of the juvenile diabetic, J. Pediat. 50:133, 1957.

Krysan, G. S.: How do we teach four million diabetics? Am. J. Nurs. 65:105, 1965.

Leiner, M., and Rahmer, A.: The juvenile diabetic and the visiting nurse, Am. J. Nurs. 68:106, 1968.

Long, P. J.: The diabetic child at home, Nurs. Outlook *12*:55, 1964.

Martin, M.: New trends in diabetes detection, Am. J. Nurs. 63:101, 1963.

———: Diabetes mellitus: current concepts, Am. J. Nurs. 66:510, 1966.

———: Insulin reactions, Am. J. Nurs. 67:328, 1967.

Moore, M. L.: Diabetes in children, Am. J. Nurs. 67:104, 1967.

Rosenthal, H., and Rosenthal, J.: Diabetic Care in Pictures, ed. 4, Philadelphia, Lippincott, 1968.

Watkins, J., and Moss, F.: Confusion in the management of diabetes, Am. J. Nurs. 69:521, 1969.

27

Nursing Care of Children With Allergic and Collagen Diseases

ALLERGIC DISEASES

General Considerations

The term "allergy" connotes an altered or abnormal degree of sensitivity to certain protein substances (antigens) with which the body comes in contact. Antigens gain access to the body as foods (ingestants), respiratory dust (inhalants), skin contaminants (contactants) or injected medications (injectants). In addition, they may be introduced as part of an infectious agent which has invaded the tissues.

Within the body, antigens stimulate the lymphatic structures to produce antagonists—antibodies. An allergic individual has more than the usual capacity to produce or react to certain antigen-antibody combinations. The union of the two antagonists releases histamine, a tissue poison, which in turn produces increased capillary permeability, edema, itching and contraction of smooth muscle of various internal organs. The response of different allergic individuals can take a number of clinical forms—eczema, asthma, hay fever, hives, headaches, abdominal pain and others.

If a material such as horse serum is given parenterally, antibody to the foreign protein* may develop. If a large amount of serum has been given, antibody may develop in quantity before all the foreign protein has been excreted or destroyed. In such an instance, the period required to develop antibody in quantity is from 8 to 13 days. Thus, an allergic reaction may develop as a result of a single injection. The reaction thus produced is called a *delayed reaction*. Subsequent injections of serum are likely to produce an immediate or early reaction because of the presence of antibody at the time of injection. Smaller initial injections may produce no symptoms, but sub-

sequently injections may cause a reaction because of the antibody produced by the first injection. This type of reaction is not limited to serum; serum is used as an example. When the allergic state develops as a result of a previous introduction of antigen in a person whose capacity to become susceptible is not a hereditary constitutional trait, the allergic response to further introduction of antigen is known as *anaphylaxis*. Often the term "atopy" is used synonymously with allergy, but it is more nearly correct to restrict its use to certain allergies present in those with a hereditary constitutional capacity to develop allergy. In the restricted atopic group belong hay fever, asthma, some urticarias (hives) and certain of the eczemas.

Another type of allergy is that associated with certain infections. For example, in tuberculosis the body becomes sensitive to tuberculoprotein in approximately 30 days after the initial infection. Thereafter a positive skin reaction is obtained with tuberculin, the reaction being an allergic one. Positive skin reactions are obtainable in a similar manner in other infectious diseases, including undulant fever, histoplasmosis and streptococcal infection. The allergy is not only manifest by a skin reaction, but in these and other infections the subsequent course of the chronic infections and the course of the acute illness of recurring infections are also altered importantly because of the allergy. The adult type of tuberculosis differs from the childhood type (primary infection) because of the allergic response of the body. The tertiary lesions of syphilis differ from the earlier lesions because of allergy.

Allergic phenomena occurring spontaneously are usually caused by sensitivity to either foods or material inhaled or in some instances to both. Hay fever (allergic rhinitis) and allergic asthma commonly are caused by inhalants. The general principles which underlie the management of allergy to inhalants are

---

* "Foreign protein" emphasizes its origin from a different animal species. Horse serum and rabbit serum are foreign proteins for man, but human plasma, convalescent human serum and gamma globulin are not.

discussed under Asthma. The general principles of the management of allergy to foods are dicussed under Eczema (see Chap. 15). Certain of the allergies in these two groups lend themselves to complete or partial desensitization; others do not. In any case, the desensitization is a slow and tedious process, and in many instances, especially in the case of foods, it is easier to avoid the offending material. Desensitization in the case of inhalants is carried out by hypodermic injections of extracts of the material in gradually increasing doses, with less than the amount which produces symptoms always being given. Food desensitization is accomplished by giving the material by mouth in gradually increasing amounts but in amounts which do not cause reactions.

Serum Disease

An allergic illness which does not occur spontaneously is that caused by the prophylactic or therapeutic injection of various serums. It may occur with the first injection as a delayed reaction or with subsequent injection as an immediate or early reaction. These reactions are anaphylactic. In certain constitutionally atopic persons, immediate illness may result from the first injection. It is most important to recognize constitutional atopy, since it is probably only persons with this condition who are likely to die as a result of serum injection.

Serum sickness occurs with various degrees of severity. In the most common variety the illness is mild. One may expect moderate fever, local redness and itching or pain at the site of injection and a generalized skin eruption which most commonly is urticarial but may be morbilliform or scarlatiniform. The child is uncomfortable but not particularly ill. A more severe and less common variety produces in addition several of the following symptoms: malaise, albuminuria, joint pains, swelling of the mucous membranes with hoarseness and cough, vertigo, nausea and vomiting. A rare and still more severe variety produces extreme weakness approaching collapse; the temperature may be subnormal and the pulse weak; catarrhal or hemorragic enteritis may be present. The most rare type of reaction is that which produces immediate shock, usually fatal. Usually the duration of the common varieties of serum sickness is 3 or 4 days. The more serious effects of serum sickness may be controlled to a large extent by the administration of epinephrine for rapid response and full dosage with antihistamines for a more prolonged effect.

Today, serums made in animals are infrequently used in the treatment of disease, but it must be remembered that testing of the individual child before giving such injections is extremely important. This can be done by instilling a diluted portion of the serum into the conjunctiva and watching for evidence of inflammation; or by giving a small dose of diluted serum intracutaneously and observing the site for the appearance of an urticarial reaction. When sensitivity is demonstrated the serum must be given in very small graduated doses at frequent intervals and with epinephrine and injectable antihistamines available.

Drug Sensitivity

The symptoms of serum disease, particularly urticaria, may occur when a child acquires sensitivity to any of several drugs. Penicillin is much the most frequent and important offender and in these circumstances the symptoms are often delayed until 10 days or even 3 weeks after the penicillin therapy is begun. Any of the features of serum disease may be mimicked. Immediate severe reactions to penicillin are almost unknown in the child but can occur in the adult.

Asthma

Asthma is really a complicated pulmonary symptom rather than a specific disease. The mechanical changes in the bronchial tree that lead to the characteristic obstruction, dyspnea and wheezing are the same in all patients, but the factors that produce the mechanical disturbances are varied and often complex.

Etiology. Children who have asthma are generally considered to be allergic subjects. This implies a constitutional predisposition toward abnormal sensitization, and in many instances the trait is clearly inherited. Among infants and young children the appearance of asthma is usually restricted to periods when there is obvious acute infection of the respiratory tract, and the symptom abates when the infection is treated adequately. Infection may play a role in older children too, but the relation between it and asthma is usually less obvious. Frequently, the obstructing mechanism is set off by specific sensitivity to an inhalant such as ragweed, house dust or an animal dander. More often, specific sensitivities are suspected but cannot be identified clearly. In some children emotional disturbances alone appear to be capable of setting off an attack of asthma; in the majority of cases emotional factors play an important role in determining the length and the severity of symptoms. Thus, one can recognize constitution, infection, specific sensitivity and emotional factors as playing a part in the production of asthma. The degree to which each participates is a matter that must be determined by study of the individual child.

Symptoms and Diagnosis. The lungs are afflicted by the same sort of disturbance as that described in Chapter 14 for obstructive bronchitis of infancy. There is widespread narrowing of the small branches of the bronchial tree due to a combination of spasm of the circular muscles surrounding them, of edema of the mucous membrane which lines them, and of thick mucus contained within their lumens. The obstruction to air flow is more marked during expiration than during inspiration. Air tends to be trapped in the alveoli, producing overdistention of the lung and requiring the child to make a forcible effort during expiration in order to push air through the narrowed bronchioles. The result is an overdistended (emphysematous) chest with rapid, shallow inspirations and prolonged wheezing expirations.

A typical asthmatic attack usually occurs in a school-age child abruptly at night and without antecedent illness. There is no fever. The child develops a hacking cough and has difficulty sleeping because of the necessity for making a conscious effort to breathe. He finds that he must push during expiration and that he is more comfortable if he is propped up in bed. Characteristically, he is quiet and less upset than his parents are about the symptoms and tends to resist efforts to assist him. He does not want to be disturbed because he is already burdened with the task of breathing. Mild cyanosis may be present. Asphyxiating asthma is rare in children, except in those who have repeated attacks over a long period of time. After the symptom has persisted for a day or two the child may produce thick tenacious secretions during coughing spells. The symptoms tend to become worse at night and to clear somewhat in the daytime. Sleep and the ingestion of food may be seriously curtailed during prolonged attacks. Single attacks may be as brief as an hour or may last for several days to be followed by an additional period of bronchitis.

The diagnosis is made by observation or from the accurate description of an attack by the parent. It is confirmed by physical examination and analysis of the character of the respirations. Prompt relief following the injection of adrenalin helps to substantiate the diagnosis. Determination of the precipitating factors for the individual child is usually a difficult and protracted process which may involve allergic technics or the services of a psychiatrist, or both.

Treatment of the Acute Attack. Adrenalin administered by injection or by inhalation usually gives relief for a brief period of time. Ephedrine and aminophylline operate more slowly but have a longer-lasting effect. Treatment is usually more effective if used early after the appearance of symptoms. Sedation with barbiturates reduces the child's anxiety and encourages sleep. The above drugs are available in combinations (Tedral, Quadrinal) which can be administered 3 or 4 times a day until the attack is controlled. If the attack is prolonged or severe, the child is usually sent to the hospital. For reasons which probably are grounded in the relief of emotional tension, treatment of asthma in a hospital setting is rapidly effective in nearly all instances, even though the same measures have been tried previously at home without much improvement. Unusually severe attacks of asthma may require oxygen administration and the intravenous use of large doses of hydrocortisone. With prolonged attacks, dehydration and severe disturbance of blood electrolytes may also be encountered.

Prevention of Future Attacks. To forestall future attacks of asthma it is necessary to understand the importance of the various factors that precipitate attacks in the individual child. Sometimes the task is relatively simple. If attacks occur only at certain seasons in the year, pollen sensitivity is likely to be responsible, and the offending agent is discovered by allergic skin testing. Treatment then depends on the individual's avoiding the pollen in question or, if this is not feasible, in receiving desensitizing injections over a period of several weeks. When asthmatic attacks are clearly related to the onset of respiratory infections, attention is directed to clearing up any existing sources of chronic infection in the nose and the throat. When the child is losing an excessive amount of sleep or is unable to attend school because of recurring respiratory infections with asthma, small doses of sulfonamide or oral penicillin are given throughout the winter months as prophylaxis against re-infection.

Although steroids will terminate acute attacks and prevent recurrences, they are not generally used in children on a long-term basis for the control of asthma. Too often the child becomes dependent upon them and requires gradually increasing doses which eventually lead to toxic symptoms.

When the factors which precipitate asthma are not so obvious, prolonged allergic or psychiatric study may be required to bring the symptoms under control. Since both of these technics are likely to be long, arduous and upsetting to both child and parents, generally they are reserved for children whose asthma is frequent, disabling or so severe that permanent damage to the structure of the lung is threatened if they continue. Severe prolonged asthma almost always stems from an emotional conflict between the child and some member of his immediate family. The most careful and extensive program of desensitization, drug management or change of climate may be unavailing if no consideration is given to the psychological implications of the disorder.

Nursing Care. The child who has to be hospitalized because of chronic asthma presents both a challenge and an opportunity for the knowledgeable nurse who is concerned in his care. Children with asthma may often be anxious, fearful of death and poorly equipped to master normal developmental tasks. Their disease may have interfered with the development of normal social relationships with others. The necessary environmental protection may have kept the boy from normal participation in sports, so important to the school-age child and thus have damaged his self-esteem and emphasized his differentness from other children. His school attendance may have been frequently disrupted, thus weakening his motivation toward intellectual progress.

The nurse working with such a child must understand that he may have unsatisfied longings for love which could not be met in his earlier years because of the emotional climate within his home. When hospitalized, such children may demonstrate a need for clinging possessiveness with their nurse and indicate a wish for close and perpetual care. However, when such care is denied them, normal expression of aggression and hostility may be modified by an anticipation of danger or fear of loss of the needed affection. Because of this conflict, large amounts of normal activity may be forfeited, causing regression to a more passive level.

The nurse caring for such a child must provide evidence of her constant affection and concern, while on the other hand avoiding overprotectiveness and encouraging activity and social intercourse with peers. Through provision of acceptable means of expression of hostility, she may release energy for healthy emotional and intellectual growth.

Many children with asthma improve physically to a marked extent while hospitalized, because of a temporary release from the emotional tension within the home. Concomitant fulfillment of their dependency needs and needs for shelter and protection without the need to deal with an intense emotional milieu or the arousal of dangerous aggressive impulses makes possible the effectiveness of therapeutic intervention. The nurse who is knowledgeable and patient can take advantage of this opportunity through cooperating with the efforts of the psychiatrist and social worker in supporting healthy growth of the child's ego and toward his emotional maturation.

Chronic Neurodermatitis

A few infants who suffer from eczema (Chap. 15) will have a persistence of lesions beyond the third year of life. Older children occasionally develop a similar eruption without having had the infantile form of the disease. The etiology is variable, but constitutional, allergic and emotional factors influence the course. The eruption in its mildest form is a dry transverse cracking about the flexor surfaces of joints, particularly the wrist, the elbow and the knee. From these areas erythema and weeping may extend to involve adjacent areas of skin. In severe cases most of the skin of the extremities, the face and the neck may be affected, but the trunk is usually spared. The eruption tends to improve in summer and with exposure to ultraviolet light. It is aggravated by emotional disturbances which also increase the degree of scratching. Specific food and contact sensitivities are often demonstrated in an individual child, and an important part of the treatment is to shield the child from such allergens insofar as is feasible. Constitutionally, these individuals are usually energetic, ambitious and sensitive. It seems as if their problems are converted into itching and eruption of the skin. Sedation with phenobarbital is used but has little effect unless ordered in an amount which produces drowsiness. Partial relief of itching is obtained through the use of ointments

and protective dressings. Steroid therapy is almost always beneficial but cannot be given for long without hazard. Improvement can be expected with maturation, since many of these children learn their limitations and organize their lives in a way which keeps their skin troubles minimal. Psychiatric treatment has been successful in reducing the symptoms.

THE COLLAGEN DISEASES

The term "collagen disease" is applied to a group of disorders which have as their common feature destruction and degeneration of the supporting connective tissue of the body. The name "collagen" refers to the fibers that can be seen under the microscope. There is evidence that the ground substance between and among fibrils also is disturbed. The etiology of each of these disorders is under debate at the present time. They all improve under the influence of adrenal cortical steroid therapy. In general their symptomatology is sufficiently distinctive to permit sharp grouping into diagnostic entities, but in a few cases it is difficult for the physician to decide which diagnosis to apply to an individual child. In pediatric medicine, rheumatic fever is much the most common representative of the group; rheumatoid arthritis and disseminated lupus erythematosus are uncommon; dermatomyositis, scleroderma and periarteritis nodosa are distinctly rare. These diseases are grouped with the allergic diseases because they appear to be unusual (or allergy-like) responses of the body to infection, to stress, or to its own components.

Rheumatic Fever

Rheumatic fever is a systemic disease that causes characteristic involvement of many organs and tissues, most important of which is its effect on the heart. The common manifestations are migratory joint pains, various skin eruptions, subcutaneous nodules, chorea and carditis.

Etiology. The causative mechanism in rheumatic fever is the subject of controversy. The facts seem to be sufficient to warrant certain tentative conclusions. The primary underlying factor is infection in the throat with Group A beta-hemolytic streptococci. As a result of chronic infection or repeated acute infections, the body becomes sensitized to the organism. Continued infection or repeated infection after sensitization leads to allergic response, the response varying in nature and degree according to the degree of sensitization. Before sensitization, the throat infection has only locally apparent effects. After sensitization, the systemic phenomena consist of certain proliferative and exudative changes with their accompanying symptoms (carditis, arthritis, skin eruptions, rheumatic nodules).

Incidence. The stated cause of rheumatic fever explains its age incidence. Rheumatic fever is rare in the first years of life, not because infections are uncommon, but because the development of allergy requires time. The curve of incidence of onset gradually rises. It has reached a fair height by 5 years of age and is at its peak between 7 and 10. ·After this time it declines. Rheumatic fever is most prevalent in those parts of the world (temperature zones) and in those seasons of the year in which respiratory infections are most frequent. Rheumatic fever has a relatively high family incidence. A hereditary predisposition to the disease is recognized. The environment and the living conditions are often such that respiratory infections are induced easily, and the causative organism is transferred easily. It is well recognized that rheumatic fever is more frequent in the low-income than in the high-income levels. No doubt this difference is explained in part by living conditions, but nutritional status also is known to be important.

Symptoms. The symptoms of rheumatic fever are extremely variable in type and severity. Some children are affected so mildly that the symptoms are vague, and even the most careful and extensive study by laboratory methods leaves some doubt about the validity of the diagnosis. Other children are assailed by a severe, fulminating disorder that rapidly threatens life.

Unlike many of the infectious diseases, the medical problem in rheumatic fever involves more than the management of a single episode of disease, for the child who has experienced one attack is vulnerable to recurrences. Each return of rheumatic activity carries with it the threat of additional cardiac damage. Consequently, it is important to know which children have suffered from rheumatic fever in order to shield them from additional attacks, even though the first one may have been mild. Conversely, it is undesirable to classify a child as rheumatic unless good evidence is available, for in some instances this leads to unnecessary anxiety and restriction of activity, which hamper normal physical and psychosocial development.

The symptoms of rheumatic fever may be grouped into major and minor manifestations. If present in characteristic form and accompanied by evidence of recent beta-hemolytic streptococcus infection, any two of the major manifestations is presumptive evidence of rheumatic fever. The minor manifestations may or may not be due to rheumatic fever, but when several of them are present in conjunction with a major manifestation they add to the suspicion. The major manifestations are polyarthritis, carditis, chorea and subcutaneous nodules. In the young child carditis is apt to be the presenting manifestation, with polyarthritis present in mild degree. In the older child polyarthritis and chorea are more common as presenting complaints.

POLYARTHRITIS. The arthritis of rheumatic fever tends to involve the larger joints such as the knee, the elbow, the ankle, the wrist and the shoulder. However, it may be present in any joint, including the spinal articulations and the mandibular joint. Pain, tenderness and restriction of motion are present. In the young child these symptoms tend to be mild and to last for only a few days but they may return in a different joint. More severe joint manifestations usually are seen in older children, in whom the part may be swollen, visibly inflamed and exquisitely tender to touch or manipulation. Spontaneous subsidence within a few days even without treatment is characteristic, but migration to other joints may persist over a period of weeks.

The arthritis of rheumatic fever has two distinctive characteristics: it is relieved rapidly by salicylates and it never results in permanent deformity of the joint. The pathologic changes are those of exudation of fluid into the joint and inflammation of the surrounding structures.

The problem of differentiating rheumatic pains from "growing pains" is often a difficult one. Usually the latter are limited to the night hours after the child has fallen asleep. They seldom interfere with his daytime play or provide visible evidence of pain or restricted motion. They tend to recur nightly for long periods of time and are not associated with other manifestations of the rheumatic state.

CARDITIS. Acute rheumatic carditis is discussed in detail in the next section.

CHOREA (SYDENHAM'S CHOREA). Chorea is considered in a following section.

SUBCUTANEOUS NODULES. Nodules are not a common manifestation of rheumatic fever, but when they do occur they are almost certain confirmation of the diagnosis. They consist of accumulations of fibrous tissue proliferation which are located beneath the skin near the larger joints or along the spine or in the scalp. Small ones are difficult to find and are easily missed unless careful palpation is carried out. The larger ones are often visible through the skin (Fig. 27-1). They are painless and persist for weeks or months before they disappear gradually.

MINOR MANIFESTATIONS. Rheumatic fever is accompanied by a number of other symptoms which by themselves are not necessarily rheumatic. Lassitude, pallor, fatigability and loss of appetite are seen frequently.

Fever is usually present, but its degree may be variable. In severe rheumatic fever it is regularly

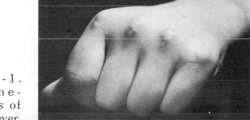

FIG. 27-1. Subcutaneous nodules of rheumatic fever.

present and may be high. Sometimes it is present only during the period when arthritis is evident. At other times it may appear as a low-grade protracted elevation which extends over many weeks during the activity of the rheumatic process. However, absence of fever cannot be regarded as equivalent to absence of rheumatic activity, for the two features are not always parallel.

Muscle pains which are transient or mild may or may not have a rheumatic basis.

Nosebleed is a traditional but not a common symptom. Bleeding is usually mild and creates no significant problem, except as it may distress the child.

Abdominal pain is an important symptom because it may be severe enough to lead to the diagnosis of

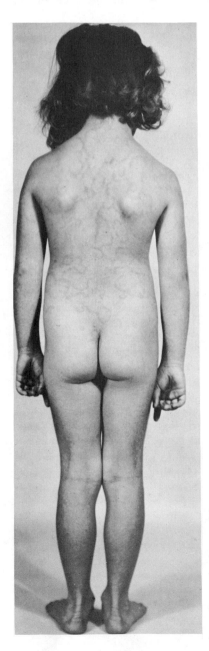

FIG. 27-2. Erythema marginatum.

appendicitis and an exploratory operation. The exact mechanism of such pain is not clearly understood but ordinarily is attributed to peritoneal inflammation or mesenteric lymph node enlargement.

Erythema marginatum (Fig. 27-2) is a faint, changing skin eruption which consists of small red circles, wavy lines or portions of circles which appear and disappear rapidly on the trunk and the abdomen. The characteristic eruption seldom is seen except during the progress of rheumatic fever and is regarded by many physicians as proof of rheumatic activity. It creates no symptoms and is not necessarily associated with fever.

Laboratory Aids to Diagnosis. The clinical task of deciding whether an individual child does or does not have rheumatic fever is a difficult one. Unfortunately, no specific test is available to detect the presence of the disease and the degree of its activity, although several give useful nonspecific information. Each such test is interpreted in the light of the patient's entire clinical picture.

SEDIMENTATION RATE. An increase in the sedimentation rate of the red blood cells indicates the presence of an inflammatory reaction or a disturbance of the plasma proteins. It is a relatively simple procedure which is widely used as a way of following the course of rheumatic activity after the diagnosis has been established by other means. Of course, it can be influenced by inflammatory processes that have nothing to do with rheumatic fever.

C-REACTIVE PROTEIN. Determination of the C-reactive protein of the blood is a similar indicator of the presence of an inflammatory reaction.

LEUKOCYTOSIS. Leukocytosis also indicates inflammation but is a less sensitive index than the other tests named.

Since it now is believed that rheumatic fever almost invariably follows beta-hemolytic streptococcus infection, the detection of evidence of such an infection adds weight to the suspicion that symptoms are being produced by rheumatic fever. Usually the streptococcal infection is sufficiently distant or has been treated adequately, so that the organisms are not present in the throat culture at the time that rheumatic symptoms appear. However, certain antibodies may have been formed against the streptococcus products; by laboratory means it is possible to detect *antistreptolysin, antifibrinolysin* or *antihyaluronidase*. Of course, their presence merely proves that the person has suffered a streptococcal infection and does not indicate the presence of rheumatic fever specifically.

ELECTROCARDIOGRAM. The electrocardiogram provides valuable evidence of the presence of carditis. The most frequent alteration is a prolongation of the P-R interval.

Course and Prognosis. The prognosis for children with rheumatic fever depends entirely on the effect that the disease has on the heart. Except for the carditis, none of the other manifestations is likely to be lethal or to leave any permanent after-effects. The common form of first attack (monocyclic) consists of a period of activity which lasts from 1 to 4 months and during which about half of the children will have evidence of cardiac involvement. More serious is the polycyclic form of the disease in which continuing waves of activity keep the disease process going for many months or even a year or two. It appears as though treatment is able to suppress the activity temporarily but not to shorten the course of the disease.

Once the child has passed through an initial attack he is a candidate for a recurrence if he suffers another beta-hemolytic streptococcal infection. Studies indicate that the risk of recurrence is greatest during the first 5 years after an initial attack and that it declines rapidly thereafter. Each attack or period of prolonged rheumatic activity carries with it the threat of additional heart damage from carditis.

Prophylaxis. Once the child has been identified as a rheumatic subject it becomes very important to prevent future episodes of infection. Since recurrence will depend on reinfection with beta-hemolytic streptococci, this objective can be attained if he is protected adequately against these organisms. It now is recognized that children with rheumatic fever may be so protected by administering a small daily dose of sulfadiazine or penicillin by mouth or by monthly injections of long-acting penicillin preparations. Administration is continued so that the child has a constant low level of the drug present in his tissues to protect him from the very first minimal exposure to streptococci. Many clinicians recommend that such prophylactic drugs be taken during the 5 years following the first attack.

General Treatment. In the main, the treatment of rheumatic fever is the treatment of acute rheumatic carditis, which is discussed fully in the following section. Even when the child has little or no evidence of cardiac involvement during a first attack, usually he is given suppressive treatment with salicylates or steroids in the hope of warding off any important cardiac damage, and at the same time he is kept relatively inactive until it can be demonstrated that the stage of rheumatic activity has passed.

Acute Rheumatic Carditis

The term "rheumatic carditis" is used in preference to "rheumatic endocarditis," which was employed formerly, for the reason that the changes in the heart never are limited to the endocardium in the acute stages of the disease. The myocardium always is affected, and often the pericardium also. Rheumatic carditis is an inflammation of the heart which occurs as a part of rheumatic fever, not as a complication.

Incidence. The mechanism that causes rheumatic carditis is the same as that which produces rheumatic fever. Fully nine tenths of all the acquired heart disease that occurs in the first 4 decades of life is rheumatic, and in nearly three fourths of these cases the cardiac disease has its onset before 15. It is rare in the first years of life, common after 5 and has its greatest incidence of onset between 7 and 10. Its distribution between the sexes is approximately equal. The frequency of its occurrence varies with the geographic location. In surveys of hospital admissions, the proportion has varied from 0.1 to 5.5 per cent. Among college students, a mean average of 1.2 per cent has been found. The seriousness, as well as the frequency, of the disease is indicated by mortality statistics, which are more accurately known than is the morbidity. The mortality formerly varied from 5 to more than 9 for each 100,000 population, according to the area of the country. In the last year for which reports are available (1959), the mortality rate in the United States as a whole dropped to 1.3 per 100,000 for children in the age range of 5 to 14. During the last decade deaths from rheumatic fever and heart disease have fallen from third to fifth place as a cause of death among children.

Pathophysiology. At the onset of rheumatic carditis and during exacerbations, microscopic rheumatic nodules form in the various heart structures. Subsequently, some localized endothelial proliferation takes place, and frequently small excrescences, consisting largely of fibrin (vegetations), occur on the heart valves and the chordae tendinae. The left atrioventricular (mitral) valve is the one most often affected; the aortic valve is the next. The vegetations interfere with good closure and function of the valves, thus throwing an added load on the heart muscle in order to maintain circulation. The function of the myocardium is disturbed directly by the inflammatory changes within its structure. Thus, frequently the work demanded of the heart muscle exceeds its capacity, with the result that the heart may increase in size by dilatation. The circulatory inadequacy which results is reflected in the symptoms exhibited by the child.

Symptoms. The symptoms of rheumatic carditis are proportionate quantitatively and qualitatively to the severity of the carditis. In cases of mild disease, the symptoms are in part those of a prolonged low-grade infection. The usual picture is one of irregular low-grade fever, pallor, moderate anemia and poor nutrition, with a history of preceding poor appetite, loss of weight and easy fatigue. All these symptoms are vague as far as indicating carditis is concerned. If other rheumatic manifestations are present, the significance of the symptoms may become apparent, but mild carditis easily may escape recognition when a careful physical examination is lacking. On closer observation one may find slight dyspnea on exertion and pulse and respiration rates out of proportion to the temperature. A soft systolic murmur usually is to be heard over the apex of the heart, the point where murmurs produced by lesions of the mitral valve are heard best. Often epistaxis occurs in the early stage of the disease.

When the carditis is more severe, the child is definitely ill, restless and apprehensive (Fig. 27-3). He finds it necessary to remain in bed. Usually the face is flushed, with perhaps some cyanosis. The temperature may be high in the very acute disease or range up to 101° or 102° F. with disease of moderate severity. The temperature is always irregular. The white blood cell count is increased, sometimes greatly. Cardiac damage is severe, and pain over the precordium is frequent. Abdominal pain also is often present. Because of the myocardial weakness and the concomitant valvular lesions, the heart dilates, and evidences of inadequate circulation appear. Failure of the heart in this manner is known as decompensation. Decompensation causes rapid pulse and respiration rates, dyspnea, pallor, a hacking cough and cyanosis. It also permits a back pressure of the blood in the venous system, which causes enlargement of the liver and, in more severe decompensation, edema and ascites.

When the cardiac valves are involved, the sounds produced by the heart are modified, causing murmurs. From the timing and the location of the murmur the physician may determine the valve affected; from the character of the murmur the condition of the valve may be estimated. The stronger the action of the heart and the greater the scarring of the valve, the louder and rougher the murmur will be. The amount of myocardial inflammation is indicated by the weakening, the spacing and the rapidity of the heart

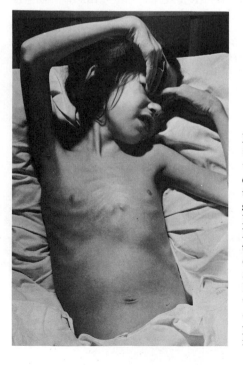

FIG. 27-3. Physiologic threat associated with cardiac decompensation leads to despondency unless the child has the continued support of his parents and the staff. Note the way in which this child expresses her physical discomfort and misery.

sounds, as well as by the amount of dilatation. Enlargement of the heart may be caused by stretching of weakened heart muscle, or it may be the result of hypertrophy consequent to cardiac damage by preceding attacks of carditis. An associated pericarditis may cause accumulation of fluid around the heart, simulating cardiac enlargement.

Prognosis. The normal healing powers of the body tend to check the cardiac inflammation, particularly if outlying infections subside and cardiac work is kept at a minimum. Thus, children may become cured after a period of several months. Recovery from the first attack is usual. However, carditis, like other rheumatic manifestations, has a strong tendency to recur. The child may die as a result of failing circulation in the midst of one of these attacks, or, if he recovers from the illness, the summation of damage to the valves with associated scarring may lead to permanent valve deformity and dysfunction with its consequent invalidism because of inability to withstand the effects of even moderate exercise. On the other hand, from apparently severe valvular lesions in the absence of further recurrences he may recover ultimately to the extent that no dysfunction exists and even the murmurs largely disappear.

Treatment and Nursing Care. The treatment of active rheumatic carditis attempts to spare the heart as much work as possible until the acute inflammatory reaction in its muscle has subsided completely. The measures which reduce cardiac work include (1) continuous and absolute bed rest, (2) the relief of pain, fever and anxiety insofar as possible, and (3) appropriate treatment of cardiac failure when it is present.

Measures that suppress the rheumatic inflammatory process are an important adjunct to the treatment outlined above. Salicylates or steroids or ACTH terminate fever and pain and reduce cardiac activity in most instances. What effect these measures have in limiting the ultimate degree of cardiac damage is still a matter of dispute. Their withdrawal before the end of the usual period during which spontaneous subsidence of rheumatic activity might be expected results in an immediate return of symptoms. Whether suppression of rheumatic activity does or does not limit the ultimate damage to cardiac valves and muscle, it is an important temporary expedient which lessens cardiac work by the reduction of fever and the relief of pain and anxiety.

Both the salicylates and the steroids have undesirable side-effects which must be recognized and eliminated before the disturbances which they create add to the burden of cardiac work. High dosage of salicylates may result in gastrointestinal upsets, ringing in the ears, headaches or disturbances of mental state. Stimulation of respiration can cause alkalosis through hyperventilation. Acidosis also may occur when there is excessive accumulation of salicylates in the blood. The manner in which children respond to salicylate dosage is a highly individual matter. Some can tolerate large doses without disturbance; others are easily upset by relatively small quantities.

Administration of steroids and ACTH also is restricted by toxic manifestations. The bodily appearance may change through the rounding of facial contours (moon face), localized fat deposits, the appearance of acne or excessive hair and by weight increase with linear marks appearing in the stretched skin (striae). More serious to the child with rheumatic carditis are hypertension and the tendency to accumulate sodium and water within the tissues. The latter may be counteracted by restricting the dietary intake of salt and by the periodic administration of mercurial or other diuretics. When mental or emotional disturbances occur during steroid therapy, they must be regarded as a serious complication which will probably require withdrawal of the drug. Steroid therapy also diminishes the child's resistance to some of the contagious diseases such as chickenpox and measles. When he acquires such an infection it may be unusually severe.

During the acute stage of rheumatic carditis the maintenance of nutrition presents a serious problem. The sick child eats poorly, yet needs essential nutrients to combat his disease. Steroid therapy usually is attended by an increase in appetite which is superior to that observed when salicylates are used. Blood or plasma transfusions in small amounts are sometimes given to improve nutrition. The medical management of cardiac decompensation is the same as that described for congenital heart disease in Chapter 22.

Every measure possible should be taken to alleviate the child's anxiety about the functioning of his heart, because anxiety utilizes energy and produces fatigue. Peace of mind and assurance that his needs will be anticipated make it more possible for the child to relax. He will need to be forewarned before procedures are begun to avoid apprehensiveness. Preventing interruptions in rest after sedatives are given is also of great importance.

Comfortable and frequent changes of body position aid in relaxation and in prevention of tissue breakdown or joint stiffness. Elevation of the back rest may relieve dyspnea and support of the arms with pillows will prevent the tendency to fold them over his abdomen, which restricts chest expansion. The legs should be kept in good alignment to prevent external rotation of the hips and the feet should be supported with a foot board or cradle to prevent footdrop. If the child's joints are painful and swollen, they should be supported carefully when he is moved and protected from the weight of the bedclothes by a cradle.

Pressure areas of the skin may form swiftly unless daily care is given to combat the effects of continual pressure, fever, increased perspiration and edema. The back and buttocks should be washed and rubbed with lotion several times daily and the elbows protected by long sleeves and lubricating lotion.

Good mouth care is comforting, especially if the child is receiving limited fluids or is breathing primarily through his mouth. After cleansing the mouth, teeth and gums, a solution of lemon juice and glycerine may be applied to prevent dryness and cracking.

Careful recording of the temperature and the pulse and respiration rates is an important part of good nursing care. The pulse rate indicates the progress of the child, and it should be counted for a full minute. When the sleeping pulses are requested, the nurse must take care lest she awaken the child.

Administration of oxygen is usually the next remedial measure after rest is instituted. An oxygen tent maintains a good concentration of oxygen, and the child can see the personnel; yet his motion is not too restricted. He should wear appropriate body covering so that he will feel comfortable when the proper temperature of 65° to 70° is maintained. He should know the purpose of the tent before he is put into it. A bell which he can use to bring the nurse to him also is helpful in alleviating fears associated with confinement inside a tent.

A pericardial tap usually gives immediate relief to the heart if pericarditis has caused a large amount of fluid to collect in the pericardial sac. Paracentesis of the abdominal cavity also may be indicated for relief of respiratory difficulty caused by ascites. The nurse can give support to the child and assist the physician in preparing for these procedures.

Digitalis slows and strengthens the heart and so improves circulation. The pulse rate should be counted carefully before administration of digitalis, and if it has gone down markedly or has changed in quality, the physician should be notified before the next dose is given. The chief toxic symptoms of digitalis overdose are anorexia, nausea and vomiting.

The toxic manifestations of overdosage with salicylates, steroids and ACTH have been described under Acute Rheumatic Carditis. The nurse must be thoroughly familiar with the untoward reactions of these drugs which may necessitate a change in the plan of medical care. Even though the child is on prophylactic antibiotic therapy, he must be shielded from personnel and visitors who have respiratory infections.

As the acute stage subsides and the heart becomes compensated, less rigorous restriction of activity is required, but confinement to bed is continued for as long as any evidence of activity of the disease persists or for as long as compensation is incomplete. The criteria for determining persistence of activity of the disease are stated under Rheumatic Fever. After the child has been permitted out of bed for brief periods and has been given bathroom privileges, the pulse rate is a fairly good criterion as to the degree of compensation of the heart. Other tests of cardiac function may be applied, such as noting how quickly the pulse rate returns to its former level after a brief period of exercise. Restriction of bodily activity for many months has been a common custom. Such radical restriction is unnecessary, provided that all evidence of infection, including laboratory evidence, has disappeared and provided that the state of nutrition is excellent. In most instances, unlimited activity may be allowed 6 weeks after the child has been permitted to be out of bed. When heart damage persists, the activity of the child always must be restricted within the limits of easy tolerance, as discussed subsequently.

The measures for the prevention of recurrences of rheumatic episodes are of utmost importance for children who have suffered from carditis.

Chronic Valvular Disease

Damage to the heart valves, usually produced by rheumatic carditis, leads to changes which alter the normal functioning of the valves. When the child has recovered from the active or the acute inflammation of carditis, the residual heart damage with scarring of the valves is termed "chronic valvular disease." It results in changes in the remainder of the circulatory system to compensate for the valvular changes.

Two types of valvular damage may be produced. One of these consists of a puckering or a partial destruction or a binding down of the valve leaves, which results in an inability of the valve to close tightly and so allows a leakage of the blood in the circulation in the direction opposite to that in which it normally goes. This type of defect occurs most frequently at the mitral valve. At this site the condition is known as mitral insufficiency, and the backward flow of blood is spoken of as mitral regurgitation.

The other type of valve damage consists of a narrowing of the valve orifice by scar contraction or fusion of valve leaflets so that the leaflets cannot open completely. Such a lesion constitutes a stenosis and prevents easy passage of blood through the heart.

As a result of these changes, the heart must do more work. This goal is accomplished usually by increase of musculature or hypertrophy. If hypertrophy is insufficient, the heart rate also is increased.

Symptoms. When compensation is adequate, chronic valvular disease produces no symptoms. Examination reveals cardiac murmurs and an enlarged heart. Symptoms arise when for any reason compensation is inadequate. Decompensation is discussed in Chapter 22. In the absence of cardiac insufficiency or decompensation, children with chronic valvular disease need only to avoid exertion beyond their cardiac capacity and to guard against further cardiac damage.

Management. It is necessary for some children with heart disease to lead a guarded and restricted life. However, it is always desirable that they lead a life as nearly normal as possible. Such children should be examined at suitable intervals to determine whether the regimen followed is adequate or unnecessarily restrictive. They should have such supervision as would detect at their onset any deleterious conditions. The mental attitude toward life needs careful consideration and adjustment. The chief function of childhood is preparation for adult life, and an important part of the preparation is formal education. A lack of understanding between medical supervisor and educator may result in unnecessary neglect of the child's education.

Too often the instruction to the parent or the child is of a negative type with admonition as to what not to do, for example, "Do not run up the stairs and do not play hard." Instruction of this type may well produce cardiac invalidism. Help is required to develop the child's resources and at the same time conserve his energy and prevent overburdening of his cardiovascular system. When restrictions are necessary, the child's participation must be elicited in planning the time for rest periods so that his plans for activity are not disrupted.

Chorea (Sydenham's Chorea; St. Vitus' Dance)

Symptoms. Chorea is characterized by involuntary, purposeless, irregular movements commonly involving all the voluntary musculature but occasionally affecting one side of the body more than the other.

The greatest incidence of chorea is between the ages of 6 and 15 years. It is much more frequent in girls than in boys and more frequent in the spring than at other seasons. Chorea is said to be more frequent in families with emotional problems, and it has been assumed that heredity plays a role.

The most prominent symptom in chorea consists of peculiar body movements. These are jerking, spasmodic, incoordinated and without regularity. They cannot be suppressed by volition; in fact, they are made worse by attempts to inhibit them and by embarrassment. In severe chorea, these movements may be so extreme that the child may be bruised and injured by tossing and jerking against the sides of the bed unless the bed is padded. Such children cannot walk, talk, sit or feed themselves and are incontinent. Fortunately, in most instances the disease is not so severe. To be seen are all grades of severity from that described to such mildness that recognition of the condition requires close observation. Frequently, one half of the body is affected so much more than the other half that the condition is spoken of as "hemichorea."

All attacks begin gradually, with signs of increased nervousness. Difficulty in the finer movements such as writing or buttoning clothing is evident early. The child stumbles easily and often drops articles being handled. Food is spilled, and soon, because of the jerky movements, self-feeding becomes impossible. The involvement of the muscles of the face causes grimaces. Incoordinate movements affecting the mouth

Fig. 27-4. Spindle-shaped swelling of finger joints characteristic of rheumatoid arthritis.

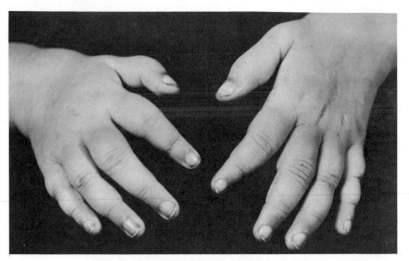

and the tongue make speech difficult or impossible. When one part of the body is involved more than the remainder, as in hemichorea, the chief complaint often is stated as "paralysis." The paralysis is apparent but not real and is due to inability to use the parts purposefully. Choreic movements are absent during sleep.

Treatment and Nursing Care. The treatment of chorea is largely palliative and symptomatic. Neither the salicylates nor the steroids have any effect on this aspect of rheumatic fever. In the milder attacks, no specific care is required. When the disease is more severe, bed rest, sedative drugs, warm baths and avoidance of stress are indicated.

Children with chorea have uncontrolled body movements, sometimes to the point of helplessness, but they do not feel ill. Not only must all their needs be supplied by others, but also in many instances their needs must be anticipated because they have lost their ability to talk. They must be fed, and the process must be a slow and safe one because of the incoordinate movements of the head, the mouth and the muscles of swallowing. If movements are severe, a fork should never be used to feed a child with chorea.

Special attention must be given to the skin of the elbows, the knees and other points of contact which are constantly being rubbed and chafed. Massaging the skin over the joints with soothing ointment and keeping the extremities covered with flannel pajamas will protect these areas from irritation. When chorea is severe, the nurse must perform the many duties required by a helpless but mentally active child. He should be cared for in a crib bed with padded sides, and those toys that could injure him should be eliminated.

These children are usually malnourished. Their constant movements use energy, and though their appetites are usually good, they are underweight and anemic. Frequent feedings of foods which are high in protein, calories, vitamins and iron should be provided.

Children improve faster if they are out of bed and permitted a fair amount of liberty and activity. This is especially true if the attack has been prolonged, laboratory evidence of infection has vanished, and the manifestations of the disease have subsided. Children with chorea often rest better if they are in a room by themselves where there is protection from stimuli. Occasionally, however, a child may react adversely to being separated from other children and may begin to show signs of improvement when he has the companionship of another child.

Often the physical symptoms of chorea are preceded by a period of emotional instability which has caused family conflicts. The child may have persistently quarrelled with his siblings, been inattentive and fearful at school and had frequent temper outbursts. A good relationship between the child and his parents needs to be re-established before he can receive maximum benefit from his parents' visits. It is important that the nurse observe the child's reactions during visiting hours and after the parents leave the ward. The parents may welcome a chance to discuss any problems in relationships with the social worker. Guilt from misinterpretation of the child's behavior is prevalent. When it is alleviated parents become able to regain their child's trust.

Understanding of the cause of the child's instability helps the nurse to exercise patience in the care of the child. An intelligent, sensitive child who develops chorea may be upset by his own instability and troubled by his parents' failure to understand him. Tendencies toward introspection continue unless the nurse succeeds in helping him to find interests outside of himself. A poised, unhurried nurse who listens to the child's defective speech, reads to him and talks with him about his favorite subjects will help the child to rebuild confidence in himself.

Play materials can be introduced when movements are controlled. At first, play things that require the use of large muscles are more appropriate. Later, as improvement continues, materials requiring fine coordination can be presented. Children appreciate help

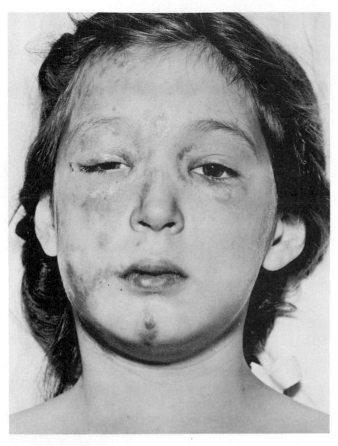

Fig. 27-5. The facial rash seen in lupus erythematosus.

in regaining skills lost during acute illness, and well-directed activity programs help to restore the former image that they had of themselves.

Rheumatoid Arthritis

Rheumatoid arthritis is a chronic systemic disease which has as its distinguishing feature protracted and deforming inflammation of the joints. It is not common among children but may be seen at almost any age. The onset-may be with joint swelling or may be in a nonspecific fashion. Fairly high fever with splenic and generalized lymph node enlargement is common in the acute stage. The small joints of the body (Fig. 27-4) are attacked most regularly, but the larger joints and the spine also may be involved. In contrast with rheumatic fever, the disease has no apparent relation to streptococcal sensitization; the arthritis is not as readily relieved with aspirin; the symptoms remain in the joints originally involved; the inflammation runs a protracted course and may result in permanent disability of the joint. Although the course of the disease is ultimately self-limited, the spontaneous subsidence of symptoms usually does not take place until the person has been sick for several years. During this period, joint deformity and muscle atrophy may progress to

a point where complete restoration to normal cannot be expected. Occasionally, the heart is involved during the course of the rheumatoid arthritis, but this is the uncommon exception rather than the expected complication that it is in rheumatic fever.

Salicylates may give symptomatic relief when the disease is mild, but in contrast to rheumatic fever, they are relatively ineffectual when the disease is at all severe and do not readily control the febrile aspect. Steroid therapy may give dramatic relief in many instances, but it must be undertaken with great caution for too often it is necessary to use increasingly larger doses over long periods of time and thus produce hyperadrenocorticism with its attendant complications. Furthermore, it is often difficult to reduce the dose of steroids when complications appear, without precipitating an exacerbation of rheumatoid symptoms. For these reasons, steroids are generally avoided in the milder cases of rheumatoid arthritis and are used in combination with other drugs such as chloroquine, Daraprim, or phenylbutazone in severe cases with the hope of keeping the steroid dosage as low as possible. Unfortunately, these adjunctive drugs also have their own toxic properties for which the child must be carefully watched. In the case of the antimalarials, cataracts and retinitis are to be feared. With phenylbutazone there may be severe gastrointestinal disorders, purpura, hepatitis or blood dyscrasia.

The symptomatic nursing care of rheumatoid arthritis includes shielding of joints from unexpected motion during the time they are acutely inflamed. This is achieved by the use of splints or bivalved lightweight casts which are applied at night while the child sleeps. During the acute stage of the disease the child may need to be fed, dressed and bathed by the nurse because of the restricted usefulness of his hands. For those with the severer forms of the disease long periods of hospitalization are often required during which they will need encouragement to use their bodies and minds to the fullest. Convalescent care is considered in a later section of this chapter.

Disseminated Lupus Erythematosus

Disseminated lupus is an uncommon disorder seen mainly in adolescent and young adult females. It is a slowly progressive and usually fatal disorder, and the multitudinous symptoms depend on a widespread abnormality of the vascular tree. Prolonged fever, recurring arthritis, pleurisy, erythematous skin eruptions on portions of the body exposed to the sun, chronic nephritis, endocarditis and hypersplenism are some of the features that may be present clinically. Diagnosis usually is suspected from the combination of some or all of these findings in a girl. The skin eruption and a persistent leukopenia are the features which most often direct attention to the correct diagnosis. Confirmation is obtained by finding characteristic polymorphonuclear leukocytes that contain large masses of amorphous substance (L. E. cells). These cells may be found in bonemarrow preparations or in leukocytes which have been incubated with the patient's serum. The underlying disturbance is thought to be an abnormality of protein metabolism which affects nucleic acid in particular. Accumulation of the same sort of material as that seen in the typical L. E. cell takes place beneath the endocardium to create a verrucous endocarditis and beneath the endothelium of small vessels anywhere in the body, resulting in occlusion of such vessels. The body also makes antibodies against DNA and other products of destroyed cells. Such antibodies detected in the circulating blood are important confirmation of the clinical diagnosis. Renal biopsy may also give strong evidence of the presence of lupus erythematosus.

Treatment with steroid hormones is temporarily effective in obtaining remission of symptoms. Unfortunately, these persons tend to become easily sensitized by sulfonamides and other substances, including the hormones. Eventually, therapy becomes less effective or progression of the renal disease takes place, and the child succumbs to it. Nursing care is similar to that which is required for the child with any protracted and ultimately fatal disease.

Other Collagen Diseases

Other collagen diseases which are seen infrequently among children are dermatomyositis, scleroderma and periarteritis nodosa. The reader is referred to sources listed in the bibliography for full description and discussion of these disorders which, like lupus, involve widespread changes in many tissues with a progressive and usually fatal course.

CONVALESCENT CARE OF CHILDREN WITH CHRONIC ILLNESS

Skill, patience, knowledge and ingenuity are required to help the child adapt as constructively as possible to prolonged periods of bed rest. Although bed rest provides the restriction which is necessary to protect his cardiovascular system, it also entails dangers to his physical, intellectual and emotional functioning and developmental progress. The concomitant abatement in normal activity may produce loss of muscle tone and reduction of normal intestinal and urinary activity. Decreased respiration may influence mental alertness and the ability to sustain intellectual concentration. The decline of perceptual efficiency and of sensory stimulation may diminish normal contact with the environment and weaken the usual behavioral controls.

Such changes in usual functioning and control of his body are frightening to the child in addition to the anxiety caused by his illness. Since he may not feel fatigue, he can see no valid reason for adhering to the restrictions which he senses are increasing his problems. The loss of independence, of caring for himself, and the reduction of involvement in learning new skills are difficult for the school age child and adolescent to bear. As a consequence, the disregard of proscriptions against activity may become more pronounced as the period of confinement lengthens.

With some children however, flaunting of rules may come at an early period in the illness when the load on the heart must be minimized to prevent serious damage. Disregard of the physician's judgment may stem from a need for attention, to annoy the nurse or to get relief from unbearable tension. More often, however, the causes of the child's behavior are deeply buried and, therefore, are out of his control.

Resistance to prescribed regulations may hide the longing for dependency or the meaning which a damaged heart has for the child personally, or it may be the means by which he copes with anxiety related to problems which are not associated with his illness. Children who have an unconscious wish to regress may resist bed rest because it violates their concept of their own adequacy. Being "good" patients means losing respect for themselves. To prove their independence, they violate the rules made by the very persons on whom they should be dependent for help in getting well. They often display a pseudomaturity which they cannot maintain and should not even if they could because it would lead to further self-destruction.

The nurse's task in such situations is not easy because the child is apt to arouse feelings which make her want to berate his intelligence and expose his immaturity. Instead, she has to redirect her energy toward finding ways in which she can prove her respect for the maturest parts of his personality. Encouraging participation in plans for his care and in formulating rules which he can use when he is tempted to defy authority will restore his self-confidence and prove his strength. He will rise to the occasion when his opinions are sought about the events of the day and move toward cooperation when he is given the chance to grouse about the restrictions he longs for but cannot accept emotionally. With this support he can begin to abandon his injurious guise and tolerate the care which is necessary for his recovery.

Resistance to restrictions may also manifest the child's attempt to maintain the image he had of himself before he became ill. Self-esteem in the school age child is greatly influenced by self judgments as a reflection of the judgments of peers in attainment of physical skills and in control of bodily coordination in addition to competent intellectual functioning. Functional limitations are therefore threatening to the former burgeoning sense of "I" and of his position among his peers. Physical weakness motivates protection of his sense of former adequacy by denial of symptoms and unauthorized activity with the purpose

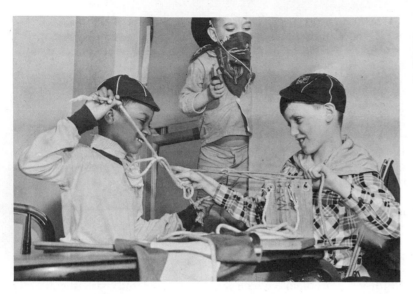

Fig. 27-6. The play of boys with cardiac disease is similar to the play of normal children. (La Rabida Jackson Park Sanitarium for Children with Cardiac Disease, Chicago, and The Chicago Daily Sun Times)

of proving to himself that his capabilities are intact. Failure in physical performance however, may increase his frustration and fear, and further threaten his positive sense of self. The effect may be to strengthen his defenses of denial or rationalization and to increase his anger. Failure with repeated trials may initiate a feeling of humiliation and intensify withdrawal.

Attempts to convince the hyperactive school age child or adolescent that he is injuring himself are fruitless in winning his cooperation. Instead, they force him to deepen his defenses and prevent him from rebuilding an image of himself which he can respect. The nurse who can extend her interest from the cardiac functioning of the child to the child as a personality who must become actively involved in making his own adjustment to heart disease can lessen his self concern and the anxiety stemming from old conflicts refocused on his heart.

Children who have lost hope, ceased to fight against frustration and withdrawn from their environment may sit passively, demonstrate little feeling and remain partially mute. The child who is able to express resentment overtly may receive reassurance that his feelings are understandable if his aggression does not produce retaliation. The child who is withdrawn is also denied proof that he has the right to resent his illness and treatment and the relief of tension which self expression can produce. He is unable to reach out for recognition and love but instead waits for it to be given unsolicited. When his needs are not recognized, his hope dwindles rapidly to the point of loss of contact with his environment. If he is encouraged to express himself, however, he may be able to view his feelings in a more realistic light, begin to cope

with them and thus release energy into constructive mastery.

A short résumé of Shirley's behavior after a prolonged period of stress is given to show the depth of despair which is hidden behind helpless submission.

There was always a look of complete inertia about 11-year-old Shirley. After a long period of bed rest for rheumatic fever, she spent most of her time rolling her wheelchair in the corridor or into the playroom where the children congregated. Her eyes were continually watchful, and her facial expression rarely changed. She was a child who "sat and waited" with patience but with little hope. She rarely had visitors because her family lived in another city. When she was in her room, her TV was on continually, and she appeared to be absorbed in the pictures. She had roommates, but she never became "one of the girls."

Three days before discharge, Shirley was in the playroom where a group of children were making placemats for luncheon. Shirley fringed the end of one lethargically and then rolled herself about the room touching playthings but never stopping long enough to play with them.

When Shirley learned that her bedridden roommates were remaining in the playroom for rest hour and that she had to rest in her room alone, she did not protest or beg to stay there but instead quickly vanished from the room. A few minutes later the nurse found her in her room with her back to the door watching TV. Her spindly legs were drawn up under her and her "pouty" countenance betrayed the loneliness and the frustration which she was enduring. Shirley could not ask for the comfort she needed. Nor could the nurse be sure that she could accept it if it were offered. But because she knew that Shirley was facing reunion with a family she had not seen for months, the nurse suspected that rejection of her wish to remain with the group in the playroom for rest had stirred up the feelings of loneliness which she had had since she was admitted to the hospital. She also surmised that Shirley might be worrying about her return home. The nurse shared her thoughts with Shirley

FIG. 27-7. Scout activities are a part of the activity program at the La Rabida Jackson Park Sanitarium. (La Rabida Sanitarium, Chicago, and The Chicago Daily Sun Times)

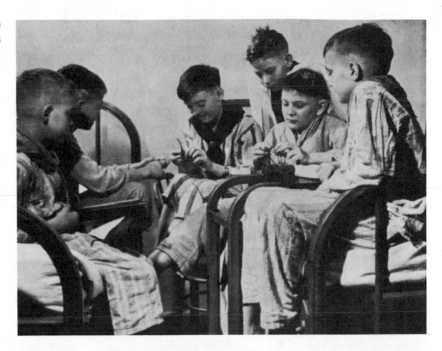

in the hopes that it would give her the courage to talk with her: "You have been disappointed so many times, Shirley, and you were disappointed again when you couldn't stay with your friends. I wonder if you might also be worrying about going home." Shirley's eyes filled with tears as she nodded her head. Because it was obvious that Shirley needed gratification, the nurse asked her if she would like to sit on her lap for awhile. Shirley fairly leaped into her lap, buried herself as tightly against the nurse's body as she could and sobbed disconsolately. It had been so long since Shirley had been able to let herself cry that when she once broke down, her feelings poured out in a stream. Then, finding comfort as a little child, she gradually became able to relax quietly.

As previously mentioned, enforced bed rest may decrease the amount of oxygen in brain tissues thus reducing normal alertness, affecting perception and limiting ability to concentrate on the mastery of intellectual tasks so important in the normal development of the school age child. In addition, the reduction of a normal amount of sensory input resulting from a restricted environment affects the arousal mechanisms of the reticular activating system of the brain. The decline in the rate of former arousal may influence the lack of ability to sustain attention, result in a distorting of perception and thought processes and culminate in disorganized behavior and loss of contact with reality. The cognitive effect of reduced and repetitive stimuli results from the static quality of the hospital experience as opposed to the dynamic effects of prehospitalization experience. Habituation to repetitive stimuli is thus also involved in the passivity so often encountered in the child who is hospitalized for long periods of time even though there is a fairly high, constant level of sensory input.

When a minimum of bed rest is enforced and pa-

tients are observed carefully to determine physiologic limits, many of the dangers to emotional and intellectual progress can be prevented. "Don't" should be used sparingly to reduce anxiety, antagonism and the personality problems which can be more defeating than the heart disease. The acutely ill child can benefit from the warmth of human companionship and varied stimulation when the nurse tells him stories, reads to him, introduces pictures or allows manual exploration of toys of varying shapes and colors. As he recuperates, activity and stimulation can be increased by allowing him to hold the book, turn the pages, cut pictures from magazines or design a scrapbook. Later he can color, fingerpaint, mold clay, work simple puzzles, use paper dolls, dress dolls and do school work.

At first play periods need to be short, without strain and interspersed with quiet periods of music, stories and movies. With physical progress, a graduated program of activity and exercise is introduced.

A child who has had prolonged bed rest cannot maintain quiet when he is tempted with a chair which can transport him to places he has wanted to explore. When he is first placed in a chair without wheels, locating him in front of a window or near a table of appropriate play materials will encourage relaxation. Later, excursions in a wheel chair will revive his spirits and stimulate interests outside himself. The pulse rate should be counted before and after new activities are introduced. If his pulse rate does not return to normal within 5 minutes, bed rest should be resumed. Rise in the evening temperature, disturbed sleep and fatigue usually mean that activity has been started prematurely.

The location for convalescent care is determined

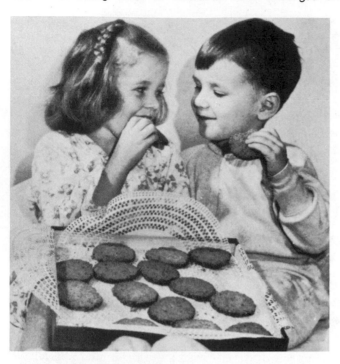

FIG. 27-8. Two children with cardiac disease enjoying party food and the company of each other. (La Rabida Jackson Park Sanitarium, Chicago, and The Chicago Daily Sun Times)

through casework study of the child's particular needs, his home and family circumstances. Care is provided in the child's own home whenever his family can meet his physical and emotional needs. However, care in a convalescent home or hospital may be preferable

for some children. Group activity and school work can be continued more easily (Figs. 27-6 to 27-10), and association with a group of children with similar limitations helps some children to become better prepared for life in the community. Early symptoms of respiratory infection can be detected more quickly, and, as a result of prompt care, recurrences of rheumatic fever can be reduced. Foster home care is sometimes indicated when convalescent home care is unavailable or when the child has not had a stable home life which has given him security.

Fortunately, many children of this age have the resources and ego strength to utilize a hospital experience constructively when conditions are optimum. They are able to sustain more prolonged periods of separation from their parents than are younger children while continuing to maintain ties of affection. Their concept of causality is more mature, so that hospital placement does not hold the same intense connotations of deprivation and punishment. Their sense of time is also more acute so that anticipation of the return of their parents is not fraught with the former acute anxiety.

For some children, hospitalization can be beneficial if relationships within the home are tenuous or filled with tension. Separation from home may then afford relief from emotional turmoil. If the child's needs are understood and demands are consistent with his abilities, emotional growth can be encouraged in this stress-reduced environment. The child can also be given an opportunity to learn constructive methods of coping with his anxiety, to understand the functioning of his body and the causation and treat-

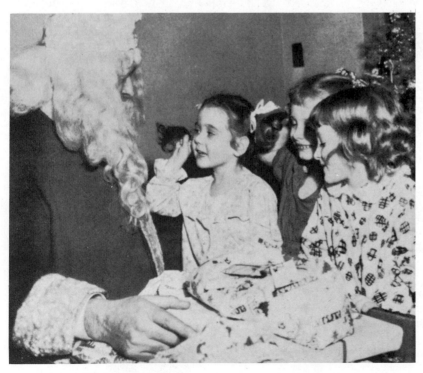

FIG. 27-9. Christmas festivities are important for children in hospitals. (La Rabida Jackson Park Sanitarium, Chicago, and The Chicago Daily Sun Times)

ment of his illness. This information can often do much toward alleviating guilt as to the source of his disability and contribute to his emotional stability. When nurses are accepting of his behavior, his self-esteem, respect and acceptance of himself can be strengthened.

Available personnel can also be utilized to evaluate the disturbing home conditions and to help in resolving the conflicts which retard the child's progress. When parents visit, nurses have an excellent opportunity to be helpful in altering parental patterns of interaction with their child.

Encouragement of the child's active participation in planning for convalescent care aids in the prevention of maladjustment. Unless he is prepared for adjustment in a strange hospital or foster home, he is apt to feel rejected by those persons he has trusted before. Adjustment into a new family situation is eased when foster parents visit the child before he is discharged. Continued supervision of the foster home is usually provided, and the child's own parents are encouraged to maintain their emotional ties to him through frequent visits. He is returned to his own home as soon as satisfactory adjustments are made in it.

Thoughtful guidance is required for the re-establishment of independence after a long period of helplessness. Those who are responsible for the child's supervision must provide emotional security, and the group activities which promote healthy psychosocial development and protection of his physical health. In some cities, visiting teachers are sent to the home when children are unable to attend school. Schools exist for severely handicapped children and provide transportation and special programs of physical supervision as well. Some children (and adults) find it difficult to give up the privileged position which they enjoyed during their acute illness. When this tendency is observed, concentration on the child's wish to grow up will help him to overcome residual regressive tendencies.

Preparation for Discharge and Continued Health Supervision

Announcement that discharge is planned usually arouses mixed feelings in the child and sometimes in the parents as well. Pleasant thoughts about going home are intermingled with fears about starting something new. Discharge terminates an experience which has caused a profound change in the child's patterns of living. Therefore, difficulties may be encountered in readjusting to family life. Some children are depressed on return home. Others may express overtly those feelings which they suppressed in the hospital. Any reactions which parents and children are unprepared for will cause worry and stress.

Insight into the child's particular needs is necessary to help the child to become readjusted to life at home

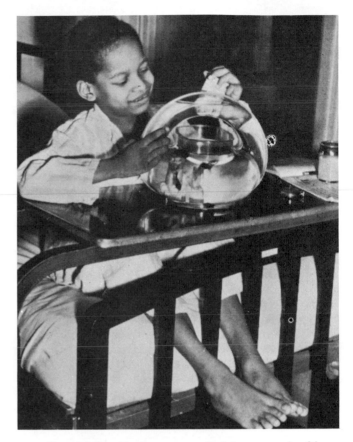

Fig. 27-10. Confinement to bed is more tolerable when interesting projects are available. (La Rabida Jackson Park Sanitarium, Chicago, and The Chicago Daily Sun Times)

and at school. It is important that teachers and parents neither push the child before he becomes ready to tackle a new experience nor retard his progress when he is ready to move ahead. Teamwork between the hospital personnel, the physician, the school nurse, the teacher and the child and his parents is essential in the provision of health supervision. The teacher will need the school nurse's help in implementing the health team's recommendations in the classroom.

Consideration is often given to the advantages and the disadvantages of special school arrangements for the child with cardiac disease. These children have limitations, but usually they are temporary. Most authorities believe that they should be placed in classes with healthy children as soon as they can meet the requirements without stress.

Recurrence of disease is prevented through continuous health supervision. Parents and children need understanding of the importance of clinic visits, dental care, prophylactic drug therapy, rest, diet and protection from infection. Knowledge of the earliest signs of respiratory infection helps to alert the youngster to his need for extra rest and fluids. The child who has felt supported during hospitalization will be strengthened by the experience. He will be ready to use the advice which he has been given for home care and will want to turn to hospital personnel again when he needs further help in learning to care for himself.

SITUATIONS FOR FURTHER STUDY

1. Study a school-age child with asthma while you give him care. What are his behavioral responses to an attack and how did you react to them and to his physical symptoms? What elements of nursing care relieved his anxiety? Describe his relationship with his mother and father and with you. If he is having psychiatric therapy, what help did you get from his therapist in understanding his particular needs? What problems did you have in following suggestions for his care? What changes in behavior did you observe when you were able to use the therapist's suggestions?

2. What symptoms in a school-age child would lead you to suspect that he might have rheumatic fever?

3. What common human needs are characteristic of the school-age child with heart disease?

4. What might be possible sources of anxiety in a school-age child with rheumatic fever?

5. What problems did you encounter in nursing a child with rheumatoid arthritis? Describe the way in which you helped him to overcome his limitations during play?

6. What might have been some of the reasons why Shirley's unhappiness was not picked up early in the course of the treatment? Describe some alternate ways in which her flight from the playroom might have been handled. What might be the outcome of Shirley's mode of adjustment to hospitalization? What kind of transition do you imagine Shirley will make to adolescence?

BIBLIOGRAPHY

Apemow, M. L., and Odenal, J.: Lupus erythematosus, Am. J. Nurs. 51:383, 1951.

Birchfield, M. O.: Easier said than done, Am. J. Nurs. 59:1566, 1959.

Brewer, E. J.: Rheumatoid arthritis in childhood, Am. J. Nurs. 65:66, 1965.

Burgin, L. B.: Emotion as an allergen, Pediat. Clin. N. Am. 6:657, 1959.

Cluster, P. F.: One-room school for hospitalized children, Nurs. Outlook, 15:56, 1967.

Coolidge, J. C.: Asthma in mother and child as a special type of communication, Am. J. Orthopsychiat. 26:165, 1956.

DiMaggio, G.: The child with asthma, Nurs. Clin. N. Am. 3:453, 1968.

Dubo, S., et al.: A study of relationships between family situations, bronchial asthma and personal adjustment in children, Pediatrics 59:402, 1961.

Dutcher, I., and Hakerem, H.: Mother-child interaction in psychosomatic illness, Nurs. Forum 7:173, 1968.

Erickson, F. H.: Helping the sick child to maintain behavorial control, Nurs. Clin. N. Am. 2:695, 1967.

Feinberg, S. M.: Allergies and air conditioning, Am. J. Nurs. 66:1333, 1966.

Itkin, I. H.: The pros and cons of exercise for the person with asthma, Am. J. Nurs. 66:1584, 1966.

Jessner, L., et al.: Emotional impact of nearness and separation for the asthmatic child and his mother, Psychoanal. Stud. Child 10:353, 1955.

Johnstone, D. E., and Crump, L.: Value of hyposensitization therapy for perennial bronchial asthma in children, Pediatrics 27:39, 1961.

Josselyn, I. M., et al.: Anxiety in children convalescing from rheumatic fever, Am. J. Orthopsychiat. 25:120, 1955.

Kelsey, W. M.: Rheumatoid disease in juvenile patients, J. Pediat. 59:227, 1961.

Long, R. T., Lamont, J. H., et al.: A psychosomatic study of allergic and emotional factors in children with asthma, Am. J. Psychiat. 114:890, 1958.

Mansmann, H.: Management of the child with bronchial asthma, Pediat. Clin. N. Am. 15:357, 1968.

Miller, H., and Baruch, D. W.: A study of hostility in allergic children, Am. J. Orthopsychiat. 20:506, 1950.

————: Psychotherapy of parents of allergic children, Ann. Allergy 18:990, 1960.

Mitchell, J. H.: The emotional factors in eczema and urticaria, Ann. Allergy 18:170, 1960.

Olson, Edith: The hazards of immobility, Am. J. Nurs. 67:4, p. 780, 1967.

Prugh, D. G.: Toward an Understanding of Psychosomatic Concepts in Relation to Illness in Children, in Solnit, A. J., and Provence, S. (eds.), Modern Perspectives in Child Development, New York, Internat. Univ. Press, 1963.

Ross Roundtable on Maternal Child Nursing: Patients with Sensory Disturbances—Implications for Nursing Practice and Research, Ross Laboratories, 1966, Columbus, Ohio.

Rubin, R.: Body image and self-esteem, Nurs. Outlook 16:20, 1968.

Sather, Mary: Environmental care of an asthmatic child, Am. J. Nurs. 68:816, 1968.

Sears, F. F.: Relation of early socialization experiences to aggression in middle childhood, J. Abnorm. and Social Psychol. 63:466, 1961.

Shore, M., Geiser, R., and Walman, H. M.: Constructive uses of a hospital experience, Children 12:3, 1965.

Thompson, R. M.: The cardiac child at home, Nurs. Outlook 9:77, 1961.

Vaughn, V. C.: The place of drug therapy in childhood asthma, Am. J. Nurs. 66:1049, 1966.

Walike, B. C., Marmor, L., and Upshaw, M. J.: Rheumatoid arthritis, Am. J. Nurs. 67:1420, 1967.

Watson, H. T.: The role of the school nurse in the support of children with certain cardiovascular disorders, Nurs. Clin. N. Am. 1:31, 1966.

FILMS

The Valiant Heart, M.P.O. Productions, distributed by the American Heart Association, 44 E. 23rd St., New York 10, N. Y. (28½ minutes).

28

Nursing Care of Children with Neurologic and Psychological Disorders

The school years place the child under increased intellectual and social demands. It is important that he put his best foot forward in order to realize his maximum potential. Under the stress of the new life which he adopts for much of his waking day, physical and psychological handicaps assume increasing importance, particularly when they interfere with his school progress. It is especially important that the school nurse have an understanding of how such handicaps affect children so that she can function with them and their parents, teachers and medical and psychiatric therapists in facilitating adjustment to life at school, at home and in the community.

VISUAL DEFECTS

In the infant or small child visual defects are usually suspected through the observation of abnormal eye movements (Chap. 13). However, many children have vision which is defective because of refractive errors which produce no unusual movement of the eyes. It is important for such defects to be recognized and corrected before the child's school work begins to suffer from his inability to identify numbers and letters on the blackboard or in his school books. For this reason school health programs include an estimation of visual acuity of all students at the beginning of school and every few years thereafter. Screening tests are performed with the usual Snellen eye charts for those children who know letters. Younger children may be tested with a similar chart in which they manipulate an "E" in their hands to match the position in which it is printed on the chart. Significant defects of vision should be more completely examined by a competent ophthalmologist. Children who are already wearing glasses are included in the testing both with and without their glasses. It is desirable to make sure that the correction obtained is satisfactory and that changes in the eye have not progressed since the last fitting of glasses. An adequate visual examination is imperative for children who are not performing adequately in school or for those who complain of headache.

HEARING LOSS

Severe degrees of hearing loss in the young child prevent proper development of speech because the child is unable to imitate the language being used around him. This situation is usually apparent by the time the child is 2 to 3 years of age. However, lesser or unilateral hearing loss may go unrecognized unless carefully sought. Screening tests of hearing are difficult in the pre-school child, since they require his understanding and cooperation. Gross tests can be made with a watch or the carefully modulated spoken voice when the child is old enough to cooperate. Such tests are only a rough measure of hearing competence, and whenever doubt exists, the more accurate method of audiometry should be employed. In this latter method the child is asked to signal when he hears single tones which are electronically controlled both as to pitch and intensity. In this fashion both the range and the extent of his hearing loss can be discovered. Personnel in many school health programs test all pupils every few years with an audiometer. If hearing defects are uncovered, the child should be referred to a competent audiologist for more refined diagnosis and for treatment. Children whose hearing loss is extensive must be taught lip-reading or fitted with hearing aids. Special classes are desirable for such children until they have mastered the hearing aids and are able to resume their places among children with normal hearing.

SPEECH DEFECTS

The most common form of speech difficulty is seen among children of the lower grade levels who retain elements of baby talk, lisping and inability to pronounce certain consonants such as l, r, w, s, th and z. In many instances this stems from a family attitude which regarded such mispronunciations as cute or unimportant. The school environment is usually less tolerant, and most children rapidly correct such speech habits in order to sound like their teachers and classmates. Some are not able to do so without special help from a speech therapist. Usually it is wise to wait for spontaneous improvement over a year or so before enlisting special help for the child with persistent speech abnormalities.

A few children suffer from speech defects which are related to structural abnormalities of the mouth such as cleft palate. Most of these receive special help before they enter school, particularly if they have had the benefit of care in a clinic designed to meet the many needs of the child with such a deformity.

Stuttering or stammering is often a transient and unimportant symptom in the preschool or early school years. It is handled most satisfactorily by ignoring it so as to prevent the child from becoming self-conscious about it. In many instances the hesitancy will disappear spontaneously and permanently. However stuttering or stammering which persists into the middle or late school years is a more complicated problem which usually involves the child's total personality and may require the services of not only a speech therapist but a psychiatrist as well.

TIC (HABIT SPASM)

A habit spasm or tic is a simple or complex muscular movement which is repeated over and over in the same manner. Tics differ from choreiform movements in that the latter are without order or purpose and never are repeated twice in the same order of progression. Tics most frequently involve the face, but often also the neck, the shoulders or some other part of the body. They may take the form of blinking of the eyes, a facial grimace, shrugging of the shoulders or other movements, or a combination of some of these.

Tics begin as voluntary movements and are repeated until they become habitual and involuntary. Even in the habitual and involuntary stage, the movements can be repeated voluntarily on request. The movements may have had their origin in imitation of another or they may have started as the result of some local irritation or psychic or physical discomfort; they continue long after the exciting cause has disappeared. A tic may leave one part of the body and appear in another. As in chorea, the movements are increased by anxiety and cease during sleep.

Drugs and disciplinary measures are ineffectual in the treatment of tics. The parents should be urged to ignore the symptom as much as possible and to expend their efforts toward relieving stress which may be contributing to the child's feelings of insecurity. If changes in environmental circumstances do not result in cessation of the tic, psychiatric therapy is probably needed. It is particularly important to differentiate the movements from those of rheumatic chorea, since the treatment of the latter disorder is quite different.

HEADACHE

Among children, headaches occur under a wide variety of circumstances. Severe or persistent complaints require careful exclusion of organic disease of the brain or meninges with accompanying increased intracranial pressure. Among older children headache may be a symptom of stress, refractive error of the eyes, chronic sinusitis, fatigue, anemia or toxic or metabolic disorder. Occasionally, it announces the presence of hypertension. Migraine headaches occur in children but with lesser frequency than in adults. They usually are associated with a family predisposition to migraine and occur more frequently in girls. They may have the features of one-sidedness and abrupt onset seen in the older individual. Sensitivity to light and sound, dizziness, spots before the eyes and vomiting are often features of the onset. Treatment with aspirin or phenobarbital or codeine is usually not sufficient to give relief. Ergotamine is sometimes effective. In many instances the headaches appear to be precipitated by emotional stress or unusual fatigue. Detailed examination of the child's environment and way of life may disclose ways in which such pressures can be relieved.

Headaches among younger children often precede the appearance of fever with an infectious illness. For some children they represent the somatic manner in which anxiety is expressed. Headaches are often projected on small, suggestible children by an anxious mother through questions such as "Are you sick? What's the matter? Does your head ache?" The child in agreeing with the suggestion finds that he receives solicitous attention and may later use the symptom of headache as a method of achieving the secondary gain.

ENURESIS

Enuresis is the involuntary passage of urine, particularly at night, in an individual whose age and medical condition are such that control could reasonably be expected. It must be distinguished from incontinence due to neurologic deficit of the brain or spinal cord or, rarely, from an anatomic abnormality of the urinary tract which makes voluntary control mechanically impossible. Children ordinarily begin to acquire daytime urinary control at about 2 to 3 years of age, but many are not dry at night until 4 to 5 years. Surveys show a varying incidence of enuresis beyond the age of 5 years ranging from 5 to 15 per cent. Boys are afflicted more often than girls, and in a significant number of cases the symptoms persist beyond puberty and into the adult years. The social handicap attending enuresis is obvious.

Etiology

Many explanations for enuresis have been advanced, and it is probably true that there is not a single theory which will account for all cases. The largest number appear to be related to emotional conflict in the home environment, sometimes originating in too early and too vigorous attempts at toilet training, sometimes in a hostile-dependent mother-child relationship. In some children there appears to be an irritable bladder which is unable to hold large quantities of urine and which automatically discharges its contents when it begins to fill. This variety of enuresis is not uncommonly transmitted through several generations. Very deep sleep on the part of the child also is blamed for failure to control nocturnal urination.

Management

Methods used to help a child with enuresis must be modified according to his age, the severity of the symptom and the appraisal of his desire to gain control. The latter factor is probably the most important determinant of success. When the child himself is uninterested and it is primarily the parents who wish the symptom terminated, suggested measures usually are futile.

It is imperative to be sure that the enuresis is not due to organic disease beyond the child's control. In most instances this is readily apparent from the fact that he exerts perfect control during the day and wets only when asleep. If there is doubt, urologic examination is sometimes indicated, and in any event a careful urinalysis should be made to be sure that infection is not present.

With an interested child in whom the symptoms are not based in deep emotional conflict, simple measures sometimes will work. These include restriction of fluids at bedtime and some arrangement for wakening the child in time to avoid enuresis. If the latter arrangement is self-directed rather than being under the control of the parents, it will work more frequently. For those with irritable bladders a system of voluntary withholding of urine during the daytime may help by gradually distending the bladder until it gains a better capacity. This scheme may be abetted by gold stars or other rewards. Drugs such as the atropine derivatives are sometimes helpful in decreasing the irritability of the bladder, and Dexedrine or imipramine (Tofranil) can be used to lessen the depth of sleep. Another simple measure which demonstrates to the child his ability to gain control is to arrange for him to sleep overnight at the house of a friend. Often, to his surprise, he will fail to wet the bed in the strange environment because of concern over the social consequences. For the same reason, older children with a history of regular enuresis often lose this symptom when admitted to the hospital.

When simple measures fail after a reasonable trial, or when there are other manifestations of disturbed family relations, the assistance of a psychiatrist is indicated.

ENCOPRESIS

Encopresis means the uncontrolled passage of stools in a child beyond the age at which bowel control is normally expected and without neurologic or anatomic cause. It is evidence of deep-seated emotional problems in most instances and cannot be managed as casually as enuresis. Persistence of involuntary defecation beyond 4 years (with the exception of the occasional accident during concentrated play) generally indicates an emotional disturbance. .

Encopresis is sometimes related to strict and demanding efforts at toilet training against which the child has rebelled. A lack of maternal affection and sympathy is often associated. In other instances, toilet training is achieved, but in the preschool or school years the child begins to withhold stool and develops a symptom complex which must be differentiated from megacolon. The abdomen enlarges as the lower bowel becomes packed with large, often hard masses of feces. Eventually a paradoxic diarrhea appears in which there is uninhibited passage of liquid feces which bypass the retained masses in the rectum and the colon. After careful exclusion of megacolon, these children should have psychiatric treatment because the cause is deep-seated and difficult to eradicate.

RECURRENT SEIZURES—CONVULSIONS

Persons who have recurring seizures of one sort or another often are said to be victims of epilepsy. To the average person this condition connotes a disease that is hereditary, incurable, socially disgraceful and a precursor of mental deterioration. While it is true that some unfortunate sufferers have an incurable disease, it is unjust to stigmatize every person with a convulsive disorder. A much larger number have infrequent seizures or are able to control their seizures completely. These individuals may have normal or even superior intelligence and may lead useful and productive lives. Epilepsy does not denote a specific disease entity. It is preferable to avoid the use of the term entirely and to speak of individual varieties of recurrent seizure patterns.

Nearly three-fourths of those who eventually suffer from recurrent seizures do so in childhood; a significant number begin to have seizures before the age of 5. Untreated seizures tend to become more frequent and more severe. However, if a therapeutic regimen can be discovered which will keep the child free of attacks over a long period of time, it is often possible to withdraw the drugs gradually without return to symptoms.

Varieties of Recurrent Seizures

Recurrent seizures may be manifested in a great variety of ways. Because the basic mechanism of a seizure still is not completely understood, there is some difference of opinion about the implications of the different types.

Generalized Convulsions, Major Convulsions or Grand Mal. The symptoms of a generalized convulsion are described in Chapter 13. Such seizures also are called major convulsions or grand mal attacks. There is always loss of consciousness and postural muscle tone, followed by tonic or clonic movements of the extremities. Older children and adults who have generalized convulsions often describe a constellation of warning symptoms known as an aura. Peculiar feelings, sights, sounds, tastes, smells or involuntary muscle contractions may occur a few seconds before consciousness is lost and may lead the victim to utter a warning cry or noise before he falls. Headache and deep sleep not infrequently follow · a generalized convulsion.

Akinetic Seizure. An akinetic seizure is similar to a generalized convulsion except that there is no clonic jerking or tonic contraction of the extremities. The child loses consciousness and postural tone and falls limply.

Focal Convulsions. In focal convulsions consciousness may be retained and postural tone preserved while involuntary convulsive movements of an extremity progress from its tip toward its connection with the body (jacksonian fit). Episodic sensory disturbances may replace the muscle movements in this type of seizure, so that it appears as a temporary disturbance of sight, smell, hearing or taste or as pallor, flushing, hypertension, abdominal pain, changes in heart rate and other manifestations. Differentiation of the last group from other varieties of bodily disorder may be very difficult.

Minor Convulsions or Petit Mal. Minor convulsions or petit mal attacks consist of very brief absences or loss of consciousness without loss of postural tone or abnormal muscle movements. The victim momentarily stops whatever he is doing for a few seconds and then resumes where he left off. He is frequently unaware that he has had a brief seizure.

Psychomotor Attacks or Epileptic Equivalents. Various abnormalities of behavior of recurrent and often bizarre type are regarded as psychomotor attacks or epileptic equivalents. The child has no memory of his peculiar behavior. Psychomotor attacks usually occur in children who have other types of seizure as well.

Recurrent seizures of more than one variety may occur in the same child. For instance, akinetic seizures may precede the appearance of generalized convulsions. A high percentage of children with uncon-trolled petit mal attacks eventually develop generalized convulsions in addition to or instead of the initial form of seizure.

Diagnostic Considerations

Children who have recurrent seizures require special study either (1) to ascertain that the episodes are really seizures or (2) to attempt to discover an anatomic or physiologic reason for them. When the child suffers from characteristic generalized convulsions there is seldom any doubt about their nature, but recognition of minor attacks and psychomotor attacks may be more difficult. Supporting evidence can usually be obtained by the use of the electroencephalograph, which records the cyclic changes in the electric potentials of the brain. Most individuals with seizures display abnormal patterns not only during the seizures but between attacks. In some instances the shape of the waves may be altered by having the child hyperventilate his lungs—a technic which occasionally precipitates an actual seizure. Although it is usually true that an individual with seizures has an abnormal pattern, this is not invariably so. Conversely, some persons who never manifest seizures may have abnormal tracings. Electroencephalograms also may be used to localize areas of abnormal brain discharges in some instances where operative correction is contemplated.

Diagnostic procedures are indicated in many children whose recurrent seizures are suspected to have an anatomic or physiologic basis. Electroencephalography is a common diagnostic procedure in convulsive disorders and may be done on an outpatient basis as well as during hospitalization. Usually some type of sedation is given to the child prior to the examination. Electrodes are placed on the scalp and connected to an apparatus which records the amplified patterns of brain activity. Abnormal patterns may be discovered by this method, and these disturbances in brain rhythm may give the physician an indication of the type of convulsive disorder present. Roentgenograms of the skull often show various abnormalities of shape, proportions and calcifications of the cranial bones which give clues to an underlying disorder. "Pneumoencephalogram" is described with nursing care.

When there is suspicion of previous infection of the nervous system, various types of specific diagnostic tests may be indicated to exclude virus encephalitis, tuberculosis, syphilis or toxoplasmosis. Abnormalities of carbohydrate metabolism leading to periods of hypoglycemia or of calcium metabolism leading to tetany require special biochemical study. Rickets and lead poisoning produce changes in the x-ray appearance of the ends of the long bones, which may afford etiologic clues.

Treatment

A small number of children with recurrent seizures will be found to have a remediable underlying condition, the correction of which will terminate the seizures. But in most instances the seizures are of unknown causation or are associated with some disturbance which cannot be modified. The main problems in therapy consist of the discovery of a drug regimen that will abolish the seizures or reduce them to a minimum and the guidance of parents and child to an acceptance of a realistic way of life.

Phenobarbital is the most widely used drug for the prevention of recurrent seizures. It is almost devoid of toxic effects and has a large factor of safety which permits liberal dosage even in small children. Its disadvantage is that it is not very effective against petit mal attacks or psychomotor seizures. In large dosage it may cause drowsiness or unsteadiness. For the control of generalized convulsions it is given in doses of 1 to 3 grains per day, depending on the size of the child and the frequency of convulsions. The total dose usually is divided into 2 or 3 portions. A level of drug is sought which will prevent attacks without producing drowsiness or unsteadiness. When there is a tendency for the child to have an attack at a certain period of the day, accurate timing of his medicine is necessary to forestall seizures. Attacks that occur during or on waking from sleep pose a difficult problem that is solved by administering enteric coated capsules the effect of which is delayed. When a successful regimen is found, it is continued for 2 years. Then, after the cessation of seizures, slow withdrawal of medication is attempted.

When phenobarbital is not effective in controlling generalized convulsions or if it produces drowsiness, other drugs are substituted or used in combination with it. Dilantin is most commonly used as an adjunct to or substitute for phenobarbital. One to 5 grains is ordered per day, depending on the age of the child. Toxic effects are observed more frequently than when phenobarbital alone is used. These include ataxia, rash and hypertrophy of the gums. A closely related drug is Mesantoin, which has the additional hazard of depressing the blood-forming elements in the bone marrow, a toxic effect which must be sought by periodic leukocyte and differential blood counts in order to terminate the use of the drug at the first sign of difficulty. Mebaral and Mysoline are also useful in the treatment of major seizures which have not responded to the more conventional drugs.

Generally, minor convulsions are controlled effectively by Tridione. The dosage ranges from 5 to 20 grains a day. Its ability to terminate petit mal is often dramatic. Disadvantages lie in the side-effects which it may produce—rashes, drowsiness, a peculiar sensation of glare and, infrequently, depression of the blood-forming organs. Paradione is a closely related compound which is often used in its place. Of the newer drugs available for treatment of minor seizures, Zarontin is the most effective and least toxic. Celontin, Valium, Diamox and Atabrine are also used for various effects.

Dilantin is usually prescribed for focal and psychomotor seizures. Phenurone is sometimes used but is a more toxic substance.

In children who suffer from both petit mal and major convulsions, a therapeutic problem arises in that Dilantin generally tends to aggravate minor convulsions while suppressing the major attacks, while Tridione may stimulate major seizures while controlling minor attacks.

Bromides and ketogenic diets are mainly of historic interest in the control of seizures. In unusual instances the former may be required for the control of major convulsions. The ketogenic diet may be used in the control of petit mal attacks but is difficult to maintain.

Nursing Care

The nurse contributes important information when she observes and records the child's behavior, response to drugs and the circumstances of each seizure in detail. Events preceding the seizure, its duration and the child's behavior and bodily reactions during and after it has ended should be recorded. Protection of the child from injury during the seizure and help in becoming reoriented to his environment when the convulsion has ended are also a part of the nurse's responsibility. Minimizing anxiety and providing constructive activity is of special importance.

Pneumoencephalograms are utilized in an attempt to find an anatomic cause for the seizures. Cerebrospinal fluid is replaced by air through a spinal puncture needle followed by an x-ray of the skull. One method for this procedure is to withdraw 10 ml. of fluid and replace it with 5 ml. of air; this process is repeated until no more fluid is obtained. Approximately 100 ml. of air may be injected in this manner. Normally, air will fill the ventricles and spread over the cortex of the brain. A roentgenogram shows the outline of the ventricles and the cortical convolutions. Distortions and changes from the normal outlines indicate the location and often the nature of any existing lesion.

Before the preliminary sedative, a cleansing enema and Avertin may be given, and the child must know how these procedures are done and the effects they may have on him. Headaches, prostration or shock may occur. Children cope with the after-effects of a pneumoencephalogram more easily if they have been forewarned of the discomforts they may have. A blood pressure recording should be made before Avertin is given because it lowers blood pressure and may distort the picture of the child's condition if the pre-anesthesia reading is not available.

If the air is injected on the ward, two nurses are required to assist with the procedure. The child is held on the treatment table in a sitting position to allow the injected air to rise and replace the cerebrospinal fluid. This position is maintained more easily if a tray covered with a pillow is placed over his lap and his body is bent forward to rest on it. A second nurse assists the doctor, collects samples of spinal fluid, records the amounts withdrawn and injected, and observes for changes in pulse and respiration rates.

The child is transported in an upright position to the x-ray department for skull films. Hypodermic equipment and stimulants should accompany him. Change in color, pulse, respiration or blood pressure may indicate the need for a stimulant. Vital signs must be checked frequently until stable, as symptoms of shock or increased intracranial pressure (rise in blood pressure, slowing of pulse, confusion and coma) are danger signals.

Parenteral fluids are sometimes given following the procedure to replace those lost through perspiration and because oral intake is usually low during the first 24 hours. Absorption of injected air and prevention of headache and nausea are achieved by the administration of oxygen at hourly intervals for 8 hours. Encouraging the child to remain flat in bed relieves headache to some extent.

In the presence of brain tumor a *ventriculogram* is done. Cerebrospinal fluid is replaced by air through a needle passed into the lateral ventricles through trephine openings in the skull. Postoperative care is the same as that for pneumoencephalogram.

The child, not merely his seizures, must be studied to determine his needs for care, as his personality is influenced by his response to the problems created by his symptoms. Although the distorted activity of brain tissue may affect behavior, it is chiefly the significance of the convulsions to the child that affects his psychosocial development.

Often the child with recurrent seizures is described as being emotionally unstable, egocentric, tempestuous, selfish and moody. If these traits exist in the child, they indicate a need to discover the cause of the emotional disturbance. Eliminating the cause of distress will tend to decrease the number of attacks even when the seizures are not psychogenic in origin. The above behavior traits are not peculiar to the child with seizures; they are seen as frequently in physically healthy children from environments which fail to meet their emotional needs.

Unless convulsions are severe and uncontrolled, school experience with healthy children is advised. Teachers need aid in handling their feelings about children with convulsions and concrete help in understanding the symptom complex, its treatment, prognosis and the ways in which to protect the child during seizures.

Conflicts in interpersonal relationships which produce stress at home and at school must be eliminated to give the child peace of mind. The therapeutic value of any anticonvulsant drug is lessened when the child has more anxiety than he can handle constructively.

PROBLEMS OF ADJUSTMENT IN SCHOOL

Reading Disability

The further a child progresses in school the more important his facility in reading becomes. Without this essential tool his ability to acquire knowledge in many fields is severely restricted. A significant percentage of children with otherwise normal intellectual endowment find it difficult to master the art of reading. In some, the basic difficulty lies in poor visual discrimination in which the child confuses letters such as "d" and "b" or reverses the order of short words such as "was" and "saw." In other children the language disorder is related to minimal brain damage or to a malfunctioning central nervous system. In still others there appear to be emotional disturbances which inhibit the child's ability to read. Whatever the source of the difficulty, it is highly desirable for a reading disability to be recognized early in the course of schooling and for specific treatment to be instituted.

Intellectual Competence

In Chapter 13 the recognition of the more obvious and severe forms of mental deficiency in the infant are discussed. Children with lesser degrees of intellectual handicap often are not identified until they show evidence of academic difficulties. An estimate of the severity of the intellectual deficit is acquired by the use of standardized intelligence tests such as the Binet-Simon or Welchsler-Bellevue. From these an intelligence quotient or "I.Q." is computed by dividing the mental age as measured in the test by the child's chronologic age and multiplying the result by 100.

The interpretation of such tests is not a simple matter. Repeat testing in 6 to 12 months is done to confirm the accuracy of a test. When interfering factors are suspected, a series of tests over several years is more likely to reveal the child's true capacity.

Assuming that a valid measure of intelligence has been obtained, some rough predictions of school progress can be made. Most children with an I.Q. below 70 need special arrangements made for training in self-care and in manual skills. Those with an I.Q. below 90 will generally make slow academic progress.

Whatever the child's level of intellectual competence it is desirable that his grade placement in school be high enough to challenge his ability but not so high that he is frustrated by repeated failure. Frequently parents need assistance in reducing undue pressure to succeed academically.

Behavior Disorders

More energy is now being directed into the alleviation of disabilities which prevent children from succeeding in school. In recent years increasing attention has also been devoted to those children who are indefinitely classified as minimally brain-damaged. In general this term is applied to children without obvious neurologic deficit and with normal or borderline intelligence who present signs of difficulty in grasping broad generalizations and in concentrating. Or there may be fixation on one segment of the school work and labile emotional reactions to the people and situations about them. It is presumed that these children have suffered subtle brain damage either at birth or during the course of some subsequent illness. Not all such children show disturbances in behavior, but in others management is aided by the setting of firm but fair restrictions, and sometimes by the use of drugs such as amphetamine and tranquilizers. Innumerable other types of errant behavior are seen in the school population. The reader is referred to the bibliography for source material on the further treatment of specific types.

"Cerebral Palsy" in the School-age Child

As indicated in Chapter 13, the term "cerebral palsy" signifies a wide range of disability due to abnormal motor control of the body resulting from damage to the nervous system. During infancy and the preschool years such children are usually under medical care for the purpose of controlling convulsions and relieving the effects of abnormal muscle spasms. The intellectual potential of these children is hard to estimate because of their difficulty in acquiring understandable speech and controlling their muscle movements in the performance of voluntary acts. The presence of severe athetosis or spasticity does not necessarily imply lack of normal intellectual capacity. One of the goals of care during the early years is to evaluate the child's intellectual potential so that appropriate schooling can be arranged. Sometimes education must be provided in a special school because of severe physical problems. However, whenever possible, it is desirable for them to attend regular schools if they are able to adjust to their requirements. An early start in accepting and accommodating to their handicap can prevent maladjustment in school.

HEREDITARY DEGENERATIVE NEUROMUSCULAR DISORDERS

A few of the types of hereditary disease of the nervous and muscular systems which declare their presence in infancy are discussed in Chapter 13. Another group of hereditarily transmitted disorders lie dormant during infancy and early childhood but become increasingly apparent as the child enters the school years. The hereditary nature of these disorders is established by the strong propensity to occur in more than one member of a family. Fortunately these disabilities are rare. Treatment in general is unsatisfactory, and nursing care consists in making the child's life as nearly normal as circumstances will permit. The brief descriptions appended are mainly for the purpose of orienting the reader who may happen to see examples among her clinical contacts.

Hepatolenticular Degeneration (Wilson's Disease)

Wilson's disease is a combination of degenerative changes in the liver and the central nervous system. It appears usually during the school years and is slowly progressive and ultimately fatal. It is due to a hereditary disorder, recessively transmitted, in which there is congenital absence of ceruloplasmin. This is one of the normal protein constituents of the blood and is concerned with the transport of copper within the body. Copper tends to accumulate in the tissues and slowly poisons the liver and the lenticular nuclei of the brain. Neurologic symptoms appear first and include abnormalities of speech, a fixed stare, tremor, spasticity of muscles (athetosis) and eventually convulsions and behaviorial disorganization. Jaundice and the classic signs of cirrhosis may not appear until late in the disease. A typical finding is yellow pigmentation of the margin of the cornea of the eye (Kayser-Fleischer rings). Treatment consists of limitation of the intake of dietary copper and attempts to bind the copper already in the body by the use of those chelating agents (versene, BAL) which are commonly prescribed for the treatment of lead poisoning. D-penicillamine is effective in removing copper from nervous tissue but not from liver. Thus, improvement in neurologic status may be achieved while cirrhosis progresses.

Dystonia Musculorum Deformans

This is a hereditary disturbance of muscle tone which is limited to children of Russian-Jewish descent. Symptoms start gradually before puberty with extension of one foot with its toes flexed. Later, torsion and writhing movements appear, at first involving only the legs but later spreading to the trunk and the arms. The movements are absent during sleep but gradually increase in severity until the child becomes bedridden. No treatment is known.

Huntington's Chorea

The most common variety of chorea is the type associated with rheumatic fever, which is self-limited and always has a favorable outcome before puberty. Congenital forms of chorea which are apparent in infancy and persist throughout life are seen less commonly.

Huntington's chorea is a hereditary affliction transmitted as a dominant trait. It has a delayed onset, seldom appearing in childhood. Symptoms are similar to other forms of chorea except that they progress and ultimately lead to difficulty in swallowing, in locomotion and in cerebration. The disease is eventually fatal. No treatment is known.

Friedreich's Ataxia

This is a disorder that is a genetically caused slowly progressive degeneration of some of the tracts in the spinal cord. Its symptoms usually appear before puberty and consist of high arching of the foot and unsteadiness of gait so that the child walks with his feet widely separated. Sensory changes in the legs and the arms and visual disturbances also may be found. An unusual type of myocarditis is often associated. Progression is slow so that the child may survive for one or two decades. No treatment is effective.

Pseudohypertrophic Muscular Dystrophy

This is the most common form of muscular dystrophy. It affects boys more frequently than girls. At some time during the preschool years the child begins to show weakness in his legs, generally accompanied by enlargement of the calf muscles, which feel firm and rubbery. To arise from a sitting posture on the floor such children learn that they must kneel on all fours, then straighten their legs and gain the erect posture by putting hands on knees and "climbing up the legs." This performance is typical and practically diagnostic of the disease. Weakness of the leg muscles and later of the arm and the shoulder muscles progresses gradually, and the victim usually succumbs in early adult life to some intercurrent disease.

The advancing weakness and atrophy with increasing age is illustrated in Figure 28-1. Periods of bed rest are to be avoided whenever possible, for muscle strength tends to deteriorate more rapidly unless activity is maintained. At present no useful treatment has been discovered.

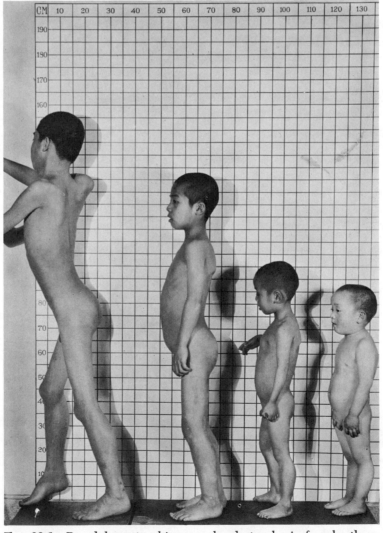

FIG. 28-1. Pseudohypertrophic muscular dystrophy in four brothers.

Myasthenia Gravis

This familial disorder is characterized by excessive fatigability of muscle, which usually is most marked in the muscles of the face and the pharynx. Drooping eyelids, a weak smile, difficulty in swallowing and severe fatigue following mild exercise are characteristic. The symptoms are relieved promptly by injection of neostigmine or Tensilon which constitutes the chief diagnostic test. Unfortunately, there is a tendency toward progression of the symptoms, so that the attacks become more frequent and severe, and the relief obtained from neostigmine or Mestinon or Tensilon is lessened. Thymectomy is occasionally effective. Death in the severely affected child or adult results from respiratory failure during an unrelieved exacerbation.

Myotonia Congenita (Thomsen's Disease)

This is a peculiar disability of muscles which is transmitted genetically. Affected individuals have stiff muscles which hold their contractions longer than normal. Repeated flexion often will warm up the muscle so that it relaxes more quickly. Movements are slow and stiff, and the child has difficulty releasing his grasp on objects. Muscles which are struck briskly with a reflex hammer can be seen to go into a state of sustained contraction. The disorder is neither fatal nor progressive and can be relieved by taking quinine.

Familial Periodic Paralysis

As the name implies, this disorder is transmitted genetically and consists of periods during which there is paralysis of voluntary muscles. Between attacks there is no discernible weakness or neurologic abnormality. The attacks vary in frequency, duration and severity from brief involvement of a small group of muscles which clears in an hour or two, to extensive paralysis involving the muscles of respiration or cardiac muscle and thus threatening life. During the episodes there is demonstrable disturbance of the level of blood potassium, and the attack can be relieved rapidly by administering potassium by mouth or intravenously. Prognosis is good, since the frequency and the severity of attacks tends to diminish in middle age. Prevention of attacks is possible by the prophylactic administration of potassium salts by mouth.

THE CHILD WITH A HANDICAP

Many children must face life with physical or mental limitations that deny them a normal childhood and which may cause, directly or indirectly, severe personality damage which is often more crippling than the original handicap. Emotional complications are inevitably part of the life of the handicapped child and his family, and the nurse must have understanding of the impact of handicapping conditions on the parents, on the child and on the nurse, herself.

Impact on the Parents

All parents hope for a normal child. The appearance of a blind, deaf, mentally retarded or otherwise defective child is a severe blow which initiates grief and mourning for the expected perfect child. Guilt for having committed or omitted acts which may have caused the defect is prominent and leads to feelings of inadequacy or failure. These feelings are intensified by the realization that the handicapped child requires sustained energy and wisdom from his parents in order to utilize fully those assets which he does possess, and even then he often will not fulfill the expectations they hold for him.

Reactions of parents may range from denying the seriousness of the handicap to the other extreme of giving up the child as hopeless (often equally unrealistic). Responses to a defective child are determined by the life style of the parents, their defenses against overwhelming anxiety and by the support they receive when the handicap becomes obvious or definite diagnosis is confirmed.

Parents cannot assimilate a diagnosis of a handicapping condition nor its implications immediately. They require the long-term support of health professionals who can allow them to express their feelings and to explore gradually, as they are able, the realistic potentials of their child. Without help the parents may continue to defend against pain by refusing to acknowledge the handicap and make demands on the child which he is unable to meet, thus denying him the special help he requires. Others may become overprotective and not allow the child the opportunity to attain independence and mastery of the developmental tasks of which he is capable.

Some observable physical handicaps in children are often more realistically perceived by parents than those that are not as readily visible. It is difficult for parents of a mentally retarded child to relinquish the hope and expectation that he will outgrow or otherwise overcome his handicap. Frequently they consult numerous physicians in the anticipation that the deficiency can be attributed to a correctable physical or emotional cause. Some parents may deny his lack of progress until the child reaches an age at which his retarded development can no longer be overlooked; he is too obviously lagging behind his peers.

The nurse who works with a handicapped child and his family can teach a great deal by explanation and example. It is important to strengthen the confidence of parents and child. In teaching parents the nurse should remember that no one will learn until he is ready and has confidence in the teacher. If parents are not receptive to constructive suggestions, the nurse must discover and attempt to alleviate their concerns before effective teaching can occur. The mother must be assured of her competence in mothering the child and must be genuinely interested in his progress before he can be given the freedom to explore and play to the extent of his ability and in a way natural to him.

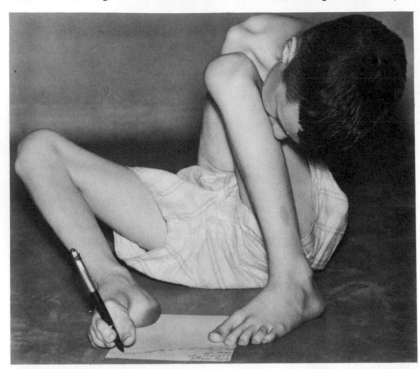

FIG. 28-2. A handicapped child who is making the most of his assets. This 7-year-old boy born with complete absence of arms has learned to feed himself, put on his clothes and manipulate objects with his feet. Although not easily visible in the picture, the foot-writing when magnified is very legible.

Practical and concrete suggestions made by the nurse will promote the parents' confidence in her. Eventually she can begin to sketch out the normal developmental picture of the child at his particular age. She can also help the mother to anticipate expected patterns of behavior and prepare her for the learning experiences that the child will require to make full use of his assets. Such instruction may also have the secondary benefit of causing the child to appear less abnormal in the eyes of his parents.

Consider the blind child, for instance. Healthy babies begin to learn at birth from contact with their mothers' bodies and from the use of their eyes and other sense organs. A blind baby who is left in his crib because contact with him arouses painful feelings in the mother cannot gain trust or learn through sensory exploration. Unless stimulation is provided when the child reaches out for it and he is helped to associate the feel of things and sounds with words, his capacities for learning about his world will be greatly limited. His opportunities for healthy personality growth will be impeded, for he will not receive the stimulation and the emotional satisfactions which are necessary to differentiate himself from his mother and to become a person in his own right. In writing of the blind child's need for self-directed explorations in contrast with direct teaching, Norris *et al.* made a statement which has implications for the guidance of all parents of handicapped children:

Freeing the parents from their anticipated responsibility for teaching specific skills unrelated to daily living is often the first step in helping them to think realistically about

the blind child and to be comfortable in their relationships with him. If this can be accomplished within the first few months of the child's life, his responsiveness gives assurance to the parents that they are on the right track. Their resulting confidence in their ability to meet the child's needs and their pleasure in his achievement then become primary factors in encouraging his further progress. Major developmental problems are avoided, in contrast to those situations where failure to understand and meet the child's needs in the early period has created difficulties which are discouragingly slow to respond to treatment.*

Impact on the Child

The child's response to his handicap is determined by the way in which his parents have met his needs throughout his life. Many handicapped children are emotionally secure and lead as nearly normal lives as their condition permits.

But many of the handicapped children the nurse sees in the hospital and in homes are troubled children with poor opinions of themselves stemming from a lack of unconditional acceptance and wise nurturing. The handicapped child usually is quite aware of his parents' feelings toward him and the problems which his birth has created. He senses their tension and often concludes that he has been a disappointment to them.

Handicapped children whose parents cannot accept them cope with rejection in the only way they are able. Some, never having been loved, are themselves unable to love. Others have withdrawn into a world of fantasy, never having learned to use the potentiali-

* Norris, M., Spaulding, P. and Brodie, F.: *Blindness in Children*, Chicago, University of Chicago Press, 1957, p. 95.

ties with which they were born. Some have denied their limitations. Others have grown discouraged as they have looked for friends while simultaneously denying their need for love; sometimes they try to hurt others as they have been hurt. A few have compensated for their difficulties and fought to overcome their limitations.

Some handicapped children defend themselves against anxiety with provocative behavior—that is, they do their utmost to strain the patience of everyone about them. Usually such children have not had systematic guidance at home, are insecure and in perpetual doubt as to what is expected of them and what they can get away with. Such a child will persistently and deliberately irritate his mother in an attempt to discover the limits of her tolerance and with that knowledge gain some measure of security.

There is a vicious circle inherent in provocative behavior. Because the child never has had the consistent discipline which would help him to give *constructive* direction to his normal aggressiveness, his misdirected attempts to express himself and to learn have brought only condemnation and he is convinced that he is bad. His conscience hurts him, and he finds relief in being punished. His provocative behavior can be considered a solicitation of punishment.

If such a pattern of behavior has been established at home, the child undoubtedly will use it in the hospital because it is a habitual way of relieving his tension and guilt. He will literally ask for punishment— not in words, because his need for punishment is unconscious, but in behavior.

Johnny was 7 years old and in the hospital for further correction of a clubbed foot. Every time the nurse came to give him care, he knocked the equipment off the table. When she pulled up his cribside he would leap over the side of the bed. He did not wait until she had left the room; he did the jumping in her presence.

The nurse might properly conclude that punishment merely serves to encourage the child with provocative behavior to repeat his misdemeanors. He can be expected to do the things that he is expressly forbidden to do. If the nurse refrains from punishing the child, he will be less likely to repeat the offense because it brings no satisfaction. Yet a major problem remains: how to teach the child the meaning of benevolent discipline and at the same time convince him that he really is not bad, so as to relieve his constantly nagging conscience.

With consistent, kind and firm guidance, the child will learn what is expected of him and what he can and cannot do. Only then will he have the security which comes from knowledge that others entertain reasonable expectations in regard to his behavior. The child who is under compulsion to provoke adults to anger is difficult to deal with; he is the way he is because he has been made that way. When he discovers

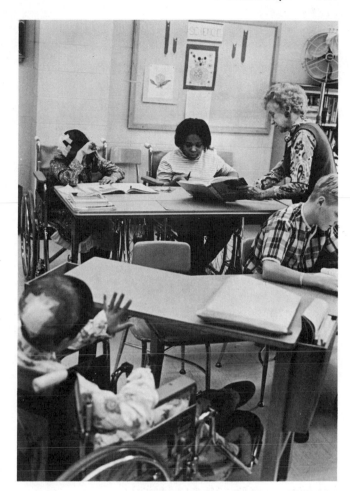

FIG. 28-3. Handicapped children make the most of their potential through individualized instruction in special classes.

that his behavior brings a response different from the retaliatory kind he previously has been accustomed to, his behavior is fairly certain to show signs of change. If it does not change, psychotherapy is probably indicated.

Children with a handicap which warrants frequent or prolonged institutionalization often exhibit symptoms of emotional and sensory deprivation. They rarely laugh, do not openly express destructive feelings nor do they develop deep, warm feelings toward other people. These children have developed unhealthy defenses against anxiety which lead to lack of feeling, superficiality and hopelessness. Nursing plans must include measures which promote normal personality development.

The handicapped child must be helped to make the most of the strengths he possesses (Fig. 28-3). Guided by the recommendations of the health team, the nurse formulates a plan of care with the object of helping the child to become independent and to win self-esteem and social acceptance. Most of these children, especially the mentally retarded, will require consistent, repeated help to learn how to care for themselves. Children almost invariably measure up to what is expected of them. Many handicapped children make remarkable progress in adaptation because of the faith and confidence of others. The handicapped child does not want pity. Like the normal child, he has a drive for autonomy and self-realization. Once a handicapped child has begun to trust himself and is able to achieve self-control, progress will become evident, although it probably will be slower than that observed in the healthy child.

Impact on the Nurse

In her work with handicapped children and their parents the nurse may find it especially difficult to maintain an objective attitude. She may feel overcome by pity, fear or revulsion in her contacts with the child, or the parents' behavior may provoke anxiety or anger. These feelings are not "bad," unusual or anything of which the nurse should be ashamed. Almost everyone experiences some negative feelings when first confronted by an incapacitated child. The best antidote for such emotions is to delve into their source, seeking to identify those which are irrational. Avoidance of the handicapped child most often stems from the helplessness which the child's afflictions provoke in the inexperienced person. With experience the nurse should find herself devoting increased attention to the child's assets rather than his liabilities.

Excerpts from the Study of Mickie

The following study illustrates several problems encountered in the nursing care of a handicapped child.

Collection of Observational Data. Mickie, age 5 years, was admitted for diagnostic studies to determine the etiology of the cataracts which partially blinded him and were first observed by his parents when he was 18 months of age. A student reported that Mickie was a "queer" child. During rest hour he walked constantly about his bed with a blanket over his head and mumbled incoherently. When he was out of bed and came upon the student who was sitting on a low chair, he tickled her face and arms and literally burrowed himself into her arms. The tickling annoyed the student. She said that she felt like running away from him. The day before the student began her care of Mickie, skull roentgenograms and blood tests had been done. Because his behavior indicated intense anxiety during these diagnostic measures, he was sedated before a catheterized specimen of urine was obtained. Although Mickie was asleep when the doctor arrived to do the catheterization, Mickie became aware of what was happening to him and shrieked and struggled so that firm restraint was necessary.

Because of Mickie's odd behavior and the difficulties the student was having in understanding him, an observational study was made to find the answers to the following questions: (1) Was Mickie psychotic, mentally retarded or disturbed because he had no one to help him to feel secure in a strange world that he could not see well or understand? (2) Would recognition of his visual defect provide the key that would open the door to a relationship with Mickie? (3) What strengths did Mickie have to solve his problems? (4) What was Mickie so desperately afraid of? The instructor predicted that a friendly and trusting relationship could be established with Mickie if someone were to help him to learn what a child with normal vision ordinarily would discover by himself, and all the while accept him as he was.

When first observed Mickie was in the playroom crawling on all fours. As the instructor entered the room, Mickie crawled into the playpen, put a blanket over his head and began to mumble quietly. At this point the instructor was called away. She saw Mickie next in the otolaryngology clinic. His respirations were rapid, his facial muscles were tensed, his pupils dilated, and he stood rigidly as if he were frozen with fear. Mickie sat in the examination chair and permitted the ear and nose examination, but clenched his teeth tight when the doctor tried to examine his throat. After the doctor left the room, Mickie was given a tongue blade and a nasal speculum to handle. He fingered them gingerly without a word or an aggressive gesture. A second doctor came in to try his hand at examining Mickie's throat. He was jovial and positive. Mickie's respirations decreased; he permitted the doctor to look into his throat but resisted the use of a tongue depressor. Immediately after this examination Mickie was scheduled to visit first the eye clinic and then the dental department. He cooperated with the eye examination but was silent and partially immobilized during it. When it was over he burrowed close to the instructor. (This showed the degree to which Mickie had regressed, but it was not massive regression by any means.)

In the dental clinic Mickie's feelings erupted. He drew back and screamed. Instead of forcing him to have the examination, another attempt at preparation was done after Mickie's control of himself had been regained. The dentist and the nurse conferred and decided that a visit the following day would be more profitable for him. Outside the dental clinic there were pictures that could be illuminated. Mickie felt these with his hands and put his face close to them in order to see. Because the instructor had observed that Mickie managed himself better when helped by a man, she obtained the dentist's help in preparing him for the dental x-ray. She knew that Mickie would feel safer if he had become acquainted with the person who would direct the study on the following day. The dentist promised Mickie that he would be there the next day. Before Mickie left the dental department, he moved close to the dentist, thus showing that he had felt his friendliness. On his return to the ward Mickie uttered his first intelligible words since admission 4 days before. He said, "I want to go to the playroom."

Mickie was taken to the playroom at once, and for 20 minutes he played as a 2-year-old child plays. He ran to the toy shelves, fingered toys, found a wind-up truck with his hands and set it in motion. Then he began to play with other vehicles. He ran one across the floor and followed the noise it made. When his hands landed on another toy he began to play with it. He used pull toys as toddlers do. All of a sudden, he picked up a toy, ran to the instructor and said, "Lady, what's this?" The instructor told him that it was a toy caterpillar. "Give me your hand, Mickie. These are the caterpillar's ears. This is its tail. This is its body. This string is used to pull it about," she said. He ran off and played enthusiastically. Next he tried to wind a mechanical toy, but he was unsuccessful. Immediately the instructor went to him and said, "Mickie, I'll show you how to make it go. Let me have your hand. Feel the winder. I'll teach you how to use it." Mickie learned at once and repeated it over and over again. During the next 15 minutes Mickie did not contact the instructor. He talked as he played, and his speech became more and more intelligible. The instructor watched for opportunities to help him the minute he showed a need for it, since he had communicated his urgent desire for recognition of his inability to see clearly when he brought the caterpillar to her.

Twenty minutes after he had requested help in learning about the caterpillar, he came to the instructor with a tiny wooden train in his hand and said, "Lady, how do you put this together?" The instructor said, "Feel the metal at the end of the train car. It's a hook. One end is open so the hook of another car can be placed into it. The hook keeps the cars together." She placed Mickie's hands on the parts and taught him how to put them together. Mickie observed that one car was upside down and remarked on it. "So it is, Mickie," said the instructor. "I'll help you fix it. When boys can't see very well, they need help to learn. Your nurse and I can help you learn, Mickie." He looked up at the instructor and the student and smiled a smile that looked as if it had come from deep down inside of him. His whole being seemed to say: "I feel better! At last I've found someone who can help me learn. I've wanted help all along, but I just didn't know how to ask for it." In a short time Mickie had learned to put away toys.

The Nursing Diagnosis; Formulation of Goals of and Plans for Nursing Care. From these initial observations the instructor and the student learned that Mickie was neither psychotic nor mentally retarded but excessively anxious when first observed. He could get along with others, use their help and learn rapidly. The instructor concluded that meeting Mickie's need to learn was a way to demonstrate friendliness. During lunch the instructor sought to help Mickie to transfer his beginning relationship with her to the student who would be caring for him each day.

At the lunch table Mickie tried to cut up his salad. He held the knife with the blade away from the tomato, demonstrating his need to be taught the use of eating utensils. Thereafter, he used the knife over and over again not only on the tomato but also on other foods. In the middle of the meal he held his bread close to the student's face and pointed to the smudge of dirt on it. The student said, "That's from your hands. I didn't show you how to turn on the faucets so you could wash your hands." Mickie said, "Let's do it now." The student took him to the sink and showed him how to manipulate the faucets. He washed meticulously. During the process, he squirmed continuously. When the student said, "Mickie, I think you are telling me you need to go to the toilet," he looked up at her, smiled and said, "Yeh, I do!"

After Mickie had eaten, he was called to the dermatology clinic for skin tests. "Mickie, the doctor is going to put medicine under your skin with a needle. It will sting for a minute. I'll help you hold yourself still," the student said. Immediately Mickie's respirations increased. The student took him in her arms where he cried and squirmed vigorously. Half way to the clinic, the student had to stop for rest. To pacify Mickie, a clerk brought out a drum, drumsticks and beads to string. Mickie pounded the drum. His crying ceased, but his respiration rate continued at a high level. He beat the drum in a beautifully rhythmic fashion and chewed chocolate mints as fast as the student could give them to him. He began to string beads and learned how to tie a knot in the cord to keep the beads from falling off. Then he said he had to go to the toilet. The student said, "Mickie, it's so scary to go for skin tests. I will stay with you and help you." Mickie put both hands on the student's face and caressed it. When he had returned from the toilet, they walked toward the clinic. Then he stopped and shrieked. The student picked him up, and he fought to prevent himself from being taken through the door. He spread his legs and put a foot on either side of the doorway in an attempt to protect himself, acting as if he expected to be murdered.

From the adult's vantage point Mickie's fear was unusually acute. It is possible that he suspected another catheterization—a procedure which can be terrifying to a preschool boy if he has not been adequately prepared for it. Preparation for the skin tests increased rather then lessened his fear. Therefore, it seemed advisable to help Mickie to learn as quickly as possible that nothing was as bad as he imagined it to be. The instructor predicted that wise, strong support during skin tests would help him to master what seemed to be an irrational fear of injury.

The nurse held Mickie firmly during the procedure which necessitated 5 intradermal injections in each forearm. He screamed at the top of his voice: "I hate you. I'm dying. I'm going to die." It was interesting to note that his screaming and respiration rate lessened with each injection. As soon as it was over, Mickie pulled himself together, enjoyed sitting on the doctor's lap and munched chocolate cookies that the doctor gave him. Mickie listened intently as the doctor talked. He made no attempt to get off his lap, but he did not burrow himself against the doctor's body as he had into the nurse's lap. After a few minutes, the doctor put him down.

The skin procedure had the effect of bringing Mickie's fears into consciousness where he could deal with them. His behavior subsequent to this experience led the instructor to believe that he had succeeded in mastering his anxiety.

On his return to the ward Mickie went willingly to bed but was unable to sleep. He kept putting his forearm close to his eyes and asked, "When will they go away?" The student said, "In a few days you won't be able to see the bumps any more. The doctor put medicine in your arms. He is trying to find out what keeps your eyes from seeing well. The medicine made your arms sting. You were scared as all boys are. I'm glad you could tell us how angry and scared you were. Did you really think you were going to die, Mickie?" His reply substantiated the student's hunch; Mickie had expected the worst. The student said, "The nurses and the doctors won't hurt you, Mickie. They want to help you so that you can see better and grow up to be big like your daddy. Those were tests. They do them to find ways to make you see better. Tomorrow the dentist will take pictures of your teeth, and then the tests will be done."

The next day Mickie walked silently to the dental clinic. At the door, he stood still and refused to enter. His respirations mounted as they had before, but this time he did not shriek. The dentist whom Mickie had met the previous day came to greet him. He told him the technician was going to take pictures, and he explained every step of the procedure to him. When the dentist invited Mickie to enter, he followed him into the room. Slowly he climbed into the chair and laid his head on the film as he was directed to do. Mickie smiled when he was given a film to hold. His cooperation was elicited by such requests as "Mickie you can help us by holding your head still on this plate." When it came time for the roentgenograms to be taken, Mickie not only opened his mouth widely for the insertion of a film but he also opened it in between times over and over again. He was able to do what he had not been able to do the day before when the doctor wanted to put a tongue blade into his mouth. (He had been given tongue blades and a flashlight the day before while the nurse sat close by to encourage his play with them.) After the film was placed in his mouth, he concentrated on holding it in place and on learning when the technician wanted him to remove it. The dentist said, "You can tell your boy friends that you had pictures made of your teeth," and Mickie replied plaintively, "But I haven't got any boy friends." Another source of Mickie's frustration was revealed to the student.

When the x-ray pictures were completed, the dentist invited Mickie into the next room, having first prepared him for a mouth examination. Mickie followed the dentist and climbed into the dental chair, opened his mouth widely and showed that he had mastered his fear of having something put into it. Mickie left the clinic clutching the films that the dentist had given him. On his return trip to the ward, there was no halting. He skipped beside the student. He carried himself more erect and kept saying, "It was fun." He seemed to have acquired a new concept of himself and the world which had been so terrifying to him only a few days before.

Evaluation of the Effects of Nursing Intervention. Mickie's situation when he was first observed was a precarious one. He came into a strange world unprepared for what he would experience there. He heard the cries of children and felt the tension in the air. Yet because he could not see the world about him, he could not understand it, nor could he question or reach out for help as many children can. When strange and painful things were done to him, he reacted with panic and marked regression, all indicative of some degree of personality disorganization.

Mickie's signals for help were respected. Between tests, play periods were provided not only to give Mickie an opportunity to work through his problems but also to enable the instructor to learn more about him as a person. Bringing the caterpillar with the question, "Lady, what is this?" could well have been his way of saying, "There is so much in this world that I don't understand. I can't see well enough to

identify the things in it, and I'm scared. Please help me to learn."

When the instructor used ways of teaching that took his limitations into account, Mickie's behavior showed that he felt understood. His ability to think was respected. When the instructor commended his observation of the upside-down car, his body language showed that his self-esteem had been heightened.

Mickie showed excellent potentialities for growth. With assistance he was able to pull himself together and perceive that tests were not what he imagined them to be. While having the tests, he was able to express with words and actions his aggression and fear. The doctor's and the nurses' friendliness helped to promote trust and cooperation. Experience that originally provoked panic became "fun." Other changes in behavior helped the student to evaluate her work with Mickie: his play became productive; he was able to rest; he began to communicate with words; his need to burrow himself into her lap vanished (and before he was discharged his need for a friend had been realized). The experience also had helped the parents to prepare Mickie for cataract extraction which was scheduled for the following month.

From this experience the student learned to overcome her initial uneasiness (and therefore dislike) in trying to work with a child who showed such odd behavior. It taught her to make an intelligent appraisal of the handicap and, recognizing the child's need for help and his inability to ask for it directly, to interpret for him the things and the events about him which were only dimly seen and not at all understood.

SITUATIONS FOR FURTHER STUDY

1. An 8-year-old child has been brought to the clinic because of enuresis. Observe the medical interview, talk with the parents and the child and consider the following points: How did the mother describe the child's problem? What attitudes did you detect toward the child and his problem? Has night control ever been established? If it was, when did enuresis begin? What methods did the mother use in helping the child to establish daytime control? Night control? How do you think the child felt about his problem? What is the basis for your conclusion? From the data you collected, what impression did you draw about the mother-child relationship? How did the child respond to the physical examination? What was the outcome of the examination? What help did the doctor give the mother? How did she respond to it? What further help do you think the mother and the child will require?

2. Study a child with seizures. How do you think he feels about them? On what do you base your impression? What were his problems in adjustment to the hospital? What impression do you have of the parent-child relationships? What impression did you

have of this child's relationships with his peers? What did you observe which leads you to draw these conclusions? How does his mother react to the fact that her child has epilepsy? Visit the child's school and talk to the school nurse to determine if he has had any problems in adjustment there. What role has the nurse assumed in facilitating the child's adjustment in school? To what community resources does the school nurse refer the family if the child is not making progress physically or emotionally? What problems has the school nurse encountered in working with the teachers of children who have seizures?

3. Write to the National Epilepsy League, 203 N. Wabash Ave., Chicago, Ill., and obtain literature concerning the needs of the child with seizures. What social problems arise for parents of children with seizures?

4. Write to the National Society for Crippled Children and Adults, Inc., 2023 W. Ogden, Chicago, Ill., for literature pertaining to the mental hygiene needs of the child with a handicapping condition. Use the literature in studying a school-age child with a handicap in the hospital. What limitations are imposed by his handicap? What is he capable of doing? How is he thwarted in solving the developmental crisis of the school-age period? What did you observe which helped you to understand the meaning of the handicap to this child? Talk with his mother to discover the problems she is having in rearing her child? What impressions did you draw about the mother-child relationship? What is the quality of his relationships with his roommates? How does he cope with the stress of medical procedures? Describe a situation in which you succeeded in teaching the child to do something he had never done before.

BIBLIOGRAPHY

Adams, M. L.: Care of the retarded child in the home, Nurs. Forum 6:403, 1967.

Barnard, K.: Teaching the retarded child is a family affair, Am. J. Nurs. 68:305, 1968.

Basara, S.: The behavioral patterns of the perceptually handicapped child, Nurs. Forum 5:24, 1966.

Bette, M.: Summer work with the retarded, Am. J. Nurs. 67:1228, 1967.

Burlingame, D. in collaboration with Goldberger, A.: The re-education of a retarded blind child, Psychoanalytic Study of the Child 23:369, 1968.

Burlingham, D.: Hearing and its role in the development of the blind, Psychoanal. Stud. Child 19:95, 1964.

————: Some problems of ego development in blind children, Psychoanal. Stud. Child 20:194, 1965.

————: Developmental considerations in the occupations of the blind, Psychoanal. Stud. Child 22:187, 1967.

Cohen, J.: The effects of blindness on children's development, Children 13:23, 1966.

Colonna, A.: A blind child goes to the hospital, Psychoanal. Stud. Child 23:391, 1968.

Connors, C.: The syndrome of minimal brain dysfunction: psychological aspects, Pediat. Clin. N. Am. 14:749, 1967.

Davis, J. A.: Headache in children, Brit. J. Clin. Pract. 14:41, 1960.

Fraiberg, S., and Freedman, D.: Studies in the ego development of the congenitally blind child, Psychoanal. Stud. Child 19:113, 1964.

Fraiberg, S., Siegel, B., and Gibson, R.: The role of sound in the search behavior of a blind infant, Psychoanal. Stud. Child 21:327, 1966.

Fraiberg, S.: Parallel and divergent patterns in blind and sighted infants, Psychoanal. Stud. Child 23:264, 1968.

Gordon, R.: A nursery school in a rehabilitation center, Children 13:145, 1966.

Haynes, V.: Nursing approaches in cerebral dysfunction, Am. J. Nurs. 68:2170, 1968.

Healy, H.: Variations in services to handicapped children, Am. J. Nurs. 68:1725, 1968.

Katz, A. H.: Parents of the Handicapped, Springfield, Ill., Thomas, 1961.

Keogh, B., and Legeay, C.: Recoil from the diagnosis of mental retardation, Am. J. Nurs. 66:778, 1966.

Knox, L., and McConnell, M.: Helping parents to help deaf infants, Children 15:183, 1968.

Legeay, C., and Keogh, B.: Impact of mental retardation on family life, Am. J. Nurs. 66:1062, 1966.

Lemkau, P. V.: The influence of handicapping conditions on child development, Children 8:43, 1961.

Livingston, S.: Antiepileptic drugs, Am. J. Nurs. 63:103, 1963.

MacQueen, J.: Services for children with multiple handicaps, Children 13:55, 1966.

Maebius, N.: The nurse as an observer, Am. J. Nurs. 68:2608, 1968.

Millichap, J. E., and Dodge, P. R.: Diagnosis and treatment of myasthenia gravis in infancy, childhood and adolescence, Neurology 10:1007, 1960.

Nagera, H., and Colonna, A.: Aspects of the contribution of sight to ego and drive development: a comparison of the development of some blind and sighted children, Psychoanal. Stud. Child 20:267, 1965.

Nilo, E.: Needs of the hearing impaired, Am. J. Nurs. 69:114, 1969.

Paine, R.: Syndrome of minimal cerebral damage, Pediat. Clin. N. Am. 15:779, 1968.

Pas Yatis, F.: Three sisters with Friedreich's ataxia, Nurs. Outlook 12:38, 1964.

Pendleton, T., and Simonson, J.: Training children with cerebral palsy, Am. J. Nurs. 64:126, 1964.

Peters, B. M.: Courage for Kim, Am. J. Nurs. 67:1200, 1967.

Shane, M.: Encopresis in a latency boy: an arrest along a developmental line, Psychoanal. Stud. Child 22:296, 1967.

Solnit, A., and Stark, M.: Mourning and the birth of a defective child, Psychoanal. Stud. Child 16:523, 1961.

Starfield, B.: Functional bladder capacity in enuretic and non-enuretic children, J. Pediat. 70:777, 1967.

Steele, S.: The nurse's role in the rehabilitation of children with meningomyelocele, Nurs. Forum 6:104, 1967.

————: Children with amputations, Nurs. Forum 7:411, 1968.

Wills, D.: Some observations on blind nursery school children's understanding of their world, Psychoanal. Stud. Child 20:344, 1965.

PAMPHLETS

Epilepsy and the School Child, Epilepsy Information Center, 73 Tremont St., Boston, Mass.

Mental Retardation, Washington, U. S. Govt. Printing Office, 1962.

Neurologically Handicapping Conditions in Children, Univ. of California, Berkeley, California, 1961.

Services for Children with Emotional Disturbances, 1790 Broadway, New York City, The American Public Health Ass., Inc., 1961.

FILMS

The Dark Wave, 20th Century Fox Film in color (26 minutes) 16 mm. Distributed by Films Inc., Wilmette, Ill.

Modern Concepts of Epilepsy, Ayerst Laboratories (23 minutes) 16 mm. Distributed by Nat'l Epilepsy League, Chicago, Ill.

29

Nursing Care of School-age Children with Surgical and Orthopedic Conditions

In this chapter no attempt has been made to include all conditions requiring surgical correction. Those described herein have been selected as typical of or peculiar to the school-age child.

TONSILS AND ADENOIDS

The term *tonsils,* when used without qualification, usually refers to the faucial tonsils which are located anteriorly in the oropharynx, one on each side. The term *adenoids* refers to a mass of lymphoid tissue of the same general structure as the faucial tonsils located in the nasopharynx posteriorly. Adenoids are known also as the pharyngeal tonsil. The lingual tonsil is located at the base of the tongue. The tubal tonsils are situated near the eustachian tube, one on each side of the pharynx. All these lymphoid tissues as a group are referred to as Waldeyer's ring.

Acute inflammation of any of these lymphoid tissues may be catarrhal, follicular or membranous, depending on the severity and the type of infection. The lingual, the pharyngeal or the faucial tonsils may be involved separately, or all may be affected at the same time. Similarly, any of these tissues may be the site of chronic infection or may be abnormally hypertrophied.

Normal faucial tonsils vary considerably in size; the pillars are not adherent; the crypt mouths are open and show no inflammatory products on pressure, and the color of the tonsil is the same as that of the mouth.

Chronic disease or abnormality of the faucial tonsils may manifest itself in several ways. The tonsils may be large and ragged from hypertrophy. They may be small and fibrous, and, in addition, they may be buried between adherent pillars. The crypts on pressure may exude pus or cheesy material. The surface of the tonsil may be redder than normal and appear to be subacutely inflamed. Enlargement of the cervical lymph glands is corroborative evidence of chronic tonsillar inflammation.

Chronic infection of the lymphoid tissues of the pharynx may be a factor in the occurrence of rheumatic fever, pyelitis, arthritis, otitis media, partial deafness, cervical adenitis, recurrent colds and infections of the nasopharynx, unexplained fever, periodic gastrointestinal and metabolic upsets, and other conditions.

Tonsillectomy

Chronic disease in the tonsil, repeatedly recurring acute disease and hypertrophy to the extent of interference with breathing are indications for tonsil removal.

Antibiotic treatment of chronic and acute respiratory disease has been responsible for a considerable decrease in the number of tonsillectomies performed.

While there is no question about the benefits of tonsillectomy for properly selected children, it does not necessarily follow that all children are better off without their tonsils and adenoids. So long as these structures remain healthy they provide a first line of defense against respiratory infection. They also probably limit the spread of such diseases so long as they function normally. The decision to remove tonsils and adenoids must also take into consideration the risks of anesthesia, silent bleeding in the small infant, and the psychic trauma to a young child who is unable to comprehend what is being done to him.

Nursing Care. Many children face hospitalization for the first time when they are admitted for tonsillectomy. Frequently it is the only instance in which the child has been placed in the care of people unfamiliar to him. He is usually admitted the day of operation or the prior evening, and has little opportunity to become acquainted with those who will be with him after surgery.

Even with the best preparation, it is doubtful that the child can realize how ill and uncomfortable he will be following surgery. The nurse must be prepared to receive a frightened and often angry child when he returns from the operating room. Recognizing that the mother can mitigate his distress, many hospitals allow parents to be with the child during the early postoperative period. It is essential that the mother know what to expect; his appearance may frighten her unless she has been told that she will see dried blood in his nose, between his teeth and possibly in his vomitus. She will not be embarrassed by his regressive or angry behavior if she understands that it is expected.

Until the child regains full consciousness, he should be kept in a prone or semiprone position. A pillow is often placed under his chest and abdomen to facilitate drainage and to prevent aspiration of blood or secretions. When alert, he may assume the position of comfort.

Fluids should be given cautiously until vomiting ceases; then they can be increased as rapidly as they are tolerated. Cold and sweetened synthetic fruit juices and milk drinks usually are tolerated a few hours postoperatively. The child's pulse rate and behavior should be observed at frequent intervals to detect early signs of bleeding. Restlessness, frequent swallowing, clearing the throat and vomiting, often accompany bleeding. Apparatus for suction and materials necessary for checking hemorrhage should be in readiness. In some instances, throat icebags relieve the pain; in others, they tend to annoy and to increase restlessness. Aspirin may be indicated for relief of discomfort.

Before the child leaves the hospital the mother should be instructed to provide soft, warm, nonirritating foods for her child until the soreness of the throat has subsided. Also, she should understand the necessity for keeping him in bed for a few days and for providing daily rest periods for a short time subsequently. Earache, not accompanied by fever, sometimes occurs after tonsillectomy, and the mother should be forewarned of this. She should also know the importance of reporting to the doctor immediately any mild or sudden bleeding during convalesence.

APPENDICITIS

Appendicitis is less frequent in children than in adults. It is uncommon under 5 years and rare under 2. In all instances the fundamental cause is the same, namely, obstruction of the lumen of the appendix. Obstruction may be due to a variety of causes.

Symptoms

In the adult, the usual findings are sudden onset of nausea, vomiting, localized tenderness, leukocytosis, fever and constipation. In the older child the symptoms may be entirely similar to those of the adult; but children in general, and the younger victims in particular, often present an insidious onset with symptoms that are difficult to evaluate. The classic localization of tenderness in the right lower quadrant of the abdomen may be obscured by poor cooperation or by general hypersensitivity. Pain may be referred elsewhere or may be overshadowed by crying and restlessness. Vomiting is frequently present but is not a very helpful symptom, since it is a common aspect of so many childhood ailments. Very often the diagnosis of appendicitis in a child remains in doubt until he has been observed and examined repeatedly over a period of several hours.

A number of conditions may be confused with appendicitis and lead to unnecessary abdominal exploration. The early symptoms of infectious hepatitis or gastroenteritis often suggest appendicitis. The mesenteric lymph nodes in children sometimes enlarge and become painful during the course of acute tonsillitis. Irritation of the peritoneum may occur in rheumatic fever. Pain may be referred to the abdomen in right-sided pneumonia, in pyelitis and occasionally in meningitis. Some of the most disconcerting patients are the number of small children who suffer from recurring bouts of afebrile abdominal pain which on repeated or close examination give inconsistent or bizarre findings. Many of these children suffer from hysterical or psychosomatic disorders which are more likely to be aggravated than helped by a fruitless operation.

Prognosis

The prognosis of appendicitis in children is generally good when the disease is recognized and treated. Delay in making the diagnosis or unusually rapid progression of the infection in a young child may increase the hazard to recovery, for diffuse peritonitis may occur within a short time of the initial symptoms.

Treatment

Once the diagnosis is made, treatment is by surgical exploration and removal of the infected appendix. Preceding the operation the child should be kept at bed rest. If postponement is necessary for some reason, an icebag will help to relieve pain and decrease peristaltic activity of the bowel. Enemas are permissible but cathartics are unwise. If operation is contemplated within a short time, usually fluids and feedings are withheld. The sulfonamides, penicillin and streptomycin are of great value in preventing or minimizing peritonitis. Postoperative care of children is usually simple, for they seldom suffer from paralytic ileus.

UNDESCENDED TESTICLE (CRYPTORCHIDISM)

Early in fetal life the testicles develop within the abdomen near and below the kidneys. In most instances, they descend into the scrotum during the last 2 months. In some instances, they are still in the inguinal canal at the time of birth and occasionally within the abdomen. Those undescended at birth usually descend during the first few weeks after birth, but may descend at any time up to the period of adolescence. When nondescent is bilateral, the testes nearly always descend before puberty. When it is unilateral, approximately half descend at puberty or soon afterward. Undescended testicle is to be found in only about 0.3 per cent of men by the time full maturity is reached.

At puberty, the testes normally increase in size and develop spermatogenic and increased androgenic activity. An undescended testis develops at puberty in the same manner for a short time, but eventually the sperm-forming cells degenerate, with sterility as a result if both testes are affected. Although slight decrease in androgenic activity may occur, the body and the secondary sexual characteristics develop normally. The temperature at which the testis is maintained seems to be the controlling factor in its spermatogenic activity, scrotal temperature being lower than that of the body.

A testicle in the inguinal canal is more subject to injury than when in the scrotum—both external injury and that from torsion and strangulation. An undescended testis may also be a psychological handicap.

There is considerable divergence of opinion about the proper treatment of undescended testis. Many physicians wait until puberty before instituting treatment. Others treat at from 10 to 11 years old, a period preceding puberty, in order to avoid the possibility of degeneration. Normal puberty is initiated by a hormone produced by the anterior pituitary gland. An active principle similar in action to the pituitary hormone can be obtained from human pregnancy urine. This material, known as chorionic gonadotropic hormone, may be responsible for descent of the testis before birth. Some physicians advocate the administration of this gonadotropin to boys with undescended testes in order to see whether this physiologic stimulus will bring them down into the scrotum. Others believe that this is a futile or unwise procedure and recommend surgical operation after a reasonable period of waiting for spontaneous descent.

Nursing Care

When a child is hospitalized for surgical repair of undescended testicle, the nurse should make every effort to determine what he has been told about his condition and the treatment. A surprising number of these children are believed by their parents to be ignorant of the absence of one or both testes from the scrotum. Many are told that they are to have a hernia repair. Parental anxieties often revolve around concerns which they do not feel comfortable in verbalizing, such as cancer, homosexuality and sterility. They may perceive the child as inadequate or defective.

In these instances, the child is usually well aware of what is wrong with him, but he has learned that it is not a subject to be discussed and frequently will deny all knowledge of his physical problem. His fantasies about what will happen in surgery are often startling. The nurse can help the child learn what will happen to him and can clarify many of his misunderstandings.

While anxiety about genital mutilation is not as dominant in the school-age child as in the younger child, the older boy with undescended testicle has increased genital concerns. Attention has been focused on his genitalia by frequent medical examinations and by parental anxiety.

When the child returns from surgery, his testicle will be held in position in the scrotal sac by means of a suture which is placed in the testis and attached to a rubber band. The rubber band is secured to the thigh by adhesive tape. The purpose is to maintain position, not to put tension on the testicle. The appliance remains in place for 5 to 7 days. Normal activity is encouraged for the child as soon as he recovers from anesthesia.

BRAIN TUMOR

Brain tumor is a result of abnormal growth of cells already present in the brain or of malignant cells transported to the brain from their origin elsewhere in the body. Most brain tumors are of the first group.

Etiology

Brain tumors are approximately one sixth as frequent in children as in adults. However, among children they are the third most common type of malignancy prior to age 5 and the second in frequency during later childhood. Most of the brain tumors of children occur in the posterior fossa of the skull cavity, whereas most of the tumors of adults occur above the tentorium. Fully three fourths of the tumors of childhood are composed of glial cells (glioma). These cells are of various types which differ in their invasive ability. The most common type is slow growing and not invasive. The type of glial cell is known as an astrocyte, and the tumor is an astrocytoma. These tumors usually are in the cerebellum.

Symptoms

Most of the symptoms are caused by increase in intracranial pressure. Tumors of the posterior fossa are almost certain to cause hydrocephalus from obstruction of the outflow of cerebrospinal fluid from the basal foramina. Increased intracranial pressure is likely to cause headache and vomiting. Among the nerve changes resulting, one easy to detect is swelling of the head of the optic nerve, as observed by ophthalmoscopic examination ("choked disk"). After a period of persistent swelling, the optic nerve atrophies, causing permanent blindness. In young children, the skull sutures are not united. Therefore, the sutures may separate as a result of the increased pressure and thus delay some of the more severe pressure effects. Increased intracranial pressure is likely to cause slowing of the pulse and may cause increase in blood pressure. Fretfulness, irritability, vomiting, and changes in disposition are common results, followed later by mental dullness and drowsiness. Older children may complain of dizziness.

Symptoms from local destructive effects of the tumor vary greatly and may be lacking. Cerebellar tumors often cause nystagmus and disturbances in gait and ability to stand. Localizing symptoms are produced more often by tumors above the tentorium. Convulsions are common with cerebral and rare with cerebellar tumors.

Diagnosis

Tumors of the brain have an insidious beginning, and often early diagnosis is impossible. The course is progressive, and soon or late symptoms suggesting the condition appear. The course of some of the slow-growing tumors at times may be as long as several years before serious symptoms appear. In other instances of tumor, perhaps only a few weeks elapse. The coexistence of headache, vomiting and choked disks is highly suggestive of brain tumor, but these 3 conditions appear together late in the disease. A ventriculogram or an encephalogram is helpful in making the diagnosis and locating the tumor. In some instances, an electroencephalogram also is helpful. Evidence of increased intracranial pressure may be obtained by direct measurement of the cerebrospinal fluid pressure and in many instances by x-ray examination of the skull. The skull may show separation of the sutures in the younger children and atrophy of bone in the same pattern as the brain convolutions in the older children. Symptoms identical with those of brain tumor may be produced by brain abscess, encephalitis and certain degenerative diseases of the brain. Examination of the cerebrospinal fluid is often helpful in making a differential diagnosis.

Treatment

The treatment of brain tumor is surgical removal when this procedure is feasible. An invasive tumor cannot be removed completely, and it is certain to recur after operation. Some of the tumors of children are enucleated easily and removed completely. With such tumors the prognosis is good if the child survives the operative procedure.

Nursing Care

When a child comes under observation because brain tumor is suspected, the nurse should watch for symptoms that may help to localize the lesion. Even when the child is unable to communicate his symptoms, the observant nurse will note behavior that results from visual disturbances, hallucinations, headache and intracranial pressure. Pulse and respiration rates, temperature and blood pressure should be noted at short intervals and changes promptly reported. It is important to observe: mental state, drowsiness, sleepiness, irritability, pupillary changes, vomiting with or without nausea, quality of speech, yawning, hiccoughing, sphincter control and details of convulsions.

Frequent feedings are important prior to operation. Vomiting usually is unaccompanied by nausea; often the child is hungry and can be refed.

A preoperative enema may be contraindicated because of the danger of increasing intracranial pressure. Preoperative drugs which depress the central nervous system are seldom used.

A crib bed or side rails should be provided for the child with brain tumor in both the preoperative and postoperative periods. When he returns from the operating room he should be positioned on his unaffected side, with his head level. The nasopharynx must be kept free of secretions and vomitus.

Knowledge of the anesthetic used will guide the nurse in understanding the significance of the temperature, blood pressure and pulse and respiration rates. Vital signs should be observed every 15 minutes until the child's condition justifies longer intervals. Symptoms of surgical shock may be striking. When external heat is indicated, warm blankets should be used. Raising the foot of the bed is considered inadvisable, because of the possibility of increasing intracranial pressure and bleeding. Emergency stimulants, oxygen inhalation, intravenous fluids, blood transfusion and ventricular tap may be necessary, and the equipment needed to carry out these measures must be immediately available.

If the dressing becomes moistened with blood or spinal fluid, the physician may wish to be notified. If the child is young or restless, elbow restraints can be applied to prevent him from disturbing his dressing. Other restraints should be avoided, for the restless child's efforts to escape them may cause an increase in intracranial pressure.

A marked rise in temperature may be due to trauma, to disturbance of the heat-regulating center or to intracranial edema. The child's temperature should be monitored hourly, and if it begins to rise, intensive nursing care is often required to control it. Removal of clothing and/or covering (except for the pubic area), the use of a cold water mattress and tepid water sponge bath are often ordered. If these measures do not reduce the temperature, ice water enemas or alcohol sponge baths may be necessary. For a markedly elevated temperature (104° F. or above), small retention enemas or rectal suppositories containing aspirin often will produce diaphoresis and temperature reduction.

It is not expected that the temperature will be reduced to the normal level, but only that it be maintained within a reasonably low range. Care must be exercised to prevent too rapid a drop; if it goes as much as 1° below the point at which it began to rise, temperature-reducing procedures should be discontinued.

Surgical trauma may produce edema of the face and eyelids, which can impair circulation of lacrimal secretion, causing dryness and subsequent infection of the eye. Gentle saline irrigations keep the eyes free of exudate, and elbow restraints prevent the child from further irritating his eyes. Swelling of the eyelids can be partially controlled by the application of cold compresses, but care should be taken to prevent dampening the dressing.

The extent of external facial and scalp edema may be indicative of the amount of intracranial edema that exists. Marked external edema, accompanied by drowsiness and pupillary change should alert the nurse to additional signs of intracranial pressure.

When nausea subsides, small sips of fluids can be given. When the swallowing reflex is known to be functioning, amounts can be increased gradually; rapid ingestion may cause vomiting. As solid foods are introduced, encouragement to eat increasingly larger amounts is often necessary.

Infusions are continued until the child's fluid and food requirements are satisfied orally. In the absence of the swallowing reflex, gavage feedings may be instituted. When tube feedings are given, the nurse must be alert for signs of distention.

To prevent pressure sores and hypostatic pneumonia, the child's position should be changed hourly, and meticulous skin care provided. When he is moved, his head must be supported, and turning should be done slowly and carefully. Rapid movements tend to produce vertigo. When paralysis or spasticity of the extremities exists, support of the parts with pillows, rolls, or other means is necessary.

Even when the child appears to be unconscious, it is vitally important that conversations that could be upsetting to him be avoided in his presence.

The child's parents need much support and consideration. In addition to the shock of the diagnosis, and the grave concern they feel about the ultimate prognosis, the present surgical procedure entails acute stress and anxiety in that the operation is itself life-threatening. If they have been prepared prior to operation, the sight of the child with his bandaged, edematous head and the emergency procedures so often required will be less frightening.

Convalescent care of the child is directed toward his return to independent functioning. Parents must be helped to see his increasing abilities and encouraged to foster independence at home.

ACUTE OSTEOMYELITIS

Pathophysiology

Infection of the bone in the absence of traumatic or operative exposure can occur only when infectious agents enter the blood stream and are transported to the inner recesses. Thus septicemia, even though it be brief, is a necessary precursor of osteomyelitis. In the small infant and young child, the septicemia itself is likely to be the major disorder with one or more foci of bone involvement as secondary complications. In the older child this circumstance is less common and the localized invasion of bone is more likely to be the primary topic of concern.

Although viruses and fungi may invade bone and produce lesions, bacterial infections are much the most common. Staphylococci are the usual offenders; streptococci are found less frequently, and other agents only rarely. The special physical characteristics of bone with its rigidity account for the fact that inflammatory reactions within generate contained pressure which in turn compresses the blood vessels and interferes with delivery of blood to the bone beyond. This may lead to thrombosis of vessels or complete occlusion with infarction of bone in the area distal to the obstruction. The peculiar anatomic arrangement of the blood supply tends to localize osteomyelitis to the ends of the long bones where blood flow is plentiful but slow. Primary localization is most commonly seen just beneath the epiphyseal plate at the ends of the bones, where growth in length is under way. Here too the cortex of the bone is thin and relatively easily eroded so that the infection makes its way out underneath the periosteum and produces an exquisitely tender localized point of inflammation. While this is the most common site of osteomyelitis, it can also occur in the flat bones of the skull, pelvis or spine.

Symptoms

Usually the onset is sudden with acute discomfort and localized tenderness near a joint—most commonly the knee, hip, elbow or shoulder. Depending upon the degree of septicemia there may or may not be associated constitutional signs of fever, chills and

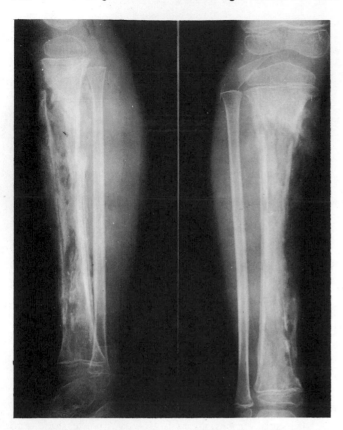

Fig. 29-1. X-ray of lower leg showing bone destruction and a little new bone formation in the tibia which is extensively involved in osteomyelitis.

general malaise. Leukocytosis is almost always present and the sedimentation rate of the blood is elevated.

Diagnosis

Although bone is being eroded by the inflammatory process, it takes time for the characteristic changes to appear in x-rays of the involved bone. Hence early films are not likely to be helpful. One to 3 weeks after the acute onset, typical changes of bone destruction just beneath the epiphyseal line with changes in the surrounding soft tissues may be found and may give a more definitive idea about the extent of bone involvement. Actually, early diagnosis and appropriate treatment must be based largely on the clinical manifestations.

To guide proper early treatment, isolation of the invading bacterium is of great importance. Hence, blood cultures must be obtained before treatment is started.

Treatment

Early and vigorous antibiotic therapy can be expected to bring acute osteomyelitis under rapid control and prevent extensive destruction of bone with its long-term deformity and multiple operative procedures. Thus, as soon as acute osteomyelitis is sus-

pected and after blood cultures have been obtained, administration of antibiotics which can be expected to stop the usual invaders is begun. The traditional use of penicillin has been improved by the addition of chloramphenicol or the substitution of ampicillin or other agents which will cover the possibility of penicillin-resistant staphylococci while still giving protection against streptococci and perhaps even the less common gram-negative bacilli which might be found in the blood culture. (Sickle-cell anemia may be complicated by osteomyelitis due to a salmonella organism.)

Relief of pain by the use of sedatives and particularly by cautious handling of the involved part or by immobilization in plaster are important aspects of the early management.

When treatment is begun late in the course of the disease after extensive bone destruction has occurred, it is necessary to remove areas of dead bone surgically since they do not absorb readily and interfere with the reformation of normal bone.

SEPTIC ARTHRITIS

Invasion of joint spaces by pyogenic bacteria occurs occasionally from extension of osteomyelitis into the joint cavity, or by direct bloodstream invasion. Diagnosis is made by aspiration of the joint with identification of purulent fluid from which the offending bacterium may be cultivated and tested for antibiotic sensitivity. The symptoms are similar to osteomyelitis but physical findings reveal evidence of excessive fluid accumulation in the involved joint. In general, therapy is the same as for osteomyelitis. If the clinical course is not rapidly improved by antibiotic therapy, surgical drainage of the joint may be necessary to prevent destruction of tissues in the joint cavity and ultimate interference with function of the joint. When the hip joint is the one involved, many orthopedic surgeons believe that surgical drainage should always be done because of the speed with which destruction of the femoral head occurs and leads to ultimate dislocation of the hip.

SYNOVITIS OF THE HIP

More common than osteomyelitis or suppurative arthritis of the hip is a relatively benign complaint whose etiology and pathogenesis are poorly understood. It affects boys in the early school years most commonly. Abrupt onset of pain in the hip, thigh or knee and difficulty in bearing weight upon the involved side are present, but the constitutional manifestations of fever, chills, leukocytosis, increased sedimentation rate of the blood or general toxicity are usually lacking. Synovitis must be differentiated from rheumatic fever, osteomyelitis, septic arthritis and infectious arthritis. The prognosis for full recovery with preservation of joint function is excellent after a

Table 26. Osteochondroses Seen in Children

Name of Disease	Site	Age (Yrs.)	Characteristics
Legg-Calvé-Perthe's	Head of femur	4-10	Boys; pain in knee or hip; limp; may deform joint.
Köhler's	Navicular of foot	5-9	Boys; pain and swelling of foot.
Apophysitis	Calcaneus	8-14	Boys; pain in heel.
Freiberg's	Metatarsal head	10-18	Girls; pain in foot.
Kienböck's	Carpal lunate	10-20	Boys; pain in wrist.
Osgood-Schlatter	Tibial tubercle	11-16	Boys; pain, swelling just below knee.
Scheuermann's	Vertebral body	13-20	Girls; pain in back; kyphosis; may need operation.

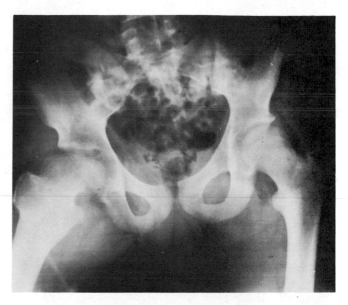

FIG. 29-2. X-ray of the hips of a teenager with osteochondrosis of the capital femoral epiphysis (Legg-Perthe's disease). Note the flattening of the head of the right femur and the distortion of the joint socket or acetabulum.

period of a week or 10 days. No therapy except rest in bed and avoidance of weight bearing is necessary.

TUBERCULOSIS OF THE HIP

The pathogenesis of tuberculosis is considered in Chapter 19. Involvement of the hip produces a chronic disorder which must be differentiated from some of the other conditions discussed here. Tuberculosis of the hip is a low-grade osteomyelitis which begins in the capital femoral epiphysis but may advance to involve other portions of the joint cavity. It occurs in boys more commonly than girls—usually before the age of 10 years. Early symptoms are vague pain in the knee or inner side of the thigh with slight limp. Nocturnal pains are characteristic. Limitation of motion at the hip joint occurs due to muscle spasm. X-ray findings show destructive changes in the femoral head early and general destruction of the joint in advanced cases. Treatment consists of the usual antibiotic therapy for tuberculosis plus bed rest and prevention of weight-bearing. In some instances surgical ankylosis of the joint is required.

OSTEOCHONDROSIS

For unknown reasons, developing epiphyseal centers in various locations of the body may undergo spontaneous degeneration which is not due to infection (aseptic necrosis). Table 26 lists the sites involved, symptoms, sex predilection, and eponymic names given to these disorders. In most instances the destruction of the epiphyseal center can be observed by x-ray as a loss of bony density followed by an increase in surrounding calcification. The process is self-limited, and if treated by relief of weight-bearing or other muscle strain upon the affected part, the localized pain is relieved and healing takes place after several months, usually without loss of function of the involved bone or joint.

SCOLIOSIS

Lateral curvature of the spine may be produced by unequal length of legs, by congenital abnormality of the spine such as hemivertebra, by paralysis of spinal muscles such as occurs in poliomyelitis or by idiopathic disturbances of muscle tone which may endure

throughout the growth period. Corrective measures may include the use of braces or body casts to limit the amount of distortion. Spinal fusion may be required when the deformity is severe.

BENIGN BONE TUMORS

A large variety of localized benign tumors and disorders of bone growth may be seen in children. Most of these entities are uncommon and all are designated by names which reveal their histologic structure; e.g., chondromyxoma, fibroma, hemangioma, neurofibroma, giant cell tumor. In most instances symptoms are lacking and the lesion is discovered either by palpation of an excresence or accidentally when the skeleton is being x-rayed for some other purpose. Their chief importance lies in the need to identify them as benign lesions and thus distinguish them from the malignant ones which require prompt treatment. A few of the more common types are briefly described below.

Osteochondroma (Osteocartilaginous Exostosis)

These lesions are disorders of bone growth in which excessive cartilage and bone are formed at the epiphyseal line during the growth process. The excrescences produced may be small, firm spurs or grow into large pedunculated masses with knobby ends. They tend to grow in such a fashion that they infrequently produce interference with the operation of muscles or joints. Most commonly they are single tumors, but a hereditary form with multiple tumors is also seen. No treatment is necessary unless they

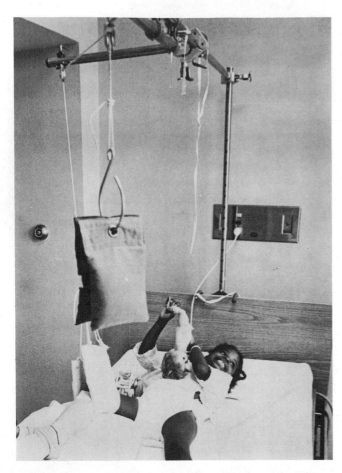

Fig. 29-3. Company and toys can lighten the long hours spent in traction while recovering from a broken tibia.

interfere with function or cosmetic appearance, or if there is doubt about their benign nature. They may be excised surgically. Occasionally they disappear spontaneously if left alone.

Enchondroma

These too are probably disturbances of bone growth rather than true neoplasms. They differ from osteochondromas in that they are within the normal architecture of the bone rather than excrescences from its surface. Unless accidentally discovered, they usually announce their presence when the involved bone fractures from relatively minor stress owing to the thinning of the cortex overlying the enchondroma. Treatment consists of curettage of the lesion and insertion of bone chips within the cavity.

Solitary Bone Cyst

These lesions are similar to enchondromas but have a different appearance on x-ray and contain only fluid and old blood. They are generally located at the ends of the long bones, beneath and not invading the epiphyseal plate but expanding and thinning the cortex of the bone around them. They are asymptomatic until a pathologic fracture results. Treatment is by curettage and implantation of bone chips.

Osteoid Osteoma

This entity is a painful localized region of abnormal bone formation with osteoid formation in the center and sclerosis around it. It occurs usually along the shaft of long bones and must be distinguished from osteomyelitis. Cure is achieved by surgical excision of the lesion.

MALIGNANT TUMORS OF BONE

Next to leukemia and lymphoma, malignant bone tumors are the most common cause of neoplastic death in older children. All but a small number of such tumors are either osteogenic sarcomas or Ewing's tumor of bone. Unfortunately, the prognosis is poor and treatment generally unsatisfactory even when the tumor is discovered early. Psychologic management of the child and his family faced with a probably incurable disorder and often associated with the necessity for amputation of an extremity, poses a very difficult and uncomfortable problem for the medical attendants.

Osteogenic Sarcoma

About half of the malignant bone tumors of childhood are osteogenic sarcomas. Most often they appear about the knee as rapidly appearing swellings which are painful. Metastasis to the lungs takes place early in the course and such metastases yield only transiently to radiation or drug therapy. Only about 10 to 20 per cent of the victims can expect to survive even when early amputation and a combination of radiation therapy and antinomycin-D is given.

Ewing's Tumor

Although histologically different from osteogenic sarcoma, the clinical course and symptoms of Ewing's tumor are often similar. The prognosis is equally poor although the tumor responds initially to radiation therapy. Between them, Ewing's tumor and osteogenic sarcoma account for more than 90 per cent of malignant bone tumors in children.

An occasional child will suffer from a malignant bone tumor which histologically is found to be a *reticulum cell sarcoma* or *fibrosarcoma*. Both of these entities carry a somewhat better prognosis for survival.

RECONSTRUCTIVE SURGERY AND REHABILITATION

A wide variety of surgical and orthopedic procedures are available for the improvement of the function of limbs and bodies which have been damaged by congenital maldevelopment, by burns, by trauma, and by the ravages of disease such as poliomyelitis, cerebral palsy, chronic osteomyelitis and arthritis.

Technical details of operative procedures must be sought in surgical and orthopedic texts. Whatever the corrective procedure, the nurse caring for such children should be prepared to deal with the pre- and postoperative anxieties of her patients and should be skilled in the physical care of restraining apparatus such as traction, casts and braces. In addition she should have an understanding of the realistic objectives of rehabilitative procedures which attempt muscle re-education and the acquisition of new skills to open the way toward gainful occupations or satisfying recreation.

Reconstructive surgery often entails frequent or prolonged hospitalization, multiple operative procedures and immobilization of affected parts for long periods. Extensive nursing care is frequently required in order to maintain skin intactness and optimal function of uninvolved body parts. Understanding the meaning that the physical problem has to the child is essential if the nurse is to supply the psychological support so urgently needed by these children.

SITUATIONS FOR FURTHER STUDY

1. How would you prepare a child for tonsillectomy? How would the preparation for a child whose mother will be with him after surgery differ from that of a child whose mother could not be present?

2. If, while talking with a mother of a child with undescended testicle, you found that he had not been told the truth about the surgery he was to have, how would you handle the situation? With the boy? With the mother?

3. What methods might you use to allay the anxiety and quiet a very restless child who has recently undergone brain surgery?

4. Observe a child who is having reconstructive surgery. How might his physical problem affect his future? What are his limitations now? To what extent can they be corrected? How much does he understand about the treatment and what it can or cannot accomplish? How does he perceive himself in relation to other children? Is his perception realistic? If not, how can you help him raise or lower his expectations to fit the reality of his situation?

BIBLIOGRAPHY

Boegli, E., and Steele, M.: Scoliosis: spinal instrumentation and fusion, Am. J. Nurs. 68:2399, 1968.

Cytryn, L., Cytryn, E., and Reiger, R. E.: Psychological implications of cryptorchidism, J. Am. Acad. Child Psychiat. 6:131, 1967.

Dison, N.: A mother's view of tonsillectomy, Am. J. Nurs. 69:1024, 1969.

Jessner, L., Blom, G. E., and Waldfogel, S.: Emotional implications of tonsillectomy and adenoidectomy on children, Psychoanal. Stud. Child 7:126, 1952.

Keiser, R.: Treatment of scoliosis, Nurs. Clin. N. Am. 2:409, 1967.

Minor, C.L.: The empty scrotum, Pediat. Clin. of N. Am. 6:1137, 1959.

Robertson, J.: A mother's observations on the tonsillectomy of her four-year-old daughter, Psychoanal. Stud. Child 12:410, 1956.

Rousseau, O.: Mothers do help in pediatrics, Am. J. Nurs. 67:798, 1967.

UNIT 6

Growth, Development and Care During Puberty and Adolescence (13 to 18 Years)

During puberty and adolescence the child is being transformed into an adult. It is an age period of paradox: Growth is rushing to a halt. Strivings for independence and individuality are submerged in conformity to the group. Meticulous concern over personal appearance and normality is counterbalanced by extremes in fashion, custom and forms of entertainment. Although the disease level is low, there is an almost hypochondriacal preoccupation with bodily complaints, mixed at the same time with reckless exuberance in sports, in social life and in the use of that lethal weapon—the motor vehicle.

Adolescence is confused and unpredictable. Though general trends in growth, development and disease can be stated, the individual variations from average performance tend to be more marked than at other stages of life. The chief threat to life is from accidents. Major disease is at a low level of incidence, but when it does occur it often has unusual implications for the adolescent.

In many aspects of his life the teen-ager is struggling with the problem of transition. He is attached to and identified with his past but anxious to break away from it into a new world of independent relationships —a world which he both covets and fears. The same uncertainty has marked his source of medical care. Too often he has fallen into neglect between the waning responsibility of the pediatrician and the children's hospital, and the yet unrealized supervision of adult medicine. A growing acceptance of the importance of continuing medical supervision is creating a trend toward the extension of pediatric care at least to the college age. Recognition of the unique needs of adolescents has given birth to a class of medical specialists—the ephebiatrists—who concentrate their attention on the problems of children during these transition years. Wards and clinics for teen-agers have been established so that their particular problems and needs can be studied. Personnel with interest in youth in transition are finding that adolescents appreciate health services that are specially designed to meet their requirements. When the teen-age patients can have the companionship of their age-mates without the interference of younger children, problems are lessened for them and also for the staff.

30

Growth, Development and Care During Puberty and Adolescence (13 to 18 Years)

The relatively serene, steady advance which characterized the school years is disrupted by the appearance of pubertal changes. Coming at an earlier age in girls than in boys, and at an unpredictable age in both sexes, the process of sexual maturation governs the growth and the physical development of each individual. The hormonal changes also affect emotional development. They probably have little or no effect on intellectual growth.

The interaction between puberty and growth is somewhat different in the two sexes. For simplicity of presentation they will be considered separately. An approximate time schedule of the main sexual changes is given in Table 27.

FEMALE GROWTH

Height and Weight

The menarche (first menstrual period) provides a convenient maturational milestone from which to date the growth changes in girls. Among American girls the menarche occurs, on the average, at 13 years of age, but the range of normal is so wide that in some girls it will appear as early as 9 and in others as late as 17 years. For a year or two preceding the menarche most girls show the preliminary bodily changes of growth of breasts and nipples, appearance of pubic hair and enlargement of the external genitalia. At the same time there is often a significant rise in the direction of the height curve of the Iowa graph (Fig. 25-2) as the increased influence of growth and gonadotropic hormones is felt. An accompanying upswing of the weight curve is due not only to the increase in height but also to the deposition of fat in breasts, shoulders, hips and thighs which is mediated by estrogenic hormone. The initial spurt is followed by a tapering off in both height and weight so that the girl approaches her final measurements within about 3 years after the onset of menstruation. Hidden from view, changes are taking place in the

skeletal system where, as the excretion of growth hormone wanes, the ends of the long bones knit firmly to their shafts and further elongation becomes impossible.

The age of menarche has an important effect on the girl's final stature for it dates the terminal 3 to 5 years during which significant increases in height can occur. Thus a girl who has her menarche at 10 years may move ahead of her classmates temporarily, but she will do little further growing after 13. The girl whose menarche appears at 16 may still have 2 or 3 years in which to become taller. Of course, another important determinant of final height is the height which the girl has reached when menarche begins. In a general, but not highly exact fashion, it is possible to guess the final height from these two pieces of information.

The range of variation of height for girls between 13 and 18 years of age is as follows: Average height at 13 years is 62 inches (157 cm.). About two-thirds of all girls at this age fall between 59 and 64 inches (150-163 cm.) in height. At the upper point of the age range, 18 years, the average height is 64 inches (162.5 cm.), and the corresponding range runs from 62 to 66 inches (157-168 cm.). Thus it can be seen that most girls add a final 2 to 3 inches in height after they pass the menarche. Few girls grow more than 4 inches in height after menarche.

Variations in the weights of girls during this age period are considerably greater than those for height. Unfortunately, the changes of puberty make it easy for girls to gain weight excessively, a disadvantage which will be discussed in more detail in the next chapter. At 13 years the average weight of American girls is about 100 pounds (45 Kg.) with a range from 85 pounds (38 Kg.) to 120 pounds (54 Kg.); about two-thirds of them fall within this range. By the conclusion of adolescence at 18 years, the average weight is about 120 pounds (54 Kg.), and the two-thirds

Table 27. Approximate Age of Primary and Secondary Sexual Development*

	Age

	8	9	10	11	12	13	14	15	16	17	18	19	20	21
Maturation Changes—Girls														
Beginning of Growth Spurt														
Beginning of Breast Enlargement														
Appearance of Pubic Hair														
Menarche														
Appearance of Axillary Hair														
Ovulation														
End of Skeletal Growth														
Maturation Changes—Boys														
Beginning of Growth Spurt														
Early Growth of External Genitalia														
Appearance of Pubic Hair														
Change in Voice														
Spermatogenesis (?)														
Transient Enlargement of Nipples														
Appearance of Axillary Hair														
Heavy Facial Hair—Beard														
End of Skeletal Growth														

* Bars indicate the age range within which the phenomena usually appear. The vertical line indicates the median, or most frequent age of appearance. (Compiled from several sources.)

range extends from 107 pounds (48 Kg.) to 136 pounds (62 Kg.).

Body Proportions and Configuration

With the spurt in growth in early puberty, the most dramatic change takes place in the length of the legs so that the girl tends to become longer-legged and higher-hipped, an appearance commonly described as "gangling." After making their major contribution to the increase in height, however, the legs stop growing before the trunk does. Thus, eventually some of the original body proportion is restored before all growth finally ceases during the early adult years.

The sex hormones are chiefly responsible for those changes which convert the girl from the indifferent body shape of childhood to the distinguishing contours of womanhood. In greater or lesser degree all girls experience these changes in predictable sequence. Early in puberty there is an increase in the width of the bony pelvis—an important biologic change looking ahead to the time when reproduction may require the passage of a baby's head through this bony ring. At the same time, the breadth of hips is exaggerated by the laying down of more subcutaneous fat around the pelvic girdle. To a lesser extent, fat tends to deposit in other areas of the body such as the shoulder girdle, back, abdomen and legs. Later, the development of the breasts begins to increase the apparent depth of the chest, which is further enhanced by growth changes in the bony and the muscular structure of the chest beneath.

The Head and the Face

During this final push, growth of the bones of the face may produce a temporary thickening and coarsening of the features as the bony ridges and the subcutaneous tissues enlarge. In some adolescents the result is a rather marked change in physiognomy. In many instances the exaggeration of the features will be toned down by the smoothing out of contours which takes place in early adult life. But for many teen-age girls this change in personal appearance is a potential source of unhappiness, particularly if accompanied by facial acne.

Skin

Puberty is accompanied by a rapid increase in the activity of the glands in the skin which secrete both perspiration and sebaceous material. Increased sweating, greasiness of the skin and acne are so common during this period of life that they can scarcely be considered abnormal. Some girls have an increase in general body hair as well as the growth of sexual hair about the genitalia and in the axillae. However, increase in facial hair is uncommon. Pigmentation of the skin increases generally with particular accentuation about nipples, axillae and labia.

Reproductive Organs

The internal organs of reproduction begin to grow rapidly in size at about the time of the prepubertal growth spurt and achieve adult status by the conclusion of adolescence. However, the onset of menstruation does not mark the onset of ovulation and the beginning of fertility. Most girls spend a year or two in a preliminary type of menstruation before ova are extruded. Thus, pregnancy is seldom possible until 1 or 2 years after the first menstrual period.

MALE GROWTH

As in the female, puberty produces rapid and drastic changes in the rate of growth and pushes the boy into the physical mold he will occupy as a man. However, there is no specific point in time, like the menarche, from which puberty and its phenomena can be dated. Those changes which are comparable to female phenomena appear later, on the average, by almost 2 years. Boys, as well as girls, vary considerably in the age at which they enter the transition. Some start as early as 11 years; others are still immature at 18 and yet capable of completing maturation. Of course, the quality of change is different and depends on the predominating influence of the androgenic or male sex hormones in contrast to the estrogenic or female sex hormones which guide the process in adolescence in girls.

Height and Weight

The prepubertal height spurt starts on the average at about 11 years in boys, but a significant number of the younger members of the 13 to 18 year age group are still growing at the rate of the school-age child. Most of the girls are already spurting and have temporarily advanced in height beyond their male classmates. This situation is reflected in the graphs (Figs. 25-1 and 25-2) which show that 13-year-old boys have an average height of 60 inches (152 cm.) which is about 2 inches shorter than the girls of the same age. The range for two-thirds of the boys extends from 57½ inches (146 cm.) to 63½ inches (162 cm.). At the conclusion of the age period, however, the boys have not only passed the girls but have outstripped them, and many still have additional growing to do. At 18 years the average height for boys is 68½ inches (174 cm.), a figure which is now more than 2 inches greater than the female average for the age. The two-thirds range extends from 66 inches (167 cm.) to 72 inches (183 cm.).

The changes in weight parallel the growth in height. At 13 years the average boy is only 93 pounds (42 Kg.) in weight—distinctly lighter than his female classmate. The range in weight extends from 79 pounds (35 Kg.) to 110 pounds (50 Kg.). Because of the deposition of larger and firmer muscles superimposed on the increase in size of the skeletal system, the average boy at 18 weighs 140 pounds (63½ Kg.) and the two-thirds range extends from 124 pounds (57 Kg.) to 155 pounds (70 Kg.).

Body Proportions and Configuration

As it does among the girls, the growth spurt begins in boys with an increase in the length of the legs producing the high-hipped, gangling appearance which will be partially corrected in late puberty by continued elongation of the trunk after the legs have ceased to grow. Although there is some widening of the hips in boys, the more striking development is taking place in the shoulder girdle, where an increase in depth and the appearance of large pectoral muscles lend an air of sturdiness and solidity not seen in the school-age child. Fat deposition occurs to a lesser degree in boys than in girls. Much of the contour filling is due to the rapid increase in muscle size rather than to the accumulation of subcutaneous fat. The changes in the facial features and the skin which were described for the girls also take place, usually with greater intensity. One striking evidence of maturity which occurs in boys is the change in the voice, which follows a rapid increase in the size of the larynx, produced by the androgenic hormones. The lengthening vocal cords are for a time poorly controlled so that the boy in midpuberty vacillates in his speaking from the high pitch of boyhood to the deep bass of adult man.

The Reproductive Organs

Early enlargement of the external genitalia may begin as early as the 10th year and is usually apparent by the age of 13 to 14. Growth may be slow and erratic, and the adult configuration often is not achieved before 18 to 20 years of age. The time at which sperm are produced marks the beginning of male fertility. It is difficult to obtain precise information on this point, but, on the average, boys are thought to be capable of reproduction at about 15 years.

NUTRITIONAL REQUIREMENTS OF ADOLESCENCE

Several aspects of adolescence increase energy requirements and call for supervision of the diet in respect to quality as well as quantity. Because the age period is marked by great individual differences it becomes impossible to set uniform requirements. The factors which must be taken into consideration are the stage of sexual maturation, the rate of physical growth, and the amount of athletic and social activity which the individual is pursuing.

Those children who have not yet felt the effect of a growth spurt continue to have appetites and energy requirements similar to those described for the school-age child. Caloric intakes of 1,600 to 2,400 per day with 1½ to 2 Gm. of protein per kilogram of body weight and the same vitamin intake as previously recommended are appropriate. Boys require somewhat more food than girls in general.

However, when the effects of rapid growth appear, there is almost inevitably a corresponding increase in appetite and an upswing in the daily energy requirements. For the pubertal girl who is moderately active, an allowance of 2,200 to 2,800 calories per day is reasonable. However, a very athletic boy in the similar stage of growth may need between 3,000 and 4,000 calories per day. Since much of the growth is taking place in muscle and bone, it is desirable to be sure that protein, vitamin and mineral intakes are plentiful. The protein requirement approaches 80 to 100 Gm. per day. Calcium should be supplied at the rate of at least 1.5 Gm. per day. Vitamin D is needed in the amount of 400 to 800 units; vitamin C in quantities of 50 to 100 mg. per day.

Obesity occurs in some adolescents when growth and appetite are increased but are not accompanied by physical activity. Another problem may arise, particularly among girls who consider that they are becoming too heavy for their own ideals of body proportions and place themselves on diets which are deficient in the essentials needed for proper growth. These are a few of the nutritional problems which must be considered and dealt with on an individual basis during this period of rapid transition.

PSYCHOSOCIAL AND INTELLECTUAL DEVELOPMENT OF THE ADOLESCENT

Adolescence begins with the onset of physical maturity and ends when the individual has reorganized his personality, achieved the level of adult intellectual functioning and found satisfying, constructive and mature resolutions of his conflicts. At no other stage of development are changes so extreme and varied in effect as they are in adolescence.

During a few years the adolescent must reaffirm his identity and take his place as an interdependent member of a society which expects a great deal of its citizens. The adolescent has many tasks: he must adapt to a rapidly changing body and resolve old problems intensified by physical maturation; he must emancipate himself from attachment to and dependence on his parents and make a heterosexual adjustment; and finally he must modify his conscience for adult living and begin to prepare himself for a vocation or career.

The adolescent's response to his core problem (identity vs. role diffusion) is determined by the quality of his past relationships with significant persons and by the guidance which he receives throughout this period. The adolescent who believes in himself and others and has a strong, flexible ego approaches his problem with confidence. Of course, he has periods of stress, because the transition from childhood to adolescence is full of problems, but he is able to meet his own expectations and those of his society.

The youngster who has suffered repeated defeats which resulted in doubts about his competence and sexual identity is burdened with more than the usual number of problems during adolescence. Consequently he needs more understanding and support than the individual who approaches the period with sound preparation by his family.

Intellectual Functioning in Adolescence

During the period of middle childhood, the child became capable of cooperation, empathy and reflection and began to structure reality through the use of reason and logical thinking. At the same time, however, he was dependent on concrete experience for immediate learning, dealt with problems in isolation, and his thought was situation-focused. During this time concrete phenomena aroused curiosity which motivated further investigation and inquiry.

In contrast, the adolescent transcends everyday realities and becomes interested in theoretical problems and questions. He is now concerned with the *possible,* versus the *real,* builds abstract theories regarding the future of the world and is interested in philosophy, art and politics. Adolescents together argue endlessly, beginning with the problem at hand and branching outwards toward all possible solutions.

After the age of 12, the child enters the stage of intellectual development which Piaget has termed the phase of *formal operations.* During this period, a fundamental reorientation to cognitive problems occurs. He is no longer exclusively preoccupied with organizing and understanding phenomena which are examined directly through his sense receptors, but his thought now ranges into all the possibilities of what might be there. He can consider the hypothetically possible as well as the real and this potentiality now directs his perception and behavior. The process of thought and mental activity dominates over his sense perceptions so that he no longer needs to confine his attention to immediate reality. This type of thinking is primarily *hypothetico-deductive* in character; i.e., he is capable of entertaining a set of possible hypotheses which can then be confirmed or discarded, to draw conclusions from pure hypotheses and not merely from personal observation. Unlike the child who lives in the present, the adolescent moves into the nonpresent or the world of the future, spatially removed, and the domain of the hypothetical which permits the building of theory. Spontaneous reflection, not tied to concrete experience, characterizes the transition from childhood thinking to mature, logical reflection. With the potential for abstract thought, verbally presented conceptions and arguments become an important source for further learning and to some degree can make up for lack of concrete experience.

With the ability for hypothetical and reflective thought, the adolescent now considers future plans, both for himself and for society in general, which implies a simultaneous centering upon the self and a focus on ideation and humanity that goes beyond his immediate situation. Disequilibrium induced by the multitude of current changes and the possibilities for the future also contributes to the egocentricity of adolescence.

Through the utilization of hypotheses and imagination related to the future, the adolescent can examine a world of personally relevant possibilities in adult roles, occupational choices, marital choices and ideational convictions. Value systems are built and re-examined in terms of a life plan. These values and ideational stances also condemn the present society and underlie proposals for the reforming and re-shaping of reality.

Maturity—the Adolescent's Goal

The emotionally mature adult's interests lie outside himself. He knows who he is, what he believes in, what he wants and is able to accomplish. In other words he has searched for and found his identity, his own standards and values and prepared himself to contribute to society. He is secure, self-understanding, honest with himself, free of the fetters which bind him to his parents and emotionally liberated for creative work. He is free from exaggerated competitiveness, inferiority or egotism and can use his creative powers without being threatened.

The mature person is discriminating and wise in his judgment. He is able to choose and remain loyal to a mate and to provide a home which supports the personal growth of each family member. He can face life with confidence and enjoys both independent and shared activities. He can balance responsibility with recreation and thus prevent tension from curtailing his productivity. He can love and values the devotion bestowed on him by others. He is reality-oriented and adapts constructively to changes in himself and in the outer world. He has control of his instinctual drives, is in harmony with himself and society and has no hesitancy in drawing on the strengths of others when he is ill or faced with problems in adjustment to everyday life. Although he is master of himself, he is also humble and able to accept his own limitations and those that he perceives in others.*

An entire lifetime is needed to gain all the attributes of emotional maturity. Individuals are constantly confronted with periods of stress, but as problems are solved constructively, strength and wisdom for future hurdles are accumulated. When the personality reorganization of adolescence results in the formation of a strong, flexible ego, the individual can grow with every new relationship. But if he builds a rigid character structure or takes flight from his problems at adolescence, he will have little freedom to experiment with new problem solving methods.

The adolescent has not attained emotional maturity, but he values it and struggles relentlessly to attain it. The influx of energy from hormonal stimulation intensifies the strength of his impulses and produces many of his problems, but it also supplies the forces for mastering his conflicts.

Life in adolescence has its challenges and pleasures, but it also presents new complex problems which arouse bewilderment and anxiety. The adolescent feels the weight of his problems in growing up in a competitive, war-threatened and ever-changing society. He is uncertain of his status in his family and frightened lest he not measure up to his ego-ideal and to the expectations of others.

Adolescents in primitive societies often have fewer problems in adjustment than do the youth of America. In cultures where rites of passage confer adult status and where the adolescent is given precise and definite rules to follow, there is less confusion about cultural standards and infrequent rebellion since conformity assures adult status and security in relationships with others.

In contrast, in societies such as Japan, which are undergoing rapid change from a long history of cultural stability and continuity, youth are conflicted and in identity diffusion. The push to change versus tradition and the interplay between inertia and the flux of growth alienate the individual from his personal and cultural heritage. In a postwar world, the adolescent often becomes confused in his beliefs and attempts to blend the old and the new, the past and the future, and is critical of reality and current social structure. In order to maintain an ideology and cultural identity, experiences must be compartmentalized —a necessity which adds to the pressures for the adolescent in defining an acceptable self-hood.

In other cultures, such as in pre-Communist China, overt rebellion against authority was minimal because the maturing male was initiated into the adult world gradually and imperceptibly. Participation in adult activities began early through accompanying the parent in the performance of his adult role in the business and social sphere. Through such activities, he gradually became acquainted with adult behavior patterns and accepted his place in society and a realistic view of life. Sudden changes of status did not occur and parents did not strive to provide their children with a world which was qualitatively different from the one they had experienced. In such societies

---

* Saul, Leon: Emotional Maturity, ed. 2, Philadelphia, Lippincott, 1960, p. 3.

there is less adolescent turbulence and a smoother transition from childhood to adulthood.

In our own society as contrasted with many older and more stable cultures, the adolescent is less involved in a vertical line with his elders than on the horizontal plane with his peers. The route from childhood to maturity has few precise guideposts. In addition, self-reliance and the rights of the individual are stressed, communicating to the adolescent that he must choose his own pattern of self-development. Unsure of his identity, insecure in relationships and personally inexperienced in observance of adult roles, the adolescent faces great frustrations and considerable anxiety in adjusting to the transition to adult behavior patterns. The discontinuity between early and late experience in our society, however, is not entirely a disadvantage: American youths may retain an idealism, a passionate wish for change and improvement, a tendency to fight toward a better way of living, and a lack of acceptance of compromise.

Parental Problems

The Necessity for Change. The period of adolescence is also difficult for parents. Many are confused by the shift from the rigid discipline which they experienced in their childhood to permissiveness and by the current trend toward a balance between these extremes. Some are unsure of their own opinions and confused by conflicting patterns of child rearing. Others have strong convictions about their standards and values but worry for fear they will be too severe in enforcing them. With the present stress on the societal value of fulfillment of individual potential, they hesitate to exert their authority lest it may interfere with the development of individuality and independence. A few parents resent adolescent growth and change because of resulting clashes with their authority in the home. They are resistant to the change in themselves which is necessary to accommodate to their adolescent's changing role.

Many parents have experienced heartaches and rebellion in their own adolescence which are painful to remember. They have forgotten all the stages they passed before they established a true interdependent relationship with their parents and assumed the responsibility in their family which this mature role implies. As a consequence they are apprehensive about the behavior which reflects the adolescent's healthy struggle for emotional maturity and fear failure as parents. They know their adolescent is bewildered. Parental worry about the consequences of this bewilderment and their concentration on him makes the adolescent more anxious than ever.

The adolescent cannot be entirely submissive to adult authority without forfeiting his right to growth. He must be ready to make some adjustments, but parents also must be prepared to examine their behavior and to determine whether they are exerting effort to adjust to change or clinging to old, satisfying patterns of behavior. Such change is difficult for both parents, and particularly for mothers, because it involves finding substitute satisfactions for the loss of the child's dependence on her.

Substitute satisfactions, such as work outside the home, help many mothers bear the period of waiting until her offspring has developed enough security to establish a new and more satisfying relationship with her. Those parents who prepare themselves for their children's adolescence by encouraging increasing independence during childhood can deliver them into the adult world more painlessly than those who have held tightly to the reins of control. If parents are not ready for the changes of adolescence, they will need as much understanding as their children do. Unless they have help which makes it possible for them to become emotionally closer to one another, they may inflict an unreasonably strict regimen of discipline on their teen-agers or give up in despair, leaving them alone and unsupported.

External Control. Value systems, standards and conscience have developed throughout childhood, so that during the adolescent period there are many unspoken understandings between parent and child. Although the norms of the peer culture gain increased importance, frequently the discrepancy from the norms of parents are less serious than meet the eye and conflict may be enacted around peripheral issues of the social code. The peer group is also a moralizing and limit-setting group, and in many areas their standards reinforce and overlap those of the adult generation. When the cultural heritage and social norms of parents and peer group are seriously deviant, as may occur in immigrant families, much emotional turmoil may be generated. In such situations, attempts to integrate conflicting values may be abandoned with resolution involving adherence to either the peer or adult standards or dissociation in living between the two.

Because the adolescent must loosen family ties and dependence on his parents, they are frequently the target for conflict and hostility. The degree of conflict engendered will depend upon the parents' ability to accept the child's anger and on their security in exerting rational authority and understanding guidance.

Although adolescents fight against delimitation, they also resent extreme permissiveness and desire assistance in decision making as to the degree of responsibility they are able to assume. Despite frequent derogation of their parents, adolescents basically need adults as models, since their self-esteem is dependent on the regard they hold for their families.

Neither rigidity in discipline nor undue permissiveness prepares the adolescent for life in our complex society. Nor do either of these solutions satisfy his parents. If their youngster does not reach maturity, they can never realize the pleasure of an adult rela-

Fig. 30-1. Sustained parental interest during early adolescence when the youngster is hardest to live with because he is so unsure of himself is a boost to his self-esteem. Gathering together before bedtime to discuss the day's events helps to further the family's understanding of each other. (Photographer Ken Heyman)

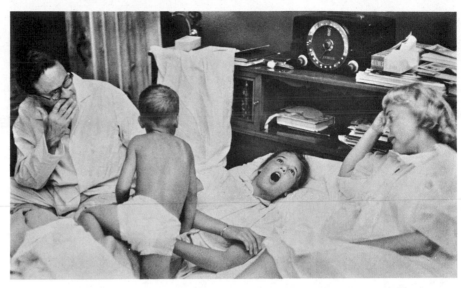

tionship with him. The problem that parents face is in the regulation of loosening control; neither exerting authority so tightly as to force resistance, nor relaxing it so as to endanger the child's security. The adolescent needs many and varied real life experiences to give him security in his new role and to prepare him to become a responsible member of society. His parents must be able to evaluate his strengths and allow him to enter into activities which strengthen his motivation to grow. Experimentation and the testing of his adequacy are necessary for the adolescent in order to learn how to deal with the frustrations and hazards of maturity and to learn to deal with reality. Through achievement of satisfaction in assuming responsibility, he will be motivated to leave the dependent gratifications of childhood.

The adults in the adolescent's world must also understand his immaturity and must have the strength to restrict him from activities for which he is not ready. After careful study of the adolescent's current level of adjustment, restrictions should be introduced and carried out *consistently* and *persistently* until he can control himself independently. Authority must not ebb and rise like the ocean's tide; it must remain steadfast when the adolescent needs it and then be modified gradually as he builds his own controls. Complaining about restrictions helps to reduce his tensions and to maintain the illusion that he is more independent than he feels himself to be.

His parents' limits are a comfort and a source of reassurance to the adolescent. They indicate to him that his parents have the strength of their convictions and care enough about him to show him the way to adulthood. He may wish for unlimited freedom and pretend that he has himself under control, but actually he does not know where he stands in his family or what his parents will allow until they tell him. Nor does he know the sexual role behavior which is appropriate in his community. His needs are too vague to

define, but he hungers for his parents' help in meeting them.

The adolescent's rebellion against the limits set for him can also benefit his parents and the adults who guide him. If they listen to his viewpoint concerning their restrictions, they can get valuable cues to assist them in evaluating his readiness for more flexible rules and independence. When the adolescent finds that his opinions are considered from his point of view, he in turn will become increasingly more receptive to those of the adult.

More than anything else the adolescent needs understanding and faith in himself. If his family background of experience is known, it is possible to visualize the world through his eyes and gain insight into his behavior. To support the adolescent wisely, the adults guiding him need understanding of the forces which produce his unstable, aggressive and unpredictable behavior. They must be ready to let him stand on his own two feet when he is ready for independence or to permit him to lean temporarily on them when he is frightened or has overextended himself and failed to attain his aspirations. In addition, the adults who work with adolescents must have found constructive solutions to their own problems and remained flexible enough to allow the adolescent freedom to solve his problems. When an adolescent feels loved and respected, he takes himself less seriously, does not feel hurried in working through his problems and has energy to gain the maturity which he desires.

Steps in Reaching Maturity

Adapting to Natural Bodily Changes. The increased hormonal activity which initiates puberty affects the adolescent's whole being. It produces physical changes, affects his feelings about himself and others, creates new conflicts and interests and causes marked changes in his behavior.

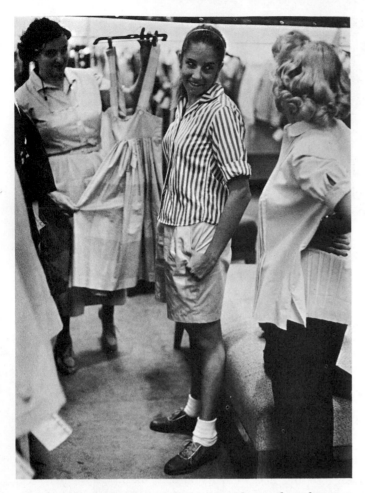

Fig. 30-2. The transition from the tomboyishness of preadolescence to interest in feminine attire is furthered by the mother's approval. (Photographer Ken Heyman)

In preadolescence the well adjusted girl looks forward to the time when she will be adult.

However, anticipating menstruation is different from experiencing it. Many girls are embarrassed by the menstrual flow. Some are disgusted and afraid that others will detect it. Attitudes toward body functions are the outgrowth of preschool experiences. The toddler observes that feces, urine, saliva and vomitus create feelings of disgust in his parents. At the onset of menstruation feelings about body discharges are revived, and additional problems in dealing with the menstrual flow also arise.

Most girls have ambivalent feelings about menstruation when it begins. They view it as a burden and resent their inability to control their bodies. However, they are also happy to find proof that they have become women. The girl's response to menstruation reflects her feelings about femininity and growing up.

Anne Frank's moving diary provides insight into her early adolescent trials, loves, hates and triumphs.

She described her feelings as she entered womanhood and established adolescent relationships with those persons who shared the "Secret Annexe" which was their hiding place from the Nazis during the Second World War. Her reactions to menstruation were ambivalent, but her acceptance of her femininity and her pleasure in growing up are evident. She says:

I think what is happening to me is wonderful, and not only what can be seen on my body, but all that is taking place inside. I never discuss myself or any of these things with anybody; that is why I have to talk to myself about them.

Each time I have a period—and that has only been three times—I have the feeling that in spite of all the pain, unpleasantness, and nastiness, I have a sweet secret, and that is why, although it is nothing but a nuisance to me in a way, I always long for the time that I shall feel that secret within me again.[*]

Many girls must see advantages in growing-up before they can accept menstruation. Emotional reactions to body functions are evident in adolescents' description of menstruation. They call it "the curse" or "falling off the roof." The word "menstruation" cannot be uttered because of its emotional connotation. Often it suggests something which the girl has not digested emotionally, or it arouses sexual feelings which are uncomfortable and misunderstood.

The girl longs for a close friend with whom she can share her feelings about her body. She also needs her parents' approval of her "coming of age" and further accepts her femininity when her parents admire her enhanced beauty without solicitation.

Many boys need help in understanding the physical changes of puberty. Seminal emissions may worry the boy who has not had parental explanations about body changes. He, too, may be embarrassed and react to body discharge as though it were something about which he should be ashamed. He may be concerned about the changes in his voice because he cannot control them and may be laughed at. He must also accept temporarily an unwieldy, unattractive body. The period of orientation to his new self often is accompanied by self-consciousness and uncertainty. Like the girl, he also appreciates his parents' admiration of the changes which are taking place in him.

A period of self-absorption is necessary before the adolescent adjusts to and understands the changes which are occurring in his body and personality. First, he must come to grips with his changed body. He studies himself in the mirror and examines every inch of himself with the same fascination he displayed when he first discovered himself in babyhood. Now he searches in the mirror to find out what he is really like and works hard to accept what he sees. He created an image of the type of adult he wanted to

---

[*] Frank, A.: Anne Frank: The Diary of a Young Girl. Copyright 1952 by Otto H. Frank. Reprinted by permission of Doubleday & Company, Inc., p. 143.

be during preadolescence and now may become concerned because the picture in the mirror is different from his ideal. He exaggerates the physical characteristics he thinks are "poor qualities" and becomes afraid that they may prevent his becoming popular with the opposite sex. If he is markedly different from his friends, his sense of security becomes weakened.

Adults can further the process of self-orientation by respecting his absorption in himself, by helping him to acquire a realistic opinion of himself and by assuring him that he is developing into an attractive person. However, unless assuring words are accompanied by such tangible evidence of approval as listening to the boy's dreams for the future or helping the girl to highlight her most attractive features and develop her talents, the words will go unheard. When the adolescent becomes proud of his body, he will cease to be preoccupied with it and invest his energy in solving more weighty problems.

The rate of maturation can be a significant factor in adolescent personality and behavior and in his self-image. Early maturing boys are more attractive to their peers and to adults, whereas the physically retarded are often seen as less assured, less realistic and more affected and tense. Social experiences are different for early and late maturing boys, a fact contributing to the more positive self-image of the physically accelerated. The latter is given responsibility earlier, has a heterosexual advantage and often excels in athletics which is a source of prestige. Such differential experiences may have long lasting effects on successful vocational choice and adult emotional adjustment.

On the other hand, for girls there are social disadvantages to early maturation in that they are more "out of step" in the heterosexual peer culture. Physically accelerated girls may be lonely as they outstrip their friends in maturation and corresponding interests.

Differential rates of maturation are an added burden in adolescence. Even though physical development proceeds within normal limits, many boys are concerned about late development and lack understanding regarding the normality of differences. Both information and understanding of their concern can help to reduce this added tension.

Awareness of the concerns which beset adolescents is necessary for the nurse who works with them in clinics, schools and hospitals. When the adolescent girl is examined or treated by a male physician she wants protection and support to lessen her embarrassment. Signs of uncertainty are easily discernible in most adolescents. When these signs are observed and used to make it easy for adolescents to talk about and question the findings of an examination, for example, they appreciate the interest which is shown in them.

During the period in which the adolescent is becoming oriented to his new physical self, he may complain excessively about vague, ill-defined symptoms which arise from increased sensitivity to body sensations that he had ignored before adolescence and from fear lest he is not developing normally. Such symptoms must be investigated, for they may have real physical significance or they may be a camouflage for problems that he would like to talk about if he were convinced that they would be taken seriously. Anxiety is usually relieved after he has voiced his fears and discovered that no pathology exists. If anxiety persists after this support, it usually means that he is having trouble in adjusting to adolescence.

Adapting to Pathologic Body Changes. The hospitalized adolescent needs a tremendous amount of help from the staff because the reality he faces includes more problems than those faced by the healthy adolescent. If he has had a background of wise nurturing he has many more strengths to use during hospitalization than the younger child. A comparison of the adolescent's inner resources with those of the toddler is presented because adult recognition of his

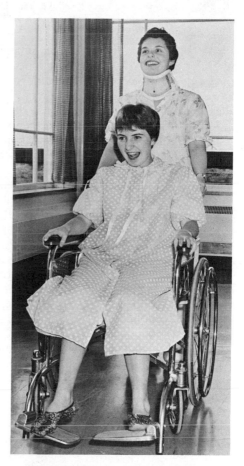

Fig. 30-3. Living with the discomforts of braces and temporary confinement in a wheelchair is made easier for adolescents in wards where care is specially designed for them. (Mr. P. R. Hanson, Administrator, Emanuel Hospital, Portland, Oregon)

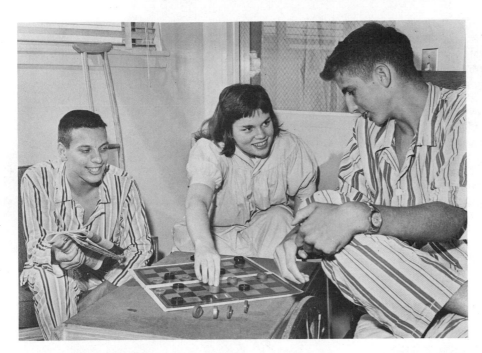

Fig. 30-4. Continued relationships with members of the opposite sex offset the burdens of hospitalization. (Mr. P. R. Hanson, Administrator, Emanuel Hospital, Portland, Oregon)

personality strengths is so important to him in maintaining his self-esteem. This is followed by a discussion of the range of meanings which illness and hospitalization may have for the adolescent.

The adolescent is able to make full use of preparation for hospitalization and for the treatments he will require. He has a background of pleasant memories to draw on in periods of loneliness and discouragement. He has had a succession of experiences which have given him trust that his family and friends will visit him. He can differentiate more accurately between reality and fantasy. He can do and think for himself. He has a much wider range of defenses and manual and mental skills to use in expressing himself, in mastering anxiety and in getting his needs met. Unlike the toddler, he can relate himself to many people rather than to only one or two. He enjoys the companionship of people other than his parents. In fact, relationships with peers and adults outside his family are required by the adolescent, and he can use them for his personal growth. The toddler has problems in relating to strangers. He has not completely found himself yet, and separation from his mother is a major threat to the self-identity he has already established.

The hospitalized adolescent has many other personality strengths, but he also has problems and limitations, not only because he is ill but also because he has not yet solved his core problem and the myriad developmental tasks associated with it. If illness strikes when he is already overburdened with the natural problems of adolescence, it can be expected that he will resent his misfortune deeply. In addition, he cannot help but respond with anger and disappointment to curtailment of his school and social life. He will

also hate interference with his struggle to emancipate himself from his parents.

The child who has been handicapped since birth or early childhood has become adjusted to his limitations. He has new problems in adolescence as he appraises himself and considers his potentialities for successful adjustment to adult life. However, he is not faced with the sudden impact of being physically handicapped at a time when his ego is already burdened with anxiety from strengthened instinctual drives.

The adolescent longs to feel "whole," proud of himself and like others. Disease is a major threat to his ego because it creates an image which is different from the self-image he has treasured. It is also different from the fantasied one he hopes to attain before he reaches adulthood. His body has become more important to him than it has ever been before, and he magnifies the damage that can be done to it by disease. He also tends to exaggerate the effects that his disease may have on his dreams for the future. Illness may also be viewed as a punishment for feelings he has not mastered or for breaking the rules that his parents or doctor have imposed. It may also be a blow to his pride which makes him feel depreciated and weak. The adolescent is infinitely more threatened by helplessness than the young child even though he has more resources to cope with it. He worries constantly that others will discover his inadequacy, dependency and confusion and hides it even from himself.

Support to sustain the adolescent's active involvement in the solution of his problems is one of his greatest needs during hospitalization. When sensitivity to the emotional impact of illness on him personally is combined with the careful physical care that he cannot give to himself, he will regain hope and self-respect and have courage to face reality. If the nurse protects his body, succeeds in bolstering his shaken ego and is unthreatened by the defenses he uses to make himself believe that he is "master of his own ship," he sees his environment in a more favorable light. Then she is in a position to influence him should he have difficulty in cooperating with the staff as they plan his treatment regimen.

Adapting to Uncertainty About the Self as a Person. Investment of energy is also made in achieving a new status in his family and community. Unfortunately, parents and teachers often expect the adolescent to define his goals and take responsibility in achieving them before he has had time to determine the direction in which he wants to go. First, he must test his powers, master his fears and establish his identity as an adult. In early adolescence he has all he can do to keep himself in emotional equilibrium.

However, the adolescent is not only interested in solving his day-to-day problems; he also thinks seriously about the future. Throughout adolescence he questions himself: "Who am I?" "What will I become?" For the boy, concerns revolve about masculine functions and job or career selection. Identity formation for the girl involves not only preparation for a career but also her sexual adjustment and aspirations toward her feminine goal of motherhood.*

The adolescent evaluates his intelligence, personality and potentials for success. He thinks about marriage and wonders if he will find a mate and be capable of establishing a home and rearing a family. He reflects on the degree of self-reliance he has attained and searches for a philosophy which will give him direction for his life and sustain his struggle for maturity.

Life in adolescence is a succession of testing experiences which frighten even those who are well prepared. Regression as a defense against anxiety is used commonly during the early part of adolescence because heavy demands are being made on the teen-ager

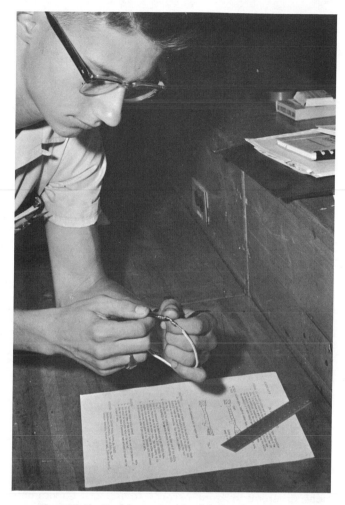

Fig. 30-5. Problems at school help the adolescent to test his aptitudes, find his special interests and consider them in terms of the opportunities they present for a career.

at a time when he is unsure of himself, unfamiliar with his new role and feeling acutely the importance of success. It may also be used during late adolescence (or throughout the rest of life, for that matter) when he has a new set of problems to tackle. Periods of regression are not only the result of environmental pressures; they may also be the means by which the adolescent handles anxiety generated from strengthened instinctual drives, physiologic instability and from his conflict between independence and dependence.

Periods of regression are not pathologic provided that they are temporary, do not hamper school work and social life and are followed by improved adjustment to problems. Under such circumstances they are in the service of the ego and therefore a healthy means of solving problems. Childish traits such as irritability, aggressiveness, demandingness, negativism and disorderliness are characteristic even though they are reminiscent of the two earliest periods of development.

---

* At the onset of puberty, the girl's wish for a child is revived. In adolescence the wish is frightening and even dangerous because of social standards. Because reality limitations exist, the wish is again submerged and becomes sublimated into constructive channels such as baby-sitting, for instance. In these situations she can get an outlet for her maternal feelings and further preparation for parenthood. In adolescence the girl's receptiveness to knowledge of child care is at its peak. She is an apt pupil because instruction fulfills a need which has deep meaning for her. During the first year or two after marriage the wish for a child is not usually the woman's most prominent wish because she is actively engaged in solving the core problem of young adulthood. When this crisis is resolved, energy becomes available for realization of her wish for a child. During the maternity cycle final identification with her mother is accomplished. Then she makes full use of her childhood preparation for motherhood. When pregnancy occurs before the core problem of adolescence is resolved, it can be expected that the ego will be grossly threatened by the additional demands for adjustment being made on it. If the pregnancy occurs out of wedlock, the woman's problems will depend on society's response to it and the purpose it serves in maintaining her emotional equilibrium.

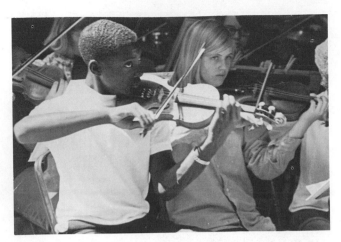

Fig. 30-6. During adolescence artistic creativity is often expressed through music. (Carol Baldwin)

Regression provides a temporary respite from pressures and gives the teen-ager another chance to discover why he cannot relinquish the remnants of baby-ishness within him. It also makes known his need for less stringent expectations. Through the use of this defense, he can complete the resolution of old conflicts that he began in preadolescence. He can also discard those methods of mastering anxiety which conflict with his ego-ideal and work out new ways to meet his goals.

Tension can also be reduced by shifting the energy formerly invested in the parents to parent substitutes or to the peer group. In early adolescence, displacement of emotion from parents to leaders is common and temporarily the adolescent feels free and independent. This independence is spurious, however, since the shift in allegiance has been abrupt and the underlying issues remain unresolved. The value of this defense depends on the personality and characteristics of the substitute or ego-ideal of the adolescent's identification.

Compulsive opposition to the parent occasionally occurs in a reversal of all positive affect to predominately negative feelings. Dependence may turn into revolt, respect into contempt, love into hate. Although again the adolescent may feel temporarily free, his tie to his parents continues without basic resolution of his conflict and anxiety. When this defense proves inadequate, the adolescent may withdraw energy from all object relationships in a return to narcissism and intense involvement with himself.

Another method often utilized to reduce anxiety during the period of puberty is intellectualization, which has the adaptive quality of focusing instinctual energy into nonconflictual areas of ego activity. Constructive coping mechanisms are adaptive in that they reduce tension in the interests of productivity and growth. Creativity, particularly artistic creation, increases the sense of self-esteem while utilizing excess

energy. A focus on the development of special endowments may compensate for felt physical shortcomings. Action expended in constructive purposes may relieve tension, integrate new abilities and rechannel inner drives.

Mastering Instinctual Anxiety. With the advent of puberty, the adolescent has increased energy which stimulates new bodily sensations and strengthens his instinctual drives. The adolescent's reawakened sexuality produces what Freud calls *instinctual anxiety.***** An adolescent whose development has progressed normally does not have to be warned about the danger of his drives; his ego senses it. He needs help to understand his sexuality and to sublimate his drives until he is emotionally ready for marriage and parenthood. Anne Frank wrote about her feelings after she found companionship with Peter, the young man who shared the "Secret Annexe" with their families.

The sun is shining, the sky is deep blue, there is a lovely breeze and I'm longing . . . so longing—for everything. To talk, for freedom, for friends, to be alone. And I do so long . . . to cry! I feel as if I'm going to burst, and I know that it would get better with crying; but I can't, I'm restless, I go from one room to the other, breathe through the crack of a closed window, feel my heart beating, as if it is saying, "Can't you satisfy my longing at last?"†

Learning to cope with strengthened instinctual drives is one of the adolescent's most difficult problems. He cannot yield to infantile impulses to prevent frustration as he did in earlier years because his super-ego and society will not permit it. In early adolescence when his anxiety level is highest, his ego struggles to balance the demands of the id with the requirements of the super-ego and to keep the balance as satisfying as it was before disorganization of personality occurred in preadolescence. Freud describes the manner in which the adolescent's ego attempts to maintain harmony between the three parts of his personality:

In this struggle to preserve its own existence unchanged the ego is motivated equally by objective anxiety [fear of persons in the outer world] and anxiety of conscience and employs indiscriminately all the methods of defence to which it has ever had recourse in infancy and during the latency-period. It represses, displaces, denies and reverses the instincts and turns them against the self; it produces phobias and hysterical symptoms and binds anxiety by means of obsessional thinking and behavior.‡

The adolescent may also use asceticism to defend himself from anxiety. If he is afraid that his instincts will overpower him, he may renounce them and all wishes for wholesome and needed pleasure. He may

---

* Freud, Anna: *The Ego and The Mechanisms of Defence,* New York, International Universities Press, 1946, p. 166.
† Frank, A.: *Op. cit.,* p. 164.
‡ Freud, A.: *Op. cit.,* p. 160. The words interpolated within the brackets are the authors'.

refuse an adequate diet or diversion and may concentrate on punishing himself for his wishes in other ways. Usually, however, this defense is discarded quickly, when he becomes confident of his inner controls.

Until the adolescent discovers ways in which he can obtain socially approved substitute satisfactions, he will be frustrated and direct his aggression toward his parents. When his parents understand the reasons for his aggression and encourage his interests in arts, music, athletics and community activities, he can sublimate his sexual drive and lessen his frustration. Then adolescent-parent conflicts will become less acute.

Emancipation from Parents. The urge to emancipate himself from his parents became intensified during preadolescence and becomes progressively stronger until the individual resolves his conflict between independence and dependence or abandons the struggle and regresses to a stage of development which is less frightening. In order to make a mature heterosexual adjustment, the individual must complete the resolution of the Oedipal conflict, free his conscience of sexual inhibitions and discover that interdependent relationships are more satisfying than childhood dependence.

Dissolving the Family Romance. At the onset of puberty the Oedipal conflict is re-experienced until the adolescent has mastered his ambivalence toward the parent of the same sex and broken his childish ties of love to his parent of the opposite sex. Then he is free to invest his love in a mate.

The revival of the Oedipal conflict gives rise to another threat to the adolescent's ego. He cannot tolerate a repetition of his earlier disappointment. Flights into fantasy do not relieve him of anxiety as they did in early childhood. In preschool years he was sexually immature. Now he is sexually mature, and again he must deal with his feelings of love for his parent of the opposite sex.

Whenever the sexual aspects of his parental relationship threatens to emerge from his unconscious, the adolescent defends himself from anxiety with denial, compensatory braggadocio and exaggerated competitiveness. Outwardly he acts as if he hated his parent of the opposite sex, but actually he is defending himself against his unconscious desires. When he was a child, he attributed his failure in winning his parent to inadequacy but he quickly repressed this conclusion because it was too painful to endure. Now, when he is threatened with conscious awareness of these old feelings, he must act against them to maintain his self-respect. The boy, for example, criticizes his mother, rebuffs her affectionate overtures and denies her physical attractiveness. At other times he struggles to outdo his father to prove his superiority. Such behavior makes it possible for him to retrieve the love he has invested in his mother and make it available for a wife.

Another way in which the adolescent relieves himself of fear of his own inadequacy is to project it outside of himself. He does not understand why he is disturbed and ambivalent and cannot talk these feelings over with anyone because they are unconscious. He is secretive with his parents because he wants to overcome his dependence on them and is fearful lest his real desires will be discovered. The behavior his parents see is defensive; it hides his unconscious feelings and fantasies from himself. He cannot bear to believe that he does not understand himself so he projects these feelings onto his parents and says that they do not understand him.

Problems also arise in freeing himself from dependence on his rival parent. The adolescent studies his parent of the same sex and compares himself with him or her. He must see his positive attributes because his unconscious knows that this parent has been the model from which he has fashioned himself. Yet he must deny his likeness to this parent and criticize the attributes he has admired and attained through

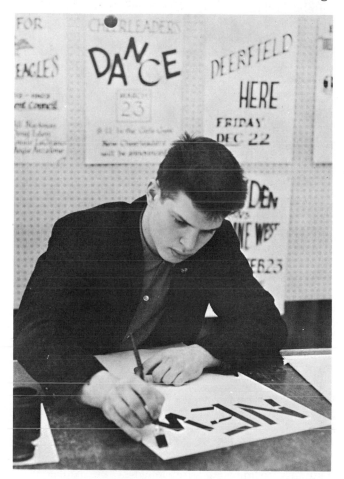

Fig. 30-7. Participation in extracurricular activities is serious business and an important outlet for the adolescent.

identification with him. He fears his rival's hostility, his own competitive attitudes and he must move away from dependence on him. However, to win a mate like the one he unconsciously desires, he thinks he must have his rival's personality characteristics. This dilemma confuses him and causes vacillation in his behavior; one minute he copies the rival parent; the next minute he searches for ways to prove he is different from, superior to and independent of this parent.

To dissolve the family romance the adolescent must enact the drama of adolescence within his home and reach maturity by working through his problems in relation to his parents. He has grown up within his family and studied his parent's ideals and personality characteristics. Now his emotions include both love and hate and are bound to his parents. Therefore, it is natural that his battle for freedom from ambivalence toward and dependence on his rival parent and from attachment to his parent of the opposite sex must be waged in his home, the place where his conflicts developed. If maturity is to be reached, these painful conflicts must be resolved.

Relinquishing the Wish to Remain a Child. The adolescent values freedom more highly when he can resolve his conflict between independence and dependence at his own pace. Too much freedom overwhelms the adolescent and causes him to cling to the comforts of childhood. In preadolescence the child asserted his independence and denied his need for dependent gratifications. The girl received it from her friends and from her mother when she regressed and demanded care from her. In adolescence, the teen-ager's assertion of independence is stronger, but he is frightened by it because he does not quite know how to use it. He cannot admit his fear, so he projects it onto his parents.

Although the move toward autonomy has been important throughout childhood, it becomes a significant issue in adolescence. The variety and insistence of demands increases and autonomy acquires a meaning beyond the specific arguments at hand. These issues contain symbolic value in terms of the adolescent's need for liberation and freedom which to him signifies the acquisition of adult status.

Frequently, the adolescent correctly senses his parent's reluctance to grant him the autonomy he so earnestly desires, yet fears. Parents are often ambivalent and uneasy regarding the use the adolescent will make of his freedom. The child's approach to adult status also signifies to parents the encroachment of middle age, so that they may be reluctant to recognize the child's increasing powers of self-regulation.[*]

Marked extremes in behavior ranging from childish petulance to unusual competence in the management of his own affairs are characteristic of the adolescent before he becomes confident of his ability to assume responsibility. One minute he refuses all advice; the next minute he demands more help than he needed since he entered school. When he receives help, he is afraid that its acceptance will make him feel infantile. When he feels strong, he berates his parents and calls them "old-fashioned" because he does not feel needful of them. Then when he becomes frightened again and seeks comfort, he thinks his parents can do no wrong; he submits to them childishly and feels protected. But this behavior makes him feel immature and defeats him because he wants so much to prove that he is adequate to the job of growing up. He repeats the cycle of self-assertion, fear and retreat until experience strengthens his ego and proves his worth.

In the interim, the healthy adolescent verbally violates the mores of his family but simultaneously lives by his parents' standards. Josselyn says that his verbal violations are attacks on his own conscience. He knows that his conscience must be modified before he can formulate a personal stand on political, social and moral issues. On this subject Josselyn writes:

His verbalization and his actual behavior are, from day to day, characteristically contradictory. He seems to be an idealist and yet his behavior does not always bear this out. At one time he too rigidly follows an idealized code of conduct and then, as if by sudden metamorphosis of character, he violates—or more often *talks* of violating—every acceptable code of behavior.

His relationship with other people is confusing. One minute he hates, the next he loves. The object of this emotional response may be the same person or it may be a different person.

He rejects his parents as if they were lepers in a community of healthy people. In almost the next breath, he idealizes them, picturing them as more saintly than the saints, more learned than the sages, more omnipotent than God.[*]

Before hormonal balance is achieved and his personality is reorganized, the adolescent must be able to depend on steady, supportive relationships. He needs the strength of others because he does not have consistent stability in himself. There is no formula for the guidance of adolescents. Their needs vary tremendously, and chronologic age is a poor index to their level of psychosocial maturity. The adult must have intuitive capacity in identifying the adolescent's particular need of the moment and be willing to modify his approach when he learns that his actions have not been helpful. When the adolescent is ready for independence, he should have the privilege of using his judgment. When he needs protection and dependent gratification, it must be given

---

[*] Douvan, E. and Adelson, J.: The Adolescent Experience, N.Y., John Wiley and Sons, 1966.

[*] Josselyn, Irene: Psychological problems of the adolescent, Part I, Social Casework 32:183-184, 1951. Quoted with permission of the Family Service Association of America.

FIG. 30-8. Daydreaming is not a waste of time if it leads to better preparation for and participation in constructive activities. (Photographer Ken Heyman)

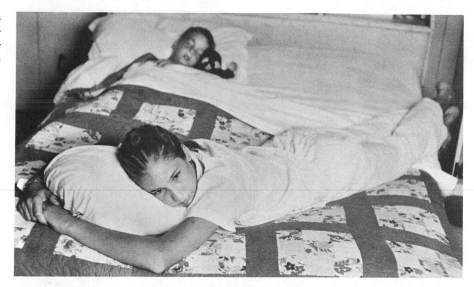

in a way which maintains his self-esteem. The adolescent is strengthened when the adult maintains his poise throughout periods of erratic, disorganized behavior. Poise communicates the adult's understanding of the adolescent's behavior and his faith in his powers to get himself under control. When repeated successes increase his confidence in the management of himself and his world, seeking help in time of need will not wound his pride any longer. Then he will have access to additional support which will hasten the maturation process. The example which follows illustrates application of these principles of guidance.

Mary was a 14-year-old who often flew into rages whenever her whims were not gratified. Her outbursts made her mother anxious, and she retaliated with similar behavior. As a consequence Mary's anxiety increased because she could not rely upon her mother's strength. Nor did she receive any help in channeling her strong feelings into socially acceptable forms of behavior. She could not apply herself in school and the interest she had had in church activities during preadolescence began to wane.

Mary wanted limits which would help her to control her impulsiveness. Her provocative behavior was her way of seeking them but instead of kindly imposed restrictions, she became the target of her mother's aggression. Their quarrels generally ended when Mary went off to do as she pleased. Neither really knew what the other was angry about. (If they could have told each other why they were angry at one another, they could have gained understanding of each other's viewpoint and found compromise solutions.)

Mary was far from ready for independence. She was actually less able to handle it than she had been in preadolescence. (This was not at all unusual in light of the new problems that she had to face.) When Mary's impulses grew stronger, she wanted help to control herself, but she did not receive it, so she became more anxious than ever. She also felt deserted and thought no one cared about her. These feelings deepened her hatred of her mother which made her guilty. Her guilt was relieved by her mother's punishing hostility, but she got no help in controlling herself.

Through the suggestion of a public health nurse, Mary's

mother sought psychiatric help. During this experience she gained understanding of herself and the reasons why she used Mary's behavior to gain emotional release for herself. She also gained understanding of Mary's behavior which relieved her anxiety and made it possible for her to remain poised during Mary's tirades. With control of herself, Mary's mother was free to consider Mary's goals. When Mary needed limits, she got them. As their tension subsided, it was possible for them to talk over situations together. Then Mary's mother was in a better position to gauge the amount of freedom that she was ready for. With this change in relationship, Mary became increasingly more able to make constructive use of her mother in growing up.

Coping with Loneliness. During the period when the adolescent is loosening his ties to his parents, he is lonely and sometimes feels unloved. To prevent unbearable emotional isolation, the adolescent must make some temporary compromise solutions to his problems. When he finds that these solutions do not take the place of close intimate relationships with others, he acquires the courage to test himself out in a mixed group of teen-agers. Then begins a period of dating, followed by "going steady." Generally he narrows his field of interest and finds a mate with whom he would like to establish a home and rear a family.

Daydreaming and swooning over heroes and heroines tide the adolescent over a rough transitional period before he finds a close friend of the opposite sex. They also help him to appraise himself and to master his fears. In the early years of life the child acted out experiences overtly; during adolescence he wants periods of solitude to act out life experiences in his mind. His introspective daydreaming serves many purposes and is not connotative of emotional illness unless it is not accompanied by *active* participation in social life. It helps him to establish a new identity and solve current problems; it gives him a chance to test himself out imaginatively in situations he has never met; it helps him to focus on the future. In solitude he can dream, formulate his goals and ex-

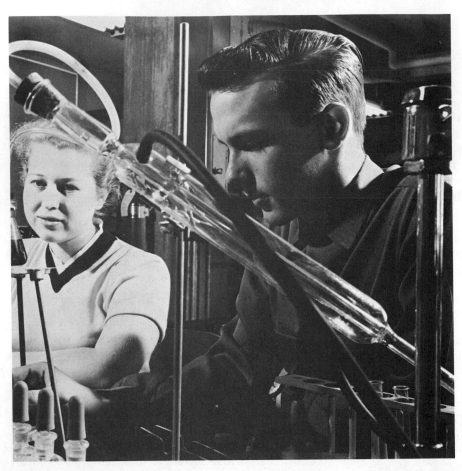

perience imaginatively how he will go about reaching them. By dreaming himself more capable than he is, he can also escape momentarily from fear of the unknowns which plague him.

Daydreams also provide a safety valve for the expression of strong feelings. It is better to imagine the kiss of a beloved person than to really experience it before the readiness to cope with the feelings the kiss arouses is acquired! Of course, daydreams which are attached to reality are infinitely more satisfying. This is the reason why teen-age girls fall in love with movie stars and singers and are seen engrossed in movie magazines, pushing their way through crowds to catch a glimpse of their latest idol or in their rooms dreamily musing to the hit songs of a popular singer. The young teen-age boy's collection of pin-up girls serves a similar purpose; he can act out imaginatively his newly discovered attraction to the opposite sex and become better prepared to handle himself when he is with them. One would hope that this period of fanhood would be short lived and become replaced with real-life activities which provide more constructive outlets for the adolescent's talents.

Another temporary compromise solution for his problem of loneliness is continued relationships with members of the same sex. During adolescence there are other advantages in being associated with a group of the same sex. He can discuss the problems he is having with the opposite sex and learn that others have similar worries which they need to share with friends.

The adolescent cannot give up parental codes of behavior without a substitute, so he incorporates those he and his group formulate. The codes of the group are usually strict, and he is a slave to them until he masters his fear of instincts and becomes self-assured. He also wants the sense of belonging and the approval that he gains from conformity. Furthermore, a sounding board for the expression of his developing philosophy helps him to get it in tune with reality. He learns from his contemporaries more easily than from his parents, and he knows that he must become adept at maintaining relationships with them if he is to succeed in a career.

This phase of adolescence may be prolonged if the teen-ager fears the opposite sex or his own reawakened sexuality. In such a case he needs more help than his group can provide. He will profit from knowledge about the psychology of the opposite sex and from concrete help in acquiring social skills. He also may need more understanding of his sexual impulses and help to know how to deal with situations which arouse him sexually. Many young adolescents do not know how to act with the opposite sex, and initial experiences cast doubts on their adequacy. They need a sounding board while they are trying to decide how they want to use their creative power and to learn about the responsibilities associated with it. In addition they need experiences with members of the opposite sex to become acquainted with and comfortable in their relationships with them and secure in the knowledge that they can think instead of reacting impulsively.

Growth in relationship to the opposite sex shows patterned progression toward maturity. In early adolescence the boy is driven to test his powers of conquest. The girl wants to prove that she is attractive and desired. A great deal of her behavior is motivated by a need for companionship. If the adolescent cannot compete with his parent of the same sex and take his mate from him or her, he can compete with his friends, and he does unless he has a problem in this area. The adolescent's conversations are full of his conquests and successes. When a teen-ager has succeeded in "stealing" his friend's girl or boy friend, his rivalry with his parents becomes partially mastered.

In late adolescence, when the person has proved his popularity, tenderness and love supplant his feelings of rivalry and competitiveness. Then he uses his energy in appraising the qualities he would like in a mate. He will also be free to recognize the advantages in postponing marriage until he finds someone whom he loves and respects and with whom he would like to share his life. When he finds this person he goes "steady," "gets pinned" or engaged and prepares himself for his role as a husband or a wife. After marriage, when he has solved his next core problem (intimacy vs. isolation),* his love becomes more encompassing, and he wants children to nurture. When the developmental tasks of the child-bearing and child-rearing stages of development are mastered, his interests expand to the needs of humanity.

The fashion of "going steady" from the beginning of adolescence causes concern to most parents who question whether it will help the adolescent to master his sexual drive and to develop discrimination in the choice of a mate. Parental advice is usually not welcomed by the teen-ager. Pointed questioning which stimulates the adolescent to think for himself and guides him in the study of his friend's character and aptitudes for successful marriage is infinitely more helpful than criticism of him. When his current love object is frowned on, he may prolong the relationship to defy his parents. Many hasty marriages are rooted in defiance rather than love and respect and, therefore, are doomed to failure.

Later in adolescence when the threat of seeking advice has diminished, it is wise to ask the adolescent's opinion before airing one's views about the subject

_____
* See Duvall, E. M.: Family Development, ed. 3, Philadelphia, Lippincott, 1967, and the references at the end of Chapter 6.

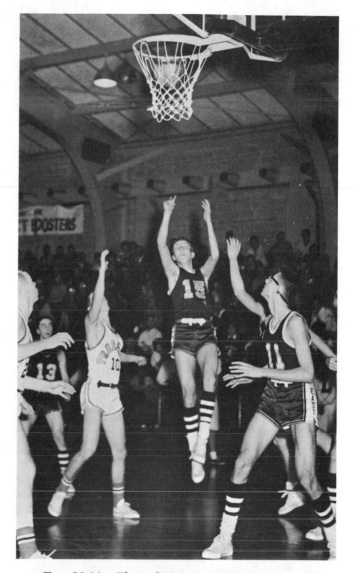

Fig. 30-10. Through participation in sports and other kinds of group activities the adolescent gets the pleasure of reaching a goal through the co-operation of all members of the team.

of his inquiry. This gives him a chance to look at his problem in a new way and also gives the adult insight into the adolescent's values and current depth of thinking. This kind of responsiveness to the adolescent's bid for advice is appropriate when helping him deal with any of his problems, including the choice of a mate. When the adult point of view is shared with him, the adolescent learns the value of differing opinions and will use the information to test the validity of his own solution before advice was sought. A genuine sharing of points of view gives him gratification in a palatable and easily digested form. More importantly, it strengthens his capacity to make wise decisions and proves to him that he has attained the status of an adult. When he feels respected by the person to whom he has turned for advice, his opinions are valued and influence the course he takes in solving his problems.

In hospital wards and residential hospital schools there are adolescents who spend months or years in becoming rehabilitated. The teen-ager cannot make a heterosexual adjustment unless he has gratifying social experiences with the opposite sex. The hospitalized adolescent has fewer opportunities to make friends of the opposite sex and more fears about acceptance by them. These adolescents must have the privilege of planning ward activities which give them a chance to work and play together. Supervision is needed to assist in the planning of activities, but so is trust in their ability to have fun with each other in socially acceptable ways.

Preparing for a Career. During adolescence the individual evaluates his interests, ideals, aspirations, strengths and limitations in order to become secure as a person and prepared for his future role in society. Some adolescents come to this phase of growth with clearly defined vocational or professional goals. However, many more do not know what they want to become and flounder about in a maze of indecision long after they have left high school and college. Some adolescents have their life work mapped out for them by their parents. From early childhood they have sensed their parents' ambitions for them and have not dared to question their expectations.

The possibilities for success and self-realization in work are greater when the person selects it independently and enjoys it. The adolescent needs help in appraising his abilities and in learning about various fields of endeavor. He needs the dreams of his elders shared with him—dreams which, although never realized, have not shattered their faith in the power of youth to accomplish more than they have been able to do. He also needs encouragement and recognition when he succeeds in defining his goals and the means by which he expects to achieve them. Youth is heartened by challenge and confidence which is placed in them. Trust in their potentialities for success motivates them to stretch themselves so that they may transcend heights for humanity never before realized by their parents or teachers. This is the stuff of which cultural progress is made.

THE CHALLENGE OF MODERN YOUTH

Much publicity and attention in recent years have been centered on student revolts, the hippie movement, the revolution in sexual mores, preadolescent runaways, and the "hang-loose" ethic. In all eras, late adolescents have banded together into a subculture and many of the ideas expressed by modern youth have a long tradition; these are now becoming more prominent because of larger numbers of adolescents in our society, the reduction in age of participation and because more are engaging in "rebellious" activities. Despite the recurrent theme of the ideas expressed by each generation of youth, the current movement has social significance in that the young people today are calling attention to problems in our society which have become urgent. Although most teen-agers remain fundamentally the same and make a healthy adjustment to the transition to adulthood, and there is danger in stereotyping and lumping teenagers as a group, the numbers of nonconforming adolescents today signal a troubled generation.

There are massive new problems in our society to which adolescents are responding. Because of accelerated social change never before seen in our culture, the experiences of parents and their children are diverging seriously, thus adding to the conflict of generations and the lack of understanding within families. Violence stemming from war, the anger of mobs and racial conflict has been a part of the earliest memories of adolescents. Youngsters today are shaped by mass media as never before in our history. Middle class youth have been spared their parents' experiences with depression or deprivation and are accustomed to an affluent society of material abundance. There are massive problems concerning overpopulation, pollution, traffic congestion, urban crises, and war. With an increasingly technological society, and the promise of an automated future, many of the stabilizing influences and prior values are losing their effectiveness. The world of work and leisure is altering drastically and rapidly so that adolescents today have no clear picture of their future and of the preparation necessary to fit them for participation in such a society. The tradition of future orientation in our society is breaking down with decline of religious values and an undercurrent of grave doubts about the future.

Many adolescents are reacting to a society which is failing to make an appropriate and meaningful place for them. Participation in adult activities is denied to them in many areas; yet the pressures on middle class youth are increasing for ever higher scholastic achievement. In order to complete educational programs, the years of adolescent dependence have increased and the time lengthened until he has voice and responsibility in societal tasks and "real living." The penalties for lack of education also increase so that for others, because of lack of opportunities or increased difficulty in admission to college, many doors are closed and the future is uncertain.

Like all of us, the teen-agers today have the threat of mass annihilation constantly hanging over their heads. Every generation has faced the prospect of war and premature death, but our present youth are the first generation to fear the possibility of death of society which lends an aura of absurdity to human life.

Because of better nutritional status, teen-agers today are reaching physical maturity at a somewhat earlier age. With the constant exposure of the mass media and the emphasis in our society on youth and sexual

symbolism, they are bombarded with more erotic stimulation than ever before. Every child today is aware
that love and sex are part of the real world. With the
additional pressures, many youngsters may seek the
security of intense companionship which leads to ultimate sexual expression. The post-World War II generation is also more open and less guilt ridden regarding sex.

With the affluence of our society more youth than
ever before have the means to buy the material things
which symbolize adulthood. The mobility given by
the automobile has become increasingly important as
a symbol of freedom and of adult status.

Teen-agers are also responding to the hostility they
receive from an adult society which continues to view
nonconformism with fear and anxiety. The threat of
disruption of established social arrangements and the
spontaneity of youth is disquieting to it. There is
also an unconscious resentment and envy of youth itself and an unprecedented fear of aging and death
in our society today. Fear of loss of control is basic
to the standards of most adults so that treatment of
the adolescent generation is often harsh.

Many parents, particularly fathers, are no longer
freely available as role models to their children. The
sense of connection with the past, the meaning of
maleness and femaleness, the gradual induction into
work roles is no longer possible for many youth so
that the problems of identification and identity are
more serious. Incomplete or selective identifications
with numbers of people may lead to alienation, difficulty in synthesizing desired characteristics into an
harmonious identity or identity diffusion.

These problems which are facing many young
people today result in a renewed and increased
emphasis on drawing the ultimate through experiencing the present. The seeking of freedom to be an
individual is expressed in reaction against the middle
class scheme of life and rejection of values and symbols of the "good life." Immediate expressive fulfillment, doing vs. passivity, the need to participate and
"get involved," "letting go" vs. control, risk taking,
new expressiveness in art forms, the merging of sex
roles and change in the ethical bases for human relationships have become the values of many youth
today and their way of saying, "I object" to the depersonalization of modern life. Adolescents are also
very action oriented people and the combination of
their need and the indifference of the adult generation
contribute to this behavior.

The vast majority of teen-agers find constructive adjustments to the increased pressures of our society.
Nonconforming adolescents, however, are teaching
their elders that there needs to be greater attention
than ever before toward facing both the individual
problems of our youth and the problems of society
in general. The challenge to the older generations to
reconsider the goals and values of our society, to re-

appraise the distribution of responsibility between
generations, to create a pattern for meaningful participation for our youth, to plan opportunities for
them to prove their competence in work and love is
serious. Meeting this challenge can prevent the numbers of our young from withdrawing from our society.

In addition, the principles outlined in the previous
sections of this chapter have a heightened significance.
Young people need warmly firm parents who admire
them, experiences which help to fit them for productive living, increased closeness and communication
within the family, acceptance and understanding of
expression of their feelings and help in handling their
anger and conflict. There is no reason for believing
that the generation gap is insurmountable. Although
the current nonconformist scene may change or be
transformed, the values emphasized should be noted.
These include a desire for openness in personal relations, a new and growing interest in the life of the
spirit, emphasis on self-awareness, self-expression and
idealism, and a willingness to speak with unabashed
feeling.

SITUATIONS FOR GROUP DISCUSSION

1. How do males and females differ in their attitudes toward discipline, rules and in the formation of
an identity?

2. How does the current "car culture" and the emphasis on mobility in our society affect the development of autonomy in the present day teen-ager?

3. Why might anesthesia pose more threat to the
adolescent than to the young child? If you believe
that it might, how would you work with him preoperatively to minimize the threat?

4. In what ways might illness and hospitalization
pose more of a threat to the adolescent than to the
school-age child?

5. Observe adolescents in a ward of adults and
describe the behavior which reflects problems in adjustment to the environmental milieu. Why do you
suppose that adolescents have such a difficult time
handling themselves to their satisfaction in a ward of
adults?

6. Observe one or two adolescents in a ward where
the majority of patients are under 6 years of age and
see if you can identify behavior which is being provoked by their environment. What suggestions can
you make for the management of the ward which
would make it a more comfortable place for adolescents?

7. Eric, a 14-year-old boy with hemophilia, was
admitted to the ward in shock from internal bleeding.
Three hours after intravenous fluids were begun, he
responded overtly to his environment. During the remainder of the afternoon, his mother stayed in the
waiting room. The nurse reacted with anger to the
mother's withdrawal from her critically ill son and
from her lack of interest in helping her to carry out
the many procedures which had to be done. When

his mother, Mrs. P., finally returned to the room, the following conversation between mother and son took place:

Mrs. P.: "Aren't we lucky to have Miss J. here to give you special care?"

Eric: "You're telling me! Scram! I don't need you. Why don't you go home?" (His tone of voice betokened anger, and he acted as if he meant what he said.)

Later when the nurse and Eric's mother were alone together, Mrs. P. said, "Eric and I have a closer relationship than most mothers and sons. He has needed so much more care than most children. We react so strongly to each other, I thought it was better if I limited my stay with him."

What might have been the reasons why Eric reacted the way he did to his mother's question? What needs does his behavior disclose? What do you think the nurse's role should be in the care of an acutely ill adolescent boy? What problems might the nurse have in fulfilling it?

8. What purposes do limits serve for the adolescent? Why is the adolescent boy less able to acquiesce passively to limits than is the girl? Describe one of your patient's responses to a ward regulation which displeased him. How did you respond to his behavior?

9. Jim, age 15, was convalescing from rheumatic fever. He resisted afternoon rest periods and kept his TV on long past the time when it was to be turned off in the evening. As the nurse pulled his shades down for rest hour, he bellowed, "You needn't think I'm going to sleep. I'm captain of my own ship and don't you think I'm not." The nurse was irritated with Jim's dictatorial manner and said, "Oh no you're not. Dr. C. is the captain of your ship."

How do you imagine Jim responded to the nurse's remark? When Jim's bellowing irritated the nurse, how might she have handled her feelings to preserve her equilibrium and help Jim get the rest that he needed?

10. Read Chapter 7 in the pamphlet "Care of Children in Hospitals" and be prepared to discuss the principles advanced which, if applied, would strengthen the adolescent's ego in coping with illness and care in a hospital. What attitudes in the nurse would help the adolescent to see her as a person from whom he could get support? In this chapter the writer says that death cannot be faced with equanimity by the adolescent. He describes the behavior which might result when death is feared and suggests ways in which his powers of adjustment might be strengthened. Be prepared to discuss in class your reactions to these suggestions. What attitudes might prevent the staff from making use of these suggestions in the ward?

BIBLIOGRAPHY

Aichhorn, A.: Delinquency and Child Guidance, N. Y., Internat. Univ. Press, 1964.

American Academy of Pediatrics: Meeting the needs of the hospitalized adolescent *in* Care of Children in Hospitals (pamphlet), Evanston, Ill., American Academy of Pediatrics, 1960.

Baldwin, J.: Go Tell It on the Mountain, Signet Books, N. Y., New Am. Lib. of World Lit., Inc., 1963.

Barclay, A., and Cusumano, D.: Father absence, cross-sex identity and field dependent behavior in male adolescents, Child Development 38:243, 1967.

Bealer, R., Willits, F., and Maida, P.: The rebellious youth subculture—a myth, Children 11:43, 1964.

Bier, W.: The Adolescent: His Search for Understanding, N. Y., Farnham Univ. Press, 1963.

Blos, P.: On Adolescence, Glencoe, Ill., The Free Press of Glencoe, 1963.

————: Character formation in adolescence, Psychoanalytic Study of the Child 23:245, 1968.

Brown, C.: Manchild in the Promised Land, Signet Books, N. Y., New Am. Lib., Inc., 1966.

Calderone, M.: Sex and social responsibility, J. Home Economics 57:499, 1965.

Checkering, S.: How we got that way, American Scholar 36:602, 1967.

Cohen, Y.: The Transition from Childhood to Adolescence, Chicago, Aldine Publ. Co., 1964.

Committee on Adolescence, Group for the Advancement of Psychiatry: Normal Adolescence: Its Dynamics and Impact, N. Y., Scribner, 1968.

Conant, J.: The American High School Today, N. Y., McGraw-Hill 1960.

Crow, L., and Crow, A.: Adolescent Development and Adjustment, N. Y., McGraw-Hill, 1965.

Douvan, E., and Adelson, J.: The Adolescent Experience, N. Y., Wiley, 1966.

Eisenberg, L.: A developmental approach to adolescence, Children 12:131, 1965.

Eissler, K. (ed.): Searchlights on Delinquency, N. Y., Internat. Univ. Press, 1965.

Elkind, D.: Egocentrism in adolescence, Child Development 38:1025, 1967.

Erikson, E.: The problems of ego identity, Psychological Issues 1:101, 1957.

Erikson, E.: Young Man Luther, N. Y., Norton, 1958.

———— (ed.): The Challenge of Youth, Garden City, N. Y., Anchor Books, Doubleday, 1965.

Espy, H. E.: Quiet, Yelled Mrs. Rabbit, Philadelphia, Lippincott, 1958.

Frank, A.: The Diary of a Young Girl, N. Y., Pocket Books, Inc., 1953.

Freud, A.: The Ego and The Mechanisms of Defence, N. Y., Internat. Univ. Press, 1946.

Gallagher, J. R.: Medical Care of the Adolescent, N. Y., Appleton-Century Crofts, Inc., 1960.

Glaser, K.: Masked depression in children and adolescents, *in* Chess, S., and Thomas, A. (eds.), Annual Progress in Child Psychiatry and Child Development, 1968, N. Y., Brunner/Mazel, 1968.

Goldfarb, A.: Understanding physiologic change, Pediat. Clin. of N. Am. 16:395, 1969.

Goodman, P.: Growing Up Absurd, Vintage Books, N. Y., Random House 1960.

Grinder, R. (ed.): Studies in Adolescence, N. Y., Macmillan, 1965.

Hammar, S.: Nursing Care of the Adolescent, N. Y., Springer, 1966.

Josselyn, I.: Psychological changes in adolescence, Children 6:43, 1959.

————: The Adolescent and His World, N. Y., Family Service Association of America, 1952.

Konapka, G.: The Adolescent Girl in Conflict, Englewood Cliffs, New Jersey, Prentice-Hall, Inc., 1966.

Kugelmass, S., and Breznitz, S.: Intentionality in moral judgment: Adolescent development, Child Development 39:249, 1968.

Laufer, M.: The body image, the function of masturbation and adolescence; problems of the ownership of the body, Psychoanalytic Study of the Child, 23:114, 1968.

Levin, M.: Healthy sexual behavior, Pediat. Clin. of N. Am. 16:329, 1969.

Masland, R.: Understanding physical change, Pediat. Clin. of N. Am. 16:407, 1969.

Maxwell, W.: They Came Like Swallows, N. Y., Harper Bros., 1957.

Mead, M.: Coming of Age in Samoa, N. Y., Mentor Books, 1928.

Peckos, P., and Heald, F.: Nutrition of adolescents, Children 11:24, 1964.

Piaget, J.: Six Psychological Studies, N. Y., Random, 1967.

Randall, A., and Randall, J.: Sex education in the schools, Pediat. Clin. of N. Am. 16:371, 1969.

Rosenberg, M.: Society and the Adolescent Self-image, Princeton, Princeton Univ. Press, 1965.

Rothchild, E.: Emotional aspects of sexual development, Pediat. Clin. of N. Am. 16:415, 1969.

Ruark, R.: Old Man and the Boy, N. Y., Henry Holt, 1957.

Shellow, R., Schamp, J., Liebow, E., and Unger, E: Suburban runaways of the 1960's, Monographs of the Society for Research in Child Development Vol. 32. No. 3, 1967.

Short, J.: Juvenile delinquency: the socio-cultural context, *in* Hoffman, L., and Hoffman, M. (eds.) Review of Child Development Research, Vol. 2, N. Y., Russell Sage Foundation 1966.

Shulman, M.: I Was a Teen-age Dwarf, N. Y., Bantam Books, 1960.

Simmons, J., and Winograd, B.: It's Happening, Santa Barbara, Calif., Marc-Laird Pub. Co., 1966.

Sorrel, P.: Teenage pregancy, Pediat. Clin. of N. Am. 16: 347, 1969.

31

Disorders of Puberty and Adolescence

The age of transition from childhood to adulthood is one of the healthiest periods of life from a statistical point of view. The mortality rate is low. Most children have acquired immunity to the infectious diseases. The impact of congenital abnormalities has been felt at a previous age. Only the rate for accidental death and injury shows an increase in this segment of the population. However, the emotional uncertainty described in the last chapter endows many of the disorders of the period with an abnormal aura of importance to the adolescent's welfare. A few of the disorders that present real threats of physical and emotional disability are considered in this chapter.

ACNE

In late childhood or during adolescence a disturbance of the pilosebaceous apparatus of the skin occurs in such a high percentage of children that it (acne) can almost be considered a normal aspect of sexual development.

Under the influence of the androgenic hormones of the maturing person an activation of the sebaceous glands occurs which results in an increased production of oily sebum. At the same time there is a tendency for the orifices of the glands to become blocked by dark inspissated material (blackheads or comedones), around which may develop an inflammatory reaction, often with pustule formation. Acne vulgaris is usually prominent about the forehead, the face and the neck. It also may be present on the shoulders and the back and occasionally on the chest. Its extent is variable. Some children have little or none during their adolescence and early adult lives. Others are affected severely, with permanent scarring as a consequence of the repeated formation of pustules. Administration of cortisone or ACTH often produces a similar eruption even in young children, but there is seldom any associated infection.

Treatment of mild acne consists of frequent bathing of the skin to remove oil and bacteria and to encourage drying. For the latter purpose various washes that cause mild peeling are useful. Exposure to ultraviolet light is also beneficial, either from the sun or from a lamp. The diet is of some importance in the aggravation of lesions, and the natural tendency of the adolescent to gorge himself with carbohydrate foods must be discouraged if the inflammatory reaction is to be controlled adequately. Expression of the contents of comedones and pustules usually is done by the physician. In severe cases, judicious use of x-ray treatment may be required.

GYNECOMASTIA

Gynecomastia is the development of breast enlargement in the male similar to the early pubertal growth of the female breast. In boys it usually consists of the appearance of a flat pad of glandular tissue beneath a nipple which becomes tender at the same time. The changes may be unilateral or bilateral. Rarely there is continued growth of breast tissue; ordinarily the process is of brief duration and stops short of the production of permanent enlargement of the breast.

Gynecomastia depends on the excretion of estrogenic hormone in the male. The fact is often overlooked that both sexes have an increase in the production of both types of hormone during the onset of puberty. Thus, girls produce androgen in increased quantity which in some of them leads to the appearance of acne. Similarly, boys produce more estrogen than formerly, and in some of them the breast responds temporarily to this stimulus.

No treatment is necessary for gynecomastia under ordinary circumstances. However, boys must be reassured that the changes are not going to be progressive. Discomfort from the tender nipple can be alleviated by wearing a band-aid or simple gauze dressing over the nipple. In the rare circumstances where growth continues to produce an embarrassingly large breast-like structure, surgical removal is indicated to restore masculine appearance and relieve embarrassment.

FAILURE OF SEXUAL DEVELOPMENT

The complicated and poorly understood sequence of events which governs sexual development is presented in oversimplified form in Figure 31-1. Failure of sexual development occurs when the sequence is distorted by (1) delay in the trigger mechanism, (2) disease of the hypothalamus, (3) disease of the pituitary, or (4) abnormality of the target organs, the gonads.

The most common reason for delay in sexual development is tardiness of the trigger mechanism in the brain which stimulates the hypothalamus, which in turn signals the pituitary to increase its production of gonadotropic hormone, and thus set the rest of the latent mechanism into operation. Disease of the hypothalamus prevents transmission of the stimulus to the pituitary but is an uncommon cause of delay in sexual development. If the pituitary itself is deficient it will not be able to elaborate the necessary hormones to affect the peripheral organs. Finally, the sex organs themselves may be deficient and consequently unable to respond to the stimulus directed at them through the pituitary hormones.

Delayed Adolescence

For a variety of reasons, delayed puberty in girls is infrequently a cause of parental concern, whereas the failure of a boy to keep up with his age-mates in sexual development is very commonly a topic of unnecessary worry. While the average male begins puberty by 13 or 14 years, some normal boys may wait until the age of 16 or 17 before the first changes occur. A particularly common cause of concern is the high-hipped, mildly or moderately obese boy who matures late. The rare Fröhlich's syndrome referred to below has unfortunately become too popular as a lay and even medical diagnosis which is pinned unjustly on normal boys of this body build. Treatment of delayed adolescence is usually not done, although, occasionally, psychological reasons may prompt the doctor to initiate maturation by the use of androgens.

Hypothalamic Lesions

Disorders of the hypothalamus, the portion of the brain immediately adjacent to the pituitary gland from which it receives nervous stimulation, may be responsible for failure of sexual development. Tumors, congenital defects and cysts known as craniopharyngiomas may interfere with the production of gonadotropic hormone by the pituitary. This combination of circumstances due to a tumor prompted the original description of the Fröhlich syndrome which combined sexual infantilism with diabetes insipidus and a feminine type of obesity.

Pituitary Abnormalities

If the pituitary gland itself is abnormal and unable to produce gonadotropic hormone, sexual maturation fails to occur. It is usually part of a general failure of the pituitary gland (panhypopituitarism) which also leads to dwarfism. Occasionally, it occurs as an isolated defect of the gland in a person of normal stature.

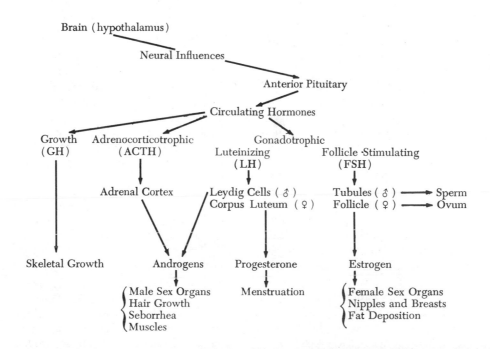

FIG. 31-1. Pathway of influences which control sexual maturation.

Gonadal Dysgenesis (Turner's Syndrome)

If the end-organs (the gonads) which the gonadotropic hormone is destined to stimulate are absent or defective it is obvious that sexual development cannot take place. Defective embryonic development of the gonads is now recognized as leading most commonly to a clinical picture in which female external genitalia are associated with a boyish appearance that does not change at the age of puberty. Other defects are usually present. Short stature is regularly found, and webbed neck, hypertension and various skeletal abnormalities are frequent. The latter characteristics may lead to the suspicion of gonadal defect even during infancy. The diagnosis can be confirmed during the prepubertal years when the urinary excretion of gonadotropic hormone (FSH) rises to high levels as the pituitary tries vainly to initiate puberty. A number of variations of the general pattern are recognized.

The most common or classical variety of the syndrome of gonadal dysgenesis is associated with an XO chromosome pattern and total number of 45 instead of 46. Because of the presence of only a single X chromosome, Barr bodies are not found in the cells of the leukocytes or on buccal smear in spite of the fact that the patient has a female body constitution. The variant types of gonadal dysgenesis in which the typical features are missing and there is greater, but incomplete development of secondary sex characteristics have been found to have mosaic chromosomal patterns with two types of cell—the usual XO cell plus one or more other types such as XX, XXY, XY, XXX, or XYY.

MENSTRUAL DISORDERS

Disturbances in menstruation are relatively common among adolescent girls. A very large percentage of the complaints that are brought to the attention of doctors and nurses stem from (1) more or less normal variations occurring during the establishment of first the anovulatory cycles and later the ovulatory cycles, and (2) exaggeration and overconcern which are a reflection of the girl's labile emotional adjustment. Thus, most doctors handle many of the complaints with a conservative approach and reassurance rather than subject an already upset patient to an extensive gynecologic examination. Unfortunately, mixed in with the more or less normal functional complaints are a few which stem from significant abnormalities of structure or hormone production. In addition, the menstrual cycle also may be affected by disease outside the generative tract. Many delicate problems in clinical judgment arise which cannot be treated adequately in the brief discussion which follows. In some instances the girl's anxieties cannot be allayed until she has had the benefit of what *she* considers to be an adequate gynecologic examination.

Amenorrhea

The preceding discussion of failure of sexual development emphasized that the most common cause of failure to menstruate was a delay in the onset of puberty, and that rarely disease of the hypothalamus, the pituitary or the ovaries might be responsible. In the latter instances there are usually other associated abnormalities which direct attention to the reason for menstrual failure. Girls with chronic or debilitating physical disease usually do not menstruate. Inadequate diets, self-imposed reducing schedules, hypothyroidism and significant emotional upsets are other well-recognized causes of amenorrhea.

Menstruation which has once begun and then ceases has the same spectrum of underlying causes as menstruation which fails to develop. It must be remembered that after the anovulatory period, pregnancy becomes a possible explanation for amenorrhea.

Irregular Menstruation

During the first year or two after the menarche, lack of ovulation is common. The production of estrogenic hormone often fails to follow a predictable cyclic curve, and the effect of progesterone is minimal. Thus, it is expected that many girls will have irregular menstrual patterns, often with long periods of amenorrhea lasting over several months. The duration of individual periods and the time lapse between them is also subject to wide variation. Unless these irregularities are accompanied by excessive flow or persist for more than 2 years, the girl may be reassured that regularity will appear eventually. A few women with otherwise normal reproductive organs go through life without ever establishing a repetitive menstrual cycle.

Dysmenorrhea

A high percentage of adolescent girls experience some pain from menstrual cramps. Only a small fraction of those who have pain find it necessary to interrupt school or social activities. It is sometimes difficult to evaluate the severity of symptoms because of the heightened emotional tension and the preoccupation with bodily complaints which is so commonly a part of the adolescent's make-up. Simple management includes the avoidance of chilling (particularly swimming), application of local heat to the abdomen and the use of mild sedatives or anodynes. Severe, persistent dysmenorrhea is usually investigated by a thorough gynecologic examination.

Menorrhagia

Excessive menstrual flow is seen in varying degrees of severity. It is more likely to be an indication of organic difficulty than are the other menstrual irregularities. Bleeding which is sufficiently intense or prolonged to result in fatigue or anemia obviously needs a thorough investigation. Local disease of the uterus may be responsible in some instances. Deficiency of ovarian function or of thyroid secretion is sometimes responsible and may be corrected by administration of the appropriate hormone. Bleeding dyscrasias such as purpura or leukemia may be accompanied by severe menorrhagia.

OBESITY

Obesity, the accumulation of excess body fat, is not a disorder limited to the period of adolescence. It is treated here because it acquires maximum significance at this time of life. In the infant, obesity is almost always transient and of no long-term import. During the school years, however, the accumulation of excessive fat must be regarded with concern because of its later effect on the child, and proper measures should be instituted to discover its cause and to bring it within reasonable control. But the full physical and psychological impact of obesity usually is reserved for the period of adolescence when it hampers participation in sports and social functions and, more importantly, arouses the adolescent's concern over the deviation of his physique from the normal.

Causative Factors

The simple explanation of obesity is that the individual takes in more food than his body requires for its necessary operations; i.e., basal functions, activity and growth. Without such an excess there is no material to fabricate fat. Consequently, obesity disappears when food supplies are insufficient. However, the converse is not universally true, for not all people who have plenty to eat become obese. Thus, we need some explanation of why some people become fat and others remain thin under ordinary circumstances when food intake is above subsistence levels. In part the answer lies in variations in food consumption, so that, in general obesity is seen more often among those who take large amounts of food regularly and is absent from the more abstemious. Differences in *constitutional make-up* account for the varying propensity of different children to accumulate fat on diets of similar composition. Just what these constitutional differences are is a matter of debate, but they must be related in some way to variations in the efficiency of enzyme systems which regulate the digestion, absorption and utilization of foodstuffs within the body. Abnormal activity of hormones has been blamed as a cause of obesity, but, except in rare instances, there is no evidence to support this concept. Deficiency of thyroid activity has been blamed most frequently for obesity, but the subjects almost without exception fail to show the characteristic features of hypothyroidism such as retardation in growth and bone age, anemia, sluggish circulation and low basal metabolic rates or protein-bound iodine levels. Thus, the theoretic basis for the treatment of obesity with thyroid extract is shaky at best.

From a practical point of view, obesity in the growing child should be viewed in relation to his longitudinal record of height and weight. Children who are able to eat as they choose without gaining excessively present no problem and can be regarded as lacking the constitutional make-up which leads to obesity. Children who begin to deviate from normal limits during school years or adolescence will have to limit their food intakes if they wish to avoid obesity. This is usually difficult to achieve because of psychological considerations which foster appetites that are too large for the child's nutritional health. A large part of the management of obesity lies in the analysis and control of such large appetites.

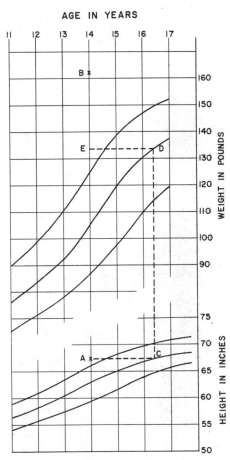

FIG. 31-2. Method of computing the percentage of overweight. The child's actual height (A) and weight (B) for the given age are plotted on the Iowa graph. A horizontal line drawn from A will intercept the average height line at C, which is the age for which the child's actual height is average. A vertical line to D shows the average weight for this height; the difference between B and D or E is the number of pounds he is overweight for his height. The formula $\dfrac{B - D}{D} \times 100$ gives the percentage over the ideal weight.

Classification of Obesity

Before considering technics of management it is desirable to have a method of grading the severity of obesity. A simple method is to calculate the percentage overweight for the child's height and age. Using the Iowa growth charts this can be done quickly by plotting the child's height (A) and weight (B) and then determining from the chart the age at which this height is average (C). The average weight for that age (D) also is read from the chart. Then B-D is the excess of the child's actual weight over the average for his height, and B-D/D × 100 will give the percentage overweight in rough terms. The rating of obesity then can be made according to the following scheme:

0-20% overweight—none or trivial obesity
20-30% overweight—mild obesity
30-40% overweight—moderate obesity
over 40% overweight—severe obesity

This purely arbitrary scheme of rating the degree of obesity is of practical value in deciding which children need attention. Those who are less than 20 percent overweight usually require no diet control; those with mild obesity require only a discussion of the social implications and the suggestion of mild dietary restrictions; those with moderate obesity require active measures; those whose obesity is rated as severe are likely to pose very difficult problems in control.

Prevention and Management of Obesity

The greater the degree of obesity the more difficult it is to bring it under control. Thus it is desirable to recognize as early as possible the tendency of a child toward the accumulation of excess fat and to discover the means of altering his diet and general way of life in order to prevent further deviation. Unfortunately, this is often impossible to achieve because neither the child nor his parents are truly interested in controlling the weight increase. Chubbiness is often regarded as a sign of health or as a mildly humorous deviation which is not worth fretting about. Unless child or parents, or both, have some desire to stem the progress of obesity, weight control measures will be futile.

In some families overweight is a general characteristic because of the cultural background. Large, starchy meals are prepared, and it is expected that adults and children alike will eat with gusto and without restraint. It is difficult to persuade a child growing up in this type of milieu to limit his food intake. Unless the family eating pattern can be altered, he will find it difficult to accept and abide by dietary restrictions.

Overweight is frequently a signal that the child is lacking other satisfactions and is concentrating on eating as the main source of pleasure and relief of anxiety. Children who are unhappy in their family lives or who are poorly adjusted in social contacts at school or elsewhere commonly take refuge in eating and in sedentary or isolated occupations. As their activity decreases and they remain around home and the refrigerator for much of the day, obesity tends to advance. The fatter they become the more difficult is participation in the physical activities of their classmates and the less willing they become to expose themselves to the expressed or implied remarks about their bodily contours. Thus, through inactivity and isolation the tendency toward overweight becomes self-perpetuating. In such situations management of the obesity must go further than the imposition of dietary restrictions. The child must be encouraged to find agreeable forms of physical activity and to move

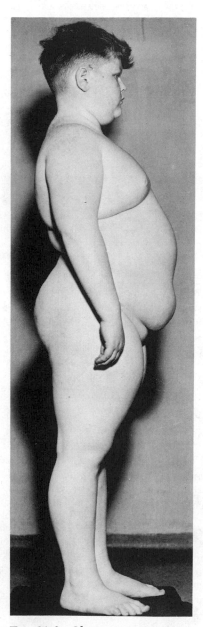

Fig. 31-3. Obesity in a teen-ager.

out into the social world. The basis for his unhappiness or anxiety must be sought. Sometimes these goals can be achieved with suggestions and encouragement; sometimes the emotional disturbance underlying the obesity is too profound to yield, and the services of a psychiatrist must be sought.

Dietary restrictions must be regulated according to the degree of obesity and the ability of the child to control his appetite. In general it is better to make modest reductions in intake and warn the child that progress will not be rapid. If too drastic a reduction in food intake is imposed, the child soon finds that his hunger is too great and he cannot conform. He becomes discouraged and gives up. Drugs which curtail appetite must be used with caution, for too often the the child jumps to the assumption that if he takes the medicine he will not have to worry about his diet. Usually anorexic agents fail except when used as an aid to the child who is strongly motivated to reduce. Thyroid generally steps up the appetite along with the metabolism so that nothing much is gained. Dietary restrictions should be monitored carefully to be sure that the child is receiving an adequate intake of protein, vitamins and minerals to support normal growth. This is particularly important to teen-age girls who may become overenthusiastic about weight reduction and impose on themselves diets which are not only low in calories but lacking in essential ingredients.

The overweight child is often the victim of continuous nagging and repeated implications that he is bad or worthless. A most important part of weight reduction is the continuing, sympathetic and encouraging interest of someone outside his family such as a nurse, or dietitian or a physician who will praise his successes, even though they are minimal at first, and overlook his lapses. If a little success can be achieved, it is likely to progress rapidly as the slenderizing subject finds it easier to engage in physical and social activities.

INFECTIOUS MONONUCLEOSIS
(Glandular Fever)

Infectious mononucleosis is a mildly contagious disease which, although it can affect younger children, produces its most important effects during the adolescent and college years. For many years it has been presumed that it is of viral origin, and although the specific agent is not surely identified, recent studies indicate that it is antigenically related to the agent which produces Burkitt's lymphoma in African children. However, no long-term relationship between infectious mononucleosis and leukemia or lymphoma has been observed in the United States.

Typically, the disease begins insidiously with general malaise, easy fatigability, mild sore throat, enlargement of cervical and other lymph nodes, and splenomegaly and hepatomegaly. In a few cases there may be a light morbilliform rash or involvement of the liver with jaundice, or severe membranous tonsillitis. In young children the disease tends to be mild. In the teen-ager it is too often a cause of prolonged fatiguing illness which in some instances lasts for months and interferes with completion of high school or college studies. There is suggestive evidence that, particularly in this age group, transmission of the disease occurs through exchange of saliva during kissing and that the incubation period is a long one—between one and two months.

Diagnosis depends upon the clinical features; the observation of an increase in large mononuclear cells in the peripheral blood, many of which have abnormally foamy cytoplasm; and, after a week or two, the appearance of heterophile antibodies in abnormally high titer.

Treatment is entirely symptomatic and, particularly in the teen-age subject, may require prolonged periods of decreased physical and social activity.

CHRONIC ULCERATIVE COLITIS

Chronic ulcerative colitis is an inflammation of the colon of unknown etiology. It is more common and more severe among adults than in children. Although it is occasionally seen as early as the second or third year of life, its appearance in the pediatric ages is generally among preadolescents and adolescents. It usually runs a protracted course with periods of increased severity and other periods of relative quiescence. In most cases psychosomatic factors appear to play an important role.

Symptoms

The presenting symptom is a chronic and persistent diarrhea with stools which contain mucus and varying amounts of blood. During acute exacerbations there may be fever, abdominal pain and tenesmus. In the well-established disease there is weight loss, growth failure, reduction of the level of plasma proteins and evidence of vitamin deficiency. The activity of the disease can be judged fairly well by the degree of anemia present, for reduction in the hemoglobin level is a regular feature of the exacerbations even when blood loss in the stools is not marked.

Many individuals with ulcerative colitis present a characteristic set of personality traits which color their social relations and complicate nursing care, especially during periods of remission of their intestinal symptoms. Typically they tend to internalize their feelings and, during periods of activity of the intestinal disorder, are subdued, dependent, anxious and depressed. However, they are prone to become demanding, to wheedle special privileges for themselves and subtly to provoke conflict among others in the social environment. Many of these adolescent victims who remain in the hospital during periods of relatively good health become the trouble-makers on the ward, fomenting disturbances, often without attracting censure to themselves.

Diagnosis

Ulcerative colitis is recognized by a characteristic appearance of the colon when examined by x-ray. These changes appear late in the course of the disease and consist of a loss of the normal haustral markings and the conversion of a portion of the colon into a smoothly outlined tube. The disease may be suspected in the absence of such findings if a persistent bloody diarrhea fails to yield etiologic agents such as dysentery bacilli or amebae. Proctoscopic examination may help to exclude other varieties of mechanical bleeding and will reveal typical changes in the appearance of the sigmoid colon.

Treatment

There is no specific treatment for ulcerative colitis. Two general approaches are adopted, one directed at symptomatic relief of the inflammation of the bowel and the other at change within the personality. The two objectives sometimes conflict with each other.

Symptomatic treatment includes diet management, antispasmodic drugs, steroids, antibiotics and transfusions. Usually, a low residue, nonlaxative, high energy, high vitamin diet is advised. Although essential during the periods of high activity of the disease, dietary restrictions often become a source of resentment during convalescence. Steroid therapy frequently is used to carry the patient through the severe stages by reducing the inflammatory reaction of the bowel, but, as with any chronic disease, it is desirable to reduce the level of dosage as rapidly as possible. Sulfonamide drugs generally are used to reduce the quantity of bacteria within the intestinal canal, since even the normal flora may invade the intestinal wall and create local abscesses. Atropine derivatives and sedatives are employed to reduce the hypermotility of the bowel and to blunt the anxiety which accompanies the disease.

Severely afflicted children usually have deep-seated emotional disturbances arising from abnormally dependent relationships with one or both parents. In many instances it is desirable for the child and the parents to have psychiatric help in resolving such interpersonal difficulties. The process is usually a protracted one.

Prognosis

During childhood the prognosis for life is generally good, but the prognosis for complete recovery is uncertain. Some children have symptoms for a few years and make a spontaneous recovery. Others continue to suffer from their disease as they progress out of the pediatric age period and retain their symptoms as adults. Few children have the severe form of the disease in which rapid advance of the process requires drastic surgery such as colectomy or ileostomy.

TUBERCULOSIS

Susceptibility to tuberculosis is highest during the early years of life (Chapter 19), and wherever small children are inadequately shielded from infected adults, the disease is a serious menace. Judged by the mortality rates at different ages this susceptibility declines so that by the age of 10 years children are relatively resistant even when protection is minimal. During adolescence the mortality rate rises sharply, and presumably the natural resistance is lowered again, probably because of the sudden increase in the rate of growth. Thus it is important to shield adolescents from contact with infectious adults and to screen them for early disease by the use of tuberculin tests and chest microfilms.

ADOLESCENT BEHAVIOR PROBLEMS

As adolescents make the transition from childhood to adulthood they pass through a period of emotionally charged conflict. On one side they are governed by the moral values and social judgments instilled by their parents during the formative years. Ranged against these standards are the powerful emotional drives which urge the adolescent toward independence from, or rebellion against, family or other authoritative control and toward the more liberal, experimental pursuits of his peer group. On some issues the adolescent will align himself firmly with his parents' viewpoint; on others he will reject their attitudes and adopt those of his peers; and on still other issues he may vacillate from one pole to the other. Most adolescents are able to weather the emotional conflict and arrive at rational decisions which maintain their behavior within reasonable bounds. But some overreact to their inner urges, defy authority, and engage in ventures which are reckless because they may warp or even terminate the prospect for a healthy, constructive adult life.

The areas of conflict are too numerous and the interplay of forces too complex to consider here in any detail. But since the nurse working with adolescents must have some understanding of the more common issues, a few of them will be discussed briefly.

Curfew. An early test of parental control centers around the question of how late the adolescent will be permitted to stay out at night. To the teen-ager, the hour at which he must report home becomes an index to his peers of the degree to which he has emancipated himself from parental authority. Whatever the limits set, he tends to regard them as unreasonably strict and as an attempt by his old-fashioned parents to restrict him unduly. The more rebellious individuals ignore the rules set up for them. In some households the parents have no control over the nocturnal activities of their youth. Many communities have set curfews to be enforced by the police because of the amount of reckless or delinquent behavior resulting from groups of high-spirited youths roaming around at night.

From the viewpoint of responsible parents, a curb on nocturnal activities is desirable for the safety, health and scholastic progress of their teen-agers. The task of maintaining amiable yet firm and reasonable relations with the teen-ager on this issue is often quite difficult.

Smoking. Our culture has traditionally frowned upon the use of tobacco by the young, partly from moralistic considerations and partly from pseudo-hygienic concerns. Today it seems clear that the real health problem centers around the acquisition of a habit which, if heavily indulged over long periods of time, results in a very significant increase in the incidence of heart disease and lung cancer in the adult. Parents, physicians and nurses may find that logical arguments fail to dissuade the teen-ager from initiating a habit which he may be unable to terminate in later years when he becomes rationally cognizant of its dangers. To him, consumption of cigarettes may provide a shield for his embarrassments and uncertainties, an aura of maturity and savoir faire, or more importantly admission to the "in" group. To him these short range benefits may outweigh the long range disadvantages.

Alcoholic Beverages. In most American communities the sale of alcoholic beverages to minors is forbidden by laws which were originally intended to protect youths until they presumably had matured enough to have sound judgment about the use of alcohol. Although the pharmacologic effects of alcohol are the same in teen-agers as in adults, the former are generally more susceptible to its intemperate use because of their emotionally powered drives toward emancipation, experimentation and the acquisition of adult status. Unfortunately the determined and resourceful teen-ager can usually find illicit sources of alcohol. For some who indulge intemperately it becomes an important factor contributing to delinquent or reckless behavior. Operation of motor vehicles while intoxicated is a tragically common cause of injury and death among the modern teen-age population.

Drugs. During the past decade there has been an enormous increase in the practice, among high school and college students, of taking various drugs for the purpose of mental stimulation, "mind expansion" or just "kicks." The great majority of such experimenters abandon the practice after one or a few trials. But some of the less stable adolescents persist in seeking escape from, or amelioration of, the psychological stresses of the age. Then they become habituated to the use of one or more of these substances in gradu-

ally increasing dosage until serious toxic effects, even including psychosis, may occur.

From the high school and college-age group some of these practices filter back to pre-teens. In addition, the younger age group may discover accidentally the stimulating effects of chemicals used for legitimate purposes or drugs taken for therapeutic reasons. Among the pre-teens the practice of sniffing the fumes from glue or "dope" used in the construction of model airplanes may develop into real addiction. Common household drugs such as aspirin, phenobarbital, antihistamines, Asthmador and amphetamines may be taken to excess in order to obtain real or fancied excitation or exhilaration. If the practice is pursued to the extent of taking toxic amounts of these substances, poisoning or even death may result. Most common among the college and high school group is the communal smoking of marijuana or "pot." Although possession of this drug is illegal, its use has become widespread through illicit sources of supply. The effects upon the smoker are said to include distortion of the sense of time, hallucinations, increased sensitivity to stimuli and euphoria. But it also has the capacity to convert anxiety into depression or panic. The use of marijuana has been defended on the grounds that its effects are transient and that it is not habit forming. However, its real hazard probably lies in its encouragement of the user to progress toward the use of more hazardous and clearly habituating drugs such as LSD, mescaline, morphine, heroin and cocaine. Adolescents who are regularly taking drugs should be guided toward psychotherapy not only for the purpose of breaking up the habit, but, more importantly, for dealing with the underlying emotional maladjustment which leads them to adopt such potentially harmful practices.

Sexual Activity. The degree to which adolescents control their normal sexual urges varies widely depending upon their individual personalities and upon the mores of the family within which they have been raised. To a lesser degree the controls imposed by the community may also play a role. Apart from moral conflicts and psychologic hazards to the participants, sexual promiscuity also carries the risk of venereal infection and unwanted pregnancy. Judged by the rising incidence of venereal disease and illegitimate pregnancy among children of high school and even grammar school age, there has been a general relaxation of sexual mores among adolescent youth, not only in the United States but in other countries as well. Control of this trend depends in part upon the development of healthier family relationships and in part upon better methods of sex education.

The management of venereal disease in the adolescent follows the same lines as in the adult. Too often the possibility of infection in the young child is overlooked and the condition neglected. Treatment of either gonorrhea or syphilis is by appropriate dosage with penicillin or another antibiotic if the child is sensitive to penicillin.

Illegitimate pregnancy among girls of high school age or younger has become a serious problem in many communities, particularly in the large cities with a central ghetto area. Among some of these families the illegitimate child is accepted into the general family and cared for by the grandmother or other female relative while the mother returns to school or takes a job. Problems of marriage, adoption and family acceptance of the pregnant adolescent are best handled through a social agency familiar with the management of such situations.

Role of the Nurse in Working with Troubled Adolescents

The behavior discussed in the previous section arises when adolescents are troubled, in conflict regarding present and future goals, unable to resolve their family relationships and confused by their feelings. Most have not had the previous warm and supportive experiences which prepare them adequately to meet the developmental tasks of transition to maturity which they are now facing and thus are ill equipped to deal with their tensions and feelings. Most are acutely aware that they are not living up to their own or their family's expectations. Many have physical problems and complaints which are symptomatic of their emotional disturbance and ambivalence.

The nurse, as a nurturing and caring individual, has a large contribution to make in helping adolescents in difficulty and in supporting their efforts to deal with their problems. Nurses are familiar figures to adolescents who have known them in school, camps, clinics and hospitals; and though they are seen as authority figures, they are less threatening to youth than are their parents or others in a disciplinary role. The nurse, as an emotionally mature adult, is a person with whom adolescent girls can identify in an atmosphere devoid of family entanglements and intense emotional conflict. Adolescents are sensitive and responsive to adults who convey genuine interest in them as individuals and respect for their values, ideas and decisions. Nurses are also knowledgeable about physical and emotional development, which is of importance to adolescents when they are intensely concerned about body functioning and physical changes. They can provide adult support necessary to youngsters who are unable to discuss problems with their parents. They also meet parents in PTA groups, health conferences and the like. Finally, nurses have access to adolescents individually and in groups in a large variety of settings within the hospital and in the community.

Although working with troubled adolescents can be challenging and rewarding, it is not always comfortable for the nurse. Discussions of sexual activity, drug use, feelings of anger and hostility, guilt and fear may be embarrassing or difficult and it takes experience for the nurse to be calm and comfortable with these expressions and in accepting values and standards which diverge from her own. To be of maximum assistance to adolescents and to their parents, nurses need to recall their own feelings during this developmental phase, to be aware of their personal values and standards and to be sensitive to their own feelings and responses. If they have resolved their own personal conflicts and can accept standards different from their own, the help they offer will be maximized. Nurses also need knowledge, regarding not only physical and emotional development, but information related to the symptomatology, treatment and consequences of smoking, drug use and venereal disease.

A warm, generous, nonjudgmental, understanding and accepting nurse can assist adolescents both individually and in groups. Through listening to them individually, she can provide a figure in whom they can confide without the threat of an intimate relationship. In a relaxed atmosphere, where the dignity of the adolescent is respected and feelings are accepted and understood, she can support him in regaining a sense of self-esteem. She can help him to work through his relationship with adults and feelings regarding his family, to identify and explore healthy aspects of his personality, to direct hostility and aggression into more appropriate and socially acceptable channels, to strengthen coping mechanisms vs. defeating defensive maneuvers, to provide basic knowledge about bodily functions and to clarify erroneous ideas, to present mature values without moralizing, and to assist and support in independent decision-making. She can bolster their self-respect through communication of her conviction that they are worthy of assistance and are understood, and therefore assist them in accepting their emotions and to deal with reality. Through respecting and honoring physical symptoms, she can help them to understand bodily changes and repair a damaged body image. She can help them also to become aware of the chemical interaction of drug use and smoking and physiologic functioning, offer support to the adolescent who is out of control and assist them in recognizing consequences so that they can make valid decisions.

Group work with adolescents can also be a rewarding experience for the nurse. The peer group is extremely important to teen-agers. In an atmosphere of support from their companions, they are often able to test and explore ideas which they are unable to do individually. They can form relationships quickly, are more aware of their feelings than are many adults and often freer and more comfortable in discussing them in group interaction. In helping them to participate, in arriving at their own decisions, the nurse leader can strengthen the healthy aspects of their personality. In doing so, it is imperative for the nurse to listen carefully, to maintain limits of reasonable behavior, to be able to express her own feelings and to be capable of accepting anger and hostility directed at her personally but as a symbol of the "establishment."

Nurses also have the opportunity for assisting parents who are bewildered by the behavior of their offspring and who often receive condemnation related to their role as parents. Often family relationships are in imbalance and disturbed and parents also feel guilty and in need of support in dealing with their child's behavior and in understanding its meaning. Many families of troubled adolescents have been disrupted and mothers are struggling alone to support their children on meager funds. They also need respect for their dignity, knowledge and understanding.

The nurse as an integral member of the health team has a responsibility to communicate her knowledge of the family dynamics to other members of the team, to initiate referrals when indicated to the social worker or psychiatrist and to work in close harmony with all members of the team.

SITUATIONS FOR FURTHER STUDY

1. After reading about children with ulcerative colitis, select for study an adolescent with this disease. Prepare an outline showing the facets of his behavior that you wish to study and record daily excerpts from your experiences with him. If he is having psychiatric therapy, get recommendations for care from his therapist. After studying his record and the data you have collected while with him, formulate a nursing diagnosis and a plan of nursing care. What changes in behavior did you note as you used his therapist's recommendations? What problems did you encounter in using them? What similarities did you see in the behavior of your patient with that which was described in the patient presented for conference by Wright and Kenward, Pediatrics 18:663, 1956?

2. Read the above-mentioned paper in preparation for a discussion of the way in which facts of physical growth and development and past history within the patient's family are correlated with changes in his physical symptoms and behavior. Also be prepared to discuss the plan of nursing care you would have designed had you been this patient's nurse at the time he was admitted to the hospital during adolescence. What additional observational data would you have needed before you completed your plan of nursing care? How would you have gone about getting it?

BIBLIOGRAPHY

Barkley, V., and Stobo, E. C.: The adolescent who smokes, Nurs. Outlook 12:25, 1964.

Blom, G. E.: Ulcerative colitis in a five-year-old boy *in* Caplan, G. (ed.): Emotional Problems of Early Childhood, p. 169, N. Y., Basic, 1956.

Byers, M.: The hospitalized adolescent, Nurs. Outlook 15:32, 1967.

Clark, A. L.: The crisis of adolescent unwed motherhood, Am. J. Nurs. 67:1465, 1967.

Daniels, A.: Reaching unwed adolescent mothers, Am. J. Nurs. 69:332, 1969.

————, and Krim, A.: Helping adolescents explore emotional issues, Am. J. Nurs. 69:1482, 1969.

Deschin, C. S.: VD and the adolescent personality, Am. J. Nurs. 63:58, 1963.

Freedman, A. M., and Wilson, E. A.: Childhood and adolescent addictions, Pediatrics 34:283, 1964.

Gallagher, J. R.: Medical Care of the Adolescent, N. Y., Appleton, 1960.

Gimpel, H.: Group work with adolescent girls, Nurs. Outlook 16:46, 1968.

Glaser, H. H., and Massengale, O. N.: Glue-sniffing in children, J.A.M.A. 181:300, 1962.

Godbout, R., Petrick, A., and Anderson, M.: Nursing and juvenile delinquency, Nurs. Forum 7:161, 1968.

Heald, Felix: Obesity in the adolescent. Pediat. Clin. N. Am. 7:207, 1960.

Konopka: Adolescent delinquent girls, Children 11:21, 1964.

Louria, D. B.: Some aspects of the current drug scene, Pediatrics 42:904, 1968.

Lowery, G. H.: Obesity in the adolescent, Am. J. Pub. Health 48:1354, 1959

Masland, R. P.: Ulcerative colitis, Pediat. Clin. N. Am. 7:197, 1960.

Mayer, J.: Obesity control, Am. J. Nurs. 65:112, 1965.

Mellinkoff, S. M.: Ulcerative Colitis, DM Disease-a-Month, Chicago, Year Book, Sept. 1961.

Menaker, J. S.: When menstruation is painful, Am. J. Nurs. 62:94, 1962.

Meyer, H.: Predictable problems of hospitalized adolescents, Am. J. Nurs. 69:525, 1969.

Michener, W.: Ulcerative colitis in children: problems in management, Pediat. Clin. N. Am. 14:159, 1967.

Miesem, M., and Wann, F.: Care of adolescents with anorexia nervosa, Am. J. Nurs. 67:2356, 1967.

Monroe, J., and Komorita, N.: Problems with nephrosis in adolescence, Am. J. Nurs. 67:336, 1967.

Nowlis, H.: Why students use drugs, Am. J. Nurs. 68:1680, 1968.

Nuffman, J. W., and Wieczorowski, E.: Gynecology of children and adolescents, Pediatrics 22:395, 1958.

Peckos, P., and Spango, J.: For overweight teenage girls, Am. J. Nurs. 64:85, 1964.

Prugh, D. G.: The influence of emotional factors on the clinical course of ulcerative colitis in children, Gastroenterology 18:339, 1951.

Sankot, M., and Smith, D.: Drug problems in the Haight-Ashbury, Am. J. Nurs. 68:1686, 1968.

Schoel, D. R.: Help for the maladjusted teenager, Nurs. Outlook 12:28, 1964.

Souza, L.: The child with ulcerative colitis in the psychiatric hospital, Nurs. Forum 3:78, 1964.

Taylor, S. D.: Clinic for adolescents with venereal disease, Am. J. Nurs. 63:63, 1963.

Vernick, J., and Lunceford, J.: Milieu design for adolescents with leukemia, Am. J. Nurs. 67:559, 1967.

Weinberg, S., Schonberg, C., and Grier, D.: Seminars in

nursing care of the adolescent, Nurs. Outlook *16*:18, 1968.

Wesseling, E.: The adolescent facing amputation, Am. J. Nurs. *65*:90, 1965.

Wright, F. H.: Preventing obesity in childhood, J. Am. Dietet. A. *40*:516, 1962.

————, and Kenward, J.: Clinical conference on ulcerative colitis. Pediatrics *18*:663, 1956.

Appendix

Appendix

ADMISSION FORM

Information collected from the mother at the time of admission should be readily available to the nurses who are assigned to the child's care. A form similar to the one on page 554, which was adapted from one developed by Bonine,* is invaluable.

PHYSICAL PROTECTIVE MEASURES

The physical safety of the child is the responsibility of the adults in his environment. Fundamental safety measures should be maintained in every pediatric unit.

1. Cribsides are kept up and securely fastened at all times unless an adult is in constant attendance.

2. Whenever the nurse turns away, however briefly, from an infant or young child she is attending, she must keep one hand on him to prevent him from rolling off the bed.

---

* Bonine, Gladys: The Role of the Nurse in the Admission of Preschool Children to Hospitals, p. 61, Unpublished Master's thesis, University of Chicago, Dept. of Nursing Education, 1950.

3. Watchfulness is necessary to protect the child from falling from scales or treatment table.

4. Safety pins and small or breakable objects are to be kept out of the child's reach.

5. Plastic sheeting is not left on a bed unless it is securely fastened in place.

6. Children should not be carried on stairs or across floors that are slippery or strewn with toys.

7. Medicine cabinets must be locked; medicines are never left on bedside tables, and all poisonous cleaning agents, disinfectants, and dangerous instruments are kept well out of reach of ambulatory patients.

8. Windows, elevators, staircases, radiators, electrical outlets and fans must be made safe.

9. The child must understand which areas of the unit he may not enter. Adults should be aware of where the child is at all times.

10. Hot water bottles must be covered and filled with water no hotter than 115° F.

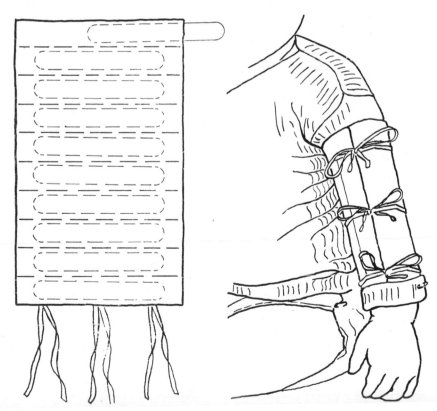

FIG. A-1. (*Left*) Elbow cuff restraint. Elbow cuff for use in treatment of eczema. (*Right*) Elbow cuff applied.

Name of Hospital

Name_____ Age_____ Date of Admission_____ Birthday_____
By what name does the child like to be called?_____ Are there other children in the family?_____
Brothers: Ages_____ Names?_____ Sisters: Ages_____ Names?_____

Patterns of Behavior Relating to Food
How is the child usually fed? Bottle?_____ Cup?_____ Spoon?_____
Feed self independently?_____ Feed self with help?_____ Food disliked?_____ Favorite foods?_____
What is his appetite like?_____

Elimination
Is the child independent in toileting?_____ To what degree?_____
What is the term used to refer to urination?_____ to defecation?_____
How does he make his needs known?_____
Is the child accustomed to a toilet chair?_____ toilet?_____
What is the approximate time of daily bowel movements?_____
Is the child taken to the toilet at night?_____ If so, at what time?_____
Does he go back to sleep quickly when awakened for toileting?_____

Patterns of Behavior Relating to Sleep
Does the child take daily naps?_____ When?_____ What is his usual bedtime hour?_____
Does the child sleep alone?_____ If not, with whom?_____
Does the child sleep in a bed with sides?_____ Does he take a favorite toy or comforter to bed with him?_____
If so what is it?_____
Does the child have a prayer that he says at bedtime?_____
Does the child have a special bedtime ritual?_____ If so, what is it?_____
Does he wake up during the night ordinarily?_____ If so, how do you help him to go back to sleep?_____

Play Interests
What type of play does the child like best?_____
Is the child accustomed to playing alone?_____ With other children?_____ With adults?_____
Does he have a pet at home?_____ If so, state name and kind_____
Favorite toys?_____ Does he enjoy being read to?_____

Personal Habits
Does the child brush his teeth?_____ Comb his hair?_____ Bathe himself?_____ Dress himself?_____
What rituals does he like used when he is cared for?_____

Responses to Stress
What does the child do when frightened?_____
What are his ways of comforting himself?_____
What seems to give him most comfort when he is frightened?_____
What does he do when he is angry?_____
How does his mother help him at these times?_____

Miscellaneous
Does the child know why he is being admitted to the hospital?_____
   What information did mother give him?_____
How did the mother react when she learned hospitalization was necessary?_____
_____

How did child respond to preparation?_____
When was he told?_____

What has mother told him about visiting?_____

Has the child fears, such as fear of unfamiliar adults?_____ Elevators?_____ People in white uniforms?_____
Needles?_____ Cuts and bruises?_____ Others?_____
Do the parents live together?_____ If not, divorced?_____ Separated?_____ Deceased?_____
At what age was the child when the parent died or became divorced or separated?_____
Have any new experiences occurred in the home recently such as birth or death of a sibling?_____
When?_____ Other?_____
Has the child attended nursery school?_____ Kindergarten?_____ Grade school?_____ Sunday school?_____
Mother's remarks?

(Record on the reverse side observations which describe the mother-child relationship, the child's and the mother's response to admission, and the kind of adjustment that the child made in the ward initially.)

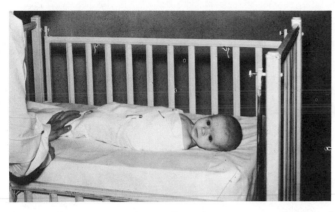

Fig. A-2. An infant "mummied" for puncture of the external and the internal jugular veins.

11. Bath water is tested by the nurse's hand before the child is placed in the bath.

12. Oral medications or feedings are never forced on children because of the danger of aspiration.

13. Medicine dropper tips must be sheathed with rubber tubing.

14. Feeding bottles are never propped.

15. Babies with teeth should be fed with spoons of non-breakable material.

16. When restraints of any kind are used, the child must be observed carefully to protect him from injury and to ascertain that the restraints are serving the purpose for which they were intended.

17. Thermometer bulbs should be inspected before insertion, and if the child cannot hold himself still, he should be held while his rectal temperature is being taken.

18. Children who cannot hold themselves still for treatments such as injections must be held by a second person.

19. Drugs and parenteral fluids must be administered with the greatest possible accuracy.

20. Each child must wear an identification band.

21. Toys must be inspected to be sure that there are no rough edges or small, breakable or removable parts which can be mouthed, swallowed or aspirated by young children.

22. Children under 6 years of age require adult supervision when they are playing together to protect them from each other's uncontrolled aggressive impulses.

23. The nurse must wash her hands thoroughly after caring for each bed patient.

VENIPUNCTURE

Because of the small size of the veins in the antecubital fossa in infants and young children, blood specimens must be obtained from the larger jugular and femoral veins. Positioning of the infant for these procedures is important to afford the operator the best chance to obtain a specimen rapidly and with minimal discomfort to the child.

Puncture of the Internal or External Jugular Veins. The mummy restraint is most frequently employed. A sheet or receiving blanket is secured about the child's body in such a manner that his arms are held to his sides, and flexion of his lower extremities is difficult (Fig. A-2).

The upper edge of the wrapping should be low enough to leave the tops of the shoulders exposed. His head is turned to the side so that his chin touches his shoulder. Then his neck is extended over the edge of a table or a small pillow so that the sternocleidomastoid muscle is well stretched. The nurse holding the infant must control his head and keep it in position without hampering the operator's approach to the vein (Fig. A-3). When the external jugular vein is used,

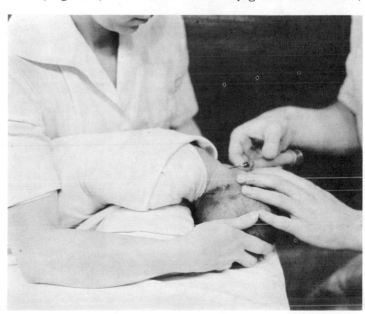

Fig. A-3. Method of using the external jugular vein for venipuncture.

it will become visible during crying and will collapse when the infant inhales. Blood flows most readily if the infant continues to cry during the procedure. The internal jugular vein is not visible beneath the muscle and must be approached blindly. If it is punctured accurately, rapid and easy removal of blood is achieved.

Puncture of the Femoral Veins. For puncture of the femoral vein the infant's groin is exposed, and his leg is extended on the abdomen and held firmly. The operator palpates the femoral artery as it emerges from the abdomen and punctures the vein which runs along its inner surface. The infant is usually wrapped so as to restrain his arms. Then his legs are abducted on either side of the corner of the table and held with knees flexed over the table edge. The nurse immobilizes his trunk with her forearms (Fig. A-4).

Puncture of the Longitudinal Sinus. Puncture of the longitudinal sinus of the skull for blood samples is done only in cases of emergency. The fontanel must be open in order to afford access to the sinus coursing in the leaves of the dura mater. A special short needle is used and is inserted exactly in the midline, first through the skin and then through the dura. The infant is wrapped as for other procedures, and the nurse holds his head firmly with his face straight upward. This procedure looks and is easy to perform, but the hazards of thrombosis of or hemorrhage from the cranial sinus are too great to permit its common usage.

COLLECTION OF URINE SPECIMENS

Single Specimens. When possible, single specimens are collected at the child's first voiding in the morning as the urine is more concentrated and the formed elements in a better state of preservation. For older children collection of urine samples is the same as for the adult. For infants and young children who lack

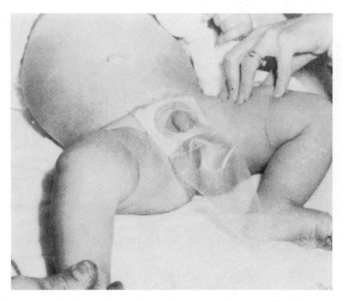

Fig. A-5. The pediatric urine collector (P.U.C.) in place. (The Sterilon Company, Buffalo, N. Y.)

bladder control, several methods of collecting specimens may be employed.

Before any collecting device is applied, the perineum

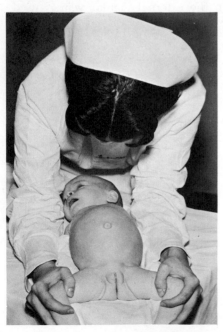

Fig. A-4. Method of restraint for femoral puncture.

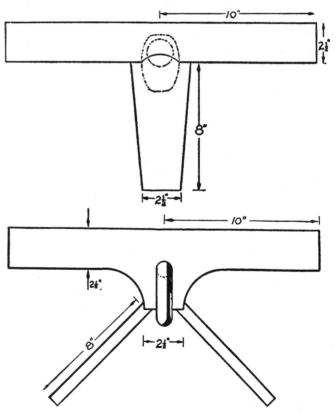

Fig. A-6. (*Top*) T-binder with bird-seed cup for collection of urine from female infant. (*Bottom*) T-binder with test tube attached for collection of urine from male infant.

FIG. A-7. Collecting single specimen of urine from male infant when binder is used. Receptacle for female also is shown.

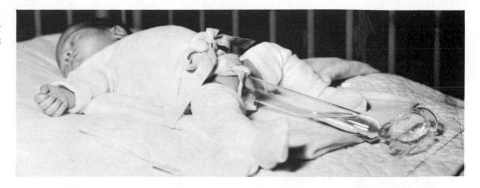

should be cleansed, rinsed and dried to prevent extraneous excretions from contaminating the specimen.

The plastic pediatric urine collector (Fig. A-5) has an opening which is surrounded by sponge rubber with an adhesive surface. It adheres to clean, dry skin, can be removed without discomfort and is suitable for collection from boys and girls. In many instances minimal restraint is required. A diaper may be applied over the plastic collector, often preventing the child from dislodging it.

When plastic collectors are not available, glass test tubes may be used to collect urine from males and bird-seed cups similarly used for females. These can be held in place with adhesive tape or with specially designed binders (Fig. A-6). The application of binders to hold the receptacles is more time consuming than the use of adhesive tape, but it avoids the discomfort and fear which are often associated with the removal of tape.

Before glass receptacles are applied, the rims must be covered with adhesive tape to protect the child's skin. The binder with the attached receptacle is pinned securely around the lower abdomen, the test tube or bird-seed cup placed over the genitals, and the binder tapes brought across the perineum and pinned to the binder where it encircles the body. Raising the head of the crib facilitates the collection of urine by gravity. For older, active infants restraint in the frog position is necessary in order not to lose the urine and to prevent breakage of the receptacle.

Clean Voided Specimen. When clean specimens are desired, the receptacles to be used are sterile and the genitalia and the perineum should be washed thoroughly. If the child is old enough to co-operate, a sample of urine can be collected directly into a sterile receptacle after the stream is well started. Encouraging oral fluids during the hour preceding the collection makes it easier for the child to void after the cleansing has been completed. Examination of a clean specimen collected in this manner provides a rough guide for estimating the number of bacteria present in the urine.

Specimen for Culture. When urine for culture is desired, catheterization may be necessary. The equipment is the same as that for an adult except that smaller catheters are used (No. 8 or 10 French).

Catheterization of the young child is often a problem for the inexperienced nurse. In the young infant the bladder is higher and more anterior than in the adult (Fig. A-8). The bladder descends rapidly during the first 3 years, then slowly. It has the adult position at 20 years. In the female adult, the urethra is relatively short and straight; in the infant it hooks around the symphysis in a "C" shape. When the meatus is located, the catheter should be introduced and directed downward instead of in the direction necessary to reach the bladder of an adult patient.

FIG. A-8. Showing the relative position of the bladder and the direction of the course of the urethra (heavy lines) in the infant and the mature female.

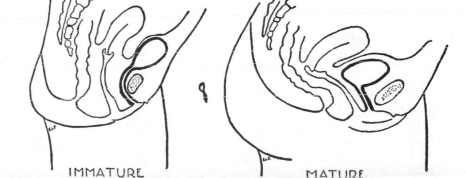

IMMATURE   MATURE

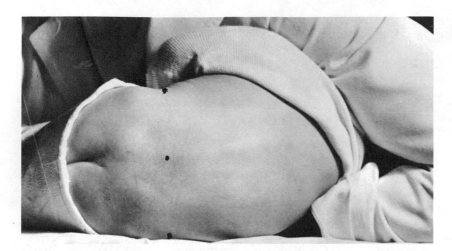

FIG. A-9. Illustrating spinal puncture. This shows a method of holding the child and the puncture site.

Continuous Collection. During certain illnesses and surgical procedures it is important to have an accurate measure of the amount of urine excreted within a certain period of time, either to determine the rate of urine formation or to measure the excretion of various chemical substances from the body. When a timed specimen is collected, the first voiding is discarded, and at that point the timing begins. All urine excreted during the specified time is saved and the last voiding, collected at the end of the period, is added to the total specimen. Older children can be handled in the same fashion as adults but must be impressed with the necessity of saving *all* the urine produced and keeping it distinct from the stool.

Procedures for continuous urine collection from children unable to cooperate vary according to the equipment available. Some hospitals have beds which have been modified to allow urine to pass through a hole in the mattress into a collection bottle below. The child may be restrained in a position to ensure direct voiding into the receptacle, or a urine collecting device may be applied to the genitalia and connected to the collection bottle by tubing. The latter method is also utilized when modified beds are not available. The collection bottle is located at the side of the bed and below the level of the mattress.

The collection apparatus must be inspected frequently to ensure that leakage and loss of urine does not occur. Skin care to prevent irritation is vital, as are nursing measures to reduce the effects of prolonged restraint.

When it is necessary to delay examination of the sample, urine must be refrigerated. At room temperature the chemical composition changes and bacteria multiply, rendering the specimen useless.

LUMBAR PUNCTURE

The sterile equipment required consists of lumbar puncture needles, spinal manometer and 3-way stopcock, hypodermic syringes and needles, local anesthetic, medicine glass, sponges, dressing, drape sheet, gloves

Table A-1. Normal Values of Body Chemical Constituents

Substance	Source	Range for Children	Range for Newborns
Albumin	Plasma	4.6-5.8 Gm.%	2.0-4.0 Gm.%
Alkaline Phosphatase	Serum	10-20 King-Armstrong units 5-13 Bodansky units	4.5-10 Bodansky units
Bicarbonate (HCO_3)	Serum	19-30 mEq./L.	17-23 mEq./L.
Bilirubin	Serum	<1.0 mg.%	1-10 mg.%
Butanol-extractable iodine (BEI)	Serum	3.0-8.0 μg.%	3.5-11.5 μg.%
Calcium (Ca)	Serum	10-12 mg.% (5-6 mEq./L.)	9-11.5 mg.% (4.5-5.8 mEq./L.)
Chloride	Serum Spinal fluid	98-106 mEq./L. 112-130 mEq./L.	104-116 mEq./L. 109-133 mEq./L.
Cholesterol	Serum	70-250 mg.%	50-100 mg.%
CO_2 Tension (pCO_2)	Arterial blood	35-45 mm. Hg	
Creatinine	Serum	0.4-1.2 mg.%	
Fibrinogen	Plasma	200-400 mg.%	200-400 mg.%
Globulin	Plasma	1.7-3.0 Gm.%	0.6-2.0 Gm.%
Glucose	Whole blood Spinal fluid	60-120 mg.% 50-90 mg.%	20-80 mg.% 20-60 mg.%
Iron (Fe)	Serum	.04-.18 mg.%	.03-.20 mg.%
Iron-binding capacity	Serum	.187-.650 mg.%	
Lead (Pb)	Serum	<.06 mg.%	
Magnesium (Mg)	Serum	1.7-2.5 mEq./L.	1.3-2.5 mEq./L.
NPN	Plasma	18-30 mg.%	30-60 mg.%
Oxygen tension (pO_2)	Arterial blood	85-100 mm. Hg	
pH	Serum	7.3-7.45	7.3-7.45
Phosphorus (P)	Serum	4.0-6.5 mg.% (2.3-4 mEq./L.)	4-8 mg.% (2.3-4.6 mEq./L.)
Potassium (K)	Serum Sweat	4.1-5.6 mEq./L. 7-14 mEq./L.	4-7 mEq./L. 9-14 mEq./L.
Protein, total	Plasma Spinal fluid	6.5-8.0 Gm.% 15-40 mg.%	4.0-7.0 Gm.% 20-120 mg.%
Protein-bound iodine (PBI)	Serum	4.0-8.5 μg.%	4.5-12 μg.%
Sodium (Na)	Serum Sweat	135-145 mEq./L. 8-40 mEq./L.	130-150 mEq./L. 7-14 mEq./L.
Urea nitrogen	Plasma	10-17 mg.%	3-13 mg.%
Uric acid	Serum	2.0-6.0 mg.%	2.0-6.0 mg.%
17-hydroxycortico-steroids	Plasma	10-16 μg.%	

Compiled from many sources.
"%," in this usage, means "per 100 cc."

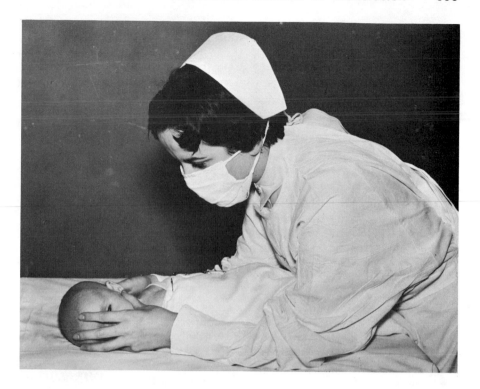

Fɪɢ. A-10. Method of holding an infant for scalp vein technic. The nurse cups her hands over the occiput and the face, holds the infant's head rotated at 90° and immobilizes his trunk with her forearms.

and medication as desired by the physician. Test tubes for collecting spinal fluid samples should be available.

The technic for spinal puncture in the child is the same as that in the adult. The puncture usually is made between the 3rd and 4th or between the 4th and 5th lumbar vertebrae. The appropriate site may be located by drawing a line across the back at the level of the iliac crests (Fig. A-9). The vertebral space nearest this line is used.

Even when the child is able to co-operate during the procedure, it is desirable to hold him in position in order to avoid trauma that may result from unexpected and involuntary movement, and to provide him with security and support. The child is usually in a recumbent position on the right side, with his thighs and legs flexed and his back arched in a curve. Restraint in optimal position is accomplished effectively when the nurse places her right arm about his thighs and her left arm about his neck, locking her hands in front of the child. A struggling child may be restrained further, if necessary, by the nurse leaning forward and placing some weight on his body.

INTRAVENOUS INFUSION OR TRANSFUSION

Older Children. The same sort of apparatus and method of immobilization which is used for the adult is satisfactory for the older child who is able to co-operate and has a good vein in the antecubital region. The arm is immobilized by taping it to a padded splint or a sandbag. With adequate taping the child will not

have to concentrate on maintaining a fixed position during the infusion. Pressure on the arm proximal to the point of needle insertion must be avoided, or flow through the vein may be hampered. Veins on the back of the hand, the flexor surfaces of the wrist or the medial side of the ankle may be used.

When fluids are injected directly into the venous system, careful observation of the patient, the apparatus and the rate at which the solution is flowing is essential. The physician must designate the speed of infusion which he desires. If an infusion is shut off completely, even for a few minutes, it may be impossible to start the flow again because of the formation of clots in the needle. If the nurse finds that the infusion will no longer run or that so much has gone in that she thinks it should be stopped, she should consult the physician at once. Air bubbles must not be permitted to enter the vein. Pain accompanied by swelling at the point of insertion of the needle usually means that the needle has slipped out of the vein.

When blood is being administered, the nurse has additional responsibilities. If the child complains of generalized discomfort, chilly sensations or backache, it may be a forewarning of a transfusion reaction. The young child, who cannot verbalize his discomfort, will manifest his feelings in his behavior. He may grow restless and cry; close observation probably will show changes in color, respiration and heart rate. Whenever any of these symptoms are noted, the flow should be stopped, and the physician notified.

Infants. The smaller the child the more difficult and potentially dangerous is intravenous fluid therapy. Special problems are created by the infant because he is harder to immobilize, his veins are smaller and less accessible, and often there is a very narrow margin between a safe speed of infusion and one that will keep the channels open.

In addition to the veins commonly used for infusions in the older child, the infant presents relatively large channels over the temporal region of his scalp which offer the best opportunity for successful entry. When such veins are to be used, the scalp is shaved, and the infant is mummied. His head is held firmly turned to one side (Fig. A-10). By pressing his head steadily and firmly against the table top it is possible to prevent slight movements which may disturb the operator's aim or dislodge the needle. Care must be taken to allow the infant ample breathing space while he is being restrained.

The nurse who is charged with watching a continuous infusion in a small infant has a very important responsibility which demands accurate recording of the fluid level, frequent observation of the rate at which the fluid is flowing, and prompt notification of the physician when the rate cannot be adjusted in a satisfactory manner. Permitting fluids to enter the vascular system too rapidly may result in serious overloading or even fatal heart failure.

Pediatric Infusion Sets

An additional safeguard to prevent fluid overload is provided by the use of infusion sets designed for the administration of fluids to children. A small chamber which holds up to 100 cc. of fluid is inserted between the solution bottle and the drip chamber. The small chamber is filled from the solution bottle, which is then clamped off. Should the rate of flow suddenly increase, only the amount in the chamber is permitted to enter the vascular system.

Subcutaneous Infusion or Clysis

The equipment for subcutaneous infusion or hypodermoclysis consists of the solution to be infused, a clysis administration set, 2 needles of gauge No. 19 to 21 and 2½ to 3 in. long, antiseptic sponges, adhesive tape and an irrigating pole.

The tubing of the administration set is filled with solution, clamped off and the needles are attached. After careful cleansing of the skin of the outer part of the anterior portion of the thigh, a needle is inserted into each thigh and the tubing secured to the thighs with adhesive tape. The clamps are opened so as to allow a flow of fluid which will not result in uncomfortable distention of the tissues.

The precautions to be observed are that careful sterile technic is maintained until the apparatus is finally removed; that the needle points lie between the skin and the muscle layers of the leg and not within the substance of either; that the needles are not near the course of the femoral or the saphenous vessels along the inner aspect of the thigh; and that restraint is maintained adequately so that the needles do not come out before the treatment is concluded.

Other places into which clyses may be given are the pectoral region and the back. If the pectoral region is used, the arms must be pinioned behind the back to prevent removal of the needles. The needles are inserted below and lateral to the nipples, and fluid is permitted to distend the loose space of the axilla. Frequently, the back is used as a site for single injections of fluid into premature or small infants, in which case a large syringe is used rather than the apparatus mentioned above. Sometimes the back is used in older children when the thighs are not accessible. A child who is restrained on his face must be watched carefully to prevent suffocation.

Close observation is necessary to prevent the solution from running too rapidly; blanching of the skin from internal pressure is to be avoided. At the completion of the procedure, the needles are removed, and the injection sites are covered with small dressings.

INTRAMUSCULAR INJECTION

Method of Injection. The length and gauge of the needle used for intramuscular injection depends on the characteristics of the material to be injected and on the size of the child.

After filling the syringe accurately, 0.2 cc. of air can be drawn into the syringe. Upon injection, the air bubble leaves the syringe last, clearing the needle and preventing deposit of medication in subcutaneous fat upon withdrawal of the needle.

Table A-2. Composition of Common Fluids used for Intravenous Therapy

Solution	Milliequivalents per Liter of				
	Na	K	Cl	HCO₃	Ca
0.2% NaCl (saline)	34		34		
0.33% NaCl (saline)	56		56		
0.9% NaCl (normal saline)	154		154		
3% NaCl	500		500		
5% NaCl	850		850		
Ringer's solution	147.5	4	156		4.5
Lactated Ringer's	130	4	109	28	3
M/6 Na lactate	167			167	
Plasma (with A.C.D.)	146	5	75	60	

The above solutions, except plasma, have no caloric value. Glucose is often combined with them, providing 40 calories per liter for each percentage of glucose in the final mixture, e.g. 5% glucose = 200 cals/L.

Many commercially and locally prepared combinations of solutions are available whose composition must be learned from the package label. Additives are also available in ampoule form which must be given in appropriate dilution. DISTILLED WATER ALONE SHOULD NEVER BE GIVEN PARENTERALLY.

Deficit Calculation Formula

mEq. required = (Normal conc.—Patient's conc.) × (DF) × (Wt.).

Where the normal and patient's concentrations are blood serum values in mEq./L.; DF is the distribution factor; and the body weight is expressed in kilograms.

Distribution factors for the main electrolytes are:

HCO₃	0.5-0.6	Cl	0.2-0.3
HCO₃ (lactate)	0.7	Na	0.6-0.7

Special considerations govern the replacement of potassium which must be monitored frequently.

The nurse should avoid last-minute manipulation of the syringe in the presence of the child. The skin must be thoroughly cleansed with an antiseptic sponge, working circularly from the center outward.

Discomfort is minimized when the site of injection is varied, the skin pulled taut and the needle inserted quickly. After aspiration to determine that the needle is not in a blood vessel, injection of the material is accomplished with care taken that the needle is in place before injection begins and that it is not withdrawn until the syringe is empty. These precautions are necessary to avoid depositing medication along the entire injection tract. Immediate massage and subsequent use of the muscle aid absorption of the drug.

The site of injection must be recorded carefully so that rotation of sites can be ensured.

Site of Injection. Four injection sites are available for use in all but the infant and the very young child.

Dorsogluteal. In older children, the upper outer quadrant provides a safe site if the needle is inserted properly. If it takes a downward and inward course, even though correctly located in the upper outer quadrant, the sciatic nerve may be injured.

The gluteal muscles do not develop until walking begins and it is generally considered unsafe for intramuscular injections until the child has been walking for a year or more. Recent information suggests that the dorsogluteal site may be utilized with safety in infants and young children provided that 1.) the needle is no longer than 1 inch, 2.) the child is positioned in a completely prone position, 3.) the needle is inserted perpendicular to *the surface on which he is lying, and not to the skin.**

Ventrogluteal. This site presents a dense muscle mass which is relatively free of hazards of injury to the nervous and vascular systems. With the patient on his back, the nurse places her index finger on the anterior superior iliac spine. With the middle finger moving dorsally, she finds the iliac crest and drops her finger below the crest. The triangle formed by the iliac crest, index finger and middle finger is the injection area. This site is visible to the child.

Deltoid. Unless the needle is carefully placed in the deltoid site, injury to the radial nerve may result.

Lateral and anterior thigh. There are no major nerves in this area and it is particularly useful in infants, small children and children difficult to restrain. This site, however, is not entirely free from hazard when used in the infant. Greater safety is ensured when 1.) the needle is no longer than 1 inch, 2.) the upper outer quadrant of the thigh is chosen, 3.) the needle is inserted at a 45° angle and pointing toward the knee.†

---

* Hill, L. F.: Sites for intramuscular injections. J. Pediat. 70: 158, 1967.
† Talbert, J. L., Haslam, R. H., and Haller, J. A., Jr.: Gangrene of the foot following intramuscular injection in the lateral thigh: A case report with recommendations for prevention. J. Pediat. 70: 110, 1967.

CARE OF THE CHILD WITH A TRACHEOSTOMY

Normally, air is filtered, warmed and moistened in the upper respiratory tract before it is taken into the lungs. After tracheotomy, nursing measures must provide warm, moist and filtered air for the child to breathe. A croup tent or humidifier is usually employed to loosen mucus and secretions and reduce chances of a mucus plug. Respiration must be watched constantly, especially for unequal chest expansion that might indicate the development of pneumothorax.

A tray with the following sterile equipment should be at the child's bedside; duplicate tracheostomy tubes, with tapes attached, obturator, scissors, 2 curved clamps, pipe cleaners, medicine dropper, gauze dressings, tongue depressors, applicators and catheters (No. 8 or 10 French) which have additional holes near the tip to facilitate aspiration. Catheters for nasal aspiration and for aspiration through the tracheostomy should be kept separate. Other necessary equipment includes 2 covered jars of sterile normal saline solution, a jar of hydrogen peroxide, a jar of sterile petrolatum and suction apparatus with a glass Y-tube inserted into the system.

During the adjustment period when the child is learning to breathe through the tube, the nurse must be in constant attendance to keep the tracheostomy tube free of mucus and drainage, to allay anxiety associated with respiratory distress, general discomfort and loss of power to use his vocal apparatus. Losing the capacity to speak and cry is a terrifying experience for a child. Vocalization has not only been a source of pleasure; it has also been the means by which he has released tension and signaled his need for help. Every means possible must be used to help him to regain and retain his trust in himself and in others.

During the first 48 hours after tracheotomy, the tube must be cleansed frequently by aspiration. The frequency depends on the amount of drainage and the needs of the individual child. Before aspiration a few drops of normal saline should be put into the tracheostomy tube to stimulate coughing and to moisten and loosen mucus so that it can be aspirated. Aspiration produces excitement, fear and coughing until the child learns that the procedure makes him more comfortable. Some form of comforting must be provided while the procedure is being carried out. After the lock of the tube has been turned upward toward the face, the inner cannula should be removed and placed in hydrogen peroxide.

The use of sterilized catheters and care in aspirating are of prime importance in protecting the fragile mucous membranes of the respiratory tract. Plum and Dunning* devised an apparatus and a method of aspiration that fulfill these criteria. A Y-glass connecting tube inserted into the suction line allows the vac-

---

* Plum, Fred, and Dunning, M.: Technics for minimizing trauma to the tracheobronchial tree after tracheotomy, New Engl. J. Med. 254:193, 1956.

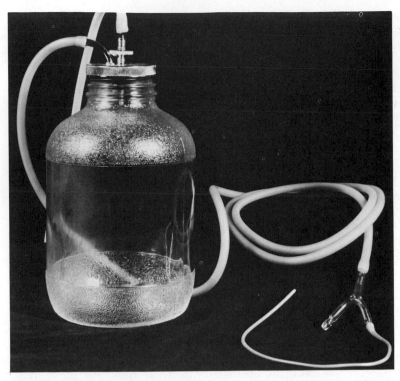

FIG. A-11. Illustrating assembly of a Y-glass connector for use in tracheal aspiration.

uum to be released immediately by fingertip control (Fig. A-11). To aspirate the right main stem bronchus, the child's head is turned to the left; to aspirate the left stem his head is turned to the right. During insertion of the catheter to the full depth of the bronchi, the Y-tube should be left open. Before closing off the Y-tube with the fingertip to create a vacuum, the catheter should be withdrawn 1 or 2 centimeters to move the tip away from the delicate mucus membrane. To aspirate, the catheter should be withdrawn slowly with a rotary movement as the pressure is controlled with the fingertip on the opening of the Y-tube. Aspirations should be limited to 15 seconds. If the catheter sucks tightly against membranes during aspiration, the vacuum must be released before it is drawn away from the tracheobronchial wall. The catheter should be withdrawn when coughing begins. Forced expiration against the partial obstruction of the catheter may increase positive pressure within the chest, which can lead to impairment of cardiac circulation. Unless the quantity of secretions threatens to suffocate the child, a 3-minute rest period between aspirations should be provided to prevent hypoxia. Each time the catheter is removed, it should be flushed with normal saline solution.

After aspirating, the inner cannula of the tracheostomy tube should be cleaned with pipe cleaners and hydrogen peroxide rinsed and inspected carefully to ensure cleanliness before reinsertion. If aspiration and cleansing of the inner cannula does not give the child relief from respiratory distress, the physician should be notified at once.

The area around the tube and the dressing should be kept scrupulously clean. Applicators dipped in hydrogen peroxide should be used to cleanse the skin before it is coated with sterile petrolatum. A gauze square cut to the center should be placed around the tube and under the tapes that hold the tube in position. Any bleeding from or signs of infection in the wound should be reported. Before the dressing is changed and before aspirating the tube, the nurse's hands should be washed thoroughly. If the tracheostomy tube should be coughed or pulled out, the nurse should spread the incision open with a sterile clamp to establish an airway.

Fluids and food may be given to the child as he tolerates them. In the early period after tracheostomy, the child may be afraid to swallow for fear that it will hurt. However, as he finds that it causes him no discomfort, he will begin to take fluids and food more eagerly. Any coughing associated with swallowing should be reported.

When drainage and respiratory difficulty have ceased, a plug is inserted in the inner cannula to obstruct the tube partially. Gradually, the opening is obstructed completely, and breathing takes place entirely around the tube, the trachea being much larger than the tube. If no respiratory embarrassment occurs during the ensuing 24 hours, the tracheostomy tube is removed, and the wound is closed and covered with a sterile dressing. The tray containing the duplicate tracheostomy tube and obturator should be kept at the bedside until respiratory difficulty has subsided completely. Continued observation is always imperative during this period. Whenever possible, constant nursing care should be provided.

ISOLATION TECHNIC—MEDICAL ASEPSIS

It may be necessary to isolate a child to prevent the spread of disease or infection to other patients and personnel or to prevent infection of the child himself (reverse isolation). The extent to which complete isolation technic is modified in the care of the child depends upon the mode of transmission of the infection and hospital policy.

When a mask is necessary, it is worn over both the nose and mouth. A new mask must be worn for each patient contact and one mask should not be used for longer than 30 minutes, as after that period the effectiveness is drastically reduced. *It must never be allowed to hang around the neck.*

To be truly effective, gowns should be worn only once and discarded rather than hung up for re-use. When used more than once, they must be handled in such a way that the inside remains clean. The gown must be worn with the edges of the back opening well overlapped and tied securely in place.

Thorough hand washing is essential and in the event of gross contamination of the hands, scrubbing with a brush may be necessary.

Furniture and equipment in isolation units should be kept to a minimum. Personnel and visitors must clearly understand which areas are considered to be clean and those designated as contaminated. Anyone entering the unit must be instructed in the procedures to be followed.

Toys should be secured to the bed so that they cannot fall to the floor. They should be made of materials that can be readily disinfected.

Concurrent Disinfection. Contaminated articles must be disinfected before being used again. Articles that are not damaged by heat are sterilized. Others are cleaned with soap and water and an appropriate disinfectant. Contaminated articles which are sent to another hospital department for disinfection or disposal must be placed in clean bags, carefully secured and clearly labeled as coming from an isolation unit. The method of disposal of body wastes varies with the facilities of the institution. If they cannot be put directly into the sewage system, they are immersed in an appropriate disinfectant. Sweeping and dusting are carried out with a damp technic to limit dispersion of infected materials.

Terminal Disinfection. After cleaning, the room should be aired for at least 24 hours before being used again. The period may be shortened by the use of ultraviolet lamps or a disinfectant fog.

PLAY EQUIPMENT

With an understanding of the emotional and intellectual development of children, their problems, interests and needs, it is comparatively easy to select toys for them when they are hospitalized. Play has a definite purpose for hospitalized children and has therapeutic aspects. Through the utilization of toys they can counteract sensory deprivation, relieve tension and feelings of hostility and aggression, "work through" problems and conflicts related to the hospitalization and developmental tasks and relieve the monotony of long days on the pediatric ward.

Discarded household equipment often makes excellent play equipment. The toys which children like best are those which make possible independent and group dramatic and imaginative play. Hospitalized children frequently are well able to utilize equipment which is available to dramatize hospital play and thus work through painful treatments, identify with hospital personnel, and counteract feelings of abandonment.

Raw materials encourage creativity. A square of cloth may become, among other things, a bandage, a sheet to restrain a doll, a dress, material that can be torn into shreds, a mask or something that is merely pleasant and stimulating to touch. Small, simple, lightweight toys are better for a bedridden child than mechanical toys.

Excellent play materials for the young child include: tin pans, small saucepans, a set of measuring spoons, small wooden bowls, a string of spools and napkin rings, clothespins and boxes. These will give the baby as much or more delight than an expensive silver rattle or commercially made toys. Bathtub toys are also a delight to the baby and incite him to reach out and splash. As a child learns to walk, things that he can push or pull about will interest him. Large blocks, a small wagon or doll carriage, animals on wheels or other pull toys will stimulate pushing and pulling activity. Nests of blocks, tin cans (which have had all sharp edges removed by a can opener designed for that purpose) and sand toys which can be filled and emptied are all popular with toddlers.

The list of equipment which appears below includes those things that would be desirable in a hospital playroom. Low shelves which make toys accessible to children encourage freedom of choice.

Blocks, large and small
Simple puzzles
Sand box on wheels, pail, shovel, etc.
Galvanized tub on wheels for water play, or rubber wading pool.
Inflatable water toys
Wagon, kiddie car, tricycle
Record player and records
Blackboard
Piano
Costumes—policeman, physician's jacket, nurse's cap, etc.
Large wooden beads for stringing
Balls, large
Toys for dramatic play—wood, dolls depicting the family, baby dolls, doll buggy, doll bed, toy cooking set, tea set, telephone, toy cleaning equipment, toy laundry equipment, bottles and nipples, over-night cases, adult clothing for dressing up
Equipment for dramatic hospital play—baby crib, rubber dolls, bedside table and equipment, physician's bag, bandage, bandage scissors, adhesive tape, other discarded (clean and safe) hospital equipment

Toys for dramatic transportation play—trains, trucks, automobiles, airplanes, fleet of boats, fire engines.
Toys for store play, farm and barn-yard animals
Pounding toys
Painting easel and long handled brushes
Raw materials for creative self-expression—crayons, paint, chalk, clay, finger paint, scissors, construction paper, bells, rhythm sticks, tambourines, cymbals, xylophones and drums.
Pets—birds, rabbits, hamsters, fish and turtles

In addition to the play materials listed above, the following equipment should be available to meet the play needs of the older child:

Puzzles of graded complexity
Construction equipment for making buildings, etc.
Construction equipment for making airplanes, space ships, vehicles and mobiles.
Materials for pottery, leather, papier-maché, jewelry, block printing, crepe-paper crafts.
Materials for making doll clothes
Materials for scrapbooks of collector's items
Paper dolls
Marionettes
Card games, and games which require skill, such as Monopoly and chess.

THE USE OF CHILDREN'S LITERATURE DURING HOSPITALIZATION

Children's literature has great potential in preparing children for hospitalization, in reducing traumatic effects of separation, in maintaining ties with the past, in counteracting sensory deprivation and in assisting mastery of events occurring throughout the hospitalization.

Many hospitals have recognized the value of preparation of the young child for hospitalization and have developed materials for parents to read prior to the child's admission. Other books are available commercially. The best of such literature are the picture books featuring a young child with whom the potential patient can identify. They should be factual stories, reports of what to expect with further elaboration of areas specific to the child. These books can be read to the child repeatedly, shortly before the hospitalization is to occur, and thoroughly digested through opportunities for discussion and dramatization of the expected experiences. Also valuable are stories that emphasize the humanity of medical personnel, such as:

Gilbert, H.: Dr. Trotter and His Big Gold Watch. Abingdon, 1941.
Averiel, E.: Jenny's Bedside Book. Harper & Row, 1959.
Jubelier, R.: Jill's Checkup. Melmont, 1957.
Kunharat, D.: Dr. Dick. Harper & Row, 1962.
Rey, M., and Rey, H.: Curious George Goes to the Hospital. Houghton Mifflin, 1966.
Viason, P.: Willie Goes to the Hospital. Macmillan, 1956.

Books and stories about mothers and children may assist the child to keep ties to home alive, to talk about his longings and to prevent denial of the need for mothering which may accompany separation. Familiar stories which have been read to the child at home are particularly suitable in maintaining ties and may provide a bridge between the nurse and the mother. Suggested books are:

Chalmers, M.: Take a Nap, Harry. Harper & Row, 1964.
Dr. Suess, Horton Hatches the Egg. Random House, 1940.
Kuskin, K.: Alexander Soames: His Poems. Harper & Row, 1962.
Lonergan, J.: When My Mother Was a Little Girl. Franklin Watts, 1961.
McCloskey, R.: Make Way for Ducklings. Viking, 1941.
Jolotow, C.: When I Have a Little Girl. Harper & Row, 1965.
Potter, B.: The Tale of Peter Rabbit. Warne, 1963.

Since the young child uses identification in his relationship with his parents and as a defense against threat, stories of people and animals fighting against odds and winning through in the end are eminently valuable in keeping the child's will to struggle alive, to prevent apathy and withdrawal, to keep hope going and to facilitate goal directed behavior. Books which can be of assistance are:

Bemelmans, L.: Madeline. Simon and Schuster, 1939.
Bulla, C.: The Sugar Pear Tree. Crowell, 1960.
Lexan, J.: Benjie. Dial, 1964.
Hewett, A.: The Tale of the Turnip. Wittlesey, 1961.
Piper, W.: The Little Engine that Could. Platt, 1954.
Anglund, J.: The Brave Cowboy. Harcourt, 1959.
Ardizzone, E.: Tim All Alone. Oxford, 1957.
Brown, M.: Dick Whittington and His Cat. Scribner, 1950.
Cameron, P.: I Can't, Said the Ant. Coward-McCann, 1961.
Dalgleish, A.: Bears on Hemlock Mountain. Scribner, 1952.
Groves-Raimes, A.: The Tidy Hen. Russell Sage, 1964.

Selected stories and books also have the potential for facilitating expression of aggression, hostility and loneliness and for dealing with such feelings openly. Suggested books to assist in this respect are:

Bemelmans, L.: Madeline in London. Viking, 1961.
Brown, M.: Little Lost Lamb. Doubleday, 1945.
Byrd, M.: Loneliest Chicken. Macmillan, 1953.
Eastman, P.: Are You My Mother? Random House, 1960.
Lexan, J.: Maria. Dial, 1964.
Zolotow, C.: The Poodle Who Barked at the Wind. Lothrop, 1964.
Sendak, M.: Where the Wild Things Are. Harper, 1963.
Udry, J.: Let's Be Enemies. Harper, 1961.
Ardizzone, E.: Tim All Alone. Oxford, 1957.
MacDonald, G.: Little Frightened Tiger. Doubleday, 1953.

Several factors must be kept in mind in the choice and use of reading material. The attention span may be shorter than the age and previous developmental level of the child would indicate. In addition, because of expected regression and utilization of energy in dealing with physical and emotional stressors, the child may respond more favorably to literature which is less difficult than that which they are accustomed to reading or having read to them.

Table A-3. Dosage of Commonly Used Pediatric Drugs*

Drug	Route	Dosage	Frequency	Form Available
Acetaminophen	O	30 mg/kg/24 hrs.	4-6 i.d.	tablets, drops, syrup, elixir
Acetazolamide	O	5 mg/kg/24 hrs.	single	tablets
Acetyl salicylic acid	O, R	65 mg/kg/24 hrs.	4-6 i.d.	tablets, suppositories
Achromycin—see tetracycline				
ACTH—see corticotropin				
Adrenalin—see epinephrine				
Aerosporin—see polymyxin B sulfate				
Albamycin—see novobiocin				
Aldactone—see spironolactone				
Aminophyllin	I.V., I.M.	12 mg/kg/24 hrs.	4 i.d.	ampules, suppositories
	R	12 mg/kg/24 hrs.	4 i.d.	
Amino salicylic acid—see para-amino salicylic acid				
Ammonium mandelate	O	250 mg/kg/24 hrs.	4 i.d.	soln., syrup
Amobarbital—same dose as phenobarbital				
Amphetamine sulfate	O	2-20 mg/24 hrs.	3 i.d. single	tablets, Spansule
Amphotericin B	I.V.	0.25-1.0 mg/kg/24 hrs.	single	vials
		(Given as drip over 6 hrs.)		
Ampicillin	O	50-200 mg/kg/24 hrs.	4 i.d.	capsules, vials
	I.V., I.M.	100-200 mg/kg 24 hrs.		
Amytal—same dose as phenobarbital				
Antepar—see piperazine				
Apresoline—see hydralazine				
Aspirin—see acetyl salicylic acid				
Atabrine—see quinacrine				
Atarax—see hydroxyzine				
Atropine sulfate	S.C.	0.01 mg/kg/dose	single	tablets, vials
Aureomycin—see chlortetracycline				
Avertin—see tribromethanol				
Azulfidine—see salicylazosulfapyridine				
BAL—see dimercaprol				
Banthine—see methantheline				
Belladonna Tincture	O	0.1 ml/kg/24 hrs.	3-4 i.d.	U.S.P. tincture
		(maximum = 3.5 ml)		(1 ml = 0.3 mg. atropine)
Benadryl—see diphenhydramine				
Benzathine penicillin G	I.M.	0.6-1.2 million units	single	vials, syringes, Tubex
Benzedrine—see amphetamine				
Bisacodyl	O	0.3 mg/kg	single	enteric tablets, suppositories
	R	0.3 mg/kg	single	
Bicillin—see benzathine penicillin G				
Brompheniramine maleate	O, S.C., I.M., I.V.	0.5 mg/kg/24 hrs.	3-4 i.d.	tablets, elixir, injectable soln.
Butabarbital—same dose as phenobarbital				
Butisol—same dose as phenobarbital				
Caffeine Na benzoate	S.C., I.M., I.V.	8 mg/kg/dose	p.r.n. 4 i.d.	ampules
		(maximum 500 mg)		
Calcium disodium edetate	I.V.	< 70 mg/kg/24 hrs.	2 i.d. for 5 days	tablets, ampules
Calcium gluconate	O	0.5 gms/kg/24 hrs.	1-3 i.d.	powder, ampules
	I.V.	(same diluted and slowly)		
Calcium lactate	O	0.5 gms/kg/24 hrs.	4-6 i.d.	powder
Caprokol—see hexylresorcinol				
Carbarsone	O	10 mg/kg/24 hrs.	2-3 i.d.	tablets, capsules
Carbinoxamine maleate	O	0.4 mg/kg/24 hrs.	3-4 i.d.	tablets
Carisoprodol	O	25 mg/kg/24 hrs.	4 i.d.	capsules, tablets
Cascara	O	1-8 ml/dose	single	fluid extract U.S.P.
Castor oil	O	1-15 ml/dose	single	oil, emulsion
Celontin—see methsuximide				
Chel-iron—see ferrocholinate				
Chloral hydrate	O, R	25-50 mg/kg/24 hrs.	3-4 i.d.	capsules, syrup, solution, elixir, suppositories
Chloramphenicol	O	50-100 mg/kg/24 hrs.	4-6 i.d.	capsules, suspension solutions
	I.V., I.M.	(premature and n.b. half dosage)		
Chlorcyclizine HCl	O	1.5 mg/kg/24 hrs.	2 i.d.	tablets
Chlorothiazide	O	20 mg/kg/24 hrs.	2 i.d.	tablets, syrup
Chlorpheniramine maleate	O	0.35 mg/kg/24 hrs.	4 i.d. single	tablets, syrup, Repetabs
Chlorpromazine	O	2 mg/kg/24 hrs.	4-6 i.d.	tablets, syrup, Spansule
Chlortetracycline—same dose as tetracycline				
Chlorthalidone	O	2 mg/kg/dose	single q. 2-3 days	tablets
Chlor-trimeton—see chlorpheniramine maleate				
Clistin—see carbinoxamine maleate				
Codeine	O, S.C.	1-3 mg/kg/24 hrs.	q. 4 h. p.r.n.	tablets, syrup
Colace—see dioctyl sulfosuccinate				

(Note—Because of wide dosage range or specialized usage the following types of drugs have been omitted—adrenal steroids, digitalis, anti-neoplastic and immuno-suppressive agents.)

* Table compiled mainly from Shirkey, H. C.: Drug Therapy *in* Nelson, W. E. (ed.), Textbook of Pediatrics, ed. 9, Saunders, Philadelphia, 1969, by permission of the authors.

Table A-3. Dosage of Commonly Used Pediatric Drugs   (Continued)

Drug	Route	Dosage	Frequency	Form Available
Colistin	0	4 mg/kg/24 hrs.	3 i.d.	suspension
Compazine—see prochlorperazine				
Corticotropin	I.V., I.M., S.C.	1.6 units/kg/24 hrs.	3-4 i.d. 1-2 i.d.	aq. vials, ampules, gel
Cotazyme—see pancreatins				
Cyclizine	0, I.M.	3 mg/kg/24 hrs.	3 i.d.	tablets, ampules
Cyproheptadine HCl	0	0.25 mg/kg/24 hrs.	3-4 i.d.	tablets, syrup
Cytomel—see liothyronine				
Darvon—see propoxyphene				
Declomycin—see demethylchlortetracycline				
Delvex—see dithiazanine				
Demerol—see meperidine				
Demethylchlortetracycline	0	10 mg/kg/24 hrs.	2-4 i.d.	capsules, syrup
Dexedrine—see dextroamphetamine				
Dextroamphetamine sulfate	0	2-15 mg/24 hrs.	3 i.d. single	elixir, tablets, Spansule
Diamox—see acetazolamide				
Diethyl carbamazine	0	15 mg/kg/24 hrs.	once i.d.	tablets, syrup
Di-iodohydroxyquin	0	40 mg/kg/24 hrs.	2-3 i.d.	tablets
Dilantin—see diphenylhydantoin				
Dimenhydrinate	0, I.M. R	5 mg/kg/24 hrs. (maximum = 300 mg/24 hrs.)	4 i.d.	tablets, liquid, ampules, suppositories
Dimercaprol	I.M.	15-5 mg/kg/24 hrs.	6-2 i.d.	ampules
Dimetane—see brompheniramine				
Dioctyl Na sulfosuccinate	0	5 mg/kg/24 hrs.	3-4 i.d.	capsules, soln, syrup
Diodoquin—see di-iodohydroxyquin				
Diphenhydramine HCl	0 I.M.	5 mg/kg/24 hrs. 5 mg/kg/24 hrs.	4 i.d. 4 i.d.	tablets, elixir, ampules, vials
Diphenylhydantoin	0 I.M., I.V.	3-8 mg/kg/24 hrs. 3-8 mg/kg/24 hrs.	1-3 i.d. 1-3 i.d.	tablets, capsules, suspension, vials
Dithiazanine	0	8 mg/kg/24 hrs.	3 i.d.	tablets
Diuril—see chlorothiazide				
Dramamine—see dimenhydrinate				
Dulcolax—see bisacodyl				
EDTA—see calcium disodium edetate				
Ephedrine sulfate	0 S.C., I.V.	3 mg/kg/24 hrs. 3 mg/kg/24 hrs.	4-6 i.d. 4-6 i.d.	capsules, syrup, tablets, ampules
Epinephrine HCl	S.C. I.M. Inhal.	.01 ml/kg/dose, aqueous 1:1000 .01-.02 ml/kg/dose, 1:500 in oil 1:100 aqueous	1-6 i.d. 1-2 i.d. p.r.n.	ampules ampules Nebulized liquid
Epsom salt—see magnesium sulfate				
Erythromycin	0 I.V., I.M.	25-40 mg/kg/24 hrs. 10 mg/kg/24 hrs.	4 i.d. 4 i.d.	tablets, drops, suspension ampules
Equanil—see meprobamate				
Ethosuximide	0	.25-.5 gm/24 hrs.	2 i.d.	capsules
Ethotoin	0	80 mg/kg/24 hrs.	4 i.d.	tablets
Feosol—see ferrous sulfate				
Fer-in-sol—see ferrous sulfate				
Ferrocholinate	0	1-6 mg/kg/24 hrs.	3 i.d.	tablets, syrup, liquid, drops
Ferrous sulfate	0	1-6 mg/kg/24 hrs.	3 i.d.	tablets, capsules, syrup, elixir, drops
Fungizone—see amphotericin B				
Furadantin—see nitrofurantoin				
Furazolidone	0	6 mg/kg/24 hrs.	4 i.d.	tablets, suspension
Furoxone—see furazolidone				
Gantrisin—see sulfisoxazole				
Gemonil—see metharbital				
Glucagon	S.C., I.M., I.V.	10 mg/kg/24 hrs.	single	ampules
Griseofulvin	0	20 mg/kg/24 hrs.	2-4 i.d.	tablets, suspension
Hetrazan—see diethyl carbamazine				
Hexylresorcinol	0	0.1 gm/year of age	single	Crystoids
Histadyl—see methapyrilene				
Hydralazine HCl	0 I.V.	0.75 mg/kg/24 hrs. 1.7-3.5 mg/kg/24 hrs.	4 i.d. 4-6 i.d.	tablets, ampules
Hydrochlorothiazide	0	2 mg/kg/24 hrs.	2 i.d.	tablets
Hydrodiuril—see hydrochlorothiazide				
Hydroxyzine	0	2 mg/kg/24 hrs.	4 i.d.	tablets, syrup
Hygroton—see chlorthalidone				
Hyoscine—see scopolamine				
Humatin—see paromomycin				
Ilosone—see propionyl erythromycin ester				
Ilotycin—see erythromycin				
Ipecac	0	10-15/ml/dose	single	syrup
Isoniazid (INH)	0 I.M.	15-40 mg/kg/24 hrs. 15-40 mg/kg/24 hrs.	2-3 i.d. 2-3 i.d.	tablets, capsules, syrup, ampules

Table A-3.   Dosage of Commonly Used Pediatric Drugs   (Continued)

Drug	Route	Dosage	Frequency	Form Available
Isoproterenol	Inhal.	Nebulized	3-4 i.d.	vials, mist
Isuprel—see isoproterenol				
Kanamycin sulfate	O	50 mg/kg/24 hrs.	4 i.d.	capsules
	I.M.	6-15 mg/kg/24 hrs.	2 i.d.	vials
Konakion—see Vitamin K₁				
Levallorphan	I.V., I.M.	.02 mg/kg/dose	single	ampules, vials
Levothyroxin Na	O	.006 mg/kg/24 hrs.	single	tablets
Liothyronine	O	2.5-7.5 mcgm/24 hrs.	single	tablets
Liquiprin—see salicylamide				
Lorfan—see levallorphan				
L-tri-iodothyronine—see liothyronine				
Luminal—same as phenobarbital				
Magnesium hydroxide	O	0.5 ml/kg/dose	single	magma
Magnesium sulfate	O	0.25 gm/kg/dose	single	crystals, 50% soln
	I.M.	0.2 ml/kg/dose	4-6 i.d.	
Marezine—see cyclizine				
Mellaril—see thioridazine HCl				
Menadiol—see Vitamin K				
Menadione—see Vitamin K				
Meperidine HCl	O	6 mg/kg/24 hrs.	p.r.n.	tablets, elixir, ampules, vials,
	I.M., S.C.	6 mg/kg/24 hrs. (maximum = 100 mg/dose)	p.r.n.	Tubex
Mephenesin	O	175 mg/kg/24 hrs.	3-5 i.d.	tablets, capsules
Mephenytoin	O	3-15 mg/kg/24 hrs.	3 i.d.	tablets
Mephobarbital	O	9-12 mg/kg/24 hrs.	3 i.d.	tablets
Mephytoin—see Vitamin K₁				
Meprobamate	O	25 mg/kg/24 hrs.	2-3 i.d.	tablets
Meralluride Na	I.M.	.125-1.0 ml/dose	1-2/week	ampules, vials
Mercaptomerin	I.M.	.125-1.0 ml/dose	1-2/week	vials, suppositories
	R	.125-1.0 ml/dose	1-2/week	
Mercuhydrin—see meralluride				
Mesantoin—see mephenytoin				
Mestinon—see pyridostigmin				
Methadone HCl	O	0.7 mg/kg/24 hrs.	4-6 i.d.	tablets, syrup, elixir, ampules,
	S.C.	0.7 mg/kg/24 hrs.	4-6 i.d.	vials
Methantheline Br	O	6 mg/kg/24 hrs.	4 i.d.	tablets, ampules
	I.M.	6 mg/kg/24 hrs.	4 i.d.	
Methapyrilene HCl	O	5 mg/kg/24 hrs.	5 i.d.	capsules, syrup, ampules, vials
	S.C., I.M.	1-2 mg/kg/24 hrs.	5 i.d.	
Metharbital	O	50-100 mg/24 hrs.	1-3 i.d.	tablets
Methdilazine	O	0.3 mg/kg/24 hrs.	2 i.d.	tablets, syrup
Methenamine mandelate	O	.05-0.1 gm/kg/24 hrs.	3 i.d.	tablets, suspension
Methicillin	I.M., I.V.	100 mg/kg/24 hrs.	4-6 i.d.	vials
Methimazol	O	0.2-0.4 mg/kg/24 hrs.	3 i.d.	tablets
Methocarbamol	O	60 mg/kg/24 hrs.	4 i.d.	tablets
Methsuximide	O	0.3-1.2 mg/kg/24 hrs.	single	capsules
Methylene blue	I.V., I.M.	2 ml/kg/dose	single	1% soln ampules
Methylphenidate HCl	I.V., I.M.	0.75 mg/kg/dose	single	tablets, vials
Milk of Magnesia—see magnesium hydroxide				
Milontin—see phensuximide				
Miltown—see meprobamate				
Morphine sulfate	S.C.	0.1-0.2 mg/kg/dose (maximum = 15 mg.)	single	tablets, soln
Mycostatin—see nystatin				
Mysoline—see primidone				
Nafcillin	O	25-50 mg/kg/24 hrs.	4 i.d.	capsules, injectable soln
	I.V., I.M.	25-50 mg/kg/24 hrs.	4 i.d.	
Nalline—see nalorphine				
Nalorphine HCl	I.V., I.M.	0.1 mg/kg/dose	single	ampules
Nembutal—same dose as phenobarbital				
Neomycin sulfate	O	50 mg/kg/24 hrs.	4 i.d.	tablets, vials
	I.V.	4-15 mg/kg/24 hrs.	4 i.d.	
Neostigmine	O	2 mg/kg/24 hrs.	6-8 i.d.	tablets
Neo-synephrine—see phenylephrine				
Nitrofurantoin	O	6 mgm/kg/24 hrs.	4 i.d.	tablets, suspension
Norethandrolone	O	0.5 mg/kg/24 hrs.	single	tablets
Novobiocin	O	20-45 mg/kg/24 hrs.	2-3 i.d.	capsules, syrup, vials
	I.M., I.V.	20-45 mg/kg/24 hrs.	2-3 i.d.	
Nystatin	O	400,000-2,000,000 units/24 hrs.	3-4 i.d.	tablets, suspension
Oxacillin Na	O	25-100 mg/kg/24 hrs.	4 i.d.	capsules
Oxytetracycline	O	20-40 mg/kg/24 hrs. (Newborn = 100 mg/kg/24 hrs.)	4 i.d.	capsules, syrup, drops
	I.V., I.M.	10-12 mg/kg/24 hrs.	2 i.d.	vials
Pancreatins	O	Adjustable with meals		granules, tablets, capsules

Table A-3. Dosage of Commonly Used Pediatric Drugs   (Continued)

Drug	Route	Dosage	Frequency	Form Available
Para-aminosalicylic acid (PAS)	O	0.3-0.5 gm/kg/24 hrs.	3 i.d.	tablets, crystals, powder
Paradione—see paramethadione				
Paraldehyde	O, R, I.M.	0.15 ml/kg/dose	single	U.S.P. liquid, 5% glucose in
	I.V.	0.15 ml/kg/dose	single	saline
Paramethadione	O	0.3-0.9 gm/24 hrs.	3-4 i.d.	capsules, tablets
Paregoric	O	0.25-0.5 ml/kg/24 hrs.	single	U.S.P. tincture
Paromomycin sulfate	O	25 mg/kg/24 hrs.	3 i.d.	capsules, syrup
Peganone—see ethotoin				
Penicillin G	O	25,000-50,000 units/kg/24 hrs.	4-6 i.d.	many preparations
	I.M., I.V.	25,000-50,000 units/kg/24 hrs.	2 i.d.	many preparations
Pentobarbital—same dose as phenobarbital				
Pen—V—see phenoxymethyl penicillin				
Perazil—see chlorcyclizine				
Periactin—see cyproheptadine				
Permapen—see benzathine penicillin G				
Perphenazine	O	4-12 mg/24 hrs.	3 i.d.	tablets, syrup
	R	2-6 mg/24 hrs.	3 i.d.	suppositories
Phenacemide	O	0.25 gm/dose	1-3 i.d.	tablets
Phenergan—see promethazine				
Phenethicillin—see phenoxymethyl penicillin				
Phenoxymethyl penicillin	O	25,000-50,000 units/kg/24 hrs.	4 i.d.	tablets, syrup, drops
Phenobarbital	O	6 mg/kg/24 hrs.	3 i.d.	tablets, elixir, ampules,
	I.M.	6 mg/kg/24 hrs.	3 i.d.	suppositories
	R	6 mg/kg/24 hrs.	3 i.d.	
Phensuximide	O	1-3 gm/24 hrs.	2-3 i.d.	capsules, suspension
Phenurone—see phenacemide				
Phenylephrine HCl	S.C., I.M.	0.1 mg/kg/dose	single	ampules
Phytonadione—see vitamin K_1				
Piperazine	O	0.25-2.0 gm	once for 7 days	tablets, wafers, syrup
Pitressin—see vasopressin				
Polycillin—see ampicillin				
Polymyxin B sulfate	O	10-20 mg/kg/24 hrs.	4 i.d.	tablets, powder
	I.M., I.V.	1-2.5 mg/kg/24 hrs.	4 i.d.	
Povan—see pyrvinium pamoate				
Primidone	O	0.125-2.0 gms/24 hrs. (increase weekly to tolerance)	1-4 i.d.	tablets, suspension
Pro-banthine—see propantheline				
Procaine penicillin G	I.M.	300,000-500,000 units/dose	1-2 i.d.	injectable soln
Procaineamide HCl	O	50 mg/kg/24 hrs.	4-6 i.d.	capsules
Prochlorperazine	O	0.4 mg/kg/24 hrs.	3-4 i.d.	tablets, syrup, suppositories,
	R	0.4 mg/kg/24 hrs.	3-4 i.d.	ampules, vials
	I.M.	0.2 mg/kg/24 hrs.	3-4 i.d.	
Promethazine HCl	O	0.5 mg/kg/dose	single	tablets, syrup, suppositories,
	R	0.5 mg/kg/dose	single	ampules
	I.M.	0.5 mg/kg/dose	single	
Pronestyl—see procaineamide				
Propantheline Br	O	1.5 mg/kg/24 hrs.	4 i.d.	tablets
Propionyl erythromycin ester	O	25-40 mg/kg/24 hrs.	4 i.d.	capsules, suspension, drops
Propoxyphene HCl	O	3 mg/kg/24 hrs.	4-6 i.d.	capsules
Propylthiouracil	O	50-300 mg/24 hrs.	3 i.d.	tablets
Prostaphlin—see oxacillin				
Prostigmine—see neostigmine				
Pseudoephedrine	O	5 mg/kg/24 hrs.	4 i.d.	tablets, syrup
Pyribenzamine HCl—see tripelennamine				
Pyridostigmin Br	O	7 mg/kg/24 hrs.	5-6 i.d.	tablets, elixir
Pyronil—see pyrrobutamine				
Pyrrobutamine	O	0.6 mg/kg/24 hrs.	2 i.d.	tablets
Pyrvinium pamoate	O	5 mg/kg	once	tablets, suspension
Quinacrine HCl	O	8 mg/kg/24 hrs.	3 i.d.	tablets
Quinidine sulfate	O	30 mg/kg/24 hrs.	5 i.d.	tablets, capsules, ampules
	I.V., I.M.	30 mg/kg/24 hrs.	5 i.d.	
Reserpine	O	0.02 mg/kg/24 hrs.	1-2 i.d.	tablets, elixir, ampules, vials
	I.M.	0.07 mg/kg/24 hrs. (hypertension)	1-2 i.d.	
Ritalin—see methylphenidate				
Robaxin—see methocarbamol				
Salicylamide	O	65 mg/kg/24 hrs.	6 i.d.	tablets, suspension
Salicylazosulfapyridine	O	150 mg/kg/24 hrs.	6 i.d.	tablets
Scopolamine HBr	O	0.006 mg/kg/dose	single	tablets
	S.C.	0.006 mg/kg/dose	single	vials, ampules
Secobarbital—same dose as phenobarbital				
Seconal—same dose as phenobarbital				
Soma—see carisoprodol				
Spironolactone	O	60 mg/M^2/24 hrs. (M^2 = square meter of surface area)	3-4 i.d.	tablets

Table A-3. Dosage of Commonly Used Pediatric Drugs (Continued)

Drug	Route	Dosage	Frequency	Form Available
Stanozolol	O	0.1 mg/kg/24 hrs.	3 i.d.	tablets
Staphcillin—see methicillin				
Streptomycin	I.M.	10-40 mg/kg/24 hrs.	2-3 i.d.	ampules, vials
Sulfadimethoxine	O	15-30 mg/kg (Max. = 2 Gm.)	once a day	tablets, suspension, drops
Sulfadiazine	O	150 mg/kg/24 hrs.	4-6 i.d.	tablets, suspension
Sulfasuxidine	O	250 mg/kg/24 hrs.	6 i.d.	tablets, powder
Sulfathalidine	O	125 mg/kg/24 hrs.	3-6 i.d.	tablets, suspension
Sus-phrine base	S.C.	.004 ml/kg/dose	2-3 i.d.	1:200 suspension
Sulfisoxazole	O	180 mg/kg/24 hrs.	6 i.d.	tablets, suspension, syrup
	I.M., I.V.	100 mg/kg/dose	2-3 i.d.	ampules
Synkavite—see vitamin K				
Synthroid—see levothyroxin Na				
Tacaryl—see methdilazine				
Tapazol—see methimazol				
Temaril—see trimeprazine				
Tempra—see acetaminophen				
Terramycin—see oxytetracycline				
Tetracycline	O	20-40 mg/kg/24 hrs.	4 i.d.	tablets, capsules, suspension, vials
	I.V., I.M.	10-12 mg/kg/24 hrs.	2 i.d.	
Theophylline	O	10 mg/kg/24 hrs.	2-3 i.d.	tablets, elixir
Thiomerin—see mercaptomerin				
Thioridazine	O	1 mg/kg/24 hrs.	3-4 i.d.	tablets, oral concentrate
Thorazine—see chlorpromazine				
Thyroid U.S.P.	O	4 mg/kg/24 hrs.	once a day	tablets
Tolserol—see mephenesin				
Triacetyloleandomycin (TAO)	O	30 mg/kg/24 hrs.	4 i.d.	capsules, drops, suspension, 3% solution
Tribromethanol	R	75 mg/kg/dose	single	
Tridione—see trimethadione				
Trilafon—see perphenazine				
Trimeprazine tartrate	O	4-7 mg/24 hrs.	3 i.d.	tablets, capsules, syrup
Trimethadione	O	40 mg/kg/24 hrs.	3-4 i.d.	capsules, tablets, soln
Tripelennamine HCl	O	5 mg/kg/24 hrs. (maximum = 300 mg/24 hrs.)	4-6 i.d.	tablets, elixir
Tylenol—see acetaminophen				
Unipen—see nafcillin				
Vancomycin	I.V.	10-45 mg/kg/24 hrs.	2-4 i.d.	ampules
Vasopressin	S.C.	1-3 ml/dose	3 i.d.	aq. U.S.P. 20 u/ml, tannate in oil, 5 u/ml
	I.M.	0.2-2.0 ml/dose	single	
V-cillin—see phenoxymethyl penicillin				
Viokase—see pancreatins				
Vistaril—see hydroxyzine HCl				
Vitamin K (synthetic)	I.M.	1 mg/dose	single	tablets, ampules
Vitamin K₁ (natural)	O	0.5-10 mg/dose	single	tablets, ampules, vials
	I.V., I.M., S.C.	0.5-10 mg/dose	single	
Winstrol—see stanozolol				
Zarontin—see ethosuximide				

BIBLIOGRAPHY

Blumgart, E., and Korsch, B.: Pediatric recreation: An approach to meeting the needs of hospitalized children, Pediatrics 34:133, 1964.

Brooks, M.: Constructive play experiences for the hospitalized child, J. of Nursery Ed. 12:122, 1957.

Flandorf, V.: Books to help children adjust to a hospital situation, The American Library Assoc., Chicago, 1967.

Friedrich, H.: Common sense in intramuscular injections, Nurs. Clinics N. Amer. 1:333, 1966.

Hanson, D.: Intramuscular injection injuries and complications, Amer. J. Nurs. 63:99, 1963.

Hill, L.: Sites for intramuscular injections, J. Pediat. 70:158, 1967.

Hymovich, D.: ABC's of pediatric safety, Amer. J. Nurs. 66:1768, 1966.

Kernick, J.: Needle puncture; Health asset or menace, Nursing Clinics N. Amer. 1:269, 1966.

Lewis, B., and Gunn, I.: Tracheostomy, O₂ administration and expiratory air flow resistance, Nurs. Research 13:301, 1964.

Loome, P.: Isolating patients with staphylococcal infections, Amer. J. Nurs. 65:102, 1965.

Mohammed, M.: Urinalysis, Amer. J. Nurs. 64:87, 1964.

Noble, E.: Play and the Sick Child, London, Faber and Faber, 1967.

Play Schools Association: Why—Play in a Hospital—How, New York (no date given).

Pitel, M., and Wemett, M.: The intramuscular injection, Amer. J. Nurs. 64:104, 1964.

Sato, F.: New devices for continuous urine collection in pediatrics, Amer. J. Nurs. 69:804, 1969.

Sylvester, M., and Bruno, P.: Factors associated with infiltration during continuous intravenous therapy, Nursing Research 15:255, 1966.

Talbert, J., Haslam, R., and Haller, J.: Gangrene of the foot following intramuscular injection in the lateral thigh: A case report with recommendations for prevention, J. Pediat. 70:110, 1967.

World Organization for early childhood education: Play in Hospital, Housing Centre Trust, London, E. T. Heron and Co. Ltd., 1966.

Index

Index